Pharmacology

A Nursing Process Approach

Pharmacology

A Nursing Process Approach

SECOND EDITION

Joyce LeFever Kee, RN, MS

Associate Professor Emerita
College of Nursing
Department of Nursing Science
University of Delaware
Newark, Delaware

Evelyn R. Hayes, RN, PhD

Professor
College of Nursing
Department of Nursing Science
University of Delaware
Newark, Delaware

W.B. SAUNDERS COMPANY

A Division of Harcourt Brace & Company

Philadelphia   London   Toronto   Montreal   Sydney   Tokyo

W.B SAUNDERS COMPANY
A Division of Harcourt Brace & Company

The Curtis Center
Independence Square West
Philadelphia, Pennsylvania 19106

Library of Congress Cataloging-in-Publication Data

Kee, Joyce LeFever.
    Pharmacology: a nursing process approach / Joyce LeFever Kee, Evelyn R. Hayes.—2nd ed.

    p.   cm.

    Includes index.

    ISBN 0–7216–6057–6

    1. Pharmacology.   2. Nursing.   I. Hayes, Evelyn R.   II. Title.
    [DNLM: 1. Pharmacology—nurses' instruction.   2. Drug Therapy—nurses' instruction.   QV 4 K26p 1997]
RM301.K44   1997   615.5'8—dc21

DNLM/DLC   96–46545

PHARMACOLOGY: A NURSING PROCESS APPROACH, Second Edition   ISBN 0–7216–6057–6

Printed in the United States of America.

Last digit is the print number: 9   8   7   6   5   4   3   2

To My Father

SAMUEL H. LeFEVER

for his continuous love and support

Joyce LeFever Kee

To My Parents

MARGARET and **JUSTIN HAYES**

for their ever-present love and confidence

Evelyn R. Hayes

Contributors

Anne E. Lara, RN, MS, OCN, CS
Nursing Manager
Radiation Oncology
Medical Center of Delaware
Wilmington, Delaware
Chapter 29

Linda Laskowski-Jones, RN, MS, CS, CCRN, CEN
Trauma Clinical Specialist
Trauma Service
Medical Center of Delaware
Wilmington, Delaware
Chapter 47

Nancy C. Sharts-Hopko, RN, PhD
Professor
Villanova University
Villanova, Pennsylvania
Chapters 45 and 46

Jane Purnell Taylor, RN, MSN
Associate Professor
Department of Nursing
Neumann College
Aston, Pennsylvania
Chapters 42, 43, and 44

Allison Bailey, BA
Illustrator
Chapters 3 and 38

Sandra Taccone, BA
Illustrator
Unit X and Chapter 38

Consultants

John Barron, PharmD
Resident, Ambulatory Care
Philadelphia College of Pharmacy and
    Science
Philadelphia, Pennsylvania

Diane Baughman, RN, EdD, CS
Nursing Department
Weber State University
Ogden, Utah

Michele Bockrath-Welch, RNC, MSN
Senior Clinical Scientist
Wyeth-Ayerst Laboratories
Philadelphia, Pennsylvania

Ilene Borze, RN, MS, CEN
Gateway Community College
Phoenix, Arizona

Richard L. Bragdon, RPh, MS, MBA
Director of Pharmacy
St. Francis Healthcare System
Hartford, Connecticut

Mark Cziraky, PharmD
Resident, Ambulatory Care
Philadelphia College of Pharmacy and
    Science
Philadelphia, Pennsylvania

Anna T. Eaton, RNC, BSN, MN
Assistant Chief Nurse: Recruitment, Education,
    and Research
King Health Center
U. S. Soldiers' and Airmen's Home
Washington, DC

Sheila Grossman, PhD, RN
Associate Professor
Fairfield University
Fairfield, Connecticut

Ronald J. Lefever, RPh
Pharmacist
Medical College of Virginia
Richmond, Virginia

Betty B. Laliberte, RN, MSN
Assistant Professor
School of Nursing
University of Connecticut
Storrs, Connecticut

Anne E. Lara, RN, MS, OCN, CS
Nursing Manager, Radiation Oncology
Medical Center of Delaware
Wilmington, Delaware

Linda Laskowski-Jones, RN, MS, CS, CCRN,
    CEN
Trauma Clinical Specialist
Trauma Service
Medical Center of Delaware
Wilmington, Delaware

Christie Marsh, RPh
Pharmacist
Kaiser Permanente
Northampton, Massachusetts

Brenda Millette, PhD, RN
Associate Professor
University of Massachusetts
Amherst, Massachusetts

Nancy G. M. Miner, RNC, MSN
Director, Bridgeport Community Mental Health
    Center
Bridgeport, Connecticut

Joseph Peoples, RPh
Clinical Pharmacist
Alfred I. duPont Institute
Wilmington, Delaware

Lisa Plowfield, PhD, RN
Assistant Professor
College of Nursing
University of Delaware
Newark, Delaware

Nancy C. Sharts-Hopko, RN, PhD
Associate Professor
Villanova University
Villanova, Pennsylvania

Rebecca A. Sisson, RN, PhD
Assistant Professor
University of Southern Florida
Tampa, Florida

Robert Thornton, RPh, BSC
Director, Pharmacy Services
St. Francis Hospital and Medical Center
Wilmington, Delaware

Judith A. Torpey, RN, MSN
Assistant Director
Visiting Nurse Association of Manchester
Manchester, Connecticut

Carol H. Tyree, RN
Piedmont Orthopedic Surgery
Lynchburg, Virginia

Mary Webb, PhD, RN
Assistant Professor
University of South Florida
College of Nursing
Tampa, Florida

Kathleen S. Whalen, RN, MN, CCRN
Community College of Denver
Denver, Colorado

Marcus D. Wilson, PharmD
Assistant Professor of Clinical Pharmacy
Philadelphia College of Pharmacy and
    Science
Philadelphia, Pennsylvania
Consultant, Health Outcomes and Clinical
    Research
HealthCare Center at Christiana
Newark, Delaware

Jonathan J. Wolfe, PhD
Pharmacy Practice
College of Pharmacy
University of Arkansas
Little Rock, Arkansas

Sue W. Young, PhD, RN
Associate Dean, Academic Affairs
University of South Carolina

Preface

This unique clinical pharmacology textbook contains complex pharmacologic principles that are organized in a readable and understandable presentation. *Pharmacology: A Nursing Process Approach*, Second Edition, focuses on the understanding of pharmacologic principles for practice, the administration of medications, and the evaluation of the client response. These foci are essential to the foundations of professional nursing practice. The book is designed for nursing students in a variety of nursing programs, for review for NCLEX preparation, for nurses in refresher programs, and for the practicing nurse in diverse settings.

The textbook is organized into 13 units and 47 chapters. Illustrations throughout the book enhance the understanding of the concepts. The drug tables found throughout the chapters provide drug names (generic and brand), dosages, and uses and considerations, including pregnancy category and pharmacokinetics.

The chapter layout promotes easy accessibility to information. Each chapter provides a content outline, objectives, related terminology, prototype drug charts, drug pharmacokinetics and pharmacodynamics, nursing process, and study questions. In addition, most chapters include case studies to illustrate applications to practice and stimulate critical thinking.

We incorporated a variety of features to support the role of the nurse in drug therapy. The drug chart format illustrates basic and comparative data for prototype drugs in selected categories. The nursing process parallels this drug chart format and can be applied to the drug therapy of each client.

We also integrated the use of the nursing process throughout the text. The nursing process includes assessment, nursing diagnoses, planning, nursing interventions including client teaching, and evaluation. With client and family teaching, we suggest helpful teaching tips that relate to general information, skills, diet, and side effects.

Calculation of drug dosages for adults and children is presented in Chapter 4, which consists of five sections: Systems of Measurement with Conversion; Methods for Calculation; Calculations of Oral Dosages, Including for Pediatrics; Calculations of Injectable Dosages, Including for Pediatrics; and Calculations of Intravenous Fluids. In this chapter, we use clinical practice problems and actual drug labels in full color for examples of calculating drug doses. The variety and large number of practice problems can eliminate the need for an additional dosage calculation textbook. Also, the study guide that accompanies this text contains additional practice problems with answers and a basic math review.

Pharmacology has kept pace with the knowledge explosion. Thus, we include innovative chapters and/or approaches in this book, such as biological response modifiers (BRMs), the role of the nurse in drug research, nutritional support, emergency drugs for both the pediatric and the adult client, drugs for gender disorders and during the maternity cycle, cultural influences, and special considerations for clients throughout the life span.

Throughout the text, we use tables, figures, and drug charts extensively to facilitate learning. A glossary of over 600 terms and the appendices assist in highlighting important information. The appendices include generic drugs with corresponding Canadian drug names, a temperature conversion chart, alternate methods of pediatric drug calculations, recommended daily allowances for vitamins and minerals, drugs that discolor urine and feces, vaccines, laboratory tests related to drug use, and therapeutic drug monitoring (TDM).

At the back of the book, we include "tear-out" cards that provide handy pocket references in the clinical area. These cards contain commonly used conversions and abbreviations, sample dosage calculations, intravenous flow rates, a blank sample of the prototype drug format, and a list of commonly used therapeutic serum values for TDM.

The changes that we have made to *Pharmacology: A Nursing Process Approach*, Second Edition, include the following:

- Chapter 1, Drug Action: Pharmaceutic, Pharmacokinetic, and Pharmacodynamic Phases, provides expanded information on pharmacologic principles of pharmacokinetics and pharmacodynamics. This chapter contains numerous illustrations and tables, and it clearly presents the material to promote student learning of basic pharmacologic concepts for practice.
- Chapter 3, Principles of Drug Administration, provides new coverage of the "10 Rights" for drug administration. We also added many new illustrations to this chapter.
- Chapter 4, Medications and Calculations, now includes additional practice problems in Sections C, D, and E; "true to life" drug labels in full color; and a section on intravenous solutions with practice problems related to direct intravenous injection, IV flow rate, and rate by IV pump.
- Content of drug considerations for both children and older adults has been enhanced.
- Twice as many case studies have been added since the first edition.
- More pharmacologic data have been included related to vitamins, antipsychotics and antidepressants, anesthetics, anticoagulants, electrolytes, gender-related drugs, and first-line emergency drugs for adults and children.
- A new chapter, Nutritional Support (Chapter 11), describes enteral nutrition and medication, including drug administration and total parenteral nutrition (TPN).
- New content has been added within chapters on fluid replacement, cultural considerations, Canadian regulations, multiple sclerosis, and anthelmintics.
- The number of chapters has been increased by four, for a total of 47 chapters, including an increase in the number of chapters on antibacterials (to five) and on cardiac drugs (to four).
- More than 100 new terms have been added to the glossary.
- New tear-out cards have been created, including selected therapeutic drug monitoring and a sample of the new drug prototype chart used in the textbook.
- Abbreviations have been listed inside the front cover for quick reference.
- New appendices include generic drug names and their corresponding Canadian drug names and drugs that affect the color of urine and feces.

Pharmacology: A Nursing Process Approach, Second Edition, is accompanied by ancillary resourses to provide instructors and students with a complete pharmacology package. These resources include:

- A study guide that contains outlines, objectives, exercises with applications of nursing process to clinical situations, and case studies to stimulate critical thinking.
- A pharmacology handbook that provides numerous prototype drug charts, application of nursing process, and drug charts annotating more than 1,500 drugs.
- An instructor's manual with objectives, outlines, and teaching strategies to promote critical thinking. The instructor's manual also includes a basic math test and answers.
- A test bank of more than 800 questions for instructors. An ExaMaster computerized test bank will be available to programs that adopt the textbook.

The students' knowledge of pharmacology and its application to the therapeutic regimen would be enhanced by the use of the recommended comprehensive pharmacology package accompanying *Pharmacology: A Nursing Process Approach*, Second Edition.

Joyce LeFever Kee
Evelyn R. Hayes

Acknowledgments

We wish to extend our sincere appreciation to the many professionals who assisted in the preparation of *Pharmacology: A Nursing Process Approach,* Second Edition, by contributing chapters, reviewing chapters, or offering suggestions. These professionals include the following pharmacologists: John Barron, PharmD; Richard L. Bragdon, RPh, MS, MBA; Mark Cziraky, PharmD; Ronald J. Lefever, RPh; Christie Marsh, RPh; Joseph Peoples, RPh; Robert Thornton, RPh, BSc; Marcus D. Wilson, PharmD; and Jonathan J. Wolfe, PhD. The clinical nurse specialists and nurse educators who provided their expertise are: Diane Baughman, RN, EdD,CS; Ilene Borze, MS, CEN, RN; Michele Bockrath-Welch, RNC, MSN; Anna T. Eaton, RNC, BSN, MN; Sheila Grossman, PhD, RN; Betty B. Laliberte, RN, MSN; Anne E. Lara, RN, MS, OCN, CS; Linda Laskowski-Jones, RN, MS, CS, CCRN, CEN; Brenda Millette, PhD, RN; Nancy G. M. Miner, RNC, MSN; Lisa Plowfield, PhD, RN; Nancy C. Sharts-Hopko, RN, PhD; Rebecca A. Sisson, RN, PhD; Judith A. Torpey, RN, MSN; Carol H. Tyree, RN; Mary Webb, PhD, RN; Kathleen S. Whalen, RN, MN, CCRN; and Sue W. Young, PhD, RN.

We wish to thank especially our contributing authors and illustrators: Anne E. Lara wrote Chapter 29, Biologic Response Modifiers; Jane Purnell Taylor wrote Chapter 42, Drugs Associated with the Female Reproductive Cycle: Pregnancy, Preterm Neonate, Labor, and Delivery; Chapter 43, Drugs Associated with the Postpartum and the Newborn; and Chapter 44, Drugs Related to Women's Health and Disorders; Nancy C. Sharts-Hopko wrote Chapter 45, Drugs Related to Male Reproductive Health: Male Reproductive Disorders, and Chapter 46, Drugs Related to Reproductive Health: Infertility and Sexually Transmitted Diseases; Linda Laskowski-Jones wrote Chapter 47, Adult and Pediatric Emergency Drugs. Allison Bailey created numerous illustrations for Chapters 3 and 38, and Sandra Taccone added illustrations to Unit X and Chapter 38.

Of course we are deeply indebted to the many clients and students we have had throughout our many years of professional nursing practice. From them we have learned many fine points about the role of therapeutic pharmacology in nursing practice.

Our deepest appreciation goes to pharmaceutical companies for permission to use their drug labels. Pharmaceutical companies that extended their courtesy to this book include:

Bristol-Myers Squibb Company
Squibb and Sons Inc.
Apothecon Laboratories
Princeton Pharmaceutical Products
Mead Johnson Pharmaceuticals
Burroughs Wellcome Company (Reproduced with permission of Burroughs Wellcome Company)
Eli Lilly and Company
Lederle Laboratories (Drug labels: Copyright, Lederle Laboratories, Division of American Cyanamid Company, all rights reserved. Reprinted with permission)
Marion Merrell Dow, Inc.
Merck and Company, Inc.
The DuPont/Merck Pharmaceuticals
Warner-Lambert Company
Warner Chilcott Laboratories
Parke-Davis Company
SmithKline Beecham Pharmaceuticals
Wyeth-Ayerst Laboratories (Courtesy of Wyeth-Ayerst Laboratories)

We extend our sincere thanks to the companies and publishers who gave us permission to use photographs, illustrations, and other materials in the text. These include:

American Association of Critical Care Nursing
American Lung Association
Appleton & Lange
Ciba-Geigy Pharmaceuticals
F. A. Davis Company
IMED Corporation
W. B. Saunders Company
Wyeth-Ayerst Laboratories

Thanks are also due to the staff at W. B. Saunders, especially Maura Connor, Editor, Nursing Books; Linda R. Garber, Senior Production Manager; and the editorial and production staffs, for their suggestions and assistance; and to Don Passidomo, librarian at the Department of Veterans Affairs, Elsmere, Delaware, for the help with library research.

We extend our appreciation and love to my husband, Edward D. Kee, and father, Samuel H. LeFever [JLK], and to my parents, Margaret K. and Justin F. Hayes [ERH], for their support.

To the Reader

Consult the product information contained in the package insert of each drug before administering the medication.

Apothecon Laboratories
Bristol-Myers Squibb Company
Burroughs Wellcome Company
The DuPont/Merck Pharmaceuticals
Eli Lilly and Company
Lederle Laboratories, Division of American Cyanamid Company
Marion Merrell Dow, Inc.
Mead Johnson Pharmaceuticals

Parke-Davis Company
SmithKline Beecham Pharmaceuticals
Squibb and Sons, Inc.
Summit Pharmaceuticals/Ciba-Geigy Corporation
Warner Chilcott Laboratories
Warner-Lambert Company
Wyeth-Ayerst Laboratories

Contents

INTRODUCTION TO PROTOTYPE DRUG CHART USE xxi

Unit I

A NURSE'S PERSPECTIVE OF PHARMACOLOGY

1 Drug Action: Pharmaceutic, Pharmacokinetic, and Pharmacodynamic Phases 3

2 Nursing Process and Client Teaching. 14

3 Principles of Drug Administration. 22

4 Medication and Calculations 40
   Section A: Systems of Measurement with Conversion 41
   Section B: Methods for Calculation 52
   Section C: Calculations of Oral Dosages, Including for Pediatrics 65
   Section D: Calculations of Injectable Dosages, Including for Pediatrics 87
   Section E: Calculations of Intravenous Fluids. 111

Unit II

CONTEMPORARY ISSUES IN PHARMACOLOGY

5 The Drug Approval Process (U.S. and Canadian), Resources, and
   Cultural Considerations. 131

6 Drug Interaction and Drug Abuse 138

7 Drug Therapy Considerations Throughout the Life Span 147

8 The Role of the Nurse in Drug Research 157

Unit III

NUTRITION AND ELECTROLYTES

9 Vitamin and Mineral Replacement. 165

10 Fluid and Electrolyte Replacement. 177

11 Nutritional Support 194

Unit IV

NEUROLOGIC AND NEUROMUSCULAR AGENTS

12 Central Nervous System Stimulants. 207

13 Central Nervous System Depressants 214

14 Nonnarcotic and Narcotic Analgesics. 228

15 Anticonvulsants 242

16 Antipsychotics, Anxiolytics, and Antidepressants 251

17 Autonomic Nervous System 274

18 Adrenergics and Adrenergic Blockers 279

19 Cholinergics and Anticholinergics 292

20 Drugs for Neuromuscular Disorders: Parkinsonism, Myasthenia Gravis, Multiple
Sclerosis, and Muscle Spasms 305

Unit V

ANTIINFLAMMATORY AND ANTIINFECTIVE AGENTS

21 Antiinflammatory Drugs 326

22 Antibacterials: Penicillins and Cephalosporins. 341

23 Antibacterials: Macrolides, Tetracyclines, Aminoglycosides, Fluoroquinolones 355

24 Antibacterials: Sulfonamides 370

25 Antitubercular Drugs, Antifungal Drugs, Peptides 376

26 Antiviral, Antimalarial, and Anthelmintic Drugs. 386

27 Drugs for Urinary Tract Disorders. 396

Unit VI

ANTINEOPLASTIC AGENTS

28 Anticancer Drugs. 407

29 Biologic Response Modifiers 424
  Anne E. Lara

Unit VII
RESPIRATORY AGENTS

30 Drugs for Common Upper Respiratory Infections 444

31 Drugs for Acute and Chronic Lower Respiratory Disorders 455

Unit VIII
CARDIOVASCULAR AGENTS

32 Drugs for Cardiac Disorders 473

33 Diuretics 489

34 Antihypertensive Drugs. 502

35 Drugs for Circulatory Disorders 518

Unit IX
GASTROINTESTINAL AGENTS

36 Drugs for Gastrointestinal Tract Disorders. 541

37 Antiulcer Drugs. 563

Unit X
EYE, EAR, AND SKIN AGENTS

38 Drugs for Disorders of the Eye and the Ear. 581

39 Drugs for Dermatologic Disorders. 596

Unit XI
ENDOCRINE AGENTS

40 Endocrine Pharmacology: Pituitary, Thyroid, Parathyroids, and Adrenals. 610

41 Antidiabetic Drugs. 628

Unit XII

REPRODUCTIVE AND GENDER-RELATED AGENTS

42 Drugs Associated with the Female Reproductive Cycle: Pregnancy, Preterm Neonate, Labor, and Delivery 643
Jane Purnell Taylor

43 Drugs Associated with the Postpartum and the Newborn 680
Jane Purnell Taylor

44 Drugs Related to Women's Health and Disorders 697
Jane Purnell Taylor

45 Drugs Related to Reproductive Health: Male Reproductive Disorders 718
Nancy C. Sharts-Hopko

46 Drugs Related to Reproductive Health: Infertility and Sexually Transmitted Diseases . . 731
Nancy C. Sharts-Hopko

Unit XIII

EMERGENCY AGENTS

47 Adult and Pediatric Emergency Drugs 751
Linda Laskowski-Jones

Appendix A: Generic Drugs with Corresponding Canadian Trade Drug Names 767

Appendix B: Temperature Conversion: Celsius and Fahrenheit 771

Appendix C: Alternative Pediatric Drug Calculations 772

Appendix D: Recommended Daily Allowances for Vitamins and Minerals During
 Pregnancy 773

Appendix E: Drugs That Discolor Urine and Feces 775

Appendix F: Vaccines 777

Appendix G: Laboratory Tests Related to Drug Use 782

Appendix H: Therapeutic Drug Monitoring 791

References 795

Glossary 801

Index 819

Introduction to Prototype Drug Chart Use

Nursing interventions related to drug therapy are based on pregnancy category, dosages, contraindications for drug use, drug–lab–food interactions, pharmacokinetics, pharmacodynamics, therapeutic effects/uses, mode of action, side effects, and adverse reactions, including those that are life-threatening. The nursing process correlates with selected aspects of the drug chart as illustrated in the drug chart format. Sample (not inclusive) activities are provided for each step of the nursing process. A more comprehensive application of the nursing process is detailed further in the chapters following each drug group.

The following is the basic format for prototype drug charts found in the chapters throughout Units III to XIII.

PROTOTYPE DRUG

Drug Name	Dosage	**NURSING PROCESS** Assessment and Planning
Pregnancy Category:		
Contraindications	**Drug-Lab-Food Interactions**	
Pharmacokinetics	**Pharmacodynamics**	Interventions
Absorption: *Distribution:* PB: *Metabolism:* t½: *Excretion:*	PO: Onset: Peak: Duration:	

Therapeutic Effects/Uses: *Mode of Action:*	Evaluation

Side Effects	**Adverse Reactions**
	Life-threatening:

KEY: PO: by mouth; PB: protein-binding; t½: half-life.

For the selected drug category, one to two drugs are listed and compared according to dosage; contraindications for drug use; interactions (drug–drug, drug–food, drug–laboratory); pharmacokinetics; pharmacodynamics; therapeutic effects and mode of action; side effects; and adverse reactions. Based on these data, the nursing process can be applied for each drug. The nurse assesses contraindications for use related to the patient's past and present health, illness, and drug history. Relevant laboratory test results, food, and other drugs the client is taking should be assessed and recorded. Based on assessment data, a plan for drug use is developed. Nursing interventions include administering the drug by the appropriate route, in the appropriate amount, and at the appropriate time (influenced by protein-binding and half-life); obtaining specimens such as blood and urine; monitoring the effects with vital signs; observing for any untoward reactions; and client teaching (how drug is to be taken, side effects to report, drug compliance). The nurse evaluates the effects of the drug and any side effects or adverse reactions the client experiences with the drug therapy. Then further assessment and nursing interventions follow.

The nurse may use this format to map out a specific drug and then proceed to identify the specific implications for that drug in the nursing process format that is located on the right side of the drug chart. The drug chart is an ideal format to use with clinical assignments. After initial preparation of the drug chart, the nurse may decide to save it to be used again when administering the same drugs to other clients. The nursing process section may be "penciled in" so it can be easily removed when used for another client.

There are a total of 92 drug charts in this text, some of which compare pharmacologic data for two drugs. For individual use in a clinical setting, one drug may be mapped out according to the drug chart format.

The following drug charts are included in this text:

Unit III

9 Vitamin and Mineral Replacement
Figure 9–2: Fat-Replacement Soluble Vitamin: Vitamin A
Figure 9–3: The Water-Soluble Vitamin: Vitamin C
Figure 9–4: Antianemia, Mineral: Iron

10 Fluid and Electrolyte Replacement
Figure 10–2: Potassium Chloride
Figure 10–3: Calcium

Unit IV

12 Central Nervous System Stimulants
Figure 12–1: Amphetamine-like Drugs

13 Central Nervous System Depressants
Figure 13–2: Sedative-Hypnotic: Barbiturate
Figure 13–3: Sedative-Hypnotic: Benzodiazepine

14 Nonnarcotic and Narcotic Analgesics
Figure 14–1: Analgesic: Acetaminophen
Figure 14–2: Narcotic: Morphine
Figure 14–3: Narcotic: Meperidine
Figure 14–4: Narcotic: Agonist-Antagonist, Pentazocine

15 Anticonvulsants
Figure 15–1: Anticonvulsant: Phenytoin

16 Antipsychotics, Anxiolytics, and Antidepressants
Figure 16–1: Antipsychotics (Neuroleptics): Chlorpromazine and Prochlorperazine
Figure 16–2: Antipsychotic: Nonphenothiazine: Haloperidol
Figure 16–3: Anxiolytics: Diazepam
Figure 16–4: Antidepressants: Amitriptyline and Amoxapine
Figure 16–5: Antimanic: Lithium

18 Adrenergics and Adrenergic Blockers
Figure 18–3: Adrenergic Agonist: Epinephrine
Figure 18–4: Beta-Adrenergic Agonist: Albuterol
Figure 18–5: Beta-Adrenergic Blocker (Sympatholytic): Propranolol

19 Cholinergics and Anticholinergics
Figure 19–3: Cholinergic: Bethanechol
Figure 19–5: Anticholinergic: Atropine Sulfate
Figure 19–6: Antiparkinsonism: Anticholinergic: Trihexyphenidyl HCl

20 Drugs for Neuromuscular Disorders: Parkinsonism, Myasthenia Gravis,
Multiple Sclerosis, and Muscle Spasms
Figure 20–2: Antiparkinsonism: Dopaminergic: Carbidopa-Levodopa
Figure 20–3: Myasthenia Gravis (Drugs for): Pyridostigmine
Figure 20–4: Muscle Relaxants: Carisoprodol and Dantrolene

Unit V

21 Antiinflammatory Drugs
Figure 21–1: Analgesic and Antiinflammatory Drug: Aspirin
Figure 21–2: Antiinflammatory: Nonsteroidal Antiinflammatory Drug (NSAID)
Figure 21–3: Antiinflammatory Agent: Gold
Figure 21–4: Antigout: Allopurinol

22 Antibacterials: Penicillins and Cephalosporins
Figure 22–2: Penicillin Derivatives: Amoxicillin and Cloxacillin
Figure 22–3: Cephalosporins: Cefazolin and Cefaclor

23 Antibacterials: Macrolides, Tetracyclines, Aminoglycosides, Fluoroquinolones
Figure 23–1: Antibacterials: Erythromycin
Figure 23–2: Antibacterials: Tetracyclines
Figure 23–3: Antibacterials: Aminoglycosides
Figure 23–4: Antibacterials: Fluoroquinolones (Quinolones)

24 Antibacterials: Sulfonamides
Figure 24–1: Antibacterials: Sulfonamides (Trimethoprim-Sulfamethoxazole)

25 Antitubercular Drugs, Antifungal Drugs, Peptides
Figure 25–1: Antitubercular Drugs: Isoniazid
Figure 25–2. Antifungals: Nystatin

26 Antiviral, Antimalarial, and Anthelmintic Drugs
Figure 26–1: Antivirals: Acyclovir sodium
Figure 26–2: Antimalarials: Chloroquine HCl

27 Drugs for Urinary Tract Disorders
Figure 27–1: Urinary Antiinfectives: Nitrofurantoin
Figure 27–2: Urinary Analgesics: Phenazopyridine

Unit VI

28 Anticancer Drugs
Figure 28–2: Antineoplastic: Alkylating Drug: Cyclophosphamide
Figure 28–3: Antineoplastic: Antimetabolite: Fluorouracil
Figure 28–4: Antitumor Antibiotics: Doxorubicin and Plicamycin

29 Biologic Response Modifiers
Figure 29–5: Biologic Response Modifiers: Erythropoietin
Figure 29–6: Granulocyte Colony-Stimulating Factor: Filgrastim
Figure 29–7: Granulocyte Macrophage Colony-Stimulating Factor: Sargramostim

Unit VII

30 Drugs for Common Upper Respiratory Infections
Figure 30–1: Antihistamine: Diphenhydramine HCl
Figure 30–2: Antitussive: Dextromethorphan hydrobromide

31 Drugs for Acute and Chronic Lower Respiratory Disorders
Figure 31–2: Bronchodilator: Adrenergic: Metaproterenol
Figure 31–4: Bronchodilator: Methylxanthine: Theophylline

Unit VIII

32 Drugs for Cardiac Disorders
Figure 32–1: Cardiac Glycoside: Digoxin
Figure 32–2: Antianginal: Nitroglycerin
Figure 32–4: Antidysrhythmics: Procainamide HCl

33 Diuretics
Figure 33–2: Thiazide: Hydrochlorothiazide
Figure 33–3: Loop (High Ceiling): Furosemide
Figure 33–4: Potassium-Sparing: Triamterene

34 Antihypertensive Drugs
Figure 34–3: Beta-Adrenergic Blocker: Metoprolol

Figure 34–4: Alpha-Adrenergic Blocker: Prazosin HCl
Figure 34–5: Angiotensin Antagonist: Captopril

35 Drugs for Circulatory Disorders
Figure 35–2: Anticoagulants: Heparin and Warfarin
Figure 35–3: Thrombolytic Drugs: Streptokinase
Figure 35–4: Antilipemics: Lovastatin
Figure 35–5: Vasodilators: Isoxsuprine HCl

Unit IX

36 Drugs for Gastrointestinal Tract Disorders
Figure 36–2: Antiemetics: Phenothiazine: Perphenazine
Figure 36–3: Emetics: Ipecac syrup
Figure 36–4: Antidiarrheals: Diphenoxylate with atropine
Figure 36–5: Laxatives: Contact: Bisacodyl
Figure 36–6: Laxatives: Bulk-forming: Metamucil

37 Antiulcer Drugs
Figure 37–3: Antiulcer: Antacids
Figure 37–4: Antiulcer: Histamine$_2$ blockers
Figure 37–5: Antiulcer: Pepsin Inhibitor: Sucralfate

Unit X

38 Drugs for Disorders of the Eye and the Ear
Figure 38–2: Direct Acting Miotic: Pilocarpine

39 Drugs for Dermatologic Disorders
Figure 39–1: Topical Antiinfectives: Burns: Mafenide acetate

Unit XI

40 Endocrine Pharmacology: Pituitary, Thyroid, Parathyroids, and Adrenals
Figure 40–1: Pituitary Hormone: Adrenocorticotropic Hormone (ACTH)
Figure 40–2: Thyroid Hormone: Levothyroxine sodium
Figure 40–3: Parathyroid Hormone Replacement: Calcitriol
Figure 40–4: Adrenal Hormone: Prednisone

41 Antidiabetic Drugs
Figure 41–2: Injectable Insulins: Regular and NPH
Figure 41–3: Oral Hypoglycemic Drug: Acetohexamide

Unit XII

42 Drugs Associated with the Female Reproductive Cycle: Pregnancy, Preterm Neonate, Labor, and Delivery
Figure 42–2: Beta$_2$-Adrenergic Agonist: Ritodrine
Figure 42–3: Oxytocic: Pitocin

45 Drugs Related to Reproductive Health: Male Reproductive Disorders
Figure 45–7: Androgens: Testosterone

46 Drugs Related to Reproductive Health: Infertility and Sexually Transmitted Diseases
Figure 46–3: Ovulation Stimulant: Clomiphene Citrate

Unit XIII

47 Adult and Pediatric Emergency Drugs
Figure 47–1: Emergency Treatment of Cardiac States: Antidysrhythmics
Figure 47–2: Emergency Treatment of Neurosurgical States: Diuretic
Figure 47–3: Emergency Treatment of Poisoning
Figure 47–4: Emergency Treatment of Shock
Figure 47–5: Emergency Treatment of Hypertensive Crisis

Unit I

A Nurse's Perspective
of Pharmacology

Assessing a client's response to drug therapy is an ongoing nursing responsibility. To adequately assess, plan, intervene, and evaluate drug effects, the nurse needs to have knowledge of the pharmaceutic, pharmacokinetic, and pharmacodynamic phases of drug action. A drug chart—see Introduction to Drug Chart Use—organizes specific drug data that are needed for preparation and application of the nursing process. Client teaching is essential to promote client and family adherence to the drug regimen and therapy.

In addition to understanding the three phases of drug action, nursing process, and client teaching, the application of principles of drug administration and calculation of drug doses are important functions in nursing practice. Chapter 3, Principles of Drug Administration, contains basic learning material for the administration of medications. It describes the "ten rights" in drug administration, drug orders, drug distribution, drug charting, guidelines for drug administration, and routes for drug administration with illustrated parenteral sites.

Chapter 4, Medications and Calculations, provides practice in drug calculation for adult and child dosages. This chapter could be assigned as an overall review of drug calculation. Chapters 3 and 4 may be used for drug administration and calculation in place of a nursing fundamentals text or a drug calculation text.

Chapter 1

Drug Action: Pharmaceutic, Pharmacokinetic, and Pharmacodynamic Phases

OUTLINE

Objectives
Terms
Introduction
Pharmaceutic Phase
Pharmacokinetics
    Absorption
    Distribution
    Metabolism, or Biotransfor-
      mation
    Excretion, or Elimination

Pharmacodynamics
    Onset, Peak, and Duration
      of Action
    Receptor Theory
    Therapeutic Index and
      Therapeutic Range
    Peak and Trough Levels
    Loading Dose
    Side Effects, Adverse Reac-
      tions, and Toxic Effects

Summary
Nursing Process
Study Questions

OBJECTIVES

Define the three phases of drug action.

Identify the two processes that occur before tablets are absorbed into the body.

Describe the four processes of pharmacokinetics.

Explain the meaning of pharmacodynamics, the receptor, and nonreceptors in drug action.

Define the terms *protein-bound drugs, half-life, therapeutic index, therapeutic drug range, side effects, adverse reaction, and drug toxicity.*

Check drugs for half-life, percentage of protein-binding effect, therapeutic range, and side effects in a drug reference book.

TERMS

active absorption
adverse reactions
agonists
antagonists
bioavailability
creatinine clearance
disintegration
dissolution
distribution
duration of action
elimination
first-pass effect
free drugs

half-life
high therapeutic index
loading dose
low therapeutic index
metabolism
nonselective drug response
nonspecific drug response
onset of action
passive absorption
peak action
peak level
pharmaceutic phase
pharmacodynamic phase

pharmacokinetic phase
pinocytosis
protein-binding
rate limiting
receptor
side effects
therapeutic index
therapeutic window
therapeutic range
time–response curve
toxicity
trough level

INTRODUCTION

A drug taken by mouth goes through three phases—pharmaceutic (dissolution), pharmacokinetic, and pharmacodynamic—in order for drug action to occur. In the pharmaceutic phase the drug goes into solution so that it can cross the biologic membrane. When the drug is administered parenterally by subcutaneous, intramuscular, or intravenous routes, there is no pharmaceutic phase. The second phase, the pharmacokinetic, comprises four processes: absorption, distribution, metabolism (or biotransformation), and excretion. In the pharmacodynamic or third phase, a biologic or physiologic response results.

PHARMACEUTIC PHASE

Approximately 80% of drugs are taken by mouth. **Pharmaceutic** (dissolution) is the first phase of drug action. In the gastrointestinal (GI) tract, drugs need to be in solution to be absorbed. A drug in solid form (tablet or capsule) must disintegrate into small particles in order for it to dissolve into a liquid, a process known as dissolution. Drugs in liquid form are already in solution. Figure 1–1 displays the pharmaceutic phase of a tablet.

Tablets are not 100% drug. Fillers and inert substances, generally called excipients, are used in drug preparation to allow the drug to take on a particular size and shape and to enhance dissolution of the drug. Some additives in drugs, such as the ions potassium (K) and sodium (Na) in penicillin potassium and penicillin sodium, increase the absorbability of the drug. Penicillin is poorly absorbed from the GI tract because of gastric acid. By making the drug a potassium or sodium salt, penicillin can be absorbed. An infant's gastric secretions have a higher pH (alkaline) than those of adults, so babies absorb more penicillin.

Disintegration is the breakdown of the tablet into smaller particles. **Dissolution** is the dissolving of the smaller particles in the gastrointestinal fluid prior to absorption. **Rate limiting** refers to the time it takes the drug to disintegrate and dissolve to become available for the body to absorb it. Drugs in liquid form are more rapidly available for GI absorption than are solids. Generally, drugs disintegrate faster and are absorbed faster in acidic fluids

that have a pH of 1 or 2 than in alkaline fluids. The young and the elderly have less gastric acidity, so drug absorption is generally slower for those drugs absorbed primarily in the stomach.

Enteric-coated (EC) drugs resist disintegration in the gastric acid of the stomach, so disintegration does not occur until the drug reaches the alkaline environment in the small intestine. Enteric-coated tablets can remain in the stomach for a long time; therefore, their effect may be delayed in onset. Enteric-coated tablets or capsules and sustained-release (beaded) capsules *should not be crushed.*

Food in the GI tract may interfere with the dissolution and absorption of certain drugs. However, food can enhance absorption of other drugs; thus, some drugs should be taken with food. Some drugs are irritating to the gastric mucosa, so fluids or food may be necessary to dilute drug concentration and act as protectants.

PHARMACOKINETICS

Pharmacokinetics is the process of drug movement to achieve drug action. The four processes are: absorption, distribution, metabolism (or biotransformation), and excretion (or elimination).

By using the knowledge of the four pharmacokinetic processes of the drug's make-up, the prescriber promotes safety of drug therapy. The nurse needs to be alert to possible adverse drug effects that can result from the pharmacokinetics of the drug, and to report promptly such findings.

ABSORPTION

Absorption is the movement of drug particles from the GI tract to body fluids by passive absorption, active absorption, or pinocytosis. Most oral drugs are absorbed into the surface area of the small intestine through the action of the extensive mucosal villi. If the villi are decreased in number because of disease, drug effect, or removal of small intestine, absorption is reduced. Protein-based drugs, such as insulin and growth hormones, are destroyed in the small intestine by digestive enzymes. **Passive absorption** occurs mostly by diffusion (movement from higher concentration to lower concentration). With the process of diffusion, the drug does not require energy to move across the membrane. **Active**

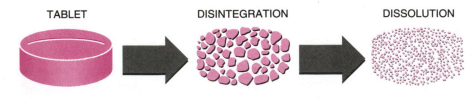

TABLET   DISINTEGRATION   DISSOLUTION

FIGURE 1–1 The two pharmaceutic phases are disintegration and dissolution.

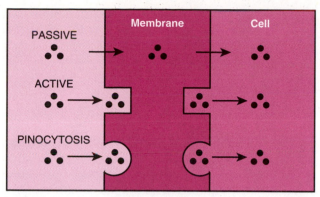

FIGURE 1–2 The three major processes for drug absorption through the gastrointestinal membrane are passive absorption, active absorption, and pinocytosis.

absorption requires a carrier such as an enzyme or protein to move the drug against a concentration gradient. Energy is required for active absorption. **Pinocytosis** is a process by which cells carry drug across their membrane by engulfing the drug particles (Fig. 1–2).

The GI membrane is composed mostly of lipid (fat) and protein, so drugs that are lipid soluble pass rapidly through the GI membrane. Water-soluble drugs need a carrier, either enzyme or protein, to pass through the membrane. Large particles pass through the cell membrane if they are nonionized (no positive or negative charge). Weak acid drugs, such as aspirin, are less ionized in the stomach, and they pass through the stomach lining easily and rapidly. Hydrochloric acid destroys some drugs, such as penicillin G; therefore, a large oral dosage of penicillin is needed because of partial dose loss due to the gastric juices.

REMEMBER: Drugs that are lipid soluble and nonionized are absorbed *faster* than water-soluble and ionized drugs.

Drug absorption is affected by blood flow, pain, stress, hunger, fasting, food, and pH. Poor circulation due to shock, vasoconstrictor drugs, or disease hampers absorption. Pain, stress, and foods that are solid, hot, and fatty can slow gastric emptying time, so the drug remains longer in the stomach. Exercise can decrease blood flow by causing more blood to flow to the peripheral muscle, decreasing blood circulation to the GI tract.

Drugs given intramuscularly can be absorbed faster in muscles that have more blood vessels, such as the deltoid, than those that have fewer blood vessels, such as the gluteal. Subcutaneous tissue has fewer blood vessels, so absorption is slower in such tissue.

Some drugs do *not* go directly into the systemic circulation following oral absorption but pass from the intestinal lumen to the liver, by the portal vein.

In the liver, some drugs may be metabolized to an inactive form, which may then be excreted, thus reducing the amount of active drug. Some drugs do not undergo metabolism at all in the liver, and others may be metabolized to drug metabolite, which may be equally or more active than the original drug. The process in which the drug passes to the liver first is called the **first-pass effect,** or **hepatic first pass.** Examples of drugs with first-pass metabolism are warfarin (Coumadin) and morphine. Lidocaine and some nitroglycerins are *not* given orally, because they have extensive first-pass metabolism, and so the majority of the dose would be destroyed.

Bioavailability is a subcategory of absorption. It is the percentage of the administered drug dose that reaches the systemic circulation. For the oral route of drug administration, bioavailability occurs after absorption and hepatic drug metabolism. The percentage of bioavailability for the oral route is always less than 100%. Bioavailability for the intravenous route is usually 100%. Oral drugs that have a high first-pass hepatic metabolism may have a bioavailability of 20% to 40% upon entering systemic circulation. To obtain desired drug effect, the oral dose could be three to five times larger than the drug dose for intravenous use.

Factors that alter bioavailability include (1) the drug form (tablet, capsule, sustained-release, liquid, transdermal patch, rectal suppository, inhalation); (2) route of administration (oral, rectal, topical, parenteral); (3) GI mucosa and motility; (4) food and other drugs; and (5) changes in liver metabolism due to liver dysfunction or inadequate hepatic blood flow. A decrease in liver function or a decrease in hepatic blood flow can increase the bioavailability of a drug, but only if the drug is metabolized by the liver. Less drug is destroyed by hepatic metabolism in the presence of liver disorder.

With some oral drugs, rapid absorption increases the bioavailability of the drug and can cause an increase in drug concentration. Drug toxicity may result. Slow absorption can limit the bioavailability of the drug, thus causing a decrease in drug serum concentration.

DISTRIBUTION

Distribution is the process by which the drug becomes available to body fluids and body tissues. Drug distribution is influenced by blood flow, its affinity to the tissue, and **protein-binding** effect (Fig. 1–3).

As drugs are distributed in the plasma, many are bound to varying degrees (percentages) with pro-

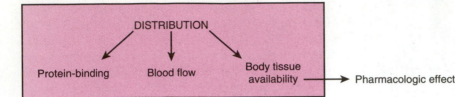

FIGURE 1–3 Drug distribution.

tein (primarily albumin). Drugs that are greater than 89% bound to protein are known as highly protein-bound drugs; drugs that are 61% to 89% bound to protein are moderately highly protein-bound; drugs that are 30% to 60% bound to protein are moderately protein-bound; and drugs that are less than 30% bound to protein are low protein-bound drugs. Table 1–1 lists selected highly protein-bound drugs and moderately highly protein-bound drugs. The portion of the drug that is bound is inactive because it is not available to receptors, and the portion that remains unbound is free, active drug. Only **free drugs (drugs not bound to protein)** are active and can cause a pharmacologic response. As the free drug in the circulation decreases, more bound drug is released from the protein to maintain the balance of free drug.

When two highly protein-bound drugs are given concurrently, they compete for protein-binding sites, thus causing more free drug to be released into the circulation. Drug accumulation and possible drug toxicity can result in this situation. Also, a low protein level decreases the number of protein-binding sites, and can cause an increase in the amount of free drug in the plasma. Drug overdose may then result. Drug dose is prescribed according to the percentage in which the drug binds to protein.

With some health conditions that result in a low serum protein level, excess free or unbound drug goes to nonspecific tissue binding sites until needed. When this occurs, excess free drug in the circulation would not occur.

Some drugs bind with a specific protein component such as albumin or globulin. Most anticonvulsants bind primarily to albumin. Some basic drugs such as antidysrhythmics (lidocaine, quinidine) bind mostly to globulins.

Clients with liver or kidney disease or who are malnourished may have an abnormally low serum albumin level. This results in fewer protein-binding sites, which in turn leads to excess free drug and eventually to drug toxicity. The elderly are more likely to have hypoalbuminemia.

Checking the protein-binding percentage of all drugs administered to a client is important in order to avoid possible drug toxicity. The nurse should also check the client's plasma protein and albumin levels, because a decrease in plasma protein (albumin) decreases protein-binding sites, permitting more free drug in the circulation. Depending on the drug(s), the result could be life-threatening.

Abscesses, exudates, body glands, and tumors hinder drug distribution. Antibiotics do not distribute well at abscess and exudate sites. In addition,

TABLE 1–1 Protein-Binding Percentage and Half-Life of Specific Drugs

Drug	Protein-Bound (%)	Half-Life (t½) (h)
Highly Protein-Bound Drugs (>89%)		
Amitriptyline	97	40
Chlorpromazine	95	30
Diazepam	98	30–80
Dicloxacillin	95	0.5–1
Digitoxin	90	8
Furosemide	95	1.5
Ibuprofen	98	2–4
Lorazepam	92	15
Piroxicam	99	30–86
Propranolol	92	4
Rifampin	89	2
Sulfisoxazole	85–95	4.5–7.5
Valproic acid	92	15
Moderately Highly Protein-Bound Drugs (61%–89%)		
Erythromycin	70	3
Nafcillin	86	2–20
Phenytoin	88	10–40
Quinidine	70	6
Trimethoprim	70	11
Moderately Protein-Bound Drugs (30%–60%)		
Aspirin	49	0.25–2
Lidocaine	50	2
Meperidine	56	3
Pindolol	40	3–4
Theophylline	60	9
Ticarcillin	45–65	1–1.5
Low Protein-Bound Drugs (<30%)		
Amikacin	4–11	2–3
Amoxicillin	20	1–1.5
Atenolol	6–16	6–7
Cephalexin	10–15	0.5–1.2
Digoxin	25	36
Neostigmine bromide	15–25	1–1.5
Terbutaline sulfate	25	3–11
Timolol maleate	<10	3–4
Tobramycin sulfate	10	2–3

Key: >: greater than; <: less than; h: hour.

some drugs accumulate in particular tissues, such as fat, bone, liver, eyes, and muscle.

METABOLISM, OR BIOTRANSFORMATION

The liver is the primary site of **metabolism.** Most drugs are inactivated by liver enzymes and are then converted or transformed by hepatic enzymes to inactive metabolites or water-soluble substances for excretion. A large percentage of drugs are lipid soluble; thus, the liver metabolizes the lipid-soluble drug substance to a water-soluble substance for renal excretion. However, some drugs are transformed into active metabolites, causing an increased pharmacologic response. Liver diseases, such as cirrhosis and hepatitis, alter drug metabolism by inhibiting the drug-metabolizing enzymes in the liver. When the drug metabolism rate is decreased, excess drug accumulation can occur, which can lead to toxicity.

The **half-life,** symbolized as $t\frac{1}{2}$, of a drug is the time it takes for one-half of the drug concentration to be eliminated. Metabolism and elimination affect the half-life of a drug. For example, with liver or kidney dysfunction, the half-life of the drug is prolonged and less drug is metabolized and eliminated. When a drug is taken continually, drug accumulation may occur. Table 1–1 gives the half-life of selected drugs.

A drug goes through several half-lives before more than 90% of the drug is eliminated. If the client takes 650 mg (milligrams) of aspirin and the $t\frac{1}{2}$ is 3 h (hours), then it takes 3 h for the first half-life to eliminate 325 mg, and the second half-life (at 6 h) for an additional 162 mg to be eliminated, and so on until the sixth half-life (or 18 h), when 10 mg of aspirin is left in the body (Table 1–2). A short half-life is considered to be 4 to 8 h and a long one is 24 h or longer. If the drug has a long half-life (such as digoxin: 36 h), it takes several days until the body completely eliminates the drug.

By knowing the half-life, the time it takes for the drug to reach a steady state of serum concentration can be computed. Administration of the drug for three to five half-lives saturates the biologic system to the extent that the intake of drug equals the amount metabolized and excreted. An example is digoxin, which has a half-life of 36 hours with normal renal function. It would take approximately 5 days to 1 week (three to five half-lives) to reach a steady state for digoxin concentration. Steady-state serum concentration is predictive of therapeutic drug effect. The half-life of drugs is also discussed in the next section on pharmacodynamics.

EXCRETION, OR ELIMINATION

The main route of drug **elimination** is through the urine. Other routes include bile, feces, lungs, saliva, sweat, and breast milk. Free, unbound drugs, water-soluble drugs, and drugs that are unchanged are filtered by the kidneys. Protein-bound drugs cannot be filtered through the kidneys. Once the drug is released from the protein, it is a free drug and eventually is excreted in the urine. The lungs eliminate volatile drug substances and products metabolized to CO_2 and H_2O.

The urine pH influences drug excretion. Urine pH varies from 4.5 to 8. Acid urine promotes elimination of weak base drugs, and alkaline urine promotes elimination of weak acid drugs. Aspirin, a weak acid, is excreted rapidly in alkaline urine. If a person takes an overdose of aspirin, sodium bicarbonate may be given to change the urine pH to alkaline in order to help potentiate excretion of the drug. Large quantities of cranberry juice can decrease the urine pH, causing an acid urine, thus inhibiting the elimination of the aspirin.

With a kidney disease that results in decreased glomerular filtration rate (GFR) or decreased renal tubular secretion, drug excretion is slowed or impaired. Drug accumulation with possible severe adverse drug reactions can result. A decrease in blood flow to the kidneys can also alter drug excretion.

The most accurate test to determine renal function is **creatinine clearance (CL_{cr}).** Creatinine is a metabolic byproduct of muscle that is excreted by the kidneys. Creatinine clearance varies with age and gender. Lower values are expected in the elderly and in the female due to decreased muscle mass. A decrease in renal GFR results in an increase in serum creatinine level and a decrease in urine creatinine clearance.

With renal dysfunction due to kidney disorders or in the elderly, drug dosage usually needs to be

TABLE 1–2 Half-Life of 650 mg of Aspirin

Number $t\frac{1}{2}$	Time of Elimination (h)	Dosage Remaining (mg)	Percentage Left
1	3	325	50
2	6	162	25
3	9	81	12.5
4	12	40	6.25
5	15	20	3.1
6	18	10	1.55

decreased. In these cases, the creatinine clearance needs to be determined in order to determine the appropriate drug dosage. When the creatinine clearance is decreased, drug dosage may need to be decreased. Continuous drug dosing according to a prescribed drug dose could result in drug toxicity.

The creatinine clearance test consists of a 12- or 24-hour urine collection and a blood sample. Normal creatinine clearance is 85 to 135 mL/min. This number decreases with age, because aging decreases muscle mass and results in a decrease in functioning nephrons. The elderly may have a creatinine clearance of 60 mL/min. For this reason, drug dosage in the elderly may need to be decreased.

PHARMACODYNAMICS

The study of a drug's effect on cellular physiology and biochemistry and the drug's mechanism of action is known as **pharmacodynamics.** Drug response can cause a primary or secondary physiologic effect, or both. The primary effect is desirable and the secondary effect may be desirable or undesirable. An example of a drug with a primary and secondary effect is diphenhydramine (Benadryl), an antihistamine. The primary effect of diphenhydramine is to treat the symptoms of allergy, and the secondary effect is a central nervous system depression that causes drowsiness. The secondary effect is undesirable when driving a car, but at bedtime, it could be desirable by causing a mild sedation.

ONSET, PEAK, AND DURATION OF ACTION

Onset of action is the time it takes to reach the minimum effective concentration (MEC) after a drug is administered. **Peak action** occurs when the drug reaches its highest blood or plasma concentration. **Duration of action** is the length of time the drug has a pharmacologic effect. Figure 1–4 illustrates the areas in which onset, peak, and duration of action occur.

Some drugs produce effects in minutes, but others may take hours or days. A **time–response curve** evaluates three parameters of drug action: the onset of drug action, peak action, and duration of action. Figure 1–4 indicates these parameters by using T (time) with subscripts $_{0, 1, 2, 3}$.

It is necessary to understand the time–response in relationship to drug administration. If the drug plasma or serum level drops below threshold or MEC, adequate drug dosing is *not* achieved; too high a drug level, above the minimum toxic concentration (MTC), can result in toxicity.

RECEPTOR THEORY

Most **receptors,** protein in structure, are found on cell membranes. Drugs act through receptors by binding to the receptor to produce (initiate) a response or to block (prevent) a response. The activity of many drugs is determined by the ability of the drug to bind to a specific receptor. The better the drug fits at the receptor site, the more biologically active the drug is. It is similar to the fit of the right key in a lock. Figure 1–5 illustrates a drug binding to a receptor.

Drugs that produce a response are called **agonists,** and drugs that block a response are called **antagonists.** Isoproterenol (Isuprel) stimulates the $beta_1$ receptor, and so it is an agonist. Cimetidine (Tagamet), an antagonist, blocks the H_2 receptor, thus preventing excessive gastric acid secretion.

Almost all drugs, agonists and antagonists, lack specific and selective effects. A receptor produces a

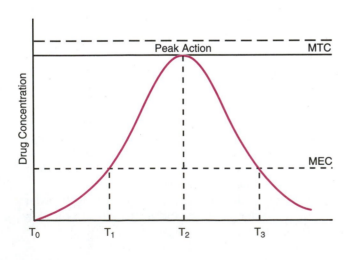

Key:

T_0-T_1 = onset

T_0-T_2 = peak

T_1-T_3 = duration

FIGURE 1–4 The time-response curve evaluates three parameters of drug action: (1) onset, (2) peak, and (3) duration. MEC: minimum effective concentration; MTC: minimum toxic concentration.

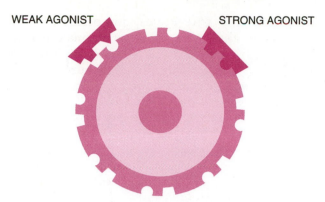

WEAK AGONIST   STRONG AGONIST

FIGURE 1–5 Two drug agonists attach to the receptor site. The drug agonist that has an exact fit is a strong agonist and is more biologically active than the weak agonist.

variety of physiologic responses, depending on where in the body that receptor is located. Cholinergic receptors are located in the bladder, heart, blood vessels, lungs, and eyes. A drug that stimulates or blocks the cholinergic receptors affects all anatomic sites of location. Drugs that affect various sites are considered to be **nonspecific** or have properties of **nonspecificity.** Bethanechol (Urecholine) may be prescribed for postoperative urinary retention in order to increase bladder contraction. This drug stimulates the cholinergic receptor located in the bladder, and urination occurs by strengthening bladder contraction. Because bethanechol affects the cholinergic receptor, other cholinergic sites are also affected. The heart rate decreases, blood pressure decreases, gastric acid secretion increases, the bronchioles constrict, and the pupils of the eye con-

strict (Fig. 1–6). These other effects may or may not be desirable, and may or may not be harmful to the client. Drugs that evoke a variety of responses throughout the body have a nonspecific response.

Drugs may act at different receptors. Drugs that affect various receptors are **nonselective** or have properties of **nonselectivity.** Chlorpromazine (Thorazine) acts on the norepinephrine, dopamine, acetylcholine, and histamine receptors, and a variety of responses result from these receptor sites (Fig. 1–7). Another example is epinephrine. It acts on the alpha$_1$, beta$_1$, and beta$_2$ receptors.

Drugs that produce a response but do *not* act on a receptor may act by stimulating or inhibiting enzyme activity or hormone production.

The four categories of drug action include (1) stimulation or depression, (2) replacement, (3) inhibition or killing of organisms, and (4) irritation. Drug action that stimulates increases the rate of cell activity or increases the secretion from a gland. Those drugs that depress reduce cell activity and reduce function of a specific organ. Replacement drugs, such as insulin, replace essential body compounds. Drugs that inhibit or kill organisms interfere with bacterial cell growth; i.e., penicillin exerts its bactericidal effects by blocking the synthesis of the bacterial cell wall. Drugs also can act by the mechanism of irritation: laxatives can irritate the inner wall of the colon, thus increasing peristalsis and defecation.

Drug action might last hours, days, weeks, or months. The length of action depends upon the half-life of the drug, so half-life is a reasonable guide for determining drug dosage intervals. Drugs

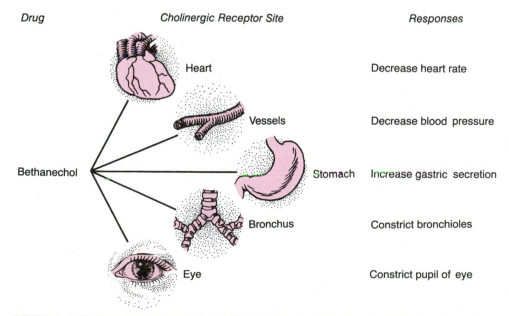

Drug	Cholinergic Receptor Site	Responses
	Heart	Decrease heart rate
	Vessels	Decrease blood pressure
Bethanechol	Stomach	Increase gastric secretion
	Bronchus	Constrict bronchioles
	Eye	Constrict pupil of eye

FIGURE 1–6 Cholinergic receptors are located in the heart, blood vessels, stomach, bronchi, and eyes.

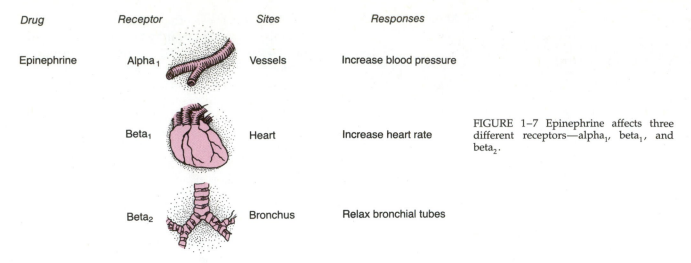

Drug	Receptor		Sites	Responses
Epinephrine	Alpha₁		Vessels	Increase blood pressure
	Beta₁		Heart	Increase heart rate
	Beta₂		Bronchus	Relax bronchial tubes

FIGURE 1–7 Epinephrine affects three different receptors—alpha$_1$, beta$_1$, and beta$_2$.

with a short half-life, such as penicillin G (t½ is 2 h), are given several times a day. Drugs with a long half-life, such as digoxin (36 h), are given once a day. If a drug with a long half-life is given twice or more times a day, drug accumulation in the body and drug toxicity are likely to result. If there is liver or renal impairment, the half-life of the drug increases. In these cases, high doses of the drug or too-frequent dosing can result in drug toxicity.

THERAPEUTIC INDEX AND THERAPEUTIC RANGE (THERAPEUTIC WINDOW)

The safety of drugs is a major concern. The **therapeutic index** (TI), calculated below, estimates the margin of safety of a drug by using a ratio that measures the effective therapeutic dose in 50% of animals (ED_{50}) and lethal dose in 50% of animals

(LD_{50}) (Fig. 1–8). The closer the ratio is to 1, the greater the danger of toxicity.

$$TI = \frac{LD_{50}}{ED_{50}}$$

Drugs with a **low therapeutic index** have a narrow margin of safety (Fig. 1–9A). Drug dosage might need adjustment and plasma (serum) drug levels need to be monitored because of the small safety range between effective dose and lethal dose. Drugs with a **high therapeutic index** have a wide margin of safety and less danger of producing toxic effects (Fig. 1–9B). Plasma (serum) drug levels do not need to be monitored routinely for drugs with a high therapeutic index.

The **therapeutic range (therapeutic window)** of a drug concentration in plasma should be between the MEC (minimum effective concentration) in the plasma for obtaining desired drug action and the minimum toxic concentration (MTC), the toxic effect. When the therapeutic range is given, it includes both protein-bound and unbound portions of the drug. Drug reference books give many plasma (serum) therapeutic ranges of drugs. If the therapeutic range is narrow, such as for digoxin (0.5 to 2 ng/mL [nanograms per milliliter]), the plasma drug level should be monitored periodically in order to avoid drug toxicity. Monitoring the therapeutic range is not necessary if the drug *is not* considered highly toxic. Table 1–3 lists the therapeutic ranges and toxic levels for anticonvulsants.

PEAK AND TROUGH LEVELS

Peak drug level is the highest plasma concentration of drug at a specific time. If the drug is given

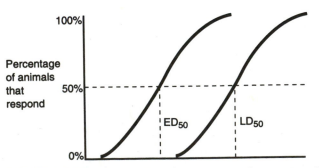

FIGURE 1–8 The therapeutic index measures the margin of safety of a drug. It is a ratio that measures the effective therapeutic dose and lethal dose.

FIGURE 1–9 (*A*) A low therapeutic index drug has a narrow margin of safety, and the drug effect should be closely monitored. (*B*) A high therapeutic index drug has a wide margin of safety and carries less risk of drug toxicity. (*Source:* Adapted from A. K. Swonger and M. P. Matejski: *Nursing Pharmacology,* 2nd ed. Philadelphia, JB Lippincott, 1991, p 37.)

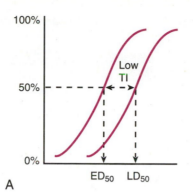

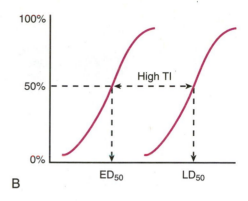

orally, the peak time might be 1 to 3 h after drug administration. If the drug is given intravenously, the peak time might occur in 10 min. A blood sample should be drawn at the proposed peak time, according to the route of administration.

The **trough level** is the lowest plasma concentration of a drug and measures the rate at which the drug is eliminated. Trough levels are drawn immediately before the next dose of drug is given, regardless of route of administration. Peak levels indicate the **rate of absorption** of the drug, and the trough levels indicate the **rate of elimination** of the drug. Peak and trough levels are requested for drugs that have a narrow therapeutic index and are considered toxic, such as the aminoglycosides (antibiotics) (Table 1–4). If either the peak or trough level is too high, toxicity can occur. If the peak is too low, no therapeutic effect will be achieved.

LOADING DOSE

When immediate drug response is desired, a large initial dose, known as the **loading dose,** of drug is given to achieve a rapid MEC in the plasma. After a large initial dose, a prescribed dosage per day is ordered. Digoxin, a digitalis preparation, requires a loading dose when first prescribed. *Digitalization* is the term used to achieve the MEC level for digoxin in the plasma within a short time.

SIDE EFFECTS, ADVERSE REACTIONS, AND TOXIC EFFECTS

Side effects are physiologic effects not related to desired drug effects. All drugs have side effects, desirable or undesirable. Even with a correct drug dosage, side effects occur and are predicted. Side effects result mostly from drugs that lack specificity, such as bethanechol (Urecholine). In some health problems, side effects may be desirable, such as the use of diphenhydramine HCl (Benadryl) given at bedtime: its side effect of drowsiness is beneficial. At times, however, side effects are called adverse reactions. The terms *side effects* and *adverse reactions* might be used interchangeably. **Adverse reactions** are more severe than side effects. They are a range of untoward effects (unintended and occurring at normal doses) of drugs that cause mild to severe side effects, including anaphylaxis (cardiovascular collapse). Adverse reactions are always undesirable. Adverse effects must always be reported and documented, because they represent variances from planned therapy.

Toxic effects, or **toxicity,** of a drug can be identified by monitoring the plasma (serum) therapeutic range of the drug. However, for drugs that have a wide therapeutic index, the therapeutic ranges are seldom given. For those drugs with a narrow therapeutic index, such as aminoglycoside antibiotics and anticonvulsants, the therapeutic ranges are

TABLE 1–3 Anticonvulsants: Therapeutic Ranges and Toxic Levels

Drug	Therapeutic Range (μg/mL)	Toxic Level (μg/mL)
Carbamazepine	6–12	>12–15
Ethosuximide	40–80	>80–100
Phenytoin	10–20	>30
Primidone	5–10	>12–15
Valproic acid	50–100	>100

TABLE 1–4 Aminoglycoside Antibiotics: Peaks and Troughs

Drug	Peak (μg/mL)	Trough (μg/mL)	Toxic Peak Level (μg/mL)	Toxic Trough Levels (μg/mL)
Amikacin	15–30	5–10	>35	>10
Gentamicin	5–10	<2	>12	>2
Tobramycin	5–10	<2	>12	>2

Pharmaceutic	Pharmacokinetics	Pharmacodynamics
Solid form Liquid form	Absorption Distribution Metabolism/Bio- transformation Excretion	Drug Action: Onset, Peak, and Duration Receptors Enzymes Hormones

FIGURE 1–10 Three phases of drug action.

closely monitored. When the drug level exceeds the therapeutic range, toxic effects are likely to occur from overdosing or drug accumulation.

SUMMARY

The phases of drug action are pharmaceutic, pharmacokinetic, and pharmacodynamic. Figure 1–10 illustrates these three phases for drugs given orally, but drugs given by injection are involved only in the pharmacokinetic and pharmacodynamic phases. Nurses should be aware that tablets must disintegrate and go into solution (the pharmaceutic phase) to be absorbed.

To avoid toxic effects, the nurse needs to know the half-life, protein-binding percentage, normal side effects, and therapeutic ranges of the drug. This information can be obtained from drug reference books.

NURSING PROCESS

ASSESSMENT

- Recognize that drugs in liquid form are absorbed faster than those in solid form.
- Assess for signs and symptoms of drug toxicity when giving two drugs that are highly protein-bound. The drugs compete for protein-binding sites and displacement of drugs occurs. More free drug is in circulation because there are not enough protein-binding sites. Too much of a free drug can result in drug toxicity.
- Assess for side effects of drugs that are non-specific (same receptor at different tissue and organ sites), such as atropine, for tachycardia, dry mouth and throat, constipation, urinary retention, and blurred vision. If nonspecific drugs are given in large doses or at frequent intervals, many side effects are likely to occur.
- Assess for side effects of drugs that are nonselective (drugs that affect different receptors).
- Check peak levels and trough levels of drugs that have a narrow therapeutic range, such as aminoglycosides. If the trough level is high, toxic effects can result.

NURSING INTERVENTION

- Advise the client not to eat fatty food prior to ingesting an enteric-coated tablet, because fatty foods decrease absorption rate.

- Check the drug literature for the drug's protein-binding percentage. Those drugs with a high protein-binding effect have a large portion of drug bound to protein, causing the drug to become inactive until it is released from the protein. The portion that is not bound to protein is free drug.
- Report to the health care provider if drugs with a long half-life (greater than 24 h) are given more than once a day. Some drugs with a long half-life, such as the anticoagulant warfarin (Coumadin), can be more dangerous than others and should be monitored frequently.
- Monitor the therapeutic range of drugs that are more toxic or have a narrow therapeutic range, such as digoxin.

EVALUATION

- Evaluate the determinants affecting drug therapy according to Figure 1–11.

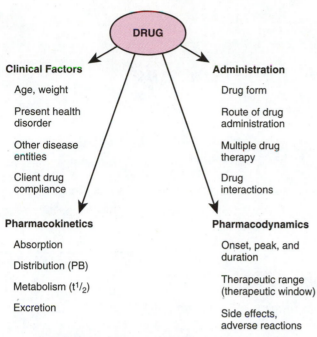

FIGURE 1–11 Determinants affecting drug therapy.

STUDY QUESTIONS

1. What are the three phases of drug action?
2. What are the two processes that a tablet undergoes before it is absorbed? Describe each process.
3. What is the purpose of pharmacokinetics? Name the four processes involved and describe each.
4. Explain the term *first-pass effect* or *hepatic metabolism* of the drug. What effect does first-pass have on drug bioavailability and activity?
5. What is the purpose of pharmacodynamics? What is the role of receptors in this phase? Of what importance is the location of the receptor? Differentiate between nonspecific and nonselective drug responses.
6. Define the following: bioavailability, protein-bound drugs, half-life, therapeutic index, therapeutic drug range, therapeutic window, side effects, adverse reaction, and toxicity. What are the implications of these terms to your nursing practice?
7. A drug that is 75% protein-bound is considered to be _____ protein-bound.

Chapter 2

Nursing Process and Client Teaching

OUTLINE

Objectives

Terms

Introduction

Nursing Process

Assessment

Nursing Diagnosis

Planning

Implementation

Evaluation

Special Teaching Tips for Over-
the-Counter Drugs

Study Questions

OBJECTIVES

Identify the steps of the nursing process and their purpose in relation to drug therapy.

Identify the components of a goal.

State at least eight principles for health teaching related to drug therapy plans.

Identify at least five precautions to be practiced with over-the-counter drugs.

TERMS

assessment

evaluation

goal setting

holistic nursing approach

implementation

nursing diagnosis

over-the-counter (OTC)
drugs

planning

INTRODUCTION

Nurses have a significant role in the management of drug therapy. Influences on this role include technology, increased longevity of the citizenry, and survival of those with multiple and varied biopsychosocial needs. Variables in drug therapy are numerous and, at times, unknown. A **holistic nursing** **approach** to care is crucial to the success of drug therapy initiation, maintenance, and evaluation.

This chapter explores the use of the nursing process as it relates to drug therapy. Careful detail to each step of the process will foster the client's success with the prescribed medication regimen. Considerations in the use of over-the-counter (OTC) drugs also are explored.

NURSING PROCESS

The steps of the nursing process are assessment (including nursing diagnosis), planning, implementation, and evaluation. Each step is discussed as it relates to health teaching in drug therapy.

ASSESSMENT

Assessment, the first step of the nursing process, is particularly important because the data provided by the assessment are the basis on which care is planned, implemented, and evaluated. Data collection involves both subjective and objective information.

Subjective Data
  Current health history
    Client symptoms as verbalized by client
  Current medications
    Dosage, frequency, route, prescribing health care provider, if any
    Client knowledge about drug and its side effects, and for what diagnosis/symptoms is taking the drug
    Client expectation and perception of drug effectiveness
    Client compliance with regimen and reasons for deviations. Are deviations based on valid data/rationale and clinically sound?
    Drug allergies or reactions, both past and present; also food/dye intolerance and reactions
    Street drugs—frequency of use
  Past health history
    Past illnesses, major injuries, and drug therapy, including reactions
    Medications saved from previous use; how stored; expiration date
    Street drugs
  Client's environment
    History of compliance with drug therapy as prescribed; i.e., were prescriptions filled and finished?
    Does client read and follow instructions from the pharmacy?
    Availability, willingness, and ability to administer or assist in the administration of medications; this is essential information for third-party payment in order to continue home visits or for an extended care facility
  Household members, neighbors, friends, and their roles; ages of household members
  Activities of daily living (ADL) capabilities
  Dietary patterns, cultural and economic influences, safety
  Financial resources (drugs can be quite expensive)
  Mental status

Remember that clients, even those who do not intend to withhold information, do not always tell you about all their medications. Therefore, in addition to asking about prescription drugs, ask specifically about vitamin, birth control, aspirin or acetaminophen, and antihistamine or decongestant usage. Also identify caffeine and nicotine use. Ask to see what is in the medicine chest at home and if a pharmacist is used as a consultant.

Objective Data
  Laboratory tests   } Baseline data for future
  Diagnostic studies   }   comparisons
  Physical assessment

Focus on symptoms and those organs most likely to be affected by drug therapy. For example, if you were aware that a drug is nephrotoxic, you would want to assess the client's creatinine clearance. Assess major body systems for any signs of reaction or interaction of drugs or ineffectiveness of therapy.

NURSING DIAGNOSIS

A **nursing diagnosis** is made based on the analysis of the assessment data. More than one applicable nursing diagnosis may be generated, and a nursing diagnosis may be actual or potential. The registered nurse formulates nursing diagnoses and uses them, with the assistance of others, to guide the care

TABLE 2–1 Nursing Diagnoses Accepted by NANDA 1994

- ACTIVITY/REST
  Activity intolerance
  Activity intolerance, high risk for
  Disuse syndrome, high risk for
  Diversional activity deficit
  Fatigue
  Sleep pattern disturbance
- CIRCULATION
  Cardiac output, decreased
  Dysreflexia
  Tissue perfusion, altered (specify); cerebral, cardiopulmonary renal, gastrointestinal, peripheral
- EGO INTEGRITY
  Adjustment, impaired
  Anxiety (specify level)
  Body image disturbance
  Coping, defensive
  Coping, ineffective individual
  Decisional conflict (specify)
  Denial, ineffective
  Fear
  Grieving, anticipatory
  Grieving, dysfunctional
  Hopelessness
  Personal identity disturbance
  Post-trauma response
  Powerlessness
  Rape trauma syndrome
  Rape trauma syndrome: compound reaction
  Rape trauma syndrome: silent reaction
  Relocation stress syndrome
  Self-esteem, chronic low
  Self-esteem disturbance
  Self-esteem, situational low
  Spiritual distress
- ELIMINATION
  Bowel incontinence
  Constipation
  Constipation, colonic
  Constipation, perceived
  Diarrhea
  Incontinence, functional
  Incontinence, reflex
  Incontinence, stress
  Incontinence, total
  Incontinence, urge
  Urinary elimination, altered patterns of
  Urinary retention [acute/chronic]
- FOOD/FLUID
  Breastfeeding, effective
  Breastfeeding, ineffective
  Breastfeeding, interrupted
  Fluid volume deficit [active loss]
  Fluid volume deficit [regulatory failure]
  Fluid volume deficit, high risk for
  Fluid volume excess
  Infant feeding pattern, ineffective
  Nutrition, altered: less than body requirements
  Nutrition, altered: more than body requirements
  Nutrition, altered: high risk for more than body requirements
  Oral mucous membranes, altered
  Swallowing, impaired
- HYGIENE
  Self-care deficit: feeding, bathing/hygiene, dressing/grooming, toileting
- NEUROSENSORY
  Peripheral neurovascular dysfunction, high risk for
  Sensory-perceptual alterations (specify): visual, auditory, kinesthetic, tactile, olfactory
  Thought processes, altered
  Unilateral neglect
- PAIN/COMFORT
  Pain [acute]
  Pain, chronic
- RESPIRATION
  Airway clearance, ineffective
  Aspiration, high risk for
  Breathing pattern, ineffective
  Gas exchange, impaired
  Ventilation, spontaneous: inability to sustain
  Ventilatory weaning response, dysfunctional
- SAFETY
  Body temperature, altered, high risk for
  Health maintenance, altered
  Home maintenance management, impaired
  Hyperthermia
  Hypothermia
  Infection, high risk for
  Injury, high risk for
  Physical mobility, impaired
  Poisoning, high risk for
  Protection, altered
  Self-mutilation, high risk for
  Skin integrity, impaired
  Skin integrity, impaired, high risk for
  Suffocation, high risk for
  Thermoregulation, ineffective
  Tissue integrity, impaired
  Trauma, high risk for
  Violence, high risk for: directed at self/others
- SEXUALITY (COMPONENT OF EGO INTEGRITY AND SOCIAL INTERACTION)
  Sexual dysfunction
  Sexuality patterns, altered
- SOCIAL INTERACTION
  Caregiver role strain
  Caregiver role strain, high risk for
  Communication, impaired verbal
  Family coping, compromised
  Family coping, disabling
  Family coping, potential for growth
  Family processes, altered
  Parental role conflict
  Parenting, altered
  Parenting, altered, high risk for
  Role performance, altered
  Social interaction, impaired
  Social isolation
- TEACHING/LEARNING
  Growth and development, altered
  Health-seeking behaviors (specify)
  Knowledge deficit [learning need] (specify)
  Noncompliance [compliance, altered] (specify)
  Therapeutic regimen (individuals), ineffective management of

plans. A list of nursing diagnoses accepted by the North American Nursing Diagnosis Association (NANDA) is presented in Table 2–1.

Common nursing diagnoses related to drug therapy include:

- Knowledge deficit about drug action, administration, and side effects related to language difficulties
- Potential for injury related to side effects of drug, such as dizziness and drowsiness related to a cerebral vascular accident

- Alteration in thought processes related to forget-fulness, affecting whether the client takes medication as prescribed

The benefit to the client of the nursing diagnosis is that it facilitates development of an optimum quality care plan.

PLANNING

The **planning** phase of the nursing process is characterized by **goal setting,** or expected outcomes. Effective goal setting has the following qualities:

- Client-centered and clearly states the expected change
- Acceptable to both client and nurse (dependent on client decision-making ability)
- Realistic and measurable
- Shared with other health care providers
- Realistic deadlines
- Prescriptive for evaluation

Examples of a goal are (1) E.C. (client) will independently administer prescribed dose of insulin by the end of the fourth session of instruction; (2) D.Z. will prepare a medication recording sheet that correctly reflects prescribed medication schedule within 3 days.

IMPLEMENTATION

The **implementation** phase includes the nursing actions necessary to accomplish the established goals or expected outcomes. Client education and teaching are key nursing responsibilities during this phase. In most practice settings, administration of drugs and assessment of drug effectiveness are also important nursing responsibilities.

Client education is an ongoing process. Teaching is more effective in an environment free of distractions, and the information should be tailored to the client's interests and level of understanding. Assessment data suggest the complexity, number, and length of teaching sessions that may be required. Be sensitive to the client's motivation to learn, attention span, and level of frustration. Readiness to learn is paramount. Assess readiness before information is presented to the client. Use a positive approach; for example, "This narcotic is usually effective in relieving the type of pain that you have." Be an *active* listener and observer.

The inclusion of a family member or friend in the teaching plan is an excellent idea. Provide simple written materials. Assessment data guide the nurse to the appropriate person(s) to be included. This other person may act as a psychological support, actually administer all or part of the drug therapy, observe the effectiveness and side effects of drug therapy, and implement other changes, such as shopping or new methods of food preparation. Health professionals should be available for the client to call with any questions or concerns.

Client teaching is a complex activity. As such, it might be helpful for the nurse to use an outline format. Suggested headings related to pharmacotherapeutics might include:

(1) *General.* Instruct the client to take drug as prescribed. Compliance is of utmost importance, because discontinuing the drug before the course is completed may result in relapse or future ineffectiveness of the drug. Do not adjust dose, frequency, time of day taken, etc., unless first checking with health care provider. Advise women contemplating pregnancy to check first with health care provider before taking the antitubercular drugs ethambutol or rifampin. Advise the client to consult with health care provider regarding laboratory tests such as liver enzymes, blood urea nitrogen (BUN), creatinine, and electrolytes, which should be monitored when taking drugs such as antifungal agents.

(2) *Skill.* Instruct the client on administration of drug according to prescribed route, such as eye or nose drops, subcutaneous insulin injections, suppositories, swish and swallow suspensions, and metered-dose inhalers with and without spacers. Include demonstration and return demonstration where appropriate and written instructions for the sighted client or audio instructions for the visually impaired. Instruct more than one person, where possible, because this aids in reinforcement and retention of information.

(3) *Diet.* Instruct the client about what foods to include in diet and foods to avoid. Advise client to eat foods rich in potassium (e.g., bananas) when taking most diuretics, unless on a KCl supplement, and to avoid large amounts of green, leafy vegetables if taking warfarin (Coumadin) preparations.

(4) *Side effects.* Instruct the client to immediately report to the designated health care provider, usually a nurse, physician, or pharmacist, if he or she experiences unusual symptoms. Also, give the client instructions that help to minimize any side effects, such as avoiding direct sunlight in order to de-

crease the risk of photosensitivity/sunburn. Inform the client of any expected changes in the color of urine or stool. Advise the client who has dizziness caused by orthostatic hypotension to rise slowly from a sitting to a standing position.

A teaching plan with interventions that involve stimulation of several senses and active participation by the client enhances learning. Inclusion of return demonstrations by the client and others, where applicable, gives the nurse important feedback about the client's learning and gives the client confidence in carrying out the regimen or selected aspects of the regimen. Additional teaching tips include:

- Provide written instructions in addition to other teaching aids.
- Use colorful charts and graphs.
- Teach with audiocassette tapes; obtain a tape recorder.
- Encourage client and family questions; provide time for this. Do not rush.
- Use materials and language appropriate to the client's level of understanding.
- Space instruction over several sessions, if appropriate.
- Review community resources related to the client's nursing diagnosis.
- Support multiagency collaboration in mobilization of resources.

The use of Teaching Drug Cards is helpful. These cards provide information about a specific drug or drug group. They may be developed by the health care provider or obtained from drug manufacturers. Cassette tapes and videos are now available from many drug companies. Group classes are useful for clients with certain diagnoses or who require certain drugs. A variety of formats can be developed. Be creative! Helpful components might include:

- Name of drug
- Reason you are taking drug
- Your dose is
- Specific time(s) to take the drug
- What specific things you should or should not do while you are taking the medication; e.g., tablets may or may not be crushed, etc.
- Possible side effects of medication

In addition to the individualized component of the teaching drug card, there are some general helpful

TABLE 2–2 Helpful and Healthful
Points to Remember

1. Take medication as prescribed by your health care provider. If you have questions, call.
2. Keep medication in original labeled container and store as instructed.
3. Keep all medicines **out of reach** of children. Remind grandparents and visitors to monitor their purses and luggage when visiting.
4. **Before** using any OTC drugs, check with your health care provider. This includes use of aspirin, laxatives, and so on. Pharmacists are good resources before buying or using a product.
5. Bring all medications with you when you visit the health care provider.
6. Know why you are taking each medication and under what circumstances to notify the health care provider.
7. Alcohol may alter the action and absorption of the medication. Use of alcoholic beverages is discouraged around the time you are taking your medications and absolutely contraindicated with certain medications.
8. Smoking tobacco also alters the absorption of some medications (e.g., theophylline-type drugs, tranquilizers, antidepressants, and pain medications). Consult your health care provider/pharmacist for specific information.

and healthful points to remember. These pointers are presented in Table 2–2.

Enhancing client compliance with the drug therapy regimen is an essential component of health teaching. The client and family response to the following three questions provides the nurse with critical information unique to each client's teaching situation.

1. What things help you take your medicine as you should?
2. What things prevent you from taking your medicine as you should?
3. What would you or do you do when you forget to take a medication?

Frequently cited factors for noncompliance include forgetfulness, knowledge deficit, side effects, low self-esteem, depression, lack of trust in the health care system, family problems, language barriers, high cost of medications, anxiety, value systems (religious and other), and lack of motivation.

Many people are taking multiple medications simultaneously several times each day, presenting a challenge to the client, his or her family, and the nurse. This complex activity can be segmented into several simple tasks, including:

(1) Preparation of a day's or week's supply of medication. The day's medication can be put in one container. Sorting of a day's supply allows the

client and the nurse to see at a glance what medications have and have not been taken. Keep in mind that a missing pill may have been dropped and not actually taken. A variation in accomplishing this task is to take a day's medication and sort or package the pills according to the time each is to be taken. Multicompartment dispensers (available at the local drug or variety stores) or an egg carton may help some clients to sort their drugs.

(2) A recording sheet may be helpful. The client or a family member marks when each medication is taken. The sheet is designed to meet the client's individual needs; for example, the time can be noted by the client or could be preentered, with the client marking when each dose is taken. A generic format might be:

Medication	Dosage (mg q.d.)	Day of Week						
		S	M	T	W	T	F	S
Captopril (Capoten)	12.5							
Digoxin	0.25							
Furosemide (Lasix)	40							

Alternatives to recording sheets are also available. Mechanical alarm reminder devices may be helpful to some clients.

(3) A combination of daily supply and recording may be helpful. Consider color coding. Visual acuity, manual dexterity, and mental processes have a major effect on which system works best for each client.

Throughout the teaching plan, the nurse promotes client independence. The nurse should not lose sight of the goals or outcomes and become immersed in the intervention process; i.e., teaching a client with short-term memory loss. Table 2–3 pre-

TABLE 2–3 Checklist for Health Teaching in Drug Therapy

- Comprehensive drug and health history
- Reason for medication therapy
- Expected results
- Side effects and adverse reactions
- When to notify physician, pharmacist, or health care provider
- Drug–drug, drug–food, drug–laboratory, drug–environment interactions
- Required changes in ADL
- Demonstration of learning; may take several forms, such as listening, discussing, or return demonstration of psychomotor skills (insulin administration)
- Medication schedule, associated with ADL and drug level of action as appropriate
- Recording system
- Discussion and monitoring of access to financial resources, medication, and associated equipment
- Development and support of back-up system
- Community resources

sents suggestions for a checklist for health teaching in drug therapy.

EVALUATION

The effectiveness of health teaching about drug therapy and attainment of goals are addressed in the evaluation phase of the nursing process. The time at which the **evaluation** of a goal occurs is dependent on the time frame specified in the statement of a goal. Evaluation should be ongoing and related to progress as well as to attainment of the final goal.

If goals are not met, the nurse needs to determine the reasons for this and revise the plan accordingly. This includes additional assessment data and the setting of new goals. If the goals are met, the plan of care has been completed.

To complete the care for any current client, follow these recommendations:

- Review with the client and family the need for follow-up care, if required.
- Encourage choices in ADL.
- Refer the client to community resources, as necessary.

SPECIAL TEACHING TIPS FOR OVER-THE-COUNTER DRUGS

Over-the-counter (OTC) drugs, drugs available without a prescription, are found in most households today. Nurses need to be aware of these products and the implications of their use for clients' drug therapy. OTC drugs provide both advantages and potential serious complications for the consumer.

The Food and Drug Administration (FDA) has the responsibility of monitoring the safety of drug therapy. This group of professionals is charged with (1) identifying standards for known active ingredients and (2) establishing mandatory labeling to assist the consumer in the proper use of the drug. The FDA OTC drug categories are shown in Table 2–4.

As a result of the review by the FDA panel, drugs are placed in one of three categories:

Category I: Drugs judged to be both safe and effective

Category II: Drugs judged to be either unsafe or ineffective, and which should not be included in nonprescription products

Category III: Drugs for which there are insufficient data to judge safety or efficacy

The FDA has recommended that drugs in category II be reformulated to be included in category I or removed from the market. (Note: Manufacturers can maintain the brand name after changing the components of an OTC product.) The FDA also has recommended that selected prescription drugs be reclassified so that they can be sold over the counter. As a result, it is vitally important that nurses be aware of current drug information, any changes in FDA recommendations, and the implications of this information for an informed client population.

It is important that both consumers and health care providers be knowledgeable about OTC products. The following cautions may assist you as you consider OTC preparations for your client:

- Delay in professional diagnosis and treatment of serious or potentially serious conditions may occur if client self-prescribes OTC drugs.
- Symptoms may be masked, thereby making diagnosis more complicated.
- Labels and instructions should be followed carefully.
- The client's health care provider or pharmacist should be consulted before OTC preparations are taken.
- Ingredients in OTC products may interact with medications that are prescribed by the health care provider or are self-prescribed by the client.
- Inactive ingredients (e.g., alcohol, dyes, and preservatives) may result in adverse reactions.
- A placebo effect could occur that fosters needless use of a potentially dangerous substance.
- Potential for overdose exists because of the use of several preparations with similar active ingredients. A double dose does not equal quicker recovery.
- Multiple medication users, whether prescription or OTC, are at increased risk as more medications are added to a therapy regimen.
- Interactions of selected prescription medications and OTC preparations are potentially dangerous. Many individuals routinely reach for aspirin, acetaminophen, and ibuprofen to relieve a discomfort or pain without being aware of these interactions. For example: an individual taking digoxin should avoid taking ibuprofen because it may increase the serum digoxin level, thereby resulting in digoxin toxicity; ibuprofen increases fluid retention, which could worsen the condition of a client with congestive heart failure; use of ibuprofen on a long-term basis may decrease the effectiveness of antihypertensive drugs.

Clients with asthma need to be aware that aspirin can trigger an acute asthma episode. Furthermore, aspirin is not recommended for children with flu symptoms or chicken pox because it has been associated with Reye's syndrome.

Clients with impaired renal function should avoid aspirin, acetaminophen, and ibuprofen because each can further decrease renal function, especially with long-term use. Aspirin and ibuprofen increase the effects of oral anticoagulants, so clients taking these medications may be at increased risk for bleeding.

The above examples are not inclusive. Caution is advised before using any OTC preparations, including antacids, decongestants, and laxatives. Clients should check with their health care

TABLE 2–4 FDA Over-the-Counter Drug Categories

Allergy treatment products (internal)
Analgesics–antipyretics (internal)
Antacids and antiflatulents
Antidiarrheal products
Antimicrobials
Antiperspirants
Antirheumatic products
Antitussives
Bronchodilators and antiasthmatic products
Cold remedies, decongestants
Contraceptive products
Dandruff products
Dentifrices and other dental products
Dermatologic products
Emetics and antiemetics
Hematinics
Hemorrhoidal products
Laxatives and cathartics
Ophthalmic products
Oral hygiene drug products
Sedatives and sleep aids
Stimulants
Sunburn prevention and treatment products
Vitamin–mineral supplements
Weight-loss aids
Miscellaneous products (OTC products not covered in above categories)

providers and read the drug labels before taking OTC medications in order to be aware of possible contraindications and adverse reactions.

Good information sources for OTC drugs include *The Handbook of Nonprescription Drugs*, 13th ed., 1995, American Pharmaceutical Association, Washington, DC (phone # 1-800-237-2742); and *Facts and Comparisons*, 1995 (updated monthly), JB Lippincott, St. Louis. Both provide comprehensive comparisons on nonprescription drug products written for use by health care providers.

STUDY QUESTIONS

1. What are the steps of the nursing process and the primary purpose of each step?

2. Explain how the nursing process relates to administration of medications.
3. What are the essential components of a goal? Write a goal that incorporates all the essential components. How and when would you know if a goal or outcome is realistic for client?
4. What is the basis of a nursing diagnosis?
5. List at least five principles of health teaching about drug therapy regimens.
6. List at least five potential disadvantages to the use of OTC preparations.
7. List three ways to evaluate whether a client is compliant with a drug therapy regimen.

Chapter 3

Principles of Drug Administration

OUTLINE

Objectives
Terms
Introduction
The "Ten Rights" in Drug Administration
    Self-Medication Administration
    Special Considerations: Factors that Modify Drug Response

Guidelines for Drug Administration
Forms and Routes for Drug Administration
    Tablets and Capsules
    Liquids
    Transdermal
    Topical
    Instillations
    Inhalations

Nasogastric and Gastrostomy Tubes
Suppositories
Parenteral
Nursing Implications
Study Questions

OBJECTIVES

Describe the "ten rights" of drug administration.

List safety guidelines for drug administration.

Identify factors modifying drug response.

Describe routes of administration.

Identify the various sites for parenteral therapy.

Explain the equipment and technique used in parenteral therapy.

Explain the method for charting medications.

Describe the nursing interventions related to administration of medications by various routes.

TERMS

absorption
buccal
canister
cumulative effect
distribution
inhalation
instillation
intradermal
intramuscular
intravenous
meniscus
metabolism

metered-dose inhaler
parenteral
pharmacogenetics
right assessment
right client
right documentation
right dose
right drug
right to education
right evaluation
right to refuse
right route

right time
spacer
subcutaneous
sublingual
suppositories
tolerance
topical
toxicity
transdermal
unit dose
Z-track technique

INTRODUCTION

Administration of medications is a basic activity in nursing practice. As a result of the transition from hospital/institution to community-based services, an increasing number of nurses are practicing in a variety of settings. Nurses must be knowledgeable about the actual drugs, their administration, client response, and related resources.

Nurses are accountable for the safe administration of medications. Nurses must know all the components of a drug order and question those orders that are not complete or clear or that give a dosage outside the recommended range. Nurses are legally liable if they give a prescribed drug and the dosage is incorrect or the drug is contraindicated for the client's health status. In some health care settings, interns and medical students write drug orders; these orders must be countersigned by an attending or staff physician or other prescribing health care provider before they are considered official. Once the drug has been administered, the nurse becomes liable for the predicted effects of that drug. Drug references such as the *United States Pharmacopeia (USP)*, *National Formulary (NF)*, *Physicians Desk Reference (PDR)*, and *American Hospital Formulary* and human resources, such as pharmacists, must be consulted when the nurse is unclear about the expected therapeutic effect, contraindications, dosage, potential side effects, or adverse reactions of a medication.

This chapter describes selected, essential content related to administration of medications, a multifaceted activity. Selected content areas include the "rights" of drug administration, factors that modify drug response, guidelines for various routes of administration, and related nursing implications.

THE "TEN RIGHTS" IN DRUG ADMINISTRATION

To provide safe drug administration, the nurse should practice the **ten rights:** the right client, the right drug, the right dose, the right time, the right route, the right assessment, the right documentation, the client's right to education, the right evaluation, and the client's right to refuse.

The **right client** can be assured by checking the client's identification bracelet and by having the client state her or his name. Some clients answer to any name or are unable to respond, so client identification should be verified *each* time a medication is administered. In the event of a missing identification bracelet, the nurse must verify the client's identity prior to any drug administration.

Nursing implications include:
- Verify client by checking the identification band. Some facilities put the client's photo on his or her health record.
- Distinguish between two clients with the same last name; have warnings in bright color on ID such a med cards, bracelet, Kardex.

In settings where clients are not wearing ID bands (school, occupational health, outpatient departments, provider's office), the nurse also has the responsibility of accurately identifying the individual when administering a medication.

The **right drug** means that the client receives the drug that was prescribed. Medication orders may

FIGURE 3–1 Prescription pad medication order.

Jennifer A. Smith, M.D.
Health Street
Hope, Pennsylvania 98765

(123) 456-7891

NAME _____ Age _____

Address _____ Date _____

R$_X$

Label_____

Safety Cap_____

Refill _____times

_____ M.D.

be prescribed by a physician (MD), dentist (DDS), podiatrist (DPM), or a licensed health care provider such as an advanced practice registered nurse (APRN) with authority from the state to order medications. Prescriptions may be written on a prescription pad and filled by a pharmacist at a drug store or hospital pharmacy (Fig. 3–1). For institutionalized clients, the drug orders are written on "doctors' order sheets" and signed by the duly authorized person (Fig. 3–2). A telephone order (TO) or verbal order (VO) for medication must be cosigned by the health care provider within 24 h. The nurse must comply with the institution's policy regarding a telephone order, which sometimes requires that two licensed practitioners listen to and sign the order.

The components of a drug order are:

1. Date and time the order is written
2. Drug name (generic preferred)
3. Drug dosage
4. Route of administration
5. Frequency and duration of administration, such as times seven days, times three doses
6. Any special instructions for withholding or adjusting dosage based on effectiveness or laboratory results
7. Physician or provider's signature or name if TO/VO
8. Signature(s) of licensed practitioner taking TO/VO

Although the nurse's responsibility is to follow an appropriate order, if any one of the components is missing, the drug order is incomplete and the drug should not be administered. Clarification of the order must be obtained; the health care provider is usually contacted. The following is an example of a drug order and its interpretation:

6/4/97 10:10A Lasix 40 mg, PO, q.d. (signature)
(Give 40 mg of Lasix by mouth daily.)

To avoid drug error, the drug label should be read three times: (1) at the time of contact with the drug bottle or container, (2) before pouring the drug, and (3) after pouring the drug. One-time and PRN medication orders should be checked against original orders. Nurses should be aware that certain drug names sound alike and are spelled similarly. Examples are digoxin and digitoxin; quinidine and quinine; Keflex and Kantrex; Demerol and dicumarol; and Percocet and Percodan. More specifically, Percocet contains oxycodone and acetaminophen, whereas Percodan contains oxycodone and aspirin. A client may be allergic to aspirin, so it is important that this client receive Percocet. **Read the labels carefully.**

Nursing implications include:
- Check that the medication order is complete and legible. If the order is not complete or legible, notify nurse manager and health care provider.
- Know the reason for which the client is receiving the medication.
- Check the drug label three (3) times before administering the medication(s).
- Med card / Kardex should include the date the medication was ordered and any last date; e.g., for controlled substances and antibiotics, limited / specific number of doses.

FIGURE 3–2 Client's orders.

There are four categories of drug orders:

1. Standing
2. One-time (single)
3. PRN
4. STAT

Table 3–1 summarizes the drug order categories with examples of each.

The **right dose** is the dose prescribed for this particular client. In the vast majority of cases, this dose is within the recommended range for that particular drug. Nurses must calculate each drug dose accurately, considering the variables: drug availability and the prescribed drug dose. In selected situations, the client's weight range must also be considered, such as 3 mg / kg / day. Refer to Chapter 4A through 4E for drug calculations.

Prior to calculating a drug dose, the nurse should have a general idea of the answer based on a knowledge of the basic formula or ratios and proportions. Calculation of drug doses should be rechecked if a fraction of a dose or an extremely large dose has been calculated. Consultation with a peer or a pharmacist should occur whenever doubt exists.

The stock drug method and unit dose method are the two most frequently used methods of drug distribution. Table 3–2 describes these methods and the advantages and disadvantages of each.

In the traditional stock drug method, the drugs are dispensed to all clients from the same containers. In the **unit dose** method, drugs are individually wrapped and labeled for single doses. The unit dose method is popular today in many institutions and community settings. Unit dosing has eliminated many drug dosage errors.

TABLE 3–1 Categories of Drug Orders

Category Description	Examples
Standing Orders	
May be an ongoing order or may be given for a specific number of doses or days	Digoxin 0.2 mg PO q.d. Colace 100 mg PO q.d., PRN
May have special instructions to base administration on lab values	
May include PRN orders	
One-Time or Single Orders	
Given once and usually at a specific time	Versed 2 mg IM at 7 AM
PRN Orders	
Given at the client's request and nurse's judgment concerning need and safety	Tylenol 650 mg q3 to 4h PRN for headache
STAT Orders	
Given once, immediately	Morphine sulfate 2 mg IV STAT

TABLE 3–2 Drug Distribution Methods

Stock	Unit Dose
Description	
Drugs are stored on unit and dispensed to all clients from the same container	Drugs are packaged in doses for 24 h by the pharmacy
Advantages	
Always available, cost efficiency of large quantities	Saves time for nurse; no dose calculation required Billed for specific doses More accountability Less chance for contamination
Disadvantages	
Drug errors are more prevalent with multiple "pourers"	Potential delay in receiving drug
More risk of abuse by health care workers	Not immediately replaceable if contaminated
Less accountability for amount used; unable to track usage	More expensive

The nursing implications include:

• Calculate the drug dose correctly. When in doubt, the drug dose should be recalculated and checked by another nurse. In many settings, the first nurse to administer the particular drug to the client must calculate the dose according to the stated formulary doses and sign in the nurse's signature space once the safety parameter has been established.

• Check the *PDR*, *American Hospital Formulary*, drug package insert, or other drug references for recommended range of specific drug doses.

The **right time** is the time at which the prescribed dose should be administered. Daily drug dosages are given at specified times during a day, such as b.i.d. (twice a day), t.i.d. (three times a day), q.i.d. (four times a day), or q6h (every 6 h), so that the plasma level of the drug is maintained. When the drug has a long half-life (t½), the drug is given once a day. Drugs with a short half-life are given several times a day at specified intervals (see Chapter 1). Some drugs are given before meals, and others are given with meals or with food.

Many nursing settings currently are using military time. Military time has the advantages of reducing administration errors and decreasing documentation.

Nursing implications include:

• Administer drugs at the specified time(s). Drugs may be given 0.5 h before or after the time prescribed if the interval is >2 h.

• Administer drugs that are affected by foods, such as tetracycline, before meals.

• Administer drugs that can irritate the stomach (gastric mucosa), such as potassium and aspirin, with food.

- The drug administration schedule may sometimes be adjusted to fit schedule of client's lifestyle, activities, tolerances, or preferences.
- It is the nurse's responsibility to check whether the client is scheduled for any diagnostic procedures, such as endoscopy or fasting blood tests, that would contraindicate the administration of medications. Determine per policy if the medication should be given after test is completed.
- Check the expiration date. Discard the medication or return it to the pharmacy (depending on policy) if the date has passed.
- Antibiotics should be administered at even intervals (e.g., q8h rather than t.i.d.) throughout a 24-hour period in order to maintain therapeutic blood levels.

The **right route** is necessary for adequate or appropriate absorption. The more common routes of absorption include oral (by mouth): liquid, elixir, suspension, pill, tablet, or capsule; sublingual (under tongue for venous absorption); buccal (between gum and cheek); topical (applied to the skin); inhalation (aerosol sprays); instillation (in nose, eye, ear); suppository (rectal, vaginal); and four parenteral routes: intradermal, subcutaneous, intramuscular, and intravenous.

Nursing implications include:
- Assess the client's ability to swallow prior to administering oral medications.
- Do not crush or mix medications in other substances before consulting a pharmacist.
- Use aseptic technique when administering drugs. Sterile technique is required with the parenteral routes.
- Administer the drugs at the appropriate sites.
- Stay with the client until oral drugs have been swallowed.

The **right documentation** requires that the nurse immediately record the appropriate information about the drug administered. This includes the **name** of the drug, the **dose,** the **route** (injection site if applicable), the **time** and **date,** and the nurse's **initials** or **signature.** Documentation of the client's response to the medication is required with a variety of medications, such as (1) narcotics—how effective was the pain relief?—(2) non-narcotic analgesics, (3) sedatives, (4) antiemetics, and (5) unexpected reactions to the medication, such as gastrointestinal (GI) irritation or signs of skin sensitivity. Delay in charting could result in forgetting to chart the medication or in another nurse's administering the drug because she or he thought the drug was not given.

To assist in the accurate and timely recording of drugs administered, many health care facilities are using a graphic format (Fig. 3–3) or computerized systems.

The **right assessment** requires that appropriate data are collected prior to administration of the drug. Examples of assessment data may include taking the apical heart rate prior to administering digitalis preparations or serum blood sugar levels prior to the administration of insulin.

The **right to education** requires that the client receive accurate and thorough information about the medication and how it relates to his or her particular situation. Client teaching also includes therapeutic purpose, possible side effects of the drug, any diet restrictions or requirements, skill of administration, and laboratory monitoring. This right is a principle of **informed consent,** which is based on the individual's having the knowledge necessary to make a decision.

The **right evaluation** requires that the effectiveness of the medication be determined by the client's response to the medication. Evaluation in this context asks, Did the medication do for the client what it was supposed to do? It is also appropriate to determine the extent of side effects, and adverse reactions, if any.

The **right to refuse the medication.** Clients can and do refuse to take a medication. It is the nurse's responsibility to determine, when possible, the reason for the refusal and to take reasonable measures to facilitate the client's taking the medication. Explain the risk to the client of refusing to take the medication and reinforce the reason for the medication. When a medication is refused, this refusal must be documented immediately. The nurse manager, primary nurse, or health care provider should be informed when the omission may pose a specific threat to the client, such as with insulin. Follow-up is also required when a change is expected in the lab values, such as with insulin and warfarin (Coumadin).

SELF-MEDICATION ADMINISTRATION

Self-medication is a common practice in the home and in many community-based settings, such as the workplace. However, self-medication administration (SMA) is relatively new to clients and staff in institutional settings. In practical terms, SMA means that the nurse gives the client a packet of appropriate medications and instructions that are kept at the bedside and that the client takes home on discharge. The client is responsible for taking the medications according to the instructions when she or he feels they are needed. The client has a key role in his or her care and exercises control associated with taking of selected medications. SMA helps clients to manage medications during the hospital stay and prepares them to keep as comfortable as possible at home. For example, refer to

UNIVERSITY HOSPITAL			CLIENT'S NAME				
			ROOM #				

Nurse's Signature/Title		Initial					
Evelyn Hayes	RN	EH					
Joyce Kee	RN	JK					
Rodney Brown	LPN	RB	Allergies:				
Jody Smith	LPN	JS		Codeine			

Continuing Medication Record

Date Order	Stop Date	Medication/ Dosage/Route/Frequency	Time	Date	Initials		
				8/14	8/15	8/16	8/17
8/14 EH		Digoxin 0.125 mg po qd	0900	EH AR=74	EH AR=70	JK AR=70	
8/14 EH		Capoten 12.5 mg po bid	0900 2100	EH RB	EH RB	JK RB	
8/15 EH 1100	8/22 LD 0600	Amoxicillin 250 mg q6h x7d	0600 1200 1800 2400	X	X EH RB JS	JS JK RB JS	

One-Time/PRN/STAT Medications

Date	Medication/Dose Route/Frequency	Time/ Initial	Reason	Result
8/14	Nitroglycerin 1/150 gr PRN Chest pain	1600 EH	Chest pain	Relief of pain

FIGURE 3–3 Medication record.

Chapter 42 for a thorough description of SMA for the maternity client.

SPECIAL CONSIDERATIONS: FACTORS THAT MODIFY DRUG RESPONSE

The pharmacologic response to a drug is complex. Nurses must be mindful of the number and variety of factors that influence an individual's response to a drug. (Refer to Chapters 6 and 7 for comprehensive information.) Examples of factors that modify drug responses include:

1. **Absorption:** A major variable is the route of administration of the drug. Oral absorption takes place as drug particles move from the GI tract (stomach and small intestine) to body fluids.

Any GI disturbances, e.g., vomiting or diarrhea, affect drug absorption.

2. **Distribution:** Protein-binding is a major modifier of drug distribution in the body. Propranolol (Inderal) is 90% protein-bound. Another factor is the blood–brain barrier, which allows only lipid-soluble drugs, such as general anesthetics and barbiturates, to enter into the brain and cerebral spinal fluid. Compounds that are strongly ionized and poorly soluble in fat are barred from entry into the brain. Neoplastic agents are examples of drugs that do not cross the blood–brain barrier. The placental barrier is a membrane that for the most part keeps the blood of the mother and fetus separate. However, both lipid-soluble and lipid-insoluble drugs can diffuse across the placenta. Some drugs have teratogenic effects if taken during the first trimester of pregnancy; that is, they may induce aberrant development of fetal organs or body systems. This is especially true if the drugs are taken during the fourth through eighth weeks of gestation.

3. **Metabolism, or Biotransformation:** The liver is the primary organ for drug metabolism. All infants, especially neonates and low-birthweight infants, have immature liver and kidney function. Influences on liver function, such as the aging process, also affect the metabolism of a medication.

4. **Excretion:** The main route of drug excretion is via the kidney. Through the normal aging process, there is a decrease in the functioning cells of the kidney with the result of decreased excretion of drugs. Bile, feces, respiration, saliva, and sweat are also routes of drug excretion.

5. **Age:** Infants and the elderly are more sensitive to drugs. The elderly are hypersensitive to barbiturates and central nervous system (CNS) depressants. Such clients have poor absorption through the GI tract because of decreased gastric secretion. Infant doses are calculated based on weight in kilograms, rather than on biologic or gestational age.

6. **Body Weight:** Drug doses (e.g., of antineoplas-

TABLE 3–3 Guidelines for Correct Administration of Medications

Preparation
Wash hands before preparing medications.
Check for drug allergies; check the assessment history and Kardex.
Check medication order with health care provider's orders, Kardex, medicine sheet, and medicine card.
Check label on drug container three (3) times.
Check expiration date on drug label, card, Kardex; use only if date is current.
Recheck drug calculation of drug dose with another nurse.
Verify doses of drugs that are potentially toxic with another nurse or pharmacist.
Pour tablet or capsule into the cap of the drug container. With unit dose, open packet at bedside after verifying client identification.
Pour liquid at eye level. Meniscus, lower curve of the liquid, should be at the line of desired dose (see Fig. 3–4).
Dilute drugs that irritate gastric mucosa (potassium, aspirin) or give with meals.

Administration
Administer only those drugs that you have prepared. Do not prepare medications to be administered by another.
Identify the client by ID band or ID photo.
Offer ice chips to numb taste buds when giving bad-tasting drugs. When possible, give bad-tasting medications first, followed by pleasant-tasting liquids.
Assist the client to an appropriate position, depending on the route of administration.
Stay with the client until the medications are taken.
Administer no more than 2.5–3 mL of solution intramuscularly at one site. Infants receive no more than 1 mL solution intramuscularly at one site and no more than 1 mL subcutaneously. *Never* re-cap needles (universal precautions).
When administering drugs to a group of clients, give drugs last to clients who need extra assistance.
Discard needles and syringes in appropriate containers.
Discard drugs in the sink or toilet, *not* in the trash can. Controlled substances must be returned to the pharmacy. Some disposals need signed witnesses.
Discard unused solutions from ampules. Appropriately store (some require refrigeration) unused stable solutions from open vials. Write date and time opened and your initials on label.
Keep narcotics in a double-locked drawer or closet. Medication carts must be locked at all times when not in attendance.
Keys to the narcotics drawer must be kept by the nurse and *not* stored in a drawer or closet.
Keep narcotics in a safe place, out of reach of children and others in the home.
Avoid contamination of one's own skin or inhalation to minimize chances of allergy or sensitivity development.

Recording
Report drug error immediately to client's health care provider and to the nurse manager. Complete an incident report.
Charting: record drug given, dose, time, route, and your initials.
Record drugs promptly after given, especially STAT doses.
Report to health care provider and record drugs that were refused with reason for refusal.
Record amount of fluid taken with medications on I & O chart; provide only liquids allowed on the diet.

tics) may be ordered according to body weight. Obese people may need increased drug doses, and very thin persons may need decreased doses.

7. **Toxicity:** This term refers to the *first adverse symptoms* that occur at a particular dose. Toxicity is more prevalent in those persons with liver or renal impairment and in the young and old.

8. **Pharmacogenetics:** This term refers to the influence of genetic factors on drug response. If your mother or father has an adverse reaction to a drug, you may also; some are associated with ethnicity.

9. **Route of Administration:** Drugs administered intravenously act more rapidly than those administered orally.

10. **Time of Administration:** The presence or absence of food in the stomach can affect the action of some drugs.

11. **Emotional Factors:** Suggestive comments about the drug and its side effects may influence its effects.

12. **Preexisting Disease State:** Liver, kidney, heart, circulatory, and GI disorders are examples of preexisting states that can affect a response to a drug. For instance, diabetics should not be given elixirs or syrups that contain sugar.

13. **Drug History:** The use of the same or different drugs may reduce or intensify the effects of the drug.

14. **Tolerance:** The ability of a client to respond to a particular dose of a certain drug may diminish after days or weeks of repeated administration. A combination of drugs may be given to decrease or delay the development of tolerance for a specific drug.

15. **Cumulative Effect:** This occurs when the drug is metabolized or excreted more slowly than the rate at which it is being administered.

16. **Drug–Drug Interaction:** The effects of a combination of drugs may be greater than, equal to, or less than the effects of a single drug. Some drugs may compete for the same receptor sites. An adverse reaction may lead to toxicity or complications, such as anaphylaxis.

GUIDELINES FOR DRUG ADMINISTRATION

General guidelines for administering drugs are listed in Tables 3–3 and 3–4. These guidelines are summarized as the "dos" and "don'ts" of drug administration. Follow these guidelines to enhance safety when administering medications.

FORMS AND ROUTES FOR DRUG ADMINISTRATION

There are a variety of forms and routes for the administration of medications, including oral (tablets, capsules, liquids, suspensions, elixirs); sublingual; buccal; transdermal; topical; instillation (drops and sprays); inhalations; nasogastric and gastrostomy tubes; suppositories; and parenteral. A brief description of each follows.

TABLETS AND CAPSULES

- Oral medications are **not** given to clients who are vomiting, lack a gag reflex, or who are comatose. Clients who gag may need a brief rest before proceeding with further intake of medications.
- Do not mix with a large amount of food or with contraindicated food.
- Enteric-coated and timed-release capsules *must* be swallowed whole to be effective.
- Administer irritating drugs *with food* to decrease GI discomfort.
- Administer drugs on an empty stomach if food interferes with medication absorption.
- Drugs given **sublingually** (placed under tongue) or **buccally** (placed between cheek and gum) remain in place until fully absorbed. No food or fluids should be taken while the medication is in place.
- Encourage the use of child-resistant caps. The Consumer Public Safety Commission has ordered a redesign of these caps because the current caps are difficult for seniors. This has contributed to a

TABLE 3–4 The "Don'ts" of Administration of Medication

Do *not* be distracted when preparing medications.
Do *not* give drugs poured by others.
Do *not* pour drugs from containers with labels that are difficult to read, or whose labels are partially removed or have fallen off.
Do *not* transfer drugs from one container to another.
Do *not* pour drugs into your hand.
Do *not* give medications for which the expiration date has passed.
Do *not* guess about drugs and drug doses. Ask when in doubt.
Do *not* use drugs that have sediment, are discolored, or are cloudy (and should not be).
Do *not* leave medications by the bedside or with visitors.
Do *not* leave prepared medications out of sight.
Do *not* give drugs if the client says he or she has allergies to the drug or drug group.
Do *not* call the client's name as the sole means of identification.
Do *not* give drug if the client states the drug is different from the drug he or she has been receiving. Check the order.
Do *not* re-cap needles. Use universal precautions.
Do *not* mix with large amount of food or foods that are contraindicated.

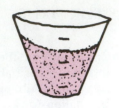

FIGURE 3–4 To read meniscus, locate the lowest fluid mark.

safety hazard for children and others because many people, in an effort to have easy access to their medications, leave the caps off. The new design requires you to lightly squeeze the two side bottle tabs and turn the cap. Nonchild-resistant caps are available on request.

LIQUIDS

- There are several forms of liquid medication, including elixirs, emulsions, and suspensions.
- Read the labels to determine if dilution or shaking is required.
- The **meniscus** is at the line of desired dose (Fig. 3–4).
- Many liquids require refrigeration once reconstituted.

TRANSDERMAL

- **Transdermal** medication is stored in a patch placed on the skin and absorbed through skin, thereby having systemic effect. There was widespread use of such patches beginning in the 1980s. Patches for cardiovascular drugs, neoplas-

TABLE 3–5 Administration of Eye Drops

WASH HANDS

Instruct client to lie or sit down and to look up toward the ceiling.

Gently draw skin down below the affected eye to expose the conjunctival sac.

Administer the prescribed number of drops into the center of the sac. Medication placed directly on the cornea can cause discomfort and/or damage. Do not touch eyelids or eye lashes with dropper.

Gently press on lacrimal duct with sterile cotton ball or tissue for 1–2 min after instillation to prevent systemic absorption through lacrimal canal.

Client should keep eyes closed for 1–2 min following application to promote absorption.

tic drugs, hormones, drugs to treat allergic reactions, and insulin are in production or being developed. Transdermal drugs provide more consistent blood levels and avoid GI absorption problems associated with oral products (Fig. 3–5).

TOPICAL

- **Topical** medications can be applied to the skin in a number of ways, such as with a glove, tongue blade, or cotton-tipped applicator. Never apply with one's own skin unprotected.
- Use appropriate technique to remove medication from container and apply to clean, dry skin, when possible. Do not contaminate medication in container; use gloves or an applicator.
- Observe sterile technique when the skin is broken. Take precautions to avoid medication stains.
- Use firm strokes if medication is to be rubbed in.

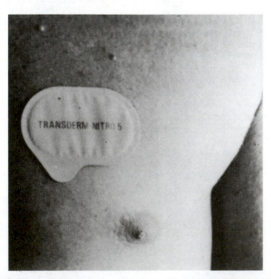

FIGURE 3–5 Transdermal patch (e.g., Transderm-Nitro). (Courtesy of Summit Pharmaceutical.)

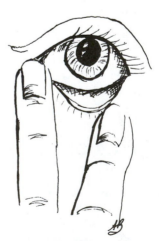

FIGURE 3–6 To facilitate administration of eye drops, gently pull down the skin below the affected eye to expose the conjunctival sac.

TABLE 3–6 Administration of Eye Ointment

WASH HANDS
Instruct client to lie or sit down and to look up toward the ceiling.
Gently draw skin down below the affected eye to expose the conjunctival sac.
Squeeze strip of ointment (about 1/4 inches unless stated otherwise) onto conjunctival sac. Medication placed directly on cornea can cause discomfort or damage.
Instruct client to close eyes for 2–3 min.
Instruct client to expect blurred vision for a short time. Apply at bedtime, if possible.

TABLE 3–7 Administration of Ear Drops

WASH HANDS
Medication should be at room temperature.
Client should sit up with head tilted slightly toward the unaffected side. To straighten the external ear canal for better visualization and to facilitate drops reaching the affected area (see Fig. 3–8).
Child: pull down and back on auricle. Same as adult after 3 years of age, since canal has straightened.
Adult: pull up and back on auricle.
Instill prescribed number of drops.
Take care not to contaminate dropper.
Have client maintain position for 2–3 min.

INSTILLATIONS

• **Instillations** are liquid medications usually administered as drops, ointment, or sprays in the following forms:

Eye drops (Table 3–5, Fig. 3–6)
Eye ointment (Table 3–6, Fig. 3–7)
Ear drops (Table 3–7, Fig. 3–8)
Nose drops and sprays (Table 3–8, Figs. 3–9 and 3–10)

INHALATIONS

• Hand-held nebulizers
• Hand-held metered-dose devices are a convenient method of administration of these medications. See Figure 3–11.
• Preferred client position is semi- or high Fowler's.
• Teach client correct use of equipment.
• Nebulizer (aerosol) changes a liquid medication into a fine mist.
• **Metered dose inhaler** (MDI). See Table 3–9 for correct use of inhaler.
• **Spacers** are devices used to enhance the delivery of medications from the MDI. Figure 3–12 illus-

trates the distribution of medication with and without a spacer. AeroChamber (distributed by Forest Pharmaceuticals) and Inspirease (distributed by Key Pharmaceuticals) are examples of spacers available.

NASOGASTRIC AND GASTROSTOMY TUBES

• Check for proper placement of tube.
• Pour drug into syringe without plunger or bulb, release clamp, and allow medication(s) to flow in properly, usually by gravity.

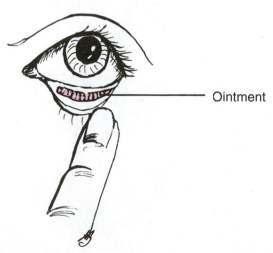

FIGURE 3–7 To facilitate administration of eye ointment, squeeze strip of ointment, about ¼ inch, onto conjunctival sac.

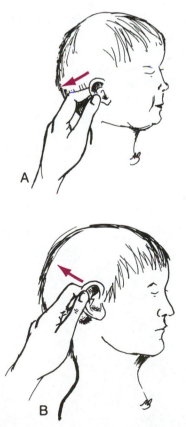

FIGURE 3–8 To facilitate administration of ear drops, straighten the external ear canal by pulling down on the auricle in children (*A*) or by pulling up and back in adults (*B*).

TABLE 3–8 Nose Drops and Sprays

Have client blow nose.

Have client tilt head backwards.

Administer prescribed number of drops or sprays. Some sprays have instructions to close one nostril, tilt head to closed side, and hold breath or breathe through nose for a minute.

Have client keep head tilted backward for 5 min after instillation of drops.

- Flush tubing with 50 mL of water. (Refer to agency policy for exact amount.)
- Clamp tube and remove syringe.

SUPPOSITORIES

Rectal

- Medications administered as **suppositories** or enemas can be given rectally for both local and systemic absorption. The numerous small capillaries in the rectal area promote absorption.
- The foil around the suppository is removed, and the suppository may be lubricated before insertion. When medications such as antipyretics and bronchodilators are given, the clients must be reminded to retain the medication and not to expel it.
- Suppositories tend to soften at room temperature and, therefore, need to be refrigerated.
- Explain the procedure to the client and provide for privacy.
- Use glove for insertion.
- Instruct client to lie on left side and breathe through the mouth to relax the anal sphincter.
- Apply a small amount of water-soluble lubricant to tip of the unwrapped suppository and gently insert the suppository beyond the internal sphincter.

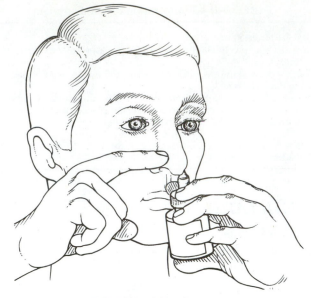

FIGURE 3–10 Nasal sprays.

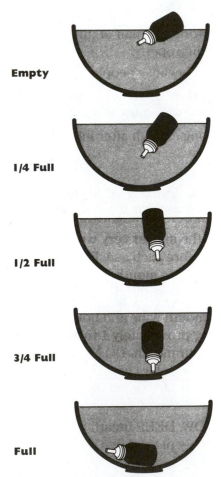

Empty

1/4 Full

1/2 Full

3/4 Full

Full

FIGURE 3–11 Testing canister for amount of medication. (*Source: Understanding Lung Medications: How They Work—How to Use Them.* American Lung Association, 1993, p 4.)

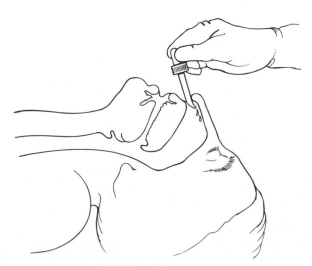

FIGURE 3–9 Nose drops.

TABLE 3–9 Correct Use of MDI

1. Insert the medication canister into the plastic holder.
2. Shake the inhaler well before using. Remove cap from mouthpiece.
3. Breathe out through the mouth. Open mouth wide and hold the mouthpiece 1–2 inches from the mouth. Do *not* put mouthpiece in the mouth unless using a spacer. Discuss techniques with the health care provider.
4. With mouth open, take slow, deep breath through mouth and at same time push the top of the medication canister once.
5. Hold breath for a few seconds; exhale slowly through pursed lips.
6. If a second dose is required, wait 2 min and repeat the procedure by first shaking the canister in the plastic holder with the cap on.
7. If the inhaler has not been used recently or when it is first used, "test spray" before administering the metered dose.
8. If a glucocorticoid inhalant is to be used with a bronchodilator, wait 5 min before using the inhaler containing the steroid.
9. Teach client to monitor pulse rate.
10. Caution against overuse, because side effects and tolerance may result.
11. Teach client to monitor amount of medication remaining in the canister (see Fig. 3–11).
12. Instruct client to avoid smoking.
13. Teach client to do daily cleaning of the equipment including wash hands; take apart all washable parts of equipment and wash with warm water; rinse; place on clean towel and cover with another clean towel to air dry; store in clean plastic bag when *completely* dry. It is a good idea to have two sets of washable equipment to make this process much easier!

- Have the client remain on his or her side for 20 min after insertion.
- If indicated, teach the client how to self-administer suppositories and observe return demonstration for effectiveness.

Vaginal

- Vaginal suppositories are similar to rectal suppositories. They are generally inserted into the vagina with an applicator. Wear gloves. Client should be in lithotomy position. After insertion of medication, provide client with sanitary pad.

PARENTERAL

Intraderm

Intradermal

Action

- Local effect
- Small amount is injected so that volume does not interfere with wheal formation or cause a systemic reaction.
- Used for observation of an inflammatory (allergic) reaction to foreign proteins. Examples include tuberculin testing, testing for drug and other allergic sensitivities, and some immunotherapy for cancer.

Sites

- Locations are chosen so that an inflammatory reaction can be observed. Preferred areas are lightly pigmented, thinly keratinized, and hairless, such as ventral mid-forearm, clavicular area of chest, scapular area of back, and medial aspect of thighs.

Equipment

- Needle: 26 to 27 gauge
- Syringe: 1 mL calibrated in 0.01-mL increments Usually 0.01 to 0.1-mL injected

Technique

- Cleanse area using circular motion; observe sterile technique.
- Hold skin taut.

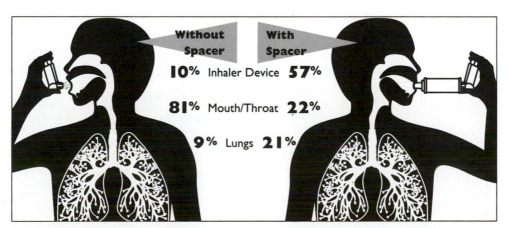

FIGURE 3–12 Distribution of medication with and without a spacer. (*Source: Understanding Lung Medications: How They Work—How to Use Them.* American Lung Association, 1993, p 5.)

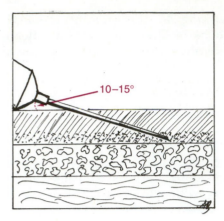

FIGURE 3–13 Needle–skin angle for intradermal injection.

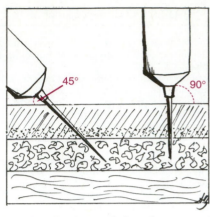

FIGURE 3–14 Needle–skin angle for subcutaneous injection.

- Insert needle, bevel up, at a 15-degree angle; out-line of needle under skin should be visible (Fig. 3–13).
- Inject medication slowly to form a wheal (blister or bleb).
- Remove needle slowly.
- Do *not* massage area; instruct client not to do so.
- Mark area with pen and ask client not to wash it off until read by health care provider.
- Assess for allergic reaction in 24 to 72 h; measure diameter of local reaction. For tuberculin, measure only indurated area—do not include redness.

Subcutaneous (SC)

Action

- Systemic effect
- Sustained effect; absorbed mainly through capillaries. Usually slower in onset than with intramuscular route.
- Used for small doses of nonirritating, water-soluble drugs.

Sites

- Locations for subcutaneous injection are chosen for adequate fat-pad size and include the abdomen, upper hips, upper back, lateral upper arms, and lateral thighs.

Equipment

- Needle: 25 to 27 gauge
      ½ to ⅝ inches in length
- Syringe: 1 to 3 mL
      Usually 0.5 to 1.5 mL injected
- Insulin syringe measured in units for use with insulin only.

Technique

- Cleanse area with circular motion using sterile technique.
- Pinch the skin.
- Insert needle at angle appropriate to body size: 45 to 90 degrees (Fig. 3–14).
- Release skin.
- Aspirate, except with heparin.
- Inject medication slowly.
- Remove needle quickly; do not re-cap.
- Gently massage area, unless contraindicated as with heparin.
- Apply Band-Aid if needed.

TABLE 3–10 Preferred Intramuscular Injection Site: Ventrogluteal

Volume of Drug Administered
Usual: 1.0–4.0 mL
Maximum: 5.0 mL

Common Needle Size
20–23 gauge, 1.25–2.5 inches

Client Position
Supine lateral (with appropriate restraint, if pediatric)

Angle of Injection
Angle the needle slightly toward the iliac crest

Special Considerations
Serves as alternative to dorsogluteal and vastus lateralis for deep IM or Z-track injections. Considered secondary to vastus lateralis site for infants and children.

Advantages
Relatively free of major nerves and vascular branches
Well defined by bony anatomic landmarks
Thinner layer of fat than dorsogluteal site
Sufficient muscle mass for deep IM or Z-track injections
Readily accessible from several client positions

Disadvantages
Should a hypersensitivity reaction occur, tourniquet cannot be applied to delay absorption
Health professional's unfamiliarity with site

Adapted from Tubex/Wyeth-Ayerst, Intramuscular Injections, A Guide to Sites and Technique (1989), Philadelphia: Wyeth-Ayerst Laboratories. Permission granted.

Intramuscular (IM)

Action

- Systemic effect
- Usually more rapid effect of drug than with subcutaneous
- Used for irritating drugs, aqueous suspensions, and solutions in oils

Sites

- Locations are chosen for adequate muscle size and minimal major nerves and blood vessels in the area. Locations include ventrogluteal, dorsogluteal, deltoid, and vastus lateralis (pediatrics) (Tables 3–10 through 3–13). A section on each site is shown in the diagrams of the sites (Figs. 3–15 through 3–18) and includes the volume of drug administered, needle size, angle of injection, client position, advantages and disadvantages of site, and additional considerations, if any. Clients with low weight should be evaluated for sites with adequate muscle. The ventrogluteal is the preferred site for adults and infants older than 7 months.

TABLE 3–11 Intramuscular Injection Site: Dorsogluteal

Volume of Drug Administered
Usual: 1.0–3.0 mL
Maximum: 3.0 mL
       5.0 mL gamma globulin

Common Needle Size
18–23 gauge; 1.25–3.0 inches
Longer for obese clients

Client Position
Prone

Angle of Injection
90-degree angle to flat surface, upon which client is lying prone

Additional Considerations
Requires strict adherence to correct anatomic site location and injection technique

Advantages
Large muscle mass accommodates deep IM or Z-track injections
Injection not visible to client

Disadvantages
Boundaries of the upper outer quadrant are arbitrarily selected and may exceed margin of safety
Danger of injury to major nerves and vascular structures if incorrect site or technique
Fat is often very thick; an injection intended for muscle may be subcutaneous
If hypersensitivity reaction occurs, tourniquet cannot be used
Difficult area to maintain antisepsis
I & D (incision and drainage) of any abscesses complicated by proximity of large nerves and vascular structures

Adapted from Tubex/Wyeth-Ayerst, Intramuscular Injections, A Guide to Sites and Technique (1989), Philadelphia: Wyeth-Ayerst Laboratories. Permission granted.

TABLE 3–12 Intramuscular Injection Site: Deltoid

Volume of Drug Administered
Usual: 0.5 mL
Maximum: 1.0 mL

Common Needle Size
23–25 gauge; ⅝–1.5 inches

Client Position
Sitting, prone, supine, lateral

Angle of Injection
90-degree angle to skin surface (or angled slightly toward acromion)

Additional Considerations
Preferred site for administration of vaccines in infants older than 7 months

Advantages
Easily accessible
General acceptance by client
In hypersensitivity reaction, tourniquet can be applied above

Disadvantages
Small muscle mass relative to other sites
Close proximity to nerves and vascular structures; small margin of safety with any deviation from site
Not suitable for repeated or large-volume (>2.0 mL) injections

Adapted from Tubex/Wyeth-Ayerst, Intramuscular Injections, A Guide to Sites and Technique (1989), Philadelphia: Wyeth-Ayerst Laboratories. Permission granted.

Equipment

- Needle: 18 to 21 gauge
  1 to 1.5 inches in length

Technique

- Same as for subcutaneous injection, with two exceptions: flatten the skin area using the thumb and index finger, injecting between them; insert the needle at 90-degree angle into the muscle (Fig. 3–13).
- Syringe: 1 to 3 mL
  Usually 0.5 to 1.5 mL injected

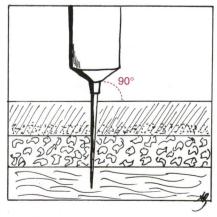

FIGURE 3–15 Needle–skin angle for intramuscular injection.

TABLE 3–13 Preferred Intramuscular Injection Site: Vastus Lateralis (Pediatric, Younger than 7 months)

Volume of Drug Administered
Usual: <0.5 mL infants
          1.0 mL pediatric
Maximum: 1.0 mL infants
          2.0 mL pediatric

Common Needle Size
22–25 gauge; ⅝–1 inch

Client Position
Supine, sitting

Angle of Injection
45-degree angle to frontal, sagittal, and horizontal planes of the thigh (directed toward the knee)

Additional Considerations
IM site of choice for infants younger than 7 months

Advantages
Relatively large muscle mass at birth; suitable site for infants
Area of sufficient size for several injections
Free of major nerves and vascular branches

Disadvantages
Use of long needle relative to small extremity may reach sciatic nerve or femoral vascular structures if improper technique is used

Adapted from Tubex/Wyeth-Ayerst, Intramuscular Injections, A Guide to Sites and Technique (1989), Philadelphia: Wyeth-Ayerst Laboratories. Permission granted.

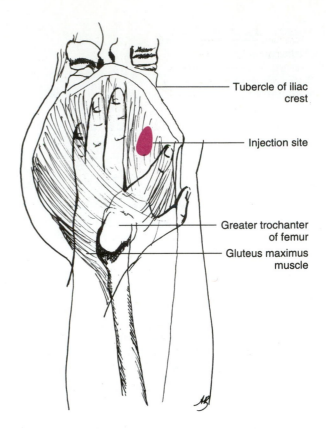

FIGURE 3–16 Ventrogluteal injection site.

Preferred Intramuscular Injection Sites

• Ventrogluteal (Table 3–10, Fig. 3–16)
• Dorsogluteal (Table 3–11, Fig. 3–17)
• Deltoid (Table 3–12, Fig. 3–18)
• Vastus lateralis (pediatric [Table 3–13, Fig. 3–19])

Z-Track Injection Technique

Z-track technique prevents medication from leaking back into the subcutaneous tissue. It is frequently advised for medications that cause visible and permanent skin discolorations (e.g., iron dextran). The gluteal site is preferred. Following medication order policy and aseptic technique, draw up the medication. Replace the first needle with a second needle of appropriate gauge and length to penetrate muscle tissue and deliver the medication to the selected site. Removal of the first needle prevents the medication that is adhering to the needle shaft from being taken into the subcutaneous tissue. If removal is not possible, gently wipe needle with sterile source; this does present a chance for contamination and also for "self-sticks." Consider having medication prepared in the pharmacy.

Z-track injection technique is presented in Figure 3–20.

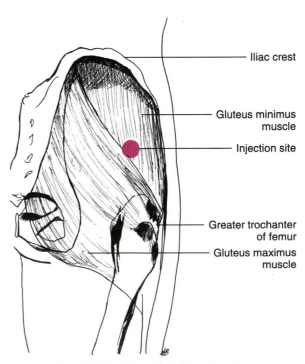

FIGURE 3–17 Dorsogluteal injection site.

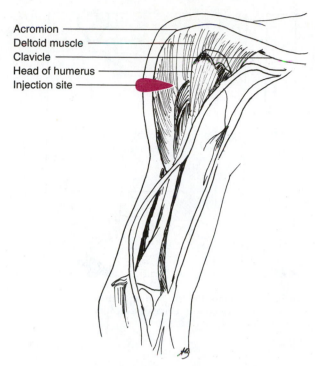

FIGURE 3–18 Deltoid injection site.

Intravenous (IV)

Action

- Systemic effect
- More rapid than IM or SC

Sites

- Accessible peripheral veins (e.g., cephalic or cubital vein of arm; dorsal vein of hand) are preferred (Fig. 3–21). When possible, ask client for preference. Avoid needless restriction. In newborns, the veins of the feet, lower legs, and head may also be used after the previous sites have been exhausted.

Equipment

- Needle: 20 to 21 gauge; 1 to 1.5 inches
  24 gauge; 1 inch for infants
  22 gauge; 1 inch for children
  Larger bore for viscous drugs, whole blood or fractions; large volume for rapid infusion

Technique

- Apply a tourniquet.
- Cleanse area using aseptic technique.
- Insert butterfly or catheter, and bend up into vein until blood returns. Remove tourniquet.

- Stabilize needle and dress site.
- Monitor flow rate, distal pulses, skin color and temperature, and insertion site.
- Consult agency policy regarding addition of medications to bottle or bag, piggyback technique, IV push, and so on.

NURSING IMPLICATIONS

SITES

- Ventrogluteal site is preferred for adults and infants older than 7 months.
- Do not use the dorsogluteal site for IM injections in children. For infants younger than 7 months, the vastus lateralis is preferred.

EQUIPMENT

- Use a needle size and syringe appropriate to the client's needs.
- Size of syringe should approximate volume of medication to be administered.
- Use tuberculin syringe for amounts <0.5 mL.
- Use filter needle to draw up medication from glass vial or ampule. Change the needle prior to administration to prevent tissue irritation from any medication left on the needle.

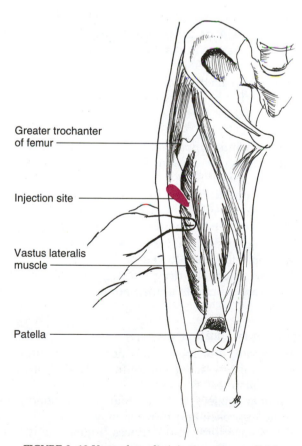

FIGURE 3–19 Vastus lateralis injection site—pediatric.

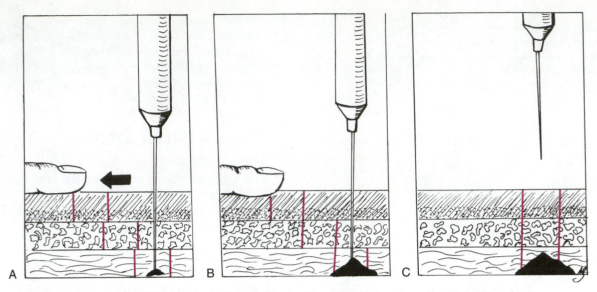

FIGURE 3–20 Z-track injection. (A) Pull skin to side and hold; insert needle; (B) holding skin to side, inject medication; (C) withdraw needle and release skin. This technique prevents medication from entering the subcutaneous tissues.

TECHNIQUE

- Explain what you are going to do. Gain the client's cooperation. Allow the client time to co-operate.
- Demonstrate empathy and concern for every client, as well as using proper technique.
- Allay anxiety. Encourage expression of feelings.
- Position the client.
- Administer medication only via ordered route.
- Inspect skin prior to each injection.
- Inject medication slowly to minimize tissue damage.
- Do not administer injections if sites are inflamed, edematous, or lesioned (moles, birth marks, scars).
- Rotate injection site to enhance absorption of drug (e.g., insulin). Document injection site.
- Chart fluids taken with medications if the client is being monitored for intake and output. Provide only liquids allowed on the diet.
- Observe client for drug effectiveness. Report any untoward reactions immediately.

FOR PEDIATRIC CLIENTS

Anticipate developmental needs. Examples of these needs associated with administration of medications include:

- Stranger anxiety (infant): Maintain a nonthreatening approach and move slowly.
- Hospitalization and illness/injury may be viewed as punishment (3 to 6 years old): Allow control where appropriate, obtain child's view of situation, encourage positive relationships and expression of feelings in acceptable manner/activities.
- Fear of mutilation (3 to 6 years old): Explain procedures carefully, use less intrusive routes whenever possible, such as oral medication, allow children to give "play injections" to a doll or stuffed animal.

Medications are administered by various routes. Figure 3–22 illustrates selected routes.

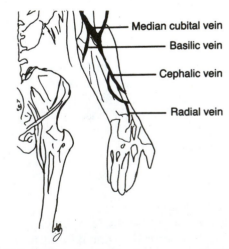

Median cubital vein

Basilic vein

Cephalic vein

Radial vein

FIGURE 3–21 Common sites for intravenous administration.

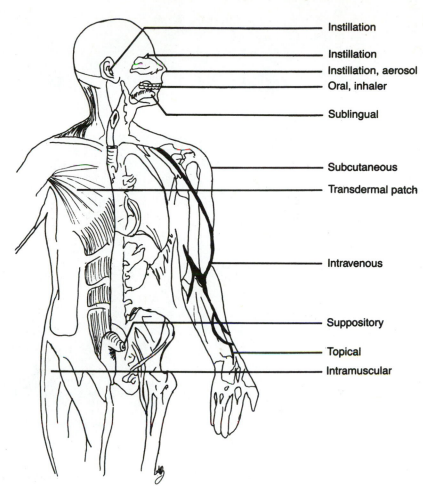

Instillation

Instillation

Instillation, aerosol

Oral, inhaler

Sublingual

Subcutaneous

Transdermal patch

Intravenous

Suppository

Topical

Intramuscular

FIGURE 3–22 Many of the routes for the administration of medications.

STUDY QUESTIONS

1. What is the meaning of the "rights" of medication administration to your nursing practice? What precautions must you take to ensure them?
2. List 10 safety guidelines for safe administration of medications.
3. What are the sites for administration of medication via parenteral routes? What factors influence the selection of the site?
4. What are the nursing implications for each route of medication administration?
5. What is the preferred angle of needle insertion for each type of parenteral injection?
6. What are the essential items to be charted for the administration of each medication? What do you record when an ordered medication is not given?
7. What do you need to do when a client refuses to take a medication?
8. Describe at least 10 factors that modify client response to a drug.
9. List at least three nursing interventions specific to the pediatric client associated with the administration of medications.
10. Describe the purpose of self-medication administration.

Chapter 4

Medications and Calculations

OVERVIEW

This chapter on medications and calculations is subdivided into five sections: (A) systems of measurement; (B) methods for calculation; (C) calculations of oral doses, including for pediatrics; (D) calculations of injectable dosages, including for pediatrics; and (E) calculations of intravenous fluids. The nurse may proceed independently through Sections A–E to practice and master calculation of drug doses during the fundamental nursing or pharmacology course. This chapter also serves as a review of drug calculation for nurses in practice settings.

Numerous drug labels are used in the drug calculation problems in order to familiarize the nurse with important information on a drug label. That information is then used in correctly calculating the drug dose.

There are four calculation methods explained; two are general methods (nurse selects one of the methods), and the other two methods are used for individualizing drug dosing by body weight and body surface area. The drug calculation charts, 4A–4 and 4B–1, may be used in the clinical setting. Abbreviations for drug dosing are found inside the front cover. The nurse might find it helpful to review Chapter 3, Principles of Drug Administration.

Keeping in mind that your goal is to prepare and administer medications in a safe and correct manner, we offer the following recommendations:

- **Think.** Focus on each step of the problem. This applies to simple as well as to difficult problems.
- **Read accurately.** Pay particular attention to the location of the decimal point and to the operation to be done, such as conversion from one system of measurement to another.
- **Picture the problem.**
- **Identify an expected range** for the answer.
- **Seek to understand the problem,** not merely the mechanics of how to do it.

Chapter 4

Systems of Measurement with Conversion

OUTLINE

Objectives
Terms
Introduction
Metric System
   Conversion within the
    Metric System

Metric Conversion
Apothecary System
   Apothecary Conversion
Household System
   Household Conversion

Conversion between the Metric,
   Apothecary, and Household
   Systems
    Metric, Apothecary, and
    Household Equivalents

OBJECTIVES

Name the three systems of measurement.

Convert measurements within the metric system, larger units to smaller units, and smaller units to larger units.

Convert measurements within the apothecary system, larger units to smaller units, and smaller units to larger units.

Convert measurements within the household system, larger units to smaller units, and smaller units to larger units.

Convert metric, apothecary, and household measurements among the three systems of measurement as appropriate.

TERMS

apothecary system
dram
grain
gram

household measurement
liter
meter

metric system
minim
ounce

INTRODUCTION

Three systems of measurement (metric, apothecary, and household) are used in measuring drugs and solutions. The metric system, developed in the late 18th century, is the internationally accepted system of measure. It is replacing the apothecary system, which dates back to the Middle Ages and had been used in England since the 17th century. It is proposed that the apothecary system will phase out by the end of this century. Household measurement is commonly used in community and home settings in the United States.

METRIC SYSTEM

The **metric system** is a decimal system based on the power of 10. The basic units of measure are: **gram** (g, gm, G, Gm) for weight; **liter** (l, L) for volume; and **meter** (m, M) for linear measurement, or length. Prefixes indicate the size of the units in multiples of 10. Table 4A–1 gives the metric units of measure in weight (gram), volume (liter), and length (meter), in larger and smaller units that are commonly used.

Kilo is the prefixed used for larger units (e.g., kilometer), and centi, milli, micro, and nano are the prefixes for smaller units (e.g., milligram). The prefix stands for a specific degree of magnitude; for instance, kilo stands for thousands, milli for one-thousandth, centi for one-hundredth, and so forth. Because the difference between degrees of magnitude is always a multiple of 10, converting from one magnitude to another is relatively easy.

CONVERSION WITHIN THE METRIC SYSTEM

The metric units most frequently used in drug notation are:

1 g = 1000 mg
1 L = 1000 mL
1 mg = 1000 μg (mcg)

To be able to convert a quantity, one of the values must be known, such as gram or milligrams, liter or milliliters, and milligrams or micrograms. Gram, liter, and meter are larger units; milligram, milliliter, and millimeter are smaller units.

METRIC CONVERSION

A. When converting *larger* units to smaller units in a metric system, move the decimal point one space to the **right** for each degree of magnitude change.
Note: It does not apply to micro and nano units.

TABLE 4A–1 Metric Units of Measurements

Unit	Names and Abbreviations	Measurements
Gram (weight)	1 kilogram (kg, Kg)	1000 g
	1 gram (g, gm, G, Gm)	1 g
	1 milligram (mg)	0.001 g
	1 microgram (μg, mcg)	0.000001 g
	1 nanogram (ng)	0.000000001 g
Liter (volume)	1 kiloliter (kL, KL)	1000 L
	1 liter (L, l)	1 L
	1 milliliter (mL)	0.001 L
Meter (length)	1 kilometer (km)	1000 m
	1 meter (m, M)	1 m
	1 centimeter (cm)	0.01 m
	1 millimeter (mm)	0.001 m

Note: 1 mL (milliliter) = 1 cc (cubic centimeter). Values are the same in drug and fluid therapy.
1 mg (milligram) = 1000 μg (micrograms)

EXAMPLE:

Change 1 gram to milligrams.
   Grams are three degrees of magnitude **greater** than milligrams (see Table 4A–1). Move the decimal point three spaces to the right.

$$1 \text{ g} = 1.000 \text{ mg} \quad \text{or} \quad 1 \text{ g} = 1000 \text{ mg}$$

   B. When converting *smaller* units to larger units in the metric system, move the decimal point one space to the **left** for each degree of magnitude of change.

EXAMPLE:

Change 1000 milligrams to grams.
   Milligrams are three degrees of magnitude **smaller** than grams. Move the decimal point three spaces to the left.

$$1000 \text{ mg} = 1\,000. \text{ g} \quad \text{or} \quad 1000 \text{ mg} = 1 \text{ g}$$

   Remember: When changing larger units to smaller units, move the decimal point to the *right*, and when changing smaller units to larger units, move the decimal point to the *left*.

I. PRACTICE PROBLEMS: METRIC CONVERSION

Larger to Smaller Units

1. Change 2 g to mg

2. Change 0.5 (½) g to mg

3. Change 2.5 L to mL

Smaller to Larger Units

4. Change 1500 mg to g

5. Change 3 g to kg

6. Change 500 mL to L

APOTHECARY SYSTEM

The **apothecary system** uses Roman numerals instead of ordinary Arabic numbers to express the quantity, and the Roman numeral is placed after the symbol or abbreviation for the unit of measure. The Roman numerals are written in lowercase letters; for example, gr x stands for 10 grains. The letters $\overline{ss}$ indicate one-half; for example, gr $\overline{ss}$ stands for ½ grain.
   In the apothecary system, the unit of weight is the **grain** (gr), and the units of fluid volume are the **ounce** (fluidounce, or f ʒ), the **dram** (fluidram, or f ʒ), and the **minim** (m, min). Today drams are not used frequently.
   In clinical practice, ounce and dram are more frequently used for measurement of fluid vol-

TABLE 4A–2 Apothecary Equivalents in Weights and Fluid Volume

Dry Weight		Fluid Volume*	
Larger Units	**Smaller Units**	**Larger Units**	**Small Units**
1 ounce (oz)	= 480 grains (gr)	1 quart (qt)	= 2 pints (pt)
1 ounce (oz)	= 8 drams (ʒ)	1 pint (pt)	= 16 fluid ounces (fl oz or fl ʒ)
1 dram (ʒ)	= 60 grains (gr)	1 fluid ounce	= 8 fluid dram (fl dr or fl ʒ)
1 scruple	= 20 grains (gr)	1 fluid dram	= 60 minims (m, min)
		1 minim	= 1 drop (gt)

Fluid volume units are more commonly used than dry weight and should be remembered.

ume than for dry weights. Therefore, when writing fluid volume, the word fluid (f) in front of an ounce or dram is usually dropped. Table 4A–2 gives the apothecary equivalent of larger and smaller units of measure in drug weight and fluid volume.

APOTHECARY CONVERSION

A. When converting a larger unit to a smaller unit, *multiply* the measurement that is requested by the basic equivalent value.

EXAMPLES:

1. 3 Fluidounces (f℥) = _____ fluid dram (f℥).
   The equivalent value is 1 f℥ = 8f℥

$$3f℥ \times 8 f℥ = \underline{24} f℥.$$

2. 2 fluidrams (f℥) = _____ minims (m, min).
   The equivalent value is 1f℥ = 60m.

$$2 f℥ \times 60m = \underline{120m}$$

B. When converting a smaller unit to a larger unit, *divide* the requested number by the basic equivalent value.

EXAMPLES:

1. 8 fluidounces (f℥) = _____ pint (pt).
   The equivalent value is 1 pt = 16 f℥.

$$8 \div 16 = 0.5 \text{ pt, or } \frac{1}{2} \text{ pt}$$

2. 12 drams (℥) = _____ ounce (℥).
   The equivalent value is 1 f℥ = 8 f℥.

$$12 \div 8 = 1.5℥$$

II. PRACTICE PROBLEMS: APOTHECARY CONVERSION

Refer to Table 4A–2 as needed.

Larger to Smaller Units

1. Change 3 qt to pt

2. Change 1.5 pt to f℥

3. Change 2 f℥ to f℥

Smaller to Larger Units

4. Change 3 pt to qt

5. Change 32 f℥ to qt

6. Change 4 f℥ to f℥

HOUSEHOLD SYSTEM

The household system of measurement is not as accurate as the metric system because of the lack of standardization of spoons, cups, and glasses. The measurements are approximate. A teaspoon (t) is considered to be equivalent to 5 mL according to the official USP. Remember mL (milliliters) is the same as cc (cubic centimeters) in value (Fig. 4A–1). Three teaspoons

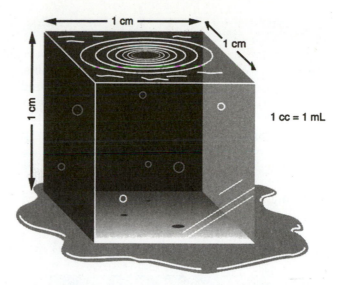

FIGURE 4A–1 One cubic centimeter equals one milliliter.

1 cm

1 cm

1 cm

1 cc = 1 mL

equal 1 T (tablespoon). Ounces are fluid ounces in the household measurement; the word "fluid" in front of ounce is usually not used.

One milliliter of water fills a cubic centimeter exactly.

Table 4A–3 gives the household equivalents in fluid volume. The measurements having asterisks are frequently used in drug therapy and should be remembered.

HOUSEHOLD CONVERSION

A. When converting larger units to smaller units within the household system, *multiply* the requested number by the basic equivalent value.

> **EXAMPLE:**

Change 2 glasses of water to ounces.
   The equivalent value is 1 medium-size glass = 8 oz.

$$2 \text{ glasses} \times 8 \text{ oz} = \underline{16} \text{ oz.}$$

B. When converting a smaller unit to a larger unit, *divide* the requested number by the basic equivalent value.

> **EXAMPLE:**

Change 6 teaspoons to tablespoons.
   The equivalent value is 1 T = 3 t.

$$6 \div 3 = \underline{2} \text{ T}$$

TABLE 4A–3 Household Equivalents in Fluid Volume

1 measuring cup = 8 ounces (oz)
1 medium-size glass = 8 ounces (oz)
   (tumbler size)
   1 coffee cup (c) = 6 ounces (oz)
                      (varies with cup size)
      1 ounce (oz) = 2 tablespoons (T)
   1 tablespoon (T) = 3 teaspoons (t)
      1 teaspoon (t) = 60 drops (gtt)*
         1 drop (gt)* = 1 minim (𝑚, min)

Varies with viscosity of liquid and dropper opening.

III. PRACTICE PROBLEMS: HOUSEHOLD CONVERSION

Remember: To change larger units to smaller units, *multiply* the requested number of units by the basic equivalent value. To change smaller units to larger units, *divide* the requested number of units by the basic equivalent value. Refer to Table 4A–3 as needed.

Larger to Smaller Units

1. Change 3 oz to T

2. Change 5 T to t

3. Change 3 coffee cups to oz

Smaller to Larger Units

4. Change 3 T to oz

5. Change 16 oz to a measuring cup

6. Change 12 t to T

IV. SUMMARY PROBLEMS: METRIC, APOTHECARY, AND HOUSEHOLD MEASUREMENTS

1. *Metric System:* Refer to Table 4A–1 as needed.
   1. 2 g = _____ mg
   2. 1.2 kg = _____ g
   3. 5 mg = _____ μg
   4. 2.5 L = _____ mL
   5. 1.5 km = _____ m
   6. 500 mg = _____ g
   7. 10,000 μg = _____ mg
   8. 2400 mg = _____ g
   9. 1500 mL = _____ L
   10. 1200 cm = _____ m

2. *Apothecary System:* Refer to Table 4A–2 as needed.
   1. 5 qt = _____ pt
   2. 2 pt = _____ f℥
   3. f℥v = _____ f℥
   4. f℥iiss (2½) = _____ ♏ (minims)
   5. 1.5 pt = _____ f℥
   6. 8 f℥= _____ pt
   7. 3 pt = _____ qt
   8. 12 f℥ = _____ f℥
   9. 32 f℥ = _____ qt
   10. 5♏ = _____ gtt

3. *Household System:* Refer to Table 4A–3 as needed.
   1. 5 glasses = _____ oz
   2. 3 T = _____ t
   3. 2 c = _____ oz
   4. 4 oz = _____ T
   5. 15 t = _____ T
   6. 5 T = _____ oz

CONVERSION BETWEEN THE METRIC, APOTHECARY, AND HOUSEHOLD SYSTEMS

Drug doses are usually ordered in metric units (grams, milligrams, liters, or milliliters), but some physicians still use the apothecary units of measurement (grain) when prescribing med-

TABLE 4A–4 Approximate Metric, Apothecary, and Household Equivalents

	Metric System		Apothecary System	Household System
Weight				
	*1 g;	1000mg	15 (16) gr	
	0.5 g;	500 mg	7½ gr	
	0.3 g;	300 (325) mg	5 gr	
	0.1 g;	100 mg	1½ gr	
	*0.06 g;	60 (65) mg	1 gr	
	0.03 g;	30 (32) mg	½ gr	
	0.01 g;	10 mg	⅙ gr	
		0.6 mg	⅟₁₀₀ gr	
		0.4 mg	⅟₁₅₀ gr	
		0.3 mg	⅟₂₀₀ gr	
Volume				
	1 L; 1000 mL (cc)		1 qt; 32 oz f ʒ (f ʒ)	1 qt
	0.5 L; 500 mL		1 pt; 16 oz f ʒ	1 pt
	0.24 L; 240 mL		8 ʒ (f ʒ)	1 glass
	0.18 L; 180 mL		6 ʒ	1 c
	*30 mL		1 ʒ; 8 ʒ (f ʒ)	2 T; 6 t
	15 mL		½ ʒ; 4 ʒ	1 T; 3 t
	†5 mL			1 t
	4 mL		1 ʒ; 60 ɱ (min)	1 t
	1 mL		15 (16) ɱ	15–16 gtt
Other				
	1 kg; 1000 g			2.2 lb

* *Equivalents commonly used for computing conversion problems by ratio.*
† *5 mL = 1 t (teaspoon); Official USP measurement.*
Key: *g = gram; mg = milligram; gr = grain; L = liter; mL = milliliter; f ʒ = fluidounce; T = tablespoon; t = teaspoon;*
gtt = drops; ɱ = minim; kg = kilogram; cc = cubic centimeter; ʒ = dram.

ication. To calculate drug doses, the same unit of measure (grams, milligrams, or grains) must be used. The nurse needs to be familiar with the three systems of measure and their equivalents (Table 4A–4). Note that the metric and apothecary equivalents are approximate; thus, the equivalents should be rounded off to a whole number, for example, 1 g = 15.432 gr, or 1 g = 15 gr.

Some authorities indicate that it is easier to convert to the unit used on the bottle or container. The answer is in the system of the drug to be dispensed. If the label on the bottle reads in milligrams and the order is in grains, the conversion should be from grains to milligrams.

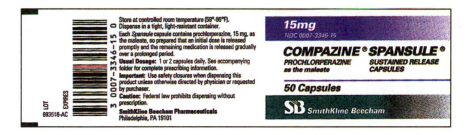

EXAMPLE:

Order: Compazine spansule gr ¼.
Available: Compazine spansule 15 mg. Convert grains to milligrams, gr ¼ = 15 mg.

METRIC, APOTHECARY, AND HOUSEHOLD EQUIVALENTS

Conversion to one unit of measure is essential in administering drugs. With discharge teaching for a client who requires liquid medication(s) at home, the nurse may find it necessary to

SECTION A

convert metric to household measurements. Table 4A–4 gives the metric and apothecary equivalents by weight, and the metric, apothecary, and household equivalents by volume.

V. PRACTICE PROBLEMS: METRIC, APOTHECARY, HOUSEHOLD CONVERSION

Change measurements by conversion. Refer to Table 4A–4 as needed.

1. 3 g to gr.

2. 7½ gr (gr viiss) to g.

3. 2.5 g to mg.

4. 0.5 g to gr.

5. 0.1 g to gr.

6. 4 gr to mg.

7. 3 gr to g.

8. 7½ gr to mg.

9. 150 gr to g.

10. 10 mg to gr.

11. 1.5 ℨ to mL.

12. 15 mL to t.

13. 2t to mL.

14. 8 ℨ to mL.

15. 60 mL to oz.

16. 75 mL to T.

17. 2 coffee cups to mL.

18. 9 t to T.

19. 3 oz. to T.

20. ½ oz to t.

ANSWERS TO PRACTICE PROBLEMS

I. Practice Problems: Metric Conversion

1. 2.0 g = 2.000 mg   or   2.0 g = 2000 mg.

   The gram is three degrees of magnitude greater than the milligram, so the decimal point is moved three spaces to the right.

2. 0.5 g = 0. 500 mg   or   0.5 g = 500 mg.

The gram is three degrees of magnitude greater than the milligram, so the decimal point is moved three spaces to the right.

3. 2.5 L = 2. 500 mL   or   2.5 L = 2500 mL.

The liter is three degrees of magnitude greater than the milliliter, so the decimal point is moved three spaces to the right.

4. 1500 mg = 1 500. g   or   1500 mg = 1.5 g.

The milligram is three degrees of magnitude smaller (less) than the gram, so the decimal point is moved three spaces to the left.

5. 3 g = 003. kg   or   3 g = .003 kg.

The gram is three degrees of magnitude smaller than the kilogram, so the decimal point is moved three spaces to the left.

6. 500 mL = 500. L   or   500 mL = 0.5 L.

The milliliter is three degrees of magnitude smaller than the liter, so the decimal point is moved three spaces to the left.

II. Practice Problems: Apothecary Conversion

1. 3 qt × 2 pts = 6 pt
   The equivalent value is 1 qt = 2 pt
2. 1.5 pt × 16 = 24 f℥
   The equivalent value is 1 pt = 16 f℥
3. 2 f℥ × 8 f℥ = 16 f℥
   The equivalent value is 1 f℥ = 8 f℥
4. 3 pt = 1.5 qt
   The equivalent value is 1 qt = 2 pt

$$3 \text{ pt} \div 2 = 1.5 \text{ qt}$$

5. 32 f℥ = 2 pt or 1 qt
   The equivalent values are 1 pt = 16 f℥ or 1 qt = 2 pt

$$32 \text{ f℥} \div 16 \text{ f℥} = 2 \text{ pt (2 pt = 1 qt)}$$

6. 4 f℥ = 0.5 or ½ f℥
   The equivalent value is 1 f℥ = 8 f℥

$$4 \text{ f℥} \div 8 \text{ f℥} = 0.5 \text{ f℥}$$

III. Practice Problems: Household Conversion

1. 3 oz = 6 T
   The equivalent value is 1 oz = 2 T

$$3 \text{ oz} \times 2 = 6 \text{ T}$$

2. 5 T = 15 t
   The equivalent value is 1 T = 3 t

$$5 \text{ T} \times 3 = 15 \text{ t}$$

3. 3c = <u>18</u> oz
   The equivalent value is 1 c = 6 oz

$$3 \text{ c} \times 6 = 18 \text{ oz}$$

4. 3 T = <u>1½</u> oz
   The equivalent value is 1 oz = 2 T

$$3 \text{ T} \div 2 = 1½ \text{ or } 1.5 \text{ oz}$$

5. 16 oz = <u>2</u> c
   The equivalent value is 1 measuring cup = 8 oz

$$16 \text{ oz} \div 8 = 2 \text{ c}$$

6. 12 t = <u>4</u> T
   The equivalent value is 1 T = 3 t

$$12 \text{ t} \div 3 = 4 \text{ T}$$

IV. Summary Problems: Metric, Apothecary, and Household Measurements

Metric
1. 2000 mg

$$1 \text{ g} = 1000 \text{ mg}$$

$$2 \times 1000 \text{ mg} = 2000 \text{ mg}$$

or 2 000 mg
(three spaces to the right)
2. 1200 g
3. 5000 μg

$$1 \text{ mg} = 1000 \text{ μg}$$

4. 2500 mL
5. 1500 meters
6. 0.5 g

$$1000 \text{ mg} = 1 \text{ g}$$

$$500 \div 1000 = 0.5$$

or 500 g = 0.5 g
(three spaces to the left)
7. 10 mg
8. 2.4 g
9. 1.5 L

10. 1.2 m

Apothecary
1. 10 pt

$$1 \text{ qt} = 2 \text{ pt}$$

$$5 \times 2 = 10$$

2. 32 f℥
3. 40 f℥

$$v = 5 \text{ (Roman numeral)}$$

4. 150 ♏
5. 24 f℥
6. ½ pt

$$16 \text{ f℥} = 1 \text{ pt}$$

$$8 \div 16 = 0.5 \text{ or } ½$$

7. 1½ qt
8. 1½ f℥
9. 1 qt

$$32 \div 32 = 1 \text{ qt}$$

10. 5 gtt

Household
1. 40 oz
2. 9 t
3. 12 oz
4. 8 T
5. 5 T
6. 2½ oz

V. Practice Problems: Metric, Apothecary, Household Conversion

1. 45 gr
2. 0.5 g
3. 2500 mg
4. 7½ gr
5. 1½ (1.5) gr
6. 240 mg
7. 0.2 g
8. 500 mg
9. 10 g
10. ⅙ gr
11. 45 mL
12. 3 t
13. 10 mL
14. 240 mL
15. 2 oz
16. 5 T
17. 360 mL
18. 3 T
19. 6 T
20. 3 t

Chapter 4

Methods for Calculation

OUTLINE

Objectives

Terms

Introduction

Interpreting Oral and Injectable
Drug Labels

Basic Formula

Ratio and Proportion

Body Weight

Body Surface Area

OBJECTIVES

Select a formula, the basic formula or the ratio-and-proportion method, for calculating drug dosages.

Convert all measures to the same system, and same unit of measure within the system, prior to calculating drug dosage.

Calculate drug dosage using one of the general formulas.

Calculate drug dosage according to body weight and body surface area.

List meanings for abbreviations used in drug therapy.

TERMS

basic formula

body surface area

body weight

ratio and proportion

INTRODUCTION

Two general methods for calculating drug doses are the basic formula and ratio and proportion. These methods are used for calculating oral and injectable drug doses. The nurse needs to select one of the methods to calculate drug doses and use that method consistently.

For drugs that require individualized dosing, calculation by body weight (BW) or by body surface area (BSA) may be necessary. In the past these two methods have been used for calculating pediatric dosage and for drugs used in the treatment of cancer (antineoplastic drugs). Today we calculate by body weight and body surface area especially for those individuals whose body weight is low, who are obese, or who are older adults.

Before calculating drug doses, all units of measure must be converted to a single system (see Section 4A). It is most helpful to convert to the system used on the drug label. If the drug is ordered in grains (gr) and the drug label gives the dose in milligrams (mg), convert grains to milligrams, the measurement on the drug label, and proceed with the drug calculation. Table 4B–1 gives the metric and apothecary conversions most frequently used for dry and liquid measurements.

INTERPRETING ORAL AND INJECTABLE DRUG LABELS

The pharmaceutical companies usually label their drugs with the brand name of the drug in large letters and the generic name in smaller letters. The dose per tablet, capsule, or liquid (for oral and injectable doses) is printed on the drug label. Two examples of drug labels are given below, one for an oral drug and the second for an injectable drug.

EXAMPLE I: ORAL DRUG

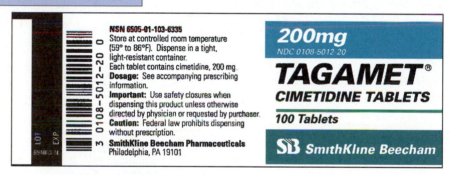

Tagamet is the brand name, cimetidine is the generic name, and the dose is 200 mg/tablet.

EXAMPLE II: INJECTABLE DRUG

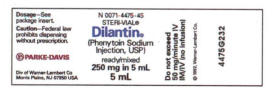

Dilantin is the brand name, phenytoin sodium is the generic name, and the dose is 250 mg/5 mL.

BASIC FORMULA

The **basic formula** is easy to recall and is most frequently used in calculating drug dosages. The formula is:

$$\frac{D}{H} \times V = A$$

TABLE 4B–1 Metric and Apothecary Conversions

Metric		Apothecary
Grams *(g)*	*Milligrams* *(mg)*	*Grains* *(gr)*
1	1000	15
0.5	500	7½
0.3	300 (325)	5
0.1	100	1½
0.06	60 (64)	1
0.03	30 (32)	½
0.015	15 (16)	¼
0.010	10	⅛
0.0006	0.6	1/100
0.0004	0.4	1/150
0.0003	0.3	1/200

Liquid (approximate)
30 mL (cc) = 1 oz (fl ℥) = 2 tbsp (T) = 6 tsp (t)
15 mL (cc) = 0.5 oz = 1 T = 3 t
1000 mL (cc) = 1 quart (qt) = 1 liter (L)
500 mL (cc) = 1 pint (pt)
5 mL (cc) = 1 tsp (t)
4 mL (cc) = 1 fl dr (f℥)
1 mL (cc) = 15 minims (♏) = 15 drops (gtt)

where *D* is the desired dose: drug dose ordered by the physician,
H is the on-hand dose: drug dose on label of container (bottle, vial),
V is the vehicle: drug form in which the drug comes (tablet, capsule, liquid), and
A is the amount calculated to be given to the client.

EXAMPLES:

1. Order: ampicillin 0.5 g, PO, b.i.d.
   Available (drug label):

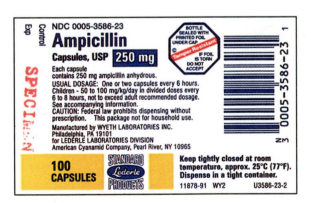

   a. The unit of measure that is ordered, grams, and the unit on the bottle, milligrams, are from the same system of measurement, the metric system. Conversion to the same unit is necessary to work the problem. Since the bottle is in milligrams, convert grams to milligrams.
   To convert grams (large value) to milligrams (smaller value), move the decimal point three spaces to the right (see Section 4A: Conversion within the Metric System).

$$0.5 \text{ g} = 0.500 \text{ mg or } 500 \text{ mg}$$

   b.
$$\frac{D}{H} \times V = \frac{500 \text{ mg}}{250 \text{ mg}} \times 1 \text{ capsule} = \frac{500}{250} = 2 \text{ capsules}$$

2. Order: codeine gr i (1), PO, STAT
   Available: see drug label

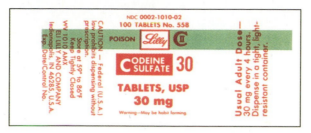

a. Grains need to be converted to milligrams before you can calculate drug dose (see Table 4A–4 or 4B–1).   1 gr = 60 mg

b.
$$\frac{D}{H} \times V = \frac{60 \text{ mg}}{30 \text{ mg}} \times 1 \text{ tablet} = \frac{60}{30} = 2 \text{ tablets}$$

RATIO AND PROPORTION

The **ratio-and-proportion** method is the oldest method currently used in calculating drug dosage. The formula is:

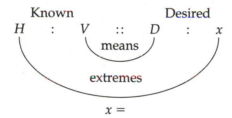

where H is the drug on hand (available),
   V is the vehicle or drug form (tablet, capsule, liquid),
   D is the desired dose (as ordered),
   x is the unknown amount to give, and
   ∷ stands for "as" or "equal to."

Multiply the means and the extremes. Solve for *x*; *x* is the divisor.

EXAMPLES:

1. Order: amoxicillin 100 mg, PO, q.i.d.
   Available:

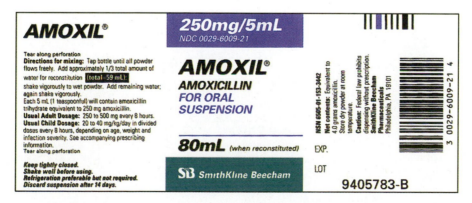

a. Conversion is not needed since both are expressed in the same unit of measure.

b.

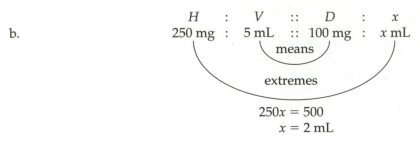

$$250x = 500$$
$$x = 2 \text{ mL}$$

Answer: amoxicillin 100 mg = 2 mL.

2. Order: aspirin/ASA gr x, q4h, PRN
   Available: aspirin 325 mg/tablet

   a. Convert to one system and unit of measure. Change grains to milligrams (see Table 4A–4 or 4B–1).

   $$325 \text{ mg} = 5 \text{ gr} \quad 600 \ (650) \text{ mg} = 10 \text{ gr}$$

   b.

   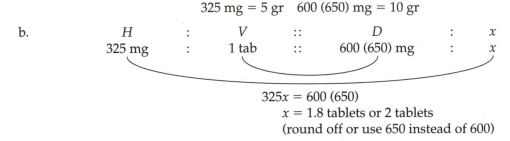

   $$325x = 600 \ (650)$$
   $$x = 1.8 \text{ tablets or 2 tablets}$$
   (round off or use 650 instead of 600)

Answer: Aspirin gr x = 2 tablets.

BODY WEIGHT

The **body weight** method of calculating allows for individualizing the drug dose and involves three steps.

1. Convert pounds to kilograms if necessary (lb ÷ 2.2).
2. Determine drug dose per body weight by multiplying:

$$\text{Drug dose} \times \text{body weight} = \text{Client's dose per day.}$$

3. Follow the basic formula or ratio-and-proportion method to calculate drug dosage.

> **EXAMPLES:**

1. Order: fluorouracil (5-FU), 12 mg/kg/day intravenously, not to exceed 800 mg/day. The adult weighs 132 lb.

   a. Convert pounds to kilograms by dividing the number of pounds by 2.2 (1 kg = 2.2 lb).

   $$132 \div 2.2 = 60 \text{ kg}$$

   b. mg × kg = client's dose
      12 × 60 = 720 mg IV/day

Answer: fluorouracil 12 mg/kg/day = 720 mg.

2. Order: cefaclor (Ceclor) 20 mg/kg/day in three divided doses. The child weighs 31 lb.
   Drug label: cefaclor 125 mg/5 mL

   a. Convert pounds to kilograms.

   $$31 \div 2.2 = 14 \text{ kg}$$

b. 20 mg × 14 kg = 280 mg per day

$$280 \text{ mg} \div 3 \text{ divided doses} = 93 \text{ mg/dose}$$

c. $$\frac{D}{H} \times V' = \frac{93}{125} \times 5 = \frac{465}{125} = 3.7 \text{ mL}$$

or:

H	:	V	::	D	:	x
125 mg	:	5 mL	::	93 mg	:	x mL

$$125x = 465$$

$$x = \frac{465}{125} = 3.7 \text{ mL}$$

Answer: cefaclor 20 mg/kg/day = 3.7 mL per dose.

BODY SURFACE AREA

The **body surface area** (BSA) method is considered to be the most accurate way to calculate the drug dose for infants, children, older adults, and clients who are on antineoplastic agents or whose body weight is low. The body surface area, in square meters (m²), is determined by where the person's height and weight intersect the nomogram scale (Figs. 4B–1 [children] and 4B–2 [adults]). To calculate the drug dosage by the BSA method, multiply the drug dose ordered by the number of square meters.

$$100 \text{ mg} \times 1.8 \text{ m}^2 \text{ (BSA)} = 180 \text{ mg per day}$$

EXAMPLES:

1. Order: cyclophosphamide (Cytoxan) 100 mg/m²/day, IV.
   Available:

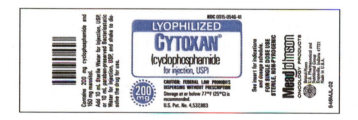

   Client is 5 ft 10 in. (70 in.) tall and weighs 160 lb.

   a. 70 in. and 160 lb intersect the nomogram scale at 1.97 m² (BSA).

   b. 100 mg × 1.97 = 197 mg.

Answer: Administer cyclophosphamide 197 mg or 200 mg/day.

2. Order: mephenytoin (Mesantoin) 200 mg/m², PO, in three divided doses. The child is 42 in. tall and weighs 44 lb.

   a. 42 in. and 44 lb intersect the nomogram scale at 0.8 m².

   b. 200 mg × 0.8 = 160 mg/day or 50 mg (53) t.i.d. (three times a day).

Answer: Administer mephenytoin 50 mg, t.i.d.

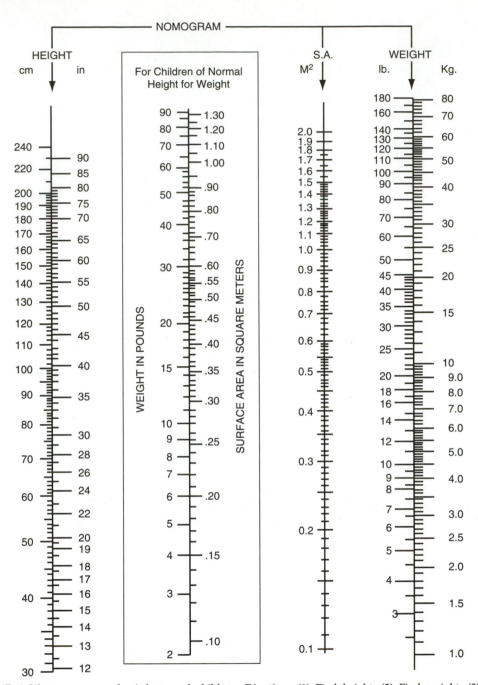

FIGURE 4B–1 West nomogram for infants and children. *Directions:* (1) Find height. (2) Find weight. (3) Draw a straight line connecting the height and weight. Where the line intersects on the SA column is the body surface area (m²). (Modified from data of E. Boyd and C. D. West, in Behrman, R. E. and Vaughan, V. C. (1992). *Nelson Textbook of Pediatrics*, 14th ed. Philadelphia: W. B. Saunders.)

PRACTICE PROBLEMS

Additional practice problems are given in Sections 4C and 4D (orals and injectables).

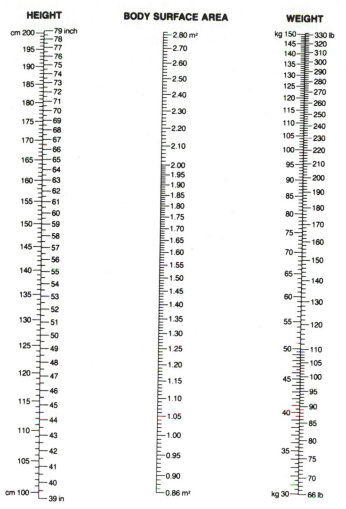

HEIGHT

BODY SURFACE AREA

WEIGHT

FIGURE 4B–2 Nomogram of body surface area for adults. *Directions:* (1) Find height. (2) Find weight. (3) Draw a straight line connecting the height and weight. (4) Where the line intersects on the BSA column is the body surface area (m^2).

(*Sources:* Deglin, Vallerand, and Russin: *Davis's Drug Guide for Nurses,* 2nd ed. Philadelphia: F. A. Davis, 1991, p. 1218. Used with permission. From C. Lentner (ed.) *Geigy Scientific Tables,* 8th ed., Vol. 1, Ciba-Geigy, Basle, Switzerland: 1981, pp 226–227. Used with permission.)

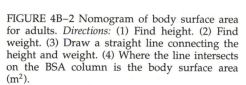

SECTION B

I. DRUG DOSAGE USING A GENERAL FORMULA:

Solve the problem and determine the drug dose given the following:

1. Order: cimetidine (Tagamet) 0.4 g, PO, q6h (every 6 h).
   Available (drug label):

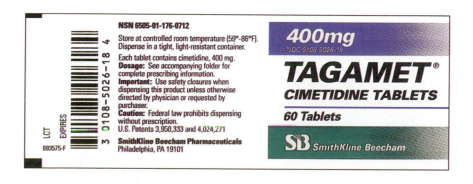

How many tablet(s) of Tagamet should the client receive? _____

2. Order: dexamethasone (Hexadrol) 1 mg, PO, q.d.
   Available: dexamethasone 0.5 mg tablet
   How many tablet(s) should the client receive? _____

3. Order: phenobarbital gr ½, PO, t.i.d.
   Available: phenobarbital 15 mg tablet
   How many tablet(s) should the client receive? _____

4. Order: hydrochlorothiazide (HydroDIURIL) 25 mg, PO, q.d.
   Available: hydrochlorothiazide 50 mg tablet
   How many tablet(s) should the client receive? _____

5. Order: cefadroxil (Duricef) 500 mg, PO, b.i.d.
   Available (drug label):

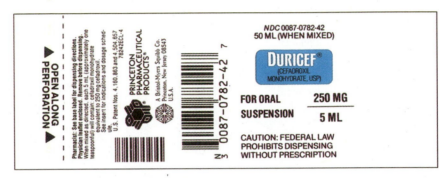

   How many mL should the client receive? _____

6. Order: dicloxacillin 100 mg, PO, q8h
   Available: dicloxacillin 62.5 mg / 5 mL
   How many mL should the client receive? _____

7. Order: meperidine (Demerol) 35 mg, IM, STAT
   Available:

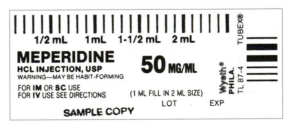

   How many mL should the client receive? _____

8. Order: atropine sulfate gr ½₀₀, SC, on call.
   Available (drug label): atropine sulfate 0.4 mg / 1 mL

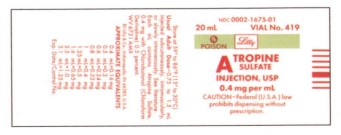

   How many mL should the client receive? _____

II. DRUG DOSAGE USING BODY WEIGHT

9. Order: phenytoin (Dilantin) 5 mg/kg/day, P.O., in two divided doses.
   Client weighs 55 lb.
   How many milligrams (mg) should the client receive per day? _____
   Per dose? _____

10. Order: sulfisoxazole (Gantrisin) 50 mg/kg/day, P.O., in four divided doses (q6h).
    Child weighs 44 lb.
    How many mg should the client receive per day? _____ Per dose? _____

11. Order: albuterol (Proventil) 0.1 mg/kg/day, P.O., in four divided doses.
    Client weighs 86 lb.
    How many mg should the client receive per dose? _____

12. Order: cephalexin 40 mg/kg/day, P.O., in four divided doses.
    Child weighs 33 lb.
    Available (drug label):

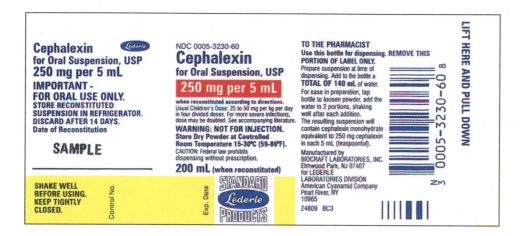

   a. How many milligrams should be given per day?

   b. How many milliliters should the child receive per dose?

III. DRUG DOSAGE USING BODY SURFACE AREA

13. Client's height is 62 in. and weight is 130 lb. The BSA is _____

14. Order: bleomycin sulfate 20 Units/m², IV. Client is 70 in. tall and weighs 160 lb.
    How many unit(s) should the client receive? _____

15. Order: sulfisoxazole (Gantrisin) 2 g/m² in four divided doses. Child's height is 50 in. and weight is 60 lb.
    Available: sulfisoxazole 500 mg/5 mL.

   a. What is the child's BSA? _____

   b. How many gram(s) should the child receive per day? _____

   c. How many mL should the child receive per dose? _____

ANSWERS TO PRACTICE PROBLEMS

Practice Problems: Drug Dosage Using a General Formula

1. a. Convert grams to milligrams by moving the decimal point three spaces to the right.

$$0.4 \text{ g} = 0.400 \text{ mg}$$

   b.
$$\frac{D}{H} \times V = \frac{400 \text{ mg}}{400 \text{ mg}} \times 1 \text{ tablet} = 1 \text{ tablet}$$

   or:

H	:	V	::	D	:	x
400 mg	:	1 tab	::	400 mg	:	x tab

$$400x = 400$$

$$x = 1 \text{ tablet}$$

2. 2 tablets.

$$\frac{1 \text{ mg}}{0.5 \text{ mg}} = 0.5 \,\overline{)1.0}^{\;2.0 \text{ tablets}}$$

3. a. Convert grains to milligrams. Table 4A–4 or 4B–1 gives 30 mg = ½ gr, or 60 mg = 1 gr

60 mg	:	1 gr	::	x mg	:	½ gr

$$x = 60 \times 0.5 \; (½)$$

$$x = 30 \text{ mg}$$

   b.
$$\frac{D}{H} \times V = \frac{30}{15} \times 1 = 2 \text{ tablets}$$

   or:

H	:	V	::	D	:	x
15 mg	:	1 tab	::	30 mg	:	x tab

$$15x = 30$$

$$x = 2 \text{ tablets}$$

4. ½ tablets

5. 10 mL

6.
$$\frac{D}{H} \times V = \frac{100}{62.5} \times 5 = \frac{500}{62.5} = 8 \text{ mL}$$

   or:

H	:	V	::	D	:	x
62.5 mg	:	5 mL	::	100 mg	:	x mL

$$62.5x = 500$$

$$x = 8 \text{ mL}$$

7. 0.7 mL

8. a.   The drug label shows 0.4 mg = 1 ml. Change ½₀₀ gr to milligrams (see Table 4A–4 or 4B–1).

$$\tfrac{1}{200}\text{ gr } = 0.3\text{ mg}$$

b.
$$\frac{D}{H} \times V = \frac{0.3}{0.4} \times 1\text{ mL} =$$

$$0.4\overline{)0.3.0}^{\,0.75} = 0.75\text{ mL}$$

or:
H	:	V	::	D	:	x
0.4 mg	:	1 mL	::	0.3 mg	:	x mL

$$0.4x = 0.3$$

$$x = \frac{0.3}{0.4} = 0.75\text{ mL}$$

Practice Problems: **Drug Dosage Using Body Weight**

9. a.   55 lb ÷ 2.2 kg = 25 kg

   b.   5 mg × 25 kg = 125 mg/day, or 62.5 mg b.i.d.

10. a.   20 kg

   b.   50 mg × 20 kg = 1000 mg/day
      1000 ÷ 4 times a day = 250 mg q.i.d., or q6h

11. a.   86 ÷ 2.2 = 39 kg

   b.   0.1 mg × 39 = 3.9 mg, or 4 mg
      4 ÷ 4 = 1 mg q6h

12. 33 ÷ 2.2 = 15 kg
   40 mg × 15 = 600 mg/day
   600 ÷ 4 times a day = 150 mg q6h per dose

$$\frac{D}{H} \times V = \frac{150}{250} \times 5\text{ mL} = \frac{750}{250} = 3\text{ mL q6h}$$

H	:	V	::	D	:	x
250 mg	:	5 mL	::	150 mg	:	x mL

$$250x = 750$$

$$x = 3\text{ mL q6h}$$

   a.   Administer cephalexin 600 mg/day

   b.   Administer 150 mg = 3 mL q6h.

Practice Problems: **Drug Dosage Using Body Surface Area**

13. 1.65 m^2

14. a. Client's height and weight intersect the nomogram scale at 1.97 m^2.

    b. 20 U × 1.97 = 39.4 or 39 U

15. a. Height and weight intersect the nomogram scale at 0.98 m^2.

    b. 2 g × 0.98 = 1.96 g, or 2 g/day

    c. 5 mL (convert grams to milligrams. 0.5 g = 0.500 mg)

Chapter 4

Calculations of Oral Dosages, Including for Pediatrics

OUTLINE

Objectives
Terms
Introduction
Tablets, Capsules, and Liquids
Interpreting Oral Drug Labels
Drug Differentiation

Calculation for Tablet, Capsule, and Liquid Doses
Body Weight and Body Surface Area
Percentage of Solutions
Pediatric Drug Calculations

Pediatric Dosage per Body Weight
Pediatric Dosage per Body Surface Area
Pediatric Dosage from Adult Dosage

OBJECTIVES

Calculate oral dosages from tablets, capsules, and liquids with selected formula.

Calculate oral medications according to body weight and body surface area (BSA).

Calculate the amount of tube feeding solution needed for dilution according to the percentage ordered.

Calculate the drug parameters for safe child's dose.

Calculate pediatric dosages according to body weight, body surface area, and adult dosage with BSA.

TERMS

body surface area
capsule
drug parameters

enteric-coated
sustained-release

tablet
tube feeding

INTRODUCTION

Eighty percent of all drugs consumed are given orally. Oral drugs are available in tablet, capsule, powder, and liquid form. The written abbreviation for drugs given orally is P.O. or PO (per os, or by mouth). Oral medications are absorbed by the gastrointestinal tract, mainly from the small intestine.

Oral medications have the following advantages: the client frequently can take the drug without assistance, the cost of the drug is usually less than when given via other routes, e.g., parenteral, and it is easy to store. The disadvantages include variation in absorption due to food in the gastrointestinal (GI) tract and pH variation of GI secretions, irritation of the gastric mucosa by certain drugs (potassium chloride), and destruction or partial inactivation of the drugs by liver enzymes.

TABLETS, CAPSULES, AND LIQUIDS

Tablets come in different forms and drug strengths. Most tablets are scored, and thus can be readily broken when half of the drug amount is needed. **Capsules** are gelatin shells containing powder or timed-release pellets (beads). **Sustained-release** (pellet) capsules *should not* be crushed and diluted, because the medication will be absorbed at a much faster rate than indicated by the manufacturer. Many of the medications that are in tablet form are also available in liquid form. When the client has difficulty in taking tablets or if the client is an infant, the liquid form of the medication is given. The liquid form can be in a suspension, syrup, elixir, or tincture. Some liquid medications that are irritating to the stomach, such as potassium chloride, are diluted. The tincture form is always diluted.

Enteric-coated (hard shell) tablets *must not* be crushed, because the medication could irritate the gastric mucosa. Enteric-coated drugs pass through the stomach, with the coating being dissolved in the small intestine; thus, absorption takes place in the intestine. Oral drugs (tablets, capsules, liquids) that irritate the gastric mucosa should be taken with 5 to 8 oz of fluids or taken during mealtime. Figure 4C–1 shows the different forms of tablets and capsules.

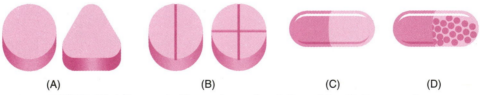

(A)   (B)   (C)   (D)

FIGURE 4C–1 Shapes of tablets and capsules. *A, B* = tablets; *C, D* = capsules.

Liquid medications are poured into a medicine cup that is calibrated in ounces, teaspoons, tablespoons, and milliliters. Figure 4C–2 shows the markings on a medicine cup.

FIGURE 4C–2 Medicine cup for liquid measurement. (*Source:* From Kee JL, Marshall SM: Clinical Calculations, 3rd ed. Philadelphia: WB Saunders, 1992, p 99.)

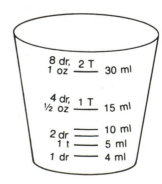

INTERPRETING ORAL DRUG LABELS

The pharmaceutical companies usually label their drugs with the brand name of the drug in large letters and the generic name in smaller letters. The dose per tablet, capsule, or liquid is often printed under the drug name. Two examples of oral drug labels are:

EXAMPLE I:

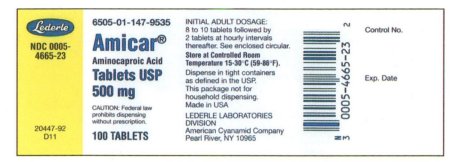

Amicar is the brand name; aminocaproic acid is the generic name; and the dose is 500 mg/tablet.

EXAMPLE II:

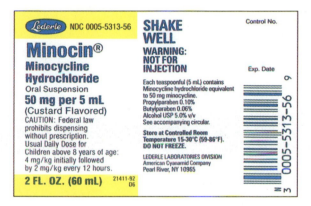

Minocin is the brand name; minocycline HCl is the generic name; and the dose is 50 mg/5 mL (liquid suspension).

DRUG DIFFERENTIATION

Some drugs with similar names, such as quinine and quinidine, have different chemical drug structures. Extreme care must be exercised when administering drugs whose names look alike. Examine the following examples.

EXAMPLE 1: PERCODAN AND PERCOCET

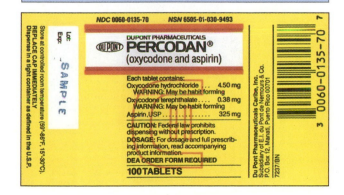
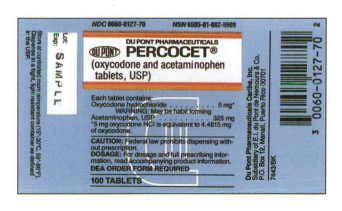

SECTION C

Percodan contains oxycodone and aspirin, and Percocet contains oxycodone and aceta-minophen. A client may be allergic to aspirin or should not take aspirin because of a stomach ulcer; therefore, it is important that the client take Percocet. *Read the drug labels carefully.*

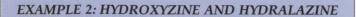

EXAMPLE 2: HYDROXYZINE AND HYDRALAZINE

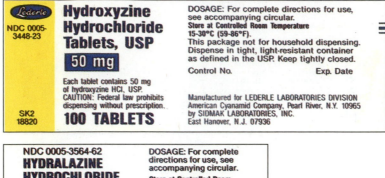

Hydroxyzine is an antianxiety drug and hydralazine is an antihypertensive drug.

CALCULATION FOR TABLET, CAPSULE, AND LIQUID DOSES

When calculating oral dosages, choose one of the methods for calculation from Section 4B. Examples will be given using the basic formula and the ratio-and-proportion methods.

Basic Formula

$$\frac{D}{H} \times V =$$

Ratio and Proportion

$$H : V :: D : x$$
$$\text{on hand} \quad \text{vehicle} \quad \text{desired dose} \quad \text{unknown}$$

means

extremes

$$x =$$

EXAMPLES:

1. Order: diltiazem (Cardizem) 60 mg, PO, b.i.d.
   Available:

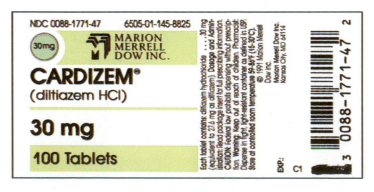

a.
$$\frac{D}{H} \times V = \frac{60}{30} \times 1 = 2 \text{ tablets}$$

b.

H	:	V	::	D	:	x
30 mg	:	1 tab	::	60 mg	:	x tab

$$30x = 60$$

$$x = 2 \text{ tablets}$$

Answer: Cardizem (diltiazem) 60 mg = 2 tablets.

2. Order: codeine sulfate 1 gr, PO STAT
   Available: Refer to the conversion tables 4A–4 or 4B–1.

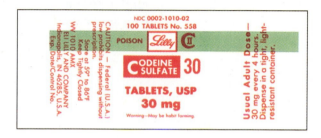

a.
$$\text{gr } 1 = 60 \text{ mg}$$

$$\frac{D}{H} \times V = \frac{60}{30} \times 1 = 2 \text{ tablets}$$

b.

H	:	V	::	D	:	x
30 mg	:	1 tab	::	60 mg	:	x tab

$$30x = 60$$

$$x = 2 \text{ tablets}$$

Answer: codeine 1 gr = 2 tablets.

3. Order: ampicillin 0.5 g
   Available:

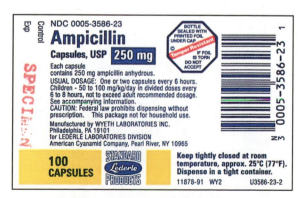

Refer to Section 4A. Grams and milligrams are in the metric system. To change grams to milligrams, move the decimal point three spaces to the right.

$$0.500 \text{ milligram}$$

a.

$$\frac{D}{H} \times V = \frac{500}{250} \times 1 = \frac{500}{250} = 2 \text{ capsules}$$

b.

$$H \quad : \quad V \quad :: \quad D \quad : \quad x$$
$$250 \text{ mg} : 1 \text{ cap} :: 500 \text{ mg} : x \text{ cap}$$

$$250x = 500$$

$$x = \frac{500}{250} = 2 \text{ capsules}$$

Answer: ampicillin 0.5 g = 2 capsules.

I. PRACTICE PROBLEMS: TABLETS, CAPSULES, AND LIQUID

Solve the drug problems for x, the unknown amount of drug to be given. Refer to Sections 4A and 4B for the conversion tables, methods of conversion, and the method chosen to solve the drug problems:

1. Order: prednisone 5 mg, PO, b.i.d.
   Available: prednisone 2.5 mg tablet
   How many tablet(s) should the client receive per dose? _____

2. Order: amantadine (Symmetrel) 0.1 g, PO, b.i.d.
   Available:

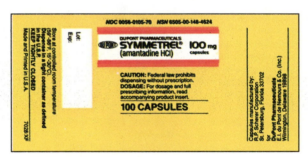

   How many capsule(s) should the client receive per dose? _____

3. Order: allopurinol (Zyloprim) 450 mg, PO, q.d.
   Available: allopurinol 300 mg tablet
   How many tablet(s) should the client receive? _____

4. Order: aspirin gr x, STAT
   Available: aspirin 325 mg tablet
   How many tablet(s) of aspirin should the nurse give? _____

5. Order: digoxin (Lanoxin) 0.5 mg, PO, q.d.
   Available:

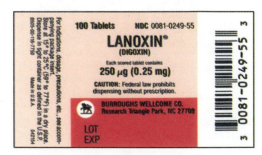

   How many tablet(s) should the nurse administer? _____

6. Order: nitroglycerin ¹⁄₁₅₀ gr, sublingual, STAT
   Available:

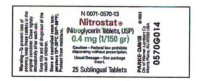

How many sublingual tablet(s) should the client take? _____

7. Order: bethanechol Cl (Urecholine) 20 mg, PO, t.i.d.
   Available:

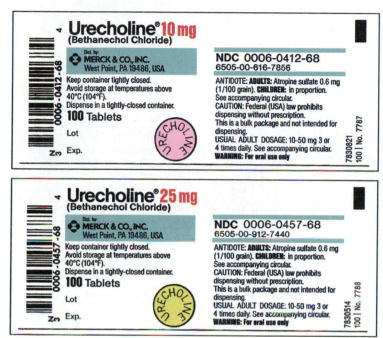

   a. Which Urecholine bottle should the nurse select? _____

   b. How many tablet(s) should the client receive per dose? _____

8. Order: tetracycline 500 mg, PO, b.i.d.
   Available:

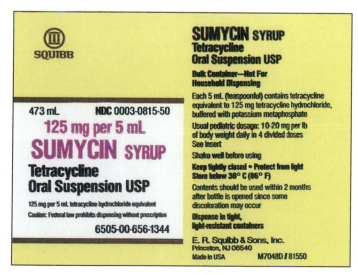

How many mL should the client receive per dose? _____

9. Order: nystatin (Mycostatin) 300,000 units, swish and swallow, t.i.d.
Available:

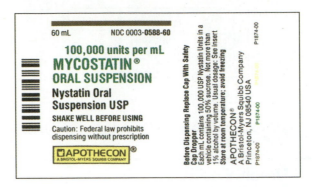

How many mL should the client receive per dose? _____

10. Order: cephalexin, 200 mg, PO, q6h
Available:

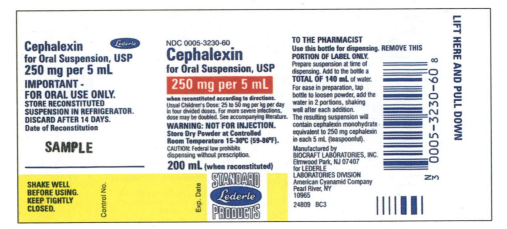

How many mL should the client receive per dose? _____

11. Order: potassium chloride (Kay Ciel) 30 mEq, PO, q.d.
Available: potassium chloride 20 mEq/15 mL (cc)
How many mL should the client receive per day? _____

12. Order: docusate sodium (Colace) 50 mg, PO, h.s.
Available: Colace syrup 20 mg/5 mL
How many mL should the client receive at bedtime? _____

13. Order: cefadroxil (Duricef) 500 mg, PO, b.i.d.
Available:

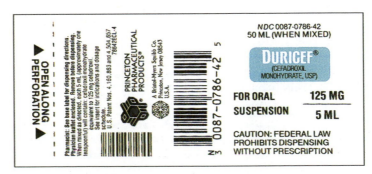

How many mL should the client receive per dose? _____

14. Order: prazosin (Minipress) 10 mg, PO, q.d.
    Available: prazosin 1 mg, 2 mg, and 5 mg tablets.
    Which tablet would you select and how much would you give? _____

15. Order: carbidopa–levodopa (Sinemet) 12.5–125 mg, PO, b.i.d.
    Available: Sinemet 25–100, 25–250, 10–100 mg tablets.
    Which tablet would you select and how much would you give? _____

BODY WEIGHT AND BODY SURFACE AREA

Calculating the drug dosage for adults by body weight and body surface area is used mostly when administering drugs to treat cancer (antineoplastic) drugs. These two individualized methods are used frequently in calculating drug dosage for children. Examples and practice problems for pediatrics are given in this section.

To use the **body weight** method, convert the person's weight in pounds to kilograms (kg). To convert, divide pounds by 2.2 to equal kilograms. In using the **body surface area** method, the person's weight and height and a nomogram are needed. (See Section 4B and the pediatric section of 4C). Daily requirements are usually divided into two to four doses per day.

> **EXAMPLE:**

Order: cyclophosphamide (Cytoxan) 2 mg / kg / day, PO
Client weighs 143 lb. How much does the client weigh in kilograms? How many milligrams (mg) should the client receive?
> *Answer:*

$$143 \text{ lb} \div 2.2 = 65 \text{ kg}$$

$$2 \text{ mg} \times 65 = 130 \text{ mg of Cytoxan daily.}$$

> **II. PRACTICE PROBLEMS: BODY WEIGHT**

1. Order: valproic acid (Depakene) 8 mg / kg / day in four divided doses. Client weighs 165 lb. How much Depakene should be administered per dose?

2. Order: cyclophosphamide (Cytoxan) 4 mg / kg / day. Client weighs 176 lb. How much Cytoxan should the client receive per day?

PERCENTAGE OF SOLUTIONS

When clients are unable to take food or fluids by mouth, they may receive nutrients through a nasogastric (NG) tube. The nutrients that are administered through NG tubes are in solution form, and the process is usually called **tube feeding.** When tube feedings are initiated, they are usually diluted with water to prevent diarrhea due to the richness of the solution. Dilutions of tube feeding are ordered in percentage. Clients tolerate tube feedings better when the feedings are started at low strength and the concentration is incrementally increased over time. When a percentage strength of solution is ordered, the nurse calculates the amount of solution and water that are to be given.

The percentage of a solution indicates its strength. Tube feeding solutions, such as Ensure, Ensure Plus, Osmolite, Isomil, and others, are considered to be 100%. Fifty percent of the solution is 50% strength of the solution or 50/100. To determine the amount (mL) of tube feeding solution to give, the basic formula or ratio-and-proportion method can be used with the following changes:

SECTION C

D stands for the desired percentage.
H represents the on-hand strength, which is 100%.
V represents the desired total volume.
x stands for the unknown amount of solution.

Following the tube feeding, 30 mL (cc) of water should be given to clear the tubing. Usually the tube is clamped for 30 min after feeding to keep fluid content from backing out of the stomach into the tube. The client should remain with head elevated at a 30 to 90-degree angle after feeding for 30 minutes.

> **EXAMPLE:**

Order: 250 mL (cc) of 30% solution, q4h × 6 feedings, via NG tube
    Calculate how much Ensure and water is needed to make 250 mL of 30% solution.
Note: 30% solution is 30 in 100 parts.

a. $$\frac{D}{H} \times \frac{\text{Desired \%}}{\text{On-hand strength}} \times V \text{ (Desired total volume)} =$$

$$\frac{30}{100} \times 250 = \frac{7500}{100} = 75 \text{ mL of Ensure}$$

b.
$$H \quad : \quad V \quad :: \quad D \quad : $$
$$100 \quad : \quad 250 \quad :: \quad 30 \quad : \quad x$$

$$100x = 7500$$
$$x = 75 \text{ mL of Ensure}$$

How much water should be added?

Total amount − Amount of tube feeding = Amount of water

250 mL   −   75 mL   =   175 mL

Answer: 75 mL of Ensure + 175 mL of water.

Oral medications can be administered through the nasogastric tube, but should *not* be mixed with the entire tube feeding solution. Mixing the medications in a large volume of tube feeding decreases the amount of drug the client receives for a specific time. The medication (**NOT** time-released or sustained-release capsules and psyllium hydrophilic mucilloid [Metamucil]) should be diluted in 1 oz, or 30 mL, of warm water unless otherwise instructed, administered through the tube, and followed with extra water to ensure that the drug reaches the stomach and is not left in the tube.

> **III. PRACTICE PROBLEMS: PERCENTAGE OF SOLUTIONS**

Refer to example as needed.

1. Order: 500 mL of 60% Ensure Plus solution three times a day through the nasogastric tube.
   How much Ensure Plus solution and water should be mixed to equal 500 mL?

2. Order: 250 mL of 70% Osmolite solution, q6h, via NG tube.
   How much Osmolite and water should be mixed to equal 250 mL?

3. Order: 400 mL of 40% Isomil solution, q6h, through the NG tube.
   How much Isomil and water should be mixed to equal 400 mL?

4. Order: 300 mL of 75% Ensure solution four times a day, through the NG tube.
   How much Ensure and water should be mixed to equal 300 mL?

PEDIATRIC DRUG CALCULATIONS

The purpose of learning how to calculate pediatric drug dosages is to ensure that children receive the correct dose within the approved therapeutic range. The two methods that are considered safe in administering drugs to children are the body weight (kg) and body surface area (BSA, or m²) methods. Many manufacturers supply information in their literature concerning drug doses for children according to body weight. Also, manufacturers might give **parameters** for safe dose ranges. It is the nurse's responsibility to check the dose ranges, given by the pharmaceutical manufacturers, to be certain that the prescribed dose is within the parameters. Children's dosage can be determined from the adult dose using the body surface area rule. Older methods used in calculating children's dosages are Fried's rule and Young's rule, which are based on the child's age, and Clark's rule, which is based on the weight of the child. These older methods are obsolete, but are occasionally used today, see Appendix C for their formulas.

PEDIATRIC DOSAGE PER BODY WEIGHT

EXAMPLE:

Order: cefaclor (Ceclor) 50 mg, q.i.d.
   Child weighs 15 lb or 6.8 kg (15 ÷ 2.2 = 6.8).
   Child's drug dosage: 20–40 mg/kg/day in three divided doses.
   Available: cefaclor 125 mg/5 mL.
   Is the prescribed dose safe?

Answer:

Drug parameters: 20 mg × 6.8 kg = 136 mg/day

                                40 mg × 6.8 kg = 272 mg/day

Dosage order: 50 mg × 4 = 200 mg/day

Dosage is within safe parameters.

a.
$$\frac{D}{H} \times V = \frac{50}{125} \times 5 = \frac{250}{125} = 2 \text{ mL}$$

b.

H	:	V	::	D	:	x
125 mg	:	5 mL	::	50 mg	:	x mL

$$125x = 250$$
$$x = 2 \text{ mL (cc)}$$

Cefaclor 50 mg = 2 mL. Give 2 mL four times a day.

PEDIATRIC DOSAGE PER BODY SURFACE AREA

To calculate pediatric dose by BSA, the child's height and weight are needed.

> **EXAMPLE:**

Order: methotrexate (Mexate) 50 mg, weekly
    Child's height: 54 inches; Weight: 90 lb (41 kg)
    Child's drug dosage: 25–75 mg/m^2/week
    Child's height and weight intersect at 1.3 m^2 (BSA).
    Is the prescribed dose safe?

Answer:
    Multiply the BSA, 1.3 m^2, by the minimum and maximum doses.

$$25 \text{ mg} \times 1.3 \text{ m}^2 = 32.5 \text{ mg}$$

$$75 \text{ mg} \times 1.3 \text{ m}^2 = 97.5 \text{ mg}$$

Dosage is considered safe within the parameters according to the child's body surface area (BSA).

PEDIATRIC DOSAGE FROM ADULT DOSAGE

To calculate the pediatric dosage from the adult dosage, determine the child's height and weight, and where they intersect on the nomogram is the body surface area in square meters. The formula for calculation is:

$$\frac{\text{Surface area (m}^2)}{1.73 \text{ m}^2} \times \text{Adult dose} = \text{Pediatric dose}$$

> **EXAMPLE:**

Order: erythromycin (E-Mycin) 125 mg, PO, q.i.d.
    Child's height is 42 inches; weight is 60 lb
    Child's height and weight intersect at 0.9 m^2.
    The adult dose is 1000 mg/day.

$$\frac{0.9 \text{ m}^2}{1.73 \text{ m}^2} \times 1000 = \frac{900}{1.73} = 520 \text{ mg/day}$$

Drug dosage: 520 mg ÷ 4 times a day = 130 mg/dose
Dosage is within safe range.

> **IV. PRACTICE PROBLEMS: PEDIATRICS**

Solve the following problems using one of these three methods: body weight, body surface area, or pediatric dosage from adult dosage. The safe dosage is given in drug reference books.

  1. Order: phenytoin (Dilantin) 50 mg, b.i.d.
     Child weighs 44 lb (20 kg).
     Child's drug dosage: 4–8 mg/kg/day in two to three divided doses

Available:

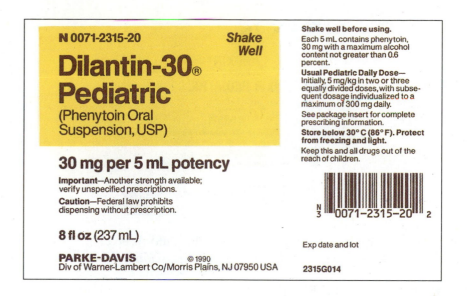

Is the prescribed dose safe? How many milliliters should the child receive for each dose?

2. Order: ethosuximide (Zarontin) 500 mg/d, PO.
   Child weighs 26 kg.
   Child's drug dosage: 20 mg/kg/day
   Available: ethosuximide syrup 250 mg/5 mL
   How many milligrams and milliliters should the child receive each day?

3. Order: cloxacillin (Tegopen) 75 mg, PO, q6h
   Child weighs 33 lb (15 kg).
   Child's drug dosage: <20 kg: 12.5–25 mg/kg/day
   Available:

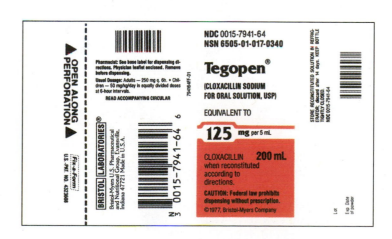

Is the prescribed dose safe? How many milliliters should be given for each dose?

4. Order: digoxin (Lanoxin), 35 μg / kg / loading dose (μg = mcg), PO.
   Child weighs 10 kg.
   Available:

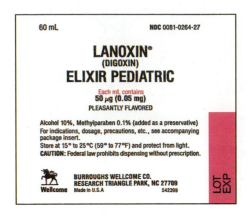

a. How many micrograms or milligrams should the child receive?
b. How many milliliters (mL) should be given for the loading dose?

5. Order: erythromycin 250 mg, PO, q6h
   Child weighs 26 lb (12 kg).
   Child's drug dosage: 30–50 mg / kg / day in three to four divided doses
   Available:

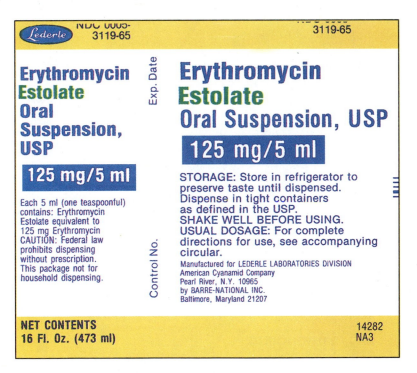

Is the prescribed dose safe? How many milliliters should be given every 6 h?

6. Order: theophylline sodium glycinate (Asbron G) 200 mg, PO, q6h
   Child is 12 years old and weighs 74 lb (34 kg).
   Child's drug dosage: 9–16 years old: 6 mg / kg / q6h
   Is the prescribed dose safe?

7. Order: amoxicillin and clavulanate potassium (Augmentin) 100 mg, PO, q8h.
   Child's weight: 28 lb.

Child's drug dosage: 20–40 mg / kg / day
Available:

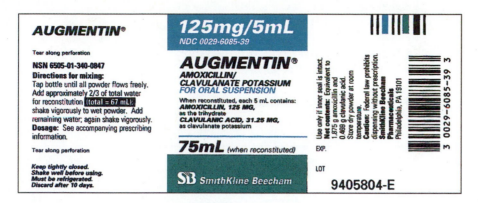

   a. Is the prescribed drug dose within safe parameters? _____

   b. How many mL should the child receive per dose? _____

8. Order: cefadroxil (Duricef) 75 mg, PO, q12h.
   Child's weight: 20 lb.
   Child's drug dosage: 30 mg / kg / day
   Available:

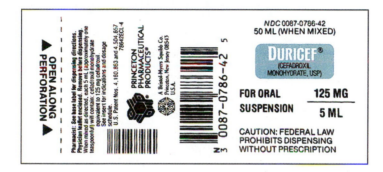

   a. Is the prescribed drug dose within safe parameters? _____

   b. How many mL should the child receive per dose? _____

9. Order: ampicillin 50 mg, PO, q6h
   Child weighs 7 kg.
   Child's drug dosage: 25–50 mg / kg / day
   Available:

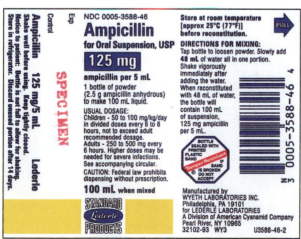

   Is the prescribed dose safe? How many milligrams per dose?

10. Order: vinblastine (Velsar)
    Child's body surface area (BSA) is 1.2 m².
    Child's drug dosage: 2.5 mg/m²
    How many milligrams should the child receive?

11. Order: penicillin V potassium in 4 divided doses/day
    Child's height is 36 inches; weight is 40 lb.
    Child's BSA is 0.7 m².
    Adult dose is 1000 mg/day in four divided doses.
    Available:

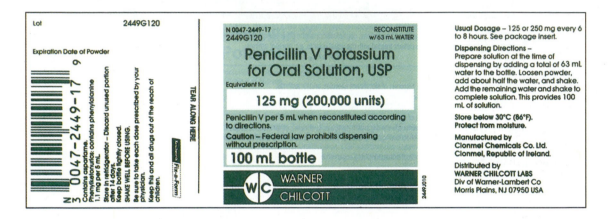

How many milligrams should the child receive per day and how many milliliters per day?

12. Order: trimethoprim–sulfamethoxazole (Septra)
    Child's BSA is 0.75 m².
    Adult dose: trimethoprim 160 mg/sulfamethoxazole 800 mg, q12h
    Available: Septra (trimethoprim 40 mg/sulfamethoxazole 200 mg) suspension/5 mL

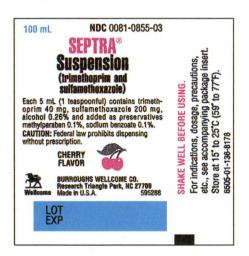

What is the correct dosage for the child and how many milliliters should be given?

ANSWERS TO ALL PRACTICE PROBLEMS

I. Practice Problems: Oral Medications (a and b are the two methods of calculation)

1. 2 tablets

a.
$$\frac{D}{H} \times V = \frac{5}{2.5} \times 1 = 2 \text{ tablets}$$

b.

H	:	V	::	D	:	x
2.5 mg	:	1 tab	::	5 mg	:	x tab

$$2.5x = 5$$

$$x = \frac{5.0}{2.5} = 2 \text{ tablets}$$

2. 1 capsule.
   Change grams to milligrams. Move decimal point three spaces to the right. Refer to Section 4A if necessary.

$$0.100 \text{ mg} = 100 \text{ mg}$$

3. 1½ tablets.

4. Convert grains to milligrams. See Table 4A–4 or 4B–1.
   5 gr = 300, or 325 mg; thus 10 gr = 650 mg (approximate value).

a.
$$\frac{D}{H} \times V = \frac{650}{325} \times 1 = 2 \text{ tablets}$$

b.

H	:	V	::	D	:	x
325 mg	:	1 tab	::	650 mg	:	x tab

$$325x = 650$$

$$x = 2 \text{ tablets}$$

5. 2 tablets

a.
$$\frac{D}{H} \times V = \frac{0.5}{0.25} \times 1 = 0.25\sqrt{0.50\,0} = 2 \text{ tablets}$$

b.

H	:	V	::	D	:	x
0.25 mg	:	1 tab	::	0.5 mg	:	x tab

$$0.25x = 0.5$$

$$x = 2 \text{ tablets}$$

6. 1 sublingual tablet.
   Convert grains to milligrams.

$$\frac{1}{150} \text{ gr} = 0.4 \text{ mg}$$

7. a.   Select Urecholine 10 mg bottle.

b.
$$\frac{D}{H} \times V = \frac{20 \text{ mg}}{10 \text{ mg}} \times 1 \text{ tab} = \frac{20}{10} = 2 \text{ tablets}$$

$$H \quad : \quad V \quad :: \quad D \quad : \quad x$$
$$10 \text{ mg} \quad : \quad 1 \text{ tab} \quad :: \quad 20 \text{ mg} \quad : \quad x \text{ tab}$$

$$10x = 20$$

$$x = 2 \text{ tablets of Urecholine}$$

8. 20 mL of tetracycline syrup.

$$\frac{D}{H} \times V = \frac{\overset{4}{\cancel{500 \text{ mg}}}}{\underset{1}{\cancel{125 \text{ mg}}}} \times 5 \text{ mL} = 20 \text{ mL}$$

9. 3 mL of Mycostatin.

10. 4 mL.

 a.

$$\frac{D}{H} \times V = \frac{200}{250} \times 5 = \frac{1000}{250} = 4 \text{ mL}$$

 b.

$$H \quad : \quad V \quad :: \quad D \quad : \quad x$$
$$250 \text{ mg} \quad : \quad 5 \text{ mL} \quad :: \quad 200 \text{ mg} \quad : \quad x \text{ mL}$$

$$250x = 1000$$

$$x = 4 \text{ mL of cephalexin}$$

11. 22.5 mL or 4½ t.

 a.

$$\frac{D}{H} \times V = \frac{30}{20} \times 15 = \frac{450}{20} = 22.5 \text{ mL}$$

 b.

$$H \quad : \quad V \quad :: \quad D \quad : \quad x$$
$$20 \text{ mEq} \quad : \quad 15 \text{ mL} \quad :: \quad 30 \text{ mEq} \quad : \quad x \text{ mL}$$

$$20x = 450$$

$$x = \frac{450}{20} = 22.5 \text{ mL of potassium chloride}$$

12. 12.5 mL (cc) of Colace syrup.

13. 20 mL of cefadroxil.

 a.

$$\frac{D}{H} \times V = \frac{500}{125} \times 5 = \frac{2500}{125} = 20 \text{ mL}$$

 b.

$$H \quad : \quad V \quad :: \quad D \quad : \quad x$$
$$125 \text{ mg} \quad : \quad 5 \text{ mL} \quad :: \quad 500 \text{ mg} \quad : \quad x \text{ mL}$$

$$125x = 2500$$

$$x = 20 \text{ mL}$$

14. Select 5 mg tablets. Give two tablets.

15. Select 25–250 mg strength. Give ½ tablet.

II. Practice Problems: Body Weight

1. 150 mg/dose. 600 mg/day.

$$165 \div 2.2 = 75 \text{ kg}$$
$$8 \text{ mg} \times 75 = 600 \text{ mg/day}$$
$$= 600 \text{ mg} \div 4 = 150 \text{ mg/dose, q.i.d.}$$

2. 320 mg/day.

$$176 \div 2.2 = 80 \text{ kg}$$

$$4 \text{ mg} \times 80 = 320 \text{ mg/day}$$

III. Practice Problems: Percentage of Solutions

1.

$$\frac{D}{H} \times V = \frac{60}{100} \times 500 = \frac{30,000}{100} = 300 \text{ mL of Ensure Plus}$$

H	:	V	::	D	:	x
100	:	500	::	60	:	x

$$100x = 30,000$$
$$x = 300 \text{ mL of Ensure Plus}$$

Total amount − Amount of tube feeding = Amount of water

| 500 mL | − | 300 mL | = | 200 mL |

300 mL of Ensure Plus + 200 mL of water.

2. 175 mL of Osmolite + 75 mL of water.

3. 160 mL of Isomil + 240 mL of water.

4. 225 mL of Ensure + 75 mL of water.

IV. Practice Problems: Pediatrics

1. Drug parameters:

$$4 \text{ mg} \times 20 \text{ kg} = 80 \text{ mg/day}$$

$$8 \text{ mg} \times 20 \text{ kg} = 160 \text{ mg/day}$$

Dosage order: 50 mg × 2 (b.i.d.) = 100 mg/day
Dosage is within safe parameters.

a.

$$\frac{D}{H} \times V = \frac{50}{30} \times 5 = \frac{250}{30} = 8.3 \text{ mL, or 8 mL}$$

b.

H	:	V	::	D	:	x
30 mg	:	5 mL	::	50 mg	:	x mL

$$30x = 250$$

$$x = \frac{250}{30} = 8.3 \text{ mL}$$

Administer 8 mL of phenytoin per dose.

2. Child's drug dosage: 20 mg × 26 kg = 520 mg, or 500 mg

a.
$$\frac{D}{H} \times V = \frac{500}{250} \times 5 = \frac{2500}{250} = 10 \text{ mL}$$

b.

H	:	V	::	D	:	x
250 mg	:	5 mL	::	500 mg	:	x mL

$$250x = 2500$$

$$x = 10 \text{ mL}$$

Administer ethosuximide 10 mL/day.

3. Drug parameters:

$$12.5 \text{ mg} \times 15 \text{ kg} = 187.5 \text{ mg/day}$$

$$25 \text{ mg} \times 15 \text{ kg} = 375 \text{ mg/day}$$

Dosage order: 75 mg × 4 times a day (q6h) = 300 mg/day
Dosage is within safe parameters.

a.
$$\frac{D}{H} \times V = \frac{75}{125} \times 5 = \frac{375}{125} = 3 \text{ mL of cloxacillin}$$

b.

H	:	V	::	D	:	x
125 mg	:	5 mL	::	75 mg	:	x mL

$$125x = 375$$

$$x = 3 \text{ mL of cloxacillin}$$

4. Child's drug dosage:

a.
$$35 \ \mu g \times 10 \text{ kg} = 350 \ \mu g, \text{ or } 0.35 \text{ mg}$$

$$350 \ \mu g = 0.350 \text{ mg}$$

b.
$$\frac{D}{H} \times V = \frac{350 \ \mu g}{50 \ \mu g} \times 1 \text{ mL} = 7 \text{ mL loading dose}$$

or

$$\frac{0.35 \text{ mg}}{0.05 \text{ mg}} \times 1 \text{ mL} = 7 \text{ mL loading dose}$$

5. Drug parameters:

$$30 \text{ mg} \times 12 \text{ kg} = 360 \text{ mg/day}$$

$$50 \text{ mg} \times 12 \text{ kg} = 600 \text{ mg/day}$$

Dosage order: 250 mg $\times$ 4 (q6h) = 1000 mg/day
Dosage is *not* within safe parameters. Dose exceeds the drug parameters.
Health care provider must be contacted.

6. Drug dosage: 6 mg $\times$ 34 kg = 204 mg, or 200 mg
Dosage of 200 mg is within safe parameters.

7. a.   Drug parameters: (28 lbs $\div$ 2.2 = 12.7 kg)

$$20 \text{ mg} \times 12.7 \text{ kg} = 254 \text{ mg/day}$$

$$40 \text{ mg} \times 12.7 \text{ kg} = 508 \text{ mg/day}$$

Dosage order: 100 mg $\times$ 4 (q8h) = 400 mg/d
Dosage is within safe parameters.

  b. $$\frac{D}{H} \times V = \frac{100 \text{ mg}}{125 \text{ mg}} \times 5 \text{ mL} = \frac{500}{125} = 4 \text{ mL of Augmentin}$$

8. 20 lbs $\div$ 2.2 = 9 kg

  a.   Drug parameters: 30 mg $\times$ 9 kg = 270 mg/day
Drug dosage order: 75 mg $\times$ 2 (q12h) = 150 mg/day
Drug dose is safe; it is below the drug parameter.

  b. $$\frac{D}{H} \times V = \frac{75 \text{ mg}}{125 \text{ mg}} \times 5 \text{ mL} = \frac{375}{125} = 3 \text{ mL of Duricef}$$

9. Drug parameters:

$$25 \text{ mg} \times 7 \text{ kg} = 175 \text{ mg/day}$$

$$50 \text{ mg} \times 7 \text{ kg} = 350 \text{ mg/day}$$

Dosage order: 50 mg $\times$ 4 (q6h) = 200 mg/day
Dosage is within safe parameters.

  a. $$\frac{D}{H} \times V = \frac{50}{125} \times 5 = \frac{250}{125} = 2 \text{ mL of ampicillin}$$

  b.

H	:	V	::	D	:	x
125 mg	:	5 mL	::	50 mg	:	x mL

$$125x = 250$$

$$x = 2 \text{ mL of ampicillin}$$

10. Drug dosage: 2.5 mg $\times$ 1.2 m^2 = 3 mg
    Administer 3 mg vinblastine.

11. Drug dosage calculated from adult dose.

$$\frac{0.7 \text{ m}^2}{1.73 \text{ m}^2} \times 1000 = \frac{700}{1.73} = 400 \text{ mg/day, or } 100 \text{ mg, q.i.d. or q6h}$$

a.
$$\frac{D}{H} \times V = \frac{100}{125} \times 5 = \frac{500}{125} = 4 \text{ mL}$$

b.

H	:	V	::	D	:	x
125 mg	:	5 mL	::	100 mg	:	x mL

$$125x = 500$$

$$x = 4 \text{ mL}$$

Administer penicillin V potassium 100 mg, or 4 mL four times a day (q.i.d.).

12. Drug dosage calculated from adult dose.

$$\frac{0.75 \text{ m}^2}{1.73} \times 160/800 = \frac{120/600}{1.73} = \begin{array}{l} 70 \text{ mg of trimethoprim and} \\ 350 \text{ mg sulfamethoxazole} \end{array}$$

$$\frac{D}{H} \times V = \frac{70/350}{40/200} \times 5 = \frac{350/1750}{40/200} = 8.75 \text{ mL, or 9 mL}$$

H	:	V	::	D	:	x
40/200 mg	:	5 mL	::	70/350 mg	:	x mL

$$40/200x = 350/1750$$

$$x = 8.75 \text{ mL, or 9 mL}$$

Administer trimethoprim–sulfamethoxazole (Septra) 9 mL, q12h.

Chapter 4

Calculations of Injectable Dosages, Including for Pediatrics

OUTLINE

Objectives
Terms
Introduction
Injectable Preparations
    Vials and Ampules
    Syringes
    Prefilled Drug Cartridges
      and Syringes
    Needles

Interpreting Injectable Drug
    Label
Intradermal Injections
Subcutaneous Injections
    Calculations: Subcutaneous
      Injections
Insulin Injections
    Types of Insulins
    Mixing Insulins

Intramuscular Injections
    Drug Solutions for Injection
    Powdered Drug Reconstitu-
      tion
    Mixing Injectable Drugs
Pediatric Calculations for
    Injectables

OBJECTIVES

Describe the difference between vials and ampules.

Describe the types of syringes and needles and their uses.

Explain how to administer intradermal, subcutaneous, and intramuscular injections.

Calculate dosage of drugs for subcutaneous and intramuscular injections.

Identify the amount of insulin dosage using an insulin syringe.

Explain the methods for mixing two insulins in one insulin syringe and for mixing two injectable drugs in one syringe.

Describe the procedure for preparing and calculating medications in powdered form for injectable use.

TERMS

ampule
bevel
diluent
gauge

insulin syringe
intradermal
intramuscular
lumen

parenteral
subcutaneous
tuberculin syringe
vial

SECTION D

INTRODUCTION

When medications cannot be taken by mouth because of an inability to swallow, a decreased level of consciousness, an inactivation of the drug by the gastric juices, or a desire to increase the effectiveness of the drug, the parenteral route may be the route of choice. **Parenteral** medications are administered intradermally (under the skin), subcutaneously (SC, into the fatty tissue), intramuscularly (IM, within the muscle), and intravenously (IV, in the vein). Intravenous injectables are discussed in Section 4E. The injectables in this section include intradermal, subcutaneous (including insulin and heparin), and intramuscular from prepared liquid and reconstituted powder in vials and ampules. Prefilled drug cartridges (syringes) are also discussed.

This section is divided into five sections: (1) injectable preparations, (2) intradermal injections, (3) subcutaneous injections, (4) insulin injections, and (5) intramuscular injections. With the four latter groups, examples and practice problems to solve for the correct dosage are given.

INJECTABLE PREPARATIONS

The appropriate drug container (vial or ampule) and the correct selection of needle and syringe are essential when preparing the prescribed drug dose. The route of administration is part of the medication order.

VIALS AND AMPULES

Vials are usually small glass containers with a self-sealing rubber top. Some are multiple-dose vials, and when properly stored they can be used over time. **Ampules** are glass containers with a tapered neck for snapping open and are used only once. Drugs that deteriorate readily in liquid form are packaged in powder form in vials and ampules for storage. Once the dry form of the drug is reconstituted (usually with sterile water, bacteriostatic water, or saline), the drug is used immediately or must be refrigerated. Check the accompanying drug circular for specific storage length and other instructions. The person reconstituting the drug should write on the label when the drug is to be discarded and include her or his initials. Usually a vial should be used within 96 h to 1 week.

Drug labels on vials and ampules provide the following information: generic and brand name of the drug, drug dose in weight (milligrams, grams, milliequivalents) and amount (milliliters), expiration date, and directions about administration. If the drug is in powdered form, mixing instructions and dose equivalents (such as milligrams equal milliliters) may be given. Figure 4D–1 is a diagram of a vial and ampule.

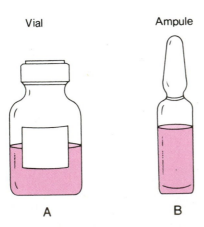

Vial

Ampule

A

B

FIGURE 4D–1 (*A*) Vial (*B*) ampule. (*Source:* From Kee JL, Marshall SM: Clinical Calculations, 3rd ed. Philadelphia: WB Saunders, 1996, p 124.)

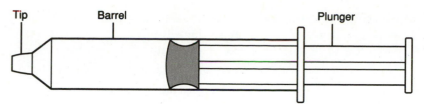

FIGURE 4D–2 Parts of a syringe. (*Source:* From Kee JL, Marshall SM: Clinical Calculations, 3rd ed. Philadelphia: WB Saunders, 1996, p 125.)

SYRINGES

The syringe is composed of a barrel (outer shell), plunger (inner part), and the tip where the needle joins the syringe (Fig. 4D–2). Syringes are available in various types and sizes, the most common of which are the 3-mL and 5-mL sizes of tuberculin, insulin, and metal and plastic syringes for prefilled cartridges. Glass syringes may be used in the operating room and on special instrument trays. Selected injectable drugs are packaged in prefilled cartridges for Tubex and the Carpuject brand syringes. The tip of the syringe and inside of plunger should remain sterile.

The 3-mL syringe is calibrated in tenths (0.1 mL) and minims. The amount of fluid in the syringe is determined by the black rubber end of the plunger (the inner end of the plunger) that is closest to the tip (Fig. 4D–3). Remember milliliter (mL) and cubic centimeter (cc) may be used interchangeably.

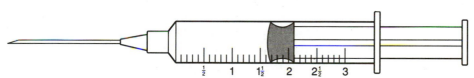

FIGURE 4D–3 Three-milliliter syringe. (*Source:* From Kee JL, Marshall SM: Clinical Calculations, 3rd ed. Philadelphia: WB Saunders, 1996, p 125.)

The 5-mL syringe is calibrated in 0.2-mL marks. A 5-mL syringe is usually used when the fluid needed is more than 2.5 mL. It is frequently used when reconstituting the dry drug form with sterile bacteriostatic water or saline. Figure 4D–4 shows the 5-mL syringe and its markings.

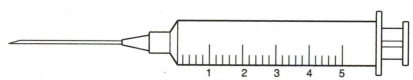

FIGURE 4D–4 Five-milliliter syringe. (*Source:* From Kee JL, Marshall SM: Clinical Calculations, 3rd ed. Philadelphia: WB Saunders, 1996, p 125.)

The **tuberculin syringe** is a 1-mL, slender syringe with markings in tenths (0.1) and hundredths (0.01). It is also marked in minims. (Fig. 4D–5). This syringe is used when the amount of drug solution to be administered is less than 1 mL and for pediatric and heparin dosages.

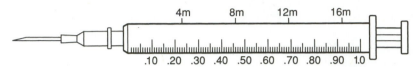

FIGURE 4D–5 Tuberculin syringe. (*Source:* From Kee JL, Marshall SM: Clinical Calculations, 3rd ed. Philadelphia: WB Saunders, 1996, p 126.)

The **insulin syringe** has the capacity of 1 mL; however, insulin is measured in units and insulin dosage *must not* be calculated in milliliters. Insulin syringes are calibrated as 2-U marks, and 100 U equal 1 mL (Fig. 4D–6). *Insulin syringes must be used for the administration of insulin.*

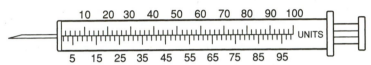

FIGURE 4D–6 Insulin syringe. (*Source:* From Kee JL, Marshall SM: Clinical Calculations, 3rd ed. Philadelphia: WB Saunders, 1996, p 126.)

PREFILLED DRUG CARTRIDGES AND SYRINGES

Many injectable drugs are packaged in prefilled, disposable cartridges. The disposable cartridge is placed into a Tubex injector or a reusable metal or plastic holder. Usually the prefilled cartridge contains 0.1 to 0.2 mL of excess drug solution. Based on the amount of drug to be administered, the excess solution must be expelled prior to administration. Figure 4D–7 illustrates the Tubex injector and cartridge.

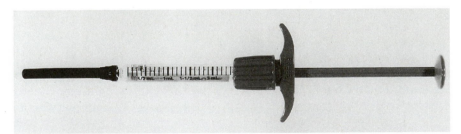

FIGURE 4D–7 Prefilled cartridge and Tubex injector. (*Source:* From Kee JL, Marshall SM: Clinical Calculations, 3rd ed. Philadelphia: WB Saunders, 1996, p 126. Courtesy of Wyeth-Ayerst Laboratories, Philadelphia.)

TABLE 4D–1 Needle Size and Length

Type of Injection	Needle Gauge	Needle Lengths (inches)
Intradermal	25, 26	⅜, ½, ⅝
Subcutaneous	23, 25, 26	⅜, ½, ⅝
Intramuscular	19, 20, 21, 22	1, 1½, 2

NEEDLES

Needle size has two components, gauge (diameter of the lumen) and length. The larger the **gauge,** the smaller the diameter of the **lumen,** and the smaller the gauge, the larger the diameter of the lumen. The more common gauge numbers of needles range from 18 to 26. Needle length varies from ⅜ to 2 in. Table 4D–1 lists the needle gauges and lengths for use in subcutaneous and intramuscular injections.

When choosing the needle length for an intramuscular injection, the size of the client and the amount of fatty tissue must be considered. A client with minimal fatty (subcutaneous) tissue may need a needle length of 1 inch. For an obese client, the length of the needle for an intramuscular injection would be 1.5 to 2 inches.

Insulin syringes and prefilled cartridges have permanently attached needles. With other syringes, the needle can be changed to the desired needle size. Needle gauge and length are indicated on the syringe package or on the top cover of the syringe. It appears as gauge/length; for example, 20 g/1½.

Figure 4D–8 illustrates the parts of a needle.

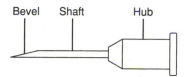

FIGURE 4D–8 Parts of a needle. (*Source:* From Kee JL, Marshall SM: Clinical Calculations, 3rd ed. Philadelphia: WB Saunders, 1996, p 126.)

Angles for Injections

For injections, the needle enters the skin at different angles. Intradermal injections are given at a 10- to 15-degree angle, subcutaneous injections at a 45- to 90-degree angle, and intramuscular injections at a 90-degree angle. Figure 4D–9 illustrates the angles for intradermal, subcutaneous, and intramuscular injections.

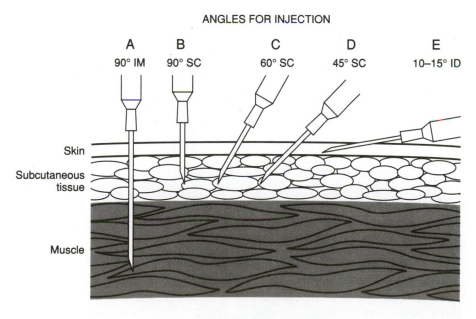

FIGURE 4D–9 Angles for injections. Key: (*A*) IM 90°; (*B*) (*C*) (*D*) SC 90°, 60°, 45°; (*E*) ID (intradermal) 10–15°. (*Source:* Adapted from Norton BA and Miller AM: *Skills for Professional Nursing Practice.* East Norwalk, CT, Appleton and Lange, 1986, p. 891.)

I. PRACTICE PROBLEMS: SYRINGES AND NEEDLES

Think through and answer each question. Correct answers are given at the end of the section.

1. To mix 4 mL of bacteriostatic water in a vial with a powdered drug, which size syringe should be used?

2. To give 0.4 mL of drug solution subcutaneously, what type of syringe would you use?

3. Meperidine (Demerol) is available in a prefilled cartridge. Half of the drug solution is used. Should the remaining solution in the cartridge be saved for future use?

4. Which has the larger needle lumen, a 21-gauge needle or a 26-gauge needle?

5. Which needle has a length of ⅝ inch, a 21-gauge needle or a 25-gauge needle?

6. Which needle is used for an intramuscular injection, a 20-gauge needle with a 1.5-inch length or a 25-gauge needle with a ⅝-inch length?

INTERPRETING INJECTABLE DRUG LABEL

Drugs for injections are stored in liquid and powder form in vials and ampules. If the drug is in liquid form, the drug dose with its equivalent in milliliters is printed on the drug label. However, drugs in powder form have to be reconstituted (liquid form for use). Usually the instructions for reconstitution are given on the drug label and drug circular. If this is not the case, consult a pharmacist.

EXAMPLE:

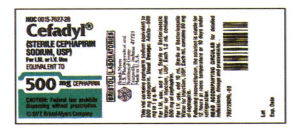

Cefadyl is the brand name; cephapirin is the generic name. The drug is for IM or IV administration. Instructions on drug label read: "For IM, add 1.0 mL of bacteriostatic or sterile water; 500 mg = 1.2 mL. For IV use, add 10 mL sterile or bacteriostatic water; 50 mg = 1.0 mL."

INTRADERMAL INJECTIONS

An **intradermal** injection is usually used for skin testing to diagnose the cause of an allergy or to determine the presence of a microorganism. The choice of syringe for intradermal testing is the tuberculin syringe with a 25-gauge needle.

The inner aspect of the forearm is frequently used for diagnostic testing because there is less hair in the area and the test results will be more visible. The upper back may also be a testing site. The needle is inserted with the **bevel** upward at a 10- to 15-degree angle. Do not aspirate. Test results are read 48 to 72 h after the intradermal injection. A reddened or raised area is a positive reaction.

SUBCUTANEOUS INJECTIONS

Drugs injected into the **subcutaneous** (fatty) tissue are absorbed slowly because there are fewer blood vessels in the fatty tissue. The amount of drug solution administered subcutaneously is generally 0.5 to 1 mL at a 45-, 60-, or 90-degree angle. Drug solutions that are irritating to the fatty tissues are given intramuscularly because they can cause sloughing of the subcutaneous tissue.

The two types of syringes used for subcutaneous injections are the tuberculin syringe (1 mL), calibrated in 0.1 mL and 0.01 mL, and the 3-mL syringe, calibrated in 0.1 mL. The needle gauge commonly used is 25 or 26, and the length is ⅜ to ⅝ inch. Insulin is also administered subcutaneously and will be discussed later in this section.

CALCULATIONS: SUBCUTANEOUS INJECTIONS

To calculate dosages for subcutaneous injections use the basic formula of $D/H \times V$ or the ratio-and-proportion method (see Section 4B). Heparin is a drug frequently administered subcutaneously. It can be given at a 60- to 90-degree angle, depending on the amount of fatty tissue (see Fig. 4D–9). The skin is lifted, and the heparin solution is injected into the subcutaneous tissue. Do not aspirate, and do not massage the injected site, because massage could cause small-vessel damage and bleeding.

Units (U) should be written out as a word and not as U only. When U is written, it may appear as O and thus the client could receive a higher dose of the drug.

> **EXAMPLE:**

Order: heparin 2500 Units, SC.
Available: heparin 10,000 Units/mL in multiple-dose vial (10 mL).

Basic Formula:

$$\frac{D}{H} \times V = \frac{2500 \text{ Units}}{10000 \text{ Units}} \times 1 \text{ mL} = \frac{25}{100} = 0.25 \text{ mL}$$

Ratio-and-Proportion Method:

$$
\begin{array}{ccccccc}
H & : & V & :: & D & : & x \\
10{,}000 \text{ Units} & : & 1 \text{ mL} & :: & 2500 \text{ Units} & : & x \text{ mL}
\end{array}
$$

$$10{,}000x = 2500$$
$$x = \frac{25}{100} = 0.25 \text{ mL}$$

Answer: Heparin 2500 Units = 0.25 mL.

> ## II. PRACTICE PROBLEMS: SUBCUTANEOUS INJECTIONS

Use the formula you have chosen for calculating drug dosages from Section 4B. The same formula should be used when calculating oral, subcutaneous, intramuscular, insulin, and intravenous dosages. Refer to the conversion Table 4A–4 or 4B–1 as needed.

1. Order: heparin 4000 Units, SC
   Available:

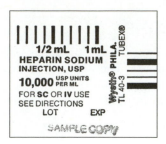

   How many mL should the client receive? _____

2. Order: heparin 7500 Units, SC
   Available:

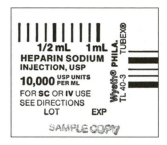

   How many mL should the client receive? _____

3. Order: atropine sulfate 0.5 mg, SC
   Available:

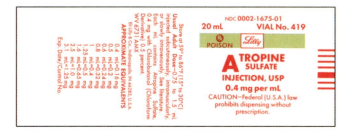

   How many mL should the client receive? _____

4. Order: epinephrine (Adrenalin) 0.2 mg, SC, STAT
   Available: epinephrine 1 mg/mL (1:1000) in ampule.
   What type of syringe would you use?

INSULIN INJECTIONS

Insulin is prescribed and measured in USP units. Today, most insulins are produced in concentrations of 100 Units/mL. Insulin should be administered with an insulin syringe, which is calibrated to correspond with the 100 Units of insulin. Insulin concentrations are also available in 40 Units and 500 Units, but these are rarely used.

Insulin bottles and syringes are color-coded to avoid error. The 100 Units/mL (or U-100) insulin bottle and the 100 Units/mL syringe are coded orange. The 40 Units/mL (or U-40) insulin bottle and the 40 Units/mL syringe are coded red. *Always* match the insulin strength with the calibrated insulin syringe; the units of the insulin bottle and syringe should match. Administering insulin with a tuberculin syringe *should be avoided.*

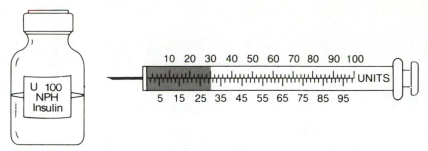

FIGURE 4D–10 Bottle of U 100 insulin and a U 100 calibrated insulin syringe. (*Source:* From Kee JL, Marshall SM: Clinical Calculations, 3rd ed. Philadelphia: WB Saunders, 1996, p 133.)

Administration of medication requires attention to detail, and insulin is no exception. Insulin is ordered in units. For example, if the prescribed insulin dosage is 30 Units, withdraw 30 Units from a bottle of 100 Units of insulin using a 100-Unit calibrated insulin syringe (Fig. 4D–10).

Insulin is administered subcutaneously at a 45-, 60-, or 90-degree angle into the subcutaneous tissue. The subcutaneous absorption rate of insulin is slower because there are fewer blood vessels in the fatty tissue than in muscular tissue. The angle for administering insulin depends upon the amount of fatty tissue. For an obese person the angle may be 90 degrees, and for a very thin person the angle may be 45 to 60 degrees.

TYPES OF INSULINS

Insulins are clear (regular or crystalline insulin) and cloudy (NPH, lente) because of the substances protamine and zinc, used to prolong the action of insulin in the body. Only clear (regular) insulin can be given intravenously as well as subcutaneously. The source of insulin is beef, pork, beef-pork, and human (Humulin). Some individuals are allergic to beef insulin, so pork insulin is used because it has biologic properties similar to those of human insulin.

Insulin is categorized as fast-acting, intermediate-acting, and long-acting. The drug labels in the following example (Fig 4D–11) are arranged according to insulin action. Chapter 41 gives the peaks and durations of action of insulins.

MIXING INSULINS

Regular insulin is frequently mixed with insulin containing protamine (NPH) and zinc (lente). The following is an example of a method for mixing insulin:

EXAMPLE:

Order: Regular insulin 10 Units and NPH insulin 35 Units, SC, q 7AM.
Available: Regular insulin 100 U/mL and NPH insulin 100 U/mL. Insulin syringe: 100 U/mL.

Method

Step 1. Clean the rubber tops of the insulin bottles.
Step 2. Draw up 35 Units of air* and inject into the NPH insulin bottle. Avoid letting the needle contact the NPH insulin solution. Withdraw the needle.
Step 3. Draw up 10 Units of air and inject into the regular insulin bottle.
Step 4. First, withdraw 10 Units of regular insulin. Regular insulin is always drawn up first.
Step 5. Insert needle into NPH bottle and withdraw 35 Units of NPH insulin. The total is 45 Units.

---

* You may draw up 45 U of air; inject 35 U into the NPH bottle and 10 U into the regular insulin bottle.

A: Fast-Acting Insulins.

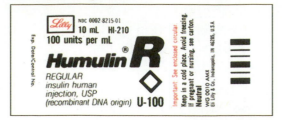
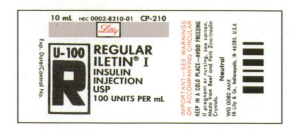

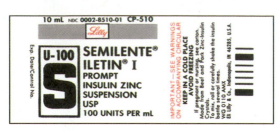

B: Intermediate-Acting Insulins.

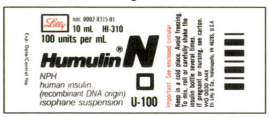
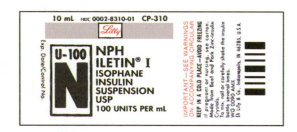

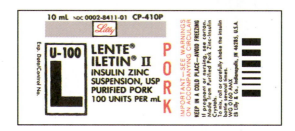

C: Long-Acting Insulins.

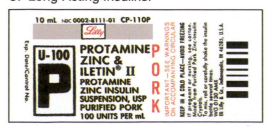
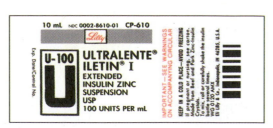

FIGURE 4D–11 Insulin types.

Step 6. Administer the two insulins immediately after mixing. Do *not* allow the insulin mixture to stand, because unpredicted physical changes may occur. Unpredicted changes are more common with protamine insulins, such as NPH and PZI, than with lente insulin.

III. PRACTICE PROBLEMS: INSULINS

Indicate on the insulin syringe the amount of insulin that should be withdrawn for each type of insulin.

1. Order: lente insulin 30 Units, SC
   Available: lente insulin 100 U/mL and insulin syringe 100 U/ml

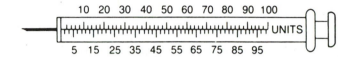

2. Order: NPH insulin 45 Units, SC
   Available: NPH insulin 100 U/mL and insulin syringe 100 U/mL

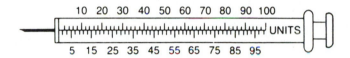

3. Order: regular insulin 15 Units and NPH insulin 25 Units, SC
   Available: regular insulin 100 U/mL and NPH insulin 100 U/mL, and insulin syringe 100 U/mL

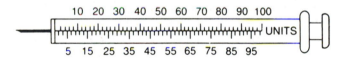

4. Order: regular insulin 6 Units and lente insulin 40 Units.
   Available: regular insulin 100 U/mL and lente insulin 100 U/mL, and insulin syringe 100 U/mL

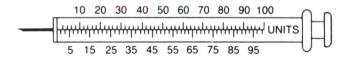

INTRAMUSCULAR INJECTIONS

Muscle has more blood vessels than the fatty tissue, so medications given by **intramuscular** (IM) injections are absorbed more rapidly than subcutaneous injections. The volume of solution for an IM injection is 0.5 to 3.0 mL, with the average being 1 to 2 mL. A volume of drug solution greater than 3 mL causes increased muscle tissue displacement and possible tissue damage. Occasionally, 5 mL of selected drugs, such as magnesium sulfate, may be injected into a large muscle, such as the dorsogluteal. A dose greater than 3 mL is usually divided and given at two different sites.

The needle gauges for intramuscular injections that contain thick solutions are 19 and 20, and for thin solutions are 20 and 21. Intramuscular injections are administered at a 90-degree angle. The needle length depends upon the amount of adipose (fat) and muscle tissues; the average needle length is 1.5 inches.

This section on intramuscular injections is divided into three subsections: (1) drug solutions for injection, (2) powdered drug reconstitution, and (3) mixing injectable drugs. An example is given for each subsection, and practice problems follow.

Sites of intramuscular injections are shown in Chapter 3.

DRUG SOLUTIONS FOR INJECTION

Commercially premixed drug solutions are stored in vials and ampules for ready use. The drug label on the container gives the drug dose by weight and its equivalent in milliliters.

EXAMPLE:

Order: gentamicin (Garamycin) 50 mg, IM.
Available: gentamicin 80 mg/2 mL in a vial.

a.
$$\frac{D}{H} \times V = \frac{50}{80} \times 2 = \frac{100}{80} = 1.25 \text{ mL}$$

b.

H	:	V	::	D	:	x
80 mg	:	2 mL	::	50 mg	:	x mL

$$80x = 100$$
$$x = \frac{100}{80} = 1.25 \text{ mL}$$

POWDERED DRUG RECONSTITUTION

Certain drugs lose their potency in liquid form; therefore, manufacturers package these drugs in powdered form. They are reconstituted using a **diluent** (bacteriostatic water or saline) prior to administration. The drug label or the instructional insert (accompanying pamphlet) frequently gives the type and amount of diluent to use. If the type and amount of diluent are not on the drug label or in the instructional insert, call the pharmacist.

Usually manufacturers determine the amount of diluent to mix with the drug powder to yield a 1 to 2 mL/dose. The powdered drug occupies space; therefore, the volume of the drug solution is increased. Once the powdered drug has been reconstituted, the unused drug solution should be dated, and initialed on the drug label. Unused drug solutions in vials are refrigerated and may be used for 48 h to 1 week according to the manufacturer's recommendation. Unused drug solutions in ampules are discarded.

EXAMPLE:

Solve the drug problem using the information on the drug label.
Order: aqueous penicillin 250,000 Units, IM, q4h.
Available: aqueous penicillin 5,000,000 Units (5 million units).
The drug is in powdered form in a vial. The drug label states:

DILUENT ADDED (mL)	UNITS/mL
18	250,000
8	500,000
3	1,000,000

Add 18 mL of diluent. The drug powder is equivalent to 2 mL. Each 250,000 Units equals 1 mL. When working the problem, add 18 mL and 2 mL (powdered drug) = 20 mL.

a.
$$\frac{D}{H} \times V = \frac{250,000}{5,000,000} \times 20 = \frac{50}{50} = 1 \text{ mL}$$

b.
H	:	V	::	D	:	x
5,000,000 Units	:	20 mL	::	250,000 Units	:	x mL

$$5,000,000x = 5,000,000$$

$$x = 1 \text{ mL}$$

MIXING INJECTABLE DRUGS

Drugs mixed together in the same syringe must be compatible to prevent precipitation. To determine drug compatibility, check drug reference texts or with a pharmacist. When in doubt about compatibility, do *not* mix drugs.

The three methods used for mixing drugs are: (1) mixing two drugs in the same syringe from two vials, (2) mixing two drugs in the same syringe from one vial and one ampule, and (3) mixing two drugs in a prefilled cartridge from a vial.

Method 1: Mixing Two Drugs in the Same Syringe from Two Vials

1. Draw air into the syringe to equal the amount of solution to be withdrawn from the first vial, and inject the air into the first vial. Do *not* allow the needle to come into contact with the solution. Remove the needle.
2. Draw air into the syringe to equal the amount of solution to be withdrawn from the second vial. Invert the second vial and inject the air. Withdraw the desired amount of solution from the second vial.
3. Change the needle, unless you will be using the entire volume in the first vial.
4. Invert the first vial, and withdraw the desired amount of solution.

Method 2: Mixing Two Drugs in the Same Syringe from One Vial and One Ampule

1. Inject air into the vial.
2. Remove the desired amount of solution from the vial.
3. Withdraw the desired amount of solution from the ampule.

Method 3: Mixing Two Drugs in a Prefilled Cartridge from a Vial

1. Check the drug dose and the amount of solution in the prefilled cartridge. If a smaller dose is needed, expel the excess solution.
2. Draw air into the cartridge to equal the amount of solution to be withdrawn from the vial. Invert the vial and inject the air.
3. Withdraw desired amount of solution from the vial. Be sure that the needle remains in the fluid, and do *not* take more solution than needed.

EXAMPLE: MIXING DRUGS IN THE SAME SYRINGE.

Order: meperidine (Demerol) 25 mg and atropine sulfate 0.4 mg, IM.
Available: meperidine in a Tubex cartridge labeled 50 mg/mL.
　　　　Atropine sulfate in a multidose vial labeled 0.4 mg/mL.
How many milliliters of each drug would you give and how are they mixed?

a. Meperidine dose

a.
$$\frac{D}{H} \times V = \frac{25}{50} \times 1 = \frac{25}{50} = 0.5 \text{ mL}$$

b.

	H	:	V	::	D	:	x
	50 mg	:	1 mL	::	25 mg	:	x mL

$$50x = 25$$
$$x = \frac{1}{2} = 0.5 \text{ mL}$$

b. Atropine dose:
   The label indicates 0.4 mg = 1 mL

Answer: Give meperidine 0.5 mL and atropine 1 mL.

PROCEDURE. Mix two drugs in the cartridge with one drug from a vial and the other drug in the prefilled cartridge.

1. Check the drug dose and volume on the prefilled cartridge.
2. Expel 0.5 mL and any excess drug solution (meperidine) from the cartridge (0.5 mL remains in the cartridge). Have another nurse witness the waste of a narcotic.
3. Draw 1 mL of air into the cartridge, and inject the air into the vial that contains the atropine.
4. Withdraw 1 mL of atropine from the vial into the meperidine solution in the cartridge.

IV. PRACTICE PROBLEMS: INTRAMUSCULAR INJECTIONS

1. Order: cefazolin (Ancef) 500 mg, IM, q6h
   Available:

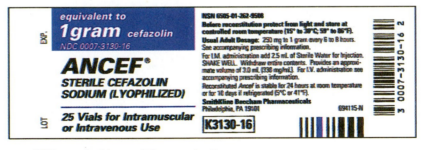

   How many milliliters (mL) would you give?

2. Order: procaine penicillin 400,000 Units, IM, q8h
   Available: procaine penicillin 300,000 Units/mL in a multiple-dose vial.
   How many milliliters (mL) of procaine penicillin would you give?

3. Order: atropine sulfate 0.3 mg, IM, STAT
   Available: atropine sulfate

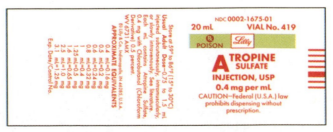

   How many milliliters (mL) of atropine would you give?

4. Order: oxacillin 250 mg, IM, q6h
   Available:

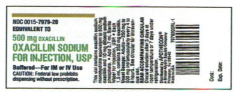

How many milliliters (mL) would you give? After the drug is reconstituted, how long can it be refrigerated?

5. Order: digoxin 0.25 mg, IM, q.d.
   Available: digoxin 0.5 mg/2 mL, in a Tubex cartridge

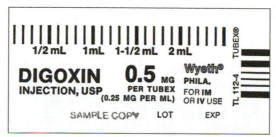

How many milliliters (mL) would you give? What should be done with the excess digoxin solution? (Usually parenteral digoxin is administered intravenously.)

6. Order: chlorpromazine (Thorazine) 50 mg, IM, STAT
   Available:

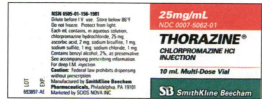

How many milliliters (mL) would you give? Can the vial be used again?

7. Order: meperidine 60 mg and hydroxyzine (Vistaril) 25 mg, IM. These two drugs are compatible.
   Available: Hydroxyzine 100 mg/2 mL in vial.

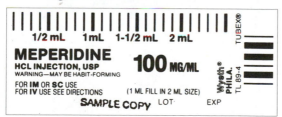

How many milliliters (mL) of meperidine and how many of hydroxyzine would you give? Explain how the two drugs would be mixed in the cartridge.

8. Order: naloxone (Narcan) 0.4 mg, IM, and repeat in 3 min if needed
   Available:

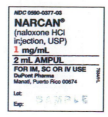

How many milliliters (mL) would you give per dose?

9. Order: clindamycin phosphate 150 mg, q6h, IM
   Available:

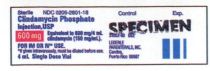 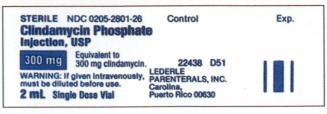

a. Which clindamycin vial would you select? _____

   Explain _____

b. How many milliliters (mL) of clindamycin would you administer per dose? _____

10. Order: ampicillin 250 mg, q6h, IM
    Available:

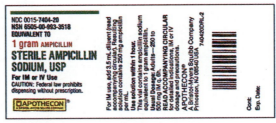

a. How many milliliters (mL) of diluent would you add to the ampicillin vial? _____

b. How many milliliters (mL) of ampicillin should the client receive per dose? _____

c. How many milligrams (mg) should the client receive per day? _____

PEDIATRIC CALCULATIONS FOR INJECTABLES

The same three methods used for calculating oral dosages for children are used for calculating injectable dosages. They include calculating from (1) body weight (kg), (2) body surface area (BSA, m^2), and (3) the adult dose. Use the nomogram for BSA. For the three methods for calculating children's dosages, see Section 4C.

V. PRACTICE PROBLEMS: PEDIATRIC INJECTABLES

Solve the following drug problems and indicate if the drug dose is within the safe parameters.

1. Order: tobramycin (Nebcin) 10 mg, IM, q8h
   Child's weight: 10 kg
   Child's drug dosage: 3 mg/kg/day in three divided doses
   Available: Nebcin

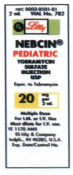

Is dose within safe parameters?

2. Order: promethazine (Phenergan) 20 mg, IM, q6h
   Child's weight: 45 kg
   Child's drug dosage: 0.25 to 0.5 mg/kg/dose, repeat every 4 to 6 h
   Available: Phenergan 25 mg/mL
   Is dose within safe parameters?

3. Order: cefamandole (Mandol) 250 mg, IM, q6h
   Child's weight: 15 kg
   Child's drug dosage: 50 to 100 mg/kg/day in three to six divided doses
   Available: Mandol

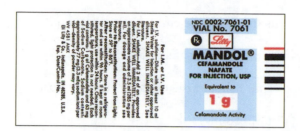

   Is dose within safe parameters?

4. Order: amikacin (Amikin) 7.5 mg/kg, q12h, IM
   Child's weight: 15 kg
   Available:

   a. How many milligrams (mg) should the child receive per dose? _____

   b. How many milliliters (mL) should the child receive per dose? _____

5. Order: ampicillin sodium 75 mg, q6h, IM
   Child's weight: 17½ pounds
   Child's drug dosage: 25 to 50 mg/kg/day
   Available:

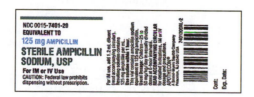

   a. How much diluent should be added? _____

   b. How many milligrams (mg) should the child receive per day? _____

   c. Is drug dosage per day within safe parameters? _____

      Explain _____

6. Order: nafcillin sodium 200 mg, q6h, IM
   Child's weight: 10 kg
   Child's drug dosage: 100 to 300 mg/kg/day in divided doses.
   Available:

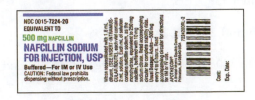

   a. How many milligrams (mg) will the child receive per day? _____

   b. Is the drug dosage per day within safe parameters? _____

   c. How many milliliters (mL) should the child receive per dose? _____

7. Order: hydroxyzine (Vistaril) 50 mg, IM
   Child's height and weight: 47 inches, 45 lb
   Child's drug dosage: 30 mg/m²
   Available: Vistaril 25 mg/mL
   Is dose within safe parameters?

8. Order: methotrexate (Mexate) 50 mg, IM, weekly
   Child's height and weight: 56 inches, 100 lb
   Child's drug dosage: 25 to 75 mg/m²/week
   Available: methotrexate 2.5 mg/mL; 25 mg/mL; 100 mg/mL.
   Is dose within safe parameters?

ANSWERS TO PRACTICE PROBLEMS

I. Practice Problems: Syringes and Needles

1. 5-mL syringe
2. Tuberculin syringe (1 mL)
3. No, it should be discarded in the sink or toilet and witnessed by another RN or LPN.
4. 21-gauge needle
5. 25-gauge needle
6. 20-gauge needle 1.5 (1½) inches in length

II. Practice Problems: Subcutaneous Injections

1. a.
$$\frac{D}{H} \times V = \frac{4000}{10,000} \times 1 = \frac{4}{10} = 0.4 \text{ mL}$$

   b.

H	:	V	::	D	:	x
10,000 Units	:	1 mL	::	4000 Units	:	x mL

$$10,000x = 4000$$
$$x = \frac{4000}{10,000} = 0.4 \text{ mL}$$

Answer: heparin 4000 Units = 0.4 mL

2. 0.75 mL
3. The drug label reads: 1.25 mL = 0.5 mg of atropine. Also, under the word *atropine*, it reads 0.4 mg/mL

a.
$$\frac{D}{H} \times V = \frac{0.5}{0.4} \times 1 = 1.25 \text{ mL}$$

b.

H	:	V	::	D	:	x
0.4 mg	:	1 mL	::	0.5 mg	:	x mL

$$0.4x = 0.5$$

$$x = \frac{0.5}{0.4} = 1.25 \text{ mL}$$

Answer: atropine sulfate 0.5 mg = 1.25 mL

4. A tuberculin syringe should be used.

$$\frac{D}{H} \times V = \frac{0.2}{1.0} \times 1 = 1.0\sqrt{0.20} = 0.2 \text{ mL}$$

H	:	V	::	D	:	x
1.0 mg	:	1 mL	::	0.2 mg	:	x mL

$$1.0x = 0.2$$

$$x = \frac{0.2}{1.0} = 0.2 \text{ mL}$$

Answer: epinephrine 0.2 mg = 0.2 mL.

III. Practice Problems: Insulins

1.

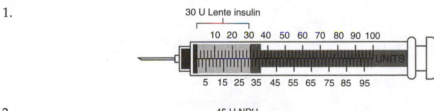

30 U Lente insulin

2.

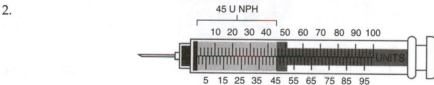

45 U NPH

3.

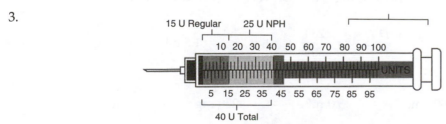

15 U Regular   25 U NPH

40 U Total

4.

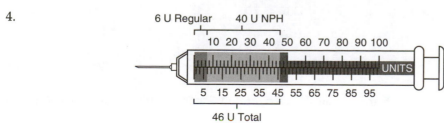

6 U Regular   40 U NPH

46 U Total

IV. Practice Problems: Intramuscular Injections

1. Instructions on the drug label read: add 2.5 mL of sterile water. The drug solution equals 3.0 mL (drug powder is equal to 0.5 mL).
   Change 1 g to mg. 1 g = 1000 mg *or*
   Change 500 mg to g. 500 mg = 0.500 g (0.5 g)

   a.
   $$\frac{D}{H} \times V = \frac{0.5}{1\,g} \times 3\;mL = 1.5\;mL$$

   b.
H	:	V	::	D	:	x
1000 mg	:	3 mL	::	500 mg	:	x mL

   $$1000x = 1500$$

   $$x = 1.5\;mL$$

Answer: cefazolin 500 mg = 1.5 mL

2. 1.3 mL of procaine penicillin

3. The atropine drug label is marked as 0.4 mg/mL. The approximate equivalent of 0.3 mg is 0.8 mL as marked on the label. If the 0.3 mg = 0.8 mL is unknown, the problem may be calculated using 0.4 mg = 1 mL.

   a.
   $$\frac{D}{H} \times V = \frac{0.3}{0.4} \times 1 = \frac{0.3}{0.4} = 0.75,\;or\;0.8\;mL$$

   b.
H	:	V	::	D	:	x
0.4 mg	:	1 mL	::	0.3 mg	:	x mL

   $$0.4x = 0.3$$

   $$x = \frac{0.3}{0.4} = 0.75,\;or\;0.8\;mL$$

4. For oxacillin sodium, the drug label indicates that 2.7 mL of sterile water should be added to the vial containing 500 mg of drug. The total volume would be 3.0 mL.

   a.
   $$\frac{D}{H} \times V = \frac{250}{500} \times 3.0 = \frac{750}{500} = 1.5\;mL$$

   b.
H	:	V	::	D	:	x
500 mg	:	3.0 mL	::	250 mg	:	x mL

   $$500x = 750$$

   $$x = \frac{750}{500} = 1.5\;mL$$

Answer: Oxacillin 250 mg = 1.5 mL. It can be refrigerated for 96 h after it has been reconstituted.

5. a.
$$\frac{D}{H} \times V = \frac{0.25}{0.50} \times 2 = \frac{0.50}{0.50} = 1 \text{ mL}$$

b.

H	:	V	::	D	:	x
0.5 mg	:	2 mL	::	0.25 mg	:	x mL

$$0.5x = 0.5$$

$$x = 1 \text{ mL}$$

Expel 1 mL of digoxin solution from the Tubex cartridge before administering 1 mL.

6. Thorazine 50 mg = 2 mL. Yes, the vial can be used for multiple doses.
7. Meperidine 60 mg = 0.6 mL; hydroxyzine 25 mg = 0.5 mL
   Meperidine

a.
$$\frac{D}{H} \times V = \frac{60}{100} \times 1 = \frac{60}{100} = 0.6 \text{ mL}$$

b.

H	:	V	::	D	:	x
100 mg	:	1 mL	::	60 mg	:	x mL

$$100x = 60$$

$$x = 0.6 \text{ mL}$$

Hydroxyzine

a.
$$\frac{D}{H} \times V = \frac{25}{100} \times 2 = \frac{50}{100} = 0.5 \text{ mL}$$

b.

H	:	V	::	D	:	x
100 mg	:	2 mL	::	25 mg	:	x mL

$$100x = 50$$

$$x = 0.5 \text{ mL}$$

PROCEDURE
1. Check the meperidine dose and volume in the prefilled cartridge.
2. Expel any excess solution from the prefilled cartridge; 0.6 mL of solution should remain.
3. Draw 0.5 mL of air into cartridge and inject into the vial.
4. Withdraw 0.5 mL of hydroxyzine from the vial into the cartridge.
5. Total volume for the injection: meperidine and hydroxyzine = 1.1 mL

8. Narcan 0.4 mg = 0.4 mL (1 mg = 1 mL). The ampule contains 2 mL of Narcan (2 mg = 2 mL).
9. a. Select 300 mg = 2 mL vial of clindamycin (either 300 mg or 600 mg vial could be used). Why? Less than 300 mg (150 mg) per dose is ordered.
   b. 1.0 mL from the 300 mg vial or 1.0 mL from the 600 mg vial (600 mg = 4 mL per label).
10. a. 3.5 mL of diluent (3.5 mL diluent + 0.5 mL of powdered drug = 4 mL of 1 g of ampicillin).
    b. 1 mL = 250 mg (1 g or 1000 mg = 4 mL)
    c. 250 mg × 4 (q6h) = 1000 mg or 1 g/d

V. Practice Problems: Pediatric Injectables

1. Tobramycin parameter: 3 mg/kg/day × 10 kg = 30 mg/day in three divided doses.
   Drug order: 10 mg × 3 (q8h) = 30 mg/day
   Dosage is within safe parameters. 10 mg = 1 mL/dose
2. Phenergan parameters: 0.25 mg/kg/dose × 45 kg = 11.25 mg/dose
   0.50 mg/kg/dose × 45 kg = 22.5 mg/dose
   Drug order: Phenergan 20 mg, IM per dose
   Dosage is within safe parameters.

$$\frac{D}{H} \times V = \frac{20}{25} \times 1 = 0.8 \text{ mL}$$

Phenergan 20 mg = 0.8 mL

3. Cefamandole parameters: 50 mg/kg/day × 15 kg = 750 mg/day
   100 mg/kg/day × 15 kg = 1500 mg/day
   Drug order: cefamandole   250 mg × 4 doses = 1000 mg/day
   Dosage is within safe parameters.

$$\frac{D}{H} \times V = \frac{250}{1000} \times 3.5 \text{ mL} = \frac{895}{1000} = 0.89, \text{ or } 0.9 \text{ mL}$$

The drug label states to add 3.0 mL of diluent, equaling 3.5 mL.
Convert 1 g to 1000 mg.

4. a. 7.5 mg × 15 kg = 112.5 mg per dose

   b. $$\frac{D}{H} \times V = \frac{112.5 \text{ mg}}{500 \text{ mg}} \times 2 \text{ mL} = \frac{225}{500} = 0.45 \text{ mL or } 0.5 \text{ mL}$$

or

H	:	V	::	D	:	x
500 mg	:	2 mL	::	112.5 mg	:	x

$$500x = 225$$

$$x = \frac{225}{500} = 0.45 \text{ mL or } 0.5 \text{ mL}$$

5. Child weighs 8 kg (17.5 lbs ÷ 2.2 = 8 kg)
   a. 1.2 mL of diluent (see label)
   b. 75 mg × 4 (q6h) = 300 mg/d
   c. Dose per day is within safe parameters
      25 mg × 8 kg = 200 mg
      50 mg × 8 kg = 400 mg (200 to 400 mg/d)
6. a. 200 mg × 4 (q6h) = 800 mg/d
   b. Dose per day is safe but not in therapeutic range. Notify health care provider.
      100 mg × 10 kg = 1000 mg
      300 mg × 10 kg = 3000 mg
   c. Add 1.8 ml diluent = 2 mL (500 mg = 2 mL)

$$\frac{D}{H} \times V = \frac{200 \text{ mg}}{500 \text{ mg}} \times 2 \text{ mL} = \frac{400}{500} = 0.8 \text{ mL}$$

Answer: nafcillin 200 mg = 0.8 mL

7. Height and weight intersect at 0.82 m^2.

     Hydroxyzine parameter: 30 mg/m^2 × 0.82 m^2 = 24.6 mg, or 25 mg

     Drug order: hydroxyzine 50 mg, IM

     Dosage ordered is *not* within safe parameters. Dosage exceeds the drug parameters. *Do not* give the medication. Notify the health care provider.

8. Height and weight intersect at 1.38 m^2.

     Methotrexate parameters: 25 mg/m^2/week × 1.38 m^2 = 34.5 mg/week

     75 mg/m^2/week × 1.38 m^2 = 103.5 mg/week

     Drug order: methotrexate 59 mg/week, IM

     Dosage is within safe parameters.

     (1) If methotrexate 25 mg/mL is used, give 2 mL (50 mg) or

     (2) If methotrexate 100 mg/mL is used, give 0.5 mL. Because of the amount of solution, it may be more desirable to give 0.5 mL of the 100 mg/mL solution.

SECTION D

Chapter 4

Calculations of Intravenous Fluids

OUTLINE

Objectives
Terms
Introduction
Continuous Intravenous
  Administration
    Intravenous Sets
    Calculating Intravenous
      Flow Rate

Mixing Drugs for Continu-
  ous Intravenous Admin-
  istration
Intermittent Intravenous
  Administration
    Secondary Intravenous Sets
      Without Controllers

Electronic Intravenous
  Regulators
Patient-Controlled
  Analgesic
Calculating Flow Rates for
  Intravenous Drugs
Critical Care Drug
  Calculation

OBJECTIVES

Describe the differences between continuous IV infusion and intermittent IV infusion.

Define macrodrip and microdrip sets, KVO, and TKO.

Calculate IV flow rate by using one of the given formulas.

Explain how IV drug solutions administered by secondary set are calculated.

Differentiate between volumetric and nonvolumetric IV regulators, and controllers and pump electronic regulators.

TERMS

bolus
drop factor
electronic IV regulators
IVPB
KVO

macrodrip set
microdrip set
nonvolumetric regulator
PCA
primary IV sets

SASH procedure
secondary IV sets
TKO
volumetric regulator

INTRODUCTION

Intravenous (IV) fluid therapy is used for administering fluids containing water, dextrose, vitamins, electrolytes, and drugs. Today there are an increasing number of drugs administered by the intravenous route for direct absorption and fast action. Some drugs are given by IV push **(bolus).** Many of the drugs administered intravenously are irritating to the veins, so these drugs are diluted in 50 to 100 mL of fluid. Other drugs are delivered in a large volume of fluid over a period, such as 4 to 8 h.

There are two methods used to administer IV fluids and drugs: continuous IV infusion and intermittent IV infusion. Continuous IV administration replaces fluid loss, maintains fluid balance, and is a vehicle for drug administration. Intermittent IV administration is primarily used for giving IV drugs.

Nurses have an important role in the preparation and administration of intravenous solutions and IV drugs. The nursing functions and responsibilities during drug preparation include:

1. Knowledge of intravenous sets and their drop factors
2. Calculating IV flow rates
3. Mixing and diluting drugs in IV fluids
4. Gathering equipment
5. Knowledge of the drugs and the expected and untoward reactions

Nursing responsibilities continue with assessment of the client for effectiveness and untoward effects of the therapy and assessment of the IV site.

CONTINUOUS INTRAVENOUS ADMINISTRATION

When IV solutions are required, the health care provider orders the type and amount of IV solution in liters over a 24-h period or in milliliters per hour. The nurse calculates the IV flow rate according to the drop factor, the amount of fluids to be administered, and the time period.

INTRAVENOUS SETS

There are various IV infusion sets marketed by Abbott, Cutter, McGaw, and Travenol. The **drop factor,** the number of drops per milliliter, is normally printed on the packaging cover of the IV set. Sets that deliver large drops per milliliter (10 to 20 gtt/mL) are referred to as **macrodrip sets,** and those with small drops per milliliter (60 gtt/mL) are called **microdrip,** or **minidrip, sets.** Examples of drop factors, macrodrip sets, and microdrip sets are listed in Table 4E–1.

In most instances, the nurse has the choice of using either the macrodrip or microdrip set. If the IV rate is to infuse at 100 mL/h or more, the macrodrip set is usually used. If the infusion rate is less than (<) 100 mL/h, or with pediatric client the microdrip set is preferred. Slow drip rates of <100 mL/h make macrodrip adjustment difficult.

At times, intravenous fluids are given at a slow rate to **keep vein open (KVO),** also called **to keep open (TKO).** The reasons for ordering KVO include a suspected or potential emer-

TABLE 4E–1 Intravenous Sets

Manufacturer	Drops (GTT/ML)
Macrodrip Sets	
Abbott	15
Cutter	20
McGraw	15
Travenol	10
Microdrip Sets	
Travenol	60
Minidrip sets	

gency situation for rapid administration of fluids and drugs and the need for an open line to give IV drugs at specified hours. For KVO, a microdrip set (60 gtt/mL) and a 250-mL IV bag may be used. KVO is usually regulated to deliver 10 mL/h.

CALCULATING INTRAVENOUS FLOW RATE

Three different methods may be used to calculate IV flow rate (drops per minute, gtt/min). The nurse should select one method, memorize it, and consistently use it to calculate IV flow rate.

Method I: Three-Step

1. $\dfrac{\text{Amount of solution}}{\text{Hours to administer}} = \text{milliliters/hour (mL/h)}$

2. $\dfrac{\text{Milliliters per hour}}{60 \text{ minutes}} = \text{milliliters/minute (mL/min)}$

3. Milliliters per minute × drops per milliliter of IV set = drops/minute (gtt/min)

Method II: Two-Step*

1. $\dfrac{\text{Amount of fluid}}{\text{Hours to administer}} = \text{milliliters/hour (mL/h)}$

2. $\dfrac{\text{Milliliters per hour} \times \text{Drops per milliliter (IV set)}}{60 \text{ minutes}} = \text{drops/minute (gtt/min)}$

If the milliliters per hour is known, then use step 2 to determine the drops per minute.

Method III: One-Step

$\dfrac{\text{Amount of fluid} \times \text{Drops per milliliter (IV set)}}{\text{Hours to administer} \times \text{Minutes per hour (60)}} = \text{drops/minute (gtt/min)}$

MIXING DRUGS FOR CONTINUOUS INTRAVENOUS ADMINISTRATION

Drugs such as potassium chloride and vitamins are frequently added to the IV solution bag for continuous IV infusion. Drugs should be added to the bag or bottle immediately before administering the intravenous fluid. Inject the drug into the rubber stopper on the IV bag or bottle and rotate the bag several times to ensure that the drug is dispersed throughout the solution (Fig. 4E–1). *Do not add the drug while the infusion is running unless the bag is rotated.* A drug solution injected into an upright infusing IV solution concentrates the drug into the lower portion of the IV bag, preventing it from being evenly dispersed. The client receives a concentrated drug solution, which may be harmful, for example, if the drug is potassium chloride. If drugs are injected into the IV bag prior to use, the bag should be refrigerated to maintain drug potency.

There are various nutrients (e.g., dextrose) and electrolytes in commercially prepared intravenous solutions. The commonly used solutions are 5% dextrose in water (D_5W), normal saline (NSS), one-half normal saline (½ NSS), and lactated Ringer's. These types of solutions are abbreviated as listed in Table 4E–2.

---

* The two-step method is the most popular method for IV calculation of the flow rate.

SECTION E

FIGURE 4E–1 Intravenous bag. (*Source:* From Kee JL, Marshall SM: Clinical Calculations, 3rd ed. Philadelphia: WB Saunders, 1996, p 166.)

IV bag

EXAMPLE:

Order: 1000 mL of 5% dextrose in water (D_5W) with potassium chloride (KCl) 20 mEq in 8h.
Available: 1000 mL of 5% dextrose in water.
  Potassium chloride 40 mEq/20 mL ampule
  IV set labeled 10 gtt/mL
Drug calculation: Using the basic formula and the ratio-and-proportion method

a.
$$\frac{D}{H} \times V = \frac{20}{40} \times 20 = \frac{400}{40} = 10 \text{ mL of KCl}$$

b.
$$
\begin{array}{ccccccc}
H & : & V & :: & D & : & x \\
40 \text{ mEq} & : & 20 \text{ mL} & :: & 20 \text{ mEq} & : & x \text{ mL}
\end{array}
$$

$$40x = 400$$
$$x = 10 \text{ mL of KCl}$$

TABLE 4E–2 Abbreviations of Solutions

Intravenous Solutions	Abbreviations
5% Dextrose in water	D_5W, 5% D/W
10% Dextrose in water	$D_{10}W$, 10% D/W
0.9% Sodium chloride, normal saline solution	0.9% NaCl, NSS
0.45% Sodium chloride, ½ normal saline solution	0.45% NaCl, ½ NSS
5% Dextrose in 0.9% sodium chloride	D_5NSS, 5% D/NSS, 5% D/0.9% NaCl
5% Dextrose in 0.45% sodium chloride,	D_5/½ NSS, 5% D/½ NSS
	5% Dextrose in ½ normal saline solution
Lactated Ringer's solution	LR

The calculation of IV flow rate will be described using the three methods outlined previously. However, it is strongly recommended that you select one method for determining IV flow rate.

Method I

1. $\dfrac{1000 \text{ mL}}{8 \text{ h}} = 125 \text{ mL/h}$

2. $\dfrac{125 \text{ mL}}{60 \text{ min}} = 2.0\text{–}2.1 \text{ mL/min}$

3. $2.1 \times 10 = 21 \text{ gtt/min}$

Method II

1. $1000 \div 8 = 125 \text{ mL/h}$

2. $\dfrac{125 \text{ mL/h} \times \overset{1}{\cancel{10}} \text{ gtt/mL}}{\underset{6}{\cancel{60}} \text{ min}} = \dfrac{125}{6} = 20\text{–}21 \text{ gtt/min}$

Method III

$\dfrac{1000 \text{ mL} \times \overset{1}{\cancel{10}} \text{ gtt/mL}}{8 \text{ h} \times \underset{6}{\cancel{60}} \text{ min}} = \dfrac{1000}{48} = 21 \text{ gtt/min}$

I. PRACTICE PROBLEMS: INTRAVENOUS FLOW RATES

Select one of the three methods for calculating IV flow rate.

1. Order: 1000 mL of $D_5/\frac{1}{2}$ NSS to infuse over 12 h
   Available: macrodrip set with 10 gtt/mL and a microdrip set with 60 gtt/mL.

   a. Would you use a macrodrip or microdrip IV set?

   b. Calculate the IV flow rate in drops per minute according to the IV set that you selected.

2. Order: 3 L of IV solutions to infuse over 24 h
   1 L of D_5W and 2 L of $D_5/\frac{1}{2}$ NSS

   a. One liter is equal to how many milliliters?

   b. Each liter should infuse for how many hours?

   c. The institution uses a set with a drop factor of 15 gtt/mL. How many drops per minute should the client receive?

3. Order: 250 mL of D_5W to keep vein open (KVO)

   a. What type of IV set would you use?
      Why?

   b. Determine how many drops per minute the client should receive.

4. Order: 1000 mL of $D_5/\frac{1}{2}$ NSS, 1 vial of MVI (multiple vitamin), and 10 mEq of KCL (potassium chloride) in 10 h
Available: 1000 mL of $D_5/\frac{1}{2}$ NSS
Macrodrip set: 15 gtt/mL; microdrip set: 60 gtt/mL
MVI: 5 mL vial
KCl: 20 mEq/20 mL vial

   a. How many milliliters of KCl should be injected into the IV bag?

   b. How many drops per minute should the client receive using the macrodrip set and microdrip set?

5. A liter (1000 mL) of IV fluid was started at 9 AM and was to infuse for 8 h. The IV set delivers 10 gtt/mL. Four hours later only 400 mL were absorbed.

   a. How much IV fluid is left?

   b. Recalculate the flow rate for the remaining IV fluids.

INTERMITTENT INTRAVENOUS ADMINISTRATION

Some IV drugs are prescribed to be administered three to six times a day in a small volume of IV fluid (50 to 100 mL of D_5W or normal saline solution [NSS: 0.9% sodium chloride]). The drug solution is usually infused over a period of 15 min to 1 h. Separate tubing for IV drugs, the secondary line, is inserted into a port (rubber stopper) of the IV connector on the continuous, or **primary, IV line.** This type of IV administration is called intermittent IV therapy.

SECONDARY INTRAVENOUS SETS WITHOUT CONTROLLERS

Two IV sets available for administering IV drugs are (1) the calibrated cylinder (chamber) with tubing, such as the Buretrol, Volutrol, and Soluset, and (2) the secondary set, which is similar to a regular IV set except that the tubing is shorter (Fig. 4E–2). The **secondary set** is used mostly for infusing small volumes—50, 100, 250 mL. The chamber of the Buretrol, Volutrol, and Soluset holds 150 mL of solution. Medication is injected into the chamber, then diluted with solution. These methods of administering IV drugs are referred to as **IV piggyback (IVPB).**

Drugs for IV infusion are diluted prior to infusion. Clinical agencies frequently have their own protocols for dilutions; the pharmacist and the drug circular are also resources for infusion guidelines. Guidelines and protocols help in preventing drug and fluid incompatibility.

When using the Buretrol, 15 to 30 mL of IV solution should be added to flush the drug out of the IV line once the infusion is completed.

When continuous IV fluid infusion is to be discontinued and intermittent drug therapy is to begin, an adapter is attached to the IV catheter or needle where the IV tubing was disconnected. Adapters have ports (stoppers) where needles or IV tubing can be inserted as needed to continue drug therapy. The use of adapters increases the client's mobility by not having an IV line "tagging along," and is cost-effective because less IV tubing, solution, and equipment are needed.

The adapter may have short tubing, which is called the heparin lock. IV catheters and needles with adapters are kept free of blood clots by administering low doses of heparin after each drug infusion. In some institutions this is known as the **SASH procedure.** SASH stands for:

S = Solution (saline) flush (2 mL)
A = Administer drug into rubber stopper
S = Solution (saline) flush (2 mL)
H = Heparin 1:100 solution (1 mL)

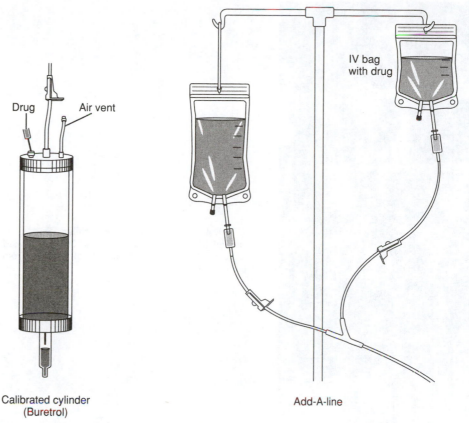

FIGURE 4E–2 Secondary intravenous sets. (*Source:* From Kee JL, Marshall SM: Clinical Calculations, 3rd ed. Philadelphia: WB Saunders, 1996, p 172.)

Before any drug is given, the IV tubing and adapter are flushed with 2 mL of saline solution for the purpose of clearing the line of heparin solution and assessing for IV patency. After the drug is administered, a 2-mL saline flush is given, followed by a low dose of heparin.

ELECTRONIC INTRAVENOUS REGULATORS

Controllers and pumps are the two basic types of **electronic intravenous regulators** used in hospitals and some community settings. The electronic IV regulators are set to deliver a prescribed rate of intravenous solution. If the flow rate is obstructed, an alarm sounds.

Controllers operate by the pressure that gravity exerts on the fluid in the IV bag. A drop sensor is attached to the drip chamber to monitor the flow rate. The controller is the metal box through which the IV tubing is fed. It is set by the nurse for a flow rate in milliliters per hour, and the rate is displayed on the front panel of the controller. Since the controllers work by gravity, the IV solution bag should be at least 36 inches above the controller. Controllers are sensitive to any restrictions, such as infiltration or obstruction when a client is lying on the tubing. An alarm sounds when the set rate cannot be maintained.

IV pumps look like controllers, but they deliver intravenous solution against resistance. The flow rate is set in milliliters per hour. Pumps do not recognize infiltration. The alarm does not sound until the pump has exerted its maximum pressure to overcome resistance.

IV pumps are recommended for use with all central lines, such as femoral and subclavian sites. Controllers are used for peripheral lines, especially if fluid overload is a concern. Ongoing nursing assessment is essential whatever type of electronic IV regulator is used.

There are two types of flow control for electronic regulators, the volumetric and nonvolumetric regulators. The **volumetric regulators** deliver a specific volume of fluid at a specific rate, in milliliters per hour. The **nonvolumetric regulators** are designed to infuse at a drop

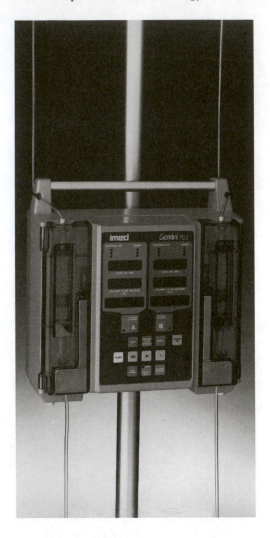

FIGURE 4E–3 IV pump and controller. (*Source:* From Kee JL, Marshall SM: Clinical Calculations, 3rd ed. Philadelphia: WB Saunders, 1996, p 174. Courtesy of IMED Corporation, San Diego, CA.)

rate in drops per minute. To determine if the machine is volumetric or nonvolumetric, check to see if the panel display is calibrated for mL/hr or gtt/min. Figure 4E–3 shows a combination IV controller and pump regulator.

PATIENT-CONTROLLED ANALGESIA

Patient-controlled analgesia (PCA) is another method of administering drugs intravenously. The objective of PCA is to provide a uniform serum concentration of drug(s), thus avoiding drug peaks and valleys. This method is designed to meet the needs of those clients who require at least 24 to 48 h of regular intramuscular narcotic injections.

Several reasons for the use of PCA include (1) effective pain control without feeling oversedated, (2) considerable reduction in the amount of narcotic used (approximately one-half that of intramuscular delivery), and (3) clients' feelings of greater control over their pain.

There are choices available in the delivery of PCA. The pump is programmed to administer the prescribed medication (1) at client demand, (2) continuously, and (3) continuously and supplemented by client demand.

The health care provider's order must include:

1. Drug ordered
2. Loading dose: administered by the health care provider to obtain baseline serum concentration of analgesic
3. PCA dose: amount to be administered each time client activates the button
4. Lockout interval: time during which PCA cannot be administered
5. Dose limit: the maximum amount the client can receive during a specified time

Client Teaching

- Inform the client that the pain should be tolerable, not necessarily absent.
- Advise the client of the pump's safety features, including the alarms.
- Instruct the client in use of control button (medication administered when button is *released*).
- Instruct the client to report any side effects or adverse reactions to the medication.
- Have naloxone (Narcan) easily accessible.

CALCULATING FLOW RATES FOR INTRAVENOUS DRUGS

Intravenous drug infusion rates depend upon the drug dosing instructions, which indicate the amount of solution for dilution, and the length of infusion time. The nurse must first calculate the drug dose from the health care provider's order, then calculate the flow rate.

1. *Secondary Sets:* To find drops per minute for IV drugs use calibrated cylinders (Buretrol, Volutrol), 50- to 250-mL bag (Add-A-Line), or any nonvolumetric regulator.

$$\frac{\text{Amount of solution} \times \text{Drops per milliliter of the set}}{\text{Minutes to administer}} = \text{Drops/minute (gtt/min)}$$

2. *Volumetric Regulators:* To find milliliters per hour

$$\text{Amount of solution} \div \frac{\text{Minutes to administer}}{60 \text{ minutes/hour}} = \text{Milliliters/hour (mL/h)}$$

Problems for calculating IV drug dosage and IV flow rate in drops per minute and in milliliters per hour are given below.

EXAMPLE I:

Order: cephapirin (Cefadyl) 1.5 g, IV, q6h
Available: Cefadyl

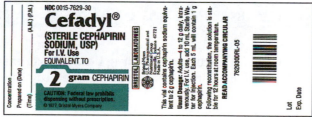

Set and solution: Cylinder set with drop factor of 60 gtt/mL; 500 mL of D_5W.
Instruction: Dilute cephapirin 1.5 g in 100 mL of D_5W and infuse over 30 min.

1. Calculate drug dosage according to drug label.
2. Calculate drops per minute for drug solution.
3. Calculate milliliters per hour using volumetric pump rate.

ANSWER:

1. Drug Calculation:
Drug label states to add 10 mL of sterile water (2 g = 10 mL)

a. $$\frac{D}{H} \times V = \frac{1.5\,\text{g}}{2.0\,\text{g}} \times 10\,\text{mL} = \frac{15}{2} = 7.5\,\text{mL of cephapirin}$$

b.

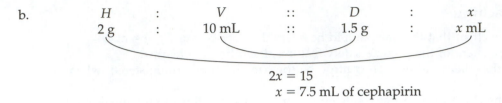

$$2x = 15$$
$$x = 7.5 \text{ mL of cephapirin}$$

2. IV Flow Calculation (Secondary Set):

$$\frac{\text{Amount of Solution} \times \text{Drops per milliliter (set)}}{\text{Minutes to administer}} = \frac{100 \text{ mL} \times \overset{2}{\cancel{60}} \text{gtt}}{\underset{1}{\cancel{30}} \text{min}} = 200 \text{ gtt/min}$$

Inject 7.5 mL of cephapirin in 100 mL of D_5W in the cylinder chamber.

Regulate IV flow rate to 200 gtt/min. It may be impossible to count 200 gtt/min. Instead of using the cylinder chamber, the nurse may use a secondary set that has a larger drop factor or a regulator. If the cylinder set is the only available secondary IV set, then the 200 gtt/min may be approximated.

3. Volumetric Pump Rate:

$$\text{Amount of Solution} \div \frac{\text{Minutes to administer}}{60 \text{ minutes per hour}} = 100 \text{ mL} + 7.5 \text{ mL (drug)} \div \frac{30 \text{ min}}{60 \text{ min}}$$

$$= 107.5 \text{ mL} \times \frac{\overset{2}{\cancel{60}}}{\underset{1}{\cancel{30}}} = 215 \text{ mL/h}$$

Set volumetric rate at 215 mL/h to deliver drug in 30 min.

II. PRACTICE PROBLEMS: INTERMITTENT INTRAVENOUS SET

Solve the IV drug problems by: (1) calculating the drug dosage according to the drug label or information given, and (2) calculating drops per minute for the drug solution.

1. Order: Clindamycin 450 mg, IV, q6h
   Available:

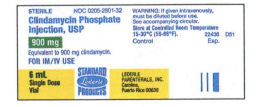

   Set and solution: Cylinder set with a drop factor of 60 gtt/mL; 500 mL D_5W
   Instruction: Dilute the drug in 75 mL of D_5W and infuse over 30 min.

2. Order: cefamandole (Mandol) 500 mg, IV, q6h
   Available: cefamandole (Mandol) is in powdered form in a vial.

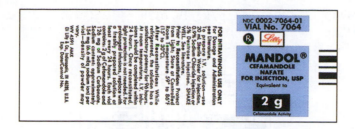

For reconstitution: Add 6.6 mL of diluent = 8 mL of drug solution (2 g = 8 mL)
Set and solution: Secondary set with 100 mL D$_5$W. Drop factor is 15 gtt/mL.
Instruction: Dilute in 100 mL of D$_5$W and infuse over 30 min.

3. Order: tobramycin (Nebcin) 50 mg, IV, q8h
   Drug parameters: 3 mg/kg/day in three divided doses. Client weighs 65 kg.
   Available: Nebcin

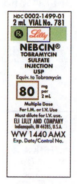

Set and solution: Cylinder IV set with drop factor of 60 gtt/mL; 500 mL D$_5$W
Instruction: Dilute tobramycin in 100 mL of D$_5$W and infuse over 40 min.
Is the tobramycin dose within safe parameters? Explain.

4. Order: piperacillin (Pipracil) 2.0 g, IV, q6h
   Available: piperacillin 4 g vial in powdered form. Add 7.8 mL of diluent to yield 10 mL of
   drug solution (4 g = 10 mL).
   Set and solution: Cylinder IV set with drop factor of 60 gtt/mL; 500 mL D$_5$W
   Instruction: Dilute piperacillin in 100 mL of D$_5$W and infuse over 45 min.
   Determine the volumetric pump rate for this problem in addition to the drug and IV flow
   calculations.

5. Order: ampicillin 500 mg, IV, q6h
   Available: Add 4.5 mL of diluent = 5 mL (2 g = 5 mL).

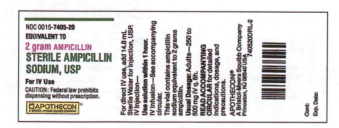

Convert grams to milligrams.
Set and solution: Cylinder set with drop factor of 60 gtt/mL; 500 mL of D$_5$W
Instruction: Dilute ampicillin in 50 mL of D$_5$W and infuse over 15 min.
Determine the volumetric pump rate for this problem in addition to the drug and IV flow
calculations.

SECTION E

6. Order: amikacin SO_4 (Amikin) 7.5 mg/kg, IV, q12h.
   Client weighs 66 kg.
   Available:

   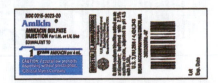

   a. How many milligrams (mg) should the client receive per dose? _____

   b. How many mL should be given per dose? _____

   Set and solution: Cylinder IV set with drop factor of 60 gtt/mL; 500 mL D_5W.
   Instruction: Dilute amikacin in 100 mL of D_5W and infuse over 45 min.

7. Order: digoxin 400 μg (0.40 mg), IV b.i.d. × 1 day.
   Drug parameter: 10 to 15 μg/kg/day (1 mg) in divided doses
   Client's weight: 75 kg
   Available:

   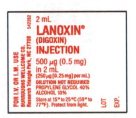

   Instruction: Administer digoxin diluted in 4 mL of D_5W or 0.9% saline solution (NaCl) by direct intravenous injection over 5 or more minutes.

   a. Is the drug dose within safe parameter? _____

   b. How many milliliters (mL) of drug should the client receive per dose? _____

8. Order: diltiazem (Cardizem) 0.25 mg/kg, IV bolus (direct intravenous) over 2 min.
   Client's weight: 178 pounds
   Available:

   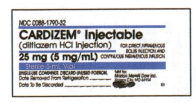
   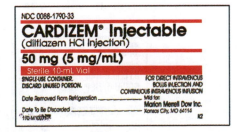

   a. Which Cardizem vial would you choose? _____

   Why? _____

   b. How many milligrams (mg) should the client receive? _____.

   c. How many milliliters (mL) should be given direct IV? _____.

ANSWERS TO PRACTICE PROBLEMS

I. Practice Problems: Continuous Intravenous Flow Rate

1. a. Microdrip set since the client is to receive 83 mL/h
   b. Two-step method: for continuous IV flow rate

   Step 1. $\dfrac{1000}{12} = 83$ mL/h

   Step 2. $\dfrac{83 \text{ mL/h} \times \overset{1}{\cancel{60}} \text{ drops}}{\underset{1}{\cancel{60}} \text{ minutes}} = 83$ gtt/min

2. a. 1000 mL
   b. 8 h

   c. Step 1. $\dfrac{1000}{8} = 125$ mL/h

   Step 2. $\dfrac{125 \text{ mL/h} \times \overset{1}{\cancel{15}} \text{ gtt}}{\underset{4}{\cancel{60}} \text{ minutes}} = \dfrac{125}{4} = 31$ gtt/min

3. a. Microdrip set

   b. Step 1. $\dfrac{250}{24} = 10$ mL/h

   Step 2. $\dfrac{10 \text{ mL/h} \times \overset{1}{\cancel{60}} \text{ gtt}}{\underset{1}{\cancel{60}} \text{ minutes}} = 10$ gtt/min

4. a. $\dfrac{D}{H} \times V = \dfrac{10}{20} \times 20 = \dfrac{200}{20} = 10$ mL KCl

   b. $\dfrac{1000}{10} = 100$ mL

   Macrodrip set $\qquad \dfrac{100 \times \overset{1}{\cancel{15}}}{\underset{4}{\cancel{60}} \text{ min}} = 25$ gtt/min

   Microdrip set $\qquad \dfrac{100 \times \overset{1}{\cancel{60}}}{\underset{1}{\cancel{60}} \text{ min}} = 100$ gtt/min

5. a. 600 mL
   b. Step 1. $\dfrac{600}{4} = 150$ mL/h

   Step 2. $\dfrac{150 \text{ mL/h} \times \overset{1}{\cancel{10}}}{\underset{6}{\cancel{60}} \text{ minutes}} = 25$ gtt/min

II. Practice Problems: Intermittent Intravenous Set

1. Use the One-Step for Intermittent IV Flow Rate
    Drug calculation:

$$\frac{D}{H} \times V = \frac{450 \text{ mg}}{900 \text{ mg}} \times 6 = \frac{2700}{900} = 3 \text{ mL of clindamycin}$$

Flow calculation:

$$\frac{75 \text{ mL} \times 60 \text{ (set)}}{30 \text{ minutes}} = \frac{4500}{30} = 150 \text{ gtt/min} \qquad \textbf{or}$$

$$\frac{3 \text{ mL} + 75 \text{ mL} \times \overset{2}{\cancel{60}}}{\underset{1}{\cancel{30}}} = 78 \times 2 = 156 \text{ gtt/min}$$

2. Drug calculation: Change 2 g to milligrams.
    2 g = 2.000 mg

$$\frac{D}{H} \times V = \frac{500}{2000} \times 8 \text{ mL} = \frac{4000}{2000} = 2 \text{ mL Mandol}$$

Flow calculation:

$$\frac{100 \text{ mL} \times \overset{1}{\cancel{15}} \text{ gtt (set)}}{\underset{2}{\cancel{30} \text{ minutes}}} = \frac{100}{2} = 50 \text{ gtt/min}$$

3. Drug calculation:

$$\frac{D}{H} \times V = \frac{50}{80} \times 2 = \frac{100}{80} = 1.25 \text{ mL of tobramycin}$$

Flow calculation:

$$\frac{100 \text{ mL} \times \overset{3}{\cancel{60}} \text{ gtt (set)}}{\underset{2}{\cancel{40} \text{ minutes}}} = \frac{300}{2} = 150 \text{ gtt/min}$$

Drug parameter: It is within safe parameters (3 kg × 65 = 195 mg/day).
Client is receiving 50 mg × 3 = 150 mg/day.

4. Drug calculation:

$$\frac{D}{H} \times V = \frac{2}{4} \times 10 = \frac{20}{4} = 5 \text{ mL of piperacillin}$$

Flow calculation: 5 mL + 100 mL = 105 mL

$$\frac{105 \text{ mL} \times \overset{4}{\cancel{60}} \text{ gtt (set)}}{\underset{3}{\cancel{45} \text{ minutes}}} = \frac{420}{3} = 140 \text{ gtt/min}$$

Volumetric pump rate:

$$\text{Amount of solution} \div \frac{\text{minutes to administer}}{60 \text{ min}} = \text{Milliliters/hour (mL/h)}$$

$$100 \text{ mL} + 5 \text{ mL (drug)} \div \frac{45 \text{ min}}{60 \text{ min}} = 105 \text{ mL} \times \frac{\overset{4}{\cancel{60}}}{\underset{3}{\cancel{45}}} = \frac{420}{3} = 140 \text{ mL/h}$$

5. Drug calculation: Convert to milligrams.
   $2 \text{ g} = 2.000 \text{ mg}$

$$\frac{D}{H} \times V = \frac{500}{2000} \times 5 = \frac{5}{4} = 1.25 \text{ mL of ampicillin}$$

Flow calculation:

$$\frac{50 \text{ mL} \times \overset{4}{\cancel{60}} \text{ gtt (set)}}{\underset{1}{\cancel{15}} \text{ minutes}} = \frac{200}{1} = 200 \text{ gtt/min}$$

Volumetric pump rate:

$$50 \text{ mL} + 1.25 \text{ mL} \div \frac{15}{60} = 51.25 \text{ mL} \times \frac{\overset{4}{\cancel{60}}}{\underset{1}{\cancel{15}}} = 205 \text{ mL/h}$$

6. a. $7.5 \text{ mg} \times 66 \text{ kg} = 495 \text{ mg or } 500 \text{ mg of amikacin per dose}$
   $1 \text{ g} = 1.000 \text{ mg}$

   b. $$\frac{D}{H} \times V = \frac{500 \text{ mg}}{1000 \text{ mg}} \times 4 \text{ mL} = \frac{2000}{1000} = 2 \text{ mL of amikacin}$$

$$
\begin{array}{ccccccc}
H & : & V & :: & D & : & x \\
1000 \text{ mg} & : & 4 \text{ mL} & :: & 500 \text{ mg} & : & x \text{ mL}
\end{array}
$$

$$1000 \, x = 2000$$

$$x = 2 \text{ mL of amikacin}$$

Flow calculation:

$$\frac{100 \text{ mL} \times \overset{4}{\cancel{60}} \text{ gtt (set)}}{\underset{3}{\cancel{45}} \text{ minutes}} = \frac{400}{3} = 133 \text{ gtt/min}$$

Volumetric pump rate:

$$100 \text{ mL} + 2 \text{ mL} \div \frac{45}{60} = 102 \text{ mL} \times \frac{\overset{4}{\cancel{60}}}{\underset{3}{\cancel{45}}} = \frac{408}{3} = 136 \text{ mL/h}$$

7. a. Drug dose is within safe parameters; 800 μg/d

$$10\ \mu g \times 75\ \text{kg} = 750\ \mu g/\text{d}$$

$$15\ \mu g \times 75\ \text{kg} = 1125\ \mu g/\text{d}$$

b. $$\frac{D}{H} \times V = \frac{400\ \mu g}{500\ \mu g} \times 2\ \text{mL} = \frac{800}{500} = 1.6\ \text{mL of digoxin}$$

H	:	V	::	D	:	x
500 μg	:	2 mL	::	400 μg	:	x

$$500x = 800$$

$$x = 1.6\ \text{mL of digoxin per dose}$$

Answer: Mix 1.6 mL of digoxin with 4 mL of diluent and administer the 5.6 mL by direct intravenous injection.

8. Client's weight: 178 lbs ÷ 2.2 = 81 kg.
   a. Either Cardizem vial could be used. The Cardizem 25 mg vial is preferred because the dose is less than 25 mg and the balance of the solution would need to be discarded.
   b. 0.25 mg × 81 kg = 20.25 mg or 20 mg.

c. $$\frac{D}{H} \times V = \frac{20\ \text{mg}}{25\ \text{mg}} \times 5\ \text{mL} = \frac{100}{25} = 4\ \text{mL of Cardizem}$$

CRITICAL CARE DRUG CALCULATION

Linda Laskowski-Jones, RN, MS, CCRN, CEN

Infusion rate to deliver medication (cross multiply):

$$\text{Formula:}\ \frac{\text{mg/mL of drug}}{60\ \text{gtt/mL}} = \frac{\text{mg/min}}{\text{gtt/min}}$$

Keep in mind that with a volumetric pump, gtt/min = mL/h.

EXAMPLE 1:

Order: Lidocaine 2 g in 250 mL D_5W; run at 2 mg/min. How many mL/h should the infusion pump be set to deliver 2 mg/min?

1. Calculate mg/mL of drug: 2 g = 2000 mg

$$\frac{2000\ \text{mg}}{250\ \text{mL}} = \frac{x\ \text{mg}}{1\ \text{mL}} \qquad x = 8\ \text{mg/1 mL}$$

2. Apply formula:

$$\frac{8\ \text{mg/mL}}{60\ \text{gtt/mL}} = \frac{2\ \text{mg/min}}{x\ \text{gtt/min}}$$

$$8x = 120$$

$$x = 15\ \text{gtt/min} = 15\ \text{mL/h}$$

EXAMPLE 2:

Order: Dopamine 800 mg in 250 mL D_5W; run at 5 $\mu g/kg/min$. Estimated weight = 70 kg.

1. Calculate mg/mL of drug:

$$\frac{800 \text{ mg}}{250 \text{ mL}} = \frac{x \text{ mg}}{1 \text{ mL}} \qquad 250\,x = 800;\ x = 3.2 \text{ mg/mL}$$

2. Convert $\mu g/kg/min$ to mg/min to use the formula:

$$5\ \mu g/1000 = .005 \text{ mg}$$

$$.005 \text{ mg} \times 70 \text{ (kg)} = 0.35 \text{ mg/min}$$

3. Apply formula:

$$\frac{3.2 \text{ mg/mL}}{60 \text{ gtt/mL}} = \frac{0.35 \text{ mg/min}}{x \text{ gtt/min}}$$

$$3.2\,x = 21$$

$$x = 6.6 \text{ or } 7 \text{ gtt/min} = 7 \text{ mL/h}$$

EXAMPLE 3:

Order: Nitroglycerin 50 mg in 250 mL D_5W; run at 20 $\mu g/min$.

1. Calculate mg/mL of drug:

$$\frac{50 \text{ mg}}{250 \text{ mL}} = \frac{x \text{ mg}}{1 \text{ mL}} \qquad 250\,x = 50;\ x = 0.2 \text{ mg/mL}$$

2. Convert $\mu g/min$ to mg/min to use the formula:

$$20\ \mu g/1000 = .020 \text{ mg}$$

3. Apply formula:

$$\frac{.2 \text{ mg/mL}}{60 \text{ gtt/mL}} = \frac{.020 \text{ mg/min}}{x \text{ gtt/min}}$$

$$0.2\,x = 1.2$$

$$x = 6 \text{ gtt/min} = 6 \text{ mL/h}$$

EXAMPLE 4:

Order: Lidocaine 2 g in 250 mL D_5W; run at 30 mL/h. Calculate mg/min of lidocaine infusion.

1. Calculate mg/mL of drug: 2 g = 2000 mg

$$\frac{2000 \text{ mg}}{250 \text{ mL}} = \frac{x \text{ mg}}{1 \text{ mL}} \qquad x = 8 \text{ mg}/1 \text{ mL}$$

2. Apply formula: (30 mL/h = 30 gtt/min with an infusion pump)

$$\frac{8 \text{ mg mL}}{60 \text{ gtt/mL}} = \frac{x \text{ mg/min}}{30 \text{ gtt/min}}$$

$$60 \, x = 240$$

$$x = 4 \text{ mg/min}$$

Unit II

Contemporary Issues
in Pharmacology

This unit is composed of Chapters 5 through 8: (5) The Drug Approval Process (U.S. and Canadian), Resources, and Cultural Considerations; (6) Drug Interaction and Drug Abuse; (7) Drug Therapy Considerations Throughout the Life Span; and (8) The Role of the Nurse in Drug Research. Chapter 5 covers drug standards and federal legislation on both American and Canadian drugs, which establish safety guidelines for drug use, drug names, and drug resources. For that reason the nurse needs to be knowledgeable about and adhere to drug regulations. Cultural considerations in the pharmacotherapeutic regimen also are addressed.

Chapter 6 covers drug interaction and abuse, two areas of special interest to nursing. Assessing drug interaction has always been and remains an ongoing function of the nurse. Because drug abuse is a national problem from which no portion of the population is immune, including health professionals, it is a topic of concern to nurses.

Drug therapy in the child and older adult is a topic of special nursing consideration. Understanding the pharmacokinetic and pharmacodynamic effects in these age groups is especially important for identifying safe drug dosing and preventing adverse reactions. Chapter 7 identifies aspects that require specific attention when administering drugs to clients in these age groups.

The role of the nurse in drug research, discussed in Chapter 8, is challenging. The nurse in general practice identifies specific needs that may be met by medications. As part of clinical drug trials, the nurse needs to be ever aware of informed consent and the client's response to drugs.

Chapter 5

The Drug Approval Process (U.S. and Canadian), Resources, and Cultural Considerations

---

OUTLINE

Objectives
Terms
Introduction
Drug Standards and Legislation
    Drug Standards
        Federal Legislation

Nurse Practice Acts
Canadian Drug Regulation
Drug Names
Drug Resources
Food and Drug Administration
    Pregnancy Categories

Cultural Considerations in the
    Pharmacotherapeutic
    Regimen
Summary
Study Questions

OBJECTIVES

Explain the Food, Drug, and Cosmetic Act of 1938 and the two amendments to it.

Explain the three Canadian schedules for drugs sold in Canada.

Describe the function of nurse practice acts.

Differentiate between chemical, generic, and brand names of drugs.

List two drug resources (reference) books.

Explain various cultural beliefs and sensitivity that the nurse should consider in relation to health care.

TERMS

American Hospital Formulary
brand name
chemical name
controlled substance
cultural beliefs

DEA
FDA
generic name
malfeasance
misfeasance

nonfeasance
PDR
pharmacology
USP-NF

INTRODUCTION

Pharmacology is the study of the effects of chemical substances on living tissues. Early drugs were derived from plants, animals, and minerals. Records of drug use date back to 2700 B.C. in the Middle East and China. The drugs most commonly used then were laxatives and emetics to induce vomiting.

In 1550 B.C., the Egyptians wrote their empirical observations of drug therapy on what is now known as the Ebers Medical Papyrus. They suggested castor oil as a laxative and opium for pain. They also suggested that moldy bread be applied to wounds and bruises 3500 years before Alexander Fleming's discovery of penicillin.

The Roman physician and writer Galen (131–201 A.D.) was considered an authority in medicine and pharmacy for hundreds of years. He initiated the common use of prescriptions and used several ingredients to treat a specific illness.

After the fall of the Roman Empire, medicine and pharmacy returned to the realms of folklore and tradition. During this time, however, Christian monks kept information on medicine and pharmacy in their monasteries and tended the sick and needy. The medicines used by the monks were derived from plants and herbs grown in the monastery gardens.

Around 1240 A.D., Arab doctors formulated the first set of drug standards and measurements (grains, drams, minims), known as the apothecary system. (Today, however, the units of the metric system are used internationally to measure drugs; the apothecary system is being phased out.) In fifteenth-century England, apothecary shops were owned by barber-surgeons, physicians, and independent merchants.

In the eighteenth century, the following breakthrough drugs were introduced: the vaccine for smallpox, digitalis from the foxglove plant for strengthening and slowing the heart beat, and vitamin C from citrus fruit. In the nineteenth century, morphine and codeine were extracted from opium; atropine, bromides, and iodine were introduced; amyl nitrite was used to relieve the pain of angina; and the anesthetics ether and nitrous oxide were discovered. In the early twentieth century, aspirin was derived from salicylic acid; and phenobarbital, insulin, and the sulfonamides were introduced. A vast majority of the drugs that are used today date back to the early 1940s. Antibiotics (penicillin, tetracycline, streptomycin), antihistamines, and cortisone were marketed in the 1940s. In the 1950s, antipsychotic drugs, antihypertensives, oral contraceptives, and the polio vaccine were introduced.

DRUG STANDARDS AND LEGISLATION

DRUG STANDARDS

The set of drug standards used in the United States is the *United States Pharmacopeia* of 1820. The **U.S. Pharmacopeia National Formulary (USP-NF)**, the current authoritative source for drug standards, is revised every 5 years by a group of experts in nursing, pharmaceutics, pharmacology, chemistry, and microbiology. Drugs included in the *USP-NF* have met high standards for therapeutic use, client safety, quality, purity, strength, packaging safety, and dosage form. Drugs that meet these standards have the initials USP following their official name.

The *International Pharmacopeia*, first published in 1951 by the World Health Organization (WHO), provides a basis for standards in strength and composition of drugs for use throughout the world. The book is published in English, Spanish, and French and, like the *USP-NF*, is revised every 5 years.

FEDERAL LEGISLATION

Through federal legislation, the public is protected from drugs that are impure, toxic, ineffective, or not tested prior to public sale. The primary purpose of this federal legislation is to assure safety. America's first law to regulate drugs was the Federal Pure Food and Drug Act of 1906, which did not include drug effectiveness and drug safety.

1938: Food, Drug, and Cosmetic Act of 1938

The Food, Drug, and Cosmetic Act of 1938 empowered a governing body, the **Food and Drug Administration (FDA),** to monitor and regulate the manufacture and marketing of drugs. It is the FDA's responsibility to ensure that all drugs are tested for harmful effects, have labels with accurate information, and that detailed literature explaining adverse effects is enclosed with the drug packaging. The FDA can prevent the marketing of any drug that it judges to be incompletely tested or dangerous. Only those drugs that are considered safe by FDA are approved for marketing.

1952: Durham-Humphrey Amendment of the 1938 Act

The Durham-Humphrey amendment to the Food, Drug, and Cosmetic Act of 1938 distinguished between drugs that can be sold with or without prescription and those that should not be refilled without a new prescription. Those drugs that should not be refilled without a new prescription, such as narcotics, hypnotics, or tranquilizers, must be so labeled.

1962: Kefauver-Harris Amendment of the 1938 Act

The Kefauver-Harris amendment to the Food, Drug, and Cosmetic Act of 1938 resulted from the widely publicized thalidomide tragedy of the 1950s, in which pregnant European women who took the sedative-hypnotic thalidomide during the first trimester of pregnancy gave birth to babies with extreme limb deformities. The Kefauver-Harris amendment tightened controls on drug safety, especially experimental drugs, and required that adverse reactions and contraindications must be labeled and included in the literature. Also included in the amendment were provisions for the evaluation of testing methods used by manufacturers, the process for withdrawal of approved drugs when safety and effectiveness were in doubt, and the establishment of the effectiveness of new drugs before marketing.

1970: The Controlled Substances Act

In 1970, the Controlled Substances Act (CSA) of the Comprehensive Drug Abuse Prevention and Control Act, Title II, was passed by Congress. This act, designed to remedy the escalating problem of drug abuse, included several provisions: the promotion of drug education and research into the prevention and treatment of drug dependence; the strengthening of enforcement authority; the establishment of

treatment and rehabilitation facilities; and the designation of schedules, or categories, for controlled substances according to abuse liability.

Controlled substances are described in five schedules, or categories, listed in Table 5–1. Schedule I drugs are *not* approved for medical use; schedule II through V drugs have accepted medical use. In addition, the abuse potential and extent of physical and psychologic dependence are greatest with schedule I drugs. This dependency decreases as one moves through the schedule, with schedule V drugs having only very limited abuse potential. Some drugs might be listed in more than one schedule category. Codeine is a schedule II drug, but when codeine is added to acetaminophen it becomes a schedule III drug, and when it is used in combination as a cough preparation, it becomes a schedule V drug.

Nursing Interventions: Controlled Substances

- Account for all controlled drugs.
- Keep special controlled substance record for required information.
- Countersign all discarded or wasted medication.
- Assure that records and drugs on hand match.
- Keep all controlled drugs locked up; narcotics must be kept under double lock.
- Be certain that only authorized persons have access to the keys.

In 1983, the **Drug Enforcement Administration (DEA)** of the Department of Justice was charged with the role of being the nation's sole legal drug enforcement agency. The Bureau of Narcotics and Dangerous Drugs, which preceded the DEA, is now defunct.

TABLE 5–1 Schedule Categories of Controlled Substances

Schedule	Examples of Substances	Description
I	Heroin, hallucinogenics (LSD, marijuana, mescaline, peyote, psilocybin)	Drugs with high abuse potential. No accepted medical use. Labeled C-I
II	Meperidine (Demerol), morphine, hydrocodone, hydromorphone, methadone, oxycodone, codeine, amphetamines, secobarbital, pentobarbital	High potential for drug abuse. Accepted medical use. Can lead to strong physical and psychological dependency. Labeled C-II
III	Codeine preparations, paregoric, nonnarcotic drugs (pentazocine, propoxyphene)	Medically accepted drugs. Potential abuse is less than that for schedules I and II. May cause dependence. Labeled C-III
IV	Phenobarbital, benzodiazepines (diazepam, oxazepam, lorazepam, chlordiazepoxide), chloral hydrate, meprobamate	Medically accepted drugs. May cause dependence. Labeled C-IV
V	Opioid controlled substances for cough and diarrhea, such as codeine in cough preparations	Medically accepted drugs. Very limited potential for dependence. Labeled C-V

KEY: C, control.

NURSE PRACTICE ACTS

Every state has its own laws regarding drug administration by nurses. Generally, nurses cannot prescribe or administer drugs without a health care provider's order, but state laws vary. A practicing nurse should request a copy of the nurse practice act in the state in which she or he is licensed. In some states, a nurse who administers a drug without a physician's order is in violation of the nurse practice act and could have her or his license revoked.

In a civil court, the nurse can be prosecuted for giving the wrong drug or dosage, omitting a drug dose, or giving the drug by the wrong route. The legal terms for these offenses are

Misfeasance: negligence; giving the wrong drug or drug dose that results in the client's death

Nonfeasance: omission; omitting a drug dose that results in the client's death

Malfeasance: giving the correct drug but by the wrong route that results in the client's death

CANADIAN DRUG REGULATION

In Canada, the Health Protection Branch, Department of National Health and Welfare is responsible for administering the two acts that are the foundation of the national drug laws. The manufacture, distribution, and sale of drugs (except narcotics) are controlled by the Canadian Food and Drug Act, amended in 1953. The manufacture, distribution, and sale of narcotic drugs are controlled by the 1961 Narcotics Control Act. Like the U.S. Controlled Substances Act, the Canadian act requires prescriptions and strict record keeping for all narcotics.

Drugs sold in Canada are assigned to one of three schedules:

- Schedule F: All prescription drugs (approximately 350) are available only with a prescription (written or verbal); thus, these drugs have essentially no potential for abuse.
- Schedule G: Fourteen drugs in this group require written or verbal prescription and refills require a written prescription. These drugs have a moderate potential for abuse and must have a "C" on the label, similar to Schedule III drugs in the United States.
- Schedule H: These drugs have no recognized medical use and are potentially dangerous, similar to Schedule I drugs in the United States. Their use is primarily limited to specialized medical research.
- Narcotics: These drugs are dispensed only with written prescription and an "N" must appear on

all advertisements and labels. Low-dose codeine (20 mg/30 mL and 8-mg tablets) is an exception and can be sold only by a pharmacist. Two additional medicinal ingredients, caffeine and acetylsalicylic acid, must be part of this codeine preparation.

Nonprescription drugs (OTC preparation) are administered by the Pharmacy Acts of the respective Canadian provinces, which identify the place and conditions of sale. These drugs are assigned to one of three categories:

1. General proprietary. These drugs are for treatment of self-limiting minor illness, injury, or discomfort. The packaging information is considered adequate and the drug can be administered without consultation with a health care provider. These drugs can be purchased at any store.
2. Availability only through pharmacies. After consultation and approval by a health care provider, drugs designed to treat minor, self-limiting conditions are available through a pharmacy. Examples are cold remedies and laxatives.
3. Recommendation of a health care provider. This category requires recommendation by a health care provider. Examples include nitroglycerin, insulin, and muscle relaxants.

To address the proliferation of a variety of provincial schedules and regulations, the Health Protection Branch has proposed to "harmonize" regulations nationwide by creating a three-schedule system:

Schedule I: All prescription drugs (Schedules F and G and narcotics)

Schedule II: Nonprescription, pharmacist-monitored drugs

Schedule III: Nonprescription drugs with no restrictions placed on location of sale

The initial harmonizing work is the development of specific criteria to identify the amount of professional involvement required for the sale and use of drug preparations. The initiation of Schedule II presents special challenges.

DRUG NAMES

Each drug may have several names. The **chemical name** describes the drug's chemical structure. The **generic name** is the official or nonproprietary name for the drug. This name is not owned by any pharmaceutical (drug) company and is universally accepted. Today most drugs are ordered by their generic name. The **brand** or **trade name**, also known as the proprietary name, is chosen by the drug company and is usually a registered trademark owned by that specific manufacturer. Drug companies market a compound using their given name (brand name). For example, Cardizem is the brand (proprietary) name registered with the manufacturer, and diltiazem HCl is the generic name recognized by the USP.

There are pros and cons to using generic drugs. Generic drugs are usually cheaper and have the same active ingredients as in brand-name, or trade-name, drugs. However, some generic drugs have inert fillers and binders that may result in variations of drug effectiveness. The FDA publishes a list of approved generic drugs that are bioequivalents to brand-name drugs. Generic drugs are less expensive because manufacturers do not have to do extensive testing, because these drugs had been clinically tested for safety and efficacy by the pharmaceutical company that first formulated the drug. The health care provider and client must exercise care in choosing generic drugs because there may be some variation in the action of or response to them. Brand-name drugs are preferred when ordering anticonvulsants for seizures, anticoagulants (such as Coumadin), medication for congestive heart failure (Lanoxin), and aspirin when giving large doses for rheumatoid arthritis. A study showed that 23 seizure-free epileptics who switched to the generic drug experienced renewed seizure activity. The nurse should check with the health care provider or pharmacist when generic drugs are prescribed.

Throughout this text, both generic and brand names are given for drugs. Because many brand names may exist for a single generic name, the generic name is given *first* in lower case letters, followed by the most commonly used brand name in parentheses. With generic drugs, the name may be long and difficult to pronounce. Brand names always begin with a capital letter. An example of a generic and brand-name drug listing is furosemide (Lasix).

DRUG RESOURCES

There are many resource reference books on drugs, including nursing texts that identify related nursing interventions and areas for health teaching.

The *American Hospital Formulary* and the *Physicians' Desk Reference (PDR)* are two such resources. The **American Hospital Formulary** Services—*Drug Information* is an excellent reference that provides accurate and complete drug information on nearly all prescription drugs marketed in the United States. It is published annually and updated regularly with monthly supplements. Additionally, many drug handbooks are available as quick drug references. Most of these include nursing implications. When more information is needed about a drug, the *PDR* or the *American Hospital Formulary* frequently is suggested.

The **Physicians' Desk Reference (PDR)** lists several thousand drugs with complete drug information given by pharmaceutical companies. The *PDR* is published yearly. It contains seven sections, two of which are the most useful to nurses: the second (pink) section, which is the drug name index, and the sixth (white) section, which gives information about the drugs. The *PDR* is a useful drug resource, but it does not provide complete pharmacologic and therapeutic information and does not include nursing interventions. The drug information is reprinted drug package inserts supplied by the pharmaceutical company, which pays to have its drug listed in the PDR.

Drug Facts and Comparisons contains information on almost all drugs marketed in the United States. The reference consists of drug actions, indications, warnings and precautions, dosage and route for administration, adverse reactions, client information, overdosage, drug interactions, contraindications, and comparison charts and tables.

The *United States Pharmacopeic—Drug Information (USP DI)* is a three-volume set that is available in the majority of hospitals and pharmacies. Monthly supplements are available. Volumes IA and IB provide drug information for the health care provider. The sections in these volumes include pharmacology, precautions to consider, side and adverse effects, client consultation, general dosing information, and dosage forms. Volume II gives drug information for the client. It is a client-oriented volume that explains information in a understandable way for the client. The sections included in Volume II are administration of drug, drug effects, indications, adverse reactions, dosage guidelines, and what to do for missed doses.

The *Handbook on Injectable Drugs* by Lawrence A. Trissel is published by the American Society of Hospital Pharmacists. It is an excellent reference for injectable medications, listing drug compatibility with other drugs, base fluids, and drugs available in large volume parenterals. Also, it includes the pH of each drug and gives some dosing administration guidelines.

FOOD AND DRUG ADMINISTRATION (FDA) PREGNANCY CATEGORIES

The FDA developed a classification system related to the effects of drugs on the unborn child (fetus). In the drug literature and drug reference books, a pregnancy category is indicated for most drugs.

TABLE 5–2 FDA Pregnancy Categories

Category	Description
A	No risk to fetus. Studies have not shown evidence of fetal harm.
B	No risk in animal studies, and well-controlled studies in pregnant women are not available. It is assumed there is little to no risk in pregnant women.
C	Animal studies indicate a risk to the fetus. Controlled studies on pregnant women are not available. Risk versus benefit of the drug must be determined.
D	A risk to the human fetus has been proved. Risk versus benefit of the drug must be determined. It could be used in life-threatening conditions.
X	A risk to the human fetus has been proved. Risk outweighs the benefit, and drug should be avoided during pregnancy.

Categories A and B are considered to be within safe limits for drug use in pregnancy, especially in the first trimester. Table 5–2 lists the FDA pregnancy categories and describes each category's effect on the fetus.

CULTURAL CONSIDERATIONS IN THE PHARMACOTHERAPEUTIC REGIMEN

Cultural beliefs contribute to health behaviors in individuals, families, and groups. Nurses and other health care professionals need to be aware of and respectful of value systems as integral parts of professional practice. Some attitudes and beliefs about health and illness are not consciously thought about on a regular basis. This is primarily because our professional education has been with the established health care system. For example, the provider–client and nurse–physician relationships portray two health care system relationships enmeshed in custom.

In addition, the health care culture tends to have its own orientations toward time, activity, human–nature, and relational values. Specifically, promptness and follow-up on schedule appointments are expected (time); accomplishments (activity) such as taking medications as prescribed are valued; acceptance of technology and the value of individual in control of environment (human–nature); and autonomy is prized and the meeting of individual's needs is fostered (relational). Operationalizing the pharmacotherapeutic regimen is reflective of these orientations. Nurses and other health care providers need to be alert to and integrate these value orientations into the client's plan of care.

An understanding of the client's health beliefs is an essential part of the planning and delivery of health care. This is especially important when the cultural beliefs of the nurse are different from or in conflict with the beliefs of the client, family, or group.

Raising cultural sensitivity to a level of awareness is very important and is the foundation of the development of cultural sensitivity. Sulc reported in Spector: *Cultural Diversity in Health and Illness* that the first step is to recognize that cultural diversity exists. He continues with the identification of seven additional steps for the development of cultural sensitivity, including (1) demonstrating respect for people as unique individuals; (2) respecting the unfamiliar; (3) identifying and examining one's own cultural beliefs; (4) recognizing that some cultural groups have definitions of health, illnesses, and practices that may differ from the nurse's; (5) modifying health care in keeping with client's cultural background; (6) not expecting all members of a given cultural group to behave in the same way; and (7) appreciating that cultural values are ingrained and thus difficult to change.

The concept of equilibrium is part of a variety of illnesses. Two examples of common imbalances are yin (cold) and yang (hot) in traditional Chinese belief. "Hot" and "cold" are restored by the use of opposing forces, by applying a "cold" remedy to treat a "hot" illness and vice versa. Of special relevance to this text is the use of appropriate "hot" or "cold" remedies, including medications and foods, to treat the imbalance.

Armed with a knowledge of cultural factors and influence, the nurse has another dimension for understanding behaviors and thereby planning and delivering of care to meet the client, family, or group needs.

Complex and comprehensive cultural assessments are beyond the scope of this chapter. Consult cultural-specific reference such as Spector: *Cultural Diversity in Health and Illness* or Geissler: *Guide to Cultural Assessment*.

SUMMARY

The nurse should be aware of the various federal acts and amendments related to the use and administration of drugs. The FDA sends out quarterly reports on new drugs, drugs that have been recalled, and other information regarding drug administration. Controlled substances should be checked according to the scheduled drug category of the Controlled Substances Act of 1970. There are many drug resource (reference) books on the market, and these books should be available to nurses in the practice setting. When the client is pregnant, the nurse is also responsible for checking the pregnancy category of the drug in a drug reference book before administering it.

Nurses should be cognizant of the various cultures that clients come from and adapt the client's health care to meet the client's cultural needs. The nurse should not try to impress her or his cultural background or behavior on others.

STUDY QUESTIONS

1. What are the provisions in the Food, Drug, and Cosmetic Act of 1938? What additional safeguards are included in the Durham-Humphrey amendment of 1952 and the Kefauver-Harris amendment of 1962?

2. Which controlled substance has the higher potential for drug abuse, controlled substance Schedule II or Schedule IV? Explain.

3. The Canadian Food and Drug Act of 1953 has identified three schedules for drug regulation. How does Schedule F differ from Schedule G?

4. What are the characteristics of the chemical name, generic name, and brand or trade name of a drug?

5. What are the titles of two drug resource books that are helpful in nursing practice?

6. Your client is taking a drug that is in pregnancy category B. Would this drug be safe? Explain.

7. Client's cultural sensitivity is a nursing responsibility of the nurse. Give examples of nursing considerations related to cultural sensitivity.

Chapter 6

Drug Interaction and Drug Abuse

OUTLINE

Objectives
Terms
Introduction
Drug Interaction
　　Pharmacokinetic Interaction
　　Pharmacodynamic Interac-
　　　tions

Drug–Food Interactions
Drug–Laboratory Interactions
　　Nursing Process: Drug
　　　Interactions
Drug-Induced Photosensitivity
Drug Abuse

Chemical Impairment in
　Nurses
　Nursing Process: Drug
　　Abuse
Study Questions

OBJECTIVES

Define the term *drug interaction*.

Explain the four pharmacokinetic processes related to drug interaction.

Explain the three effects associated with pharmacodynamic interactions.

Explain the effects of drug-food interactions.

Explain the meaning of drug-induced photosensitivity.

Define the terms *drug abuse, drug misuse, addiction, physical dependence*, and *psychological dependence*.

Identify the drugs associated with drug abuse.

TERMS

addiction
additive effect
adverse drug reaction
antagonistic effect

drug abuse
drug interaction
habituation
photosensitivity

psychological dependence
synergistic effect
withdrawal

INTRODUCTION

Drug therapy has become complex because of the number of prescribed drugs. Drug–drug, drug–food, and drug–laboratory interactions have also become an increasing problem. Because of the possibility of numerous interactions, the nurse should be knowledgeable about drug interactions and should closely monitor client responses. Communication among members of the health team is essential.

DRUG INTERACTION

A **drug interaction** can be defined as an altered or modified action or effect of a drug as a result of interaction with one or more other drugs. It should not be confused with adverse drug reaction or drug incompatibility. An **adverse drug reaction** is an undesirable drug effect ranging from mild untoward effects to severe toxic effects, including hypersensitivity reaction and anaphylaxis. **Drug incompatibility** is a chemical or physical reaction that occurs among two or more drugs in vitro (outside the body).

Drug interactions can be divided into two categories: (1) pharmacokinetic interactions and (2) pharmacodynamic interactions. These two categories of drug interaction are discussed individually.

PHARMACOKINETIC INTERACTION

The pharmacokinetic interaction is a change that occurs in the absorption, distribution, metabolism or biotransformation, or excretion of one or both drugs.

Absorption

When a person takes two drugs at the same time, the rate of absorption of one or both drugs can change. One drug can block, decrease, or increase the absorption rate of another drug. It can do this in one of three ways: by decreasing or increasing gastric emptying time, by changing the gastric pH, or by forming drug complexes.

Drugs that increase the speed of gastric emptying, such as laxatives, increase gastric and intestinal motility and cause a decrease in drug absorption. Most drugs are absorbed primarily in the small intestines; exceptions include barbiturates, salicylates, and theophylline. Narcotics and anticholinergic drugs (atropine-like drugs) decrease gastric emptying time and decrease gastrointestinal (GI) motility, thus causing an increase in absorption rate. The longer the drug remains in the stomach or intestine, the greater the amount of drug absorption (only for those drugs absorbed in the stomach).

When the gastric pH is decreased, a weak acid drug, such as aspirin, is less ionized and is more rapidly absorbed. Drugs that increase the pH of gastric juices decrease absorption of weak acid drugs. Antacids, such as Maalox and Amphojel, raise the gastric pH and block or slow absorption. Some drugs may react chemically. For example, tetracycline and the heavy-metal ions (calcium, magnesium, aluminum, iron) found in antacids form a complex, and the tetracycline is not absorbed. Tetracycline also can form complexes with dairy products. Milk products and antacids should be avoided for 1 h before and 2 h after consuming tetracycline.

Other drugs that can cause complexes with drugs besides antacids are kaolin-pectin, certain hypocholesterol drugs such as cholestyramine and colestipol, and activated charcoal. Due to the formed complexes, the drugs are less soluble, which results in less drug absorption.

Certain broad-spectrum antibacterials (antibiotics) such as erythromycin affect the GI flora, thereby causing an increase in absorption of digoxin, which depends on the flora in the intestine to metabolize digoxin.

Distribution

Drug distribution to tissues can be affected by its binding to plasma/serum protein. Only drugs unbound to protein are free, active agents and can enter body tissues. Two drugs that are highly protein-bound and administered simultaneously can result in drug displacements. Factors that influence displacement of drugs are (1) the drug concentration in the blood, (2) protein-binding power of the drugs, and (3) volume of distribution (V_d).

Two drugs that are highly bound to protein or albumin compete for protein or albumin sites in the plasma. The result is a decrease in protein binding of one or both drugs; therefore, more free drug circulates in the plasma and is available for drug action. This effect can lead to drug toxicity. Drugs that are unbound to protein are free, active drugs and can cause a pharmacologic response. When two highly protein-bound drugs need to be taken concurrently, drug dosage of one or both drugs may need to be decreased in order to avoid drug toxicity.

Examples of drugs that are highly protein-bound include warfarin (anticoagulant); certain anticonvulsants, such as phenytoin and valproic acid; clofibrate; most nonsteroidal antiinflammatory drugs

(NSAIDs); sulfonamides; tolbutamide; and quinidine. Warfarin is 99% protein-bound, thus allowing only 1% to be free drug. If 2% to 3% of warfarin is displaced in the albumin, the amount of free warfarin would be 3% to 4% instead of 1%. This increases the anticoagulant effect, and thus excess bleeding may result.

Metabolism or Biotransformation

Many drug interactions of metabolism occur with the induction (stimulation) or inhibition of the hepatic microsomal system. A drug can increase the metabolism of another drug by stimulating (inducing) liver enzymes. Drugs that promote induction of enzymes are called enzyme inducers. An example of an enzyme inducer is the barbiturates (e.g., phenobarbital). Phenobarbital increases the metabolism of beta blockers (propranolol [Inderal]), most antipsychotics, and theophylline. Increased metabolism promotes drug elimination and decreases plasma concentration of the drug. The result is a decrease in drug action. Sometimes liver enzymes convert drugs to active or passive metabolites. The drug metabolites may be excreted or may produce an active pharmacologic response. Also, there are some drugs that are enzyme inhibitors.

The anticonvulsant drugs phenytoin and carbamazepine, alcohol, and rifampin are hepatic enzyme inducers that can increase drug metabolism, e.g., the anticoagulant drug warfarin. A larger dose of warfarin is usually needed while the client is taking a hepatic inducer. The metabolism aids in decreasing the amount of drug. If the drug inducer is withdrawn, warfarin dosages need to be decreased because less drug is being eliminated by hepatic metabolism. Usually, interaction occurs after 1 week of drug therapy and can continue for 1 week after the drug inducer is discontinued. Drugs with narrow therapeutic ranges should be closely monitored.

Cigarette smoking increases hepatic enzyme activity and can increase theophylline clearance. For smokers who are taking theophylline, the theophylline dose should be increased. With chronic alcohol use, hepatic enzyme activities are increased, whereas with acute alcohol use, metabolism is inhibited.

The antiulcer drug cimetidine is an enzyme inhibitor that decreases the metabolism of certain drugs, such as theophylline (antiasthmatic). As the result of decreasing theophylline metabolism, there is an increase in the plasma concentration of theophylline. The theophylline dose needs to be decreased to avoid toxicity. If cimetidine or any enzyme drug inhibitor is discontinued, the theo-

phylline dosage should be adjusted. Certain drugs alter hepatic blood flow, causing a decrease in liver metabolism. Table 6–1 describes the effects of drug enzyme inducers and inhibitors.

Excretion

Most drugs are excreted in the urine and are filtered through the glomeruli. With some drugs, the excretion occurs in the bile, which passes into the intestinal tract. Drugs can increase or decrease renal excretion and have an effect on the excretion of other drugs. Drugs that decrease cardiac output, decrease blood flow to the kidneys, and decrease glomerular filtration can also decrease or delay drug excretion. The antidysrhythmic drug quinidine decreases the excretion of digoxin (a digitalis preparation); therefore, the plasma concentration of digoxin is increased and digitalis toxicity can occur. Furosemide (Lasix) decreases the glomerular filtration rate (GFR), which reduces clearance of drugs such as digoxin. A decrease in digoxin excretion could lead to an increase in serum digoxin levels. With a decrease in serum potassium level and a decrease in digoxin excretion, digoxin toxicity could occur (see Drug–Laboratory Interactions).

Probenecid (Benemid), a drug for gout, decreases penicillin excretion by competing for tubular reabsorption of penicillin in the kidneys. In some cases this may be desirable in order to increase or maintain the plasma concentration of penicillin, which has a short half-life, for a longer time.

Changing urine pH affects drug excretion. The antacid sodium bicarbonate causes the urine to be alkaline. Alkaline urine promotes the excretion of

TABLE 6–1 Drugs: Enzyme Inducer or Enzyme Inhibitor

Drug Category	Drug Effect
Drug enzyme inducer	Onset and termination of drug effect is slow, approximately 1 week.
	Drug dosage may need to be increased with use of drug inducer.
	Drug dosage should be adjusted after termination of drug inducer.
	Monitor serum drug levels, especially if the drug has a narrow therapeutic drug range.
Drug enzyme inhibitor	Onset of drug effect usually occurs rapidly.
	Half-life ($t^{1/2}$) of the second drug may be increased, causing a prolonged drug effect.
	Interaction may occur related to the dosage prescribed.
	Disease entities affect drug dosing.
	Monitor serum drug levels, especially if the drug has a narrow therapeutic range.

TABLE 6–2 Pharmacokinetic Interactions of Drugs

Process	Drug	Effect
Absorption	Laxatives	Speeds gastric emptying time Increases gastric motility Decreases drug absorption
	Narcotics Anticholinergics	Slows gastric emptying time Decreases gastric motility Increases drug absorption or decreases absorption depending on where the drug is delayed (gastric vs. intestinal)
	Aspirin	Decreases gastric pH Increases drug absorption
	Antacids	Increases gastric pH Slows absorption of acid drugs
	Antacids and tetracycline	Forms drug complexes Blocks drug absorption
Distribution	Anticoagulant and antiinflammatory (sulindac)	Competes for protein-binding sites Increases free drug; e.g., increases anticoagulant
Metabolism or biotransformation	Barbiturates	Promotes induction of liver enzymes Increases drug metabolism Decreases drug plasma concentration of the second drug
	Antiulcer (cimetidine)	Inhibits liver enzymes release Decreases drug metabolism of Valium, Dilantin, morphine, etc. Increases drug plasma concentration of the second drug
Excretion	Antidysrhythmic (quinidine)	Decreases renal excretion of second drug; e.g., digoxin Increases digoxin concentration
	Antigout (probenecid)	Decreases excretion of penicillin by competing for tubular reabsorption Increases penicillin concentration
	Antacid (sodium bicarbonate)	Promotes excretion of weak acid drug; e.g., aspirin, barbiturates, sulfonamides
	Aspirin, ammonium chloride	Promotes excretion of weak base drugs; e.g., quinidine, theophylline
Other: Decrease cardiac output and renal blood flow	Most drug categories	Decreases drug excretion Increases drug plasma concentration

drugs that are weak acids, such as aspirin and barbiturates. Alkaline urine also promotes reabsorption of weak base drugs. Acid urine promotes the excretion of drugs that are weak bases, such as quinidine.

With clients who have decreased renal or hepatic function, there is usually an increase in free drug concentration. It is essential to closely monitor such a client for drug toxicity when he or she is taking multiple drugs. Checking serum drug levels (therapeutic drug monitoring [TDM]) is especially important for drugs that have a narrow therapeutic range and are highly protein-bound, such as digoxin and phenytoin. Table 6–2 summarizes the drug interactions that affect pharmacokinetics.

PHARMACODYNAMIC INTERACTIONS

Pharmacodynamic interactions are those that result in an additive, synergistic (potentiation), or antagonistic drug effects. When two drugs are given that may or may not have similar actions, the combined effect may be additive (twice the effect), synergistic (greater than twice the effect), or antagonistic (the effect of either or both drugs is decreased).

Additive Drug Effect

When two drugs with similar action are administered, the drug interaction is called an **additive effect** and is the sum of the effects of the two drugs. Additive effect can be desirable or undesirable. For example, a desirable additive drug effect occurs when a diuretic and a beta blocker are given for hypertension: used in combination, these drugs lower the blood pressure and act as antihypertensive drugs. As another example, two analgesics, aspirin and codeine, can be given together for increased pain relief.

An example of an undesirable additive effect is that from two vasodilators: hydralazine (Apresoline) given for hypertension and nitroglycerin prescribed for angina. The result could be a severe hypotensive response. Another example is the interaction of aspirin and alcohol taken together, from which gastric bleeding can result. Both aspirin and alcohol can prolong bleeding time.

Synergistic Drug Effect or Potentiation

When two or more drugs are given together, one drug can potentiate or have a **synergistic effect** on the other drug, meaning that sometimes the effect is greater than the combined effect of two drugs from the same category. An example is the combination of meperidine (Demerol: narcotic analgesic) and promethazine (Phenergan: antihistamine). Phenergan enhances or potentiates the effect of Demerol. Actually, less Demerol is required when it is combined with Phenergan, which can be a desirable effect. An example of an undesirable effect occurs when two drugs, alcohol and a sedative-hypnotic drug such as chlordiazepoxide (Librium) or diazepam (Valium), are combined, increasing central nervous system depression.

Some antibacterials (antibiotics) have an enzyme inhibitor added to the drug in order to potentiate the therapeutic effect of the drug. Examples are ampicillin with sulbactam, and amoxicillin with clavulanate potassium. Ampicillin and amoxicillin can be given without these inhibitors; however, the desired therapeutic effect may not occur because of the bacterial enzyme activity (e.g., beta-lactamase enzyme) causing bacteria resistance. The combination of the antibiotic with an added enzyme inhibitor (sulbactam or clavulanate potassium), will inhibit bacterial enzyme activity, thus prolonging the effect of the antibacterial agent.

Antagonistic Drug Effect

When two drugs are combined that have opposite, or **antagonistic effects,** the drugs cancel each other's drug effect. The actions of both drugs are nullified. An example of an antagonistic effect occurs when the adrenergic beta stimulant isoproterenol (Isuprel) and the adrenergic beta blocker propranolol (Inderal) are given together. The action of each drug is cancelled. Neither delivers the expected therapeutic effect.

With morphine overdose, naloxone is given as an antagonist (antidote) to block the narcotic response. This is a beneficial drug interaction of an antagonist. Table 6–3 summarizes the drug responses associated with pharmacodynamic interaction.

DRUG–FOOD INTERACTIONS

Food is known to increase, decrease, or delay drug absorption. Food can bind with drugs, causing less

TABLE 6–3 Pharmacodynamic Interactions of Drugs

Interactions	Effect
Additive	In the same drug category, the drug effect is the sum of both drug effects.
Synergistic or potentiation	One drug potentiates or enhances the effect of the other drug (greater than effect of each alone).
Antagonistic	Two drugs in opposing drug categories cancel drug effects of both drugs.

or slower drug absorption. An example of food binding with a drug is the interaction of tetracycline and dairy products. The result is a decrease in the plasma concentration of tetracycline. Because of the binding effect, tetracycline should be taken 1 h before or 2 h after meals and *should not* be taken with dairy products. There are a few drugs in which food increases drug absorption; examples include the antiinfective agent nitrofurantoin (Macrodantin), the beta blocker metoprolol (Lopressor), and the antilipemic lovastatin (Mevacor). These drugs should be taken at mealtime or with food.

The classic drug–food interaction occurs when an antidepressant (such as a monoamine oxidase [MAO] inhibitor, e.g., Marplan) is taken with tyramin-rich foods such as cheese, wine, organ meats, beer, yogurt, sour cream, or bananas. More norepinephrine is released and the result could be a hypertensive crisis. These foods must be avoided when taking MAO inhibitors.

DRUG–LABORATORY INTERACTIONS

Abnormal plasma or serum electrolyte concentrations can effect certain drug therapies. If the client is taking digoxin (a digitalis preparation) and there are decreased serum potassium and serum magnesium levels or an increased serum calcium level, digitalis toxicity may result. Certain drugs, such as those from the thiazide diuretic group, can cause abnormal electrolyte concentrations. An example is hydrochlorothiazide (HydroDiuril), which can decrease serum potassium, magnesium, and sodium levels, and can increase the serum calcium level. Because HydroDiuril promotes potassium loss, the low serum potassium increases the plasma concentration of digoxin, thereby increasing the action. The result is digitalis toxicity (intoxication). When digoxin and HydroDiuril are taken together, the nurse should observe for digitalis toxicity (nausea, vomiting, bradycardia [pulse below 60 beats per minute], and stated visual problems).

NURSING PROCESS: DRUG INTERACTIONS

ASSESSMENT

- Obtain a drug history of the over-the-counter (OTC) drugs the client is currently taking. There could be a drug interaction with the prescribed drug.
- Review all literature provided by drug companies and pharmacy.
- Assess for drug reaction when two highly protein-bound drugs are taken together daily. For example, the anticoagulant warfarin (Coumadin) and the antiinflammatory sulindac (Clinoril) have a high affinity to protein. Warfarin is displaced from the plasma protein, causing more free warfarin and possible increase in bleeding.
- Assess the client for potential drug interaction problems related to:
  - An increased or decreased absorption rate of two drugs
  - Drug enzyme inducers that increase drug metabolism may result in a decrease in drug effect (increased drug metabolism leads to increased drug excretion).
- Assess the client for drug toxicity (overdose) when a drug enzyme inducer has been discontinued or when a drug enzyme inhibitor is taken concurrently with other drugs.
- Determine if the client is a cigarette smoker. Tobacco is an enzyme inducer and can increase the metabolic rate of drugs. If a client is taking a drug such as theophylline to control asthma and also smokes, the drug dosage needs to be increased. For nonsmokers, the theophylline dosage should be less or within the suggested drug range.
- Assess renal function by checking for adequate urine output; it should be greater than 600 mL/day. The guideline is 25 mL (cc)/h for adults.

POTENTIAL NURSING DIAGNOSIS

- High risk of tissue injury related to the adverse reaction to drug interaction.

PLANNING

- The client will be aware of drug interactions and avoid drugs that may cause a severe drug reaction.
- The client will not take any OTC drugs without consultation with health care provider.

NURSING INTERVENTIONS

- Notify the health care provider if a drug dose adjustment has not been ordered when a drug enzyme inducer has been discontinued.
- Recognize drugs of the same category that might have an additive effect. The additive drug effect might be undesirable and could cause a severe physiologic response.
- Notify the health care provider of drugs ordered that have antagonistic or opposite effects, such as beta stimulants and beta blockers.
- Consult a pharmacist about processing through a drug interaction computer program.

CLIENT TEACHING

- Advise clients not to take OTC drug with prescribed drugs without first notifying the health care provider.

EVALUATION

- Evaluate the effectiveness of the drugs and determine that the client is free of side effects.

DRUG-INDUCED PHOTOSENSITIVITY

Photosensitivity is a skin reaction due to exposure to sunlight. It is caused by the interaction of a drug and exposure to ultraviolet A (UVA) light, which can cause cellular damage. Usually, the skin area that is exposed is affected.

Phototoxicity and photoallergy from drug-induced photosensitivity reactions are terms that are used interchangeably. Both are the result of light exposure but differ according to the wavelength of light and the photosensitive drug. Photosensitivity may be the result of the drug dose. The onset of phototoxicity with erythema can be rapid, occurring in 2 to 6 hours of sunlight exposure. Examples of drugs that can induce photosensitivity are presented in Table 6–4.

Most photosensitive reactions can be avoided with the use of sunscreen block (UVA protection) ≥15 and by avoiding excessive sunlight. The higher the drug doses, the more likely that drug-induced photosensitivity will occur. Decreasing drug dose may decrease photosensitivity, if treatment is necessary; discontinuing the drug may be necessary.

TABLE 6–4 Drug-Induced Photosensitivity

Drug Induced	Occurrence
Amantadine	Was confirmed by positive photopatch testing
Amiodarone	Frequency may be 10% to 75%. Sunscreen lotion with UVA can inhibit photosensitivity
Benzodiazepines	Has been reported with drugs alprazolam and chlordiazepoxide
Carbamazepine	Frequency is less than 1%; however, photocopy machines can trigger photosensitivity
Corticosteroids	Was reported with positive photopatch testing and with use of hydrocortisone
Diphenhydramine	Was reported with positive photopatch testing with topical and oral use
Fluorouracil	Avoid sunlight with topical or IV use; erythema and hyperpigmentation could occur
NSAIDs	Aspirin, ibuprofen, and indomethacin have been reported to have low phototoxin effect; however, there is possibility for photosensitive effect with ibuprofen (dose related)
Methotrexate	Avoid sunlight to prevent severe photosensitive reaction (sunburn)
Calcium blockers	Diltiazem: possible phototoxic reaction Nifedipine: may cause phototoxicity with high drug doses
Phenothiazines·	Reported cases of phototoxic reaction with chlorpromazine and other phenothiazines at high drug doses
Piroxicam	Was confirmed with positive photopatch testing; photosensitive reaction occurs after few days of piroxicam and exposure to sunlight
Pyrazinamide	Skin color may change to reddish-brown; usually occurrence is dose-related
Quinolones (Fluorquinolones)	Phototoxicity occurs with lomefloxacin enoxacin, ofloxacin, and nalidixic acid; ciprofloxacin causes less photosensitivity
Sulfonamides	Photosensitive reaction has been reported
Sulfonylureas	Photosensitive reaction has been reported
Tetracyclines	Highly photosensitive; demeclocycline and doxycycline have a higher degree of photosensitive reaction than minocycline
Thiazines	Thiazide-induced photosensitivity has been reported; hydrochlorothiazide has a greater photosensitivity than bendroflumethiazide
Triamterene	Was confirmed by positive photopatch testing
Trimethoprim	Photosensitivity has been reported
Vinblastine	Photosensitivity of drug has been reported

Key: NSAIDs: nonsteroidal antiinflammatory drugs.

DRUG ABUSE

The definition of drug (or substance) abuse can differ among socioeconomic, ethnic, and cultural groups. It is not the misuse of drugs such as self-medicating with OTC drugs or taking prescription drugs other than as prescribed; sometimes, however, drug misuse could result in drug abuse. A broad definition of **drug abuse** is excessive self-administration of a drug that could result in **addiction** (physical dependence) and that could be detrimental to the individual's health. Some health professionals might find exceptions even with this broad definition.

A terminally ill cancer patient who takes large doses of opiates to control pain is not considered to be abusing drugs; however, an otherwise healthy person self-administering large doses of opiates is. Two major substance abuse problems today are the use of alcohol and nicotine (cigarette smoking). Ingesting an ounce or two of alcohol daily or weekly may not be considered a drug abuse problem by some, but in certain cultures and religions it could be.

Some of the categories of abused drugs include (1) central nervous system (CNS) depressants (such as alcohol, marijuana, narcotics [opiates]), analgesics (such as pentazocine [Talwin]), sedatives and hypnotics, antipsychotics, and antianxiety drugs; (2) CNS stimulants (such as cocaine, amphetamines, caffeine); and (3) mind-altering or "psychedelic" drugs (such as lysergic acid diethylamide [LSD] and mescaline). Prescribed large doses of an antipsychotic drug to maintain well-being is not considered drug abuse. The Controlled Substances Act of 1970 set regulations for use of narcotics, such as record keeping. This act has been a help in reducing and detecting drug abuse.

With drug abuse, addiction frequently occurs and is a serious physical and behavioral problem. Characteristics of **addiction** include compulsive drug use, drug craving, and drug seeking. Addiction is physical dependence. **Withdrawal** is the physical effects, such as nausea and convulsions, that result when the drug is discontinued.

Psychological dependence, or **habituation,** is an intense desire or craving for the drug when it is not available. The person does not experience any physical or withdrawal effects. If the drug has been stopped and the psychological need is strong, the use of the drug could be reactivated by the abuser, initiating the cycle of drug abuse.

CHEMICAL IMPAIRMENT IN NURSES

Of the 2.4 million nurses in the United States, it is estimated that 40,000 to 80,000 are chemically impaired; 20% may be chemically dependent. This problem frequently carries a stigma and is characterized by denial by the nurse.

The impaired nurse (1) is usually an adult at the onset of addiction, (2) most commonly initiates the behavior as an escape from life's problems, (3) is seldom "mainlining" the drug(s), and (4) continues to work. Indeed, chemically impaired nurses are considered to be capable and respected by their colleagues. Risk factors for drug abuse among nurses include overwork, chronic fatigue, physical illness, marital problems, insomnia, pending retirement, professional dissatisfaction, and the availability of drugs.

Evidence of impaired practice may involve behaviors related to the effects of the drug while under its influence and while in a state of withdrawal. Signs and symptoms depend on the particular drug being abused. Drug diversion (deliberate redirecting of a drug from a client or facility to the employee for his or her own or other use) is frequently a behavior of chemically impaired nurses. The most commonly abused chemicals include alcohol, meperidine (Demerol), oxycodone (Percodan), diazepam (Valium), alprazolam (Xanax), and flurazepam (Dalmane).

As a rule, coworkers and employers ignore or miss cues for some time about the abuse behaviors. Managers often fail to address the problem, and when they do, it is in a detrimental way.

Society generally and the health professions specifically are shifting their perspective on the chemical impairment of nurses from one of being a moral weakness to that of being a disease. This shift has facilitated the development of prevention and treatment programs. Education intervention can take many formats or directions; for example, incorporation of content on chemical impairment in the curricula of all nursing and staff development programs and the preparation of nurse specialists in addiction nursing.

Abbott (1987) outlines three approaches taken in the workplace when a chemically impaired nurse is identified: (1) administrative—involving dismissal, (2) enforcement—involving referral to narcotics division and being treated like a criminal, and (3) cooperative—involving support and treatment. There is no agreement about how to deal with chemical abuse that is acceptable both personally and institutionally.

The tragedy of allowing a treatable disease to go untreated is very costly in both human and economic terms. La Godna and Hendrix (1989) noted that the partial approximate cost of identifying an impaired nurse and filing a complaint to a board of nursing was $55,000, and it was a $32,000 economic loss to the identified nurse. Human costs may include a lowered self-esteem for both the impaired nurse and the informant, shame, and guilt. There may also be a loss of life. Boards of nursing have developed nondisciplinary programs to assist the impaired nurse and to protect the public safety. Some state nurses' associations offer support services.

The following questions pose many ethical dilemmas: What is the role of the regulatory board? Should the impaired nurse be reported? Whose responsibility is it to report the nurse? Should licenses be suspended or revoked when there is impaired practice?

It is incumbent on each and every nurse to know the rules and regulations of the state nurse practice act and its abuse component. Forty-eight state nurses' associations have peer assistance programs (PAPs) that provide one or all of the following services: information, referral, consultation, support groups, reentry, and monitoring. PAPs advocate that colleagues are more apt to report an impaired nurse if they know that help, rather than discipline, is the result.

NURSING PROCESS: DRUG ABUSE

ASSESSMENT

- Assess behavioral changes, such as lethargy or combativeness, that may suggest drug abuse.

POTENTIAL NURSING DIAGNOSIS

- Situational low self-esteem related to personal problems.

PLANNING

- Person will become aware of drug habit and seek professional help.

NURSING INTERVENTIONS

- Notify the charge nurse or health care provider if client has been receiving drugs, such as narcotics or hypnotics, over a long period of time, possibly resulting in drug abuse.
- Observe the client for physical withdrawal symptoms when a drug that creates physical dependence is discontinued. A mild symptom may be nausea, and severe symptoms include hallucination and convulsions.

CLIENT TEACHING

- Encourage the client to seek professional help in alleviating the drug habit.

- Encourage the family to be supportive of the client at all times.
- Encourage any health professional to seek help if a drug problem is suspected. Protecting a fellow employee or health professional suspected of drug abuse or drug diversion may result in serious complications for the individual and the nurse.
- Remind the client that professionals have a responsibility to protect public safety and health.

EVALUATION

- Evaluate the effectiveness of identifying individuals who need professional help for their substance abuse and make appropriate reports and referrals.

STUDY QUESTIONS

1. What is the meaning and importance of drug interaction?

2. What are the four pharmacokinetic processes related to drug interaction? Describe each process.
3. What are the three main effects associated with pharmacodynamic interaction?
4. What are the effects of drugs in food interactions? What are the implications for your nursing practice?
5. Define drug-induced photosensitivity. What are five drugs or drug groups that are attributed to photosensitivity?
6. Define the following: drug abuse, drug misuse, addiction, physical dependence, and psychological dependence. What is potential effect of each on your practice?
7. Which drugs are frequently associated with drug abuse? For what reasons?
8. List factors that contribute to chemical impairment in nurses.
9. Cite resources available to assist chemically impaired nurses. What rights do they have under most nurse practice acts?
10. What would you do if you discovered a peer taking drugs that he or she obtained illegally from the institution?

Chapter 7

Drug Therapy Considerations Throughout the Life Span

OUTLINE

Objectives
Terms
General Introduction
Pediatric Pharmacology
   Introduction
   Pharmacokinetics

Pharmacodynamics
   Nursing Process: Pediatrics
Geriatric Pharmacology
   Introduction
   Physiologic Changes
   Pharmacokinetics

Pharmacodynamics
Selected Drug Groups That
   Affect the Older Adult
Noncompliance
Nursing Process: Geriatrics
Study Questions

OBJECTIVES

Apply principles of pharmacokinetics of children to drug dosage and dosing interval.

Explain drug dosage parameters for children and where dose ranges can be found.

Explain the pharmacokinetics of the older adult (elderly) related to drug dosage.

List reasons for noncompliance to drug regimen in the older adult.

Give nursing implications related to drug therapy in children and the older adult.

TERMS

compliance
noncompliance

older adult
pharmacodynamics

pharmacokinetics

GENERAL INTRODUCTION

Drug dosages are adjusted according to the client's age, weight, serum protein, and adipose tissue. Change in drug therapy is needed for low-birth-weight infants, newborns, infants, and older adults. A client's body water, fat, and protein are factors that need to be considered when determining drug dosage for the young and the old. Because of immature organs (infants) and declining organ functions (older adult), the effect of drug therapy should be closely monitored in order to prevent the risk of adverse reactions to drugs and possible drug toxicity.

Drug therapy changes throughout the life span, beginning with the infant and continuing through to the frail older adult. Traditionally, drug therapy focused on the middle-aged adult, but today emphasis needs to be placed on the growing population of older adults. This chapter describes the physiologic changes, pharmacokinetics, and pharmacodynamics for drug therapy, bearing in mind these two ends of the continuum.

PEDIATRIC PHARMACOLOGY

INTRODUCTION

The majority of drugs administered to adults are also useful for children; however, the dosages are different. Drug doses for children may be adjusted according to the adult drug dose formula. Usually, a child's dose is calculated according to body weight or body surface area. Children's dosages are based on the maturation of the functions of the body's organs, body weight, and body surface area. Neonates (<1 month old) and infants (1 month to 1 year old) have alkaline gastric juices and an immature liver and kidneys, which cause a decrease in the metabolism and excretion of drugs. The liver and kidneys mature by the age of 1 year, and the pH of gastric juices drops to the normal adult level of pH 1 to 2.5 by the age of 3 years.

There are some drugs used for children with which the drug dosage is based on age. Fluoroquinolones or quinolones are potent antibacterials and should be avoided for children under 17 years of age because of their effect on skeletal bone growth. Verapamil, a calcium channel blocker or antagonist, should not be administered to children under 1 year of age because acute cardiorespiratory failure may occur. Adenosine is considered a safer drug for infants and children than verapamil. Valproic acid, an anticonvulsant, should not be given to a child 2 years of age or younger. Hepatic toxic-

TABLE 7–1 Selected Drugs to Avoid in Children Based on Age

Drug	Age to Avoid Drugs	Possible Effects
Fluoroquinolones	<17 y	Less skeletal bone growth
Verapamil	<1 y	Acute cardiorespiratory failure
Valproic acid	<2 y	Hepatic toxicity

ity is a serious adverse reaction of valproic acid (Table 7–1).

PHARMACOKINETICS

Pharmacokinetics in children differs from that of adults. Selection of drug dose and dosing interval is based on the effects of absorption, blood volume distribution, protein binding, drug metabolism, and drug elimination in children. Table 7–2 identifies the pharmacokinetics in infants and children. Pediatric dose ranges (parameters) have been established for many drugs, and the ranges are reported in drug references such as the *Physician's Desk Reference (PDR)*, *American Hospital Formulary*, and drug handbooks. The nurse should check the dose ranges and specifically question those doses that are outside the range. Body weight and body surface area are the two most commonly used methods for calculating infants' and children's dosages (see Chapter 4C and 4D for drug calculations).

PHARMACODYNAMICS

The immaturity of the organs in newborns and infants affects drug action, and drug dosage frequently needs to be adjusted accordingly. Receptor site sensitivity differs with the neonate, infant, and young child, and so drug dosing may need to be decreased or increased.

Some drugs, such as aspirin, morphine, and phenobarbital, are more toxic to children than to adults. Likewise, other drugs have either the same effect or are less toxic than in adults. These include atropine, codeine, digoxin, meperidine (Demerol), and phenylephrine.

The rapidly developing tissues of infants and small children can be more sensitive to certain drugs. Tetracycline given during the last trimester of pregnancy and through early childhood (to age 8 years), can cause permanent discoloration of the teeth. Corticosteroid therapy given to the young child can result in suppression of growth. The child's height should be measured and his or her weight monitored. A dehydrated child runs the risk of developing toxic accumulations of drugs.

TABLE 7–2 Pharmacokinetics in Infants and Children

Phases	Body Effects and Possible Drug Responses
Absorption	Reduced gastric acid production; gastric pH is higher than in adults. Drugs, such as penicillin, are absorbed poorly in a low gastric pH. Smaller drug dose may be required. Slow gastric emptying time due to a slow or irregular peristalsis may slow drug absorption. Drugs given orally usually take longer to reach peak plasma levels. Adults and older children have a faster absorption rate. First-pass elimination by the liver is reduced. More drug is available for distribution, thus a smaller drug dose is required for those drugs with an extensive hepatic first-pass. Topical drugs may be absorbed faster than in adults because infants have a proportionally greater body surface area. In addition, their skin is thin and drugs pass through more readily. The increased systemic absorption could result in adverse effects. Steroid creams for dermatitis should be used sparingly.
Distribution	Infants and children have lower blood pressure, which affects blood flow to tissues. The liver and brain are proportionally larger and receive more blood flow; the kidneys receive less. Infants are composed of 65% to 75% water; premature infants are 85% water. Water-soluble drugs are diluted in the large volume of their body fluid. Due to drug dilution from the large volume of water, a larger drug dose is needed to achieve the desired plasma drug level. Since infants have decreased plasma protein-binding sites, lower doses are needed. With fewer available binding sites, there is more free drug. The serum albumin level is lower in infants. Protein-binding capacity usually is not the same as adult until age one. Drug doses should be decreased with most antibiotics, including cephalosporins and sulfonamides; as well as with phenobarbital and theophylline. All drugs should be checked for recommended pediatric dose range. The blood–brain barrier is not completely developed in the infant, so more drug passes into the cerebral cells.
Metabolism or biotransformation	There is a decreased activity of liver enzymes due to the immaturity of the infant liver; thus, the hepatic metabolism of drugs in infants is low until the age of one. The half-life of drug may be more prolonged than it would be in an older child or adult; therefore, drug accumulation can occur. Drug dosage and dosing intervals should be considered when drug dosing for infants. Drug half-life in the older child can be shorter due to the increased metabolic rate. Higher doses for the older child might be needed to offset the increased metabolic rate.
Excretion	Drug elimination via the kidneys is decreased until after the first year of life. Blood flow volume through the kidneys is less than in adults, and the glomerular filtration rate is approximately 30% to 40% of the adult rate. A decrease in drug excretion leads to a longer half-life of the drug and possible drug toxicity. Many of the antibiotics and analgesics are slowly excreted. Children have a decreased ability to concentrate urine. Renal excretion of a drug is the net effect of glomerular filtration, active tubular secretion, and passive tubular reabsorption. In the presence of renal disease, a child may be unable to excrete a drug, leading to drug accumulation and possible toxicity. In childhood, the serum creatinine is less than the adult, <0.08l mg/dL. This is because of a lower muscle mass in children. Creatinine clearance test (estimated if necessary) is a better indicator of renal function.

NURSING PROCESS: PEDIATRICS

ASSESSMENT

- Record the height, weight, and age of the child. Drug calculations are based on these three factors.

POTENTIAL NURSING DIAGNOSES

- Altered growth and development
- Altered (possible) tissue perfusion
- Altered patterns of urinary elimination
- Knowledge deficit

PLANNING

- The child receives drug dosage based on age, weight, and height. Most drug calculations for

children are related to weight in kilograms or body surface area (BSA) (see Chapter 4B and 4C).

NURSING INTERVENTIONS

- Use appropriate drug references to obtain the drug parameters or ranges, side effects, and contraindications for use of the drug when administering drugs to children.
- Monitor infants closely for side effects of drugs due to their immature liver and kidneys. Because infants and young children have limited communication skills, changes in their usual behavior pattern may be indicative of side effects.
- Communicate with the health care provider about drug dosages that are questionable for in-

fants because of the drug's prolonged half-life due to decreased drug excretion.
- Calculate the child's drug dose according to weight in kilograms or body surface area.

- Instruct the responsible family member not to give over-the-counter (OTC) drugs to children without asking the health care provider.
- Instruct the family member to report side effects of the medication immediately to the health care provider.
- Advise mothers who are breast feeding their newborn or infant to avoid taking OTC drugs or another person's medication because a portion of most drugs are excreted in breast milk.
- Advise the family member to keep medications out of reach of children.
- Instruct the family member to use child-resistant medication containers.

EVALUATION

- Evaluate the family member's knowledge concerning the drug, drug dosage, schedule for drug administration, and side effects.
- Evaluate child's response to drug regimen physiologically and psychologically.

GERIATRIC PHARMACOLOGY
INTRODUCTION

Twelve percent of the population is represented by persons over 65 years old, but this age group consumes approximately 25% of all medications. It is projected that by the year 2000, older adults will constitute 18% of the population and will consume 40% of all medications.

Approximately 70% of clients over 65 years old take at least one prescribed drug yearly. Older adults take over-the-counter (OTC) drugs more frequently than the general population. About 15% of clients over 65 years old, at the time of hospital admission, are not taking any medications. During hospitalization, older adults take an average of three to five drugs. At the time of discharge from the hospital, approximately 30% of older adults are given three to five drug prescriptions. One-third of clients in nursing homes receive six to 12 drugs daily.

The adverse reactions and drug interactions that occur in the older adult are three to seven times greater than those for middle-aged and young adults. Older adults consume numerous drugs because of chronic and multiple illnesses; they are, therefore, prone to adverse reactions and interactions. Additional problems that can cause adverse reactions from drugs include: self-medication with OTC drugs, taking drugs that were prescribed for other health problems, consuming drugs ordered by several different health care providers, overdosing when symptoms do not subside, using drugs that were prescribed for another person and, of course, the ongoing physiologic aging process.

The older adult may develop drug toxicity for drug doses that are within therapeutic range for the average adult. These therapeutic drug ranges are usually safe for young and middle-aged adults but are not always within safe range for older adults. It has been suggested for the elderly that the drug dose should initially be at a low to low average and then gradually increased according to tolerance and lack of adverse reactions. This allows the older adult to avoid having a toxic reaction to the drug.

PHYSIOLOGIC CHANGES

The physiologic changes associated with the aging process have a major effect on drug therapy. Table 7–3 describes the physiologic changes occurring in the gastrointestinal (GI), cardiac and circulatory, hepatic (liver), and renal (kidney) systems of the older adult and how these changes can affect pharmacologic response to drug therapy.

PHARMACOKINETICS

Pharmacokinetic parameters for the older adult are described in Table 7–4. Drug absorption from the

TABLE 7–3 Physiologic Changes in the Older Adult

System	Physiologic Change
Gastrointestinal	↑ pH (alkaline) gastric secretions ↓ peristalsis with delayed intestinal emptying time
Cardiac and circulatory	↓ cardiac output ↓ blood flow
Hepatic	↓ enzyme function ↓ blood flow
Renal	↓ blood flow ↓ functioning nephrons (kidney cells) ↓ glomerular filtration rate

KEY: ↓: decrease, ↑: increase

TABLE 7–4 Pharmacokinetics in Geriatrics

Phases	Body Effects and Possible Drug Responses
Absorption	A decrease in gastric acidity (increased gastric pH) alters absorption of weak acid drugs, such as aspirin.
	A decrease in blood flow to the gastrointestinal tract (40%–50% less) is due to a decrease in cardiac output. Because of the reduction of blood flow, absorption is slowed but not decreased.
	A reduction in gastrointestinal motility rate (peristalsis) may delay onset of action.
	A reduction in gastric emptying time.
Distribution	Due to a decrease in body water in the older adult, water-soluble drugs are more concentrated. There is an increase in fat-to-water ratio in the older adult; fat-soluble drugs are stored and are likely to accumulate.
	Older adults have a decrease in circulating serum protein. The two most common proteins are albumin and alpha$_1$ acid glycoprotein. Acidic drugs (e.g., nonsteroidal antiinflammatory drugs [NSAIDs] including aspirin, benzodiazepines, phenytoin, and warfarin) bind to albumin, and the basic drugs (e.g., beta-adrenergic blockers, tricyclic antidepressants, lidocaine) bind to alpha$_1$ acid glycoprotein. With fewer protein-binding sites, there is more free drug. It is the free, unbound drug that is available to body tissue at receptor sites.
	Drugs with a high affinity for protein, >90%, compete for protein-binding sites with other drugs. Drug interactions result due to a lack of protein sites and an increase in free drugs.
Metabolism	In the older adult, there is a decrease in hepatic enzyme production, hepatic blood flow, and total liver function. These decreases cause a reduction in drug metabolism.
	With a reduction in metabolic rate, the half-life (t½) of drugs increases, and drug accumulation can result. Metabolism of a drug inactivates the drug and drug metabolite and prepares it for elimination via the kidneys.
	When drug clearance by the liver is decreased, the drug half-life (t½) is prolonged, and when drug clearance is increased, the drug half-life is shortened. With prolonged t½, drug accumulation can result and drug toxicity could occur.
Excretion	The older adult has a decrease in renal blood flow and a decrease in glomerular filtration rate of 40%–50%. With a decrease in renal function, there is a decrease in drug excretion, and drug accumulation results. Drug toxicity should be assessed continually while the client is on the drug.

GI tract is slowed in the older adult because of a decrease in blood flow and decrease in GI motility.

In the older adult, acidic drugs are poorly absorbed due to the alkaline gastric secretions. Drugs remain in the GI tract due to a decrease in gastric motility. Cardiac output and blood flow throughout the circulatory system is decreased, affecting blood flow to the liver and kidneys. After the age of 65 years, nephron function may be decreased by 35%, and after the age of 70 years, blood flow to the kidneys may be decreased by 40%. Liver dysfunction due to the aging process decreases enzyme function, which decreases the liver's ability to metabolize and detoxify drugs, increasing the risk of drug toxicity.

Hepatic blood flow in the older adult may be decreased by 40% to 45%. Also, there is a decrease in liver size with age. Drug clearance by hepatic metabolism is affected more in older adult males than in females.

With liver and kidney dysfunction, the efficacy of a drug dose is usually reduced. Multiple drug use may intensify drug effect in the older adult.

The liver and the kidneys are the two major organs responsible for drug clearance from the body. *Biotransformation* refers to drug metabolism that occurs in the liver (hepatic cells) and contributes to the clearance of drugs. Biotransformation can occur either in phase I by oxidation reaction or in phase II by conjugation reaction. The hepatic microsomal enzymes are responsible for phase I, oxidation reaction. The hepatic microsomal oxidation can be impaired due to aging process, liver diseases (cirrhosis, hepatitis), and drugs that reduce oxidation capability. Drug clearance by the liver is then reduced. An example of a drug that undergoes a phase I biotransformation oxidation reaction is diazepam (Valium). Diazepam is biotransformed to its active metabolites, desmethyldiazepam. In the elderly, the plasma–serum diazepam level would remain high because of an impaired phase I oxidation reaction. Other drugs that are biotransformated by phase I include barbiturates, codeine, ibuprofen, phenytoin, meperidine, lidocaine, certain benzodiazepines (alprazolam, flurazepam, midazolam, prazepam), and warfarin (Coumadin).

Phase II of biotransformation involves the conjugation or attachment of the drug to an inactive state. The hepatic conjugation is usually *not* influenced by older age, liver diseases, or drug interaction, so the drug is inactivated and excreted in the urine. Examples of drugs that are biotransformed or metabolized by phase II are aspirin, acetaminophen, certain benzodiazepines (lorazepam, oxazepam, temazepam), procainamide, and sulfanil-amide. The benzodiazepines lorazepam, oxazepam, and temazepam that undergo conjugation reaction do not have active metabolites. The drug metabolic process, phase I or II, for drug clearance for the elderly client is an important consideration with drug selection.

To assess liver function, the liver enzymes need to be checked. Elevated levels indicate possible liver dysfunction. However, normal liver enzyme results may not indicate normal drug metabolism. The elderly could have normal liver function test results and still have impaired hepatic microsomal enzyme–drug oxidation reactions.

When the efficiency of the hepatic and renal systems are reduced, the half-life of the drug is prolonged and drug toxicity is probable. The nurse needs to assess kidney function by monitoring urine output, laboratory values of blood urea nitrogen (BUN) and serum creatinine (Cr), and the creatinine clearance (Cl_{cr} or CrCl) test (estimated). Creatinine clearance is an indicator of glomerular filtration rate (GFR). To evaluate renal function based on serum creatinine alone may not be accurate for the elderly because of the decrease in the elderly's muscle mass. Creatinine is a byproduct of muscle catabolism; however, creatinine is primarily excreted by the kidneys. A decrease in muscle mass can cause a decrease in serum creatinine. With the elderly clients, serum creatinine may be within normal values because of lack of muscle mass, but still there could be a decrease in renal function. With the young or middle-aged adult, serum creatinine would be increased with a decrease in renal function.

The 24-hour creatinine clearance test and the serum creatinine level should be used to evaluate renal function. If a 24-hour creatinine clearance (Cl_{cr}, CrCl) test is not feasible, there are formulas that can be used to estimate Cl_{cr} result such as:

$$Cl_{cr} \text{(males)} = \frac{(140 - age) \times kg}{72 \times serum\ Cr\ level} = mL/min$$

$$Cl_{cr} \text{(females)} = \text{value of males} \times 0.85 = mL/min$$

The normal creatinine clearance value for an adult is 80 to 130 mL/min.

Factors contributing to adverse reactions in the older adult include a loss of protein-binding sites, which increases the amount of free circulating drug; a decline in hepatic first-pass metabolism; and a prolonged half-life of the drug due to decreased liver and kidney function. The time interval between doses of a drug may need to be increased for the older client. Assessment for adverse effects should be an ongoing process when caring for the older adult.

PHARMACODYNAMICS

Pharmacodynamics refers to how a drug interacts at the receptor site or at the target organ. Because there is a lack of affinity to receptor sites throughout the body in the older adult, the pharmacodynamic response may be altered. The older adult could be more or less sensitive to drug action because of age-related changes in the central nervous system, changes in the number of drug receptors, and changes in the affinity of receptors to drugs. Frequently, the drug dose needs to be lowered. Changes in organ functions are important to consider in drug dosing.

With the older adult, the compensatory response to physiologic changes is decreased. When a drug with vasodilator properties is administered and the sympathetic feedback does not occur quickly, orthostatic hypotension (rapid drop in blood pressure when standing up quickly) could result. In the younger adult, the sympathetic response of vasoconstriction "kicks in" to avert a severe hypotensive effect.

SELECTED DRUGS THAT AFFECT THE OLDER ADULT

Hypnotics, diuretics and antihypertensives, cardiac glycosides, anticoagulants, antibacterials (antibiotics), GI drugs (antiulcer, laxatives), antidepressants, and narcotic analgesics are drug categories that can have a drug effect on the elderly. The number of drugs taken, drug interactions (see Chapter 6), and physical health of the elderly (cardiac, renal, and hepatic function) are factors that cause drug effects in the elderly population. Drug selection is extremely important. Drugs with a shorter half-life are less likely to cause problems due to drug accumulation than drugs with a long half-life. If severe side effects occur, the drug with a shorter half-life will be eliminated more quickly than the drug with a longer half-life.

Drugs that are classified as phase II biotransformation are tolerated and eliminated more quickly than those that are from phase I (oxidation). If phase I drugs are used, the drug selection should be from those agents that have fewer active metabolites. Evaluation of hepatic and renal functions is imperative, especially if the older adult is taking multiple drugs. When side effects and adverse reactions occur, prescription and nonprescription drugs should be assessed.

Hypnotics

Insomnia is a frequently occurring problem for the older adult. Sedatives/hypnotics are the second most common group of drugs prescribed or taken OTC. Insomnia may be described as having difficulty in falling asleep, frequent awakenings during the night, or early morning awakenings with difficulty in falling back to sleep. Types of hypnotics differ according to the cause of insomnia. There are five benzodiazepine hypnotics (flurazepam, quazepam, temazepam, triazolam, and estazolam) that have been approved by the Food and Drug Administration (FDA) as hypnotics to control insomnia. For the elderly client, low doses of benzodiazepines with short or immediate action or half-lives usually are prescribed. Short-term therapy is suggested. Usually, benzodiazepines are prescribed at higher doses for sedative/hypnotic effects and at lower doses for the antianxiety effect. Approximately 35% of the older adult population takes a hypnotic.

Flurazepam HCl (Dalmane), the first benzodiazepine hypnotic, was introduced in 1970. It has three metabolites; thus, it is considered to be a short- and long-acting hypnotic. Its principal metabolite is desalkylflurazepam, which is long-acting, has a long half-life, and is slowly eliminated. This drug is not suggested for those over 65 years old. Drug hangover is a problem. Quazepam (Doral) has similar effects as flurazepam. It is a precursor of desalkylflurazepam and has a prolonged half-life.

Temazepam (Restoril) was introduced in 1981. It is biotransformed in the liver by conjugation and not by oxidation; thus, it is prescribed frequently for the elderly client. Its principal metabolite, glucuronide, is conjugated with no pharmacologic effects and is excreted in the urine. Temazepam is slowly absorbed, so it should be taken 1 to 2 h before bedtime. It is classified as an intermediate-acting benzodiazepine. Food delays its action. Temazepam is more effective for frequent awakenings during the night than for those who have a problem falling asleep.

Triazolam (Halcion) is an intermediate-acting benzodiazepine. It has a short half-life and is considered safe for the older adult at low doses (0.0625 to 0.125 mg). It is metabolized by hepatic microsomal oxidation, although the drug does differ from oxidized benzodiazepines. Triazolam helps with falling asleep and it also decreases frequent awakenings during the night. When stopping the drug, doses should be tapered rather than abruptly discontinued in order to avoid rebound insomnia. Estazolam is a new benzodiazepine. It is an intermediate- to long-acting drug. It is metabolized in the liver to two metabolites that are not highly potent.

Other benzodiazepines, lorazepam and oxazepam, can be used for insomnia. These agents have an intermediate half-life and should be taken 1 hour before bedtime. Other benzodiazepines are more effective as anxiolytics than as hypnotics.

Diuretics and Antihypertensives

Diuretics are frequently prescribed for treatment of hypertension or congestive heart failure (CHF). For the older adult, the dose is usually reduced because of dose-related side effects. Hydrochlorothiazide (HydroDIURIL) is prescribed in low doses of 12.5 mg. Doses of 25 to 50 mg daily with chronic use can cause electrolyte imbalances (hypokalemia, hyponatremia, hypomagnesemia, hypercalcemia), hyperglycemia, hyperuricemia, and hypercholesterolemia.

Many older adults are hypertensive (blood pressure >140/90 mmHg). Nonpharmacologic methods are suggested (see Chapter 34), such as exercise, weight reduction if obese, reduction of salt intake and alcohol, and adequate rest. It could reduce the systolic and diastolic pressures by 8 to 10 mmHg. Drugs such as diuretics, beta-adrenergic blockers or antagonists, calcium channel blockers, angiotensin-converting (ACE) inhibitors, and centrally acting alpha$_2$ agonists are used as antihypertensive drugs. Calcium blockers and ACE inhibitors are frequently the agents of choice because of their low incidence of electrolyte imbalance and CNS side effects. Usually antihypertensive dosing for the elderly begins with reduced doses that are gradually increased according to need, tolerance, and adverse reactions. Alpha$_1$ blockers or antagonists (prazosin, terazosin) and centrally acting alpha$_2$ agonists (methyldopa, clonidine, guanabenz, guanfacine) infrequently are prescribed for elderly clients because of their adverse reactions such as orthostatic hypotension.

Cardiac Glycoside

Digoxin is not always prescribed for long-term use because of its narrow therapeutic range (0.5 to 2 ng/mL) and the possibility of digitalis toxicity occurring. It is given for left ventricular failure, chronic atrial fibrillation, and for atrial tachycardia. Its half-life is doubled (70 h) in clients who are >80 years old. Most of the digoxin is eliminated by the kidneys, so a decline in kidney function (decreased GFR) could cause digoxin accumulation. With close monitoring of serum digoxin levels, creatinine clearance test, and vital signs (pulse should *not* be less than 60 bpm), digoxin is considered to be safe for the elderly.

Anticoagulants

Bleeding may occur with chronic use of anticoagulants for elderly clients. Warfarin (Coumadin) is 99% protein-bound; with a decrease in serum albumin, which is common among older adults, there is an increase in free, unbound circulating warfarin. There is a potential risk for bleeding. Elderly clients should have their prothrombin time (PT) or international normalized ratio (INR) checked periodically and the nurse should check for signs of bleeding.

Antibacterials

Penicillins, cephalosporins, tetracyclines, and sulfonamides are considered to be safe for the elderly. If the elderly client has a decrease in renal drug clearance and the drug has a prolonged half-life, there should be a reduction of drug dose. Aminoglycosides, fluoroquinolones (quinolones), and vancomycin are excreted in the urine. These drug agents are not frequently prescribed for clients older than 75 years and, if prescribed, the drug dose is usually reduced.

Gastrointestinal Drugs

Histamine$_2$ (H$_2$) blockers and sucralfate are safer drugs than other antiulcer agents for the treatment of peptic ulcers. Cimetidine (Tagamet) was the first H$_2$ blocker or antagonist and is not suggested for the older adult because of its side effects and multiple drug interactions. Ranitidine, famotidine, and nizatidine should be prescribed for the elderly client instead of cimetidine.

Laxatives are frequently taken by the elderly. In long-term facilities such as nursing homes, 75% of the elderly clients take laxatives on a daily basis. Fluid and electrolyte imbalances may occur with excessive use. Increased GI motility with laxative use could decrease other drug absorptions. Nonpharmacologic measures should be encouraged, such as an increase in fluid intake, consuming fiber foods such as prunes, and exercise.

Antidepressants

The antidepressant drug dose for the older adult is normally 30% to 50% of the dose for the young and middle-aged adults. Drug dose should be gradually increased according to the client's tolerance and the desired therapeutic effect. There should be close monitoring for possible adverse reactions.

The tricyclic antidepressants are effective for the elderly client. They do have anticholinergic properties that can cause the following side effects: dry mouth, tachycardia, constipation, and urinary retention; they also can contribute to narrow-angle glaucoma. Fluoxetine, a bicyclic antidepressant, has fewer side effects than the tricyclics; the side effects are mostly dose-related. The monoamine oxidase (MAO) inhibitors are not often prescribed for the elderly because of their adverse reactions, such as drug–food interactions, which could result in hypertensive crisis and severe orthostatic hypotension (see Chapter 16).

Narcotic Analgesics

Narcotics when taken by the older adult can cause dose-related adverse reactions. Hypotension and respiratory depression may result from narcotic use. Close monitoring of vital signs is important while the elderly client is taking narcotic analgesics.

NONCOMPLIANCE

Noncompliance with a drug regimen is a problem in all client categories, but especially with the older adult. Frequently, the older adult fails to ask questions during interactions with health care providers. Noncompliance can cause underdosing or overdosing that could be harmful to the elderly client's health. Some of the reasons for noncompliance are listed in Table 7–5.

Working with the older adult is an ongoing nursing responsibility. The nurse should plan strategies with the older adult and family or friends to alleviate these potential problems. Daily contact with the client may be necessary at first. Mere ordering of medication does not mean that the client is able to get the drugs or is taking them correctly. Older adults many times do not have the insurance to pay for medications and choose buying food instead of medications. Some older adults will delay purchasing or never purchase the drugs. The older adult is more apt to experience serious side effects from drug administration than the young or middle-aged adult. If a drug such as ibuprofen (Motrin) is irritating to the GI tract, the older adult frequently will *not* take the drug. However, another drug, such as magnesium hydroxide (Maalox), may be given prior to the ibuprofen dose to decrease the side effects. Food can also decrease gastric irritation from ibuprofen.

TABLE 7–5 Noncompliance to Drug Regimen in the Older Adult

Causes	Nursing Actions
Taking too many medications at different times	Develop a chart indicating times to take drugs. Provide space to place a mark for each drug taken. Use an organizer device to mark with days and weeks.
Failure to understand the purpose or reason for drug	Explain the purpose, drug action, and importance of the medications. Provide time for questions and reinforcement. Reinforce with written information.
Impaired memory	Encourage family members or friends to monitor drug regimen.
Decreased mobility and dexterity	Advise family members or friends to have drugs and water or other fluid accessible. Assist older adult as needed.
Visual and hearing disturbances	Suggest eye and ear examinations (glasses or hearing aids).
Diminished finances	Contact the social services department of your institution.
Child-resistant drug bottles	Ensure that client has access to medications as appropriate.
Side effects or adverse reactions from the drug.	Educate client and family about side effects to report to health care provider.

NURSING PROCESS: GERIATRICS

ASSESSMENT

Assess the older adult's sensorium or mental awareness. Is the person confused or disoriented? Is this state transitory?

Obtain a history of kidney, liver, or GI disorder, and determine if eyesight is failing. Kidney or liver disorders can cause a decrease in the function of these organs and can increase the half-life of drugs. Longer drug half-life and frequent drug dosing can result in drug toxicity. Assess the older adult's use of eyeglasses and check the date of the last eye examination.

Determine if the older person is taking OTC drugs, how often, and for what length of time. Specifically ask about laxatives and antacids, which can affect gastric pH, electrolyte balance, and GI motility; many people do not think of these agents as drugs. Remind the older adult or the family to tell the pharmacist about prescribed drugs when contemplating the purchase of OTC preparations.

Assess for compliance of taking drugs correctly and reasons for noncompliance.

POTENTIAL NURSING DIAGNOSES

- Perceived constipation
- Urinary retention related to drug therapy
- Nutrition, altered: less than body requirements
- Altered health maintenance
- Knowledge deficit
- Noncompliance

PLANNING

- The older adult will take the prescribed medications as ordered.
- The drug therapy will be effective with no or few side effects.

NURSING INTERVENTIONS

- Monitor the older adult's laboratory results in relationship to kidney and liver function. Are the BUN and serum creatinine levels within normal range (reference values)? Are the liver enzymes within normal range? Discuss the findings with the health care provider.
- Check the older adult's serum drug levels as ordered and report abnormal findings to the charge nurse or health care provider. Because of their reduced body water, elderly persons taking water-soluble drugs such as digoxin are likely to have higher blood levels.
- Communicate with the pharmacist or health care provider when the drug dose is in question. Check drug reference books for recommended drug doses for older adults.
- Observe the client for adverse reactions when multiple drugs are being taken. An older adult with hypertension and a failing heart (CHF) might be taking a diuretic (hydrochlorothiazide [HydroDIURIL]) and digoxin. The diuretic may cause potassium loss and, if potassium replacement is not ordered, digitalis toxicity may occur. Hypokalemia (low serum potassium) enhances the action of digoxin, causing the

toxicity. The symptoms of digitalis toxicity may be a slow or irregular pulse rate (bradycardia, <60 bpm), nausea and vomiting, and blurred vision.

- Recognize a change in usual behavior or an increase in confusion associated with the drug regimen. Report these changes to the nurse or health care provider. In the elderly, who have possible decreases in cognitive ability, drug reactions and side effects may be difficult to detect. Communication skills may be poor.

CLIENT TEACHING

- Review the medications with the older adult and the family, including the reason for the medication, its route of administration, how often it is to be taken, common side effects, and when to notify the health care provider.

- Explain to the older adult or the family the importance of compliance with the drug regimen. Emphasize taking the drug as prescribed, discarding unused or old drugs, and keeping a record of medication taken for reference. Remember: the drugs are the property of the client and may not be disposed of without his or her permission.
- Be available to answer the client's questions. Be supportive of the older adult and the family. Discuss problems related to the medications.

EVALUATION

- Evaluate the older adult's compliance to the drug regimen, and answer any questions the older adult may have.
- Evaluate the drug effect and the lack of side effects or adverse reactions.

STUDY QUESTIONS

1. Are infants and children small adults? Explain. What are drug dose parameters for children and where can that information be obtained?
2. If a water-soluble drug is given to an infant, should the drug dose be increased or decreased? Explain.
3. Do infants have an increased or decreased number of protein-binding sites? When giving a drug that is highly protein-bound, would there be less or more free drug available? Explain.
4. Growing tissue in infants and small children can be more sensitive to certain drugs. With that in mind,
   a. What effect do corticosteroids have on infants?
   b. What effect does tetracycline have on children under 8 years old?
5. Explain the following pharmacokinetics related to children and drug therapy:
   a. Gastric emptying time
   b. Protein-binding sites
   c. Liver function
   d. Kidney function
6. Explain the following pharmacokinetics related to older adults and drug therapy:
   a. GI absorption
   b. Body water and water-soluble drugs
   c. Fat-soluble drugs
   d. Effect of liver function and metabolism on half-life
   e. Renal function
7. Noncompliance to the drug regimen is common in the older adult. Give reasons for the noncompliance. What are some nursing measures that might help to improve drug regimen compliance?
8. Cite major differences between children and adults that affect drug therapy.
9. Cite major factors that influence the effect of drugs on older adults.

Chapter 8

The Role of the Nurse in Drug Research

OUTLINE

Objectives
Terms
Introduction
Basic Ethical Principles
    Respect for Person
    Beneficence
    Justice

Informed Consent
Risk-to-Benefit Ratio
Objectives and Phases of Human Clinical Experimentation
    Preclinical Testing
    Human Clinical Experimentation

Study Designs
Nursing Process: Clinical Drug Trials
Recently Approved Drugs
Study Questions

OBJECTIVES

Identify basic ethical principles

Relate three basic ethical principles governing informed consent and risk-to-benefit ratio

Describe the objectives of each phase of human clinical experimentation

Describe the role of the nurse in clinical drug trials using the nursing process

TERMS

beneficence
control group
double-blind

experimental group
informed consent
open-label study

placebo
single-blind
triple-blind

INTRODUCTION

We often hear news broadcasts or read headlines announcing a new drug for the treatment of acquired immunodeficiency syndrome (AIDS) or multiple sclerosis, or transplants to be released, an increase in a drug company's research and development budget, Food and Drug Administration (FDA) approval granted for promising drugs, or similar pharmacology-related news. Such news items signal increasing awareness of the importance of drug research.

Drug research and development is a complex process and one of interest and importance to professional nursing practice. The nursing process facilitates the integration of cutting-edge research.

This chapter is devoted to a description of basic ethical principles governing informed consent and risk-to-benefit ratio; preclinical testing and human clinical experimentation; and the role of the nurse in clinical drug trials using the nursing process.

BASIC ETHICAL PRINCIPLES

Three basic ethical principles are relevant to research involving human subjects: (1) respect for persons, (2) beneficence, and (3) justice.

RESPECT FOR PERSON

Individuals being treated in any health care system should be treated as independent persons who are capable of making decisions in their own interest. Individuals whose decision-making capability is diminished are entitled to protection. The nurse can determine this with consistent reassessment of the client's cognitive state. Clients should be made aware of the alternatives available to them in their health care, as well as the consequences that flow from those alternatives. Furthermore, the client's choice should be honored whenever possible. It is imperative that the nurse recognize when the client is not capable of rational decision making and is therefore entitled to protection.

BENEFICENCE

Beneficence is the duty to not harm others, to maximize possible benefits, and to minimize possible harm that might occur in research. It is often not possible to know if something is beneficial unless it is tested and individuals have been exposed to the risks. A central question to this issue is: Who makes this decision—the client or those caring for the client?

JUSTICE

The principle of justice in the context of clinical drug trials means that social benefits and burdens can be allocated objectively and that those with equivalent circumstances should be treated equally.

The principles of respect for person, beneficence, and justice are integral to the issues of informed consent and risk-to-benefit ratio in research involving human subjects.

INFORMED CONSENT

Informed consent has dimensions beyond protection of the individual client's choice and includes

1. Promotion of individual autonomy
2. Protection of clients and subjects from harm
3. Avoidance of fraud and duress in health care
4. Encouragement for professionals to scrutinize their efforts in communicating information
5. Promotion of rational decision making among clients
6. Promotion of self-determination as a general social value.

RISK-TO-BENEFIT RATIO

The risk-to-benefit ratio is one of the most complex problems faced by the researcher. All possible consequences of a clinical study must be analyzed and balanced with the inherent risks and the anticipated benefits. Physical, psychological, and social risks must be identified and weighed against the benefits. A requirement of the Department of Health and Human Services (DHHS) is that institutional review boards (IRBs) determine that "risks to subjects are reasonable in relation to anticipated benefits, if any, to subjects" (DHHS, 1981). No matter how noble the intentions, the calculation of risks and benefits by the researcher cannot be totally accurate or comprehensive.

Varying amounts of time are required for the process of identifying a potentially useful chemical and having it become available to the general population; in many cases, 10 years may elapse. It is noteworthy that only 1 in 10,000 potential drugs

TABLE 8–1 Basic Sequence of the Development of a New Drug

Identification of potentially clinically useful chemical
Preclinical testing
Study designs
Human clinical experimentation
   Phase I
   Phase II
   Phases III and IV

---

survives the research and development process and is used in the clinical situation. Table 8–1 lists the basic sequence of the development of a new drug.

OBJECTIVES AND PHASES OF HUMAN CLINICAL EXPERIMENTATION
PRECLINICAL TESTING

Preclinical testing consists of in vitro and in vivo systems. In vitro experimentation is generally conducted in a test tube or other laboratory equipment, and in vivo testing is conducted using living organisms. This testing is followed by toxicity screening for the purposes of identifying abnormal changes in animal organs related to drug administration and the parameters of the safe therapeutic dose. Control and experimental groups of animals are compared. Participants in the **experimental group** receive the experimental intervention or treatment. Those in the **control group** do not receive the experimental intervention or treatment and provide a baseline against which to measure the effects of the treatment. Prior to initiating human studies, an assessment is made of the seriousness of the disease to be treated using this drug in relation to the drug's toxicity.

HUMAN CLINICAL EXPERIMENTATION

Clinical experimentation in drug research and development encompasses four phases, each with its own objectives. A brief description of each phase follows.

Phase I

The objectives of phase I are to determine the human dosage range based on response in healthy human subjects and to identify the pharmacokinetics (absorption, distribution, metabolism/biotransformation, excretion/elimination) of the drug. Progression to the next phase occurs if there are no serious adverse effects demonstrated, the drug is eliminated in a reasonable amount of time, and the dose range is below that known to induce pathology in animals.

Phase II

The objective of phase II is to demonstrate the safety and efficacy of the drug in subjects ($N = 100$) who have the disease that the drug is designed to treat. A multidisciplinary team approach (nurses, physicians, pharmacologists, statisticians, and research associates) is required to ensure data collection that will answer the clinical questions. Phase III is initiated only when acceptable efficacy and safety data are generated and clearly documented.

Phases III and IV

The objectives of phases III and IV are to demonstrate the safety and efficacy of the drug for a wide client population and to include long-term data if a chronic regimen is under consideration. The sponsor submits all relevant and analyzed data in a new drug application (NDA) to the FDA. In time, the FDA decides to approve, reject, or recommend withdrawal or resubmission. After the NDA research has been approved, phase IV addresses the long-term use of the drug.

STUDY DESIGNS

An experimental design is required to determine cause and effect questions about the safety and efficacy of a drug. The experimental design must demonstrate that the researcher controls the method of treatment, uses different groups of subjects—some that receive treatment and control groups that receive no treatment or an alternative method of treatment—and assigns subjects randomly to treatment or control groups.

The following examples illustrate selected research designs.

A *descriptive* design would be a chart review of all clients hospitalized at University Hospital in 1995 who received digoxin. In this situation, there is no control group, random assignment, or researcher manipulation of the treatment.

A *quasi-experimental* design would be comparison of intermittent IV device patency of those hospitalized clients who received heparin flushes and those who received saline flushes. This study has a nonmatched comparison group, but had no random assignment to treatment group. Such quasi-experimental designs may contribute valuable information but lack the power to ascribe cause because the variables are uncontrolled and potentially influential. Ethical decisions do not permit the use of the experimental design in all situations. For example, an experimental study to determine if nicotine causes cancer would be unethical because individuals would have to be exposed to a carcinogenic substance.

The researcher designs the study to show the effect of the independent variable (the drug) on the dependent variables (clinical responses or reactions). Intervening variables are specific to the research question and may include age, sex, weight, disease and its state of severity, diet, and the subject's social environment. Controlled treatment groups in drug research trials can receive no drug, a different drug, a **placebo** (pharmacologically inert substance), or the same drug with a different dose, route, or frequency of administration.

A *crossover* design uses each subject in several different situations. In the first instance, the experimental group receives the drug and the control group receives an alternative form of treatment or no treatment. Then both groups receive no therapy. Finally, the experimental group receives the control form of therapy and the control group receives the drug. In this design, the subject serves as his or her own control.

The researcher wants to be able to generalize the findings from the sample of subjects to the larger target population, such as all women with breast cancer. A statistical method called probability sampling (subjects are randomly selected from the entire population) is recommended to provide relative confidence in the generalization of findings.

Various designs and techniques assist the researcher in reaching valid and generalizable conclusions. In a *matched-pair* design, the researcher identifies several variables that may influence the outcome, such as age, weight, or family history; then the subjects are matched for these variables. One of the pair is randomly assigned to the experimental group and the other to the control group. A less effective technique is nonrandom assignment to treatment group.

The **double-blind** technique is a powerful tool wherein neither the health care provider nor subject knows whether the subject is receiving the experimental or control form of therapy. In **triple-blind** studies, a researcher other than the prescribing health care provider collects data and is also unaware of the subject's treatment group. In a **single-blind** study, only the subject is unaware of which group he or she is assigned to. An **open-label study** indicates that all parties—data collectors, prescribing health care provider, and subject—know the treatment group assignment. The double-blind and triple-blind techniques are preferred for drug research because those involved in the study are not aware of the subject's treatment group, thereby removing a source of bias.

NURSING PROCESS: CLINICAL DRUG TRIALS

ASSESSMENT

- Explore own beliefs about clinical trials.
- Recruit subjects.
- Assess subjects.
- Assess protocol.
- Demonstrate thorough knowledge of all inclusion/exclusion criteria for subjects (Table 8–2).
- Articulate observations and concerns to health care providers, sponsors, and pharmaceutical company.

TABLE 8–2 Inclusion–Exclusion Criteria for a Hypothetical Protocol for an Experimental Diuretic Medication

Inclusion

Males and females between the ages of 18 and 65 years
Weight between 50 and 100 kg
Subjects receiving cardiac medications only if dose has been stable for past 3 months
Subjects on sodium-restricted diet

Exclusion

Pregnant or nursing females
All females in childbearing years not responsibly using birth control pill
Severe damage or disease of cardiac, hepatic, renal, neurologic, or musculoskeletal system
Clinically significant laboratory values

- Communicate need for drug to address a specific need with the appropriate individuals.

PLANNING

- Develop fact sheet of protocol guidelines.
- Educate involved staff about protocol requirements.
- Provide input into budget negotiations.
- Coordinate personnel and budget, including office visits, special tests, and laboratory work.
- Ensure that subject consent is informed (Table 8–3).
- Respond to subject's questions.

TABLE 8–3 Informed Consent Checklist

Client participation is voluntary
Identifies related drugs, treatments, and techniques
Describes benefits and risks
Describes laboratory tests to monitor client's reactions
Identifies extent of confidentiality of results
Describes availability of emergency treatment for illness/injury, if any
States compensation for study-related injury, if any
States compensation for participation, if any
Consent is written clearly and understood easily at the 10th grade reading level
Provides name and telephone number of contact person for client questions and concerns

NURSING INTERVENTIONS

- Screen subjects accurately and thoroughly based on established protocol.
- Adhere to protocol guidelines, including administration of drug.
- Monitor selected parameters. Observe and report toxicities promptly.
- Collect all data required by the sponsor (e.g., drug company).
- Communicate information in a complete, concise, accurate, and timely manner to the principal investigator and sponsor.
- Document data in a clear and timely manner.
- Record subjects' own evaluation; *seemingly unrelated responses may be significant.* At times a drug is actually marketed for a different indication than the original testing.
- Report *all* deaths to physician, sponsor, IRB, and FDA, whether or not the cause of death is drug-related.

EVALUATION

- Consider the clarity of the research statement.
- Determine if the research design is appropriate to answer research question(s).
- Evaluate subject selection; for example, in an experimental design, were subjects randomly selected and randomly assigned? Were intervening variables identified and used when a matched-pair design was used?
- Determine the validity and reliability of measurement instruments.
- Are the actual sample and the target population comparable?
- Are the conclusions valid and based on data?
- Are the clinical findings significant?

The nurse has a pivotal role in drug clinical trials. The research and development process for drug research requires the multifaceted roles of professional nursing practice. The nurse is both the client/family advocate and liaison between the client, health care provider, and research nurse responsible for the specific protocol. Nursing involvement is essential to the successful completion of clinical trials.

RECENTLY APPROVED DRUGS

Recent drug research and development has yielded few amazing cures for disease but has contributed new uses for some old medicines. For example, aspirin was reported to reduce the risk of colon cancer by almost 50%, and low doses of aspirin were found to be as effective as higher doses in preventing strokes. Ticlopidine (Ticlid), a platelet inhibitor, is now available for individuals who cannot tolerate aspirin. Specific dosages of once prescription medications are now available OTC, such as Pepcid AC and Axid AR.

Ondansetron (Zofran) has improved the quality of life for many cancer clients by controlling the nausea often associated with chemotherapy. Additional potential applications for Zofran include treatment of schizophrenia, anxiety, memory impairment, or alcohol and drug abuse. Zofran's claim to fame is its ability to modulate reaction to serotonin, a brain chemical.

Withdrawal from nicotine has been made easier by nicotine skin patches, such as Nicoderm and Habitrol. Individuals who have problems controlling their blood pressure may be aided by ramipril (Altace), fosinopril (Monopril), and felodipine (Plendil). New options for those who suffer with arthritis include etodolac (Lodine) and nabumetone (Relafen). Nabumetone is less likely to cause stomach ulcers. Pravastatin (Pravachol) and simvastatin (Zocor) are used to lower high cholesterol levels. A boon to pediatric medicine is Acel-Imune, a vaccine developed to protect against diphtheria, whooping cough, and tetanus, which is expected to have fewer adverse reactions than the traditional DPT immunization.

Asking relevant questions about informed consent and risk-to-benefit ratio is a major role of the nurse. Awareness of initial indicators of change in the client and prediction of increased risk for adverse drug reaction are also dimensions of professional nursing practice.

STUDY QUESTIONS

1. In what ways are informed consent and risk-to-benefit ratio related to drug research?
2. What are the objectives of the four phases of human experimentation?
3. What are the advantages and disadvantages of the various research designs?
4. What are the implications of clinical drug research for your nursing practice? Apply the nursing process.

Unit III

Nutrition and Electrolytes

The body requires vitamins, minerals, and electrolytes for cellular function. When there is a lack of these chemical components, replacement drug therapy is necessary. With regular nutritional dietary intake, vitamin, mineral, and electrolyte replacements are not needed.

Multiple vitamins have the highest sales volume of any over-the-counter (OTC) drugs. Usually, vitamin replacements are *not* necessary, especially for those who maintain a nutritionally balanced daily diet.

The vitamins discussed in Chapter 9 include the fat-soluble vitamins (vitamins A, D, E, and K) and the water-soluble vitamins (vitamin B complex—B_1, B_2, B_3, and B_6—and C). Iron is the primary mineral described. Other minerals of importance to good nutrition are iodine, copper, manganese, and zinc.

Body electrolytes are plentiful in extracellular fluid, intracellular fluid, and in the gastrointestinal mucosa. The cations (positively charged ions or electrolytes)—potassium (K), sodium (Na), calcium (Ca), and magnesium (Mg)—promote transmission and conduction of nerve impulses, and contractibility of muscles. Inadequate dietary intake and many disease entities contribute to electrolyte imbalances.

Drug replacements for potassium, sodium, calcium, and magnesium are discussed in Chapter 10. Implications for the nursing process are detailed for each of these electrolytes.

Nutritional support is discussed in Chapter 11.

Chapter 9

Vitamin and Mineral Replacement

OUTLINE

Objectives
Terms
Introduction

Vitamins
    Fat-Soluble Vitamins
    Water-Soluble Vitamins
    Nursing Process: Vitamins

Minerals
    Nursing Process: Antianemia,
      Mineral: Iron
Study Questions

OBJECTIVES

List the four groups into which vitamin supplements are divided.

Differentiate between water- and fat-soluble vitamins.

Identify food sources and deficiency conditions associated with each vitamin.

Define the term *recommended dietary allowance* (RDA).

Explain the need for iron and foods that are high in iron content.

Describe the nursing interventions including client teaching related to vitamin and mineral uses.

TERMS

fat-soluble vitamins
iron

megavitamin
minerals

RDA
water-soluble vitamins

INTRODUCTION

This chapter discusses two topics: vitamins and the mineral iron. These substances are needed in correct portions for normal body function. Overuse of vitamins and minerals, particularly fat-soluble vitamins and iron, may lead to vitamin or iron toxicity.

VITAMINS

Vitamins are organic chemicals that are necessary for normal metabolic functions and for tissue growth and healing. Actually, the body only needs a small amount of vitamins daily, which can be easily obtained through one's diet. A well-balanced diet has all the vitamins and minerals needed for body functioning. The intake of vitamins should be increased during periods of rapid body growth, by those who are pregnant or are breastfeeding, by those with a debilitating illness, and by those with inadequate diets, for example, alcoholics and some geriatric clients. Children who have poor nutrient intake or are malnourished may need vitamin replacement. Persons on fad or restrictive diets frequently have vitamin deficiencies.

The sale of vitamins in the United States is a multibillion dollar business. Some people take vitamins to relieve tiredness or to improve general overall health, both of which are inappropriate indications for vitamin therapy. Vitamins are not necessary if the individual consumes a well-balanced daily diet. Vitamin deficiencies can cause cellular and organ dysfunction that may result in a slow recovery from illness. Vitamin supplements are nec-

TABLE 9-1 Justification For Vitamin Supplements

Categories	Deficiencies
Inadequate absorption	Malabsorption, diarrhea, infectious and inflammatory diseases
Inability to utilize vitamins	Liver disease (cirrhosis, hepatitis), renal disease, certain hereditary deficiencies
Increased vitamin losses	Fever from infectious process, hyperthyroidism, hemodialysis, cancer, starvation, crash diets
Increased vitamin requirements	Early childhood, pregnancy, debilitating disease (cancer, alcoholism), gastrointestinal surgery, special diets

essary for the vitamin deficiencies described in Table 9-1, but vitamins frequently are taken prophylactically rather than for therapeutic purposes.

The United States Daily Allowances (USDA) Food Guide Pyramid (Fig. 9-1) provides a guide to daily food choices. Eating a variety of foods and getting the appropriate number of calories and grams of fat for a healthy weight are recommended.

The pyramid recommends the following:

Bread, cereal, rice, and pasta group—6 to 11 servings
Vegetable group—3 to 5 servings
Fruit group—2 to 4 servings
Milk, yogurt, and cheese group—2 to 3 servings
Meat, poultry, fish, dry beans, eggs, and nut group—2 to 3 servings
Fats, oils, and sweets—use sparingly; limit fat to 30% of calories

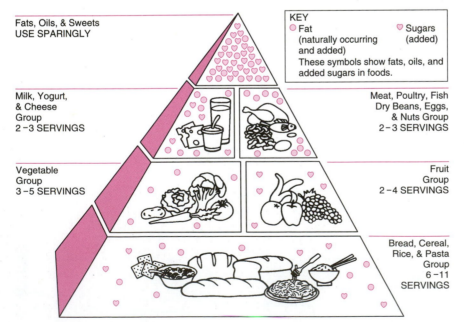

FIGURE 9-1. Food Guide Pyramid. A guide to daily food choices. (Courtesy of USDA's Food Guide Pyramid [1992]. Prepared by Human Nutrition Information Service. Home and Garden Bulletin No. 252. Used with permission.)

The National Academy of Sciences, Food and Nutrition Board, publishes the United States **recommended dietary allowance (RDA)** for daily dose requirements of each vitamin. The Food and Drug Administration (FDA) requires that all vitamin products be labeled according to the amount of vitamin content and the proportion of the RDA the vitamin product provides. Individuals should be encouraged to check the RDA listed on a vitamin container to determine if the product provides the RDA dose requirements. The recommended allowances may need to be modified for clients who are ill.

FAT-SOLUBLE VITAMINS

Vitamins fall into two general categories: fat-soluble and water-soluble. The **fat-soluble vitamins** are A, D, E, and K. They are metabolized slowly, can be stored in fatty tissue, liver, and muscle in significant amounts, and are excreted in the urine at a slow rate. Vitamins A and D are toxic if taken in excess amounts over time. Vitamin A can be stored in the liver for up to 2 years. Vitamins E and K are less toxic than vitamins A and D. Foods rich in vitamin A are fruits, yellow and green vegetables, fish, and dairy products; foods rich in vitamin D are milk, dairy products, and margarine; foods rich in vitamin E are oils, margarine, milk, grains, and meats; and foods rich in vitamin K are green leafy vegetables, meats, eggs, cheese, and milk.

Vitamin A

Vitamin A is essential for the maintenance of epithelial tissues, skin, eyes, hair, and bone growth. It has been used for the treatment of skin disorders such as acne; however, excess doses can be toxic. During pregnancy, excess amounts of vitamin A (>6000 international units [IU]) might have a teratogenic effect (birth defect) on the fetus. Figure 9–2 describes the effects of vitamin A. The nursing process can be applied as the drug data are obtained and the drug is administered.

Pharmacokinetics

When a person is deficient in vitamin A, the vitamin is absorbed faster than if there is no deficiency. Massive doses of vitamin A may cause hypervitaminosis A, symptoms of which are loss of hair and peeling skin.

The RDA for vitamin A supplement is 5000 IU. Excess use of vitamin A should be avoided because this vitamin is stored in the liver, kidneys, and fat and is slowly excreted from the body. Excess vitamin A is stored in the liver for up to 2 years. Vita-

min A toxicity affects multiple organs, especially the liver. The dose for healthy clients should not be greater than 7500 IU in order to prevent the occurrence of vitamin A toxicity.

Mineral oil, cholestyramine, alcohol, and antilipemic drugs decrease the absorption of vitamin A. Vitamin A is excreted through the kidneys and feces.

Pharmacodynamics

Vitamin A is necessary for many biochemical processes. It aids in the formation of the visual pigment needed for night vision, it is needed in bone growth and development, and it promotes the integrity of the mucosal and epithelial tissues.

Vitamin A taken orally begins to take effect in 1 to 2 h and peaks in 4 to 5 h. Its duration of action is unknown. Because vitamin A is stored in the liver, the vitamin may be available to the body for days, weeks, or months.

Vitamin D

Vitamin D has a major role in regulating calcium and phosphorus metabolism and is needed for calcium absorption from the intestines. Dietary vitamin D is absorbed in the small intestine and requires bile salts for absorption. There are two compounds of vitamin D: vitamin D_2, ergocalciferol, a synthetic fortified vitamin D; and vitamin D_3, cholecalciferol, a natural form of vitamin D influenced by ultraviolet sunlight through the skin. Once absorbed, vitamin D is converted to calcifediol in the liver. Calcifediol is then converted to an active form, calcitriol, in the kidneys.

Calcitriol, the active form of vitamin D, functions as a hormone and, with parathyroid hormone (PTH) and calcitonin, regulates calcium and phosphorus metabolism. Calcitriol and PTH stimulate bone reabsorption of calcium and phosphorus. Excretion of vitamin D is primarily in bile; only a small amount is excreted in the urine. If serum calcium levels are low, more vitamin D is activated; when serum calcium levels are normal, activation of vitamin D is decreased.

Excess vitamin D ingestion (>40,000 IU) results in hypervitaminosis D and may cause hypercalcemia (an elevated serum calcium level). Anorexia, nausea, and vomiting are early symptoms of vitamin D toxicity.

Vitamin E

Vitamin E has antioxidant properties that protect cellular components from being oxidized and red

FIGURE 9–2. Vitamin A, Fat-Soluble

Vitamin A	Dosage
Vitamin A (Acon, Aquasol A) Fat-soluble vitamin *Pregnancy Category:* A	A & C > 8 y: PO: 100,000—500,000 IU daily × 3 d; then 50,000 daily × 14 d *Maintenance:* 10,000—20,000 IU q.d. × 60 d C 1–8 y: IM: 17,000—35,000 IU daily × 10 d *Maintenance:* 4–8 y: 15,000 IU daily × 60 d 1– < 4 y: 10,000 IU daily × 60 d

NURSING PROCESS
Assessment and Planning

Contraindications	Drug-Lab-Food Interactions
Hypervitaminosis A, pregnancy (massive doses)	Decreased absorption of mineral oil, cholestyramine, oral contraceptives, corticosteroids

Pharmacokinetics	Pharmacodynamics
Absorption: PO: 1h *Distribution:* PB: UK *Metabolism:* t½: weeks–months *Excretion:* Urine and feces	PO: Onset: 1–2 h Peak: 4–5 h Duration: UK

Interventions

Therapeutic Effects/Uses: To treat vitamin A deficiency, prevent night blindness, treat skin disorders, promote bone development

Mode of action: Essential for growth, bone and teeth development, vision, integrity of skin and mucous membranes, and reproduction

Evaluation

Side Effects	Adverse Reactions
Headache, fatigue, drowsiness, irritability, anorexia, vomiting, diarrhea, dry skin, visual changes	Evident only with toxicity: leukopenia, aplastic anemia, papilledema, increased intracranial pressure, hypervitaminosis A

KEY: A: adult; C: child; <: less than; UK: unknown; PO: by mouth; PB: protein-binding; t½: half-life.

blood cells from hemolysis. Vitamin E depends on bile salts, pancreatic secretion, and fat for its absorption. Vitamin E is stored in all tissues, especially the liver, muscle, and fatty tissue. About 75% is excreted in the bile.

Vitamin K

Vitamin K occurs in four forms; vitamin K_1 (phytonadione) is the most active form, vitamin K_2 (menaquinone) is synthesized by intestinal flora, and vitamin K_3 (menadione) and vitamin K_4 (mena-

diol) have been produced synthetically. Vitamin K_2 is not commercially available. Vitamin K_1 and K_2 are absorbed in the presence of bile salts. Vitamin K_3 and K_4 do not need bile salts for absorption. After vitamin K is absorbed, it is stored primarily in the liver and in other tissues. One-half of vitamin K comes from the intestinal flora and the remaining portion comes from one's diet.

Vitamin K is needed for synthesis of prothrombin and the clotting factors VII, IX, and X. For oral anticoagulant overdose, vitamin K_1 (phytonadione) is the vitamin that is most effective in preventing hemorrhage. The commercial drugs for vitamin K_1 are Mephyton, AquaMEPHYTON, and Konakion, and the commercial drug for vitamin K_4 is Synkayvite.

WATER-SOLUBLE VITAMINS

Water-soluble vitamins are the B-complex vitamins and vitamin C. This group of vitamins is not usually toxic unless taken in extremely excessive amounts. Water-soluble vitamins are not stored by the body and are readily excreted in the urine. Protein-binding of water-soluble vitamins is minimal. Foods that are high in vitamin B are grains, cereal, bread, and meats. Citrus fruits and green vegetables are high in vitamin C.

Vitamin C

Vitamin C (ascorbic acid) is absorbed from the small intestine. Vitamin C aids in the absorption of iron and in the conversion of folic acid. Vitamin C is not stored in the body and is excreted readily in the urine. A high serum vitamin C level that results from excessive dosing of vitamin C is excreted by the kidneys unchanged. Figure 9–3 gives drug information on vitamin C.

Pharmacokinetics

Vitamin C is absorbed readily through the GI tract and is distributed throughout the body fluids. The kidneys completely excrete vitamin C, mostly unchanged.

Pharmacodynamics

Vitamin C is needed for carbohydrate metabolism and protein and lipid synthesis. Collagen synthesis also requires vitamin C for capillary endothelium, connective tissue and tissue repair, and osteoid tissue of the bone.

Large doses of vitamin C may decrease the effect of oral anticoagulants. Oral contraceptives can decrease vitamin C concentration in the body. Smoking decreases serum vitamin C levels.

The use of **megavitamin therapy,** massive doses of vitamins, is questionable at best. Megadoses of vitamins can cause toxicity and might result in minimal desired effect. Most authorities believe that vitamin C does not cure or prevent the common cold; rather, they believe that vitamin C has a placebo effect. Moreover, megadoses of vitamin C taken with aspirin or sulfonamides may cause crystal formation in the urine (crystalluria). Excessive doses of vitamin C can cause a false-negative occult

(blood) stool result and false-positive sugar result in the urine when tested by the Clinitest method. If large doses of megavitamins are to be discontinued, a gradual reduction of dosage is necessary to avoid vitamin deficiency.

Vitamin B Complex

Vitamin B_1 (thiamine), vitamin B_2 (riboflavin), vitamin B_3 (nicotinic acid, or niacin), and vitamin B_6 (pyridoxine) are four of the vitamin B complex members. This B-complex group is water-soluble. Thiamine is used to treat peripheral neuritis, which may occur from alcoholism or beriberi. Riboflavin may be given to manage dermatologic problems, such as scaly dermatitis, cracked corners of the mouth, and inflammation of the skin and tongue. Niacin is given to alleviate pellagra and hyperlipidemia, for which large doses are required. However, large doses may cause GI irritation and vasodilation, resulting in a flushing sensation. Pyridoxine is administered to correct vitamin B_6 deficiency. It may also help alleviate the symptoms of neuritis caused by isoniazid (INH) therapy for tuberculosis.

Folic Acid (Folate)

Folic acid is absorbed from the small intestine and the active form of folic acid (folate) is circulated to all tissues. One-third of folate is stored in the liver and the rest is stored in tissues. Four-fifths of folate is excreted in the bile and one-fifth in the urine.

Folic acid is essential for body growth. It is needed for DNA synthesis, and without folic acid there is a disruption in cellular division. Chronic alcoholism, poor nutritional intake, malabsorption syndromes, pregnancy, and drugs that cause inadequate absorption (phenytoin, barbiturates) or folic acid antagonists (methotrexate, triamterene, trimethoprim) are causes of folic acid deficiencies. Symptoms of folic acid deficiencies include anorexia, nausea, stomatitis, diarrhea, fatigue, alopecia, and blood dyscrasias (megaloblastic anemia, leukopenia, and thrombocytopenia). These symptoms are usually not noted for 2 to 4 months after folic acid storage is depleted.

Folic acid deficiency during the first trimester of pregnancy can affect the development of the central nervous system (CNS) of the fetus. This may cause spina bifida, defective closure of the bony structure of the spinal cord, or anencephaly, lack of brain mass formation. It is imperative that the pregnant woman take adequate folic acid supplements, 400 μg/day, starting with the first trimester of preg-

FIGURE 9–3. The Water-Soluble Vitamin: Vitamin C

Vitamin C	Dosage	NURSING PROCESS
		Assessment and Planning
Vitamin C, Ascorbic Acid (Ascorbicap, Cecon, Cevalin, Solucap C) ❦ Apo-C, Ce-Vi-Sol, Redoxon *Pregnancy Category: C*	*Prophylactic:* A: PO: 45–60 mg/d C: PO: 20–50 mg/d *Severe deficit:* Scurvy A: PO: IM: IV: 150–500 mg/d in 1 to 2 divided doses C: PO: IM: IV: 100–300 mg/d in 1 to 2 divided doses *Pregnancy and Lactation:* A: PO: 60–80 mg/d	

Contraindications	Drug–Lab–Food Interactions	
Caution: Renal calculi, gout, anemia: sickle cell, sideroblastic, thalassemia	Decreased ascorbic acid uptake taken with salicylates; may decrease effect of oral anticoagulants; may decrease elimination of aspirins	

Pharmacokinetics	Pharmacodynamics	
		Interventions
Absorption: PO: quickly *Distribution:* PB: UK *Metabolism:* t½: UK *Excretion:* In the urine; unchanged with high doses	PO: Onset: > 2d Peak: UK Duration: UK	

Therapeutic Effects/Uses: To prevent and treat vitamin C deficiency (scurvy); increase wound healing; for burns

Mode of Action: A water-soluble vitamin, essential for collagen formation and tissue repair (bones, skin, blood vessels)

Evaluation

Side Effects	Adverse Reactions
Headaches, fatigue, drowsiness, nausea, heartburn, vomiting, diarrhea	Kidney stones, crystalluria, hyperuricemia *Life-threatening:* sickle cell crisis, deep vein thrombosis

KEY: A: adult; C: child; PO: by mouth; PB: protein-binding; t½: half-life; UK: unknown; >: greater than; ❦: Canadian drug names.

nancy in order to prevent the development of CNS anomalies.

Vitamin B$_{12}$

Vitamin B$_{12}$, like folic acid, is essential for DNA synthesis. Vitamin B$_{12}$ aids in the conversion of folic acid to its active form. With active folic acid, vitamin B$_{12}$ promotes cellular division. It is also needed for normal hematopoiesis (development of red blood cells in bone marrow) and to maintain nervous system integrity, especially the myelin.

The gastric parietal cells produce an intrinsic factor that is necessary for the absorption of vitamin B$_{12}$ through the intestinal wall. Without the intrinsic factor, little or no vitamin B$_{12}$ is absorbed. After absorption, vitamin B$_{12}$ binds to the protein transcobalamin II and is transferred to the tissues. Most vitamin B$_{12}$ is stored in the liver. Vitamin B$_{12}$

is slowly excreted, and it can take 2 to 3 years for stored vitamin B$_{12}$ to be depleted and a deficit noticed.

Vitamin B$_{12}$ deficiency is uncommon unless there is a disturbance of the intrinsic factor and intestinal absorption. Pernicious anemia (lack of the intrinsic factor) is the major cause of vitamin B$_{12}$ deficiency. Strict vegetarians who do not consume meat, fish, or dairy products can develop vitamin B$_{12}$ deficiency. Other possible causes of vitamin B$_{12}$ deficiency include malabsorption syndromes (cancer, celiac disease, certain drugs), gastrectomy, Crohn's disease, and liver and kidney diseases. Symptoms may include numbness and tingling in the lower extremities, weakness, fatigue, anorexia, loss of taste, diarrhea, memory loss, mood changes, dementia, psychosis, and megaloblastic anemia with macrocytes (overenlarged erythrocytes [RBC]) in blood, and megaloblasts (overenlarged erythroblasts) in the bone marrow.

To correct vitamin B$_{12}$ deficiency, cyanocobalamin in crystalline form can be given for severe deficits intramuscularly. It cannot be given intravenously because of possible hypersensitive reactions. It also can be given orally and is found in multiple vitamin preparations.

Table 9–2 lists both the fat-soluble and water-soluble vitamins with their functions, suggested food sources, and selected deficiency conditions. Table 9–3 lists fat- and water-soluble vitamins, their RDA values, dosages for vitamin deficiencies, and therapeutic serum blood or urine ranges.

NURSING PROCESS: VITAMINS

ASSESSMENT

- Assess the client for vitamin deficiency before start of and regularly throughout therapy. Explore such areas as inadequate nutrient intake, debilitating disease, and GI disorders.
- Assess 24- and 48-h diet history.

POTENTIAL NURSING DIAGNOSES

- Altered nutrition; less than body requirements

PLANNING

- Client will eat a well-balanced diet that includes the foods and servings recommended in the food pyramid.
- Client with vitamin deficiency will take vitamin supplements as prescribed.

NURSING INTERVENTIONS

- Administer vitamins with food to promote absorption.
- Store drug in light-resistant container.
- When administering vitamins in drop form, use the supplied calibrated dropper for accurate dosage. Solution may be administered mixed with food or dropped into the mouth.
- Administer IM primarily for clients unable to take by PO route (e.g., GI malabsorption syndrome).
- Recognize need for vitamin E supplements for infants receiving vitamin A to avoid hemolytic anemia.

General
- Instruct client to take the prescribed amount of drug.
- Discourage the client from taking megavitamins over a long period unless these are prescribed for a specific purpose by the health care provider. To discontinue long-term megavitamin therapy, a gradual decrease in vitamin intake is advised to avoid a vitamin deficiency. Megadoses of vitamins can be toxic.
- Inform the client that missing vitamins for 1 or 2 days is not a cause for concern because deficiencies do not occur for some time.
- Advise the client to check the expiration dates on vitamin containers before purchasing and taking them. Potency of the vitamin is reduced after the expiration date.
- Instruct the client to avoid taking mineral oil with vitamin A on a regular basis because it interferes with the absorption of the vitamin. If needed, take mineral oil at bedtime.
- Explain to the client that there is no scientific evidence that megadoses of vitamin C (ascorbic acid) will cure a cold.
- Alert the client not to take megadoses of vitamin C with aspirin or sulfonamides since crystals may form in the kidneys and urine.
- Instruct the client to avoid excessive intake of alcoholic beverages. Alcohol can cause vitamin B-complex deficiencies.

Diet
- Advise the client to eat a well-balanced diet that includes the recommended amounts and types of

food detailed in the food pyramid. Vitamin supplements are not necessary if the person is healthy and receives proper nutrition on a regular basis.

- Instruct the client about foods rich in vitamin A, including whole milk, butter, eggs, leafy green and yellow vegetables, fruits, and liver. Foods rich in other vitamins can be found in Table 9–2.

Side Effects

- Instruct the client that nausea, vomiting, headache, loss of hair, and cracked lips (symptoms of hypervitaminosis A) should be reported to the health care provider. Early symptoms of hypervitaminosis D are anorexia, nausea, and vomiting.

EVALUATION

- Evaluate the effectiveness of the client's diet for the inclusion of the appropriate amounts and types of food from the food pyramid. Have the client keep periodic diet chart for a complete week.
- Determine if the client with malnutrition is receiving appropriate vitamin therapy.

TABLE 9–2 Vitamins: Functions, Suggested Food Sources, and Selected Deficiency Conditions

Vitamin	Function	Food Sources	Deficiency Conditions
A	Required to develop and maintain healthy eyes, gums, teeth, skin, hair, and selected glands. Needed for fat metabolism.	Whole milk, butter, eggs, leafy green and yellow vegetables and fruits*, liver	Dry skin, poor tooth development, night blindness
B_1 (thiamine)	Promotes use of sugars (energy). Required for good function of nervous system and heart.	Enriched breads and cereals, yeast, liver, pork, fish, milk	Sensory disturbances, retarded growth, fatigue, anorexia
B_2 (riboflavin)	Promotes body's use of carbohydrates, proteins and fats by releasing energy to cells. Required for tissue integrity.	Milk, enriched breads and cereals, liver, lean meat, eggs, leafy green vegetables†	Visual defects, such as blurred vision and photophobia; cheilosis; rash on nose; numbness of extremities
B_6 (pyridoxine)	Important in metabolism, synthesis of proteins, and formation of red blood cells.	Lean meat, leafy green vegetables, whole-grain cereals, yeast, bananas	Neuritis, convulsions, dermatitis, anemia, lymphopenia
B_{12} (cobalamin)	Functions as a building block of nucleic acids and to form red blood cells. Facilitates functioning of nervous system.	Liver, kidney, fish, milk	Gastrointestinal disorders, poor growth, anemias
Folic acid	Helps in formation of genetic materials and proteins for the cell nucleus. Assists with intestinal functioning and prevents selected anemias.	Leafy green vegetables, yellow fruits and vegetables, yeast, meats	Decreased WBC count and clotting factors, anemias, intestinal disturbances, depression
Pantothenic acid	Promotes body's use of carbohydrates, fats, and proteins. Essential for formation of specific hormones and nerve-regulating substances.	Eggs, leafy green vegetables, nuts, liver, kidney, skimmed milk	Natural deficiency unknown in man
Niacin	In all body tissues. Necessary for energy-producing reactions. Assists nervous system.	Eggs, meat, liver, beans, peas, enriched bread, and cereals	Retarded growth, pellagra, headache, memory loss, anorexia, insomnia
Biotin	Synthesis of fatty acids and energy production from glucose. Required by body chemical systems.	Eggs, milk, leafy green vegetables, liver, kidney	Natural deficiency unknown in man
C (ascorbic acid)	Helps tissue repair and growth. Required in formation of collagen.	Citrus fruits, tomatoes, leafy green vegetables, potatoes	Poor wound healing, bleeding gums, scurvy, predisposition to infection
D (calciferol)	Promotes use of phosphorus and calcium. Important for strong teeth and bones.	Vitamin-D fortified milk, egg yolk, tuna, salmon	Rickets, deficit of phosphorus and calcium in blood
E	Protects fatty acids and promotes the formation and functioning of red blood cells, muscle, and other tissues.	Whole-grain cereals, wheat germ, vegetable oils, lettuce, sunflower seeds	Breakdown of red blood cells
K	Essential for blood clotting.	Leafy green vegetables, liver, cheese, egg yolk	Increased clotting time, leading to increased bleeding and hemorrhage

* Yellow fruits and vegetables include apricots, cantaloupe, carrots, rutabaga, pumpkin, squash, and sweet potatoes.
† Leafy green vegetables include Brussels sprouts, chard, broccoli, kale, spinach, and turnip and mustard greens.

TABLE 9–3 Fat- and Water-Soluble Vitamins: RDA, Dosages for Vitamin Deficiencies, and Therapeutic Ranges

Vitamin	RDA	Dosages for Vitamin Deficiencies	Therapeutic Ranges
Fat-Soluble			
Vitamin A	Male: 1000 μg or 5000 IU Female: 800 μg or 4000 IU Preg: 1000 μg, 5000 IU Lact: 1200 μg, 6000 IU	10,000–20,000 IU or 3000–6000 μg/dL	30–70 μg/dL Deficit: < 20 μg/dL
Vitamin D	Male and Female: 40–80 μg; 200–400 IU	Mild: 50–125 μg/dL Moderate to severe: 2.5–7.5 mg/d; 2500–7500 μg	Unknown
Vitamin E	Male: 10 mg/d; 15 IU Female: 8 mg/d; 12 IU Preg: 10–12 mg/d	Malabsorption: 30–100 mg/d Severe deficit: 1–2 mg/kg/d or 50–200 IU/kg/d	0.5–0.7 mg/dL Deficit: < 0.5 mg/dL
Vitamin K	Male: 70–80 μg/d Female: 60–65 μg/d Taking broad–spectrum antibiotic: 140 μg/d Preg: 65 μg/d	5–15 mg/d	Based on prothrombin time (PT) results
Water-Soluble			
Vitamin C	Male and Female: 60 mg/d Preg: 70 mg/dL Lact: 95 mg/dL	150–300 mg *Burns:* 500–2000 mg/d	Serum: > 1.30 mg/dL WBC: > 15 mg/dL *Deficit:* Serum < 0.2 mg/dL WBC; < 7 mg/dL
Vitamin B₁ (thiamine)	Male: 1.5 mg Female: 1.1 mg Preg: 1.5 mg Lact: 1.6 mg	30–60 mg/d	Urine: < 50 μg/d
Vitamin B₂ (riboflavin)	Male: 1.4–1.7 mg Female: 1.2–1.3 mg Preg: 1.6 mg Lact: 1.8 mg	5–25 mg/d Prophylactic: 3 mg/d	Urine: < 50 μg/d
Vitamin B₃ (nicotinic acid or niacin)	Male: 15–19 mg/d Female: 13–15 mg/d Preg: 18 mg/d Lact: 20 mg/d	Prevention: 5–20 mg/d Deficit: 50–100 mg/d Pellagra: 300–500 mg in 3 divided doses Hyperlipidemia: 1–2 g/d in 3 divided doses	Unknown
Vitamin B₆ (pyridoxine)	Male: 2.0 mg/d Female: 1.6 mg/d Preg: 2.1 mg/d Lact: 2.2 mg/d	25–100 mg/d *Isoniazid Therapy Prophylaxis* 25–50 mg/d *Peripheral Neuritis* 50–200 mg/d	Serum: > 50 ng/mL Urine: < 1.0 mg/d
Folic acid (folate)	Male and Female: 400 μg/d Preg: 600–800 μg/d Lact: 600–800 μg/d	1–2 mg/d	Serum folate: 6–20 ng/mL RBC: 160–600 ng/mL *Deficit:* Serum: < 3–4 ng/mL RBC: < 140 ng/mL
Vitamin B₁₂	Male and Female: 3 μg/d Preg: 4 μg/d	100 mg/dL 14 d *Pernicious Anemia:* 50–100 μg/d or 1000 μg/wk × 3 wk	150–900 pg/mL *Deficit:* < 100 pg/mL *Schilling test* > 30% normal

KEY: Preg: pregnancy; Lact: lactation; d: day; wk: week; >: greater than; <: less than.

MINERALS

Various **minerals,** such as iron, copper, and zinc, are needed for body function, but **iron** (ferrous sulfate, gluconate, or fumarate) is vital for hemoglobin regeneration. Sixty percent of the iron in the body is found in hemoglobin. One of the causes of anemias is iron deficiency. A normal diet contains 5 to 20 mg of iron per day. Foods rich in iron include liver, lean meats, egg yolks, dried beans, green vegetables (such as spinach), and fruit. Food and antacids slow the absorption of iron, and vitamin C increases iron absorption.

During pregnancy, an increased amount of iron is needed, but during the first trimester of pregnancy, megadoses of iron are contraindicated because of its possible teratogenic effect on the fetus. Larger doses of iron are required during the second and third trimesters of pregnancy.

The infant and child dose of iron, ages 6 months to 2 years old, is 1.5 mg/kg. For the adult, 50 mg/day is needed for hemoglobin regeneration. The ferrous sulfate tablet is 325 mg, of which 65 mg is elemental iron. Therefore, one tablet of ferrous sulfate is sufficient as a daily iron dose when indicated. Figure 9–4 describes the effects of iron preparations.

PHARMACOKINETICS

Iron is absorbed by the intestines and goes into the plasma as heme, or it may be stored as ferritin. Although food decreases absorption by 25 to 50%, it may be necessary to take iron preparations with food to avoid GI discomfort. Vitamin C may slightly increase iron absorption, whereas tetracycline and antacids can decrease absorption.

PHARMACODYNAMICS

Iron replacement primarily is given to correct or control iron-deficiency anemia, which is diagnosed by a laboratory blood smear. Positive findings for this anemia are microcytic (small), hypochromic (pale) erythrocytes (red blood cells [RBC]). Clinical signs and symptoms include fatigue, weakness, shortness of breath, pallor and, in cases of severe anemia, increased GI bleeding. The dosage of ferrous sulfate for prophylactic use is 300 to 325 mg/day; for therapeutic use, the dosage is 600 to 1200 mg/day in divided doses.

The onset of action for iron therapy takes days,

FIGURE 9–4. Antianemia, Mineral: Iron

Iron	Dosage	NURSING PROCESS
Ferrous sulfate (Feosol, Fer-Iron) *Ferrous gluconate* (Fergon, Fetinic) *Ferrous fumarate* (Feostat, Fumerin) Mineral *Pregnancy Category:* A	A: PO: 300–325 mg q.i.d.: increase to 650 mg q.i.d. as needed and/or tolerated *Pregnancy:* PO: 300–600 mg/d C ≥ 2 y: PO 8 mg/kg q.d. in divided doses	Assessment and Planning
Contraindications	**Drug-Lab-Food Interactions**	
Hemolytic anemia, peptic ulcer, ulcerative colitis	*Increased* effect of iron with vitamin C; *decreased* effect of tetracycline, antacids, penicillamine	
Pharmacokinetics	**Pharmacodynamics**	Interventions
Absorption: PO: 5–30% intestines *Distribution:* PB: UK *Metabolism:* t½: UK *Excretion:* Urine, feces, bile	PO: Onset: 4 d Peak: 7–14 d Duration: 3–4 mon	
Therapeutic Effects/Uses: To prevent and treat iron deficiency anemia *Mode of Action:* Enables RBC development and oxygen transport via hemoglobin		Evaluations
Side Effects	**Adverse Reactions**	
Nausea, vomiting, diarrhea, constipation, epigastric pain; elixir may stain teeth	Pallor, drowsiness *Life-Threatening:* Cardiovascular collapse, metabolic acidosis	

KEY: A: adult; C: child; PO: by mouth; PB: protein-binding; t½: half-life; UK: unknown; ≥: equal to or greater than.

and its peak action does not occur for days or weeks; therefore, the client's symptoms are slow to improve. Increased hemoglobin and hematocrit levels occur within 3 to 7 days.

Iron toxicity is a serious cause of poisoning in children. As few as 10 tablets of ferrous sulfate (3 g) taken at one time can be fatal within 12 to 48 h. The child can hemorrhage because of the ulcerogenic effects of unbound iron, causing shock. Parents should be cautioned against leaving iron tablets that look like candy (M & M's) within a child's reach.

NURSING PROCESS: ANTIANEMIA, MINERAL: Iron

ASSESSMENT

- Obtain a history of anemia or health problems that may lead to anemia.
- Assess the client for signs and symptoms of iron deficiency anemia, such as fatigue, malaise, pallor, shortness of breath, tachycardia, and cardiac dysrhythmia.
- Assess the client's RBC count, hemoglobin, hematocrit, iron level, and reticulocyte count before start of and throughout drug therapy.

POTENTIAL NURSING DIAGNOSES

- Fatigue
- Altered nutrition; less than body requirements

PLANNING

- Client will consume foods rich in iron.
- Client with iron deficiency anemia or with low hemoglobin will take iron replacement as recommended by the health care provider, resulting in laboratory results within the desired range.

NURSING INTERVENTIONS

- Encourage the client to eat a nutritious diet to obtain sufficient iron. Iron supplements are not needed unless the person is malnourished, pregnant, or has abnormal menses.
- Store drug in light-resistant container.
- Administer IM injection of iron by the Z-track method to avoid leakage of iron into the subcutaneous tissue and skin because it irritates and stains the skin.

CLIENT TEACHING

General
- Instruct the client to take the tablet or capsule between meals with at least 8 oz of juice or water to promote absorption. If gastric irritation occurs, instruct to take with food.
- Advise client to swallow whole the tablet or capsule.

- Instruct client to maintain sitting upright position for 30 min to prevent esophageal corrosion from reflux.
- Do not administer the drug within 1 h of ingesting antacid, milk, ice cream, or other milk products like pudding.
- Advise client to increase fluids, activity, and dietary bulk to avoid or relieve constipation. Slow-release iron capsules decrease constipation and gastric irritation.
- Instruct adults not to leave iron tablets within reach of children. If a child swallows many tablets, induce vomiting and immediately call the local poison control center; the telephone number is in the front of most telephone books (include this number on emergency reference list). Keep ipecac available; it is an OTC drug.
- Instruct client to take prescribed amount of drug to avoid iron poisoning.
- Be alert that iron content varies among iron salts; therefore, do not substitute one for another.
- Advise client that drug treatment for anemia is generally less than 6 mon.

Diet
- Counsel the client to include iron-rich foods in diet, such as liver, lean meats, egg yolk, dried beans, green vegetables, and fruit.

Side Effects
- Instruct the client taking the liquid iron preparation to use a straw to prevent discoloration of teeth enamel.
- Alert the client that the drug turns stools a harmless black or dark green.
- Instruct client about signs and symptoms of toxicity, including nausea, vomiting, diarrhea, pallor, hematemesis, shock, and coma, and report occurrence to health care provider.

EVALUATION

- Evaluate the effectiveness of the drug therapy by determining that the client is not fatigued or short of breath and that the hemoglobin is within the desired range.

STUDY QUESTIONS

1. Vitamin A is classified in what vitamin category? What foods are high in vitamin A? How does vitamin A differ from vitamin C?
2. What are the nursing interventions when megadoses of vitamins are discontinued?
3. Why is vitamin D important? Which is the most active form of vitamin K? Where is this vitamin stored in the body?
4. What is the approved use of vitamin C (ascorbic acid)? What is the nonapproved use of the drug?

5. What are the common names of vitamins B_1, B_2, B_3, and B_6? What are the uses of these vitamin B-complex drugs?
6. How are folic acid and vitamin B_{12} similar? Why is folic acid important during the first trimester of pregnancy?
7. What is the most common cause of vitamin B_{12} deficiency? Explain.
8. List three nursing interventions and client teaching guides for clients receiving iron preparations. High doses of ferrous sulfate can result in what condition?

Chapter 10

Fluid and Electrolyte Replacement

OUTLINE

Objectives
Terms
Introduction
Body Fluids
Fluid Replacement
    Intravenous Solutions
    Nursing Process: Fluid Replacement

Electrolytes
    Potassium
    Sodium
    Calcium
    Magnesium

Case Study
Study Questions

OBJECTIVES

Define osmolality; and iso-osmolar, hypo-osmolar, and hyperosmolar intravenous fluids.

Give the iso-osmolality range for serum and intravenous solutions.

Describe the four classifications of intravenous fluids.

Differentiate between cations and anions of electrolytes.

List the major functions of cations.

List examples of oral potassium supplements.

Explain the methods for correcting potassium excess.

Describe several signs and symptoms of hypokalemia, hyperkalemia, hyponatremia, hypernatremia, hypocalcemia, and hypercalcemia.

Explain the pharmacokinetics and pharmacodynamics of oral and intravenous potassium chloride.

Describe the assessments, nursing interventions and client teaching for fluid, potassium, and calcium imbalances.

TERMS

anion	hypermagnesemia	hypomagnesemia
cation	hypernatremia	hyponatremia
electrolytes	hyperosmolar	hypo-osmolar
hypercalcemia	hypocalcemia	iso-osmolar
hyperkalemia	hypokalemia	osmolality

INTRODUCTION

Fluid replacement is based on body fluid needs. The adult body is approximately 60% water, the human embryo is 97% water, and the newborn infant is 77% water. Of the 60% adult body water (fluid), 40% of the body fluid is the intracellular fluid (cells) and 20% of the body fluid is the extracellular fluid, of which 15% is interstitial (tissue) fluid and 5% is intravascular or vascular fluid (Table 10–1).

Electrolytes in the body are substances that carry either a positive charge **(cation)** or a negative charge **(anion).** The cations and the anions are described in Table 10–2. The functions of cations are the transmission of nerve impulses to muscles and the contraction of skeletal and smooth muscles.

The cations of the electrolytes are most plentiful in the cells (potassium, magnesium, and some calcium), in the extracellular fluids (ECF) that is within the blood vessels and tissue spaces (sodium and some calcium), and in the gastrointestinal (GI) tract. Anions are attached to cations. Figure 10–1 illustrates those electrolytes that are plentiful in the stomach and in the intestines.

Fluid and electrolyte replacements based on fluid and specific electrolyte deficits and excesses are described in this chapter.

BODY FLUIDS

The concentration of body fluid is described as **osmolality** and osmolarity; these terms are frequently used interchangeably. Osmolality is the osmotic pull exerted by all particles (solutes) per unit of water, expressed as osmols or milliosmols per kilogram (mOsm/kg) of water. There are three types of fluid concentration based on the osmolality of body fluids: **iso-osmolar** (isotonic) fluid, which has the same proportion of weight of particles (e.g., sodium, glucose, urea, protein) and water; **hypo-osmolar** (hypotonic) fluid, which has fewer particles than water; and **hyperosmolar** (hypertonic) fluid, which has more particles than water. The plasma/serum osmolality (concentration of circulating body fluids) can be calculated if the serum sodium level is known or the sodium, glucose, and

TABLE 10–2 Cations and Anions

Cations	Anions
Potassium (K^+)	Chloride (Cl^-)
Sodium (Na^+)	Bicarbonate (HCO_3^-)
Calcium (Ca^{++})	Phosphate (PO_4^-)
Magnesium (Mg^{++})	Sulfate (SO_4^{--})

blood urea nitrogen (BUN) levels are known. Sodium is the main extracellular electrolyte and its major function is to regulate body fluids. The two formulas used for estimating serum osmolality are:

1) Double the serum sodium (Na) =

serum osmolality

2) $2 \times \text{serum Na} + \dfrac{BUN}{3} + \dfrac{Glucose}{18} =$

serum osmolatity

The second formula is more accurate in estimating the correct serum osmolality.

Normal serum osmolality is 275 to 295 mOsm/kg. If the serum osmolality is less than 275 mOsm/kg, the body fluid is hypo-osmolar (fewer particles than water); if the serum osmolality is greater than 295 mOsm/kg, the body fluid is hyperosmolar (more particles and less water). Hypo-osmolality of body fluid may be the result of excess water intake or fluid overload (edema) due to an inability to excrete excess water. Hyperosmolality of body fluid could be caused by severe diarrhea, increased salt and solutes (protein) intake, inadequate water intake, diabetes acidosis, or sweating.

FLUID REPLACEMENT
INTRAVENOUS SOLUTIONS

With fluid volume deficit from the extracellular body compartment, there is a loss of fluid from the interstitial (tissue) spaces and from the vascular (blood vessel) spaces. Intravenous (IV) fluids in various concentrations are available for replacing body fluid loss. The osmolalities of many IV fluids are similar to serum osmolality, with the exception that the osmolality of solutions is wider. The average serum osmolality is 290 mOsm/kg. For an IV solution, the iso-osmolar range is 240 to 340 mOsm/L. This is determined by using a factor of 50: subtract 50 from 290 mOsm to equal 240 and add 50 to 290 to equal 340. If the IV solution is <240 mOsm, it is a hypo-osmolar solution; if it is >340 mOsm, it is a hyperosmolar solution. Iso-osmolar solutions include dextrose 5% in water

TABLE 10–1 Body Fluid Volume

Fluid Compartment		Percent
Intracellular (cellular) fluid (ICF)		40
Extracellular fluid (ECF)		20
Interstitial fluid (tissue spaces)	15%	
Intravascular fluid (vascular fluid)	5%	
Total body fluid		60

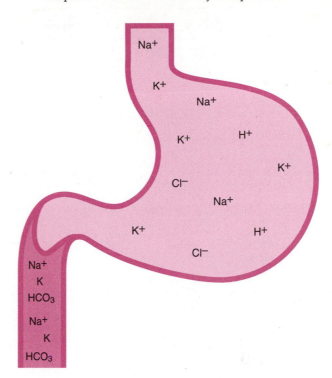

FIGURE 10–1. The electrolytes that are plentiful in the gastrointestinal tract are potassium (K), sodium (Na), hydrogen (H), bicarbonate (HCO_3), and chloride (Cl).

(D_5W), which has 250 mOsm; normal saline solution or 0.9% NaCl (sodium chloride), which has 310 mOsm; lactated Ringer's solution, which has 274 mOsm; and Ringer's solution, which has 310 mOsm. These iso-osmolar solutions have osmolalities similar to the extracellular and intracellular fluids. With fluid volume loss, iso-osmolar IV solutions are usually indicated.

Dextrose in water, when used continuously or administered rapidly, becomes a hypo-osmolar solution instead of being iso-osmolar. The dextrose is rapidly metabolized to water and carbon dioxide (CO_2). Five percent dextrose in water (D_5W) should only be given intravenously and never subcutaneously. Normal saline solution or an iso-osmolar solution of dextrose and saline may be administered subcutaneously.

There are four classifications of IV solutions used for fluid replacements: crystalloids, colloids, lipids, and blood and blood products. Crystalloids include dextrose, saline, and lactated Ringer's solutions. This group of solutions is used for replacement and maintenance fluid therapy. Colloids are volume expanders that include dextran solutions, amino acids, hetastarch, and plasmanate. Dextran is not a substitute for whole blood, because it does not have any products that can carry oxygen. Dextran 40 tends to interfere with platelet function and can prolong bleeding time. Dextran 70 tends to coat red blood cells, which makes it difficult to type and cross match blood. Hetastarch is a nonantigenic volume expander and lasts for >24 h, but it may

persist for weeks in the body. Hetastarch is a iso-osmolar solution (310 mOsm/L) that can decrease platelet and hematocrit counts, and is contraindicated for clients with bleeding disorders, congestive heart failure (CHF), and renal dysfunction. Plasmanate is a commercially prepared protein product that is used instead of plasma or albumin to replace body protein.

Blood and blood products are whole blood, packed red blood cells, plasma, and albumin. A unit of packed red blood cells contains whole blood without plasma. The advantages for using packed cells instead of whole blood are that there is a decreased chance for causing circulatory overload, a smaller risk of a reaction to plasma antigens, and a possible reduction in the risk of transmitting serum hepatitis. Whole blood should not be used to correct anemia unless the anemia is severe. A unit of whole blood elevates the hemoglobin by 0.5 to 1.0 g, and a unit of packed red blood cells raises the hematocrit by three points. Lipids are administered as fat emulsion solution and are usually indicated when IV therapy lasts longer than 5 days. Lipids add to balancing the client's nutritional needs. Total parenteral nutrition (TPN) or hyperalimentation is normally implemented for clients who require long-term IV therapy. TPN is discussed in Chapter 11.

Table 10–3 lists various IV solutions in the four classifications according to their osmolality, caloric and electrolyte compositions, and general comments.

TABLE 10–3 Intravenous Solutions

Solutions	Osmolality	Total mOsm	Dextrose mOsm	Na⁺	K⁺	Ca⁺⁺	Cl⁻	Lactate	Comments
Crystalloids									
NaCl 0.45% (sodium chloride)	Hypo	154	—	77	—	—	77	—	Helpful to establish renal function. Not to be used constantly. Could cause water intoxication.
NaCl 0.9%	Iso	310	—	154	—	—	154	—	Normal saline solution. Restores extracellular fluid volume and replaces sodium chloride deficit.
Dextrose 2.5% in 0.45% NaCl	Iso	279	125	77	—	—	77	—	Helpful in establishing renal function–urine output.
Dextrose 5% in 0.2% saline	Iso	326	250	38	—	—	38	—	Useful for daily maintenance of body fluids and when less Na and Cl are required.
Dextrose 5% in 0.33% saline	Hyper/iso	352	250	51	—	—	51	—	Same as above. May be iso-osmolar since dextrose is rapidly metabolized.
Dextrose 5% in 0.45% saline	Hyper	404	250	77	—	—	77	—	Useful for daily maintenance of body fluids and nutrition and for treating fluid volume deficits.
Dextrose 5% in saline 0.9%	Hyper	560	250	154	—	—	154	—	Replacement of fluid, sodium, chloride, and calories.
Dextrose 10% in saline 0.9%	Hyper	810	500	154	—	—	154	—	Replacement of fluid, sodium, chloride, and calories.
Dextrose 5% in water (50 g) (dextrose 10% is occasionally used)	Iso/hypo	250	250	—	—	—	—	—	Helpful in rehydration and elimination. May cause urinary sodium loss. Good vehicle for IV potassium. May be hypo-osmolar since dextrose is rapidly metabolized.
Lactated Ringer's	Iso	274	—	130	4	3	109	28	This solution resembles the electrolyte composition of normal blood serum and plasma. The amount of potassium available is not sufficient for the body's daily potassium requirement.
Dextrose 5% in lactated Ringer's	Hyper	524	250	130	4	3	109	28	Same contents as lactated Ringer's plus calories.
Ringer's solution	Iso	312	—	147	4	5	156	—	Does not contain lactate, which can be harmful to people who cannot metabolize lactic acid.
Dextrose 5% Ringer's solution	Hyper	562	250	147	4	4	156	—	Same contents as Ringer's solution plus calories.
M/6 sodium lactate	Iso	334	—	167	—	—	—	167	Supplies sodium without chloride. Lactate has some caloric value and is metabolized to CO_2 for excretion or increases bicarbonate in alkalosis.
Hyperosmolar saline 3% NaCl	Hyper	990	—	495	—	—	495	—	Helpful for severe hyponatremia by raising Na osmolality of the blood. Helpful in eliminating intracellular fluid excess.
Ionosol B with dextrose 5%	Hyper	—	250	57	25	—	49	25 (also Mg 5 and P 7)	Useful in treating clients requiring polyionic parenteral replacement, e.g., alkalosis due to vomiting, diabetic acidosis, fluid losses due to burns, and postoperative fluid volume deficit.
Ionosol D-CM with dextrose 5%	Hyper	—	250	138	12	5	108	50 (also Mg 3)	Useful for electrolyte replacement of duodenal fluid losses because of intestinal suction or biliary or pancreatic drainage and to correct mild acidosis.

Solutions	Osmolality	Total mOsm	Dextrose mOsm	Na⁺	K⁺	Ca⁺⁺	Mg⁺⁺	Cl⁻	HCO₃	Comments
Isolyte R with 5% dextrose (McGraw)	Hyper	378	250	40	16	5	3	40	24 (acetate)	For maintenance therapy. Contains multiple electrolytes. May be iso-osmolar since dextrose is rapidly metabolized.

TABLE 10–3 Intravenous Solutions *(Continued)*

Solutions	Osmolality	Total mOsm	Dextrose mOsm	Na⁺	K⁺	Ca⁺⁺	Mg⁺⁺	Cl⁻	HCO₃	Comments
Normosol M (Abbott)	Hypo	112	—	40	13	—	3	40	16 (acetate)	For maintenance therapy.
Normosol M with 5% dextrose (Abbott)	Hyper	362	250	40	13		3	40	16 (acetate)	For maintenance therapy. May be iso-osmolar since dextrose is rapidly metabolized.
Normosol R (Abbott)	Iso	296	—	140	5	—	3	98	50	For replacement therapy. Contains multiple electrolytes.
Normosol R with 5% dextrose (Abbott)	Hyper	546	250	140	5	—	3	98	50	Same as above with calories.
Isolyte E	Hyper	568	250	140	10	5	3	103	57	For replacement therapy. Is iso-osmolar without the 5% dextrose.

Solutions	Osmolality	Caloric Value	*mEq/L* (mOsm) Na⁺	K⁺	Cl⁻	Miscellaneous	Comments
Colloids							
Protein Solutions							
Aminosol 5%	Iso	175	<10	17	—*	Amino acids	Provides protein and fluid for body. Prevents shock and promotes wound healing.
Aminosol 5% with dextrose 5%	Hyper	345	<10	17	—	Amino acids	Provides protein, calories, and fluid for body; especially helpful for clients who are old and malnourished and for those with hypoproteinemia due to other causes. Not to be used in severe liver damage.
Plasma Expander							
Dextran 40 10% in normal saline (0.9%) or 5% dextrose in water (500 ml bottle)	Hyper						Dextran is a colloidal solution used to increase plasma volume. Dextran 40 is a short-lived plasma volume expander (4 to 6 hours.) Useful in early shock by correcting hypovolemia, and increasing arterial pressure, pulse pressure, and cardiac output. It improves microcirculatory flow by reducing red blood cell aggregation in the capillaries (increases small vessel perfusion). Caution: It should not be used for clients who are severely dehydrated, have renal disease, have thrombocytopenia, or are actively hemorrhaging.
Dextran 70 6% in normal saline (0.9%) or 5% dextrose in water	Hyper						Dextran 70 is a long-lived plasma volume expander (20 hours). Useful for shock or impending shock due to hemorrhage, surgery, burns. It can interfere with platelet function, thus cause prolonged bleeding. Blood for type and cross-match should be drawn before starting Dextran; it tends to coat RBC.

Solutions	Volume (mL)	Na⁺	K⁺	Cl⁻	Comments
Blood Products					
Whole blood	500–1000	142	5	103	Replacement for blood loss that is greater than 1 liter (2 pints or units). One unit of blood raises the hemoglobin by 0.5–0.75 g/dL.

Table continued on following page

TABLE 10–3 Intravenous Solutions (*Continued*)

Solutions	Volume (mL)	Na$^+$	K$^+$	Cl$^-$	Comments
Packed red blood cells	250	5	20	13	Replacement of blood loss for clients who do not require excess fluid. Prevents overload of fluid for clients with CHF. It minimizes potential risks of viral transmission.
Plasma	250	38	1	25	Volume expander. It does not require type and cross-match.
Albumin (5%–25%)	100	16	0	2	Volume expander. Helps to increase plasma oncotic (osmotic) pressure due to malnutrition, liver disease.
Lipids Fat emulsions (10% & 20%)					Contains soybean or safflower oil and egg phosphotides. Used for prolonged parenteral nutrition to provide essential fatty acids. Avoid for clients with high hyperlipemia. Use cautiously for clients with severe liver or pulmonary disease.

Source: Solution chart reviewed by Abbott Laboratories Clinical Research Associate and Baxter Laboratories Clinical Information Manager. Selected portions from Abbott Laboratories: Wall Chart, Intravenous and Other Solutions, *North Chicago, October 1968; H. Statland:* Fluid and Electrolytes in Practice, *Philadelphia, J. B. Lippincott Co., 1963; McGraw Laboratories:* Guide to Parenteral Fluid Therapy, *CA Glendale, 1963; Travenol Laboratories, Inc.:* Guide to Fluid Therapy, *Deerfield, IN, 1970:* Fluid and Electrolyte Balance, *2nd ed, Philadelphia, J. B. Lippincott Co.; J. L. Kee, B. J. Paulanka:* Fluids and Electrolytes with Clinical Applications, *5th ed, New York, Delmar Publishers, 1994; J. M. Brensilver, E. Goldberger:* A Primer of Water, Electrolyte, and Acid–Base Syndromes, *8th ed, Philadelphia, F. A. Davis, 1996.*

Daily water requirements differ according to age and medical problem(s). The approximate daily water need for a client weighing 70 kg is 30 mL per kg of body weight, or 2000 mL per day. In pounds, the calculation is 15 mL per pound. A client weighing 150 pounds should receive 2250 mL of water daily. If the client has a fever, water needs increase by 15%. A client loses water daily: 400 to 500 mL through skin by normal evaporation, 400 to 500 mL from breathing, 100 to 200 mL in feces, and 1000 to 1200 mL in urine.

When IV fluids are prescribed for 24 hours, the total amount of IV fluid ordered is usually 2000 to 3000 mL. Normally, there is more than one type of solution used. Three liters of dextrose 5% in water per day causes a hypo-osmolar state and water intoxication (intracellular fluid volume excess) can occur. If hyperosmolar IV solutions such as dextrose in normal saline solution only are used, dehydration can occur due to hyperosmolality, which pulls fluid from the cells and promotes fluid excretion. Usually there are one or two iso-osmolar solutions (this could include D$_5$W) and one or two hyperosmolar solutions administered per day.

NURSING PROCESS: FLUID REPLACEMENT

ASSESSMENT

- Assess vital signs and use for future baseline values. Report abnormal findings.
- Check the client's laboratory findings, especially the hematocrit and BUN. If both values are elevated, this may be due to fluid volume deficit (dehydration). If the BUN is >60 mg/dL, renal impairment is most likely the cause.
- Check urine output. Report if the urine output is <25 mL/h or 600 mL per day. Normal urine output should be >35 mL/h or 1000 to 1200 mL/day.
- Check urine specific gravity (SG). Normal range is 1.005 to 1.030. If the urine specific gravity is greater than 1.030, hypovolemia or dehydration may be the cause.
- Check the type(s) of intravenous fluid ordered per day. Report to the health care provider if there is continuous use of one type of IV fluid such as 5% dextrose in water (D$_5$W). This could cause hypo-osmolality.
- Check client's weight and record for a baseline level.

NURSING DIAGNOSES

- High risk for fluid volume excess related to excess volume infused, rapidly infused IV fluids, or volume infused too great for client's physical size and/or condition.

- High risk for fluid volume deficit related to inadequate fluid intake.
- Altered tissue perfusion (vascular) related to decreased blood circulation or inadequate fluid replacement.

PLANNING

Client will not develop fluid volume deficit or excess as the result of intravenous fluid replacement.

Client will be hydrated; vital signs and urine output will be within the normal ranges.

NURSING INTERVENTIONS

- Monitor vital signs and report abnormal findings. Rapid pulse rate could be indicative of hypovolemia (decrease in body fluids). Blood pressure changes should be reported. Decrease in blood pressure occurs when hypovolemia is severe and shock is occurring.
- Monitor urine output. Report if the urine output is less than 600 mL/day. This could be due to fluid volume deficit or CHF from fluid overload.
- Monitor weight daily. A gain of 2.2 to 2.5 pounds is equivalent to 1 liter of fluid. If the client gained 5 pounds in one day, it may indicate that the client is retaining 2 liters of fluid. This could be a sign of fluid overload.
- Check for signs and symptoms of fluid volume deficit (dehydration) such as excess thirst (mild dehydration). Marked thirst, dry mucous membranes, poor skin turgor, decrease in urine output, tachycardia, and slight drop in systolic blood pressure are indicators of marked dehydration.

- Check for signs and symptoms of fluid volume excess (fluid overload) such as constant, irritated cough; dyspnea; neck vein engorgement; hand vein engorgement; and moist rales in the lung.
- Monitor laboratory results daily, especially BUN, hemoglobin, and hematocrit. Elevated values can indicate dehydration.
- Monitor the types of fluids the client is receiving. Report if only one type of IV fluid is being prescribed daily. This can cause fluid imbalance (hypo-osmolality or hyperosmolality).
- Monitor IV injection site for infiltration or phlebitis.

- Instruct the client that thirst means there is a mild fluid deficit. Increasing fluid intake is important. Elderly clients' thirst mechanisms are frequently decreased. The nurse should offer fluids as needed to the elderly.
- Inform the client to report frequent vomiting or diarrhea. When vomiting and diarrhea occur constantly or over several days, severe fluid volume imbalance can result.
- Encourage the client to monitor fluid intake and output. Inform the client to report abnormal findings such as diuresis, weight gain or loss, peripheral edema, or tight shoes and rings to the health care provider.

EVALUATION

- Evaluate that the intravenous therapy has replaced the client's body fluids.
- Evaluate that the IV therapy has not caused a deficit or an excess of the client's body fluids.

ELECTROLYTES

POTASSIUM

Potassium (K^+), an important cellular cation, is 20 times more prevalent in the cells (intracellular fluids [ICF]) than in the vessels (intravascular fluid, or plasma). The normal plasma or serum level (these terms are frequently used interchangeably) for potassium is 3.5 to 5.3 milliequivalents per liter (mEq/L). A serum potassium level less than 3.5 mEq/L is called **hypokalemia,** and a serum potassium level greater than 5.3 mEq/L is called **hyperkalemia.** Potassium has a narrow normal range. Too little potassium (hypokalemia), under 2.5 mEq/L, or too much potassium (hyperkalemia), above 7.0 mEq/L, may lead to cardiac arrest.

Potassium is poorly stored in the body, so daily potassium intake is necessary. The recommended potassium intake is approximately 40 to 60 mEq daily, consumed in such foods as fruits, fruit juices, and vegetables, or in the form of potassium supplements. Bananas and dried fruits are higher in potassium content than oranges and fruit juices.

Functions

Potassium is necessary for the transmission and conduction of nerve impulses, and for the contraction of skeletal, cardiac, and smooth muscles. It is also needed for the enzyme action needed to change carbohydrates to energy (glycolysis) and amino acids to protein. Potassium promotes glycogen (energy) storage in hepatic (liver) cells. It also regulates the osmolality (solute concentration) of cellular fluids.

Hypokalemia

Whenever cells are damaged from trauma, injury, surgery, or shock, potassium leaks from the cells into the intravascular fluid and is excreted by the kidneys. With cellular loss of potassium, potassium shifts from the blood plasma into the cell to restore the cellular potassium balance. Thus, hypokalemia usually results. Vomiting and diarrhea also decrease serum potassium levels. Between 80% to 90% of potassium in the body is excreted in the urine; 8% is excreted in the feces. If the kidneys shut down or are diseased, potassium accumulates in the intravascular fluid, and hyperkalemia results.

When the serum potassium level is between 3.0 to 3.5 mEq/L, 100 to 200 mEq of potassium chloride (KCl) is needed to raise the serum potassium level 1 mEq (e.g., 3.0 to 4.0 mEq). If the serum potassium level is less than 3.0 mEq/L, then 200 to 400 mEq of KCl is needed to raise the serum potassium level 1 mEq. Potassium chloride cannot rapidly correct a severe potassium deficit.

Potassium can be given orally or intravenously and is combined with an anion, such as chloride or bicarbonate. Oral potassium can be given as a liquid, powder, or tablet. Potassium is extremely irritating to the gastric and intestinal mucosa, so it *must be given with at least a half glass of fluid* (juice or water) or, preferably, a full glass of fluid. Because cardiac arrest (standstill) results from excessive potassium, intravenous potassium must be diluted in IV fluids—it cannot be given as an IV push or IV bolus. Nurses must remember that, when administering any type of potassium, it *must be diluted*. Table 10–4 lists the potassium preparations to treat hypokalemia.

Signs and symptoms of hypokalemia include nausea and vomiting, dysrhythmias, abdominal distention, and soft, flabby muscles. If the serum potassium level is a low normal, foods high in potassium should be suggested, such as fruit juices, citrus fruits, dried fruits, bananas, nuts (peanut butter), some sodas and tea, and vegetables such as potatoes, broccoli, and green leafy vegetables.

Certain drugs promote potassium loss, such as potassium-wasting diuretics (hydrochlorothiazide [HydroDIURIL], furosemide [Lasix], ethacrynic acid [Edecrin]); and cortisone preparations. Clients receiving these drugs should increase their potassium intake by consuming foods rich in potassium or by taking potassium supplements. Their serum potassium levels should be monitored for abnormal serum potassium levels. Potassium must be used cautiously in clients with renal insufficiency. If the urine output is less than 600 mL/day, the health care provider should be notified, especially if a potassium supplement is ordered.

Figure 10–2 compares the pharmacokinetics and pharmacodynamics of oral and intravenous potassium preparations. The nursing process is based on the drug data.

Pharmacokinetics

Oral liquid potassium is absorbed faster than tablets or capsules; the pharmaceutic phase is decreased. Sustained-released capsules such as Micro-K, Slow-K, and K-Tab release the potassium over a period of time. Plenty of water, no less than 4 oz, must be taken with oral potassium preparations. The drug may be taken with a meal or immediately after eating.

Intravenous potassium is immediately absorbed in the vascular fluids. Intravenous potassium must be diluted in IV solutions and *never* given as a bolus or an IV push. Between 80% to 90% of the potassium in body fluids is excreted in the urine; 8% is excreted in feces.

TABLE 10–4 Potassium Supplements

Preparation	Drug
Oral liquid	Potassium chloride: 10% = 20 mEq/15mL, 20% = 40 mEq/15mL Kay Ciel (potassium chloride) Kaochlor 10% (potassium chloride) Kaon-Cl 20% (potassium chloride) Potassium Triplex (potassium acetate, bicarbonate, citrate). Rarely used.
Oral tablet or capsule	Potassium chloride (enteric-coated tablet) Kaon (potassium gluconate) Kaon-Cl (potassium chloride) Slow-K (potassium chloride, 8 mEq) Kaochlor (potassium chloride) K-Lyte (potassium bicarbonate-effervescent tablet) K-Lyte/Cl (potassium chloride) K-Dur (potassium chloride) Micro-K (potassium chloride) Ten-K (potassium chloride) K-Tab (potassium chloride)
Intravenous potassium	Potassium chloride in clear liquid in multidose vial or ampule (2mEq/mL)

FIGURE 10–2. Electrolyte: Potassium

Potassium	Dosage	NURSING PROCESS
		Assessment and Planning
Potassium chloride (Kaochlor, Kaon-Cl, Kay Ciel, Micro-K, K-Dur) Potassium replacement *Pregnancy Category:* A	A: *Hypokalemia (maintenance):* PO: 20 mEq in 1–2 divided doses *Hypokalemia (correction):* PO: 40–80 mEq in 3–4 divided doses IV: 20–40 mEq diluted in 1 L of IV solution	
Contraindications	**Drug-Lab-Food Interactions**	
Renal insufficiency or failure, Addison's disease, hyperkalemia, severe dehydration, acidosis, potassium-sparing diuretics *Caution:* Cardiac disorders, burns	*Increase* serum potassium level with ACE inhibitors, potassium-sparing diuretics *Lab:* May *increase* serum potassium level (> 5.5 mEq/L)	
Pharmacokinetics	**Pharmacodynamics**	Interventions
Absorption: PO: rapidly absorbed, 95% in body fluids *Distribution:* PB: UK *Metabolism:* t½: UK *Excretion:* 80–90% in urine; 10% in feces	PO: Onset: 30 min Peak: 1–2 h Duration: UK IV: Onset: Rapid Peak: 1–1.5 h Duration: UK	

Therapeutic Effects/Uses: To correct potassium deficit; strengthen cardiac and muscular activities. *Mode of Action:* Transmits and conducts nerve impulses; contracts skeletal, smooth, and cardiac muscles.	Evaluation

Side Effects	Adverse Reactions
Nausea, vomiting, diarrhea, abdominal cramps, irritability, rash (rare)	Oliguria, ECG changes (peaked T waves, widened QRS complex, prolonged PR interval), GI ulceration *Life-threatening:* Cardiac dysrhythmias, respiratory distress, cardiac arrest

KEY: A: adult; PO: by mouth; IV: intravenous; UK: unknown; PB: protein-binding; t½: half-life; >: greater than.

Pharmacodynamics

Potassium maintains neuromuscular activity; therefore, serum potassium levels should be closely monitored. Onset of action of oral potassium may be within 30 min; for intravenous potassium, it is immediate. Duration of action of potassium is not known; however, it may vary according to the dose taken. An electrocardiogram (ECG) should be closely monitored when large doses are administered.

Hyperkalemia

Hyperkalemia usually results from renal insufficiency or from the administration of large doses of potassium over time. For a mildly elevated serum potassium level, such as 5.3 to 5.5 mEq/L, restricting foods rich in potassium may correct the excess potassium level. If renal insufficiency or failure is present, additional measures must be taken.

Drugs that might be ordered for hyperkalemia (serum potassium >5.3 mEq/L) are listed in Table 10–5. To immediately decrease a temporary potassium excess in the serum potassium level, sodium bicarbonate, calcium gluconate, or insulin and glucose may be prescribed. Sodium polystyrene sulfonate (Kayexalate) with sorbital are ordered for severe hyperkalemia. This drug therapy exchanges a sodium ion for a potassium ion in the body and is a more permanent means of correcting hyperkalemia.

Signs and symptoms of hyperkalemia include nausea, abdominal cramps, oliguria (decreased urine output), tachycardia and later bradycardia, weakness, and numbness or tingling in the extremities. For mild hyperkalemia, foods rich in potassium are usually restricted.

TABLE 10–5 Correction of Potassium Excess (Hyperkalemia)

Drug Therapy	Rationale
IV Sodium bicarbonate (HCO₃)	By elevating the pH level, potassium moves back into the cells, thus lowering the serum level.
10% Calcium gluconate	Calcium decreases the irritability of myocardium resulting from hyperkalemia. It does not promote potassium loss.
Insulin and glucose	The combination of insulin and glucose moves potassium back into the cells. This lasts about 6 h. Repeating these agents is not always as effective.
Sodium polystyrene sulfonate (Kayexalate) and sorbitol 70%	Kayexalate is used as a cation exchange for severe hyperkalemia. It can be given orally or rectally. *Orally:* Kayexalate: 15 g, 1–4 × a day. Sorbitol 70%: 20 mL with each dose. *Rectally:* Kayexalate: 30–50 g. Sorbitol 70%: 50 mL. Mix with 100–150 mL of water. (Retention enema for 20–30 min.)

NURSING PROCESS: ELECTROLYTE: Potassium

ASSESSMENT

- Assess for signs and symptoms of hypokalemia (decreased serum potassium) and hyperkalemia (elevated serum potassium). Symptoms of hypokalemia include nausea, vomiting, cardiac dysrhythmias, abdominal distension, and soft flabby muscles. Symptoms of hyperkalemia include oliguria, nausea, abdominal cramps, and tachycardia and, later, bradycardia, weakness, and numbness or tingling in the extremities.
- Assess serum potassium level; normal serum potassium level is 3.5 to 5.3 mEq/L. Report serum potassium deficit or excess to the health care provider.
- Obtain baseline vital sign (VS) and ECG readings. Report abnormal findings. The VS and ECG results can be compared with future VS and ECG readings.
- Assess the client for signs and symptoms of digitalis toxicity when receiving a digitalis preparation (digoxin) and a potassium-wasting diuretic (hydrochlorothiazide, furosemide) or a cortisone preparation (prednisone). A decreased serum potassium level enhances the action of digitalis. Signs and symptoms of digitalis toxicity are nausea, vomiting, anorexia, bradycardia (pulse rate <60 or markedly decreased), cardiac dysrhythmias, and visual disturbances.

POTENTIAL NURSING DIAGNOSES

- Altered nutrition, less than body requirements.
- Impaired tissue integrity.

PLANNING

- Client's serum potassium level will be within normal range in 2 to 4 d.
- Client with hypokalemia will eat foods rich in potassium, such as fruits, fruit juices, and vegetables. Client with hyperkalemia will avoid potassium-rich foods.

NURSING INTERVENTIONS

- Give oral potassium with a sufficient amount of water or juice (at least 6 to 8 oz) or at mealtime. Potassium is extremely irritating to the gastric mucosa.
- Dilute IV potassium chloride in the IV bag and invert the bag several times to promote thorough mixing of potassium with IV fluids. Potassium *cannot* be given IM. **Potassium should never be given as an IV bolus or push.** Giving IV potassium directly into the vein causes cardiac dysrhythmias and cardiac arrest.

- Monitor the amount of urine output. If the client is receiving potassium and the urine output is <25 mL/h or <600 mL/d, potassium accumulation occurs. Remember, 80% to 90% of potassium is excreted in the urine. Report results to the health care provider.
- Monitor the serum potassium level. Hypokalemia occurs if the serum potassium value is <3.5 mEq/L; hyperkalemia occurs when the serum potassium value is >5.3 mEq/L.
- Monitor the ECG. With hypokalemia, the T wave is flat or inverted, the ST segment is depressed, and the QT interval is prolonged. With hyperkalemia, the T wave is narrow and peaked, the QRS complex is spread, and the PR interval is prolonged.
- Check the IV site for infiltration if the client is receiving potassium in the IV fluids. Potassium can cause tissue necrosis if it infiltrates into the fatty tissue (subcutaneous tissue). The IV fluid with potassium should be discontinued when infiltration occurs.
- Monitor clients receiving various medications for hyperkalemia, such as sodium bicarbonate, calcium gluconate, insulin and glucose, and Kayexalate and sorbitol, for signs and symptoms of continuing hyperkalemia or of developing hypokalemia.
- Prepare and administer Kayexalate orally or by retention enema, according to the drug circular. The client should have a cleansing enema before the retention enema. A suggested method for preparation and administration of Kayexalate retention enema is:

1. Use warm fluid to prepare (do not heat).
2. Mix with 20% dextrose in water or sorbitol.
3. Keep particles in suspension by stirring periodically and administer at body temperature by gravity.
4. Encourage the client to retain the enema for 30 to 60 min minimum.
5. Flush tubing with 50 to 100 mL of fluid before clamping for retention.

6. After completion, irrigate the colon with 2 quarts of flushing liquid and drain the fluid contents.

CLIENT TEACHING

GENERAL

- Advise the client to have serum potassium level checked at regular intervals when taking drugs that are potassium supplements or that decrease potassium levels.
- Instruct the client to drink a full glass of water or juice when taking oral potassium supplements. Potassium preparations can be taken during or after a meal. Explain to the client that potassium is very irritating to the stomach.
- Instruct the client to comply with the prescribed potassium dose, regular laboratory tests, and medical follow-up related to the health problem and drug regimen.

DIET

- Instruct the client who is taking a potassium-wasting diuretic or a cortisone preparation to eat potassium-rich foods, including citrus fruit juice, fruits (bananas, plums, oranges, cantaloupes, raisins) vegetables, and nuts.

SIDE EFFECTS

- Instruct the client to report signs and symptoms of hypokalemia and hyperkalemia. See assessment for the list. When taking large amounts of potassium supplements, hyperkalemia could result.

EVALUATION

- Evaluate the client's serum potassium level and ECG. Report to the health care provider if the level remains abnormal. Potassium replacements and diet may need modification.

SODIUM

Sodium is the major cation in the extracellular fluid (vessels and tissue spaces). The normal serum or plasma sodium level is 135 to 145 mEq/L. A serum sodium level less than 135 mEq/L is called **hyponatremia,** and a serum sodium level greater than 145 mEq/L is called **hypernatremia.**

Functions

Sodium is the major electrolyte that regulates body fluids. It promotes the transmission and conduction of nerve impulses. It is part of the sodium/potassium pump that causes cellular activity. Sodium shifts into cells as potassium shifts out of the cells, repeatedly, to maintain water balance and neuromuscular activity. When sodium shifts into the cell, depolarization occurs; when sodium shifts out of the cell, potassium shifts back into the cell and repolarization occurs. Sodium combines readily with chloride (Cl) or bicarbonate (HCO_3) to promote acid–base balance.

Hyponatremia

Sodium loss can result from vomiting, diarrhea, surgery, and potent diuretics. Signs and symptoms of hyponatremia include muscular weakness, headaches, abdominal cramps, nausea, and vomiting. The serum sodium level should be monitored as necessary.

For a serum sodium level between 125 and 135 mEq/L, normal saline (0.9% sodium chloride) may increase the sodium content in the vascular fluid. If the serum sodium level is 115 mEq/L, a hypertonic, 3% saline solution may be necessary.

Hypernatremia

When the serum sodium level is elevated above 146 mEq/L, sodium restriction is indicated. Signs and symptoms of hypernatremia are flushed skin, elevated body temperature and blood pressure, and rough, dry tongue. An increase in serum sodium can result from consuming certain drugs, such as cortisone preparations, cough medications, and selected antibiotics.

NURSING PROCESS: ELECTROLYTE: Sodium

ASSESSMENT

- Assess the client for signs and symptoms of hyponatremia and hypernatremia. See signs and symptoms in this chapter.
- Check the serum sodium level. Report abnormally low sodium levels (<125 mEq/L), because prompt medical care is required.
- Obtain history of health problems that may lead to sodium loss or excess.

POTENTIAL NURSING DIAGNOSIS

- High risk for fluid volume excess related to water retention.

PLANNING

- Client's serum sodium level will be within normal range in 3 to 5 days.
- Edema will be decreased in client with sodium retention.

NURSING INTERVENTIONS

- Monitor the medical regimen for correction of hyponatremia, such as water restriction, intravenous normal saline (0.9% sodium chloride), and 3% saline solution to correct a serum sodium level of <115 mEq/L.
- Monitor serum sodium levels. Report abnormal level.

CLIENT TEACHING

Instruct the client with hypernatremia to avoid foods rich in sodium, such as canned foods, lunch meats, ham, pork, pickles, potato chips, and pretzels. Instruct the client to avoid using salt when cooking or adding salt to food at the table. Emphasize the importance of reading labels on food products.

EVALUATION

- Evaluate the client's serum sodium level. Report if sodium imbalance continues.

CALCIUM

Calcium is found in approximately equal proportion in the ICF and ECF. The serum calcium range is 4.5 to 5.5 mEq/L, or 9 to 11 mg/dL. A calcium deficit, less than 4.5 mEq/L, is called **hypocalcemia,** and a calcium excess, greater than 5.5 mEq/L, is called **hypercalcemia.** About half of the calcium in the body fluid is bound to protein. Calcium that is unbound to protein is free, ionized calcium and can cause a physiologic response. If the serum protein (albumin) levels are decreased, there is more free circulating calcium even when the serum calcium level is decreased.

Functions

Calcium promotes normal nerve and muscle activity. It increases contraction of the heart muscle (myocardium). This cation also maintains normal cellular permeability and promotes blood clotting by

FIGURE 10–3. Calcium

Calcium	Dosage	NURSING PROCESS
		Assessment and Planning

Calcium chloride (IV)
Calcium carbonate
    (Os-cal, Tums, Caltrate, MegaCal)
Calium gluconate (Kalcinate)
Calcium lactate
Calcium replacement
Pregnancy Category: C
Drug Forms: Tab, cap, liq, inj
	Antacid use:
	A; PO: 0.5–1 g q4–6h (dose varies according to the calcium salt)
	Osteoporosis:
	A: PO: 1–2 g b.i.d.
	    IV: 0.5–1 g q.d., q.o.d.
	Tetany:
	A: IV 4–16 mEq
	C: IV: 0.5–0.7 mEq/kg t.i.d., q.i.d.
	Hypocalcemia:
	C: PO: 500 mg/d in divided doses	

Contraindications	Drug-Lab-Food Interactions	
Hypercalcemia, renal calculi, digitalis toxicity, ventricular fibrillation Caution: Renal or respiratory disorders, GI hypomotility	Increase digitalis toxicity: digoxin; Decrease calcium effect: saline solution; decrease effect of calcium channel blockers, verapamil; decrease absorption of tetracycline; increase serum calcium level: thiazide diuretics	

Pharmacokinetics	Pharmacodynamics	Interventions

Absorption: PO: 35% absorbed, requires vitamin D
Distribution: PB: UK
Metabolism: t½: UK
Excretion: 20% in urine; 70% in feces, some in saliva
	PO: Onset: UK
	        Peak: UK
	        Duration: 2–4 h
	IV: Onset: Rapid
	        Peak: UK
	        Duration: 2–3 h	

Therapeutic Effects/Uses: To correct calcium deficit or tetany symptoms, prevent osteoporosis.

Mode of Action: Transmits nerve impulses, contracts skeletal and cardiac muscles, maintains cellular permeability; promotes strong bone and teeth growth.

Evaluation

Side Effects	Adverse Reactions	
Nausea, vomiting, constipation, pain, drowsiness, headache, muscle weakness	Hypercalcemia, ECG changes (shortened QT interval), metabolic alkalosis, heart block, rebound hyperacidity Life-threatening: Renal failure, cardiac dysrhythmias, cardiac arrest	

KEY: A: adult; C: child; PO: by mouth; IV: intravenous; UK: unknown; PB: protein-binding; t½: half-life.

converting prothrombin into thrombin. In addition, calcium is needed for the formation of bone and teeth.

Vitamin D is needed for calcium absorption from the GI tract. Aspirin and anticonvulsants can alter vitamin D, affecting calcium absorption. Loop or high-ceiling diuretics (furosemide [Lasix]; see Chapter 33), steroids (cortisone), magnesium preparations, and phosphate preparations promote calcium loss. Conversely, thiazide diuretics (hydrochlorothiazide [HydroDIURIL]) increase the serum calcium level.

Hypocalcemia

Inadequate calcium intake causes calcium to leave the bone in order to maintain a normal serum calcium level. Fractures may occur if calcium deficit persists because of calcium loss from the bones (bone demineralization). Hypoparathyroidism, vitamin D deficiency, and receiving multiple blood transfusions are causes of hypocalcemia.

Signs and symptoms of hypocalcemia include anxiety, irritability, and tetany (twitching around the mouth, tingling and numbness of fingers, carpopedal spasm, spasmodic contractions, laryngeal spasm, and convulsions). If metabolic acidosis is present with hypocalcemia, tetany symptoms are absent because calcium leaves protein sites during an acidotic state; thus, more ionized calcium is available. During an alkalotic state, more calcium binds with protein. There is less ionized calcium, and tetany symptoms usually occur.

Many calcium preparations can be administered orally or intravenously. For treatment of calcium deficit, oral calcium tablets, capsules, or powder and IV calcium solutions may be given. Calcium preparations are combined with various salts, such as chloride, carbonate, gluconate, gluceptate, and lactate. Calcium for IV use should be mixed with 5% dextrose in water and *not mixed* in a saline solution. Sodium encourages calcium loss. Figure 10–3 compares the pharmacokinetics and pharmacodynamics of calcium preparations.

Pharmacokinetics

Vitamin D promotes calcium absorption from the GI tract; phosphorus inhibits calcium absorption. The pH affects the amount of circulating, free ionized calcium. When pH is decreased (acidic), there is more free calcium because it has been released from protein-binding sites. With an increased pH, more calcium is bound to protein.

Pharmacodynamics

A calcium deficit causes tetany symptoms and, if severe, can be life-threatening. Rapid administration of intravenous calcium may cause tingling and warm sensations and a metallic taste. Calcium needs to be administered at a moderate rate, and infiltration should be avoided. Calcium can be given undiluted IV in emergency situations.

Hypercalcemia

Elevated serum calcium may be due to hyperparathyroidism, hypophosphatemia, tumors of the bone, prolonged immobilization, multiple fractures, and drugs such as the thiazide diuretics. Pathologic fractures might occur because of thinning of the bone due to calcium loss from the bony structure. Calcium leaves the bone and accumulates in the vascular fluid. Signs and symptoms of hypercalcemia are flabby muscles, pain over bony areas, and kidney stones of calcium composition.

NURSING PROCESS: ELECTROLYTE: Calcium

ASSESSMENT

- Assess the client for signs and symptoms of hypocalcemia (decreased serum calcium), such as tetany (twitching of the mouth, tingling and numbness of the fingers, facial spasms, spasms of the larynx, and carpopedal spasm), muscle cramps, bleeding tendencies, and weak cardiac contractions.
- Check the serum calcium levels (normal, 4.5 to 5.5 mEq/L or 8.5 to 10.5 mg/dL) for hypocalcemia and hypercalcemia. Report abnormal test results. Serum ionized calcium (iCa) indicates free circulating calcium and is more accurate for determining calcium imbalance.
- Obtain VS and ECG readings. Report abnormal findings. VS and ECG results can be compared with future VS and ECG readings.

- Obtain a current drug history for the client. Calcium enhances the effect of digoxin. An elevated serum calcium level, when taken with digoxin, can cause digitalis toxicity. Signs and symptoms of digitalis toxicity include nausea, vomiting, anorexia, bradycardia (pulse rate <60 or markedly decreased), cardiac dysrhythmias, and visual disturbances. Thiazide diuretics can increase the serum calcium level. Drugs that decrease the effect of calcium are calcium channel blockers, tetracycline, and sodium chloride.

POTENTIAL NURSING DIAGNOSES

- Altered nutrition, less than body requirements.
- Impaired tissue integrity.

PLANNING

- Client's serum calcium level will be within normal range by 3 to 7 days.
- Tetany symptoms will cease. Client will eat foods rich in calcium or take calcium supplements as ordered.
- Client with hypercalcemia will avoid foods rich in calcium, such as milk products.

NURSING INTERVENTIONS

- Monitor VS. Report abnormal findings. Compare with baseline VS. Monitor pulse rate if the client is taking digoxin. Bradycardia is a sign of digitalis toxicity.
- Administer IV fluids slowly with 10% calcium gluconate or chloride. Calcium should be administered with D_5W and not saline solution because sodium promotes calcium loss. Calcium should not be added to solutions containing bicarbonate because rapid precipitation occurs.
- Check IV site for infiltration if the client is receiving calcium in IV fluids. Calcium can cause tissue necrosis (sloughing of the tissue) if it infiltrates into the subcutaneous tissue. Calcium gluceptate is the only calcium preparation that can be given IM.
- Monitor the serum calcium and iCa levels. Hypocalcemia occurs if the serum calcium value is <4.5 mEq/L or <8.5 mg/dL or if iCa is <2.2 mEq/L. Hypercalcemia occurs if the serum calcium value is >5.5 mEq/L or >10.5 mg/dL or if iCa is >2.5 mEq/L.
- Monitor ECGs. With hypocalcemia, the ST segment is lengthened and the QT interval is prolonged. With hypercalcemia, the ST segment is decreased and the QT interval is shortened.

General
- Instruct the client to avoid overuse of antacids and to prevent the habit of chronic use of laxatives. Excessive use of certain antacids may cause alkalosis, decreasing calcium ionization. Chronic use of laxatives decreases calcium absorption from the GI tract. Suggest fruits and foods rich in fiber for improving bowel elimination.
- Instruct the client taking calcium supplements to check that the calcium tablet is absorbable. To do this, put 1 tablet into 1 oz of white vinegar. Stir every 3 min. The tablet should break up or dissolve within 30 min.
- Take oral calcium supplements with meals or after meals to increase absorption.

Diet
- Suggest that the client consume foods high in calcium, such as milk, milk products, and protein-rich foods. Protein and vitamin D are needed to enhance calcium absorption.

Side Effects
- Instruct the client to report symptoms related to calcium excess or hypercalcemia, including flabby muscles, pain over bony areas, ECG changes, and kidney (calcium form) stones.

EVALUATION

- Evaluate the client's serum calcium level. Report if calcium imbalance continues.
- Determine if side effects due to previous untreated hypocalcemia are absent.

MAGNESIUM

Magnesium, a sister cation to potassium, is most plentiful in the intracellular fluid (ICF). When there is a loss of potassium, there is also a loss of magnesium. The normal serum magnesium level is 1.5 to 2.5 mEq/L. A magnesium deficit is called **hypomagnesemia,** and a magnesium excess is called **hypermagnesemia.** Daily magnesium requirement is 8 to 20 mEq.

Functions

Magnesium promotes the transmission of neuromuscular activity; it is an important mediator of neural transmission in the central nervous system (CNS). Like potassium, it promotes contraction of the myocardium. It activates many enzymes for the metabolism of carbohydrates and protein. It is responsible for the transportation of sodium and potassium across cell membranes.

When there is a magnesium deficit, there frequently is a potassium or calcium deficit. A serum magnesium deficit increases the release of acetylcholine from the presynaptic membrane of the nerve fiber. This increases neuromuscular excitability. A serum magnesium excess has a sedative effect on the neuromuscular system, which can result in a loss of deep tendon reflexes. Cardiac (ventricular) dysrhythmias can occur due to hypomagnesemia.

Hypotension and heart block may result from hypermagnesemia.

Hypomagnesemia is probably the most undiagnosed electrolyte deficiency. This is most likely due to the fact that hypomagnesemia is asymptomatic until the serum magnesium level approaches 1.0 mEq/L. The total serum magnesium concentration is not representative of the cellular magnesium levels.

Drugs that decrease the serum magnesium level are cortisone preparations, diuretics, and saline solutions (IV normal saline). Two groups of drugs that contain magnesium are laxatives, such as magnesium sulfate (Epsom salts), milk of magnesia (MOM), magnesium citrate; and antacids, such as Maalox, Mylanta, and Di-Gel. For severe hypomagnesemia, intravenous magnesium sulfate ($MgSO_4$) may be given. To correct hypermagnesemia, calcium gluconate may be given to decrease the serum magnesium level.

NURSING PROCESS: ELECTROLYTE: Magnesium

ASSESSMENT

- Assess the client for signs and symptoms of magnesium deficit or excess. Hypomagnesemia includes tetanylike symptoms due to hyperexcitability (tremors, twitching of the face) and ventricular tachycardia that leads to ventricular fibrillation and hypertension. Hypermagnesemia includes lethargy, drowsiness, weakness, paralysis, loss of deep tendon reflexes, hypotension, and heart block.
- Check serum magnesium levels for magnesium imbalance. Symptoms of magnesium deficit may or may not be seen until the serum level is below 1.0 mEq/L.
- Check clients receiving digitalis preparations for digitalis toxicity. A magnesium deficit, as with a potassium deficit, enhances the action of digitalis, causing digitalis toxicity.

POTENTIAL NURSING DIAGNOSIS

- Altered nutrition: less than body requirements related to insufficient intake of foods that are rich in magnesium.
- Decreased cardiac output related to hypomagnesemia or hypermagnesemia.

PLANNING

- Client's serum magnesium level will be within normal range in 2 to 5 days.

NURSING INTERVENTIONS

- Report to the health care provider if the client is NPO (nothing by mouth) and receiving IV fluids without magnesium salts for weeks. Administer IV magnesium sulfate in solution slowly to prevent a hot or flushed feeling. Monitor vital signs.
- Monitor urinary output. Most of the body's magnesium is excreted by the kidneys. Report if the urine output is less than 600 mL/day.
- Check hypomagnesemia clients who are taking digoxin for digitalis toxicity; e.g., nausea and vomiting, bradycardia. Magnesium deficit enhances the action of digoxin (digitalis preparations).
- Monitor vital signs. Report abnormal findings to the health care provider.
- Monitor serum electrolyte results. Report a low serum potassium or calcium level. Low serum magnesium levels may be attributed to hypokalemia or hypocalcemia. When correcting a potassium deficit, potassium is not replaced in the cells until magnesium is replaced. A serum magnesium level of 1.0 mEq/L or less can cause cardiac arrest.
- Check for positive Trousseau's and Chvostek's signs of severe hypomagnesemia. Tetany symptoms occur in both magnesium and calcium deficits.
- Have IV calcium gluconate available for emergency reversal of hypermagnesemia from overcorrection of a magnesium deficit.

CLIENT TEACHING

- Instruct the client to eat foods rich in magnesium (green vegetables, fruits, fish and seafood, grains, nuts, and peanut butter).
- Instruct the client with hypermagnesemia to avoid routine use of laxatives and antacids that contain magnesium. Suggest that the client check drug labels.

EVALUATION

- Evaluate the client's serum magnesium level. Report if the serum level remains abnormal.
- Observe for signs and symptoms of hypomagnesemia and hypermagnesemia.

■ CASE STUDY: Potassium

J.S., 72 years old, has been vomiting and has had diarrhea for 2 days. J.S. takes digoxin 0.25 mg/day and HydroDIURIL 50 mg/day. His serum potassium level is 3.2 mEq/L. He complains of being dizzy. His blood pressure is slightly lower than usual. The nurse assesses his physiologic status and notes that his muscles are weak and flabby, his abdomen is distended, and peristalsis is diminished.

1. What type of potassium imbalance does J.S. have?
2. Normal range of serum potassium is _____.
3. How much potassium chloride would be needed to raise J.S.'s serum potassium by 1 mEq?
4. What effect does hypokalemia have on digoxin? Explain.

J.S. was ordered intravenously one liter of 5% dextrose in water (D₅W) with 30 mEq of potassium chloride (KCl), and one liter of 5% dextrose in 0.45% NaCl (1/2 of normal saline). He was also prescribed oral KCl 15 mEq, t.i.d. × 2 days. Oral KCl is available in 15 mEq/10 mL.

5. Explain the method for diluting KCl in IV fluids.
6. Can KCl be given intramuscularly, subcutaneously or as an IV bolus (push)? Explain.
7. How should oral liquid KCl be given to J.S.?
8. What GI problem might occur if oral potassium is not properly administered? Explain.
9. Why should J.S. urine output be closely monitored? Explain.
10. What foods are rich in potassium?
11. Because J.S. is taking a diuretic and digoxin, what should the nurse include with client teaching? Give examples.

STUDY QUESTIONS

1. What is the average range of the osmolality of body fluids? If your client's serum sodium is 140 mEq/L, BUN is 12 mg/dL, and glucose is 100 mg/dL, what is your client's serum osmolality?
2. The client is receiving 1000 mL of D₅/0.9% NaCl (5% dextrose in normal saline solution). What is the osmolality of this intravenous solution? Explain.
3. What is the difference between crystalloids and colloids? Give examples of each.
4. Your client gained 15 pounds in 2 days. It is determined that the weight gain is due to body fluid retention. The weight gain could be equivalent to how many liters of fluid (water)?
5. What is the normal serum potassium range? Your client has been vomiting and has weak, flabby muscles. The client's pulse is irregular. What type of potassium imbalance would you suspect?
6. What are the nursing implications of giving oral potassium supplements and for giving IV potassium chloride? Name the groups of foods that are rich in potassium.
7. What are the drugs used to correct severe hyperkalemia? How are they administered?
8. What drugs may cause an elevated serum sodium level? What health problem may result?
9. In hypocalcemia, the serum calcium level is less than what level? What are the symptoms of hypocalcemia?
10. Why are clients with hypocalcemia and hypercalcemia at high risk of having fractures?
11. What are the functions of magnesium? Describe specific client teaching for clients with hypo/hypermagnesemia.

Chapter 11

Nutritional Support

OUTLINE

Introduction

Enteral Nutrition
    Routes for Enteral Feedings
    Enteral Solutions
    Methods for Delivery
    Complications

Enteral Medications

Nursing Process

Parenteral Nutrition
    Total Parenteral Nutrition
    Complications
    Nursing Process

Case Study

Study Questions

OBJECTIVES

Explain the differences between enteral nutrition and parenteral nutrition.

Describe the routes for enteral feedings.

Give examples of enteral solutions and explain the differences.

Explain the advantages and differences of the methods used for delivery of enteral nutrition.

Describe the complications that may occur with use of enteral nutrition and parenteral nutrition.

List the nursing interventions for clients receiving enteral nutrition and parenteral nutrition.

TERMS

bolus
continuous feeding
cyclic method
enteral nutrition

intermittent enteral feedings
intermittent infusion
parenteral nutrition
nutritional support

total parenteral nutrition
nasogastric tube
Valsalva maneuver

INTRODUCTION

Nutrients are needed for cell growth, cellular function, enzyme activity, carbohydrate-fat-protein synthesis, muscular contraction, wound healing, immune competence, and gastrointestinal (GI) integrity. Inadequate nutrient intake can result from surgery, trauma, malignancy, and other catabolic illnesses. Without adequate nutritional support, protein catabolism (breakdown), malnutrition, and diminished organ functioning affect the GI, liver, renal, cardiac, and respiratory systems. The functioning of the immune system also is decreased.

Clients who are well nourished can usually tolerate a lack of nutrients for 14 days without major health problems. However, clients who are critically ill may only tolerate a lack of nutrient support for a short period of time (a few days to a week) before signs of impaired organ function, infection, or morbidity result. If nutritional support is started within hours of an injury, as in the cases of severe trauma or burns, recovery is more rapid. In situations where the injury is due to minor surgery, there is no severe bodily effect due to lack of nutrients for days. Early nutritional support improves intestinal and liver blood flow and function, enhances wound healing, decreases the occurrence of infection, and improves the general outcome of the health situation for the critically ill as well as for the client with a minor injury. "Early fed" injured clients have a positive nitrogen balance and less chance for bacterial infections; thus, they also have a decrease in institutional length of stay.

Dextrose 5% in water (D$_5$W), normal saline, and lactated Ringer's solution are not forms of nutritional support, although these solutions do provide fluids and some electrolytes. A client requires 2000 calories per day; critically ill clients may require 3000 to 5000 calories/day. In cases of burns, the caloric need could be greater. Clients who remain NPO (nothing by mouth) for an extended period of time become malnourished. Delayed nutritional support by even 5 days for the trauma or neurologic (cervical fracture) client could hamper wound healing and risk the increase of developing an infection.

There are two routes for administering **nutritional support,** enteral or parenteral. **Enteral nutrition,** which involves the GI tract, can be given orally or by feeding tubes (tube feeding). If the client can swallow, the nutrient preparation(s) can be taken by mouth; if the client is unable to swallow, a tube is inserted into the stomach or small intestine. **Parenteral nutrition** involves administering high caloric nutrients through large veins, e.g., the subclavian vein. This method is called **total parenteral nutrition (TPN)** or hyperalimentation. Parenteral nutrition is more costly (approximately three times more expensive) than enteral nutrition, and the benefits are not significant. In fact, with TPN there is a higher infection rate. The use of TPN does not promote effective GI integrity, liver function, or body weight gain, as does enteral nutrition. Enteral feedings require a functioning small intestine. TPN is necessary when the GI tract is incapacitated, if there is intestinal obstruction, uncontrolled vomiting, high risk for aspiration, or to supplement inadequate oral intake.

This chapter is divided into enteral nutrition and parenteral nutrition. Routes for nutritional administration, nutritional preparations, methods for delivery, complications, and the nursing process are discussed for each.

ENTERAL NUTRITION

When enteral nutrition is prescribed, there should be adequate small bowel function with digestion, absorption, and GI motility. To determine if there is a lack of GI motility, the nurse assesses for abdominal distention and a decrease or absence of bowel sounds. In critically ill clients, frequently there is a decrease or absence in gastric emptying time; then TPN may be necessary. The preferred method for nutritional support is enteral feedings for clients with intact gastric emptying and with a decreased risk of aspiration.

ROUTES FOR ENTERAL FEEDINGS

Oral, gastric by **nasogastric tube** or gastrostomy, and small intestine by nasoduodenal or nasojejunal or by jejunostomy tube are the routes used for enteral feedings. Use of nasogastric tube through oral (mouth) or nasal cavities is the most common route for short-term enteral feedings. The gastrostomy, nasoduodenal/jejunal, and jejunostomy tubes are used for long-term enteral feedings. Figure 11–1 displays the four types of GI tubes used for enteral feedings. If aspiration is a concern, the small intestinal route is suggested.

ENTERAL SOLUTIONS

Several types of liquid formulas are commercially available for enteral feedings. These solutions differ according to the various nutrients, caloric values, and osmolality. There are three groups of solutions for enteral nutrition: blenderized; polymeric, which includes milk-based and lactose-free; and elemental or monomeric. The commercial preparations are listed according to their groups in Table 11–1.

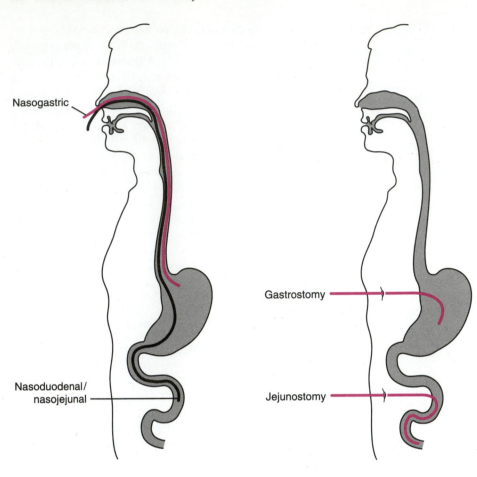

FIGURE 11–1. Types of gastrointestinal tubes for enteral feedings. *Nasogastric tube.* A tube is passed through the nose into the stomach. *Nasoduodenal/nasojejunal.* Weighted tube is passed through the nose into the duodenum/jejunum. *Gastrostomy.* Temporary or permanent opening (stoma) into the stomach for a feeding tube. *Jejunostomy.* Stoma directly into the jejunum for feeding. (*Source:* Davis, J. R., and Sherer, K.: *Applied Nutrition and Diet Therapy for Nurses,* 2nd ed. Philadelphia: W B Saunders, p. 354, 1994.)

Components of the enteral solutions include (1) carbohydrates in the form of dextrose, sucrose, lactose, starch or dextrin (the first three are simple sugars that can be absorbed quickly); (2) protein in the form of intact proteins, hydrolyzed proteins, or free amino acids; and (3) fat in the form of corn oil, soybean oil, or safflower oil (some have a higher oil content than others). With all enteral nutrition, sufficient water to maintain hydration is essential.

Blended formulas for enteral solutions are liquid in consistency to pass through the tube. These are individually prepared based on the client's nutritional need. Frequently, baby food is used with liquid added. If the food particles are too large, the tube can become clogged.

There are two groups of polymeric solutions, milk-based and lactose-free. Most of the milk-based polymeric preparations come in powdered form to be mixed with milk or water. Many of these milk-based polymeric solutions do not provide complete nutritional requirements unless given in large amounts. Frequently, they are used as a supplement to meet nutritional needs. The lactose-free polymeric solutions are commercially prepared in liquid form for replacement feedings. Many of these solutions are iso-osmolar (300 to 340

mOsm/kg) and the breakdown of nutrients includes 50% carbohydrates, 15% protein, 15% fat, and 20% other nutrients. Examples of these include Ensure, Isocal, and Osmolite. These polymeric solutions provide 1 calorie per mL of feeding.

The elemental or monomeric solutions are useful for partial GI tract dysfunction. They are available in powdered and liquid forms. The nutrients from these solutions are rapidly absorbed in the small intestine. They are more expensive than the other enteral solutions.

METHODS FOR DELIVERY

Enteral feedings may be given by bolus, intermittent drip or infusion, continuous drip, or cyclic infusion. The bolus method was the first method used to deliver enteral feedings. With the **bolus** method, 250 to 400 mL of solution is rapidly administered through a syringe or funnel into the tube four to six times a day. This method takes about 10 minutes and many times is not tolerated well due to the massive volume of solution in a short period of time. This method can cause nausea, vomiting, aspiration, abdominal cramping, and diarrhea. A healthy client can tolerate the rapidly

TABLE 11–1 Commercial Preparations for Enteral Feeding

Type	Commercial Preparations	Comments
I Blenderized	Compleat B (Sandoz) Formula 2 (Cutter) Vitaneed (Sherwood)	Blended natural foods: ready to use
II Polymeric Milk-based	Meritene (Sandoz) Instant Breakfast (Carnation) Sustacal Powder (Mead Johnson)	Pleasant tasting oral supplements: provide intact nutrients
Lactose-free	Ensure, Jevity, Osmolite (Ross) Sustacal Liquid, Isocal, Ultracal (Mead Johnson) Fibersource, Resource (Sandoz) Entrition, Nutren (Clintec) Attain, Comply (Sherwood)	May be used as tube feeding, meal replacement, or oral supplement; made with intact protein isolates, oligosaccharides and starches, and fats: provide 1 kcal/mL (others available providing up to 2 kcal): In adequate quantities meet RDIs for vitamins and minerals: ready to use: Isotonic (except Ensure and Sustacal)
III Elemental or monomeric formulas	Vital HN (Ross) Vivonex T.E.N. (Sandoz) Criticare HN (Mead Johnson) Travasorb (Clintec) Peptamen (Clintec) Reabilan (O'Brian)	Partially digested nutrients for feeding; hypertonic (except for Reabilan and Peptamen); require reconstitution (except for Peptamen, Reabilan, and Criticare)

Source: *Davis, J.R., and Sherer, K.:* Applied Nutrition and Diet Therapy for Nurses, *2nd ed. Philadelphia: W B Saunders, p. 349, 1994.*

infused solution. This method is seldom used unless the client is ambulatory.

Intermittent enteral feedings are administered every 3 to 6 hours over 30 to 60 minutes by gravity drip or pump infusion. Three hundred to 400 mL of solution is usually given at each feeding. A feeding bag is commonly used. **Intermittent infusion** is considered an inexpensive method for administering enteral nutrition.

Continuous feedings are prescribed for the critically ill or for those receiving feedings into the small intestine. The enteral feedings are given by an infusion pump, such as the Kangaroo set, at a slow rate over 24 hours. Approximately 50 to 125 mL of solution is infused per hour.

The **cyclic method** is another type of continuous feeding that is infused over 8 to 16 hours daily (day or night). The daytime hours are suggested for clients who are restless or for those who have a greater risk for aspiration. The nighttime schedule allows more freedom during the day for the clients who are ambulatory.

COMPLICATIONS

Dehydration can occur if an insufficient amount of water is given with the feedings or between feedings. Some of the enteral solutions are hyperosmolar and can draw water out of the cells to maintain serum iso-osmolality.

Aspiration may occur if the client is fed lying down or is unconscious. The head of the bed should be elevated at least 30 degrees. The nurse should check for residual feedings by gently aspirating the stomach contents before administering the next enteral feeding.

One of the major problems of enteral feeding is diarrhea. This could be due to rapid administration of feeding, high caloric solutions, malnutrition, GI bacteria (*Clostridium difficile*), and drugs. Antibacterials (antibiotics) and drugs that contain magnesium such as antacids (Maalox) and sorbitol (used as a filler for certain drugs) are associated with the occurrence of diarrhea. Many oral liquid drugs are hyperosmolar, which tends to pull water into the GI tract and cause diarrhea.

Diarrhea usually can be managed or corrected by decreasing the rate of infusion of the solution, diluting the solution, changing the enteral solution, discontinuing the drug, or increasing the water per day.

ENTERAL MEDICATIONS

Most drugs that can be administered orally can also be given via enteral tube. The drug must be in liquid form or dissolved into a liquid. Drugs that cannot be dissolved are time-release forms, enteric-coated forms, sublingual forms, and bulk-forming laxatives.

The liquid medication must be properly diluted when administered through the feeding tube. The

TABLE 11–2 Osmolality of Selected Drugs

Drug	Average mOsm
Acetaminophen elixir, 65 mg/mL	5400
Amoxicillin suspension, 50 mg/mL	2250
Cephalexin (Keflex) suspension, 50 mg/mL	1950
Cimetidine (Tagamet) solution, 60 mg/mL	5500
Digoxin elixer, 50 µg/mL	1350
Docusate sodium (Colace) syrup, 3.3 mg/mL	3900
Furosemide (Lasix) solution, 10 mg/mL	2050
Lithium citrate syrup, 1.6 mEq/mL	6850
Milk of magnesia suspension	1250
Potassium chloride liquid, 10%	3550
Prochlorperazine syrup, 1 mg/mL	3250
Theophylline solution, 5.33 mg/mL	800

drug dose is usually given as a bolus and then followed with water. Most liquid medications are hyperosmolar (>1000 mOsm/kg) when compared with the osmolality of the secretions of the GI tract (130 to 350 mOsm/kg). Although the hyperosmolality of liquid medication was once thought to be well tolerated by the GI tract, abdominal distention and cramping, vomiting, and diarrhea can result from the administration of undiluted hyperosmolar liquid medications and electrolyte solutions. Liquid medication should be diluted with water to reduce the osmolality to 500 mOsm/kg (mild hyperosmolar) in order to decrease GI intolerance. Table 11–2 lists the osmolalities of various commercial drug suspensions and solutions.

Calculation for Dilution of Enteral Medications

There are three steps that should be followed to determine the amount of water needed for diluting liquid medications.

Step 1: Calculate the drug order to find the volume of the drug.

$$\frac{D}{H} \times V \quad \text{or} \quad H : V :: D : X$$

D: Desired dose: drug dose ordered by health care provider.

H: On-hand dose: drug dose on label of container (bottle, vial, or ampule).

V: Vehicle: form and amount in which the drug is available (tablet, capsule, liquid).

Step 2: Find the osmolality of the drug (check drug literature or with pharmacist) and liquid dilution. Use 500 mOsm as a constant for the desired osmolality.

$$\frac{\text{known mOsm}}{\text{desired mOsm}} \times \text{volume of drug}$$
$$= \text{total volume of liquid}$$

Step 3: Determine the volume of water for dilution.

$$\text{total volume of liquid} - \text{volume of drug}$$
$$= \text{volume of water for dilution}$$

Order: acetaminophen 650 mg, q6h, PRN for pain
Drug Available: Acetaminophen elixir 65 mg/mL
Average mOsm/kg = 5400 (see Table 11–2)

Step 1: Calculate the volume of drug

$$\frac{D}{H} \times V = \frac{650 \text{ mg}}{65 \text{ mg}} \times 1 \text{ mL}$$
$$= \text{or } H : V :: D : X = 10 \text{ mL}$$
$$65 \text{ mg} : 1 \text{ mL} :: 650 \text{ mg} : X \text{ mL}$$
$$65 \text{ X} = 650$$
$$X = 10 \text{ mL of drug}$$

Step 2: Find osmolality of drug and total liquid dilution.

$$\frac{\text{known mOsm (5400)}}{\text{desired mOsm (500)}} \times \text{volume of drug (10)}$$
$$= \frac{5400}{500} \times 10 = 108 \text{ mL of liquid}$$

Step 3: Water for dilution

$$\text{total volume of drug (108 mL)}$$
$$- \text{volume of drug (10 mL)}$$
$$= 98 \text{ mL of water for dilution}$$

NURSING PROCESS: ENTERAL NUTRITION

ASSESSMENT

- Assess that the tape around the tube is secured.
- Assess the client's tolerance to the enteral feeding, including possible GI disturbance (nausea, cramping, diarrhea). These are common complications of enteral feeding.
- Assess urine output. Record result for future comparison.
- Obtain client's weight, which can be used for future comparisons.
- Assess for bowel sounds. Diminished or absence of bowel sounds should be reported immediately to the health care provider.

- Assess baseline laboratory values. Compare with future laboratory results.

NURSING DIAGNOSES

- High risk for fluid volume deficit related to inadequate fluid intake or excess fluid loss.
- High risk for diarrhea related to enteral feedings.
- High risk for aspiration related to enteral feedings via nasogastric tube.

PLANNING

- The client will receive adequate nutritional support through enteral feedings.
- Complication, diarrhea, related to enteral feedings will be managed.

NURSING INTERVENTIONS

- Check tube placement by aspirating gastric secretion or injecting air into the tube to listen by stethoscope for air movement in the stomach. However, injecting air to check for placement may be misleading because the tube may be in the base of the lung and air flow there produces similar sounds as when the tube is placed in the stomach. For placement of the tube for small intestine route, an X-ray confirmation may be needed.
- Check for gastric residual before enteral feeding. A residual of >50% of previous feeding indicates delayed gastric emptying. Notify the health care provider. Usually the residual is 0 to 100 mL.
- Check continuous route for gastric residual every 2 to 4 hours. If residual is >50 mL, stop infusion for 0.5 to 1 h and then recheck.
- Before feeding, raise the head of the bed to a 30-degree angle. If elevating the head of the bed is not advisable, then position the client on his or her right side.
- Deliver the enteral feeding according to the method ordered: bolus, gastric, or small intestine.

- Flush feeding tube accordingly: intermittent feeding, 30 mL before and after; continuous feeding, every 4 hours; medications, 30 mL before and after. If tube obstruction occurs, flush with warm water or cola.
- Monitor adverse effects of enteral feedings such as diarrhea. To manage or correct diarrhea, decrease flow rate for the enteral feedings and, as diarrhea lessens, gradually increase the feeding rate. Enteral solution may be diluted and then gradually increased to full strength. However, diluted solution can decrease the nutrient intake. Determine if the drug(s) could be causing the diarrhea.
- Dilute the drug solution's osmolality to 500 mOsm when giving liquid medication through the tube. Use the formula in the text. Consult with the health care provider.
- Monitor vital signs. Report abnormal findings.
- Give additional water during the day to prevent dehydration. Consult with the health care provider.
- Weigh the client to determine weight gain or loss. Compare with the baseline weight. The client should be weighed at the same time each day, with the same scale and the same amount of clothing.
- Change feeding bag daily. Do not add new solution to old solution in the feeding bag. The nutritional solution should not be ice cold, but at room temperature.

CLIENT TEACHING

- Instruct the client to report any problems related to enteral feedings such as diarrhea, sore throat, abdominal cramping.

EVALUATION

- Determine that the client is receiving prescribed nutrients daily and is free of complications associated with enteral feedings.

PARENTERAL NUTRITION
TOTAL PARENTERAL NUTRITION

Total parenteral nutrition (TPN), also called hyperalimentation or intravenous hyperalimentation (IVH), is the primary method for providing complete nutrients by the parenteral or intravenous route. TPN is an infusion of hyperosmolar glucose, amino acids, vitamins, electrolytes, minerals, and trace elements; it can meet a client's total nutri-

tional needs. TPN is indicated for clients with severe burns who are in negative nitrogen balance, clients with GI disorders, when the GI tract needs a complete rest, and debilitating diseases such as metastatic cancer or AIDS.

The average percent of dextrose in TPN is 25%. This high glucose concentration is mixed with commercially prepared protein sources. Vitamins and electrolytes are added prior to administration. Electrolytes are frequently added immediately before

TABLE 11–3 Complications of Total Parenteral Nutrition

Complication	Causes	Symptoms
Catheter Insertion		
Pneumothorax	Accidental puncture of the pleural cavity.	Sharp chest pain. Decreased breath sounds.
Hemothorax	Catheter damages the large vein.	Same as pneumothorax.
Hydrothorax	Catheter perforates the vein, releasing solution in the chest.	Same as pneumothorax.
TPN Infusion		
Air embolism	IV tubing disconnected. Catheter not clamped. Injection port fell off. Improper changing of IV tubing (no Valsalva procedure).	Coughing, shortness of breath, chest pain, cyanosis.
Infection	Poor aseptic technique when catheter inserted. Contamination when changing tubing. Contamination when solution is mixed. Contamination when dressing is changed.	Temperature > 100°F or 37.7°C. Tachycardia; chills; sweating; redness; swelling; drainage at insertion site; pain in the neck, arm, or shoulder; lethargy.
Hyperglycemia	Fluid infused too rapidly. Insufficient insulin coverage. Infection.	Nausea, headache, weakness, thirst, elevated blood glucose.
Hypoglycemia	Fluids stopped abruptly. Too much insulin infused.	Pallor, cold, clammy skin. Increased pulse rate, "shaky feeling," headache, blurred vision.
Fluid overload hypervolemia	Increased IV rate. Fluids shift from cellular to vascular spaces due to hyperosmolar solutions.	Cough, dyspnea, neck vein engorgement, chest rales, weight gain.

the infusion according to the client's serum electrolyte levels. High glucose concentrations are irritating to peripheral veins, so TPN is administered through central venous lines such as the subclavian or internal jugular.

Enteral feedings should be considered before TPN. Enteral feeding is less costly, poses less risk of sepsis, and maintains GI integrity. When enteral nutrition cannot be used because of severe GI disorders, TPN should be prescribed. TPN does enhance wound healing and provides the necessary nutrients to prevent cellular catabolism.

COMPLICATIONS

Complications associated with TPN can result due to catheter insertion and TPN infusion. Table 11–3 lists the complications associated with TPN.

Complications include pneumothorax, hemothorax, hydrothorax, air embolism, infection, hyperglycemia, and fluid overload (hypervolemia). For the prevention of an air embolism, the client should be taught the **Valsalva maneuver,** which is to take a breath, hold it, and bear down while the nurse is changing infusion bags or bottles and changing tubing. Strict asepsis is necessary when changing IV tubing and dressings at the insertion site. Gloves, masks, and antibacterial ointment usually are necessary. TPN is an excellent medium for organism growth. Most TPN solutions are prepared by the pharmacist with the use of a laminar airflow hood.

Hyperglycemia occurs primarily as the result of the hyperosmolar dextrose solution when TPN is initiated. This occurs until the pancreas adjusts to the hyperglycemic load and therefore may be transient. It also occurs when the infusion rate for TPN is administered too rapidly. In some cases, insulin is added to the TPN solution, which tends to be more effective than administering the insulin subcutaneously. Sudden interruption of TPN therapy can cause hypoglycemia. After the glucose level is decreased, the insulin level remains, causing a hypoglycemic state.

TPN solutions and tubing should be changed every 24 hours. Dressing changes are required every 48 to 72 hours, according to the hospital policy. In some institutions, the dressing is changed every 24 hours for the first 7 to 10 days.

NURSING PROCESS: TOTAL PARENTERAL NUTRITION (TPN)

ASSESSMENT

- Obtain baseline vital signs for future comparison.
- Obtain baseline weight.
- Check laboratory results. Electrolytes, glucose,

and protein levels frequently change during TPN therapy. Early laboratory results are useful for future comparison.
- Check urine output. Report abnormal findings.
- Check the label on the TPN solution. Compare the solution with the order.

POTENTIAL NURSING DIAGNOSES

- High risk for fluid volume excess related to excess fluid infusion or renal dysfunction.
- High risk for fluid volume deficit related to osmotic diuresis due to hyperosmolar TPN solution.
- High risk for infection related to TPN solution that has a high glucose concentration.
- Ineffective breathing pattern related to complication from the insertion of subclavian line.

PLANNING

- The client's nutrient needs will be met via TPN.
- The common complication from TPN therapy, infection, will be avoided.

NURSING INTERVENTIONS

- Monitor vital signs. Report changes.
- Monitor body weight and compare with baseline weight.
- Monitor laboratory results and report abnormal findings, especially electrolytes, protein, glucose. Compare laboratory changes with the baseline findings.
- Monitor intake and output. Fluid volume deficit or excess could occur. Because the TPN solution is hyperosmolar, fluid shift occurs, which can cause osmotic diuresis.
- Monitor temperature changes for possible infection or febrile state. Use aseptic technique when changing dressings and solution bottles or bags.
- Check blood glucose level periodically. When TPN therapy is started, there may be a transient elevated glucose level until the beta cells adjust to the secretion of insulin. If this occurs, the flow rate for TPN should be started slowly and gradually increased as the blood glucose level decreases. Regular insulin may be added to the TPN fluids to correct elevated glucose levels.
- Refrigerate TPN solution that is not in use. High glucose concentration is an excellent medium for bacterial growth.

- Monitor the flow rate of TPN. Start with 60 to 80 mL/h and increase the rate slowly to the ordered level to avoid hyperglycemia.
- Have the client perform the Valsalva maneuver to avoid air embolism by taking a breath, holding it, and bearing down. If the line is opened to air when changing the solution bag or bottle and IV tubing, an air embolus could occur.
- Observe cardiac status because the Valsalva maneuver can cause cardiac dysrhythmias.
- Check for signs and symptoms of overhydration, including coughing, dyspnea, neck vein engorgement, or chest rales. Report findings.
- Follow the institution's procedure for changing dressing and tubing. Usually, tubing is changed daily and the dressing is changed every 24 hours for the first 10 days and then every 48 hours thereafter.
- Do not draw blood, give medications, or check central venous pressure via the TPN line. Results could be invalid.

CLIENT TEACHING

- Provide emotional support to the client and family prior to and during TPN therapy.
- Be available to discuss the client's concerns or refer the client to the appropriate health care provider.
- Instruct the client to notify the health care provider immediately with any discomforts or reactions.
- Keep the client informed of progress and effectiveness of TPN.

EVALUATION

- Evaluate the client's positive and negative response to the TPN therapy.
- Determine periodically if the client's serum electrolytes, protein, and glucose levels are within desired ranges.
- Evaluate nutritional status by weight changes, energy level, feeling of well-being, symptom control, or healing.

■ **CASE STUDY**

M.M. had abdominal surgery and received D_5W and D_5 0.45% NaCl for 4 days. A nasogastric tube was inserted for enteral nutrition. It was determined that the function of M.M.'s GI tract was intact.

1. The route in which M.M. is receiving enteral nutrition is recommended for short-term or long-term enteral feeding? Explain.
2. What are the possible complications that could occur when using this route?
3. M.M. was given Ensure solution. What type of enteral solution is Ensure? How does it differ from a blenderized solution?
4. M.M. received Ensure by the bolus method. Explain how enteral feedings are given by this method.

5. M.M. developed diarrhea. What could be the cause(s) of diarrhea? How can this be managed or corrected?

6. M.M.'s enteral nutrition replacement was switched from the bolus method to the intermittent method. Explain how enteral feedings are administered by the intermittent method.

7. What are the specific nursing interventions in administering enteral nutrition?

M.M. was ordered amoxicillin suspension 250 mg, q.i.d., and potassium chloride solution 10% (15 mEq/10 mL), q 12 h. These medications are to be given through the enteral tubing.

8. What are the osmolalities of amoxicillin and potassium chloride? See Table 11–2.

9. How many mL of amoxicillin should M.M. receive per dose? How much water dilution is needed to reduce the drug osmolality to 500 mOsm? Refer to the chapter for calculation for dilution of liquid medications for enteral administration.

10. How many mL of potassium chloride should M.M. receive per dose? How much water dilution is needed to reduce the drug osmolality to 500 mOsm?

2. What are the four methods of delivery for enteral nutrition? How do these four methods differ from each other?

3. What are the three groups of solution used for enteral nutrition? Give an example from each group.

4. What complications can occur with the use of enteral feedings? Explain.

5. Your client is receiving cimetidine (Tagamet) solution 200 mg, t.i.d. How many mL should your client receive? How much water is needed to reduce the osmolality to 500 mOsm?

6. When is TPN therapy preferred over enteral therapy for nutritional support?

7. What is the composition of TPN solution? Normal dextrose percent is _____.

8. The osmolality of TPN solution is _____.

9. What are the major complications associated with TPN? Explain.

10. How is the Valsalva maneuver performed? What is its purpose?

11. If the blood glucose level is elevated, what are some interventions to reduce the glucose level?

STUDY QUESTIONS

1. What are the differences between enteral nutrition and parenteral nutrition? Would D_5W, normal saline solution (0.9% NaCl), and lactated Ringer's solution be a form of nutritional support? Explain.

Unit IV

Neurologic and Neuromuscular Agents

The nervous system is composed of all nerve tissues: brain, spinal cord, nerves, and ganglia. The purpose of the nervous system is to receive stimuli and transmit information to nerve centers for an appropriate response. There are two types of nervous systems: the central nervous system and the peripheral nervous system.

The **central nervous system (CNS),** composed of the brain and spinal cord, regulates body functions (Fig. IV–1). The CNS interprets information sent by impulses from the **peripheral nervous system (PNS)** and returns the instruction through the PNS for appropriate cellular actions. Stimulation of the CNS may either increase nerve cell (neuron) activity or block nerve cell activity.

The PNS consists of two divisions: the **somatic nervous system (SNS)** and the **autonomic nervous system (ANS).** The SNS is voluntary and acts on skeletal muscles to produce locomotion and respiration. The ANS, also called the visceral system, is involuntary and controls and regulates the functioning of the heart, respiratory system, gastrointestinal system, and glands. The ANS, a large nervous system that functions without our conscious control, has two subdivisions: the sympathetic and the parasympathetic.

The sympathetic nervous system of the ANS is referred to as the **adrenergic system** because its neurotransmitter is *norepinephrine*. The parasympathetic nervous system is referred to as the **cholinergic system** because its neurotransmitter is *acetylcholine*. Because organs are innervated by both the sympathetic and the parasympathetic systems they can produce opposite responses. The sympathetic response is excitability, and the parasympathetic response is inhibition.

Both the sympathetic and parasympathetic nerve pathways originate from different locations in the spinal cord. These nervous systems send information by two types of nerve fibers, the preganglionic and the postganglionic, and by the ganglion between these fibers (Fig. IV–2). The preganglionic nerve fiber carries messages from the CNS to the ganglion, and the postganglionic fiber transmits impulses from the ganglion to body tissues and organs.

The sympathetic nervous system is also referred to as the **thoracolumbar division** of the ANS because the preganglionic fibers originate from the thorax (T1 to T12) and the upper lumbar segments (L1 and L2) of the spinal cord. The sympathetic preganglionic fibers are short from the spinal cord to the ganglion, and the sympathetic postganglionic fibers are long from the ganglion to the body cells. Figure IV–3 illustrates the sympathetic preganglionic fibers from the spinal cord.

The parasympathetic nervous system is referred to as the **craniosacral division** of the ANS because the preganglionic fibers originate with the cranial nerves III, VII, IX, and X from the brain stem and the sacral segments S2, S3, and S4 from the spinal cord. The parasympathetic preganglionic fibers are long from the spinal cord to the ganglion, and the parasympa-

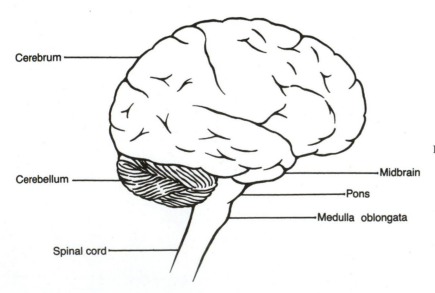

FIGURE IV–1. Brain and spinal cord.

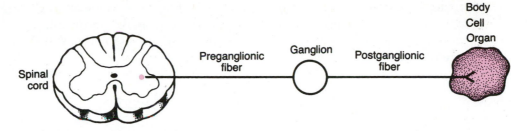

FIGURE IV–2. Preganglionic and postganglionic nerve fibers.

thetic postganglionic fibers are short from the ganglion to the body cells. Figure IV–4 illustrates the parasympathetic preganglionic fibers from the spinal cord.

Drugs that affect the sympathetic and the parasympathetic nervous systems are discussed in Chapters 17, 18, and 19. Drugs that stimulate and depress the CNS are discussed in Chapters 12, 13, and 14. Amphetamines and amphetamine-like drugs, anorexiants, analeptics, and xanthines (caffeine) stimulate the CNS. Some of these drugs are used therapeutically for narcolepsy and attention deficit disorder (ADD). The group of drugs that depress the CNS are sedatives-hypnotics, anesthetics, narcotics, and nonnarcotic agents. Drugs used to control convulsions (anticonvulsants, discussed in Chapter 15) are considered depressants of the

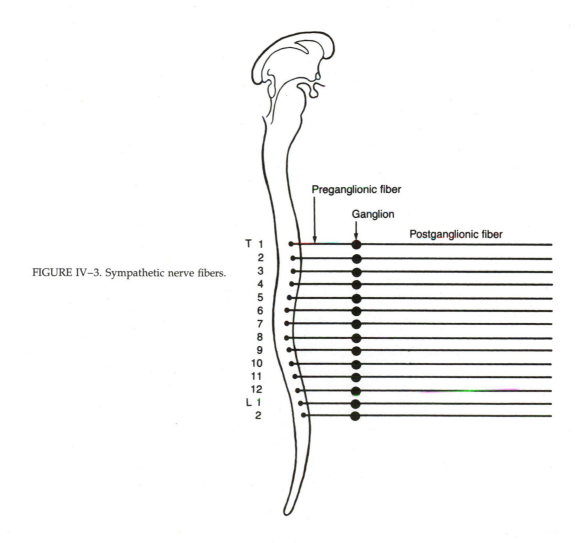

FIGURE IV–3. Sympathetic nerve fibers.

CNS. The drug groups for controlling psychiatric disorders, discussed in Chapter 16, also affect CNS response. For neuromuscular disorders, such as Parkinsonism, myasthenia gravis, and multiple sclerosis, the drugs have varying effect on the nervous system and muscles, and are discussed in Chapter 20.

Figure IV–5 is a schematic breakdown of the nervous systems in the body.

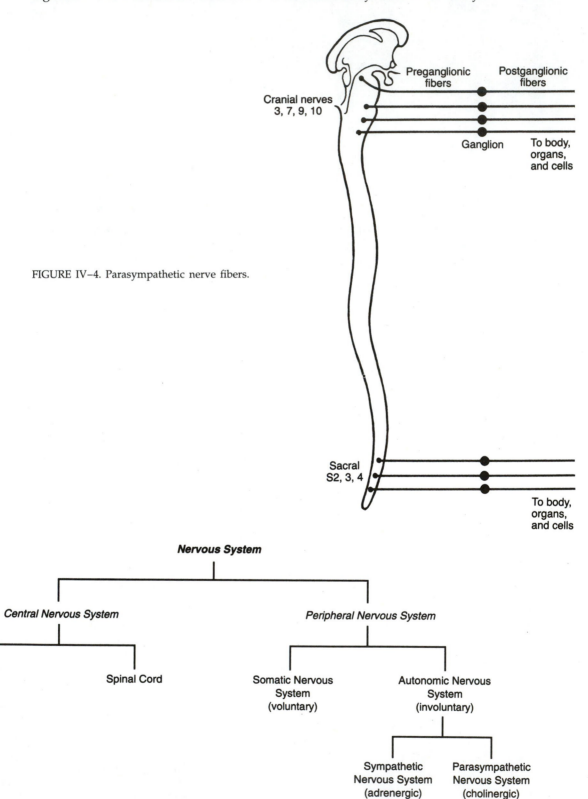

FIGURE IV–4. Parasympathetic nerve fibers.

FIGURE IV–5. Body's nervous system.

Chapter 12

Central Nervous System Stimulants

OUTLINE

Objectives

Terms

Introduction

Amphetamines

    Amphetamine-like Drugs

Anorexiants

Analeptics

Nursing Process

Study Questions

OBJECTIVES

Explain the effects of stimulants on the central nervous system.

Define narcolepsy and attention deficit disorder.

List the drugs that are used for narcolepsy and attention deficit disorder.

Identify the common side effects of amphetamines, anorexiants, analeptics, and caffeine.

Identify at least four nursing interventions when administering CNS stimulants.

TERMS

amphetamines

analeptics

anorexiants

attention deficit disorder
   (ADD)

autonomic nervous system
   (ANS)

axons

central nervous system
   (CNS)

dependence

hyperkinesis

narcolepsy

neurons

neurotransmitters

peripheral nervous system
   (PNS)

tolerance

INTRODUCTION

Numerous drugs can stimulate the **central nervous system (CNS),** but the medically approved use of these drugs is limited to the treatment of narcolepsy, attention deficit disorder (ADD) in children, obesity, and the reversal of respiratory distress. The major group of CNS stimulants includes amphetamines and caffeine, which stimulate the cerebral cortex of the brain; analeptics and caffeine, which act on the brain stem and medulla to stimulate respiration; and anorexiants, which act to some degree on the cerebral cortex and on the hypothalamus to suppress appetite. The amphetamines and related anorexiants have been greatly abused. Long-term use of amphetamines can produce psychological **dependence** and **tolerance,** a condition in which larger and larger doses of a drug are needed to reproduce the initial response. Gradually increasing a drug dose and then abruptly stopping the drug may result in depression and withdrawal symptoms.

AMPHETAMINES

Amphetamines stimulate the release of the **neurotransmitters,** norepinephrine and dopamine, from the brain and the sympathetic nervous system (peripheral nerve terminals). The amphetamines cause euphoria and alertness; however, they can also cause sleeplessness, restlessness, tremors, and irritability. Cardiovascular problems, such as increased heart rate, palpitations, cardiac dysrhythmias, and increased blood pressure, can result from continuous use of amphetamines.

The half-life of amphetamines varies from 4 to 30 h. Amphetamines are excreted faster in acid than in alkaline urine. When CNS toxicity or cardiac toxicity is suspected, decreasing the urine pH aids in the excretion of the drug. An acid urine decreases the half-life of the amphetamine. Table 12–1 lists the amphetamines and amphetamine-like drugs, their dosages, uses, and considerations.

SIDE EFFECTS AND ADVERSE REACTIONS

Amphetamines can cause adverse effects in the central nervous, cardiovascular, gastrointestinal (GI), and endocrine systems. The side effects and adverse reactions include restlessness, insomnia, tachycardia, hypertension, heart palpitations, dry mouth, anorexia, weight loss, diarrhea or constipation, and impotence.

Amphetamine-like Drugs for Narcolepsy and ADD

Amphetamine-like drugs are given for the treatment of narcolepsy and **attention deficit disorder (ADD).**

TABLE 12–1 Amphetamines and Amphetamine-like Drugs

Generic Brand	Route and Dosage	Uses and Considerations
Amphetamines		
Amphetamine sulfate CSS II	*Narcolepsy* A: PO: 5–20 mg, q.d.–t.i.d.; *max:* 60 mg/d C > 6–12y: PO: 5 mg/d *ADD* C 3–5 y: PO: 2.5 mg/d C 6–12 y: PO: 5 mg/d, *max:* 40 mg/d	For narcolepsy, attention deficit disorder (ADD). Dosage should be minimal to control symptoms in ADD. CNS and cardiac toxicity could occur. *Pregnancy category:* C; PB: UK; t½: 10–30 h.
Dextroamphetamine sulfate (Dexedrine) CSS II	*ADD* C 3–5 y: PO: 2.5 mg/d C 6–12 y: PO: 5 mg/d, *max:* 40 mg/d	Uses similar to those of amphetamines. Drug has been used for obesity and narcolepsy. *Pregnancy category:* C; PB: UK; t½: UK.
Methamphetamine HCl (Desoxyn) CSS II	C: PO: 2.5–5mg daily; increase to 20 mg as needed in 2 divided doses	For ADD. Could cause CNS and cardiac toxicity. *Pregnancy category:* C; PB: UK; t½: UK.
Amphetamine-like drugs Methylphenidate (Ritalin) CSS II	See Figure 12–1	For ADD in children. Dose is increased weekly until symptoms are alleviated. Absorption is affected by food. For narcolepsy. *Pregnancy category:* C; PB: UK; t½: 1–3 h.
Pemoline (Cylert) CSS IV	C > 6 y: PO: 37.5 mg daily and increase weekly; average: 50–75 mg/d *max:* 112.5 mg/d	For ADD in children. Less potent and fewer side effects than Desoxyn and Ritalin. Insomnia may occur; reduce dose. *Pregnancy category:* B; PB: 50%; t½: 9–12 h.

KEY: A: adult; C: child; CSS: controlled substance schedule; PB: protein-binding; PO: by mouth; t½: half-life; UK: unknown; >: greater than.

Narcolepsy is characterized by falling asleep during normal waking activity (e.g., while driving a car or talking with someone). Sleep paralysis, the condition of muscle paralysis that is normal during sleep, usually accompanies narcolepsy and affects the voluntary muscles. The person is unable to move and may collapse.

ADD is the inability to learn and to interact socially due to hyperactivity (excessive and purposeless activity) and a decrease in attention span. This condition occurs most frequently in children. The child may display poor coordination, and there may be abnormal electroencephalographic (EEG) findings. Intelligence is usually not affected. This problem has also been called minimal brain dysfunction, hyperactivity in children, **hyperkinesis,** and hyperkinetic syndrome with learning disorder. Counseling or psychotherapy as well as drug and diet therapy may be needed to decrease or alleviate the hyperactive behavior. Amphetamine and amphetamine-like stimulants are given to increase the child's attention span and improve daytime sleepiness. Sedatives are not indicated. Two amphetamine-like drugs, methylphenidate (Ritalin) and pemoline (Cylert) are usually prescribed for treating ADD and narcolepsy rather than the amphetamines, owing to their lower incidence of side effects. Figure 12–1 compares the pharmacokinetics,

FIGURE 12–1. Amphetamine-like Drugs

Amphetamine-like Drugs	Dosage	NURSING PROCESS
		Assessment and Planning
Central Nervous System Stimulants	(M) *Attention deficit disorder:* C >6 y: PO: 5 mg before breakfast and lunch; if necessary increase dosage weekly by 5–10 mg; max: 60 mg/d SR: Not recommended for initial treatment *Narcolepsy:* A: PO: 10 mg, b.i.d.-t.i.d. 30 min before meals (P) *Attention deficit disorder:* C >6 y: PO: 37.5 mg daily and increase weekly; average dose: 50–75 mg/d; max: 112.5 mg/d	
Methylphenidate HCl (M) (Ritalin, Ritalin SR) *Pregnancy Category:* C		
Pemoline (P) (Cylert) *Pregnancy Category:* B		
Contraindications	**Drug-Lab-Food Interactions**	
(M&P) Hypersensitivity (M) Hyperthyroidism, anxiety, history of seizures, motor tics, Tourette syndrome, glaucoma *Caution:* (M) Hypertension, depression, alcoholism, pregnancy (P) Impaired renal or hepatic function, psychosis (M&P) not to be used for children <6 y	(M) *Increase* hypertensive crisis with MAOIs (M) *Increase* effects of oral anticoagulants, anticonvulsants, tricyclic antidepressants (M&P) May *decrease* effects of decongestants, antihypertensives, barbiturates; may alter effects of insulin therapy. *Food:* Caffeine (coffee, tea, colas, chocolate) may *increase* effects *Lab:* (P) May *increase* AST, ALT, LDH	
Pharmacokinetics	**Pharmacodynamics**	Interventions
Absorption: (M&P) well absorbed from GI tract *Distribution:* PB: (M) UK, (P) 50% *Metabolism:* t½: (M) 1–3 h, (P) 10–14 h *Excretion:* (M) 40% excreted unchanged in urine (P) excreted in the urine	(M) PO: Onset: 0.5–1 h Peak: 1–3 h Duration: 4–6 h SR: 4–8 h (P) PO: Onset: 0.5–1 h Peak: 2–4 h Duration: 8 h	

Illustration continued on following page

FIGURE 12–1. *Continued*

Therapeutic Effects/Uses: (M&P) To correct hyperactivity caused by ADD, increase attention span, and treat fatigue

(M) To control narcolepsy

Mode of action: Acts primarily on the cerebral cortex, reticular activatory system

Side Effects	Adverse Reactions	Evaluation
(M&P) Anorexia, vomiting, diarrhea, insomnia, dizziness, nervousness, restlessness, irritability	(M&P) Tachycardia, growth suppression (M) Palpitations, transient loss of weight in children, increased hyperactivity (P) Dyskinetic movements (face, lips, tongue), hepatitis, jaundice *Life-threatening:* (M) Exfoliative dermatitis, uremia, thrombocytopenia	

KEY: PO: by mouth; PB: protein: protein-binding; t½: half-life, UK: unknown, A: adult, C: child, SR: sustained release.

pharmacodynamics, and therapeutic effects of methylphenidate and pemoline in treating ADD and narcolepsy.

Pharmacokinetics

Methylphenidate and pemoline are well absorbed from the GI mucosa. Although pemoline has a longer half-life than methylphenidate, the drugs are usually administered to children once a day before breakfast. However, methylphenidate may be given twice a day, before breakfast and lunch. Because food affects the absorption rate, the drug should be given 30 to 45 min before meals. These drugs should not be given 6 h before sleep because they may cause insomnia. Both drugs are excreted in the urine; 40% of methylphenidate is excreted unchanged.

Pharmacodynamics

Methylphenidate and pemoline help to correct ADD by decreasing hyperactivity and improving attention span. These amphetamine-like drugs are considered more effective in treating ADD than amphetamines. Amphetamines are generally avoided because they have a higher potential for abuse, habituation, and tolerance. Methylphenidate is slightly more effective than pemoline for ADD, but pemoline's side effects and adverse reactions are less severe.

Sympathomimetic drugs, such as decongestants, enhance the actions of methylphenidate and pemoline. Antihypertensives and barbiturates can decrease the action of these drugs. Foods with caffeine content should be avoided because they increase drug action.

ANOREXIANTS

Obesity has been treated with prescribed amphetamines or over-the-counter (OTC) amphetamine-like drugs. Amphetamines have been recommended as **anorexiants** (appetite suppressants) for short-term use (4 to 12 weeks). Because of tolerance, psychological dependence, and abuse, amphetamines are *not* recommended today for use as appetite suppressants. The OTC choice for short-term use of an appetite suppressant is phenylpropanolamine (Dexatrim) since it causes fewer systemic side effects and has less of a potential for abuse. Most of the anorexiants used to suppress appetite (Table 12–2) do not have the serious side effects associated with amphetamines. To lose weight, emphasis should be placed on proper diet, exercise, and behavioral modifications. Reliance on appetite suppressants should be discouraged. Those individuals who are taking anorexiants should be under a health care provider's care.

TABLE 12–2 Anorexiants and Analeptics

Drug	Route and Dosage	Uses and Considerations
Anorexiants		
Benzphetamine HCl (Didrex) CSS III	A: PO: 25–50 mg q.d.–t.i.d.	Similar to amphetamines. Potential for abuse. Avoid taking drug during pregnancy. *Pregnancy category:* X; PB: UK, t½: 6–12 h.
Dextroamphetamine sulfate (Dexedrine) CSS II	A: PO: 5–30 mg daily in divided doses 30–60 min a.c. of 5–10 mg	To treat obesity. Can cause restlessness and insomnia. For short-term use. *Pregnancy category:* C; PB: UK; t½: 30–35 h.
Diethylpropion HCl (Dospan, Tenuate, Tepanil) CSS IV	A: PO: 25 mg t.i.d.; SR: 75 mg daily	For appetite suppression by stimulating the appetite control center in the hypothalamus. Take 1 h before meals. For short-term use. *Pregnancy category:* B; PB: UK; t½: 2–3 h.
Fenfluramine HCl (Pondimin) CSS IV	A: PO: 20 mg t.i.d.; a.c. max: 120 mg/d May increase weekly	To treat exogenous obesity. Should be taken 1 h before meals. Can depress mood and motor activity, and may increase blood pressure (BP). *Pregnancy category:* C; PB: UK; t½: 20 h
Mazindol (Mazanor, Sanorex) CSS IV	A: PO: Initial: 2 mg/d A: PO: 1 mg t.i.d. a.c. or 2 mg daily	To manage obesity. To be taken 1 h before meals or daily dose before lunch. May increase heart rate. BP usually unchanged. Is a potential abuse drug. *Pregnancy category:* C; PB: UK; t½: 2.5–9 h.
Phendimetrazine tartrate (Anorex, Adipost, Trimcaps, Prelu-2) CSS III	A: PO: 17.5–35 mg 1 h a.c. b.i.d.–t.i.d.; max: 70 mg t.i.d.	To manage obesity. Should be taken 1 h before meals. Usually no change in heart rate or blood pressure. CNS stimulation (mood and motor activity). *Pregnancy category:* C; PB: UK; t½: 2–10 h.
Phenmetrazine HCl (Preludin) CSS II	A: PO: 25 mg b.i.d.–t.i.d.; SR: 75 mg daily; max: 75 mg daily	Short-term use to manage obesity. Should be taken 1 h before meals. Increases CNS, heart rate, and blood pressure. High abuse potential. *Pregnancy category:* C; PB: UK; t½: UK.
Phentermine HCl (Adipex-P, Fastin, Ionamin) CSS IV	A: PO: 8 mg t.i.d.; a.c. or 15–37.5 mg/d	To control appetite. Should be taken before meals. Increases heart rate and blood pressure. Low abuse potential. *Pregnancy category:* C; PB: UK; t½: 20h.
Phenylpropanolamine HCl (Acutrim, Control, Dexatrim, Prolamine)	A: PO: 25 mg a.c. t.i.d.; or SR: 75 mg/d in morning	To control weight gain. Should be taken before meals. OTC drugs. May increase heart rate and blood pressure. Low abuse potential. *Pregnancy category:* C; PB: UK; t½: 4–7 h.
Analeptics: Methylxanthines		
Caffeine Nō Dōz, Tirend, Vivarin)	*Neonatal apnea:* Infants and C: PO: IM-IV. 5–10 mg/kg on day 1; then 2.5–5 mg/d *Therapeutic range:* 5–20 mg/mL	Used for newborns with apnea to stimulate respiration; increases heart rate and blood pressure. Given through a nasogastric tube, intramuscularly or intravenously. *Pregnancy category:* C; PB: 25%–35%; t½: A: 3–5 h, neonate: 40–144 h.
OTC drugs (Nō Dōz, Tirend) Coffee	A: 100–200 mg q 3–4 hours as needed	Restores mental alertness. Contains citrated caffeine. Coffee contains 60–140 mg of caffeine per cup.
Theophylline	Infants: NGT; 5 mg/kg on day 1; then 2 mg in divided doses	Used for newborns with apnea to stimulate respiration. Given through a nasogastric tube.
CNS Stimulant for Migraine Sumatriptan succinate (Imitrex)	A: SC: 6 mg single dose; may repeat in 1 h; max 12 mg/d	To treat acute migraine attacks. Promotes vasoconstriction of the carotid arteries. *Pregnancy category:* C; PB: 20%; t½: 2 h.
Respiratory Stimulant Doxapram HCl (Dopram)	A: IV: 0.5–1 mg/kg; inf: 1–2 mg/min; max: 3 g/d *Neonatal apnea:* Initially: 0.5 mg/kg/h Maintenance: 0.5–2.5 mg/kg/h titrated to lowest effective rate	Used in adults only for chronic obstructive pulmonary disease (COPD). Used to treat sedative-hypnotic overdose to correct respiratory depression. It can increase blood pressure. *Pregnancy category:* B; PB: UK; t½: A: 2.5–4 h, neonate: 7–10 h.

KEY: *A: adult; C: child; CSS: Controlled Substance Schedule; max: maximum; NGT: nasogastric tube; PB: protein-binding; PO: by mouth; SC: subcutaneous; SR: sustained-release; t½: half-life; UK: unknown.*

SIDE EFFECTS AND ADVERSE REACTIONS

Children under 12 years old should *not* take anorexiants, and self-medication with anorexiants should be discouraged. Long-term use of these drugs frequently results in such severe side effects as nervousness, restlessness, irritability, insomnia, heart palpitations, and hypertension.

ANALEPTICS

Analeptics, which are CNS stimulants, mostly affect the brain stem and spinal cord but also affect the cerebral cortex. The primary use of an analeptic is to stimulate respiration. One subgroup of analeptics is the xanthines (methylxanthines), of which caffeine and theophylline are the main drugs. Depending on the dose, caffeine stimulates the CNS, and large doses stimulate respiration. Newborns with respiratory distress might be given caffeine to increase respiration. Theophylline is used mostly to relax the bronchioles; however, it has also been used to increase respiration in newborns. Table 12–2 lists the analeptics, their dosages, uses, and considerations.

SIDE EFFECTS AND ADVERSE REACTIONS

The side effects from caffeine are similar to those from anorexiants: nervousness, restlessness, tremors, twitchings, palpitations, and insomnia. Other side effects include diuresis (increased urination), GI irritation (nausea, diarrhea), and, rarely, tinnitus (ringing in the ear). More than 500 mg of caffeine affects the CNS and heart. High doses of caffeine in coffee, chocolate, and cold-relief medications can cause a psychological dependence. The half-life of caffeine is 3.5 h; however, metabolism is slowed and the half-life is prolonged in liver disease and in pregnancy. Caffeine is contraindicated during pregnancy because the effect on the fetus is not known.

NURSING PROCESS: CENTRAL NERVOUS SYSTEM STIMULANT: Methylphenidate HCl (Ritalin)

ASSESSMENT

- Determine if there is a history of heart disease, hypertension, hyperthyroidism, parkinsonism, or glaucoma; in such cases, drug is usually contraindicated.
- Assess vital signs to be used for future comparisons. Pay close attention to clients with cardiac disease as drug may reverse effects of antihypertensives.
- Assess the client's mental status; e.g., mood, affect, aggressiveness.
- Assess height, growth, weight of children.
- Assess CBC, differential WBCs, and platelets before and during therapy.

POTENTIAL NURSING DIAGNOSES

- Behavior disorders (impulsiveness, short attention span, and distractibility) that interfere with peer relationships, learning, and discipline.
- Potential for family crisis related to dysfunctional behavior.

PLANNING

- Client will be free of hyperactivity.
- Client will not experience side effects or adverse reactions to therapy. Client will increase attention span.

NURSING INTERVENTIONS

- Monitor vital signs. Report irregularities.
- Monitor height, weight, and growth of child.
- Monitor the client for withdrawal symptoms; e.g., nausea, vomiting, weakness, headache.
- Monitor the client for side effects; e.g., insomnia, restlessness, nervousness, tremors, irritability, tachycardia, or elevated blood pressure. Report findings.

CLIENT TEACHING

General
- Instruct the client to take drug before meals.
- Instruct the client to avoid alcohol consumption.
- Encourage the use of sugarless gum to relieve dry mouth.
- Instruct the client to monitor weight 2×/wk and to report weight loss.
- Instruct the client to avoid driving and using hazardous equipment when experiencing tremors, nervousness, or increased heart rate.
- Instruct the client not to abruptly discontinue the drug; the dose must be tapered off to avoid

withdrawal symptoms. Consult the health care provider before modifying the dose.

- Encourage the client to read the labels on OTC products because many contain caffeine. A high caffeine plasma level could be fatal.
- Instruct the nursing mother to avoid taking all CNS stimulants. These drugs pass into the breast milk and can cause the infant to be hyperactive or restless.
- Encourage the family to seek counseling for children with attention deficit disorder. Drug therapy alone is not an appropriate therapy program. Notify school nurse of drug therapy regimen.
- Explain to client/family that long-term use may lead to drug abuse.

Diet
- Instruct the client to avoid caffeine-containing foods.

- Instruct parents to provide children with a nutritional breakfast because drug may have anorexic effects.

Side Effects
- Instruct the client about drug side effects and the need to report tachycardia and palpitations. Monitor children for onset of Tourette's syndrome.

EVALUATION

- Evaluate the effectiveness of drug therapy. The client is not hyperactive and does not have adverse effects from drug.
- Monitor weight, sleep patterns, and mental status.

STUDY QUESTIONS

1. A 5-year-old boy was diagnosed as having attention deficit disorder (ADD). What is ADD? What drugs are effective in controlling this problem?
2. What are appetite suppressants called? Why are amphetamines not recommended today for the treatment of obesity?

3. The client has hypertension. Why are amphetamines not recommended for hypertensive clients? List the side effects of amphetamines.
4. A mother is breast feeding her infant daughter. She wants to lose 30 lb and plans to take an OTC anorexiant. What would your response be? Explain.

Chapter 13

Central Nervous System Depressants

OUTLINE

Objectives
Terms
Introduction
    Types and Stages of Sleep
Sedative-Hypnotics
    Barbiturates
    Nursing Process

Benzodiazepines
Piperidinediones
Chloral Hydrate
Nursing Process
Anesthetics
    Stages of Anesthesia
    Inhalation Anesthetics

Intravenous Anesthetics
Local Anesthesia
Spinal Anesthesia
Nursing Process
Study Questions

OBJECTIVES

Identify the types and stages of sleep.

Identify several nonpharmacologic ways to induce sleep.

Define *hangover, dependence, tolerance, withdrawal symptoms,* and *REM rebound.*

Explain which drugs might cause the above adverse effects.

List examples of short-acting and intermediate-acting barbiturates used as sedative-hypnotics.

List three benzodiazepines developed for hypnotic use.

Give the nursing interventions related to barbiturates and benzodiazepine hypnotics.

Describe the stages of anesthesia.

Identify examples of general and local anesthetics and their major side effects.

TERMS

anesthetics
balanced anesthesia
barbiturates
caudal anesthesia
dependence
epidural anesthesia

hangover
hypnotic effect
infiltration anesthesia
insomnia
nerve block anesthesia
NREM sleep

REM sleep
sedation
spinal anesthesia
tolerance
withdrawal symptoms

INTRODUCTION

Drugs that are CNS depressants cause varying degrees of depression (reduction in functional activity) within the central nervous system. The degree of depression depends primarily on the drug and the amount of drug taken. The broad classification of CNS depressants includes sedative-hypnotics, general and local anesthetics, analgesics, narcotic analgesics, anticonvulsants, antipsychotics, and antidepressants. The last five groups of drugs are presented in separate chapters. Sedative-hypnotics and general and local anesthetics are covered in this chapter.

Sleep disorders, such as **insomnia** (inability to fall asleep) occur in 5% to 10% of healthy adults, 20% to 25% of hospitalized clients, and approximately 75% of psychiatric clients. Insomnia occurs more frequently in women and increases with age. Sedative-hypnotics are frequently ordered for sleep disorders and will be discussed after the discussion on normal sleep and its major components.

TYPES AND STAGES OF SLEEP

People spend approximately one-third of their lives, or as much as 25 years, sleeping. Normal sleep is composed of two definite phases: **REM,** or **rapid eye movement,** and **NREM,** or **nonrapid eye movement.** Both REM and NREM occur cyclically during sleep at about 90-minute intervals (Fig. 13–1). The four succeedingly deeper stages of NREM sleep end with an episode of REM sleep and the cycle begins again. If sleep is interrupted, the cycle begins again with stage 1 of NREM sleep.

It is during the REM sleep phase that individuals experience most of their recallable dreams. Individuals perform better during their waking hours if they experience all types and stages of sleep. Children have few REM sleep periods, and have longer periods of stage 3 and 4 NREM sleep. Older adults (elderly) have a decrease in stage 3 and 4 of NREM sleep and have frequent waking periods.

Nonpharmacologic methods should be used for promoting sleep before using sedative-hypnotics or over-the-counter (OTC) sleep aids. Once the nurse discovers why the client cannot sleep, she or he may suggest the following ways for promoting sleep:

1. Arise at a specific hour in the morning.
2. Take few or no daytime naps.
3. Avoid drinks that contain caffeine 6 h before bedtime.
4. Avoid heavy meals or strenuous exercise before bedtime.
5. Take a warm bath, read, or listen to music before bedtime.
6. Decrease exposure to loud noises.
7. Avoid drinking copious amounts of fluids prior to sleep.
8. Drink warm milk prior to bedtime.

SEDATIVE-HYPNOTICS

The mildest form of CNS depression is **sedation,** which at lower dosages of certain CNS depressants diminishes physical and mental responses but does

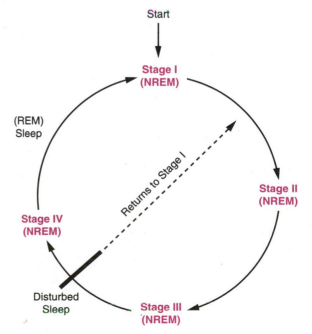

FIGURE 13–1. Types and stages of sleep. (*Key:* REM: rapid eye movement [dreaming]; NREM: nonrapid eye movement [4 stages].)

not affect consciousness. Sedatives are used mostly during the daytime. Increasing the drug dose can produce a **hypnotic effect**—not hypnosis, but a form of "natural" sleep. Sedative-hypnotic drugs are sometimes the same drug; however, certain drugs are used more often for their hypnotic effect. With very high doses of sedative-hypnotic drugs, anesthesia may be achieved. An example of an ultrashort-acting barbiturate used to produce anesthesia is thiopental sodium (Pentothal).

Sedatives were first prescribed for reducing tension and anxiety. Barbiturates were used first for their antianxiety effect, until the early 1960s when benzodiazepines were introduced. Because of the many side effects of barbiturates and their potential for physical and mental dependency, they are less frequently prescribed today. Similarly, the chronic use of any sedative-hypnotic should be avoided.

Because of the high incidence of sleep disorders, hypnotic drugs are one of the most frequently prescribed drugs. Over $35 million is spent each year for OTC sleep aids, such as Nytol, Sominex, Sleepeze, Tylenol PM. The primary ingredient in OTC sleep aids is an antihistamine, such as diphenhydramine, and not barbiturates or benzodiazepines.

There are short-acting hypnotics and intermediate-acting hypnotics. Short-acting hypnotics are useful in achieving sleep because they allow the client to awaken early in the morning without experiencing lingering side effects. Intermediate-acting hypnotics are useful for sustaining sleep; however, after using one the client may experience residual drowsiness **(hangover)** in the morning. This may be undesirable if the client is active and requires mental alertness. The ideal hypnotic promotes natural sleep without disrupting normal patterns of sleep and produces no hangover or undesirable effect. Table 13–1 lists the common side effects and adverse reactions associated with sedative-hypnotic use and abuse.

Hypnotic drug therapy should be short term to prevent drug dependence and drug tolerance. Interrupting hypnotic therapy can decrease drug tolerance. However, abruptly discontinuing a high dose of hypnotic that has been taken over a long period of time could cause withdrawal symptoms. At high doses, the dose should be tapered to avoid withdrawal symptoms. The lowest dose should be taken to obtain sleep. Clients with severe respiratory disorders should avoid hypnotics, which could cause an increase in respiratory distress. Normally hypnotics are contraindicated during pregnancy.

The category of sedative-hypnotics includes barbiturates, benzodiazepines, and piperidinediones, among others. Each of these is discussed separately. Drug charts are included for barbiturates and benzodiazepines.

BARBITURATES

Barbiturates were introduced as a sedative in the early 1900s. Over 2000 barbiturates have been developed, but only 12 are currently marketed. The barbiturates are classified as long-acting, intermediate-acting, short-acting, and ultrashort-acting. The long-acting group includes phenobarbital and mephobarbital and is used for controlling seizures in epilepsy. The ultrashort-acting barbiturate, thiopental sodium (Pentothal), is used as general anesthe-

TABLE 13–1 Common Side Effects and Adverse Reactions of Sedative-Hypnotics

Side Effects and Adverse Reactions	Explanation of the Effects
Hangover	A hangover is residual drowsiness resulting in impaired reaction time. The intermediate and long-acting hypnotics are frequently the cause of drug hangover. The liver biotransforms these drugs into active metabolites that persist in the body, causing drowsiness.
REM Rebound	REM rebound, which results in vivid dreams and nightmares, frequently occurs after taking a hypnotic over a prolonged period and then abruptly stopping. However, it may occur after taking only one hypnotic dose.
Dependence	Dependence is the result of chronic use of hypnotics. Physical and psychologic dependence can result. Physical dependence results in the appearance of specific withdrawal symptoms when a drug is discontinued after prolonged use. The severity of withdrawal symptoms depends on the drug and the dosage. Symptoms may include muscular twitching and tremors, dizziness, orthostatic hypotension, delusions, hallucinations, delirium, and seizures. The withdrawal symptoms start within 24 h and can last for several days.
Tolerance	Tolerance results when there is a need to increase the dosage over time to obtain the desired effect. It is mostly due to an increase in drug metabolism by liver enzymes. Barbiturates is one drug category that can cause tolerance after prolonged use. Tolerance is reversible when the drug is discontinued.
Excessive Depression	Long-term use of a hypnotic may result in depression, which is characterized by lethargy, sleepiness, lack of concentration, confusion, and psychologic depression.
Respiratory Depression	High doses of sedative-hypnotics can suppress the respiratory center in the medulla.
Hypersensitivity	Skin rashes and urticaria can result when taking barbituates. Such reactions are rare.

sia. Phenobarbital, introduced in 1912, is still in use today.

The short-acting barbiturates secobarbital (Seconal) and pentobarbital (Nembutal) are used to induce sleep for those who have difficulty falling asleep. These drugs may cause the person to awaken early in the morning. The intermediate-acting barbiturates amobarbital (Amytal), aprobarbital (Alurate), and butabarbital (Butisol) are useful as sleep sustainers for maintaining long periods of

TABLE 13–2 Sedative-Hypnotics: Barbiturates and Others

Generic (Brand)	Route and Dosage	Uses and Considerations
Barbiturates:		
Short Acting		
Pentobarbital sodium (Nembutal Sodium)	See Prototype Drug Chart (Fig. 13–2)	For sedative or sleep. Can be used for induction to general anesthesia. *Pregnancy category:* D; PB: 35%–45%; t½: 4 h, 30–50 h (2nd phase)
Secobarbital sodium (Seconal Sodium) CSS II	*Preoperative sedative:* A: PO: 100–300 mg before surgery C: PO: 50–100 mg or 2–6 mg/kg max: 100 mg *Hypnotic:* A: PO/IM: 100–200 mg h.s. C: IM 3–5 mg/kg; max: 100 mg *Status epilepticus:* A: IV: 5.5 mg/kg; repeat in 3–4 h *With spinal anesthesia:* A: IV: 50–100 mg; infuse over 30 sec; max: 250 mg/dose	For sedation or sleep. Also preanesthetic sedation. *Pregnancy category:* D; PB: UK; t½: 15–40 h
Barbiturates:		
Intermediate Acting		
Amobarbital sodium (Amytal Sodium)	*Sedative:* A: PO: 30–50 mg b.i.d.–t.i.d. C: PO: 2 mg/kg/d in 3–4 divided doses *Hypnotic:* A: PO/IM: 65–200 mg h.s. C: IM: 2–3 mg/kg A and C: IV: 65–200 mg	As a sedative and short-term hypnotic; to control acute convulsive episodes; and for insomnia. Take 0.5–1 h before bedtime. *Pregnancy category:* D; PB: 50%–60%; t½: 20–40 h
Aprobarbital (Alurate)	*Sedative:* A: PO: 40 mg t.i.d. *Hypnotic:* A: PO: 40–160 mg h.s.	As a sedative and short-term hypnotic; use no longer than 2 wk. *Pregnancy category:* D, PB: <50%; t½: 15–40 h
Butabarbital sodium (Butisol Sodium) CSS III	*Sedative:* A: PO: 15–30 mg t.i.d., q.i.d. *Hypnotic:* A: PO: 50–100 mg h.s. *Preoperative sedation:* A: PO: 50–100 mg, 1–1.5 h before surgery	To relieve anxiety and for short-term hypnotic for insomnia. Avoid alcohol with all barbiturates. *Pregnancy category:* D; PB: <50%; t½: 60–120 h
Other Sedative-Hypnotics		
Chloral hydrate CSS IV	*Sedative:* A: PO: 250 mg t.i.d. pc C: PO: 8.3 mg/kg t.i.d. pc; max: 1,000 mg/d or 500 mg/dose *Hypnotic:* A: PO: 500 mg–1g h.s. (15–30 min before sleep) C: PO: 50 mg/kg h.s.; max: 1,000 mg	For sedative or sleep. Used in mid 1800s. No hangover and less respiratory depression. Give with meals or fluids to prevent gastric irritation. Give 15–30 min prior to sleep. *Pregnancy category:* C; PB: 70%–80%; t½: 8–10 h
Ethchlorvynol (Placidyl)	*Sedative:* A: PO: 100–200 mg, b.i.d., t.i.d. *Hypnotic:* A: PO: 0.5–1 g, h.s. for 1 wk only	A barbiturate-like drug. For sedation and sleep. Use no longer than 1 wk. Caution: renal or liver disease and drug abuse. Give with food or fluid to decrease nausea and vomiting. It has a short duration of action. *Pregnancy category:* C; PB: UK; t½: 20–100 h
Paraldehyde (Paral) CSS IV	*Sedative:* A: PO: 5–10 mL q4–6h PRN in water or juice: max: 30 mL C: PO: 0.3 mL/kg *Hypnotic:* A: PO: 10–30 mL h.s.	Exhaled via the lungs. Strong odor and disagreeable taste. Seldom used today; had been used to control delirium tremens (DTs) in alcoholics. Can be used for drug poisoning, status epilepticus, and tetanus to control convulsions. *Pregnancy category:* C; PB: UK; t½: 7.5 h

KEY: *A: adult; C: child; PO: by mouth; IM: intramuscular; IV: intravenous; PC: after meals; UK: unknown; PB: protein-binding; t½: half-life; h.s.: hour of sleep; max: maximum; <: less than; CSS: Controlled Substance Schedule.*

sleep. Because these drugs take approximately 1 h for the onset of sleep, they are not prescribed for those who have trouble getting to sleep. Vital signs should be closely monitored while taking these two groups of barbiturates.

Barbiturates should be restricted to short-term use (2 weeks or less) because of their numerous side effects, including tolerance to the drug. In the United States, barbiturates are classified as class II in the schedule of the Controlled Substances Act. In Canada, barbiturates are classified as schedule G. The barbiturates are listed in Table 13–2 and described in more detail in Figure 13–2, with a focus on the short-acting barbiturate pentobarbital

FIGURE 13–2. Sedative-Hypnotic: Barbiturate

Pentobarbital Sodium	Dosage	**NURSING PROCESS** Assessment and Planning
Pentobarbital sodium (Nembutal Sodium), 🍁: Novopento-barb **Short-acting barbiturate** **CSS II** *Pregnancy Category:* D	*Sedative:* A: PO: 20–30 mg t.i.d. C: PO: 2–6 mg/kg/d in 3 divided doses *Hypnotic:* A: PO: 100–200 mg h.s. C: PO: 30–120 mg h.s. Also based on age and weight *Preoperative:* A: PO/IM/IV: 100 mg; repeat if needed	
Contraindications	**Drug-Lab-Food Interactions**	
Respiratory depression, severe hepatic disease, pregnancy (fetal immaturity), nephrosis	*Decrease:* respiration with alcohol, CNS depressants; incompatible in solution with numerous drugs such as codeine, insulin, penicillin G, hydrocortisone, phenytoin	
Pharmacokinetics	**Pharmacodynamics**	Interventions
Absorption: PO: 90% absorbed slowly *Distribution:* PB: 35–45% *Metabolism:* t½: 4 h (first phase); 30–50 h (second phase) *Excretion:* In urine as metabolites	PO: Onset: 15–30 min Peak: 0.5–1 h Duration: 3–6 h IM: Onset: 10–15 min Peak: 0.5–1 h Duration: 3–6 h IV: Onset: Immediate Peak: 2–5 min Duration: 15–60 min	

Therapeutic Effects/Uses: To treat insomnia; used for sedation, preoperative medication, barbiturate coma (for controlling increased intracranial pressure). *Mode of Action:* Depression of the CNS, including the motor and sensory activities.	Evaluation

Side Effects	Adverse Reactions
Nausea, vomiting, diarrhea, lethargy, drowsiness, hangover, dizziness, rash	Drug dependence or tolerance, urticaria, hypotension (rapid IV) *Life-threatening:* Respiratory distress, laryngospasm

KEY: A: adult; C: child; PO: by mouth; PB: protein-binding; t½: half-life; IM: intramuscular; IV: intravenous; 🍁: Canadian drug names.

(Nembutal). Nursing process is based on the drug data.

Pharmacokinetics

Pentobarbital (Nembutal) has been available for nearly half a century and was the hypnotic of choice until the introduction of benzodiazepines in the 1960s. It has a slow absorption rate and is moderately protein-bound. The long half-life is mainly due to the formation of active metabolites resulting from liver metabolism.

Pharmacodynamics

Pentobarbital is primarily used to induce sleep and for sedation needs. It has a rapid onset with a short duration of action; thus it is considered a short-acting barbiturate. The onset of action is slower when administered intramuscularly than when administered orally.

There are many drug interactions associated with pentobarbital. Alcohol, narcotics, and other sedative-hypnotics used in combination with pentobarbital may further depress the central nervous system. Pentobarbital increases hepatic enzyme action, thus causing an increased metabolism and decreased effect of drugs, such as oral anticoagulants, glucocorticoids, tricyclic antidepressants, and quinidine. Pentobarbital may cause hepatotoxicity if taken with large doses of acetaminophen.

NURSING PROCESS: SEDATIVE-HYPNOTIC: Barbiturate

ASSESSMENT

- Obtain baseline vital signs for future comparison.
- Determine if there is a history of insomnia or sleep disorder.
- Assess renal function. Urine output should be >600 mL/day. Renal impairment could prolong drug action by increasing the half-life of the drug.
- Assess potential for fluid volume deficit, which would potentiate hypotensive effects.

POTENTIAL NURSING DIAGNOSIS

- Sleep pattern disturbance.

PLANNING

- Client will receive adequate sleep without hangover when taking the hypnotic.

NURSING INTERVENTIONS

- Recognize that continuous use of a barbiturate might result in drug abuse.
- Monitor vital signs, especially respirations and blood pressure.
- Raise bedside rails of older adults and clients who are receiving a hypnotic for the first time. Confusion may occur, and injury may result.
- Observe the client, especially an older adult or a debilitated client, for adverse reactions to the pentobarbital; see prototype.

- Check the client's skin for rashes. Skin eruptions may occur in clients taking barbiturates.
- Observe the client for withdrawal symptoms when pentobarbital has been taken over a prolonged period of time and then discontinued.
- Administer IV pentobarbital at a rate of less than 50 mg/min. Do *not* mix pentobarbital with other medications. IM injection should be given deep in a large muscle such as the gluteus medius.

CLIENT TEACHING

General

- Instruct the client to use nonpharmacologic ways to induce sleep, such as enjoying a warm bath, listening to music, drinking warm fluids, and avoiding drinks with caffeine after dinner.
- Instruct the client to avoid alcohol and antidepressant, antipsychotic, and narcotic drugs while taking the barbiturate. Respiratory distress may occur when these drugs are combined.
- Advise the client not to drive a motor vehicle or operate machinery. Caution is always encouraged.
- Instruct the client to take the hypnotic 30 min before bedtime. Short-acting hypnotics such as pentobarbital take effect within 15 to 30 min.
- Encourage the client to check with the health care provider about OTC sleeping aids. Drowsiness may result from taking these drugs, and therefore caution in driving is advised.

Side Effects

- Advise the client to report adverse reactions, such as hangover, to the health care provider. Drug selection or dosage might need to be changed.

- Instruct the client that hypnotics such as pentobarbital should be gradually withdrawn, especially if it has been taken for several weeks. Abrupt cessation of the hypnotic may result in withdrawal symptoms (tremors, muscle twitching).

EVALUATION

- Evaluate the effectiveness of pentobarbital. Usually, this drug is given before surgery.
- Evaluate respiratory status to ensure that respiratory distress has not occurred.

BENZODIAZEPINES

Selected benzodiazepines (minor tranquilizer or anxiolytic), introduced with chlordiazepoxide (Librium) in the 1960s as antianxiety agents, are ordered as sedative-hypnotics for inducing sleep. Five benzodiazepines marketed as hypnotics are flurazepam (Dalmane), temazepam (Restoril), triazolam (Halcion), estazolam (ProSom), and quazepam (Doral) (see Table 13–2). Increased anxiety might be the cause of insomnia for some clients, so lorazepam (Ativan) can be used to alleviate the anxiety. These drugs are classified as schedule IV according to the Controlled Substances Act.

Benzodiazepines can suppress stage 4 of NREM sleep, which may result in vivid dreams or nightmares, and can delay REM sleep, except for temazepam. Benzodiazepines are effective for sleep disorders for several weeks longer than other sedative-hypnotics; however, they should not be used for longer than 3 to 4 weeks as a hypnotic to prevent REM rebound. Flurazepam (Dalmane) was the first benzodiazepine hypnotic introduced, and it is compared with temazepam in Figure 13–3. Triazolam (Halcion) is a short-acting hypnotic with a half-life of 2 to 5 h. It does not produce any active metabolites. Complaints of adverse reactions to prolonged use of triazolam, such as loss of memory, have led to it being taken off the market in Great Britain; it is being reviewed by the Food and Drug Administration (FDA). The advisory group in Great Britain is recommending that the legislative body reinstate triazolam.

Pharmacokinetics

Flurazepam is well absorbed through the gastrointestinal (GI) mucosa. Flurazepam is rapidly metabolized in the liver to active metabolites and has a long half-life of 45 to 100 h. Flurazepam is highly protein-bound, and if it is taken with other highly protein-bound drugs, more free drug is available, which increases the risk of adverse effects.

Pharmacodynamics

Flurazepam is used to treat insomnia by inducing and sustaining sleep. It has a rapid onset of action and intermediate to long-acting effects. The normal recommended dose of a benzodiazepine may be too much for the older adult; so half of the dose is recommended initially to prevent overdosing.

Alcohol or narcotics taken with a benzodiazepine may cause an additive depressive CNS response. Cimetidine (Tagamet) decreases metabolism of flurazepam, thus increasing its action. Barbiturates decrease the effectiveness of flurazepam by increasing the metabolism of the benzodiazepine. There are other drug interactions that should be carefully assessed when administering a benzodiazepine as a hypnotic.

PIPERIDINEDIONES

The piperidinediones resemble barbiturates. These sedative-hypnotics were introduced in the mid-1950s and include glutethimide, which has similar effects as the short-acting barbiturates. These drugs were marketed to be nonaddictive; however, they can be addictive and can cause severe adverse reactions, such as vasomotor collapse, serious blood dyscrasias (aplastic anemia), and allergic reactions. Gastric irritation rarely occurs.

If glutethimide is used over several weeks, a gradual tapering of the dose is necessary to avoid severe withdrawal symptoms, including hallucination and convulsion. Over the past decade, there has been a declining use of the piperidinedione group.

CHLORAL HYDRATE

Other sedative-hypnotic drugs are ethchlorvynol (Placidyl), chloral hydrate, and paraldehyde (Paral). Chloral hydrate was first introduced in the 1860s. It is used to induce sleep and to decrease nocturnal awakenings; it does not suppress REM sleep. There is less occurrence of hangover, respiratory depression, and tolerance with chloral hydrate than with other sedative-hypnotics. It has been used effectively with older adults and can be given with mild liver dysfunction, but it should be avoided if severe liver or renal disorder is present. Gastric irritation is a common complaint, so the drug should be taken with sufficient water. Drugs that interact with chloral hydrate include other CNS depressants, furosemide, and oral anticoagulants.

Table 13–3 describes the sedative-hypnotics, their dosages, uses, and considerations.

FIGURE 13–3. Sedative-Hypnotic: Benzodiazepine

Flurazepam HCl	Dosage	NURSING PROCESS
Flurazepam HCl (Dalmane), 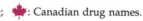: Apo-Flurazepam, novoflupam Benzodiazepine hypnotic CSS IV *Pregnancy Category:* X	A: PO: 15–30 mg h.s. Elderly: PO: 15 mg h.s.	Assessment and Planning

Contraindications	Drug-Lab-Food Interactions	
Hypersensitivity to benzodiazepine, pregnancy, lactation, intermittent porphyria *Caution:* Renal, liver, or mental disorders; elderly, debilitation	May *increase* effect with cimetidine *Decrease* effect with antacids, smoking *Decrease* CNS function with alcohol, CNS depressants, anticonvulsants *Lab: Increase* AST, ALT, ALP, bilirubin *False negatives:* Clinistix, Diastix	

Pharmacokinetics	Pharmacodynamics	
Absorption: PO: well absorbed *Distribution:* PB: 97% *Metabolism:* t½: 2–3 h; metabolites: 45–100 h *Excretion:* In urine as active metabolites	PO: Onset: 15–45 min Peak: 0.5–1 h Duration: 7–10 h	Interventions

Therapeutic Effects/Uses: To treat insomnia.

Mode of Action: Depression of the CNS, neurotransmitter inhibition.

Evaluation

Side Effects	Adverse Reactions
Drowsiness, lethargy, hangover (residual sedation), dizziness, lightedheadedness, anxiety, nausea, vomiting, diarrhea, confusion, disorientation	Tolerance, psychological and/or physical dependence, hypotension, mental depression *Life-threatening:* Coma from overdose, leukopenia (rare)

KEY: A: adult; PO: by mouth; PB: protein-binding; t½: half-life; 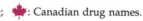: Canadian drug names.

NURSING PROCESS: SEDATIVE-HYPNOTIC: Benzodiazepine

ASSESSMENT

- Obtain baseline vital signs and laboratory tests (AST, ALT, bilirubin) for future comparisons.
- Obtain drug history. Taking CNS depressants with benzodiazepine hypnotics can depress respirations. Flurazepam is highly protein-bound. Report if the client is taking other highly protein-bound drugs such as warfarin (Coumadin). Drug displacement can occur with two highly protein-bound drugs, causing an increase in circulating drug(s).
- Ascertain the client's problem with sleep disturbance.

POTENTIAL NURSING DIAGNOSIS

- Sleep pattern disturbance

PLANNING

- Client will remain asleep for 6 to 8 h.

NURSING INTERVENTIONS

- Monitor vital signs. Check for signs of respiratory distress, such as slow, irregular breathing patterns.
- Raise bedside rails of older adults or clients receiving flurazepam for the first time. Confusion may occur, and injury may result.
- Observe the client for side effects of flurazepam, such as hangover (residual sedation), lightheadedness, dizziness, or confusion. The metabolites of flurazepam have a long half-life, so cumulative effects of the drug can occur.

CLIENT TEACHING

General

- Instruct the client to use nonpharmacological ways to induce sleep, such as enjoying a warm bath, listening to music, drinking warm fluids such as milk, and avoiding drinks with caffeine after dinner.
- Instruct the client to avoid alcohol and antidepressant, antipsychotic, and narcotic drugs while taking sedative-hypnotics. Severe respiratory distress may occur when these drugs are combined.
- Advise the client to take flurazepam before bedtime. Flurazepam takes effect within 15 to 45 min.
- Suggest that the client urinate before taking flurazepam to prevent sleep disruption.
- Encourage the client to check with the health care provider about OTC sleeping aids. Drowsiness may result from taking these drugs; therefore, caution in driving is advised.

Side Effects

- Instruct the client to report adverse reactions, such as hangover, to the health care provider. Drug selection or dosage may need to be changed if hangover occurs.

EVALUATION

- Evaluate the effectiveness of flurazepam in promoting sleep.
- Determine if side effects such as hangover occur after several days of taking flurazepam. Another hypnotic may be prescribed if side effects remain.

TABLE 13–3 Sedative-Hypnotics: Benzodiazepines-Nonbenzodiazepines

Generic (Brand)	Route and Dosage	Uses and Considerations
Benzodiazepines		
Estazolam (ProSom) CSS IV	A: PO: 1–2 mg h.s. Elderly: PO: 0.5 mg h.s.	New benzodiazepine hypnotic for treatment of insomnia. Should not be used for longer than 6 weeks. Decreases the frequency of nocturnal awakeness. *Pregnancy category:* X; PB: 93%; t½: 10–24 h
Flurazepam HCl (Dalmane)	See Prototype Drug Chart (Fig. 13–3).	For insomnia. Should not be used for longer than 4 weeks. *Pregnancy category:* X; PB: 97%; t½: 2–3 h; metabolites: 45–100 h
Lorazepam (Ativan) CSS IV	*Insomnia:* A: PO: 2–4 mg h.s.	Used as a preoperative sedative and to reduce anxiety. *Pregnancy category:* D; PB: 85%; t½: 12–14 h
Quazepam (Doral) CSS IV	A: PO: 7.5–15 mg h.s.	To treat insomnia and to decrease nocturnal awakenings. Avoid alcohol with this drug and all benzodiazepines. *Pregnancy category:* X; PB: >95%: t½: 39 h
Temazepam (Restoril) CSS IV	*Hypnotic:* A: PO: 15–30 mg h.s.	To treat insomnia and to decrease nocturnal awakenings. Also has sedative effects. *Pregnancy category:* X; PB: 96%; t½: 10–20 h
Triazolam (Halcion) CSS IV	*Hypnotic:* A: PO: 0.125–0.5 mg h.s. (0.5 mg with caution) Elderly: PO: 0.125–0.25 mg h.s.	For management of insomnia. Should not be used for longer than 7–10 d at a time to avoid tolerance. Avoid alcohol and smoking when taking triazolam. *Pregnancy category:* X; PB: 89%; t½: 2–4 h
Nonbenzodiazepines		
Zolpidem tartrate (Ambien)	A: PO: Initially 5 mg; maint: 5–15 mg h.s.; average: 10 mg h.s.; use for 7–10 d	A benzodiazepine-like drug. For treatment of insomnia. *Pregnancy category:* B; PB: 79%–92%; t½: 1.5–4 h
Piperidinediones		
Glutethimide (Doriden) CSS III	*Hypnotic:* A: PO: 250–500 mg h.s.; repeat in 4 h if necessary	For insomnia. Resembles barbiturates. Caution in use: renal disease and mental depression. Withdraw drug gradually to prevent withdrawal symptoms (rebound insomnia). *Pregnancy category:* C; PB: 50%; t½: 10–20 h

KEY: A: adult; C: child; CSS: Controlled Substance Schedule; h.s.: hour of sleep; PB: protein-binding; PO: by mouth; t½: half-life.

ANESTHETICS

Anesthetics are classified as general and local. General anesthetics depress the central nervous system, alleviate pain, and cause a great loss of consciousness. The first anesthetic, nitrous oxide (laughing gas), was used for surgery in the early 1800s. It is still an effective anesthetic and is frequently used today in dental surgery. In the mid-1800s, ether and chloroform were introduced. Ether, a highly flammable volatile liquid, has a pungent odor and can cause nausea and vomiting after it has been administered. Today it is seldom used, probably due to the hazard of possible explosion and its noxious odor. Chloroform is toxic to liver cells and is no longer used.

Today **balanced anesthesia,** a combination of drugs, is frequently used in general anesthesia. Balanced anesthesia comprises

1. A hypnotic given the night before
2. Premedication, such as a narcotic analgesic or a benzodiazepine (e.g., midazolam [Versed]) and an anticholinergic (e.g., atropine) to decrease secretions given about 1 h before surgery
3. A short-acting barbiturate, such as thiopental sodium (Pentothal)
4. An inhaled gas, such as nitrous oxide and oxygen
5. A muscle relaxant as needed

Balanced anesthesia minimizes cardiovascular problems, decreases the amount of general anesthetic needed, reduces possible postanesthetic nausea and vomiting, minimizes the disturbance of organ function, and increases recovery from anesthesia. Because the client is not receiving large doses of general anesthetics, there are fewer adverse reactions.

STAGES OF ANESTHESIA

General anesthesia proceeds through four stages (Table 13–4), during the third stage of which the surgical procedure is usually performed.

INHALATION ANESTHETICS

During stage 3 anesthesia, inhalation anesthetics (gas or volatile liquids administered as gas) are used to deliver general anesthesia. Certain gases, such as nitrous oxide and cyclopropane, are absorbed quickly, have a rapid action, and are eliminated rapidly. Cyclopropane was the popular inhalation anesthetic for 30 years (1930 to 1960), but due to its highly flammable state as ether, it is no longer used. In the late 1950s, halothane was introduced as a nonflammable alternative. Other inhalation drugs introduced as anesthetics include methoxyflurane in the 1960s, enflurane in the 1970s, isoflurane in the 1980s, and the newest, desflurane.

INTRAVENOUS ANESTHETICS

Intravenous anesthetics may be used for general anesthesia or for the induction stage of anesthesia. For outpatient surgery of short duration, an intravenous anesthetic might be the chosen form of anesthesia. Previously, thiopental sodium (Pentothal), an ultrashort-acting barbiturate, was the general anesthetic for short-term surgery. It is still used for the rapid induction stage of anesthesia and in dental procedures. Presently, droperidol (Innovar), etomidate (Amidate), and ketamine hydrochloride (Ketalar) are used intravenously as general anesthetics. Intravenous anesthetics have rapid onsets and short durations of action. Table 13–5 describes the inhalation and intravenous anesthetics used for general anesthesia.

TABLE 13–4 Stages of Anesthesia

Stage	Name	Description
1	Analgesia	Begins with consciousness and ends with loss of consciousness. Speech is difficult; sensations of smell and pain are lost. Dreams and auditory and visual hallucination may occur. This stage may be referred to as the induction stage.
2	Excitement or delirium	Produces a loss of consciousness due to depression of the cerebral cortex. Confusion, excitement, or delirium occur. Short induction time.
3	Surgical	Surgical procedure is performed during this stage. There are four phases. The surgery is usually performed in phase 2 and upper phase 3. As anesthesia deepens, respirations become more shallow and respiratory rate is increased.
4	Medullary paralysis	Toxic stage of anesthesia. Respirations are lost and circulatory collapse occurs. Ventilatory assistance is necessary.

TABLE 13–5 Inhalation and Intravenous Anesthetics

Drug	Induction Time	Considerations
Inhalation: Volatile Liquids		
Ether	Slow	Highly flammable. Has no severe effect on the cardiovascular system or liver.
Halothane (Fluothane)	Rapid	Introduced in the 1950s. Highly potent anesthetic. Rapid recovery. Could decrease blood pressure. Has a bronchodilator effect. Contraindicated in obstetrics.
Methoxyflurane	Slow	Introduced in the 1960s. Used during labor. Drug dose is usually less than other anesthetics and it does not suppress uterine contraction. Could cause hypotension. Contraindicated in renal disorders.
Enflurane (Ethrane)	Rapid	Introduced in 1970s. Similar to halothane. Can depress respiratory function; thus, ventilatory support may be necessary. Not to be used during labor because uterine contractions could be suppressed. Avoid with clients with seizure disorders.
Isoflurane (Forane)	Rapid	Introduced in 1980s. Frequently used in inhalation therapy. Has a smooth and rapid induction of anesthesia and rapid recovery. Could cause hypotension and respiratory depression. Not to be used during labor because it suppresses uterine contraction. Has minimal cardiovascular effect.
Desflurane	Rapid	The newest volatile liquid anesthetic. Similar to isoflurane. Rapid recovery after anesthetic administration has ceased. Could cause hypotension and respiratory depression.
Inhalation: Gas		
Nitrous Oxide (laughing gas)	Very rapid	Rapid recovery. Has minimal cardiovascular effect. Should be given with oxygen. Low potency.
Cyclopropane	Very rapid	Highly flammable and explosive. Seldom used.
Intravenous		
Thiopental Sodium (Pentothal)	Rapid	Has short duration of action. Used for rapid induction of general surgery. Keep client warm, for shivering and tremors may occur. Can depress respiratory center and ventilatory assistance might be necessary.
Thiamylal Sodium	Rapid	Used for induction of anesthesia and anesthesia for electroshock therapy.
Benzodiazepines		
Diazepam	Moderate to rapid	For induction of anesthesia. No analgesic effect.
Midazolam	Moderate to rapid	For induction of anesthesia and for endoscopic procedures. IV drug can cause conscious sedation. Avoid if a cardiopulmonary disorder is present.
Droperidol and Fentanyl (Innovar)	Moderate to rapid	A neuroleptic analgesic when combined with fentanyl (potent opiate narcotic). Frequently used with a general anesthetic. Can also be used as a preanesthetic drug. Also used for diagnostic procedures. May cause hypotension and respiratory depression.
Etomidate (Amidate)	Rapid	Used for short-term surgery, or as induction of anesthesia, or with a general anesthetic to maintain the anesthetic state.
Ketamine Hydrochloride (Ketalar)	Rapid	Used for short-term surgery or for induction of anesthesia. It increases salivation, blood pressure, and heart rate. May be used for diagnostic procedures. Avoid with history of psychiatric disorders.
Propofol (Diprivan)	Rapid	For induction of anesthesia and may be used with general anesthesia. Short duration of action. May cause hypotension and respiratory depression. Pain can occur at the injection site; thus, may be mixed with a local anesthetic such as lidocaine to decrease pain.

LOCAL ANESTHESIA

Local anesthetics block pain at the site where the drug is administered, allowing consciousness to be maintained. Uses for local anesthetics include dental procedures, suturing of skin lacerations, short-term (minor) surgery at a localized area, spinal anesthesia by blocking nerve impulses (nerve block) below the insertion of the anesthetic, and such diagnostic procedures as lumbar puncture and thoracentesis.

TABLE 13–6 Local Anesthetics

Anesthetics	Type	Uses and Considerations
Short-Acting (1/2–1 h)		
Chloroprocaine (Nesacaine)	Ester	For infiltration, caudal and epidural anesthesia. Onset of action is 6–12 minutes.
Procaine HCl (Novocain)	Ester	Introduced in 1905. For nerve block, infiltration, epidural and spinal anesthesias. Useful in dentistry. Caution in use for clients allergic to ester-type anesthetics.
Moderate-Acting (1–3 h)		
Lidocaine (Xylocaine)	Amide	Introduced in 1948. For nerve block, infiltration, epidural and spinal anesthesias. Allergic reaction is rare. Used to treat cardiac dysrhythmias (see Chapter 32).
Mepivacaine HCl (Carbocaine HCl; Isocaine; Polocaine)	Amide	For nerve block, infiltration, caudal and epidural anesthesias. May be used in dentistry.
Prilocaine HCl (Citanest)	Amide	For peripheral nerve block, infiltration, caudal and epidural anesthesias. May be used in dentistry.
Long-Acting (3–10 h)		
Bupivacaine (Marcaine, Sensorcaine)	Amide	For peripheral nerve block, infiltration, caudal, and epidural anesthesias.
Dibucaine HCl (Nupercainal)	Amide	For topical use (creams and ointment) to affected areas.
Etidocaine (Duranest)	Amide	For peripheral nerve block, infiltration, caudal and epidural anesthesias.
Tetracaine HCl (Pontocaine)	Ester	For spinal anesthesia (high and low saddle block). Also for topical use to affected areas, such as the eye to anesthetize the cornea; nose and throat for bronchoscopy; to the skin for relief of pain, pruritus (itching).

Most local anesthetics are divided into two groups, the esters and the amides, according to their basic structures. The amides have a very low incidence of causing an allergic reaction.

The first local anesthetic used was cocaine hydrochloride in the late 1800s. Procaine hydrochloride (Novocain), a synthetic of cocaine, was discovered in the early 1900s. Lidocaine hydrochloride (Xylocaine) was developed in the mid 1950s to replace procaine, except for dental procedures. Lidocaine has a rapid onset and a long duration of action, is more stable in solution, and causes fewer hypersensitivity reactions than procaine. Since the introduction of lidocaine, many local anesthetics have been marketed. Table 13–6 describes the various types of local anesthetics according to short-, moderate-, and long-acting effects.

SPINAL ANESTHESIA

Spinal anesthesia requires a local anesthetic be injected in the subarachnoid space at the third or fourth lumbar space. If the local anesthetic is given too high in the spinal column, the respiratory muscles could be affected, and respiratory distress or failure could result. Headaches might result following spinal anesthesia (a "spinal"), possibly due to a drop in cerebrospinal fluid pressure caused by a leak of fluid at the needle insertion. Encouraging the client to remain flat following surgery with spinal anesthesia and to take increased fluids usually decreases the likelihood of leaking spinal fluid. Hypotension also can result following spinal anesthesia.

Various sites of the spinal column can be used for a **nerve block** with a local anesthetic (Fig. 13–4). A **spinal block** is the penetration of the anesthetic into the subarachnoid membrane, the second layer of the spinal cord. An **epidural block** is the placement of the local anesthetic in the outer covering of the spinal cord, or the dura mater. A **caudal block** is placed near the sacrum. A **saddle block** is given at the lower end of the spinal column to block the perineal area. Blood pressure should be monitored during administration of these types of anesthesia, since a decrease in blood pressure due to the drug and procedure might occur. A saddle block is frequently used for clients in labor (see Chapter 42).

Nurses play an important role in client assessment prior to and following general and local anesthesia. Preparing the client for surgery by explaining the preparations and completing the preoperative orders, including premedication(s), is necessary to enhance the safety and effectiveness of the anesthesia and surgery.

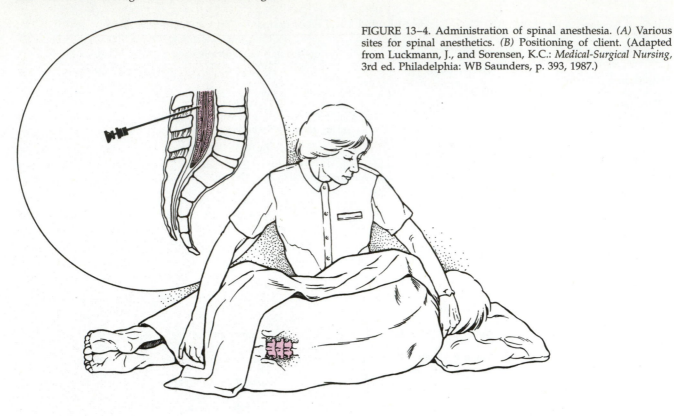

FIGURE 13–4. Administration of spinal anesthesia. (A) Various sites for spinal anesthetics. (B) Positioning of client. (Adapted from Luckmann, J., and Sorensen, K.C.: *Medical-Surgical Nursing*, 3rd ed. Philadelphia: WB Saunders, p. 393, 1987.)

NURSING PROCESS: ANESTHETICS

ASSESSMENT

- Obtain baseline vital signs.
- Obtain a drug history, noting drugs that affect the cardiopulmonary systems.

POTENTIAL NURSING DIAGNOSIS

- Pain

PLANNING

- Client will participate in preoperative preparation and understand postoperative care.
- Client's vital signs will remain stable following surgery.

NURSING INTERVENTIONS

- Monitor the client's postoperative state of sensorium. Report if the client remains nonresponsive or confused for a time.

- Check preoperative and postoperative urine output. Report deficit of hourly or eight-hour urine output.
- Monitor vital signs following general and local anesthesia; hypotension and respiratory distress may result.
- Administer an analgesic or a narcotic-analgesic with caution until the client fully recovers from the anesthetic. To prevent adverse reactions, dosage might need to be adjusted if the client is under the influence of the anesthetic.

CLIENT TEACHING

- Explain to the client the preoperative preparation and postoperative nursing assessment and interventions.

EVALUATION

- Evaluate client's response to the anesthetics. Continue to monitor the client for adverse reactions.

STUDY QUESTIONS

1. What are the advantages of using benzodiazepine hypnotics instead of barbiturates for sleep disorders?
2. Why should renal function be assessed by the nurse? What minimal daily urine output is considered adequate?
3. What is a hangover resulting from a hypnotic? What are the nursing interventions?
4. What is the meaning of withdrawal symptoms from hypnotic use? How can they be prevented? What are the symptoms and the nursing interventions for each?
5. Why should vital signs be closely monitored following general and local anesthesia?
6. What is balanced anesthesia? Give the rationale for its use.
7. What are the nursing interventions, including client teaching of a client having spinal anesthesia?

Chapter 14

Nonnarcotic and Narcotic Analgesics

OUTLINE

Objectives
Terms
Introduction
Nonnarcotic Analgesics
    Salicylates and Non-
      steroidal Antiinflam-
      matory Drugs

Acetaminophen
    Nursing Process
Narcotic Analgesics
    Morphine
    Nursing Process
    Meperidine
    Nursing Process

Narcotic Agonist-Antagonists
Narcotic Antagonists
Treatment for Narcotic-Addicted
    Persons
Case Study
Study Questions

OBJECTIVES

Define the types of pain: acute, chronic, superficial, visceral, and somatic.

Differentiate between nonnarcotic and narcotic analgesics. Explain when these drug groups are indicated.

Identify the serum therapeutic ranges of acetaminophen and aspirin.

Name the side effects of aspirin and narcotics.

Explain the methadone treatment program.

Give the nursing interventions, including client teaching, related to nonnarcotic analgesics and narcotic analgesics.

TERMS

abstinence syndrome
analgesics
methadone treatment
    program
mixed narcotic agonist-
    antagonist

narcotic
narcotic agonist
narcotic antagonist
nonnarcotic
NSAIDs
orthostatic hypotension

prostaglandins
somatic
visceral

INTRODUCTION

Analgesics, both nonnarcotic and narcotic, are prescribed for the relief of pain; the choice of drug depends on the severity of the pain. Mild to moderate pain of the skeletal muscle and joints frequently is relieved with the use of nonnarcotic analgesics. Moderate to severe pain in the smooth muscles, organs, and bones usually requires a narcotic analgesic.

There are five classifications and types of pain:

1. Acute pain, which could be mild, moderate, or severe
2. Chronic pain
3. Superficial pain
4. **Somatic** (bones, skeletal muscles, and joints) pain
5. **Visceral,** or deep, pain.

Table 14–1 lists the types of pain and the drug groups that may be effective in relieving each type of pain.

NONNARCOTIC ANALGESICS

Nonnarcotic analgesics—aspirin, acetaminophen, ibuprofen, and naproxen—are not addictive and are less potent than narcotic analgesics. They are used to treat mild to moderate pain and may be purchased over-the-counter (OTC). These drugs are effective for the dull, throbbing pain of headaches, dysmenorrhea (menstrual pain), pain from inflammation, minor abrasions, muscular aches and pain, and mild to moderate arthritis. Most of the analgesics lower an elevated body temperature, thus having an antipyretic effect. Some analgesics, such as aspirin, have antiinflammatory and anticoagulant effects as well.

SALICYLATES AND NONSTEROIDAL ANTIINFLAMMATORY DRUGS

Aspirin (ASA), a salicylate, is the oldest nonnarcotic analgesic drug still in use. Adolf Bayer marketed the original formulation in 1899, and today aspirin can be purchased under many names and with added ingredients. Examples are Bufferin, Ecotrin (enteric-coated tablet), Anacin (containing caffeine), and Alka-Seltzer. Aspirin's primary effect is as an analgesic for pain, but it also has an antipyretic effect. Aspirin should not be used and is contraindicated for any elevated temperature in a child under the age of 12 years, regardless of the cause because of the danger of Reye's syndrome (neurologic problems associated with viral infection and treated with salicylates). Acetaminophen (Tylenol) is used instead of aspirin in these circumstances.

Aspirin is also classified as an antiinflammatory drug and will be discussed with the nonsteroidal antiinflammatory drugs **(NSAIDs)** in depth in Chapter 21. Aspirin and the NSAIDs relieve pain by inhibiting the synthesis of prostaglandins. Prostaglandins accumulate at injured tissue sites, causing inflammation and pain. All NSAIDs have an analgesic effect, as well as an antipyretic and antiinflammatory action. Aspirin, ibuprofens (Motrin IB, Nuprin, Advil, Medipren), and naproxen (Aleve) can be purchased as OTC drugs. In addition to its analgesic, antipyretic, and antiinflammatory properties, aspirin decreases platelet aggregation (clotting). Some health care providers may therefore prescribe one aspirin tablet every day or every other day as a measure to prevent transient ischemic attacks (TIAs, or "small strokes"), heart attacks, or any thromboembolic episode.

TABLE 14–1 Types of Pain

Type of Pain	Definition	Drug Treatment
Acute Pain	Pain occurs suddenly and responds to treatment	Mild Pain: Nonnarcotic (acetaminophen, NSAIDs [aspirin, Motrin Advil) Moderate pain: Combination of nonnarcotic and narcotic (codeine and acetaminophen) Severe Pain: Narcotic
Chronic Pain	Pain persists for greater than 6 months and is difficult to treat or control	Nonnarcotic drugs are suggested. Narcotics if used should: 1. be by oral route 2. have a long half-life 3. include adjunct therapy 4. not cause respiratory depression
Superficial Pain	Pain from surface areas such as the skin and mucous membrane	Mild pain: Nonnarcotic Moderate pain: Combination of narcotic and nonnarcotic analgesic drug
Visceral Pain (deep pain)	Pain from smooth muscles and organs	Narcotic drugs
Somatic Pain	Pain of the skeletal muscle, ligaments, and joints	Nonnarcotics: NSAIDs (aspirin, Motrin, Advil). Also act as an antiinflammatory drug and muscle relaxants

Side Effects and Adverse Reactions

A common side effect of aspirin and NSAIDs is gastric irritation. These drugs should be taken with food, at mealtime, or with a full glass of fluid to help reduce this problem. If aspirin or a NSAID is taken for dysmenorrhea during the first two days of menstruation, excess bleeding might occur (more so with aspirin than with ibuprofen).

ACETAMINOPHEN

The analgesic acetaminophen (*para*-aminophenol derivative) is a popular nonprescription drug taken

FIGURE 14–1. Analgesic: Acetaminophen

Acetaminophen	Dosage	**NURSING PROCESS** Assessment and Planning

Acetaminophen
    (Tylenol, Tempra, Panadol),
    🍁 Robigesis, Atasol
Para-aminophenol analgesic
Pregnancy Category: B
	A: PO: 325–650 mg q4–6h PRN; max:
	    4,000 mg/d; rectal supp: 650 mg
	    q.i.d.
	C: 0–3 mo: PO: 40 mg 4–5×/d
	    4 mo–1y: PO: 80 mg 4–5×/d
	    1–2 y: PO: 120 mg 4–5×/d
	    2–3 y: PO: 160 mg 4–5×/d
	    4–5 y: PO: 240 mg 4–5×/d
	    6–8 y: PO: 320 mg 4–5×/d
	    9–10 y: PO: 400 mg 4–5×/d
	    >11 y: PO: 480 mg 4–5×/d
	C: 2–5 y: Rectal: 120 mg 4–5×/d
	    6–12 y: Rectal: 325 mg 4–5×/d	

Contraindications	**Drug-Lab-Food Interactions**	

Severe hepatic or renal disease, alco-
    holism; hypersensitivity
	Increase effect with caffeine, diflunisal
	Decrease effect with oral contraceptives,
	    anticholinergics, cholestyramine,
	    charcoal	

Pharmacokinetics	**Pharmacodynamics**	Interventions

Absorption: PO: rapidly absorbed;
    rectal: erractic
Distribution: PB: 20–50%; crosses the
    placenta, in breast milk
Metabolism: t½: 1–3.5 h
Excretion: In urine as metabolites
	PO: Onset: 10–30 min
	        Peak: 1–2 h
	        Duration: 3–5 h
	Rectal: Onset: UK
	        Peak: UK
	        Duration: 4–6 h	

Therapeutic Effects/Uses: To decrease pain and fever.

Mode of Action: Inhibition (weakly) of prostaglandin synthesis, inhibition of hypothalamic heat-regulator center.

Evaluation

Side Effects	Adverse Reactions

Anorexia, nausea, vomiting, rash	Severe hypoglycemia, oliguria,
	    urticaria
	Life-threatening: Hemorrhage, hepato-
	    toxicity, hemolytic anemia, leukope-
	    nia, thrombocytopenia

KEY: A: adult; C: child; PO: by mouth; PB: protein-binding; t½: half-life; UK: unknown: >: greater than; 🍁 : Canadian drug names.

by infants, children, adults, and older adults for pain, discomfort, and fever. It constitutes 25% of all OTC drugs sold. Acetaminophen (Tylenol, Panadol, Tempra), first marketed in the mid 1950s, is a safe, effective analgesic and antipyretic drug used for muscular aches and pains and for fever due to viral infections. It causes little to no gastric distress and does not interfere with platelet aggregation. There is no link between acetaminophen and Reye's syndrome, and it does not increase the potential for excessive bleeding if taken for dysmenorrhea, as do aspirin and NSAIDs. Acetaminophen does not have the antiinflammatory properties of aspirin, so it is not the drug of choice for any inflammatory process. See drug chart (Fig. 14–1).

Pharmacokinetics

Acetaminophen is well absorbed from the gastrointestinal (GI) tract. Rectal absorption may be erratic due to the presence of fecal material, or a decrease in blood flow to the colon. Because of acetaminophen's short half-life, it can be administered every 4 h as needed with a maximum dose of 4 g/day. Greater than 85% of acetaminophen is metabolized to drug metabolites by the liver.

Large doses or overdoses can be toxic to the hepatic cells; therefore, when large doses are administered over a long period, the level of acetaminophen in serum should be monitored. The therapeutic serum range is 5 to 20 μg/mL.

TABLE 14–2 Analgesics

Generic (Brand)	Route and Dosage	Uses and Considerations
Salicylates		
Aspirin (Bayer, Ecotrin, Astrin)	*Analgesic:* A: PO: 325–650 mg, q4h, *max:* 4 g/d C: PO: 40–65 mg/kg/d in 4–6 divided doses. *max:* 3.6 g/d	Effective in relieving headaches, muscle pain, inflammation and pain from arthritis, and as mild anticoagulant. Serum therapeutic range: headache: 5 mg/dL; inflammation: 15–30 mg/dL. Can displace other highly protein-bound drugs. If taken with acetaminophen, GI bleeding could result. Side effects: gastric discomfort, tinnitus, vertigo, deafness (reversible), increased bleeding. Should be taken with foods or at mealtime. It should *not* be taken with alcohol. *Pregnancy category:* D; 55%–90%; t½: 2–20 h (high doses)
Diflunisal (Dolobid)	A: PO: Initially: 1,000 mg; maint: 500 mg q8–12h	Used for mild to moderate pain. Considered to be less toxic than aspirin. *Pregnancy category:* C; PB: 99%; t½: 8–12 h
Para-aminophenol		
Acetaminophen (Tylenol, Panadol, Tempra)	See Prototype Drug Chart (Fig. 14–1)	Used for mild to moderate pain. Serum therapeutic range: 5–20 μm/mL. Safe to take if flu symptoms are present. Does *not* cause gastric distress or interfere with platelet aggregation. Overdose or prolonged, high dosage can cause liver toxicity. *Pregnancy category:* B; PB: 20%–50%; t½: 1–3.5 h
NSAIDs: Propionic Acid		
Ibuprofen (Motrin, Advil, Nuprin, Medipren)	*Pain:* A: PO 200–800 mg q4–6h; max: 3,200 mg/d *Fever:* A: PO 200–400 mg t.i.d-q.i.d C: 6 mo–12 y: PO: 5–10 mg/kg t.i.d.-q.i.d.	For mild to moderate muscle aches and pains. Causes some gastric distress but less than aspirin. Should be taken with food, at mealtime, or with plenty of fluids. *Pregnancy category:* B; PB: 98%; t½: 2–4 h
Miscellaneous		
Methotrimeprazine HCl (Levoprome)	*Sedative-analgesic:* A: C: >12 y: PO: 6–25 mg/d in divided doses with meals; IM: 10–12 mg q4–6h PRN (deep IM) Elderly: IM: 5–10 mg q4–6h *Postanalgesia:* A and C: >12 y: IM: 2.5–7.5 mg q4–6h PRN	Treatment of moderate to severe pain. May be used pre- and postoperatively for pain and sedation. Has properties of phenothiazines, analgesia, and sedative/hypnotic. *Pregnancy category:* C; PB: UK; t½: 20 h
Tramadol (Ultram)	A: PO: 50–100 mg q4–6h, PRN, *max:* 400 mg/d Elderly >75 y: *max:* 300 mg/d *Hepatic dysfunction:* 50 mg, q12h *Renal disorder:* Cl$_{Cr}$ (CrCl) <30 mL/min: 50–100 mg, q12h	Used for moderate to severe pain. Contraindicated in severe alcoholism or with use of narcotics. Nausea, vomiting, dizziness, constipation, headache, and anxiety may occur. *Pregnancy category:* C; PB: UK; t½: UK

KEY: A: adult; C: child; IM: intramuscular; PB: protein-binding; PO: by mouth; t½: half-life; UK: unknown; >: more than; PRN: as necessary.

Liver enzyme levels (serum glutamic-oxalo-acetic transaminase/aspartate aminotransferase [SGOT/AST], serum glutamic-pyruvic transaminase/alanine aminotransferase [SGPT/ALT], alkaline phosphatase [ALP]) and serum bilirubin should be monitored.

Pharmacodynamics

Acetaminophen weakly inhibits the prostaglandin synthesis, which decreases pain sensation. It is effective in eliminating mild to moderate pain and headaches, and is useful for its antipyretic effect. It does not possess antiinflammatory action. Its onset of action is rapid and the duration of action is 5 h or less. Severe adverse reactions may occur with an overdose, so acetaminophen in liquid or chewable form should be out of a child's reach.

Side Effects and Adverse Reactions

An overdose of acetaminophen can be extremely toxic to the liver cells, causing hepatotoxicity. Death could occur in 1 to 4 days from hepatic necrosis. If a child or adult ingests excessive amounts of acetaminophen tablets or liquid, the poison control center should be contacted immediately, or the child or adult should be taken to the emergency room. Early symptoms of hepatic damage include nausea, vomiting, diarrhea, and abdominal pain.

Table 14–2 lists the commonly used nonnarcotic analgesics, their dosage, uses, and considerations.

NURSING PROCESS: ANALGESIC: Acetaminophen

ASSESSMENT

- Obtain a medical history of liver dysfunction. Overdosing or extremely high doses of acetaminophen can cause hepatotoxicity.
- Ascertain the severity of the pain. Nonnarcotic NSAIDs such as ibuprofen or a narcotic may be necessary for relieving pain.

POTENTIAL NURSING DIAGNOSES

- High risk for injury
- Pain

PLANNING

- Client's pain will be relieved or controlled.

NURSING INTERVENTIONS

- Check liver enzyme tests such as ALT, ALP, GGPT, 5-NT, and bilirubin for elevations for clients taking high doses or overdoses of acetaminophen.

CLIENT TEACHING

- Instruct the client to keep acetaminophen out of children's reach. Acetaminophen for children is available in flavored tablets and liquid. High doses can cause hepatotoxicity. Self-medication of acetaminophen should not be used longer than 10 d for adults and 5 d for children without the health care provider's approval.
- Instruct the parent to call the poison control center immediately if a child has taken a large or unknown amount of acetaminophen. Ipecac should be available in the home.
- Check acetaminophen dosage on package level. Do *not* exceed the recommended dosage.

Side Effects
- Instruct the client to report side effects. Overdosing can cause severe liver damage and death.
- Check the serum acetaminophen level when toxicity is suspected. The normal serum level is 5 to 20 mg/μL; the toxic level is >50 μg/mL, and levels of >200 μg/mL could indicate hepatotoxicity. The antidote for acetaminophen is acetylcysteine (Mucomyst). The dosage is based on the serum acetaminophen level.

EVALUATION

- Evaluate the effectiveness of acetaminophen in relieving pain. If pain persists, another analgesic may be needed.
- Determine if the client is taking the dose as recommended and no side effects are observed or reported.

NARCOTIC ANALGESICS

Narcotic analgesics, called **narcotic agonists,** are prescribed for moderate and severe pain. In the United States, the Harrison Narcotic Act of 1914 required that all forms of opium must be sold with a prescription and could no longer be a nonprescription drug. The Controlled Substance Act of 1970 classified addicting drugs in five schedule categories according to their potential for drug abuse (see Chapter 5).

In 1803, a German pharmacist isolated morphine

FIGURE 14–2. Narcotic: Morphine

Morphine Sulfate	Dosage	NURSING PROCESS Assessment and Planning
Morphine sulfate (Duramorph, MS Contin, Roxanol SR), 🍁 Epimorph, Statex Narcotic opiate CSS II *Pregnancy Category:* B	A: PO: 10–30 mg q4h PRN SR: 30 mg, q8–12 h IM/SC: 5–15 mg PRN IV: 4–10 mg q4h PRN; diluted; inject over 5 min Epidural: 2–10 mg over 24 h C: IM/SC: 0.1–0.2 mg/kg PRN; max: <15 mg/dose	

Contraindications	Drug-Lab-Food Interactions	
Asthma with respiratory depression, increased intracranial pressure, shock *Caution:* Respiratory, renal, or hepatic diseases; myocardial infarction; elderly; very young	*Increase* effects of alcohol, sedatives-hypnotics, antipsychotic drugs, muscle relaxants *Lab: Increase* AST, ALT	

Pharmacokinetics	Pharmacodynamics	Interventions
Absorption: PO: varies; IV: rapid *Distribution:* PB: UK; crosses placenta, in breast milk *Metabolism:* t½: 2.5–3 h *Excretion:* 90% in urine	PO: Onset: variable Peak: 1–2 h Duration: 4–5 h; SR: 8–12 h SC/IM: Onset: 15–30 min Peak: SC: 50–90 min IM: 0.5–1 h Duration: 3–5 h PO: Onset: rapid Peak: 20 min Duration: 3–5 h	

	Evaluation
Therapeutic Effects/Uses: To relieve severe pain. *Mode of Action:* Depression of the CNS; depression of pain impulses by binding with the opiate receptor in the CNS.	

Side Effects	Adverse Reactions
Anorexia, nausea, vomiting, constipation, drowsiness, dizziness, sedation, confusion, urinary retention, rash, blurred vision, bradycardia, flushing euphoria, pruritus	Hypotension, urticaria, seizures *Life-threatening:* Respiratory depression, increased intracranial pressure

KEY: A: adult; C: child; PO: by mouth; SR: sustained-release; IM: intramuscular; SC: subcutaneous; IV: intravenous; PB: protein-binding; t½: half-life; UK: unknown; <: less than; PRN: as necessary; 🍁 : Canadian drug name.

from opium. Codeine is another drug obtained from opium. In the last 40 years, many synthetic and semisynthetic narcotics have been developed, with approximately 20 narcotics marketed for clinical use.

Narcotic analgesics (**narcotics**) act mostly on the central nervous system, whereas nonnarcotic analgesics (analgesics) act on the peripheral nervous system at the pain receptor sites. Narcotics not only suppress pain impulses but can suppress respiration and coughing by acting on the respiratory and cough centers in the medulla of the brain stem. One example of such a narcotic is morphine, which is a potent analgesic that can readily depress respirations. Codeine is not as potent as morphine, but it relieves mild to moderate pain and suppresses cough. It can also be classified as a cough suppressant (antitussive). Many of the narcotics possess antitussive and antidiarrheal effects, in addition to relieving pain. There are other synthetic cough suppressants on the market that are discussed in Chapter 30.

MORPHINE

Morphine, an extraction from opium, is a potent narcotic analgesic (Fig. 14–2). Morphine is effective against acute pain due to acute myocardial infarction (AMI), cancer, and dyspnea due to pulmonary edema. It may be used as a preoperative medication. Although it is effective in relieving severe pain, it can cause respiratory depression, orthostatic hypotension, miosis, urinary retention, constipation due to reduced bowel motility, and cough suppression. An antidote for morphine excess or overdose is the narcotic antagonist naxolone (Narcan).

Pharmacokinetics

Morphine may be taken orally, although GI absorption can be somewhat erratic. For severe pain such as AMI, it is given intravenously. The protein-binding power is unknown. Morphine crosses the placenta and is present in the mother's breast milk. It has a short half-life and 90% is excreted in the urine.

Pharmacodynamics

Morphine binds with the opiate receptor in the CNS. Parenterally, the onset of action is rapid, especially intravenously. Onset of action is slower for subcutaneous and intramuscular injections. Duration of action with all types of drug administration is 3 to 5 h except with sustained-release products such as MS Contin, which has a duration of action of 8 to 12 h.

NURSING PROCESS: NARCOTIC ANALGESIC I: Morphine Sulfate

ASSESSMENT

- Obtain a medical history. Contraindications to use of morphine include severe respiratory disorders, increased intracranial pressure (ICP), and severe renal disease. Morphine may increase ICP and seizures.
- Obtain a drug history. Report if a drug-drug interaction is probable. Morphine increases the effects of alcohol, sedatives or hypnotics, antipsychotic drugs, and muscle relaxants and might cause respiratory depression.
- Assess vital signs and urinary output. Note the depth and rate of respirations. Morphine can cause urinary retention.

POTENTIAL NURSING DIAGNOSES

- Pain related to surgery, injury
- Ineffective breathing patterns related to excess morphine dosage

PLANNING

- Client will be free of pain, or the intensity of pain will be lessened.

NURSING INTERVENTIONS

- Administer the narcotic before pain reaches its peak to maximize the effectiveness of the drug.
- Monitor vital signs at frequent intervals to detect respiratory changes. Respirations of <10/min can indicate respiratory distress.
- Monitor the client's urine output; urine output should be at least 600 mL/d.
- Check bowel sounds for decreased peristalsis, a cause of constipation due to morphine. Dietary change or mild laxative might be needed.
- Check for pupil changes and reaction. Pinpoint pupils can indicate morphine overdose.
- Have naloxone (Narcan) available as an antidote if morphine overdose occurs.
- Check child's dose of morphine before its administration; dose is 0.1 to 0.2 mg/kg.

General

- Instruct the client not to take alcohol or CNS depressants with any narcotic analgesics such as morphine. Respiratory depression can result.
- Suggest nonpharmacological measures to relieve pain as client is recuperating from surgery. If necessary, a nonnarcotic analgesic may be prescribed.

Side Effects

- Alert the client that with continuous use, narcotics such as morphine can become addicting. If addiction occurs, inform the client about methadone treatment programs and other resources in the area.
- Instruct the client to report dizziness or difficulty in breathing while taking morphine. Dizziness could be due to orthostatic hypotension. Advise the client to ambulate with caution or only with assistance.

EVALUATION

- Evaluate the effectiveness of morphine in lessening or alleviating the pain.
- Evaluate the stability of vital signs. Report any decrease in blood pressure.

MEPERIDINE

One of the first synthetic narcotics, meperidine (Demerol), became available in the mid-1950s. It is classified as a schedule II drug according to the Controlled Substances Act. Meperidine has a shorter duration of action than morphine, and its potency varies according to the dosage. Meperidine, which can be given orally, intramuscularly, and intravenously, is the most commonly used narcotic for alleviating postoperative pain. It does not have the antitussive property of opium preparations. It can be given during pregnancy, in contrast to the opium preparations (morphine, codeine), which are not given because of their possible teratogenic effect. Drug data related to meperidine are covered in Figure 14–3.

Pharmacokinetics

Meperidine is usually administered intramuscularly for postoperative pain because it is absorbed faster and more completely by this method than in an oral preparation. It is considered to have a moderate half-life and can therefore be administered several times a day at specified intervals. Also, its protein-binding is not prolonged. Meperidine is metabolized in the liver to an active metabolite; therefore, the dose needs to be decreased for clients with hepatic or renal insufficiency. It is excreted in the urine, mostly as metabolites.

Pharmacodynamics

Meperidine should not be taken with alcohol or sedative-hypnotics because the combination of these drugs causes an additive CNS depression. A major side effect of meperidine is a decrease in blood pressure, so blood pressure should be monitored while the client is taking meperidine, especially if the client is an older adult.

Table 14–3 lists the narcotics, their dosages, uses, and considerations.

Side Effects and Adverse Reactions

Many side effects are known to accompany the use of narcotics, and the nurse needs to be vigilant when administering these drugs. Of particular importance are signs of respiratory depression (respiration $<10/min$). Other side effects include **orthostatic hypotension** (drop in blood pressure when rising from sitting or lying position), tachycardia, drowsiness and mental clouding, constipation, and urinary retention. Also pupillary constriction (a sign of toxicity), tolerance, and psychologic and physical dependence may occur with prolonged use.

Increased metabolism of narcotics contributes to tolerance, which causes an increased need for higher doses of the narcotic. If chronic use of the narcotic is discontinued, withdrawal symptoms (called **abstinence syndrome**) usually occur within 24 to 48 h after the last narcotic dose. Abstinence syndrome is due to physical dependence. Irritability, diaphoresis (sweating), restlessness, muscle twitching, and increase in pulse rate and blood pressure are examples of withdrawal symptoms. Withdrawal symptoms from narcotics are most unpleasant but are not as severe or life-threatening as those that accompany withdrawal from sedative-hypnotics—a process that may lead to convulsions.

Contraindications

Use of narcotic analgesics is contraindicated for clients with head injuries. Narcotics decrease respiration, thus causing an accumulation of carbon dioxide (CO_2). With an increase in CO_2 retention, blood vessels dilate (vasodilation), especially cerebral vessels, which causes increased intracranial pressure.

TABLE 14–3 Narcotics: Opium and Synthetics

Generic (Brand)	Route and Dosage	Uses and Considerations
Codeine (sulfate, phosphate) CSS II	A: PO/SC/IM: 15–60 mg q4–6h PRN C: PO/SC/IM: 0.5 mg/kg dose q4–6h	Is effective for mild to moderate pain. Can be used with a nonnarcotic (acetaminophen) for pain relief. Has antitussive properties. Can decrease respiration, and cause physical dependence and constipation. *Pregnancy category:* C; PB: 70%; t½: 2.5 h.
Hydromorphone HCl (Dilaudid) CSS II	A: PO: 1–6 mg q4–6h PRN SC/IM/IV: 1–4 mg q4–6h PRN Rectal: 3 mg q6–8h PRN	For severe pain. Potent narcotic, 5–10 times more potent than morphine. Can decrease respiration, may cause constipation. Effective in controlling pain in terminal cancer. *Pregnancy category:* C; PB: 62%; t½: 1–3 h
Levorphanol tartrate (Levo-Dromoran) CSS II	A: PO/SC/IV: Initially: 2 mg PO/SC/IV: 2–3 mg q6–8 h PRN	For moderate to severe pain. Has similar side effects as morphine. *Pregnancy category:* B; PB: 50%–60%; t½: 10–16 h
Meperidine (Demerol)	See Prototype Drug Chart (Fig. 14–3)	For moderate pain. Can decrease blood pressure and cause dizziness. In head injury, can increase intracranial pressure. *Pregnancy category:* B; PB: 60%–70%; t½: 3–8 h
Morphine sulfate	See Prototype Drug Chart (Fig. 14–2)	Potent narcotic for severe pain. IV morphine is given to relieve cardiac pain due to a myocardial infarction. Can cause respiratory depression, physical dependence, orthostatic hypotension, and constipation. May cause nausea and vomiting due to increased vestibular sensitivity. *Pregnancy category:* B; PB: UK; t½: 2.5–3 h
Oxycodone HCl with acetaminophen (Percocet) and oxycodone terephthalate with aspirin (Percodan) CSS II	A: PO: 5 mg q4–6h PRN or 5–10 mg q6h PRN C: 6–12 y: 1.25 mg q6h PRN 12–17 y: 2.5 mg q6h PRN	For moderate to severe pain. Percocet contains acetaminophen; Percodan contains aspirin and can cause gastric irritation, so it should be taken with food or plenty of liquids. *Pregnancy category:* B; PB UK; t½: 2–3 h
Propoxyphene HCl (Darvon) Propoxyphene napsylate (Darvon-N) CSS IV	A: PO: HCl: 65 mg q4h PRN *max:* 390 mg/d A: PO: napsylate: 100 mg q4h PRN *max:* 600 mg/d	For mild pain. Weak analgesic. Darvon-compound contains aspirin, and Darvocet-N contains acetaminophen. Is not a constipating drug; has little effect on physical dependence. *Pregnancy category:* C; PB: >90%; t½: 12 h
Fentanyl (Duragesic, Sublimaze) CSS II	*Preoperative:* A: IM/IV: 50–100 μg q1–2h PRN (0.05–0.1 mg) C: 2–12 y: 1.7–3.3 μg/kg A: Transdermal patch: 72-h effect	Short-acting potent narcotic analgesic. It may be used with short-term surgery. Also drug is available as a transdermal patch for controlling chronic pain. *Pregnancy category:* C; PB: 80%–89%; t½: 3.6 h
Sufentanil citrate (Sufenta) CSS II	*Primary anesthetic:* A: IV: 8–30 μg/kg with 100% O_2 and muscle relaxant C: IV: 10–25 μg/kg with 100% O_2 and muscle relaxant *Adjunct to anesthesia:* IV: 1–8 μg/kg	It is a potent synthetic narcotic and is used as part of the balanced anesthesia group. Also may be used as a primary anesthetic. *Pregnancy category:* C; PB: 93%; t½: 1–3 h
For Narcotic Addiction		
Levomethadyl acetate HCl (Orlaam)	A: IM: Initially: 10–40 mg 3×/wk: maint: 60–90 mg 3×/wk; max: 140 mg 3×/wk (M, W, F regimen)	To manage narcotic addiction. *Pregnancy category:* UK; PB: UK; t½: UK

KEY: *A: adult; C: child; CSS: Controlled Substance Schedule; IM: intramuscular; IV: intravenous; PO: by mouth; PRN: as necessary; PB: protein-binding; SC: subcutaneous; t½: half-life; UK: unknown.*

Narcotic analgesics given to a client with a respiratory disorder only intensify the respiratory distress. In the asthmatic, opiates decrease respiratory drive while simultaneously increasing airway resistance.

Narcotics may cause hypotension and are not indicated for clients in shock or those who have very low blood pressure. If a narcotic is necessary, the dosage needs to be adjusted; otherwise, the hypotensive state may worsen. For the older adult or a person who is debilitated, the narcotic dose usually needs to be decreased.

FIGURE 14–3. Narcotic: Meperidine

		NURSING PROCESS
Meperidine HCl	**Dosage**	**NURSING PROCESS** Assessment and Planning

Meperidine HCl
  (Demerol HCl), Pethadol, Pethi-
  dine HCl
Synthetic narcotic
CSS II
Pregnancy Category: B
	A: PO/SC/IM/IV: 50–150 mg q3–4 h
	  PRN
	C: PO/IM/IV: 1 mg/kg q4–6 h; max:
	  <100 mg q4 h	

Contraindications	**Drug-Lab-Food Interactions**	

Alcoholism; head trauma; increased in-
tracranial pressure; severe hepatic,
renal, and pulmonary diseases, MAO
inhibitors
	Increase CNS depression with alcohol,
	  sedative-hypnotics, and other CNS
	  depressants
	Lab: *Increase* serum amylase, AST, ALT,
	  bilirubin	

Pharmacokinetics	**Pharmacodynamics**	Interventions

Absorption: PO: 50% absorbed; IM: well
  absorbed
Distribution: PB: 60–70%
Metabolism: t½: 3–8 h
Excretion: In urine, mostly as metabo-
  lites
	PO: Onset: 15 min
	       Peak: 1 h
	       Duration: 4 h
	IM/SC: Onset: 10–15 min
	       Peak: 0.5–1 h
	       Duration: 2–4 h
	IV: Onset: 1–5 min
	       Peak: 5–10 min
	       Duration: 2 h	

Therapeutic Effects/Uses: To relieve moderate to severe pain. *Mode of Action:* Synthetic morphine-like substances, depression of pain impulses by bind- ing to the opiate receptor in the CNS.	Evaluation

Side Effects	**Adverse Reactions**

Nausea, vomiting, constipation,
  headache, dizziness, drowsiness, hy-
  potension, sedation, confusion, ab-
  dominal cramps, euphoria, blurred
  vision, rash, tinnitus, tremors
	Bradycardia, severe hypotension, con-
	  vulsion, physical and/or psychologic
	  dependence, seizures
	Life-threatening: Respiratory depression,
	  cardiovascular collapse, increased in-
	  tracranial pressure

KEY: A: adult; C: child; PO: by mouth; SC: subcutaneous; IM: intramuscular; IV: intravenous;
<: less than; PRN: as necessary; : Canadian drug names.

NURSING PROCESS: NARCOTIC ANALGESIC II: Meperidine (Demerol)

ASSESSMENT

- Obtain drug history from the client of drugs he
or she is currently taking. Report if a drug-drug
interaction is probable. CNS depressants enhance

the action of meperidine; thus, respiratory depression can occur.
- Obtain baseline vital signs for future comparisons. Meperidine tends to decrease systolic
blood pressure.

- Assess type of pain, location, and duration before giving meperidine.

POTENTIAL NURSING DIAGNOSIS

- Pain related to surgery or injury

PLANNING

- Client's pain will be decreased or alleviated. Drug dosing may need to be repeated.

NURSING INTERVENTIONS

- Administer meperidine before the pain reaches its peak to maximize the effectiveness of the drug.
- Monitor vital signs to compare blood pressure with baseline pressure. Hypotension is a side effect of meperidine. Note if client is having any breathing dysfunction.
- Have naloxone (Narcan) available, which can reverse respiratory depression due to narcotic overdose.
- Check urine output and bowel sounds. Urinary retention and constipation are side effects of meperidine.
- Check older adults for side effects of meperidine. Confusion may occur, so use of side rails

and other precautions should be taken. Dosage may need to be decreased.

General

- Instruct the client not to take alcohol or CNS depressants with meperidine because of increased depression of the CNS and of respirations.
- Inform the client that drug dependence could occur with continual use of meperidine. If severe pain is still present, another narcotic analgesic or analgesic may be prescribed.

Side Effects

- Instruct the client to report side effects such as dizziness due to orthostatic hypotension, headaches, constipation, blurred vision, or decreased urine output. Report findings to the health care provider.

EVALUATION

- Evaluate the effectiveness of the narcotic analgesic in lessening or alleviating the pain. If pain persists after several days, the cause should be determined or the narcotic should be changed.
- Evaluate the stability of vital signs. Abnormal signs, such as decreased blood pressure, should be reported.

NARCOTIC AGONIST-ANTAGONISTS

In the last 20 years, **mixed narcotic agonist-antagonists,** medications in which a narcotic antagonist, such as naloxone (Narcan) is added to a narcotic agonist, were developed in hopes of decreasing narcotic abuse. Pentazocine (Talwin), the first mixed narcotic analgesic, can be given orally (tablet) and by injection (SC, IM, and IV). Pentazocine is classified as a schedule IV drug. Butorphanol tartrate (Stadol), buprenorphine (Buprenex), and nalbuphine hydrochloride (Nubain) are examples of other mixed narcotic agonist-antagonist analgesics. Reports are that pentazocine and butorphanol can cause dependence. These drug agents are considered safe during labor, but safety during early pregnancy has not been established.

Figure 14–4 details the pharmacologic behavior of pentazocine and Table 14–4 lists the various agonist-antagonist narcotics.

PHARMACOKINETICS

Pentazocine can be administered orally, intramuscularly, or intravenously. It is absorbed well from the GI tract and is rapidly absorbed parenterally. It has a short half-life and is moderately protein-bound. Pentazocine is metabolized in the liver and is excreted in the urine.

PHARMACODYNAMICS

Pentazocine is effective in alleviating moderate pain. Onset of action is rapid, and peak time occurs within 15 min for intravenous administration and 1 to 2 h for oral and intramuscular administrations. Duration of action is the same for all routes of administration, which is approximately 3 h.

Chapter 14: Nonnarcotic and Narcotic Analgesics 239

FIGURE 14–4. Narcotic: Agonist-Antagonist

Pentazocine Lactate	**Dosage**	**NURSING PROCESS** Assessment and Planning

Pentazocine lactate
  (Talwin)
Narcotic agonist-antagonist
CSS IV
Pregnancy Category: C
	A: PO: 50–100 mg q3–4 h PRN; max:
	  600 mg/d
	IM/IV: 30 mg q3–4 h PRN; max: 360
	  mg/d	

Contraindications	**Drug-Lab-Food Interactions**	
Alcoholism; head trauma; severe respi- ratory, renal, and/or hepatic disease, hypersensitivity to naloxone *Caution:* Severe heart disease	*Increase* CNS depression with alcohol, sedative-hypnotics, antipsychotics, muscle relaxants	
Pharmacokinetics	**Pharmacodynamics**	Interventions

Absorption: PO: well absorbed
Distribution: PB: 60%
Metabolism: t½: 2–3 h
Excretion: In urine (small amount ex-
creted unchanged); in feces (small
amount)
	PO: Onset: 15–30 min
	  Peak: 1–2 h
	  Duration: 2–4 h
	IM: Onset: 15–20 min
	  Peak: 1 h
	  Duration: 2–4 h
	IV: Onset: minutes
	  Peak: 15 min
	  Duration: 3 h	

Therapeutic Effects/Uses: To relieve moderate to severe pain. *Mode of Action:* Inhibition of pain impulses transmitted in the CNS by binding with the opiate receptor, pain threshold is increased.	Evaluation

Side Effects	**Adverse Reactions**
Nausea, vomiting, constipation, dizzi- ness, sedation, headaches, confusion, euphoria, rash, blurred vision, dysuria	Hallucinations, urinary retention, urticaria, tachycarda *Life-threatening:* Respiratory depression, shock

KEY: A: adult; C: child; PO: by mouth; IM: intramuscular; IV: intravenous; UK: unknown; PB: protein-binding; t½: half-life; max: maximum; CSS: Controlled Substance Schedule.

TABLE 14–4 Narcotics: Agonist-Antagonists and Narcotic Antagonist

Generic (Brand)	Route and Dosage	Uses and Considerations
Narcotic Agonist- **Antagonists**		

Buprenorphine HCl
  (Buprenex)
CSS V
	A: IM/IV: Initially: 0.3 mg q6h;
	  may increase to 0.6 mg q6h
	  PRN
		For moderate to severe pain associated with surgery, cancer, ureteral calculi, myocardial infarction, and trauma. Avoid alcohol and CNS depressants. *Pregnancy category:* C; PB: 96%; t½: 2–3 h

Butorphanol tartrate
  (Stadol)
	A: IM: 1–4 mg q3–4h PRN
	IV: 0.5–2 mg q3–4h PRN
	Nasal Spray: 1 mg (1 spray)
	  q3–4h
		Management of moderate to severe pain for cancer, renal calculi, labor, musculoskeletal, and burns. *Pregnancy category:* C; PB: >90%; t½: 2.5–4 h

Table continued on following page

TABLE 14–4 Narcotics: Agonist-Antagonists and Narcotic Antagonist *(Continued)*

Generic (Brand)	Route and Dosage	Uses and Considerations
Nalbuphine HCl (Nubain)	A: SC/IM/IV: 10–20 mg q3–4h PRN; max: 160 mg/d	To control moderate to severe pain. May be used as a supplement to surgical anesthesia. Use for clients with respiratory depression. *Pregnancy category:* B; PB: UK: t½: 5 h
Pentazocine lactate (Talwin)	See Prototype Drug Chart (Fig. 14–4)	To control moderate to severe pain. May be used as a supplement with surgery. Use with caution if hepatic, renal or respiratory dysfunction is present. *Pregnancy category:* C; PB: 60%; t½: 2–3 h
Dezocine (Dalgan)	A: IM: 5–20 mg q3–6h PRN: max: 120 mg/d IV: 2.5–10 mg q3–6h PRN	To control moderate to severe pain. *Pregnancy category:* C; PB: UK; t½: 2.2–2.6 h
Narcotic Antagonist Naloxone HCl (Narcan)	Opiate overdose; *Narcotic-induced respiratory distress:* A: IV: 0.4–2 mg; may repeat q2–3min; max: 10 mg C: IV: 0.01–0.1 mg/kg; may repeat q2–3min; max: 10 mg *Postoperative RD:* A: IV: 0.1–0.2 mg; may repeat q2–3min PRN C: IV/IM: 0.005–0.01 mg/kg; may repeat q2–3min PRN	To treat narcotic overdose. May be given rapidly IV in small amounts with repeats at 2–3 min intervals as needed. *Pregnancy category:* B; PB: UK; t½: 1–1.5 h

KEY: *A: adult; C: child; CSS: Controlled Substance Schedule; IM: intramuscular; IV: intravenous; PB: protein-binding; SC: subcutaneous; t½: half-life; UK: unknown.*

NURSING PROCESS: MIXED NARCOTIC ANALGESIC: Pentazocine (Talwin)

ASSESSMENT

- Obtain a drug history from the client. Report if a drug-drug interaction is probable. When taken with pentazocine, CNS depressants can cause respiratory depression.
- Obtain baseline vital signs for future comparison.
- Assess the type of pain, duration, and location before giving the drug.

POTENTIAL NURSING DIAGNOSIS

- Pain related to surgery or trauma.

PLANNING

- Client will be free of pain, or the intensity of pain will be lessened.

NURSING INTERVENTIONS

- Monitor vital signs. Note any changes in respirations.
- Check bowel sounds. Decreased peristalsis may result in constipation. A mild laxative may be necessary.
- Check urine output. Report if urine output is <30 mL/h or <600 mL/d.

- Administer IV pentazocine diluted in sterile water or undiluted. Do not mix with barbiturates.

CLIENT TEACHING

General
- Instruct the client not to consume alcohol or CNS depressants while taking pentazocine. Respiratory depression can occur.
- Suggest nonpharmacological methods for lessening pain, such as changing position or ambulation.

Side Effects
- Instruct the client to report side effects to pentazocine such as dizziness, headaches, constipation, dysuria, rash, or blurred vision. Hallucinations, tachycardia, and respiratory depression are adverse reactions that might occur.

EVALUATION

- Evaluate the effectiveness of pentazocine in relieving pain. If ineffective, another narcotic analgesic may be ordered.
- Evaluate the stability of the vital signs. Note if there is a change in respirations, pulse rate, or blood pressure. Report abnormal findings.

NARCOTIC ANTAGONISTS

Narcotic antagonists are antidotes for overdoses of narcotic analgesics. The narcotic antagonists have a higher affinity to the opiate receptor site than the narcotic being taken. The narcotic antagonist blocks the receptor and displaces any narcotic that would be at the receptor, thus inhibiting the narcotic action. Naloxone (Narcan), administered intramuscularly or intravenously, and naltrexone hydrochloride (Trexan), administered orally by tablet or liquid, are pure narcotic antagonists. Levallorphan tartrate (Lorfan), administered by injection, has some weak agonist properties; however, it has a strong narcotic antagonist effect. These drugs reverse the respiratory and CNS depression caused by the narcotics and are perfect examples of pharmacologic antagonists.

TREATMENT FOR NARCOTIC-ADDICTED PERSONS

Throughout the country there are many **methadone treatment programs** to help the narcotic-addicted person to withdraw from heroin or similar narcotics without causing withdrawal symptoms. Methadone is a narcotic, but it causes less dependency than the narcotics it is replacing. The half-life of methadone is longer than most narcotics, so it needs to be given only once a day. The dosage is from 40 to 120 mg/day.

There are two types of methadone programs: weaning programs and maintenance programs. In a weaning program, the person receives a dose of methadone for the first 2 days that is approximately the same as the dose of the "street" drug to which she or he is addicted. After 2 days, the methadone dose is decreased by 5 to 10 mg until the person is completely weaned from methadone. In a maintenance program, the person is given the same methadone dose every day. The dose may be less than that of the street drug, but it remains the same dose every day.

■ CASE STUDY: Client Taking a Narcotic

R.J., 79 years old, had abdominal surgery for colon resection. The narcotic analgesic meperidine (Demerol), 75 mg, q 3 to 4 h, was prescribed following the surgery. R.J. did not ask for "pain medication" because he thought he might become addicted to the narcotic. The nurse noted that he was restless and grimacing when he moved in bed. He refused to breathe deeply and cough when instructed

to do so. The nurse compared his vital signs to his baseline findings. His pulse rate had increased and his systolic blood pressure had decreased by 6 mmHg.

1. Should the nurse give the meperidine? Explain.
2. Why doesn't R.J. want to breathe deeply and cough: What nursing intervention might be taken?
3. What is the significance of the changes in the vital signs? Why should the nurse continue to monitor the vital signs?
4. What are the classic side effects of narcotic analgesics?
5. What nonpharmacologic measures might the nurse suggest to decrease the pain?

After the first day, R.J. asked for meperidine every 3 h. On the fifth day after surgery, the health care provider discontinued the meperidine and prescribed acetaminophen with codeine.

6. Why was the narcotic analgesic order changed?
7. R.J. does not want to ambulate. What is an appropriate nursing response?

STUDY QUESTIONS

1. A client has had major surgery. What type of analgesic best meets the client's needs? Explain.
2. A client is complaining of flu symptoms and is taking aspirin for fever and to relieve the achiness associated with the flu. What is an appropriate intervention? Why?
3. Aspirin is a mild nonnarcotic analgesic. Name drug categories in which aspirin is used and explain each.
4. What is the most common side effect of nonnarcotics? What nursing measures can be used to decrease or alleviate this side effect?
5. What are the advantages and disadvantages of using acetaminophen?
6. A client is physically dependent on a "street" narcotic. What type of program could be of help in decreasing or eliminating the drug addiction. How would you explain the program to the client?
7. A child took approximately 20 acetaminophen tablets. What should the parent do? What is the serious toxic effect of acetaminophen?
8. What are the serious side effects of narcotic analgesics?
9. When do withdrawal symptoms occur? Describe the symptoms.

Chapter 15

Anticonvulsants

OUTLINE

Objectives
Terms
Introduction
International Classification of
  Seizures
Anticonvulsants

Hydantoins
Barbiturates
Succinimides
Oxazolidones/Oxazolidine-
  dione
Benzodiazepines

Iminostilbenes
Valproate
Nursing Process
Summary
Case Study
Study Questions

OBJECTIVES

Describe the two international classifications of seizures and give examples of types of seizures.

Differentiate between the types of seizures.

Give the pharmacokinetics, side effects and adverse reactions, therapeutic plasma phenytoin level, contraindications for use, and drug interaction of the hydantoin, phenytoin (Dilantin).

Describe the uses for hydantoins, long-acting barbiturates, succinimides, oxazolidones, benzodiazepines, carbamazepine, and valproate.

Explain the nursing interventions, including client teaching, related to the use of hydantoins and other anticonvulsants.

TERMS

anoxia
anticonvulsants
atonic seizures
clonic seizures
electroencephalogram (EEG)

hydantoins
hyperplasia
idiopathic
seizures: grand-mal,
  petit-mal, psychomotor

status epilepticus
teratogenic
tonic seizures

INTRODUCTION

Epilepsy, a seizure disorder, occurs in approximately 1% of the population. The **seizure** associated with epilepsy results from abnormal electric discharges from the cerebral neurons, and is characterized by a loss or disturbance of consciousness and usually by a convulsion (abnormal motor reaction). The **electroencephalogram (EEG)** is useful in diagnosing epilepsy. It records abnormal electric discharges of the cerebral cortex. Fifty percent of all epilepsy cases are considered to be primary, or **idiopathic** (of unknown cause), and 50% are considered secondary to trauma, brain anoxia, infection, or cerebrovascular disorders (CVA, or stroke).

INTERNATIONAL CLASSIFICATION OF SEIZURES

There are various types of and names for seizures, such as grand-mal, petit-mal, and psychomotor. The international classification of seizures (Table 15–1) describes two categories of seizure: generalized and partial seizure. A person may have more than one type of seizure.

Drugs used for epileptic seizures are called **anticonvulsants,** or antiepileptics. Anticonvulsant drugs suppress the abnormal electric impulses from the seizure focus to other cortical areas, thus preventing the seizure but *not* eliminating the cause of the seizure. Anticonvulsants are classified as CNS depressants.

ANTICONVULSANTS

There are many types of anticonvulsants used in treating epilepsy, including the hydantoins (phenytoin [Dilantin], mephenytoin, ethotoin), long-acting barbiturates (phenobarbital, mephobarbital, primidone), succinimides (ethosuximide), oxazolidones (trimethadione), benzodiazepines (diazapam, clonazepam), carbamazepine, and valproate (valproic acid). Anticonvulsants are not used for all types of seizures; for example, the hydantoin phenytoin, is effective in treating **grand-mal** (tonic-clonic) seizures and **psychomotor** seizures but is not effective in treating **petit-mal** (absence) seizures. Anticonvulsants are usually taken throughout the person's lifetime. In some cases, the health care provider might discontinue the anticonvulsant if there has not been a seizure in the last 3 to 5 years.

HYDANTOINS

The first anticonvulsant used to treat seizures was phenytoin, a **hydantoin** discovered in 1938 that is still the most commonly used drug for controlling seizures. It has the least toxic effects, has a small effect on general sedation, and is nonaddicting. However, this drug should not be used during pregnancy because it can have a teratogenic effect on the fetus.

Drug dosage for phenytoin as well as for other anticonvulsants varies according to the age of the client. Newborns, persons with liver disease, and

---

TABLE 15–1 International Classification of Seizures

Category	Characteristics and Types of Seizures
Generalized Seizures	Involve both cerebral hemispheres of the brain. Motor changes are noted and consciousness may be lost.
	1. Tonic-clonic, or grand-mal, seizure: Most common form of seizure. In the tonic phase, the skeletal muscles contract or tighten in a spasm, lasting 3–15 sec. In the clonic phase, there is a dysrhythmic muscular contraction, or jerkiness, of the legs and arms, lasting 2–4 min.
	2. Tonic seizure: Sustained muscle contraction.
	3. Clonic seizure: Dysrhythmic muscle contraction.
	4. Absence, or petit-mal, seizure: Brief loss of consciousness, lasting less than 10 sec. Fewer than three spike waves on the EEG printout. Usually occurs in children.
	5. Myoclonic seizure: Isolated clonic contraction or jerks lasting 3–10 sec. May be secondary to a neurologic disorder, such as encephalitis or Tay-Sachs disease.
	6. Atonic seizure: Head drop; loss of posture.
	7. Infantile spasms: Muscle spasm.
Partial Seizures	No loss of consciousness in simple partial seizures, but there is a loss of consciousness in complex partial seizures. Involves one hemisphere of the brain.
	1. Simple seizure: Occurs in motor, sensory, autonomic, and psychic forms.
	Motor: Formally called the Jacksonian seizure; involves spontaneous movement that spreads; can develop into a generalized seizure.
	Sensory: Visual, auditory, or taste hallucinations.
	Autonomic response: Paleness, flushing, sweating, or vomiting.
	Psychologic: Personality changes.
	2. Complex or psychomotor (temporal lobe) seizure: Symptoms may include confusion or memory impairment, behavioral changes, and automatisms (repetitive behavior, such as chewing or swallowing motions). Client may not recall behavior after the seizure.

the older adult require a lower dosage due to a decrease in metabolism resulting in more available drug. Children and young and middle-aged adults have an increased metabolism rate. The drug dosage is adjusted according to the therapeutic plasma or serum level. Phenytoin has a narrow therapeutic range of 10 to 20 μg/mL. The benefits of an anticonvulsant become apparent when the serum drug level is within the therapeutic range; if, however, the drug level is below the desired range, the client is not receiving the required drug dosage to prevent seizures. Also, if the drug level is above the desired range, drug toxicity may result. Monitoring the therapeutic serum drug range is of utmost importance to ensure drug effectiveness. Figure 15–1 lists the pharmacologic data associated with phenytoin.

Pharmacokinetics

Phenytoin is slowly absorbed from the small intestine. It is a highly protein-bound (85% to 95%) drug; a decrease in serum protein or albumin can increase the free phenytoin serum level. With a small to average drug dose, the half-life of phenytoin is approximately 22 h; however, the range can be from 6 to 45 h. Phenytoin is metabolized to inactive metabolites, and that portion is excreted in the urine.

Pharmacodynamics

The pharmacodynamics of orally administered phenytoin include onset of action within 30 min to 2 h, peak serum concentration in 1.5 to 3 h, steady state of serum concentration in 7 to 10 days, and a duration of action dependent on the half-life. Oral phenytoin is most commonly ordered as a sustained-release capsule. The peak concentration time is 4 to 12 h (sustained-release).

Intravenous infusion of phenytoin should be administered by direct injection into a large vein. The drug may be diluted in saline solution; however, dextrose solution should be avoided because of drug precipitation. Continuous intravenous infusion should not be used. Infusion rates of more than 50 mg/min may cause hypotension or cardiac dysrhythmias, especially with elderly and debilitated clients. Local irritation at the injection site may be noted and sloughing may occur. Intramuscular injection of phenytoin is irritating to tissues and may cause damage. For this reason and its erratic absorption rate, intramuscular administration of phenytoin is discouraged.

Mephenytoin is a potent hydantoin and much more toxic than phenytoin. It is used for severe grand-mal or psychomotor seizures that do not respond to phenytoin or other anticonvulsant therapy. The newest hydantoin, ethotoin, produces similar responses as phenytoin and has a shorter half-life of 3 to 6 h, therefore, decreasing the chance of cumulative drug effects.

Side Effects and Adverse Reactions

The severe side effects of hydantoins include gingival hyperplasia, or overgrowth of the gum tissues (reddened gums that bleed easily); neurologic and psychiatric effects, such as slurred speech, confusion, depression, and thrombocytopenia (low platelet count), and leukemia (low white blood cell count). Clients on hydantoins for long periods might have an elevated blood sugar (hyperglycemia), which results from the drug inhibiting the release of insulin. Less severe side effects include nausea, vomiting, constipation, headaches, alopecia and hirsutism.

Drug-Drug Interactions

Drug-drug interaction is common with hydantoins because they are highly protein-bound. Hydantoins compete with other drugs, such as anticoagulants and aspirin, for plasma protein-binding sites. The hydantoins displace the anticoagulants and aspirin, causing more free drug and increasing their activity. Drugs, such as sulfonamides and cimetidine (Tagamet), can increase the action of hydantoins by inhibiting liver metabolism, which is necessary for drug excretion. Absorption of hydantoins can be decreased by antacids, calcium preparations, and antineoplastic drugs. Antipsychotics can lower the seizure threshold and can increase seizure activity. The client should be closely monitored for seizure occurrence.

BARBITURATES

Phenobarbital, a long-acting barbiturate, is still prescribed for treating grand-mal seizures and acute episode of seizures due to **status epilepticus** (rapid succession of epileptic seizures), meningitis, toxic reactions, and eclampsia. Possible teratogenic effects and other side effects related to phenytoin are less pronounced with phenobarbital. Problems associated with phenobarbital include its cause of general sedation and client tolerance to the drug. Discontinuance of phenobarbital should be gradual to avoid recurrence of seizures.

FIGURE 15–1. Anticonvulsants

Anticonvulsant	Dosage	**NURSING PROCESS** Assessment and Planning
Phenytoin (Dilantin) Anticonvulsant, hydantoin *Pregnancy Category:* D	A: PO: 100 mg, t.i.d. IV: LD: 10–15 mg/kg/d; infusion <50 mg/min; max: 300 mg/d C: 4–8 mg/kg/d in divided doses *Therapeutic serum range:* 10–20 μg/mL *Toxic level:* 30–50 μg/mL	

Contraindications	Drug-Lab-Food Interactions	
Hypersensitivity, heart block, psychiatric disorders, pregnancy	*Increase* effects with cimetidine, isoniazid, chloramphenicol; *decrease* effects with cisplatin, folic acid, and vinblastine *Decrease* effects of anticoagulants, oral contraceptives, antihistamines, corticosteroids, theophylline, cyclosporin, quinidine, dopamine, rifampin *Food:* Those rich in folic acid	

Pharmacokinetics	Pharmacodynamics	Interventions

Absorption: PO: slowly absorbed; IM: erratic rate of absorption
Distribution: PB: 85–95%
Metabolism: t½: 6–45 h; average: 22 h
Excretion: In urine, small amount; in bile and feces, moderate amount
	PO: Onset: 0.5–2 h
	    Peak: 1.5–3 h
	    Duration: 6–12 h
	IV: Onset: minutes–1 h
	    Peak: 2 h
	    Duration: >12 h	

	Evaluation
Therapeutic Effects/Uses: To prevent grand mal and complex partial seizures. *Mode of Action:* Reduces motor cortex activity by altering transport of ions.	

Side Effects	Adverse Reactions
Headache, diplopia, confusion, dizziness, sluggishness, decreased coordination, ataxia, slurred speech, rash, anorexia, nausea, vomiting, hypotension (IV), pink-red/brown discoloration of urine	Leukopenia, hepatitis, depression, gingival hyperplasia, gingivitis, nystagmus, hirsutism *Life-threatening:* Aplastic anemia, thrombocytopenia, agranulocytosis, Stevens-Johnson syndrome, hypotension, ventricular fibrillation

KEY: A: adult; C: child; PB: protein-binding; t½: half-life; PO: by mouth; IV: intravenous; >: greater than; <: less than.

SUCCINIMIDES

The succinimide drug group is used to treat absence or petit-mal seizures, and it may be used in combination with other anticonvulsants to treat such seizures. Ethosuximide is the succinimide of choice; the other formulations, methsuximide and phensuximide, are used mainly for petit-mal refractory seizures.

OXAZOLIDONES/OXAZOLIDINEDIONE

The oxazolidones, trimethadione and paramethadione, are also prescribed to treat petit-mal seizures. Trimethadione was the first drug developed for petit-mal and for that reason is prescribed more frequently than paramethadione. There are many severe side effects associated with this group of anticonvulsants. Trimethadione may be used in combination with other drugs or singly for treating refractory petit-mal seizures.

BENZODIAZEPINES

The three benzodiazepines that have anticonvulsant effects are clonazepam, clorazepate dipotassium, and diazepam. Clonazepam is effective in controlling petit-mal (absence) seizures; however, tolerance may occur 6 months after drug therapy starts, and consequently, clonazepam dosage has to be adjusted. Clorazepate dipotassium is frequently administered in adjunctive therapy for treating partial seizures.

Diazepam is primarily prescribed for treating acute status epilepticus and must be administered intravenously to achieve the desire response. The drug has a short-term effect; thus other anticonvulsants, such as phenytoin or phenobarbital, need to be given during or immediately following diazepam.

IMINOSTILBENES

Carbamazepine, an iminostilbene, is effective in treating refractory seizure disorders that have not responded to other anticonvulsant therapies. It is

TABLE 15–2 Anticonvulsants

Generic (Brand)	Route and Dosage	Uses and Considerations
Barbiturates		
Amobarbital (Amytal) CSS II	*Status epilepticus:* A: IM/IV: 75–500 mg; *max:* IM: 500 mg; IV: 1,000 mg Therapeutic serum range: 1–5 μg/mL	For acute convulsive episode and to control status epilepticus. Infusion rate should not exceed 100 mg/min for adult and 60 mg/m^2/min for children. *Pregnancy category:* D; PB: 50%–60%; t½: 20–25 h
Mephobarbital (Mebaral) CSS II	A: PO: 400–600 mg/d C: PO: 6–12 mg/kg/d in divided doses or C >5 y: 32–64 mg t.i.d./q.i.d. C <5 y: 16–32 mg t.i.d./q.i.d. Therapeutic serum range: 15–40 μg/mL	For grand-mal and petit-mal (absence) seizures. May be used in combination with other anticonvulsants. Also used to manage delirium tremens. May cause drowsiness and dizziness. *Pregnancy category:* D; PB: UK; t½: 34 h
Phenobarbital (Luminal) CSS IV	*Status epilepticus:* Neonate: IV: LD: 15–20 mg/kg single or divided dose A&C: IV 15–18 mg/kg; *max:* 30 mg/kg *Maintenance:* Neonate: PO/IV: 3–4 mg/kg/d in 1–2 divided doses Infant: 5–6 mg/kg/d in 1–2 divided doses C: PO: 1–5 y; 6–8 mg/kg/d in 1–2 divided doses 6–12 y: 4–6 mg/kg/d in 1–2 divided doses A: PO: 1–3 mg/kg/d; 100–300 mg/d Therapeutic serum range: 15–40 μg/mL	Long-acting barbiturate. Used for grand-mal, partial seizures, and to control status epilepticus. May be used in combination with phenytoin. High doses given to the elderly or children may cause confusion, depression, irritability. Long-term use with high doses could cause physical dependence. *Pregnancy category:* D; PB: 20%–40%; t½: A: 50–140 h; C: 35–75 h
Primidone (Mysoline)	A: PO: 125–250 mg b.i.d./q.i.d. C <8 y: PO: 1/2 of adult dose Therapeutic serum range: 5–10 μg/mL	Barbiturate-like drug. Used to manage grand-mal and psychomotor seizures. Take with food if the drug causes GI distress. *Pregnancy category:* D; PB: 99%; t½: 10–24 h
Benzodiazepines (anxiolytics)		
Clonazepam (Klonopin)	A: PO: 0.5–1 mg t.i.d.; gradually increase dose q3d until seizures are controlled C: PO: 0.01–0.03 mg/kg/d; gradually increase Therapeutic serum range: 20–80 ng/mL	For petit-mal, myoclonus, and status epilepticus. May be used when petit-mal (absence) seizures are refractory to succinimides and/or valproic acid. *Pregnancy category:* C; PB: 85%; t½: A: 20–50 h; C: 24–36 h

TABLE 15–2 Anticonvulsants *(Continued)*

Generic (Brand)	Route and Dosage	Uses and Considerations
Clorazepate (Tranxene) CSS IV	A: PO: 7.5 mg t.i.d. C >9 y: PO: 7.5 mg b.i.d.	May be used for partial seizures and as adjunctive therapy for seizures. *Pregnancy category:* D; PB: 97%; t½: 48 h
Diazepam (Valium)	*Status epilepticus:* A: IV: 5–10 mg, 2–5 mg/min C: IV: 1 mg over 3 min	For status epilepticus (drug of choice). Administer intravenously and repeat q10–15 min up to 30 mg PRN; then q2–4 h, PRN. *Pregnancy category:* D; PB: 98%; t½: 20–50 h
Lorazepam (Ativan) CSS IV	*Status epilepticus:* Neonate: IV: 0.05 mg/kg over 2–5 min; Infants & C: 0.1 mg/kg over 25 min; *max:* 4 mg/single dose A: IV: 4 mg over 2–5 min; *max:* 8 mg; may repeat in 10–15 min for all ages Therapeutic serum range: 50–240 ng/mL	To control status epilepticus. Infusion rate should not exceed 2 mg/min. *Pregnancy category:* D; PB: 85%; t½: 10–16 h
Hydantoins Ethotoin (Peganone)	A: PO: 1–3 g/d in divided doses C: PO: 0.5–1 g/d Therapeutic serum range: 15–50 µg/mL	For grand-mal, psychomotor seizures. *Pregnancy category:* D; PB: UK; t½: 3–9 h
Mephenytoin (Mesantoin)	A: PO: Initially: 50–100 mg; 100–200 mg t.i.d. C: PO: Initially: 50–100 mg; 100–400 mg/d in divided doses Therapeutic serum range: 25–40 µg/mL	For grand-mal, psychomotor, focal (simple) seizures. Severe adverse reaction may include blood dyscrasias. *Pregnancy category:* C; PB: UK; t½: 7 h; metabolite: 100–144 h
Phenytoin (Dilantin)	See Prototype Drug Chart (Fig. 15–1)	For tonic-clonic (grand-mal) and psychomotor seizures. Phenytoin is not effective for petit-mal (absence) seizures. Adverse reactions include gingival hyperplasia and CNS effects. Severe adverse reactions include aplastic anemia, agranulocytosis. *Pregnancy category:* D; PB: 85%–95%; t½: 22 h
Iminostilbene Carbamazepine (Tegretol)	A: PO: 200 mg b.i.d.; increasing doses as needed C: PO: 10–20 mg/kg/d in divided doses Therapeutic serum range 5–12 µg/mL	For grand-mal, psychomotor, mixed seizures. Used in treating seizures that do not respond to other anticonvulsants. *Pregnancy category:* C; PB: 75%–90%; t½: 15–30 h
Oxazolidones Paramethadione (Paradione)	A: PO: 300–600 mg t.i.d./q.i.d. C: PO: 13 mg/kg t.i.d. or 335 mg/m² t.i.d. or 300–900 mg/d in divided doses	For petit-mal (absence) seizures. May be used when refractory to other anticonvulsants. *Pregnancy category:* D; PB: UK; t½: 1–4 h
Trimethadione (Tridione)	Same as paramethadione	For petit-mal seizures. May be used when refractory to other anticonvulsants. It has many side effects. After prolonged use, drug should be withdrawn gradually. *Pregnancy category:* D; PB: <10%; t½: 6–12 d
Succinimides Ethosuximide (Zarontin)	A: PO: 250 mg b.i.d.; increase dose gradually C: 3–6 y: PO: 250 mg/d Therapeutic serum range: 40–100 µg/mL	For petit-mal and myoclonic seizures. Gastric irritation is common; may take with food. *Pregnancy category:* C; PB: UK; t½: A: 50–60 h, C: 25–30 h
Methsuximide (Celontin)	A&C: PO: Initially: 300 mg/d for 1 wk; may increase at intervals	For petit-mal (absence) seizures when refractory to other drugs. High occurrence of toxicity; more so than ethosuximide. *Pregnancy category:* C; PB: UK; t½: 2–4 h

Table continued on following page

TABLE 15–2 Anticonvulsants (*Continued*)

Generic (Brand)	Route and Dosage	Uses and Considerations
Phensuximide (Milontin)	A: C: PO: 0.5–1 g, b.i.d., t.i.d.	Similar to methsuximide. *Pregnancy category:* C; PB: UK; t½: 5–12 h
Valproate Valproic acid (Depakene)	A&C: PO: 15 mg/kg; *max:* 60 mg/kg/d in divided doses Therapeutic serum range: 40–100 μg/mL	For grand-mal, petit-mal, psychomotor, and myoclonic seizures. Doses may be increased weekly by 5–10 mg/kg/d until seizures are controlled. Avoid during pregnancy. *Pregnancy category:* D; PB: 90%; t½: 6–16 h
Miscellaneous Acetazolamide (Diamox)	Commonly used with other anticonvulsants: A: PO/IM/IV: 375 mg daily; *max:* 250 mg q.i.d. or PO SR: 250–500 mg daily or b.i.d. C: PO: 8–30 mg/kg in divided doses; *max:* 1.5 g/d	For grand-mal, petit-mal (absence) and focal seizures. Adequate fluid intake should be maintained to prevent kidney stones. *Pregnancy category:* D; PB: 90%; t½: 2.5–6 h
Gabapentin (Neurontin)	*Adjunctive therapy for partial seizures:* A: PO: 900–1,800 mg/d in 3 divided doses; max time between doses: 12 h	Used as adjunctive therapy for partial seizures. To avoid GI upset, give drug with food. If drug is discontinued, dose should be gradually reduced to avoid occurrence of seizures. *Pregnancy category:* C; PB: <3%; t½: 5–7 h
Magnesium sulfate	*Preeclampsia or eclampsia:* A: IV: Initially: 4 g in 250 mL D₅W; then 4 g IM; follow with 4 g IM q4h PRN or Inf: 1–4 g/h *Hypomagnesemic seizures:* A: IV: 1–2 g (19% sol) over 20 min; follow with 1 g IM q4–6h based on blood levels	To control seizures in toxemia of pregnancy due to eclampsia or preeclampsia. *Pregnancy category:* B; PB: UK; t½: UK

KEY: *A: adult; C: child; CNS: central nervous system; CSS: Controlled Substance Schedule; GI: gastrointestinal; IM: intramuscular; inf: infusion; IV: intravenous; LD: loading dose; PB: protein-binding; PO: by mouth; t½: half-life; UK: unknown; >: greater than; <: less than.*

used to control grand-mal and partial seizures and a combination of these seizures.

Carbamazepine is also used for psychiatric disorders, such as bipolar disease; as an analgesic in trigeminal neuralgia, and for treating alcohol withdrawal. However, the drug has not been approved by the Food and Drug Administration (FDA) for treatment of the above disorders.

VALPROATE

Valproic acid has been prescribed for petit-mal, grand-mal, and mixed types of seizures. Care

should be taken when giving this drug to very young children and clients with liver disorders because hepatotoxicity is one of the possible adverse reactions. Liver enzymes should be monitored.

Table 15–2 lists the various anticonvulsants, their dosages, uses, and considerations.

Anticonvulsant dosages usually start low and gradually increase over a period of weeks until the serum drug level is within therapeutic range or the seizures stop. Status epilepticus is life threatening because of its continuous seizures. If this condition is not treated immediately, respiratory arrest can occur, leading to cardiac arrest and death.

NURSING PROCESS: ANTICONVULSANTS: Phenytoin

ASSESSMENT

- Obtain a medication history from the client, including current drugs. Report if a drug-drug interaction is probable.

- Check urinary output to determine if adequate (>600 mL/d).
- Check laboratory values related to renal and liver function. If both BUN and creatinine levels are elevated, a renal disorder should be sus-

pected. Elevated serum liver enzymes, such as ALP, ALT or SGPT, γ-glutamyl transferase (GGT), and/or 5'-nucleotidase indicate a hepatic disorder.

POTENTIAL NURSING DIAGNOSES

- High risk for injury
- Altered oral mucous membranes

PLANNING

- Client will be free of seizures and will adhere to anticonvulsant therapy.
- Side effects of phenytoin will be minimal and closely monitored.

NURSING INTERVENTIONS

- Monitor serum drug levels of anticonvulsant to determine overdosing or underdosing of drug; promote compliance to regimen.
- Protect the client from hazards in the environment, such as sharp objects and table corners, during a seizure.
- Determine if the client is receiving adequate nutrients. Phenytoin may cause anorexia, nausea, and vomiting.
- Women taking oral contraceptives and anticonvulsants may need to use an additional contraceptive method.

CLIENT TEACHING

General
- Instruct the client to shake the suspension form well before pouring.
- Instruct the client not to drive or perform other hazardous activity when beginning anticonvulsant therapy. Until the client adapts to drug dosage, drowsiness is apt to occur.
- Alert female clients contemplating pregnancy to consult with the health care provider because phenytoin and valproic acid may have a teratogenic effect.
- During pregnancy, seizures frequently increase due to increased metabolism rates, and serum phenytoin levels should be closely monitored. Most anticonvulsants are classified in the D pregnancy category.

- Inform the client that alcohol and other CNS depressants can cause an added depressive effect on the body and should be avoided.
- Advise the client to obtain an alert ID card and medic alert bracelet or tag that indicate the health problem and the drug taken.
- Instruct the client not to abruptly stop the drug therapy but rather to withdraw the prescribed drug gradually under medical supervision to prevent seizure rebound (reoccurrence of seizures).
- Instruct the client of the need for preventative dental check-ups.
- Instruct the client to take the prescribed anticonvulsant, get laboratory tests as ordered, and to keep follow-up visits with the health care provider.
- Teach the client not to self-medicate with over-the-counter (OTC) drugs without first consulting the health care provider.
- Instruct the diabetic client to monitor serum glucose levels more closely than usual since phenytoin may inhibit insulin release, thus causing an increase in glucose level.
- Inform the client of the existence of national, state, and local associations that provide resources, current information, and support.

Diet
- Instruct the client to take the anticonvulsant at the same time every day with food or milk. If liquid form is used, shake well before ingesting the drug.

Side Effects
- Advise the client that urine may be a harmless pinkish-red or reddish-brown.
- Instruct the client to maintain good oral hygiene; use a soft toothbrush to prevent gum irritation and bleeding.
- Teach the client to report symptoms of sore throat, bruising, and nose bleeds, which may indicate a blood dyscrasia.
- Instruct the client to inform the health care provider of adverse reactions such as gingivitis, nystagmus (involuntary movement of the eyeball), slurred speech, rash, and dizziness.

EVALUATION

- Evaluate the effectiveness of the drug in controlling seizures.
- Continue to monitor phenytoin serum levels to determine if they are within the desired range. High serum levels of phenytoin are frequently indicators of phenytoin toxicity.

TABLE 15–3 Selected Anticonvulsants: Pharmacokinetics, Pharmacodynamics, and Therapeutic Ranges

| Drug | Pharmacokinetics | | | Pharmacodynamics | | | Therapeutic Serum Range |
	Protein-Binding (%)	*t½*	*Excretion*	*PO Onset*	*Peak Time (hours)*	*Duration of Action (hours)*	
Phenytoin (Dilantin)	85–95	6–45 h (average: 22 h)	Kidneys, bile, and GI	30 min–2 h	1.5–3	6–12	10–20 µg/mL
Phenobarbital	20–45	2–6 d	50–75% in urine	30–60 min	8–12	6–24	15–40 µg/mL
Ethosuximide (Zarontin)	UK	60 h (adult) 30 h (child)	25% in urine unchanged	UK	>4	12–60	40–100 µg/mL
Clonazepam (Klonopin)	UK	20–50 h	Kidneys and feces	20–60 min	1–2	6–12	20–80 ng/mL
Carbamazepine (Tegretol)	75	25–65 h	75% in urine, 25% in feces	Varies	4–7	6–12	5–12 µg/mL
Valproic Acid (Depakene)	90	6–16 h	kidneys	20–30 min	1–4	24	40–100 µg/mL

KEY: *GI: gastrointestinal; UK: unknown; >: greater than.*

SUMMARY

The pharmacologic behavior of specified anticonvulsants is summarized in Table 15–3.

■ CASE STUDY

S. S., age 26 years, is taking phenytoin (Dilantin) 100 mg, t.i.d. to control grand-mal seizures. S. S. and her husband are contemplating starting a family.

1. What pregnancy category is phenytoin?
2. As a nurse, what nursing action should you take?

S. S. complains of frequent "upset stomach" and "bleeding gums" when brushing her teeth.

3. To decrease GI distress, what can be suggested?
4. The dental condition causing the gums to bleed is likely _____.
5. To alleviate bleeding gums, client teaching for S. S. may include _____.
6. The nurse checks S. S.'s serum phenytoin level. Serum toxic level would be greater than _____.

STUDY QUESTIONS

1. What are the differences between generalized and partial seizures according to the international classification of seizures?
2. What are the implications of liver disease or kidney disease for a person taking anticonvulsants? Explain.
3. What is the therapeutic serum range of phenytoin? Is it considered to have a narrow or a wide range? Why should it be closely monitored?
4. What is gingival hyperplasia? Name the drug that might cause this. Give the nursing interventions for decreasing this problem.
5. What are the drug-drug interactions between hydantoins and other drugs? Give examples.
6. What drugs are used to treat status epilepticus? By what route should these drugs be given?
7. What type of seizures are benzodiazepines effective in treating? What is another classification for benzodiazepines?

Chapter 16

Antipsychotics, Anxiolytics, and Antidepressants

OUTLINE

Objectives
Terms
Introduction
Antipsychotics
    Phenothiazines
    Nonphenothiazines
    Nursing Process

Anxiolytics
    Benzodiazepines
    Nursing Process
Antidepressants
    Tricyclic Antidepressants
    Second-Generation Antidepressants

Monoamine Oxidase Inhibitors
Antimanic: Lithium
    Nursing Process
Study Questions

OBJECTIVES

Differentiate between the three groups of drugs: antipsychotics, anxiolytics, and antidepressants.

Name the general side effects associated with antipsychotics, anxiolytics, and antidepressants.

Give the nursing interventions, including client teaching, for antipsychotics, anxiolytics, and antidepressants.

Explain the uses of lithium, the serum or plasma therapeutic range, side effects and adverse reactions, and nursing interventions.

TERMS

affective disorder
akathisia
antidepressants
antiemetic
antipsychotics
anxiolytics
bipolar affective disorder
blood dyscrasias
dopamine
dyskinesia

dysphoria
dystonia
extrapyramidal reactions
    (symptoms/syndrome/
    EPS)
manic-depressive
monoamine oxidase (MAO)
    inhibitors
neuroleptic
orthostatic hypotension

parkinsonism
phenothiazines
psychosis
reactive depression
schizophrenia
second-generation antidepressants
tardive dyskinesia
tricyclic antidepressants
unipolar depression

INTRODUCTION

In Chapters 13 to 15 central nervous system (CNS) depressants were discussed: sedative-hypnotics, anesthetics, narcotic and nonnarcotic analgesics, and anticonvulsants. This chapter covers the last group of CNS depressants: antipsychotics, anxiolytics, and antidepressants, which are used to control symptoms of mental disorders. Antipsychotics are also known as neuroleptics, psychotropics, or major tranquilizers. The preferred name for this group is either antipsychotics or neuroleptics. Neuroleptic refers to any drug that modifies psychotic behavior, thus exerting an antipsychotic effect. Anxiolytics are also called antianxiety drugs or sedative-hypnotics. This group of drugs is used to treat anxiety. Antidepressants have been called mood elevators. They are used for depressive episodes with accompanying feelings of hopelessness and helplessness. Lithium, effective for bipolar affective disorder (manic-depressive illness), can be classified separately or as one of the subgroups of antidepressants.

ANTIPSYCHOTICS

Antipsychotics comprise the largest group of drugs used to treat mental illness. Specifically, these drugs improve the thought processes and behavior of clients with psychotic symptoms, especially those with **schizophrenia;** they are not used for treating anxiety or depression. The theory is that psychotic symptoms result from an imbalance in the neurotransmitter **dopamine** in the brain. Antipsychotics block D_2 dopamine receptors in the brain, thereby reducing the psychotic symptoms. Many of the antipsychotics block the chemoreceptor trigger zone and vomiting (emetic) center in the brain, producing an **antiemetic** effect. By blocking dopamine, **extrapyramidal reactions,** or **symptoms** of parkinsonism, such as tremors, mask-like facies, rigidity, and shuffling gait, may occur. Many clients taking antipsychotic drugs may require long-term medication for parkinsonian symptoms. Other extrapyramidal reactions include acute **dystonia** (facial grimacing, abnormal or involuntary eye movement), **akathisia** (restlessness, constant moving about), and **tardive dyskinesia** (protrusion of tongue, chewing motion, involuntary movement of the body and extremities). Tardive dyskinesia is a later phase of extrapyramidal reaction to antipsychotic drugs.

Antipsychotics are subdivided into four classes: the **phenothiazines** (largest class), thioxanthenes, butyrophenones, and dibenzoxazepines. The phenothiazines and thioxanthenes block norepinephrine, causing sedative and hypotensive effects early in treatment. The butyrophenones block only the neurotransmitter dopamine. But because phenothiazines represent such a large group, the antipsychotics may be classified as two groups: phenothiazines and nonphenothiazines.

PHENOTHIAZINES

In 1952, chlorpromazine hydrochloride (Thorazine) was the first phenothiazine introduced for treating psychotic behavior in clients in psychiatric hospitals. The phenothiazines are subdivided into three groups: aliphatic, piperazine, and piperidine, which differ mostly in their side effects. Chlorpromazine is in the aliphatic group. The aliphatic phenothiazines produce a strong sedative effect, decrease blood pressure, and might cause extrapyramidal symptoms (EPS) (pseudo-parkinsonism). The piperazine phenothiazines produce a moderate sedative, a strong antiemetic effect, and some decreasing of the blood pressure. They also cause more extrapyramidal symptoms than the other phenothiazines. The piperidine phenothiazines have a strong sedative effect, cause few EPS, can decrease the blood pressure, and have no antiemetic effect. Table 16–1 summarizes the effects of the phenothiazines.

A new antipsychotic drug, clozapine (Clozaril), does not have a subclassification. It is considered atypical because it does not cause the acute extrapyramidal side effects associated with other similar drugs. Manifestations are limited to mild tremors, akathisia, or occasional rigidity. Because clozapine carries the risk of agranulocytosis (decrease in production of granulocytes; decrease in body defense) and seizure, it is indicated only for the treatment of the severely ill schizophrenic client who has not responded to the accepted antipsychotic drugs.

Most of the antipsychotics can be given orally (tablet or liquid), intramuscularly, or intravenously. For oral use, the liquid form might be preferred be-

TABLE 16–1 Effects of Phenothiazines
(Varies within class)

Group	Sedation	Hypotension	EPS	Antiemetic
Aliphatic Chlorpromazine and triflupro- mazine	+++	+++	++	++ +++
Piperazine	++	+	+++	+++
Piperidine	+++	+++	+	—

KEY: —: no effect; +: mild effect; ++: moderate effect; +++: severe effect; EPS: extrapyramidal symptoms.

cause some clients hide tablets to avoid taking them. Also, the absorption rate is faster with the liquid form. The peak serum drug level occurs in 2 to 3 h. The antipsychotics are highly protein-bound (>90%), and the excretion of the drug and its metabolites is very slow. The drug is metabolized by the liver enzymes to phenothiazine metabolites. The metabolites can be detected in the urine several months after the medication has been discontinued. Phenothiazine metabolites may cause a harmless pinkish to red-brown urine color. The *full* therapeutic effects of antipsychotics may not be evident for 3 to 6 weeks following initiation of therapy; however, an observable therapeutic response may be apparent after 7 to 10 days. The dosage for the antiemetic effect is lower than for the antipsychotic effect.

Figure 16–1 compares the aliphatic phenothiazine chlorpromazine hydrochloride (Thorazine) with the piperazine phenothiazine prochlorperazine maleate (Compazine). These two phenothiazines are the early antipsychotics, and although they were marketed for treatment of psychosis, each has a different primary use today. Chlorpromazine is used to manage psychotic disorders, and prochlorperazine is used mainly for treatment of nausea and vomiting.

Pharmacokinetics

The oral absorption of chlorpromazine and prochlorperazine is variable; the liquid form has a faster absorption rate. Both drugs are strongly protein-bound and have a long half-life; the drug may accumulate. Both chlorpromazine and prochlorperazine are metabolized by the liver and are excreted as metabolites in the urine. They cross the placenta readily and are excreted in breast milk. With hepatic dysfunction, the phenothiazine dose may need to be decreased because of lack of drug metabolism in the liver, thus causing an elevation in drug level.

Pharmacodynamics

Chlorpromazine is primarily prescribed for psychotic disorders and prochlorperazine for nausea and vomiting. Prochlorperazine has anticholinergic properties and should be cautiously administered to clients with glaucoma, especially narrow-angle glaucoma. Because hypotension is a side effect of these phenothiazines, any antihypertensives being administered at the same time can cause an additive hypotensive effect. Narcotics and sedative-hypnotics administered simultaneously with these phenothiazines can cause an additive CNS depression.

Antacids decrease the absorption rate of both drugs and all phenothiazines. Give 1 h before or 2 h after giving a phenothiazine.

The onset of action of oral, intramuscular, and intravenous administration of chlorpromazine and prochlorperazine are similar. The sustained release preparations prolong the duration time of both drugs. These drugs should only be administered rectally if the oral method is not tolerated. Erratic absorption of the suppository frequently occurs. Intramuscularly, the drugs should be administered deeply in the dorsogluteal muscle. They are extremely irritating to the subcutaneous tissue.

NONPHENOTHIAZINES

A frequently prescribed nonphenothiazine is the butyrophenone haloperidol (Haldol), whose pharmacologic behavior is similar to that of the phenothiazines. Haloperidol is a potent antipsychotic drug in which the equivalent prescribed dose is smaller than drugs of lower potency; e.g., chlorpromazine. Drug dose for haloperidol is 0.5 to 5 mg, whereas the drug dose for chlorpromazine is 10 to 25 mg. Figure 16–2 provides the drug data related to haloperidol.

Pharmacokinetics

Haloperidol is absorbed well through the gastrointestinal (GI) mucosa. It has a long half-life and is highly protein-bound, so the drug may accumulate. Most of haloperidol is excreted in the urine.

Pharmacodynamics

Haloperidol alters the effects of dopamine by blocking the dopamine receptors; thus sedation and EPS may occur. The drug is used to control psychoses and decrease signs of agitation in adults as well as children. Dosages need to be decreased in the older adult due to decreased liver function and potential side effects. It may be prescribed for children with hyperactive behavior. Haloperidol has anticholinergic activity; thus, care should be taken in administering it to clients with a history of glaucoma.

Haloperidol has similar onset of action, peak time of concentration, and duration of action to those of the phenothiazines. The nurse needs to observe the client for EPS. Skin protection is necessary when taking the drug for a period of time because of the possible side effect of photosensitivity.

Side Effects and Adverse Reactions

There are several common side effects associated with antipsychotics. The most common side effect for all antipsychotics is drowsiness. Many of the antipsychotics have some anticholinergic effects, such as dry mouth, increased heart rate, urinary retention, and constipation. Blood pressure decreases with the use of antipsychotics; aliphatic and piperidine types cause a greater decrease in blood pressure than the others. EPS are most prevalent with the phenothiazines, butyrophenones, and thioxanthenes and include pseudoparkinsonism, akathisia, dystonia, and tardive dyskinesia. Twenty percent of clients taking antipsychotics for long-term therapy may develop tardive dyskinesia. Most antiparkinsonism anticholinergics are not always effective for treating tardive dyskinesia. These EPS can begin 5 to 30 days after initiation of antipsychotic therapy. Anticholinergic drugs may be given to control EPS. High dosing or long-term use of antipsychotics can cause **blood dyscrasias** (blood cell disorders), e.g., agranulocytosis.

Dermatologic side effects seen early in drug therapy are pruritus and marked photosensitivity. Use of sunscreen, hats, protective clothing, and staying out of the sun are suggested.

The side effects and adverse reactions to clozapine (Clozaril) include sustained tachycardia, with an average increase in pulse rate of 10 to 15 beats/min, hypotension (9%), and hypertension (4%). Cardiovascular effects can be minimized by starting with low doses and gradually increasing

FIGURE 16–1. Antipsychotics (Neuroleptics)

Phenothiazines	Dosage	NURSING PROCESS Assessment and Planning
Aliphatic Phenothiazine *Chlorpromazine* (C) (Thorazine), 🍁 chlorpromanyl, Largactil *Pregnancy Category:* C *Piperazine Phenothiazine* Prochlorperazine (P) (Compazine), 🍁 Stemetil *Pregnancy Category:* C	*(C) Psychoses* A: PO: 10–25 mg, b.i.d.–q.i.d.; increase by 20–50 mg/d, q3–4 d *Max:* 800 mg/d in 4 divided doses (usual dose is 200 mg/d) IM/IV: Initially: 25–50 mg; may repeat in 1 h; then q3–4h, PRN *Max:* 400 mg, q4–6 h C: PO: 0.55 mg/kg, q4–6h C: >6 mo: IM/IV: 0.55 mg/kg or 15 mg/m² q6–8 h *Max:* 6 mo–5 y: 40 mg/d; 5–12 y: 75 mg/d *(P) Severe Nausea & Vomiting, psychoses* A: PO: 5–10 mg, t.i.d., q.i.d. PO: SR: 10–15 mg, q12h PR: 25 mg, b.i.d., t.i.d. IM: 5–10 mg, q3–4h IV: 2.5–5 mg, q6–8 h *Max:* all routes: 40 mg/d C: PO: 2.5 mg, t.i.d., 5 mg b.i.d. *Max:* 15 mg/d PR: 2.5 mg, t.i.d./q.i.d. IM: 0.13 mg/kg, q3–4h	
Contraindications	**Drug-Lab-Food Interactions**	
(C & P): Coma, bone marrow depression *(C):* Hepatic, renal, or coronary disease, cerebral insufficiency, severe hypotension, CNS depression *(P):* Severe liver disease, cardiovascular disease, narrow angle glaucoma, seizures	*(C & P):* *Increase* CNS depression wth alcohol, CNS depressants, narcotics, sedative-hypnotics Tricyclic antidepressants *increase* hypotensive and anticholinergic effects *Decrease* absorption with antacids, antidiarrheals Lab: *Increase:* AST, ALT, and alkaline phosphatase; false pregnancy test, false PKU *Decrease* hemoglobin, hematocrit, leukocytes, platelets	

FIGURE 16–1. *Continued*

Pharmacokinetics	Pharmacodynamics	Interventions

Absorption: (PO) (C & P): varies
Distribution: PB:
(C): 95%
(P): >90%
Metabolism: t½:
(C): 8–30 h
(P): 23 h
Excretion: (C & P): in urine as metabolites
	(C):
	PO: Onset: 30–60 min
	  Peak: 2–4 h
	  Duration: 4–6 h
	PO: SR: Onset: 30–60 min
	  Peak: 2–4 h
	  Duration: 10–12 h
	PR: Onset: 1–2 h
	  Peak: 3 h
	  Duration: 3–4 h
	IM: Onset: 15–30 min
	  Peak: 30 min
	  Duration: 4–8 h
	IV: Onset: 5–10 min
	  Peak: 10 min
	  Duration: UK
	(P):
	PO: Onset: 30–40 min
	  Peak: UK
	  Duration: 3–4 h
	PO: SR: Onset: 30–40 min
	  Peak: UK
	  Duration: 10–12 h
	PR: Onset: 1 h
	  Peak: UK
	  Duration: 3–4 h
	IM: Onset: 10–20 min
	  Peak: UK
	  Duration: 4–12 h
	IV: Onset: 5 min
	  Peak: UK
	  Duration: UK	

Therapeutic Effects/Uses: (C): To treat psychosis (mania, schizophrenia), intractable hiccups, preoperative sedation, behavioral problems in children. Secondary use is to control nausea and vomiting. *(P):* To treat nausea and vomiting. Secondary use is to treat psychosis.

Mode of Action: Alteration in dopamine effect on CNS, depression of limbic system and cerebral cortex that controls aggression.

Evaluation

Side Effects	Adverse Reactions
(C & P): Sedation, dizziness, headaches, dry mouth and eyes, urinary retention; extrapyramidal symptoms (EPS)*; photosensitivity, skin rashes *(P):* Blurred vision, restlessness, pink-reddish urine, euphoria or depression	*(C & P):* Hypotension, tachycardia, leukopenia, tardive dyskinesia, ECG changes *(C):* Seizures *Life-threatening: (C & P):* Agranulocytosis, circulatory failure, respiratory depression, neuroleptic malignant syndrome

KEY: A: adult; C: child; PO: by mouth; PB: protein-binding; t½: half-life; UK: unknown; SR: sustained-release capsules; IM: intramuscular; IV: intravenous; 🍁: Canadian drug names.
*Extrapyramidal symptoms/reactions include symptoms of pseudoparkinsonism.

FIGURE 16–2. Antipsychotic: Nonphenothiazine

Haloperidol	**Dosage**	**NURSING PROCESS**
		Assessment and Planning

Haloperidol	**Dosage**
Haloperidol (Haldol), ❋ Peridol Antipsychotic, neuroleptic (nonphenothiazine) *Pregnancy Category:* C	A: PO: 0.5–5 mg b.i.d./t.i.d. IM: Decanoate: 50–100 mg q4wk IM: 2–5 mg, q4h, PRN C: PO: 0.15 mg/kg/d in divided doses (not for child <3 y) Elderly: Decreased doses than for younger adult; PO: 0.5–2 mg, b.i.d., t.i.d.

Contraindications	**Drug-Lab-Food Interactions**
Narrow-angle glaucoma; severe hepatic, renal, and cardiovascular diseases; bone marrow depression; Parkinson's disease; blood dyscrasias; CNS depression; subcortical brain damage	*Increase* sedation with alcohol, CNS depressants *Increase* toxicity with anticholinergics, CNS depressants, lithium *Decrease* effects with phenobarbital, carbamazepine *Decrease* effects with caffeine

Pharmacokinetics	**Pharmacodynamics**	Interventions

Pharmacokinetics	**Pharmacodynamics**
Absorption: PO: 60% absorbed *Distribution:* PB: 80–90% *Metabolism:* t½: 15–35 h *Excretion:* In urine and feces	PO: Onset: erratic Peak: 2–6 h Duration: 24–72 h IM: Onset: 15–30 min Peak: 30–45 min Duration: 4–8 h IM: Decanoate: Onset: UK Peak: 6–7 d Duration: 3–4 wk

Evaluation

Therapeutic Effects/Uses: To treat acute and chronic psychoses, for children with severe behavior problems who are combative, to suppress narcotic withdrawal symptoms, to treat schizophrenia resistant to other drugs, to treat Tourette's syndrome, to treat symptoms of dementia in elderly.

Mode of Action: Alteration of the effect of dopamine on CNS; mechanism for antipsychotic effects are unknown.

Side Effects	**Adverse Reactions**
Sedation, extrapyramidal symptoms, orthostatic hypotension, headache, photosensitivity, dry mouth and eyes, blurred vision	Tachycardia, seizures, urinary retention, tardive dyskinesia *Life-threatening:* Laryngospasm, respiratory depression, cardiac dysrhythmias, neuromalignant syndrome (NMS)

KEY: A: adult; C: child; PO: by mouth; IM: intramuscular; PB: protein-binding; t½: half-life; UK: unknown; <: less than; ❋: Canadian drug names.

the dose. Constipation, nausea, abdominal discomfort, headache, vomiting, and diarrhea are reported occasionally, and incontinence and urinary retention are reported rarely. If the WBC (leukocyte) level falls <3000 mm^3, clozapine should be discontinued.

Drug Interactions

Because phenothiazine lowers the seizure threshold, dosage adjustment of an anticonvulsant may be necessary. If either aliphatic phenothiazine or the thioxanthene group is administered, a higher dose of anticonvulsant might be necessary to prevent seizures.

Antipsychotics interact with alcohol, hypnotics, sedatives, narcotics, and benzodiazepines to potentiate the sedative effects of antipsychotics. Atropine counteracts the EPS and potentiates antipsychotic effects. Use of antihypertensives can cause an additive hypotensive effect.

Antipsychotics should *not* be given with other antipsychotic or antidepressant drugs except to control psychotic behavior for selected individuals who are refractory to drug therapy. Usually if one antipsychotic drug is ineffective, then another one is prescribed. Individuals should *not* take alcohol or other CNS depressants (such as narcotic analgesics and barbiturates) with antipsychotics because additive depression is likely to occur. Geriatric clients may require a decreased dosage to reduce side effects.

When discontinuing antipsychotics, the drug dosage should be reduced gradually to avoid sudden recurrence of psychotic symptoms. Table 16–2 lists the antipsychotic drugs (phenothiazines and nonphenothiazines), their dosages, uses, and considerations.

TABLE 16–2 Phenothiazines and Nonphenothiazines

Generic (Brand)	Route and Dosage	Uses and Considerations
PHENOTHIAZINES: **Aliphatics**		
Chlorpromazine HCl (Thorazine)	See Prototype Drug Chart (Fig. 16–1)	Effective for acute psychosis; for decreasing agitation in the elderly without causing confusion; and for intractable hiccups. It has a strong sedative effect, and can cause orthostatic hypotension. *Pregnancy category:* C; PB: 95%; t½: 8–30 h
Promazine HCl (Sparine)	A: PO: 10–200 mg q4–6h IM: 50–150 mg; may repeat × 1 C >12 y: PO: 10–25 mg q4–6h	For psychotic disorders. Not effective for an acutely agitated psychotic client. Can cause orthostatic hypotension. *Pregnancy category:* C; PB: ≥90%; t½: ≥24 h
*Triflupromazine (Vesprin)	A: PO: 10–50 mg b.i.d./t.i.d. IM: 60–150 mg/d C >2 y: PO: 0.5–2 mg/kg/d in 3 divided doses	Similar to promazine HCl. Not to be used for client with psychosis and having depression. *Pregnancy category:* C; PB: ≥90%; t½: ≥24 h
Piperazines		
Fluphenazine HCl (Prolixin)	A: PO: 1–5 mg t.i.d./q.i.d. Elderly: 1–2.5 mg/d; also long-acting weekly/biweekly dosages Therapeutic range: 5–20 ng/mL	For moderate to severe psychosis. Extrapyramidal symptoms (EPS) are likely. *Pregnancy category:* C; PB: ≥90%; t½: 5–15 h
Perphenazine (Trilafon)	A: PO: 4–16 mg, b.i.d. or t.i.d. or q.i.d.	For psychotic disorders; control severe nausea and vomiting; and treat intractable hiccups. Used also prior to chemotherapy to prevent nausea. *Pregnancy category:* C; PB: ≥90%; t½: 9.5 h
Prochlorperazine maleate (Compazine)	A: PO: 5–10 mg t.i.d./q.i.d.; *max:* 40 mg/d (can be higher for psychotic behavior)	For mild psychotic behavior. Effective antiemetic, given either orally, deep IM, or rectally. Causes less sedation and hypotension. Marked EPS. *Pregnancy category:* C; PB: ≥90%; t½: 23 h
Acetophenazine maleate (Tindal)	A: PO: 20 mg, b.i.d.–q.i.d. *max:* 120 mg/d	For psychosis. Higher doses for schizophrenia. *Pregnancy category:* C; PB: ≥90%; t½: UK
Thiothixene HCl (Navane)	A: PO: 2 mg t.i.d.; *max:* 60 mg/d IM: 4 mg b.i.d./q.i.d.; *max:* 30 mg/d	Management of psychotic disorders, especially acute and chronic schizophrenia. Can cause EPS. *Pregnancy category:* C; PB: ≥90%; t½: 24–34 h

Table continued on following page

TABLE 16–2 Phenothiazines and Nonphenothiazines (Continued)

Generic (Brand)	Route and Dosage	Uses and Considerations
*Trifluoperazine HCl (Stelazine)	A: PO: 1–5 mg b.i.d.; *max:* 40 mg/d C: PO: 1 mg q.i.d./b.i.d.	Management of psychotic disorders. To control excessive tension and anxiety. Can cause EPS. Dilute liquid in 120 mL of water, milk, or juice. *Pregnancy category:* C; PB: ≥90%; t½: ≥24 h
Piperidine Mesoridazine besylate (Serentil)	A: PO: 50 mg t.i.d.; gradually increase Optimum response: 100–400 mg/d Elderly: ⅓–½ adult dose	For psychosis and schizophrenia, severe anxiety, chronic brain syndrome (smaller doses). Few EPS. Can cause hypotensive effects. *Pregnancy category:* C; PB: 92%–99%; t½: 24–48 h
*Thioridazine HCl (Mellaril)	A: PO: 50–100 mg t.i.d.; *max:* 800 mg/d Elderly: ⅓–½ adult dose	For psychosis. Higher doses for severe psychosis. Lower doses (10–50 mg, t.i.d.) for marked depression, alcohol withdrawal, intractable pain. Few EPS. Little antiemetic effect. Can cause orthostatic hypotension. *Pregnancy category:* C; PB: ≥90%; t½: 24–34 h
NONPHENOTHIAZINES **Butyrophenone** Droperidol (Inapsine)	A: IM/IV: 2.5–10 mg 30–60 min before anesthesia C: IM/IV: 0.088–0.165 mg/kg	Primarily prescribed as a preoperative drug administered alone or in conjunction with a narcotic. Has antiemetic properties. May decrease blood pressure and increase heart rate. *Pregnancy category:* C; PB:UK; t½: 2 h
Haloperidol (Haldol)	See Prototype Drug Chart (Fig. 16–2)	For acute psychosis. Also for children with severe behavior problems who are combative. Used to suppress narcotic withdrawal symptoms and for schizophrenia that is resistant to drugs. Likely to cause EPS. Has minimal sedative, hypotensive, and anticholinergic effects. *Pregnancy category:* C; PB: 80%–90%; t½: 15–35 h
Dibenzoxazepine Loxapine (Loxitane)	A: PO: Initially: 10 mg b.i.d.; then may increase to 50–100 mg/d Elderly: ⅓–½ regular adult dose	For acute psychosis and schizophrenia. Likely to cause EPS. Overdose can cause cardiac toxicity or neurotoxicity. *Pregnancy category:* C; PB: 95%; t½: 5 h
Thioxanthenes Chlorprothixene HCl (Taractan)	A: PO: 25–50 mg t.i.d.; gradually increase to 500–600 mg/d	For psychosis and schizophrenia. Sedative effect is common. Few incidences of EPS. Can cause orthostatic hypotension. Take with food to decrease GI distress. *Pregnancy category:* C; PB: UK; t½: 3–34 h
Thiothixene HCl (Navane)		See thiothixene HCl listed with piperazine phenothiazines. Thiothixene is a piperazine-like phenothiazine drug.
Others Clozapine (Clozaril)	A: PO/IM: Initially: <50 mg/d; if tolerated, gradually increase to 300–450 mg/d in divided doses	For severely ill schizophrenic clients, especially those who do not respond to other antipsychotics. With long-term use, monitor white blood cell count. *Pregnancy category:* B; PB: 95%; t½: 8–12 h
Molindone HCl (Moban)	A: PO: Initial: 50–75 mg in 3–4 divided doses A: PO: 5–50 mg t.i.d./q.i.d. Elderly: ⅓–½ adult dose	Management of schizophrenia. Can cause EPS. Has less sedative effect. *Pregnancy category:* C; PB: UK; t½: 1.5 h
Risperidone (Risperdal)	A: PO: 1–3 mg b.i.d. Elderly: ⅓–½ adult dose	Management of psychotic disorders. Side effects include EPS, insomnia, anxiety, agitation. *Pregnancy category:* C; PB: 90%; t½: 24 h

*Avoid spilling liquid on skin. Contact dermatitis could result.
KEY: A: adult; C: child; PO: by mouth; IM: intramuscular; IV: intravenous; <: less than; ≥: equal to or greater than; PB: protein-binding; t½: half-life; EPS: extrapyramidal symptoms.

NURSING PROCESS: PHENOTHIAZINE AND NONPHENOTHIAZINE

ASSESSMENT

- Obtain baseline vital signs (VS) for use in future comparison.
- Obtain a history from the client of present drug

therapy. If client is taking an anticonvulsant, drug dose might need to be increased as antipsychotics tend to lower seizure threshold.
- Assess mental status before start of drug therapy and continue daily.

POTENTIAL NURSING DIAGNOSES

- Altered thought processes
- Activity intolerance
- Sensory-perceptual alteration

PLANNING

- Client's psychotic behavior will be controlled by drug(s) and psychotherapy.

NURSING INTERVENTIONS

- Monitor vital signs. Orthostatic hypotension is likely to occur.
- Remain with client while he or she takes the medication. Some clients hide drugs.
- Avoid skin contact with liquid concentrates to prevent contact dermatitis. Liquid must be protected from light and should be diluted with fruit juice.
- Administer oral doses with food or milk to decrease gastric irritation.
- Administer by IM route deep into the muscle because the drug is irritating to the fatty tissue. Do *not* inject into subcutaneous tissue. Check blood pressure for marked decrease 30 min after drug is injected.
- Do not mix in same syringe with heparin, pentobarbital, cimetidine, or dimenhydrinate.
- Chill suppository in the refrigerator for 30 min before removing foil wrapper.
- Observe the client for extrapyramidal syndrome (EPS): acute dystonia (spasms of the tongue, face, neck, and back), akathisia (restlessness, inability to sit still, foot tapping), pseudoparkinsonism (muscle tremors, rigidity, shuffling gait), and tardive dyskinesia (lip smacking, protruding and darting tongue, and constant chewing movement). Report these promptly to the health care provider.
- Monitor for symptoms of neuroleptic malignant syndrome (NMS): increased fever, pulse, and blood pressure; muscle rigidity; increased creatine phosphokinase and WBC; altered mental status; acute renal failure; varying levels of consciousness; pallor; diaphoresis; tachycardia; and dysrhythmias.
- Monitor urine output. Urinary retention may result.
- Monitor serum glucose level.

CLIENT TEACHING

General

- Instruct the client to take the drug exactly as ordered. In schizophrenia and other psychotic disorders, antipsychotics do not cure the mental illness but do prevent symptoms. Many clients on medication can function outside the institution setting.
- Advise the client that medication may take 6 wk or longer to achieve full clinical effect.
- Instruct the client not to consume alcohol or other CNS depressants such as narcotics; these drugs intensify the depressant effect on the body.
- Instruct the client not to abruptly discontinue the drug. Seek advice from the health care provider before making any changes in dosage.
- Encourage the client to read labels on over-the-counter (OTC) preparations. Some are contraindicated when taking antipsychotics.
- Adjust drug dose if client smokes, as necessary. Smoking increases the metabolism of some antipsychotics.
- Advise client to maintain good oral hygiene by frequent brushing and flossing.
- Encourage the client to talk with the health care provider regarding family planning. The effect of antipsychotics on the fetus is not fully known; however, there may be teratogenic effects on the fetus.
- Advise the client that phenothiazine passes into breast milk. This could cause drowsiness and unusual muscle movement in the baby.
- Instruct the client on the importance of routine follow-up examinations.
- Encourage the client to obtain laboratory tests on schedule. WBCs are monitored for 3 mon, especially during the start of drug therapy. Leukopenia, or decreased WBCs, may occur. Be alert to symptoms of malaise, fever, and sore throat, which may be an indication of agranulocytosis, a serious blood dyscrasia. Report this promptly to the health care provider, especially when taking clozapine.
- Encourage the client to wear an ID bracelet indicating the medication taken.
- Inform the client that tolerance to sedative effect develops over a period of days or weeks.

Side Effects

- Instruct the client to avoid potentially dangerous situations, such as driving, until drug dosing has been stabilized.
- Inform the client about EPS; instruct the client to promptly report symptoms to the health care provider.
- Photosensitivity may occur; instruct the client to avoid direct sunlight or to use a sun block and protective clothing. Sunbathing can cause a skin rash.

- Advise the client of orthostatic hypotension and possible dizziness.
- Advise the client who is taking aliphatic phenothiazines, such as chlorpromazine, that the urine might be pink or red-brown; this discoloration is harmless.
- Inform the client that changes may occur related to sexual functioning and menstruating. Women could have irregular menstrual periods or amenorrhea, and men might experience impotence and gynecomastia (enlargement of breast tissue).
- Suggest lozenges or hard candy if mouth dryness occurs. Advise the client to consult the health care provider if dry mouth persists for more than 2 wk.

- Advise the client to avoid extremes in temperatures and increased exercise.
- Advise the client to rise slowly from sitting or lying to standing to prevent a sudden drop in blood pressure.

EVALUATION

- Evaluate the effectiveness of the drug; the client is free of psychotic symptoms at the *lowest* dose possible.
- The client can cope with everyday living situation and attend to activities of daily living.
- Determine if any side effects of or adverse reactions to the drug have occurred.

ANXIOLYTICS

Anxiolytics, a group of antianxiety drugs, are also called sedative-hypnotic agents. The major group of anxiolytics are the benzodiazepines (a minor tranquilizer group). Long before benzodiazepines were prescribed for anxiety and insomnia, barbiturates were used. Benzodiazepines are considered more effective than barbiturates because they enhance the action of gamma-aminobutyric acid (GABA), an inhibitory neurotransmitter within the CNS. Benzodiazepines have fewer side effects and are less dangerous in overdosing. Long-term use of barbiturates causes drug intolerance and dependence and may cause respiratory distress. Today, barbiturates are not the choice of drug for anxiety.

A limited degree of anxiety might be considered normal; however, when the anxiety is excessive and could be disabling, then anxiolytics may be prescribed. The action of anxiolytics resembles that of the sedative-hypnotics, but not that of the antipsychotics.

There are two types of anxiety—primary and secondary. Primary anxiety is not caused by a medical condition or by drug use; secondary anxiety is related to selected drug use or medical or psychi-

atric disorders. The anxiolytics are not usually given for secondary anxiety unless the medical problem is untreatable, severe, and causing disability. In this case, the drug could be given for a short period to alleviate any acute anxiety attacks. Long-term use of anxiolytics is discouraged because tolerance develops within weeks or months, depending on the drug agent. Drug tolerance can occur in less than 2 to 3 months for meprobamate and phenobarbital.

Some of the symptoms of a severe or acute attack of anxiety include dyspnea (difficulty in breathing), choking sensation, chest pain, heart palpitations, dizziness, faintness, sweating, trembling and shaking, and fear of losing control. Nonpharmacologic measures should be used for decreasing anxiety before giving anxiolytics. These measures might include using a relaxation technique, psychotherapy, or support groups.

BENZODIAZEPINES

Benzodiazepines have multiple uses, such as anticonvulsants, antihypertensives, sedative-hypnotics, preoperative drugs, and anxiolytics. Most of the benzodiazepines are used mainly for severe or prolonged anxiety; examples include chlordiazepoxide (Librium), diazepam (Valium), chlorazepate dipotassium (Tranxene), oxazepam (Serax), lorazepam (Ativan), alprazolam (Xanax), prazepam (Centrax), and halazepam (Paxipam). The most commonly used benzodiazepines as a sedative and for sleep are flurazepam, temazepam, and triazolam. Benzodiazepines are lipid-soluble and are absorbed readily from the GI tract. They are highly protein-bound (80% to 98%). They could displace other highly protein-bound drugs, so the drug dosage for clients with liver or renal disease should be lowered accordingly to avoid possible cumulative effects. Traces of benzodiazepine metabolites could be present in the urine for weeks or months after the person has stopped taking the drug. These are controlled substance schedule IV (CSS IV) drugs.

In 1962, the first benzodiazepine, chlordiazepoxide (Librium), became widely used for its sedative effect. Diazepam (Valium) was the most frequently prescribed drug in the early 1970s and was called a miracle drug by many. Diazepam is the prototype drug of benzodiazepine and is described in Figure 16–3.

Pharmacokinetics

Diazepam is highly lipid-soluble and the drug is rapidly absorbed from the GI tract. The intravenous route of administration is used more frequently than the intramuscular (IM) route. IM administration results in slow, erratic absorption and lower peak plasma levels. IM administration into the deltoid muscle results in better absorption. The drug is highly protein-bound and the half-life is long (20 to 80 h). Cumulative effects may result. The drug is excreted primarily in the urine.

Pharmacodynamics

Diazepam acts on the limbic and subcortical levels of the central nervous system. The onset of action is 0.5 to 1 h by mouth and 1 to 5 min intravenously. Duration of action varies; by mouth the average is 2 to 3 h. The longest duration of action is 1 h intravenously.

It is recommended that benzodiazepines be prescribed for no longer than 3 to 4 months. Beyond the 4 months, the effectiveness of the drug lessens. Table 16–3 lists the anxiolytics, their dosages, uses, and considerations.

Before benzodiazepines, the propanediol drug meprobamate (Equanil, Miltown) was used to treat anxiety. Meprobamate was preferred over the use of barbiturates because of fewer side effects. Today, meprobamate is occasionally prescribed for short-term relief of anxiety and for its muscle relaxant properties. Alcohol should be avoided when taking meprobamate or any of the benzodiazepines.

Hydroxyzine hydrochloride (Atarax, Vistril) and diphenhydramine hydrochloride (Benadryl) are antihistamines. They cause drowsiness and have a sedative effect and are used for short-term relief of anxiety. Because they do not cause tolerance, these drugs could be used temporarily when other antianxiety drugs have been abused.

The newest anxiolytic is buspirone hydrochloride (BuSpar), developed for alleviating anxiety. It does not have many of the side effects associated with benzodiazepines, such as sedation and physical and psychological dependency. Buspirone might not become effective until 1 to 2 weeks after continuous use.

Flurazepam, temazepam, triazolam, estazolam, and quazepam are benzodiazepines used primarily as sedatives or hypnotics (see Chapter 13).

Side Effects and Adverse Reactions

The side effects associated with benzodiazepines are sedative effect, dizziness, headaches, dry mouth, blurred vision, rare urinary incontinence, and constipation. Adverse reactions include leukopenia (decreased white blood cell count) with symptoms of fever, malaise, and sore throat; tolerance to the drug dosage with continuous use; and physical dependency.

Benzodiazepines should not be abruptly discontinued because withdrawal symptoms are likely to occur. Withdrawal symptoms due to benzodiazepines are similar to those from the sedative-hypnotics (agitation, nervousness, tremor, anorexia, muscular cramps, sweating); however, they are slower to develop, taking 2 to 10 days and could last several weeks. It would depend on the half-life of the benzodiazepine. When discontinuing a benzodiazepine, the drug dosage should be gradually decreased over a period of days depending upon dose or length of time on the drug. Alcohol and other CNS depressants should *not* be taken with benzodiazepines, because respiratory depression could result. Smoking, caffeine, and sympathomimetics decrease the effectiveness of benzodiazepines. Benzodiazepines are contraindicated during pregnancy due to possible teratogenic effects on the fetus.

FIGURE 16–3. Anxiolytics

Diazepam	Dosage	**NURSING PROCESS** Assessment and Planning

Diazepam

Diazepam
   (Valium) 🍁 Apo-diazepam, Di-
   azemuls, Novodipam
Benzodiazepine
CSS IV
Pregnancy Category: D

Dosage

Anxiety:
A: PO/IM/IV: 2–10 mg b.i.d./q.i.d.
Elderly: 2.5 mg b.i.d.
C >6 mon: 1–2.5 mg t.i.d./q.i.d.
Musculoskeletal spasm:
A: PO: 2–10 mg b.i.d./q.i.d.
   IM: 5–10 mg q3–4h
Preoperative sedation:
A: IV: 5–15 mg 15 min before event
Status epilepticus:
A: IV: 5–10 mg q10–20 min; max: 30
   mg
C <6 y: 0.2–0.5 mg/kg q15–30 min;
   max: 5 mg total dose
C >6 y: 0.2–0.5 mg/kg q15–30 min;
   max: 10 mg total dose
IV: max: 5 mg/3 min

Contraindications

Hypersensitivity, CNS depression,
   shock, coma, narrow-angle
   glaucoma, pregnancy, lactation
Caution: Hepatic or renal dysfunction;
   epilepsy, elderly and infants; history
   of drug abuse; depression,
   addiction-prone, or suicidal tendency

Drug-Lab-Food Interactions

Increase effects of diazepam with
   alcohol, oral contraceptives, CNS
   depressants, cimetidine, disulfiram,
   fluoxetine, isoniazid, ketoconazole,
   levodopa, metoprolol,
   propoxyphene, propranolol, valproic
   acid; toxic effects with MAOIs;
Decrease effects with rifampin,
   cigarettes, theophylline
Increase effects of digoxin, phenytoin
Do not mix or dilute with other drugs
   in syringe
Lab: Increase bilirubin

Pharmacokinetics

Absorption: Rapid from GI tract; erratic
   from IM administration; most rapid
   and complete from deltoid muscle
Distribution: Widely PB: 98%
Metabolism: t½: 25–50 h
Excretion: In urine

Pharmacodynamics

PO: Onset: 30–60 min
       Peak: 1–2 h
       Duration: 2–3 h (varies)
IM: Onset: 15–30 min
       Peak: 1–2 h
       Duration: 1–1½ h (varies)
IV: Onset: 1–5 min
       Peak: 15–30 min
       Duration: 15–60 min

Interventions

Therapeutic Effects/Uses: To control anxiety, preoperative sedation, skeletal muscle relaxant, to treat status epilepticus, alcohol withdrawal, convulsive disorders, anterograde
amnesia.

Mode of Action: Depression of limbic and subcortical CNS and skeletal muscle relaxation,
shortens stage 4 and REM sleep.

Evaluation

FIGURE 16–3. *Continued*

Side Effects	Adverse Reactions
Drowsiness, dizziness, syncope, orthostatic hypotension, blurred vision, nausea, vomiting, fatigue, confusion	ECG changes, tachycardia, psychological and physical dependence with long-term use *Life threatening:* Laryngospasm

KEY: A: adult; C: child; PO: by mouth; IM: intramuscular; IV: intravenous; PB: protein-binding; t½: half-life; >: greater than; <: less than; 🍁: Canadian drug names.

TABLE 16–3 Anxiolytics

Generic (Brand)	Route and Dosage	Uses and Considerations
Antihistamines		
Hydroxyzine HCl (Atarax, Vistarill)	A: PO: 50–100 mg t.i.d./q.i.d. IM: 25–100 mg C <6 y: 25 mg b.i.d. C >6 y: 25 mg b.i.d./q.i.d.	For anxiety and tension; control nausea and vomiting. May be used as a preoperative and postoperative drug to reduce narcotic dose. Side effects include drowsiness, dizziness, dry mouth, hypotension. *Pregnancy category:* C; PB: UK, t½: 3-7 h
Benzodiazepines		
Alprazolam (Xanax) CSS IV	A: PO: 0.25–0.5 mg t.i.d. Elderly: 0.25 mg b.i.d./t.i.d.; *max:* 4 mg/d	Management of anxiety and panic disorders and anxiety associated with depression. Side effects include drowsiness, dry mouth, and lightheadedness. *Pregnancy category:* D; PB: 80%, t½: 12–15 h
Chlordiazepoxide HCl (Librium) CSS IV	*Anxiety disorders:* A: PO: 5–25 mg t.i.d./q.i.d. C: PO: 5 mg b.i.d./q.i.d. *Acute alcohol withdrawal:* A: PO/IM/IV: 50–100 mg; *max:* 300 mg/d Elderly: ½ adult dose	Effective for alcohol withdrawal syndrome (DTs), anxiety, and tension. Dose should be less for the older adult. *Pregnancy category:* D; PB: 90%–98%, t½: 6–30 h
Clorazepate dipotassium (Tranxene) CSS IV	A: PO: 15–60 mg/d in divided doses Elderly: 7.5 mg b.i.d.	For anxiety, alcohol withdrawal syndrome, and partial seizures. Avoid taking alcohol or CNS depressants with chorazepate. Drowsiness and dizziness may occur. *Pregnancy category:* C; PB: 80%–90%, t½: 0.5–1 h
Diazepam (Valium)	See Prototype Drug Chart (Fig. 16–3)	For anxiety disorders, alcohol withdrawal syndrome, status epilepticus, muscle spasm, sedation. Avoid alcohol intake. *Pregnancy category:* D; PB: 98%, t½: 25–50 h
Halazepam (Paxipam)	A: PO: 20–40 mg t.i.d./q.i.d. Elderly; 20 mg daily/b.i.d.	Management of anxiety disorders. Drowsiness, sedation, confusion, headaches and hypotension may occur. *Pregnancy category:* D; PB: 97%, t½: 14 h
Lorazepam (Ativan) CSS IV	A: PO: 2–6 mg/d in divided doses A: IM/IV: 2–4 mg Elderly: ½ adult dose	For short-term relief of anxiety. Can be used as preoperative drug. Has been given prior to chemotherapy. Drowsiness and dizziness may occur. *Pregnancy category:* D; PB: 90%, t½: 10–20 h
Oxazepam (Serax)	A: PO: 10–30 mg t.i.d./q.i.d. Elderly: 10–15 mg, t.i.d./q.i.d.	For mild to moderate anxiety. To control alcohol syndrome. Drowsiness, dizziness may occur. *Pregnancy category:* C; PB: 85%–95%, t½: 3.5–21 h
Prazepam (Centrax) CSS IV	A: PO: 10 mg t.i.d./q.i.d. Elderly: 10–15 mg/d in divided doses	To relieve anxiety disorders. *Pregnancy category:* D; PB: 97%, t½: 30–200 h
Propanediol		
Meprobamate (Equanil, Miltown) CSS IV	A: PO: 400 mg t.i.d./q.i.d. C: PO: 100–200 mg b.i.d./t.i.d.	An original anxiolytic drug. For short-term relief of anxiety. Promotes sleep in anxious clients. Avoid alcohol intake. *Pregnancy category:* D; PB: UK, t½: 6–16 h
Others		
Buspirone HCl (BuSpar)	A: PO: Initial: 5 mg, b.i.d./t.i.d. A: PO: 15–30 mg/d in divided doses; *max:* 60 mg/d Elderly: *max:* 30 mg/d	For anxiety and anxiety-related depression. Common side effects include drowsiness, dizziness, headache, nausea. *Pregnancy category:* B; PB: 95%, t½: 2–3 h

KEY: A: adult; C: child; CSS: Controlled Substance Schedule; PB: protein-binding, PO: by mouth, t½: half-life; UK: unknown.

NURSING PROCESS: ANXIOLYTICS

ASSESSMENT

- Assess for suicidal ideation.
- Obtain a history of the client's anxiety reaction.
- Determine the client's support system (family, friends, groups), if any.
- Obtain the client's drug history. Report possible drug-drug interaction.

POTENTIAL NURSING DIAGNOSES

- Anxiety
- Mobility, impaired physical

PLANNING

- Client's anxiety and stress will be reduced through nonpharmacologic methods, anxiolytic drugs, or support/group therapy.

NURSING INTERVENTIONS

- Administer by IM route in large muscle mass, and inject drug slowly.
- Observe the client for side effects of anxiolytics. Recognize that drug tolerance and physical and psychological dependency can result with most anxiolytics.
- Recognize that anxiolytic drug dosages should be less for the elderly and debilitated persons than for young and middle-aged adults.
- Monitor vital signs, especially blood pressure and pulse; orthostatic hypotension may occur.

- Encourage the family to be supportive of the client.

CLIENT TEACHING

General
- Advise the client not to drive a motor vehicle or operate dangerous equipment when taking anxiolytics since sedation is a common side effect.
- Instruct the client not to consume alcohol or CNS depressants such as narcotics while taking an anxiolytic.
- Instruct the client on ways to control excess stress and anxiety, such as relaxation techniques.
- Inform the client that effective response may take 1 to 2 wk.
- Encourage the client to follow drug regimen and not to abruptly stop taking the drug after prolonged use because withdrawal symptoms can occur. Drug dose is usually tapered when drug is discontinued.

Side Effects
- Instruct the client to arise slowly from the sitting to standing position to avoid dizziness from orthostatic hypotension.

EVALUATION

- Evaluate the effectiveness of drug therapy by determining if the client is less anxious and more able to cope with stresses and anxieties.
- Determine if the client is taking the anxiolytic drug as prescribed and is adhering to client teaching instructions.

ANTIDEPRESSANTS

Contributing causes of depression include genetic predisposition, social and environmental factors, and biologic conditions. It is also thought that depression may be due to insufficient monoamine neurotransmitters (norepinephrine and/or serotonin) in the brain. Some signs of major depression include loss of interest in most activities, depressed mood, weight loss or gain, insomnia or hypersomnia, loss of energy, fatigue, feeling of despair, inability to think or concentrate, and suicidal thoughts.

Three types of depression respond to **antidepressants:** reactive depression, unipolar affective disorder (unipolar depression), and bipolar affective dis-

order (manic depression). **Reactive,** or **exogenous, depression** usually has a sudden onset and precipitating event. The client knows why he or she is depressed. For these cases benzodiazepines are usually prescribed. **Unipolar,** or **endogenous, depression** is characterized by loss of interest in work and home, inability to complete tasks, and deep depression **(dysphoria).** Unipolar depression can be either primary (not related to other health problems) or secondary to a health problem, such as a physical or psychiatric disorder or drug use. Antidepressants have been effective in treating unipolar depression. **Bipolar affective disorder** involves swings between two moods, the manic (euphoric) and the depressive (dysphoria). Lithium is the drug of choice for treating this type of disorder.

Antidepressants are divided into two groups: **tricyclic antidepressants** and **monoamine oxidase (MAO) inhibitors.** Both of these antidepressant groups were marketed in the late 1950s. Recently, a new antidepressant group was introduced called **second-generation antidepressants.**

TRICYCLIC ANTIDEPRESSANTS

Tricyclic antidepressants (TCAs) block the uptake of the neurotransmitters norepinephrine and serotonin in the brain. The clinical response of TCAs follows 2 to 4 weeks of drug therapy. If there is no improvement after 2 to 4 weeks, the antidepressant is slowly withdrawn and another antidepressant is prescribed. Polydrug therapy, giving several antidepressants or antipsychotics together, is to be avoided because of possible serious side effects.

The tricyclics have been effective for treating unipolar depression. Frequently, TCAs are given at night to minimize the problems caused by their sedative action. When discontinuing TCAs, the drugs should gradually be decreased to avoid withdrawal symptoms, such as nausea, vomiting, anxiety, and akathisia. Imipramine hydrochloride (Tofranil) is used for the treatment of enuresis (involuntary discharge of urine during sleep in children).

SECOND-GENERATION ANTIDEPRESSANTS

The second-generation antidepressants were first marketed in the 1980s, but some are still in the development phase. This group of drugs is not related to tricyclics nor monoamine oxidase inhibitors. This new antidepressant group causes fewer anticholinergic symptoms than the tricyclics.

Figure 16–4 compares the tricyclic amitriptyline HCl (Elavil) with the second-generation antidepressant amoxapine (Asendin). Both drugs are antidepressants but are in different classifications.

Pharmacokinetics

Amitriptyline and amoxapine are strongly protein-bound. The half-life of amitriptyline is longer than that of amoxapine except for amoxapine metabolite; cumulative effect may therefore result from long-term use of amitriptyline. Both drugs are excreted by the kidneys.

Pharmacodynamics

Both amytriptyline and amoxapine are well absorbed; however, their antidepressant effects develop slowly over several weeks. The onset of antidepressant effect of amitriptyline and amoxapine is between 1 and 4 wk; however, the peak concentration time of amoxapine is faster than amitriptyline. The durations of action for both drugs have not been determined but they are estimated to be several weeks. The drug dose for the elderly should be decreased to reduce side effects.

Side Effects: Amitriptyline and Amoxapine

These drugs produce such anticholinergic effects as dry mouth and eyes, blurred vision, urinary retention, and constipation. Amitriptyline can cause EPS. Amoxapine may cause EPS, but it causes fewer cardiovascular symptoms. The sedative and anticholinergic effects of amoxapine are most pronounced. Care should be taken when administering these drugs to clients with a history of glaucoma.

Side Effects and Adverse Reactions: Tricyclic Antidepressants

The general side effects of tricyclics are sedation, orthostatic hypotension, and anticholinergic symptoms, such as decreased salivation, urinary retention, constipation, and increased heart rate. If the client overdoses, fatal ventricular dysrhythmia may occur. Other side effects of TCAs include allergic reactions (skin rash, pruritus, petechiae), gastrointestinal symptoms (nausea, vomiting, anorexia, diarrhea, epigastric distress), sexual dysfunction (impotence, amenorrhea, gynecomastia), and blood cell disorders or blood dyscrasias (leukopenia, thrombocytopenia, and agranulocytosis). Table 16–4 lists the tricyclic and second-generation antidepressants.

NURSING PROCESS: ANTIDEPRESSANTS

ASSESSMENT

- Assess the client's baseline vital signs (VS) and weight for future comparison.
- Check the client's liver and renal function by assessing urine output (>600 mL/d), BUN, and serum creatinine and liver enzyme levels.

- Obtain a history of episodes of depression; assess mental status.
- Obtain the client's drug history. CNS depressants can cause an additive effect. Antidepressants cause anticholinergic-like symptoms and are contraindicated if the client has glaucoma.
- Assess for tardive dyskinesia and neuroleptic

FIGURE 16–4. Antidepressants

Tricyclic Antidepressant	Dosage	**NURSING PROCESS** Assessment and Planning
Amitriptyline HCl *(E)* (Elavil), ❧ Apo-Amitriptyline, Novotriptyn *Pregnancy Category:* D **Second Generation Antidepressant** *Amoxapine (A)* (Asendin) *Pregnancy Category:* C	*(E)* A: PO: 25 mg b.i.d.–q.i.d.; increase to 150–200 mg/d; dose may be given as a single h.s. dose IM: 20–30 mg, q.i.d. C >13 y: PO: 10 mg, t.i.d., and 20 mg, h.s. Elderly: PO: 10 mg, t.i.d., 20 mg, h.s. Therapeutic Serum Range: 100–200 ng/mL *(A)* A: PO: 50 mg, b.i.d., t.i.d.; increase dose gradually to <300 mg/d or give as a single dose at h.s. *Max:* inpatient: 600 mg/d; outpatient: 400 mg/d Elderly: PO: 25 mg, b.i.d., t.i.d.; may increase to 50 mg, b.i.d. C: Not recommended for children <16 y Therapeutic serum range: 200–400 ng/mL	
Contraindications	**Drug-Lab-Food Interactions**	
(E & A): Recovery from acute myocardial infarction (AMI), taking MAO inhibitors *Caution: (E & A):* Severe depression with suicidal tendency, severe liver or kidney disease, narrow-angle glaucoma, seizures, prostatic disease	*(E & A):* *Increase* effects of CNS, respiratory depression, and hypotensive effect with alcohol and CNS depressants *Increase* sedation, anticholingeric effects with phenothiazines, and haloperidol *Increase* toxicity with cimetidine *Decrease* effect of clonidine, guanethidine Hypertensive crisis and death may occur with MAO inhibitors. *Lab:* Altered ECG readings	
Pharmacokinetics	**Pharmacodynamics**	Interventions

Absorption: PO:
(E & A): well absorbed
Distribution: PB:
(E) 95%, (A) 90%
Metabolism: t½:
(E) 10–50 h; (A): 8 h, 30 h as a metabolite
Excretion: (E & A) Excreted primarily in urine
	Antidepressant Effect
	(E):
	PO: Onset: 1–3 wk
	    Peak: 2–6 wk
	    Duration: UK
	(A):
	PO: Onset: 2–4 wk
	    Peak: 90 min
	    Duration: weeks	

Therapeutic Effects/Uses: (E & A): To treat depression with or without melancholia, depressive phase of bipolar disorder, depression associated with organic disease, alcoholism, mixed symptoms of anxiety and depression, or urinary incontinence. *Mode of Action:* Serotonin and norepinephrine increased in nerve cells due to blockage from nerve fibers.	Evaluation

Figure continues on following page

FIGURE 16–4. *Continued*

Side Effects	Adverse Reactions
(E & A): Sedation, drowsiness, blurred vision, dry mouth and eyes, extrapyramidal syndrome (EPS), urinary retention, constipation, weight gain *(E):* dizziness, nervousness	*(E & A):* Orthostatic hypotension, cardiac dysrhythmias *Life threatening: (E & A):* Agranulocytosis, thrombocytopenia, leukopenia.

KEY: A: adult; C: child; PO: by mouth; PB: protein-binding; t½: half-life; UK: unknown; <: less than; >: greater than; 🍁 ; Canadian drug names.

malignant syndrome (NMS), including hyperpyrexia, muscle rigidity, tachycardia, cardiac dysrhythmias.

POTENTIAL NURSING DIAGNOSES

- Potential for violence and injury
- Anxiety
- Social isolation

PLANNING

- Client's depression or manic-depressive behavior will be decreased.

NURSING INTERVENTIONS

- Observe the client for signs and symptoms of depression: mood changes, insomnia, apathy, or lack of interest in activities.
- Check the client's vital signs. Orthostatic hypotension is common. Check for anticholinergic-like symptoms: dry mouth, increased heart rate, urinary retention, or constipation. Check weight two or three times per week.
- Monitor the client for suicidal tendencies when marked depression is present.
- If the client is taking an anticonvulsant, observe the client for seizures; antidepressants lower the seizure threshold. The anticonvulsant dose might need to be increased.
- Provide the client with a list of foods to avoid, especially with MAOIs. These include cheese, red wine, beer, liver, bananas, yogurt, sausage, and others.
- Check the client for extremely high blood pressure when taking MAO inhibitors. Sympathomimetic-like drugs and foods containing tyra-mine may cause a hypertensive crisis if taken with MAO inhibitors.

CLIENT TEACHING

General
- Instruct the client to take the medication as prescribed. Compliance is important.
- Inform the client that the full effectiveness of the drug may not be evident until 1 to 2 wk after the start of therapy.
- Encourage the client to keep medical appointments.
- Instruct the client not to consume alcohol or any CNS depressants due to their addictive effect.
- Instruct the client not to drive or be involved in potentially dangerous mechanical activity until stabilization of drug dose has been established.
- Instruct the client not to abruptly stop taking the drug. Drug dose should be gradually decreased.
- Encourage the client who is planning pregnancy to consult with the health care provider about possible teratogenic effects of the drug on the fetus.
- Take with food if GI distress occurs.

Side Effects
- Advise the client that antidepressants may be taken at bedtime to decrease the dangers from the sedative effect. Have client check with the health care provider. Transient side effects include nausea, drowsiness, headaches, and nervousness.

EVALUATION

- Evaluate the effectiveness of the drug therapy. The client's depression is controlled or has ceased.

MONOAMINE OXIDASE INHIBITORS

The third group of antidepressants is the monoamine oxidase (MAO) inhibitors. The enzyme monoamine oxidase inactivates norepinephrine, dopamine, epinephrine, and serotonin. By inhibiting monoamine oxidase, the levels of these neurotransmitters rise. Three MAO inhibitors are currently prescribed: tranylcypromine sulfate (Parnate), isocarboxazid (Marplan), and phenelzine sulfate (Nardil). These MAO inhibitors are discussed in Table 16–4.

Today MAO inhibitors are usually prescribed when the client does not respond to tricyclic antidepressants or second generation antidepressants. However, MAO inhibitors are used for mild, reactive, and atypical depression (chronic anxiety, hypersomnia, and fear). MAO inhibitors and tricyclics should *not* be taken together for treating depression.

Drug and Food Interactions: Monoamine Oxidase Inhibitors

Certain drugs and food interactions with MAO inhibitors can be fatal. Any drugs that are CNS stimulants or sympathomimetics, such as vasoconstric-

TABLE 16–4 Antidepressants: Tricyclic Antidepressants, Second Generation Antidepressants, and Antimanic

Generic (Brand)	Route and Dosage	Uses and Considerations
Tricyclic Antidepressants		
Amitriptyline HCl (Elavil, Endep, Enovil)	See Prototype Drug Chart (Fig. 16–4) *Therapeutic serum range:* 100–200 ng/mL	For depression. Can be given at bedtime to avoid daytime drowsiness. May be used for intractable pain, eating disorders (anorexia and bulimia) associated with depression. *Pregnancy category:* D; PB: 95%; t½: 10–50 h
Clomipramine HCl (Anafranil)	A: 25–100 mg/d in divided doses; *max:* 250 mg/d; after titration; entire dose may be given h.s. Elderly: 20–30 mg/d	To treat obsessive-compulsive disorder. May be used for alleviating anxiety or panic disorder. Tremor, dizziness, weight gain, and dry mouth are common side effects. *Pregnancy category:* C; PB: 97%; t½: 20–30 h
Desipramine HCl (Norpramin, Pertofrane)	A: PO: 25 mg t.i.d. or 75 mg h.s.; increase to 200 mg/d *max:* 300 mg/d Elderly: 25–50 mg/d in divided doses *max:* 150 mg/d *Therapeutic serum range:* 150–250 ng/mL	For depression. Has been used for attention deficit disorder (ADD). Take with food if GI distress occurs. Common side effects include drowsiness, dry mouth, increased appetite, urinary retention, and postural hypotension. *Pregnancy category:* D; PB: 90%–95%; t½: 12–60 h
Doxepin HCl (Sinequan)	A: PO: 75–100 mg/d h.s. or in divided doses; *max:* 300 mg/d Elderly: 25–50 mg/d *Therapeutic serum range:* 30–50 ng/mL	For depression and anxiety related to involutional depression or manic-depressive disorder. Has less effect on cardiac status than other drugs in this group. *Pregnancy category:* C; PB: 80%–85%; t½: 6–8 h
Imipramine HCl (Tofranil)	A: PO: 75 mg/d (h.s. or 25 mg t.i.d.); *max:* 300 mg/d IM: Initially: *max:* 100 mg/d in divided doses Elderly: 25–100 mg in divided doses C <12 y: PO: 25–50 mg h.s. C >12 y: PO: 75 mg h.s. *Therapeutic serum range:* 150–250 ng/mL	For depression. Can be taken at bedtime to lessen dangers from sedative effect. Take with food if GI distress occurs. Avoid taking with alcohol or CNS depressants. Common side effects include; drowsiness, dry mouth, hypotension, delayed micturition. *Pregnancy category:* D; PB: 90%–95%; t½: 8–15 h
Nortriptyline HCl (Aventyl)	A: PO: 25 mg t.i.d./q.i.d.; *max:* 150 mg/d Elderly: 30–50 mg/d in divided doses *Therapeutic serum range:* 50–150 ng/mL	For depression. Similar to imipramine HCl. *Pregnancy category:* D; PB: 90%–95%; t½: 18–28 h
Protriptyline HCl (Vivactil)	A: PO 15–40 mg/d in divided doses; increase gradually; *max:* 60 mg/d Elderly: 5 mg, t.i.d. *max:* 20 mg/d *Therapeutic serum range:* 70–250 ng/mL	For depression. Has little sedative effect. Effects are similar to imipramine HCl. *Pregnancy category:* C; PB: 92%; t½: 60–98 h

TABLE 16–4 Antidepressants: Tricyclic Antidepressants, Second Generation Antidepressants, and Antimanic *(Continued)*

Generic (Brand)	Route and Dosage	Uses and Considerations
Trimipramine maleate (Surmontil)	A: 75–150 mg/d in divided doses or all h.s.; *max:* 200 mg/d Elderly: *max:* 100 mg/d	For depression. Similar to imipramine HCl. *Pregnancy category:* C; PB: 95%; t½: 20–26 h
Second Generation Antidepressants Amoxapine (Asendin)	See Prototype Drug Chart (Fig. 16–4)	For depression with anxiety and reactive depression. Do not take with MAO inhibitors. Side effects include drowsiness, dizziness, EPS, postural hypotension, increased appetite, urinary retention. *Pregnancy category:* C; PB: >90%; t½: 8 h
Bupropion HCl (Wellbutrin)	A: PO: Intially: 200 mg/d as b.i.d.; increase gradually to 300 mg/d in divided doses; *max* 450 mg/d	For depression. May cause increased risk of seizures. Avoid with a history of seizures. Many side effects. *Pregnancy category:* B; PB: >80%; t½: 50 h
Fluoxetine HCl (Prozac)	A: PO: 20 mg in a.m.; *max:* 80 mg/d in divided doses	For depression, anxiety, addictions, bulimia, and obsessive-compulsive disorder. Can cause insomnia and decrease appetite. Increase in suicide attempts have been reported; same as with other antidepressant drugs used. Usually takes 3 wk to become effective. *Pregnancy category:* B; PB: 95%; t½: 7–9 d
Maprotiline HCl (Ludiomil)	A: PO: 75 mg h.s. or in divided doses; *max:* 150 mg/d Elderly: 25 mg/d *max:* 75 mg/d	Same as amoxapine. Can be taken at bedtime. *Pregnancy category:* B; PB: 88%; t½: 21–25 h
Nefazodone HCl (Serzone)	A: PO: Initial: 200 mg/d in 2 divided doses *maint:* 300–600 mg/d in divided doses Elderly: PO: 50 mg b.i.d. to start	The newest antidepressant. For depression. It is effective for long-term use for longer the 6–8 wks. It should not be used with MAO inhibitors, and should not be used within 14 d after after discontinuing MAO inhibitors. *Pregnancy category:* C; PB: UK; t½: UK
Paroxetine HCl (Paxil)	A: PO: 20 mg/d in a.m. *max:* 50 mg/d Elderly: PO: Intitially: 10 mg/d *max:* 40 mg/d	For depression and obsessive-compulsive disorders. Lower dose for the elderly and those with renal and hepatic disorders. Side effects include dizziness, insomnia, headache, nausea, dry mouth, tremors, postural hypotension. *Pregnancy category:* B; PB: 90%–95%; t½: 21 h, elderly: 68 h
Sertraline HCl (Zoloft)	A: PO: 50 mg daily *max:* 200 mg/d	Management of major depression disorders. Do *not* take with MAO inhibitors or tricyclics. Take with food if GI distress occurs. Urine may be pink-red-brown color. *Pregnancy category:* B; PB: 98%; t½: 26 h
Trazodone HCl (Desyrel)	A: PO: 75 mg h.s. or 50 mg t.i.d., q.i.d.; *max:* 600 mg/d	For depression. Can be taken at bedtime to lessen dangers from sedative effect. Drowsiness, lightheadedness, orthostatic hypotension, and dry mouth might occur. Take with food to decrease GI distress. *Pregnancy category:* C; PB: 85%–95%; t½: 5–10 h
Monoamine Oxidase Inhibitors Isocarboxazid (Marplan)	A: PO: 10–20 mg/d *max:* 60 mg/d	For depression that is refractory to tricyclics. Avoid certain foods such as cheese, beer, figs, shrimp, banana, and chocolate, and avoid drugs, e.g., tricyclic antidepressants. *Pregnancy category:* C; PB: UK; t½: UK
Phenelzine sulfate (Nardil)	A: PO: 15 mg t.i.d.; 1 mg/kg in divided doses *max:* 90 mg/d Elderly: *max:* 45–60 mg/d	For depression. Avoid certain foods and drugs (see Isocarboxazid) *Pregnancy category:* C; PB: UK; t½: UK
Tranylcypromine sulfate (Parnate)	A: PO: 10 mg, t.i.d. *max:* 60 mg/d Elderly: *max:* 45 mg/d	Same as isocarboxazid and phenelzine sulfate.
Antimanic Lithium carbonate: lithium citrate	See Prototype Drug Chart (Fig. 16–5)	For manic-depressive illness (bipolar affective disorder). Monitor serum lithium levels. Toxic: 2.0 mEq/L and greater. *Pregnancy category:* D; PB: UK; t½: 21–30 h

KEY: *A:* adult; *C:* child; *PO:* by mouth; *IV:* intravenous; *UK:* unknown; *PB:* protein-binding; *t½:* half-life; *MAO:* monoamine oxidase; *EPS:* extrapyramidal symptoms; *maint:* maintenance.

tors, cold medications containing phenylephrine, pseudoephedrine, and phenylpropanolamine, can cause a hypertensive crisis when taken with an MAO inhibitor. Also foods that contain tyramine, such as cheese (cheddar, Swiss, bleu), cream, yogurt, coffee, chocolate, bananas, raisins, Italian green beans, liver, pickled herring, sausage, soy sauce, yeast, beer, and red wines, have sympathomimetic-like effects and can cause a hypertensive crisis. These types of food and drugs must be *avoided*. Frequent blood pressure monitoring is essential when the client is taking MAO inhibitors. Client teaching regarding foods and OTC drugs to avoid is an important nursing responsibility. Because of the danger associated with a hypertensive crisis, many psychiatrists will not prescribe MAO inhibitors for depression, unless they sense the client's ability to comply with the drug and food regimen. However, this group of drugs is effective for treating depression if properly taken.

Side Effects and Adverse Reactions: Monoamine Oxidase Inhibitors

Side effects of MAO inhibitors include CNS stimulation (agitation, restlessness, insomnia), orthostatic hypotension, and anticholinergic effects.

ANTIMANIC: LITHIUM

The last antidepressant drug to be discussed in this chapter is lithium, which is used to treat bipolar affective disorder, or manic-depressive illness. Lithium was first used as a salt substitute in the 1940s, but because of lithium poisoning, it was banned from the market. Some refer to lithium as an antimania drug that is effective in controlling manic behavior that arises from underlying depression. It is most effective in controlling the manic phase. Lithium has a calming effect without impairing intellectual activity. It controls any evidence of flight of ideas and hyperactivity. If the person stops taking lithium, manic behavior may return.

It is an inexpensive drug, but it has to be closely monitored. Lithium has a narrow therapeutic serum range, 0.8 to 1.5 mEq/L. Serum lithium levels greater than 1.5 to 2.0 mEq/L are toxic. The serum lithium level should be monitored biweekly until the therapeutic level has been obtained and then monitored monthly on the maintenance dose. Serum sodium levels also need to be monitored because lithium tends to deplete sodium. Use lithium with caution, if at all, in clients taking diuretics. Figure 16–5 lists the pharmacologic behavior of lithium.

Pharmacokinetics

More than 95% of the lithium is absorbed through the GI tract. The average half-life of lithium is 24 h; however, in the older adult, the half-life can be up to 36 h. Due to the long half-life, cumulative drug action may result. Lithium is metabolized by the liver and most of the drug is excreted unchanged in the urine.

Pharmacodynamics

Lithium is prescribed mostly for the manic phase of manic-depressive illness. The onset of action is fast, but the client may not receive the desired effect for 5 to 6 days. Increased sodium intake increases renal excretion, so the sodium intake needs to be closely monitored. Increased urine output can result in body fluid loss and dehydration.

Table 16–4 lists the antimanic lithium, its dosage, uses, and considerations.

Side Effects and Adverse Reactions: Lithium

Many side effects from taking lithium can be annoying to the client, such as dry mouth, thirst, increased urination (loss of water and sodium), weight gain, bloated feeling, metallic taste, and edema of the hands and ankles.

NURSING PROCESS: ANTIMANIC: Lithium

ASSESSMENT

- Assess for suicidal ideation.
- Assess the client's baseline vital signs (VS) for future comparison.
- Assess client's neurological status, including gait, level of consciousness, reflexes, and tremors.
- Check the client's hepatic and renal function by assessing urine output (>600 mL/d), whether

BUN, and serum creatinine and liver enzyme levels are within normal range. Assess for toxicity. Draw weekly blood levels initially and then every 1 to 2 mon. Therapeutic serum levels for acute mania are 1.0 to 1.5 mEq/L; for maintenance, levels are 0.6 to 1.2 mEq/L. Signs and symptoms of toxicity at serum levels of 1.5 to 2.0 mEq/L are persistent nausea and vomiting, severe diarrhea, ataxia, blurred vision, and tinnitus; at 2.0 to 3.5 mEq/L, signs and symptoms

FIGURE 16–5. Antimanic: Lithium

Antimanic	**Dosage**	**NURSING PROCESS** Assessment and Planning

Lithium carbonate
  (Eskalith, Lithane, Lithonate, Litho-
  bid), 🍁 Carbolith, Lithizine
Pregnancy Category: D
	A: PO: 300–600 mg, t.i.d.
	  maint: 300 mg, t.i.d., q.i.d.
	  max: 2.4 g/d
	  Elderly: lower dosage
	  TDR: 0.5–1.5 mEq/L	

Contraindications	**Drug-Lab-Food Interactions**	

Liver and renal disease, pregnancy, lac-
tation, severe cardiovascular disease,
severe dehydration, brain tumor or
damage, sodium depletion, children
  <12 y
Caution: Thyroid disease
	May *increase* lithium level with thiazide
	  diuretics, methyldopa, haloperidol,
	  NSAIDs, antidepressants, carba-
	  mazepine, theophylline, amino-
	  phylline, sodium bicarbonate, phe-
	  nothiazines
	Food: Increase sodium intake; lithium
	  may cause sodium depletion
	Lab: Increase urine and blood glucose,
	  protein	

Pharmacokinetics	**Pharmacodynamics**	Interventions

Absorption: PO: well absorbed
Distribution: PB: UK
Metabolism: t½: 21–30 h; >36 h with
  renal impairment or in elderly
Excretion: 98% in urine, mostly un-
  changed
	Antimanic effects:
	PO: Onset: 5–7 d
	        Peak: 10–21 d
	        Duration: days
	PO SR: Peak: 5–7 d	

Therapeutic Effects/Uses: To treat bipolar manic-depressive psychosis, manic episodes. *Mode of Action:* Alteration of ion transport in muscle and nerve cells; increased receptor sensitivity to serotonin.	Evaluation

Side Effects	**Adverse Reactions**

Headache, lethargy, drowsiness,
  dizziness, tremors, slurred speech,
  dry mouth, anorexia, vomiting,
  diarrhea, polyuria, hypotension,
  abdominal pain, muscle weakness,
  restlessness
	Urinary incontinence, clonic move-
	  ments, stupor, azotemia, leukocytosis
	Life-threatening: Cardiac dysrhythmias,
	  circulatory collapse

KEY: A: adult; C: child; PO: by mouth; PB: protein-binding; t½: half-life; UK: unknown; TDR: therapeutic drug range; 🍁: Canadian drug names.

are excessive output of dilute urine, increasing tremors, muscular irritability, psychomotor retardation, mental confusion, and giddiness; and at >3.5 mEq/L, levels are life threatening and may result in impaired consciousness, nystagmus, seizures, coma, oliguria/anuria, cardiac dysrhythmias, myocardial infarction, and cardiovascular collapse. Withhold medications and notify health care provider immediately if any of these occur.

- Obtain a history of episodes of depression or manic-depressive behavior.
- Obtain the client's drug history. Diuretics, NSAIDs (e.g., ibuprofen), tetracyclines, methyldopa, and probenecid decrease renal clearance of lithium, thus causing lithium accumulation.

POTENTIAL NURSING DIAGNOSES

- Potential for injury or violence related to excessive hyperactivity
- Ineffective individual coping
- Noncompliance

PLANNING

- Client's manic-depressive behavior will be decreased.

NURSING INTERVENTIONS

- Observe the client for signs and symptoms of depression: mood changes, insomnia, apathy, or lack of interest in activities.
- Check the client's vital signs. Orthostatic hypotension is common.
- When drawing blood to check for lithium levels, draw samples immediately before the next dose (8 to 12 h after the previous dose). Monitor for signs of lithium toxicity. Report high (>1.5 mEq/L) or toxic (>2.0 mEq/L) serum lithium levels immediately to the health care provider.
- Monitor client for suicidal tendencies when marked depression is present.
- Monitor the client's urine output and body weight. Fluid volume deficit may occur due to polyuria.
- Observe the client for fine and gross motor tremors and presence of slurred speech, which are signs of adverse reaction.
- Check the client's cardiac status. Loss of fluids and electrolytes may cause cardiac dysrhythmias.

- Monitor the client's serum electrolytes. Report abnormal findings.

General

- Instruct the client to take lithium as prescribed. Emphasize the importance of adherence to the therapy and laboratory tests. If lithium is stopped, manic symptoms will reappear.
- Encourage the client to keep medical appointments. Have client check with the health care provider before taking OTC preparations.
- Instruct the client not to drive a motor vehicle or be involved in potentially dangerous mechanical activity until stable lithium level is established.
- Advise the client to maintain adequate fluid intake: 2 to 3 L/d initially and 1 to 2 L/d maintenance. Fluid intake should increase in hot weather.
- Instruct the client to take the lithium with meals to decrease gastric irritation.
- Inform the client that the effectiveness of the drug may not be evident until 1 to 2 wk after the start of therapy.
- Encourage the client who is planning pregnancy to consult with the health care provider about possible teratogenic effects of the drug on the fetus, especially during the first 3 months.
- Encourage the client to wear or carry an ID tag or bracelet indicating the drug taken.

Diet

- Advise the client to avoid caffeine products (coffee, tea, or colas) because they can aggravate the manic phase of the bipolar disorder.
- Instruct the client to maintain adequate sodium intake and to avoid crash diets that affect physical and mental health.

Side Effects

- Instruct the client to contact the health care provider for early symptoms of toxicity: diarrhea, drowsiness, loss of appetite, muscle weakness, nausea, vomiting, slurred speech, trembling; and for late symptoms of toxicity: blurred vision, confusion, increased urination, convulsions, severe trembling, and unsteadiness.

EVALUATION

- Evaluate the effectiveness of the drug therapy. The client is free of manic-depressive behavior.
- Client verbalizes understanding of symptoms of toxicity.
- Client demonstrates a subsiding or resolution of the symptoms.

STUDY QUESTIONS

1. Your client is taking the phenothiazine promazine (Sparine). What side effects associated with phenothiazines are similar to the side effects from anticholinergics and pseudoparkinsonism? Why should the blood pressure be closely monitored? What do you tell the client about the color of the urine?

2. What group of drugs has antiemetic properties? What is the route of administration for a client who is vomiting?

3. Haloperidol (Haldol) is a drug frequently used in psychiatry. How is it different from other antipsychotics?

4. What is the major group of anxiolytics called? A client receiving a drug from this category should be observed for what side effects? Client teaching is important regarding the use of alcohol or OTC drugs and discontinuing the anxiolytic. Why?

5. The client is receiving imipramine hydrochloride (Tofranil). Imipramine is from what drug category? Why do some clients take the drug at bedtime?

6. The client is taking tranylcypromine sulfate (Parnate), an MAO inhibitor. What should the nurse teach the client regarding food and drugs? Why?

7. Lithium is effective for what type of psychiatric disorder? What is the therapeutic serum lithium level? Why should the urinary output and vital signs be closely monitored?

Chapter 17

Autonomic Nervous System

OUTLINE

Objectives
Terms
Introduction

Sympathetic Nervous System
Parasympathetic Nervous System

Summary
Study Questions

OBJECTIVES

Differentiate between the autonomic and the somatic nervous systems, sympathetic and parasympathetic nervous systems.

Explain how drugs that mimic and block the sympathetic and parasympathetic nervous systems have opposite effects and similar effects on organ tissue.

List terms that identify sympathetic stimulants and depressants, and parasympathetic stimulants and depressants.

TERMS

acetylcholine
adrenaline
adrenergic
autonomic nervous system (ANS)
central nervous system (CNS)

cholinergic
neurotransmitter
norepinephrine
parasympathetic nervous system
parasympatholytics
parasympathomimetics

peripheral nervous system (PNS)
sympathetic nervous system
sympatholytics
sympathomimetics

INTRODUCTION

The **central nervous system (CNS),** which consists of the brain and spinal cord and is the primary nervous system of the body, was previously discussed in Chapters 12 and 13. The **peripheral nervous system (PNS),** located outside the brain and spinal cord, comprises two divisions: the autonomic and the somatic. After interpretation by the CNS, the PNS receives stimuli and initiates responses to those stimuli.

The **autonomic nervous system (ANS),** also called the visceral system, acts on smooth muscles and glands. Its functions include control and regulation of the heart, respiratory system, gastrointestinal (GI) tract, bladder, eyes, and glands. The ANS innervates (acts on) smooth muscles, but it is an involuntary nervous system over which we have little or no control. We breathe, our heart beats, and peristalsis occurs without our realizing it. However, unlike the autonomic nervous system, the somatic nervous system is a voluntary system that innervates skeletal muscles, over which we do have control.

The two sets of neurons in the autonomic component of the peripheral nervous system are (1) the afferent, or sensory, neurons, and (2) the efferent, or motor, neurons. The afferent neurons send impulses to the CNS, where they are interpreted. The efferent neurons receive the impulses (information) from the brain and transmit those impulses through the spinal cord to the effector organ cells. The efferent pathways in the autonomic nervous system are divided into two branches: the sympathetic and the parasympathetic nerves, which are collectively called the sympathetic nervous system and the parasympathetic nervous system (Fig. 17–1).

The sympathetic nervous system and the parasympathetic nervous system act on the same organs but produce opposite responses in order to provide homeostasis (balance) (Fig. 17–2). Drugs act on the sympathetic and parasympathetic nervous systems by either stimulating or depressing responses.

SYMPATHETIC NERVOUS SYSTEM

The **sympathetic nervous system** is also referred to as the **adrenergic** system because at one time it was believed that **adrenaline** was the **neurotransmitter** that innervates the smooth muscle. The neurotransmitter is now known to be **norepinephrine.** Drugs that mimic the effect of norepinephrine are called adrenergic drugs, or **sympathomimetics.** They are also known as **adrenergic agonists** because they *initiate* a response at the adrenergic receptor sites. Drugs that block the effect of norepinephrine are called **adrenergic blockers** or **sympatholytics.** These are known as adrenergic antagonists since they *prevent* a response at the receptor sites.

The adrenergic receptor organ cells are of four types: $alpha_1$, $alpha_2$, $beta_1$, and $beta_2$ (Fig. 17–3). Norepinephrine is released from the terminal nerve ending and stimulates the cell receptors to produce a response.

PARASYMPATHETIC NERVOUS SYSTEM

The **parasympathetic nervous system** is referred to as the **cholinergic** system because the neurotransmitter at the end of the neuron which innervates the muscle is **acetylcholine.** Drugs that mimic acetylcholine are called **cholinergic drugs,** or **parasympathomimetics.** They are **cholinergic ago-**

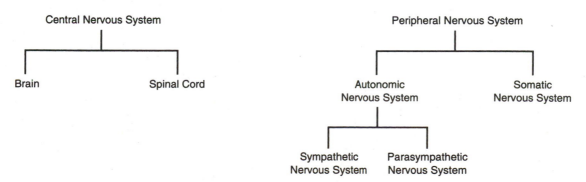

FIGURE 17–1 Subdivisions of the peripheral nervous system.

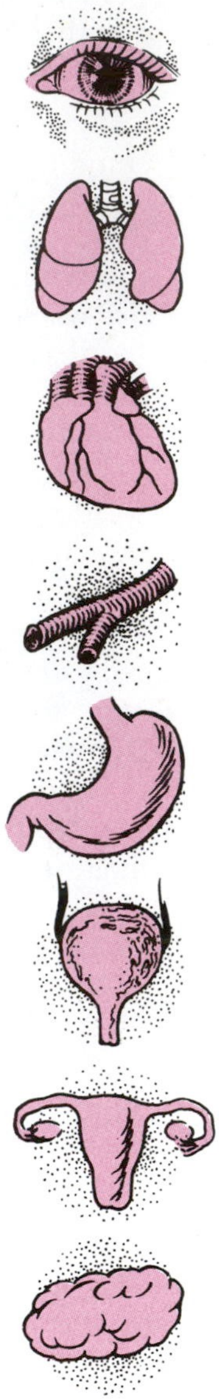

BODY TISSUE/ ORGAN		SYMPATHETIC RESPONSE*	PARASYMPATHETIC RESPONSE
Eye		Dilates pupils	Constricts pupils
Lungs		Dilates bronchioles	Constricts bronchioles and increases secretions
Heart		Increases heart rate	Decreases heart rate
Blood vessels		Constricts blood vessels	Dilates blood vessels
Gastrointestinal		Relaxes smooth muscles of GI tract	Increases peristalsis
Bladder		Relaxes bladder muscle	Contracts bladder
Uterus		Relaxes uterine muscle	
Salivary gland			Increases salivation

*The sympathetic and parasympathetic nervous systems have opposite responses on body tissues and organs.

FIGURE 17–2 Sympathetic and parasympathetic effects on body tissues.

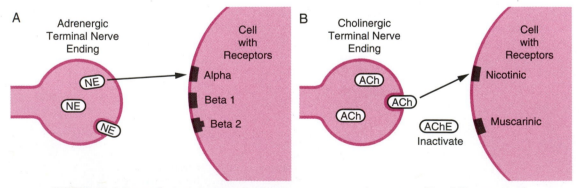

FIGURE 17–3 Sympathetic and parasympathetic transmitters and receptors. (Key: NE: norepinephrine; ACh: acetylcholine; AChE: acetylcholinesterase.)

TABLE 17–1 Autonomic Nervous Systems: Sympathetic and Parasympathetic

Sympathetic Stimulants	Parasympathetic Stimulants
Sympathomimetics (adrenergics, or adrenergic agonists) *Action:* Increase blood pressure Increase pulse rate Relax bronchioles Dilate pupils of eyes Uterine relaxation Increase blood sugar	**Direct-Acting** *Parasympathomimetics (cholinergics, or cholinergic agonists)* *Action:* Decrease blood pressure Decrease pulse rate Constrict bronchioles Constrict pupils of eyes Increase urinary contraction Increase peristalsis **Indirect-Acting** *Cholinesterase Inhibitors (anticholinesterase)* *Action:* Increase muscle tone

Sympathetic Depressants	Parasympathetic Depressants
Sympatholytics (adrenergic blockers, or adrenergic antagonists) *Action:* Decrease blood pressure Decrease pulse rate Constrict bronchioles	*Parasympatholytics (anticholinergics, cholinergic antagonists, or antispasmodics)* *Action:* Increase pulse rate Decrease mucus secretions Decrease GI motility Increase urinary retention Dilate pupils of eyes

Note: Opposite responses on organ tissue are caused by sympathomimetics and parasympathomimetics, and sympatholytics and parasympatholytics. Sympathomimetics and parasympatholytics cause similar organ responses as do sympatholytics and parasympathomimetics.

nists since they *initiate* a cholinergic response; conversely, drugs that block the effect of acetylcholine are called **anticholinergic, or parasympatholytics.** They are also known as **cholinergic antagonists** because they *inhibit* the effect of acetylcholine on the organ.

The cholinergic receptors at organ cells are either nicotinic or muscarinic, meaning that they are stimulated by the alkaloids nicotine and muscarine, respectively (see Fig. 17–3). Acetylcholine stimulates the receptor cells to produce a response, but the enzyme, acetylcholinesterase, may inactivate acetylcholine before it reaches the receptor cell.

Drugs that mimic the neurotransmitters norepinephrine and acetylcholine produce responses opposite to each other in the same organ. For ex-

ample, an adrenergic drug (sympathomimetic) increases the heart rate, whereas a cholinergic drug (parasympathomimetic) decreases the heart rate (see Fig. 17–2). However, a drug that mimics the sympathetic nervous system and a drug that blocks the parasympathetic nervous system can cause similar responses in the organ; for instance, the sympathomimetic and the parasympatholytic drugs both increase the heart rate. The adrenergic blocker and the cholinergic drug both decrease heart rate.

Many name classifications are given to drugs that mimic or block both the sympathetic nervous system and the parasympathetic nervous system (Table 17–1). The nurse needs to become familiar with these names. Drug names and specific actions will be discussed in Chapters 18 and 19.

TABLE 17–2 Sympathetic and Parasympathetic Responses to Drugs

Sympathetic	Parasympathetic	Response
Sympathomimetic	Parasympathomimetic	Opposite response
Sympatholytic	Parasympatholytic	Opposite response
Sympathomimetic	Parasympatholytic	Similar response
Sympatholytic	Parasympathomimetic	Similar response

SUMMARY

There are two subdivisions of the autonomic nervous system: the sympathetic and the parasympathetic nervous systems. These nervous systems have opposite effects on organ tissues. Drugs can either stimulate or block both of these nervous systems through their receptors. Table 17–2 illustrates the organ responses from drugs that act on these systems.

STUDY QUESTIONS

1. What are the divisions of the central nervous system and the peripheral nervous system? What is their interrelationship?

2. What does the autonomic nervous system control and regulate? What does the somatic nervous system control and regulate?

3. Drugs that mimic and block the sympathetic and parasympathetic nervous systems have opposite and similar effects on organ tissue. Explain this phenomenon.

4. What terms are used to classify sympathetic stimulants and depressants? What are their actions on the body?

5. What terms are used to classify parasympathetic stimulants and depressants? What are their actions on the body?

Chapter 18

Adrenergics and Adrenergic Blockers

OUTLINE

Objectives
Terms
Introduction
Adrenergics
   Epinephrine

Albuterol
   Nursing Process
Adrenergic Blockers (Antagonists)
   Alpha-Adrenergic Blockers

Beta-Adrenergic Blockers
Adrenergic Neuron
   Blockers
   Nursing Process
Study Questions

OBJECTIVES

Name the adrenergic receptors and give examples of their major responses.

Describe the difference between selective adrenergic drugs and nonselective drugs.

Give drug names of selective and nonselective adrenergic drugs.

List major side effects of adrenergic drugs.

Explain nursing interventions, including client teaching, associated with adrenergic drugs.

List examples of drugs that are selective and nonselective adrenergic blockers.

Describe the uses of alpha blockers and beta blockers.

List the general side effects of adrenergic blockers.

Describe nursing interventions, including client teaching, associated with adrenergic blockers.

TERMS

adrenergic blockers
adrenergic neuron blockers
adrenergic receptors
alpha blockers

beta blockers
catecholamines
nonselectivity
selectivity

sympathomimetics
sympatholytics

INTRODUCTION

Two groups of drugs that affect the sympathetic nervous system, the adrenergics (**sympathomimetics**) and the adrenergic blockers (**sympatholytics**), are discussed in this chapter. Lists of adrenergic drugs and adrenergic blockers, their dosages, and uses are also included. For explanation of the autonomic nervous system (adrenergic and cholinergic), see Chapter 17.

ADRENERGICS

Drugs that stimulate the sympathetic nervous system are called adrenergics, adrenergic agonists, or sympathomimetics because they mimic the sympathetic neurotransmitters (norepinephrine and epinephrine). They act on one or more **adrenergic receptor** sites located on the cells of smooth muscles, such as the heart, walls of the bronchioles, gastrointestinal (GI) tract, urinary bladder, and ciliary muscle of the eye. There are many adrenergic receptors. The four main receptors are alpha$_1$, alpha$_2$, beta$_1$, and beta$_2$, which mediate the major responses described in Table 18–1 and illustrated in Figure 18–1.

TABLE 18–1 Effects of Adrenergics at Receptors

Receptor	Physiologic Responses
Alpha$_1$	Increases force of contraction of heart. Vasoconstriction: increases blood pressure. Mydriasis: dilates pupils of the eyes. Glandular (salivary): decreases secretion.
Alpha$_2$	Inhibits the release of norepinephrine, dilates blood vessels, and produces hypotension; can mediate arteriolar and venous constriction.
Beta$_1$	Increases heart rate and force of contraction.
Beta$_2$	Dilates the bronchioles; promotes gastrointestinal and uterine relaxation.

The alpha-adrenergic receptors are located in the vascular tissues (vessels) of smooth muscles. When the alpha$_1$ receptor is stimulated, the arterioles and venules are constricted, thereby increasing peripheral resistance and blood return to the heart. Circulation is improved and blood pressure is increased. When there is too much stimulation, the blood flow is decreased to the vital organs. The alpha$_2$ receptor is located in the postganglionic sympathetic nerve endings, and when stimulated, it inhibits the re-

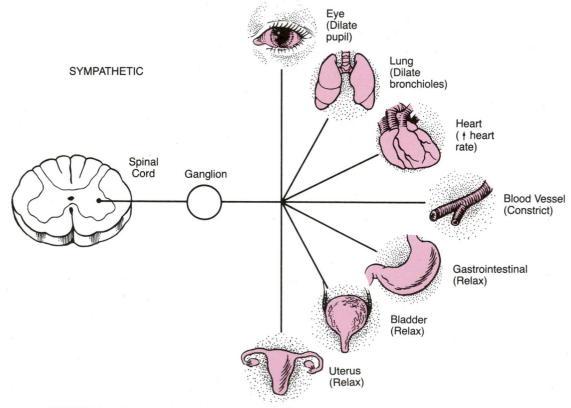

FIGURE 18–1 Sympathetic responses. Stimulation of the sympathetic nervous system or use of sympathomimetic (adrenergic) drugs can cause the pupils and bronchioles to dilate; the heart rate to increase; blood vessels to constrict; and the muscles of the gastrointestinal tract, bladder, and uterus to relax, decreasing contractions.

lease of norepinephrine, thus leading to a decrease in vasoconstriction. This results in a decrease in blood pressure.

The beta$_1$ adrenergic receptors are located primarily in the heart. Stimulation of the beta$_1$ receptor increases myocardial contractility and heart rate. The beta$_2$ receptors are found mostly in the smooth muscles of the lung, the arterioles of skeletal muscles, and the uterine muscle. Stimulation of the beta$_2$ receptor causes (1) relaxation of the smooth muscles of the lungs, resulting in bronchodilatation, (2) increase in blood flow to the skeletal muscles, and (3) relaxation of the uterine muscle, resulting in a decrease in uterine contraction.

Another adrenergic receptor is dopaminergic and is located in the renal, mesenteric, coronary, and cerebral arteries. When this receptor is stimulated, the vessels dilate and blood flow increases. Only dopamine can activate this receptor.

The sympathomimetic drugs that stimulate adrenergic receptors are classified into three categories according to their effects on organ cells: (1) direct-acting sympathomimetic, which directly stimulate the adrenergic receptor (e.g., epinephrine or norepinephrine); (2) indirect-acting sympathomimetic, which stimulate the release of norepinephrine from the terminal nerve endings (e.g., amphetamine); and (3) mixed-acting (both direct and indirect acting) sympathomimetic, which stimulate the adrenergic receptor sites and stimulate the release of norepinephrine from the terminal nerve endings (Fig. 18–2).

Catecholamines are the chemical structures of a substance (either endogenous or synthetic) that can produce a sympathomimetic response. Examples of endogenous catecholamines are epinephrine, norepinephrine, and dopamine. The synthetic catecholamines are isoproterenol and dobutamine. There are also noncatecholamines (e.g., phenyleph-

rine, metaproterenol, and albuterol) that stimulate the adrenergic receptors. Most noncatecholamines have a longer duration of action than the endogenous or synthetic catecholamines.

Many of the adrenergic drugs stimulate more than one of the adrenergic receptor sites. An example is epinephrine (Adrenalin), which acts on alpha$_1$-, beta$_1$-, and beta$_2$-adrenergic receptor sites. The responses from these receptor sites include an increase in blood pressure, pupil dilation, increase in heart rate (tachycardia), and bronchodilatation. In certain types of shock (i.e., cardiogenic, anaphylactic), epinephrine is a useful drug because it increases blood pressure, heart rate, and air flow through the lungs through bronchodilatation. Because epinephrine affects three different adrenergic receptors, it lacks **selectivity;** in other words, it is considered **nonselective** to one receptor. Side effects result when more responses occur than are desired. Figure 18–3 lists the pharmacologic behavior of epinephrine.

EPINEPHRINE

Pharmacokinetics

Epinephrine can be administered by parenteral routes, inhalation, or topically. The percentage by which the drug is protein-bound and its half-life are unknown. Epinephrine is metabolized by the liver and excreted in the urine.

Pharmacodynamics

Epinephrine is frequently used in emergencies to combat anaphylaxis, which is a life-threatening allergic response. It is a potent inotropic (force of muscular contraction) drug, causing the blood vessels to constrict, thus increasing the blood pres-

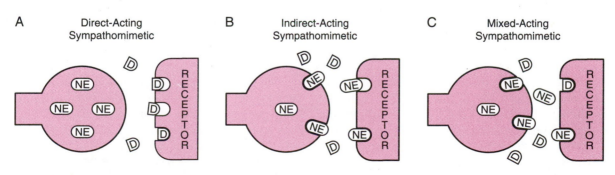

Key: Ⓓ = Sympathomimetic drug; ⓃⒺ = Norepinephrine

FIGURE 18–2 (*A*) Direct-acting, (*B*) indirect-acting, and (*C*) mixed-acting sympathomimetics.

FIGURE 18–3. Adrenergic Agonist: Epinephrine

Sympathomimetic	Dosage	NURSING PROCESS
		Assessment and Planning
Epinephrine (Adrenalin) *Pregnancy Category:* C	*Asthma anaphylaxis:* A: SC: 0.1–0.5 mL of 1:1000 PRN IV: 0.1–0.25 mL of 1:1000 C: SC: 0.01 mL/kg of 1:1000 IV: 0.01 mL/kg of 1:1000	

Contraindications	Drug-Lab-Food Interactions	
Cardiac dysrhythmias, cerebral arteriosclerosis, pregnancy, narrow-angle glaucoma, cardiogenic shock *Caution:* Hypertension, prostatic hypertrophy, hyperthyroidism, pregnancy, diabetes mellitus (hyperglycemia could result)	*Decrease* epinephrine effect with methyldopa, beta blockers, and alpha adrenergic blockers (e.g., phentolamine) *Lab: Increase* blood glucose, serum lactic acid	

Pharmacokinetics	Pharmacodynamics	
		Interventions
Absorption: SC/IM/IV: Rapidly *Distribution:* PB: UK; in breast milk *Metabolism:* t½: UK *Excretion:* In urine unchanged	SC/IM: Onset: 3–10 min Peak: 20 min Duration: 20–30 min IV: Onset: Immediate Peak: 2–5 min Duration: 5–10 min Inhal: Onset: 1 min Peak: 3–5 min Duration: 1–3 min	

Therapeutic Effects/Uses: To treat allergic reaction, anaphylaxis, bronchospasm, cardiac arrest. *Mode of Action:* Action on one or more adrenergic sites; promotion of CNS and cardiac stimulation, and bronchodilation.	Evaluation

Side Effects	Adverse Reactions
Anorexia, nausea, vomiting, nervousness, tremors, agitation, headache, pallor, insomnia, syncope, dizziness	Palpitations, tachycardia, dyspnea *Life-threatening:* Ventricular fibrillation, pulmonary edema

KEY: A: adult; C: child; SC: subcutaneous; IV: intravenous; UK: unknown; PB: protein-binding; t½: half-life.

sure, the heart rate to increase, and the bronchial tubes to dilate. High doses can result in cardiac dysrhythmias; therefore, the electrocardiogram (ECG) should be monitored. Epinephrine can also cause renal vasoconstriction, thereby decreasing renal perfusion and urinary output.

Epinephrine is usually prescribed subcutaneously or intravenously. The drug can also be administered by inhalation.

The onset of action and peak concentration times are rapid. The use of decongestants with epinephrine has an additive effect. When epinephrine is administered with digoxin, cardiac dysrhythmias may occur. Beta blockers can cause a decrease in epinephrine's action. Epinephrine is also discussed with the emergency drugs in Chapter 47.

Isoproterenol hydrochloride (Isuprel), an adrenergic drug, activates beta$_1$ and beta$_2$ receptors. It is more specific than epinephrine, because it acts on two different adrenergic receptors but is not completely selective. The response to beta$_1$ and beta$_2$ stimulation is an increase in heart rate and bronchodilation. When a client takes isoproterenol to control asthma by dilating the bronchi, an increase in heart rate also occurs due to beta$_1$ stimulation. When isoproterenol is used in excess, severe tachycardia can result.

ALBUTEROL

Albuterol sulfate (Proventil) is selective for beta$_2$-adrenergic receptors, so the response is purely bronchodilation. An asthmatic client may therefore respond better by taking albuterol than isoproterenol because its primary action is on the beta$_2$ receptor. By using selective sympathomimetics, there are fewer undesired responses (side effects).

FIGURE 18–4. Beta Adrenergic: Albuterol

Beta$_2$ Agonist	Dosage	NURSING PROCESS Assessment and Planning
Albuterol (Proventil, Salbutamol, Ventolin), 🍁 Novosalmol *Pregnancy Category:* C	A: PO: 2–4 mg, t.i.d., q.i.d. SR: 4–8 mg, q12h Inhal: 1–2 puffs, q4–6 h, PRN Nebulizer: 0.5 mL of 0.5% sol in 3 mL of 0.9% NaCl in 5–15 min C: (2–6 y): PO: 0.1 mg/kg/t.i.d. (6–12 y): PO: 2 mg, t.i.d., q.i.d. (6–12 y): Inhal: same as adult	
Contraindications	**Drug-Lab-Food Interactions**	
Caution: Severe cardiac disease, hypertension, hyperthyroidism, diabetes mellitus, pregnancy	*Increase* effect with other sympathomimetics; may *increase* effect with MAO inhibitors and tricyclic antidepressants *Antagonize* effect with beta adrenergic blockers (beta blockers) *Lab:* May *increase* glucose level slightly; may *decrease* serum potassium level	
Pharmacokinetics	**Pharmacodynamics**	Interventions
Absorption: well absorbed from the GI tract *Distribution:* PB: UK *Metabolism:* t½: PO: 2.5–6 h; Inhal: 3.5–5 h *Excretion:* 75% excreted in the urine	PO: Onset: 30 min Peak: 2–3 h Duration: 4–6 h Inhal: Onset: 5–15 min Peak: 0.5–2 h Duration: 3–6 h	

	Evaluation
Therapeutic Effects/Uses: To treat bronchospasm, asthma, bronchitis, and other COPD *Mode of Action:* It stimulates the beta$_2$ adrenergic receptors in the lungs which relaxes the bronchial smooth muscles.	

Side Effects	Adverse Reactions
Tremor, dizziness, nervousness, restlessness	Palpitations, reflex tachycardia, hallucinations *Life-threatening:* Cardiac dysrhythmias

KEY: A: adult; C: child; PO: by mouth; inhal: inhalation; PB: protein-binding; t½: half-life; UK: unknown; 🍁: Canadian drug names.

However, high dosages of albuterol may affect the beta$_1$ receptors, causing an increase in heart rate. Figure 18–4 lists the drug data related to albuterol.

Pharmacokinetics

Albuterol sulfate (Proventil, Ventolin) is well absorbed from the GI tract and is extensively metabolized by the liver. The half-life of the drug differs slightly according to the route of administration (oral route is 2.5 h and inhalation is 3.5 h).

Pharmacodynamics

The primary use of albuterol is to prevent and treat bronchospasms. With inhalation, the onset of action of albuterol is faster than with oral administration, although the duration of action is the same for both oral and inhalation preparations.

Tremors, restlessness, and nervousness may occur when high doses of the drug are taken—side effects that are most likely due to the reflex effect of beta$_1$. If albuterol is taken with a monoamine oxidase (MAO) inhibitor, a hypertensive crisis can result. Beta blockers may inhibit the action of albuterol. Albuterol and the beta$_2$ drugs are also discussed in Chapter 31.

Clonidine (Catapres) and methyldopa (Aldomet) are selective alpha$_2$-adrenergic drugs that are used primarily to treat hypertension. The accepted theory for the action of alpha$_2$ drugs is

TABLE 18–2 Adrenergic Drugs (Alpha, Beta$_1$, and Beta$_2$)

Generic (Brand)	Route and Dosage	Uses and Considerations
Epinephrine (Adrenaline) Alpha$_1$, beta$_1$, and beta$_2$	See Prototype Drug Chart (Fig. 18–3)	For nonhypovolemic shock, cardiac arrest, acute anaphylaxis, acute asthmatic attack. Pulse rate and blood pressure will greatly increase. Bronchial tubes will dilate. *Pregnancy category:* C; PB: UK; t½: UK
Ephedrine HCl Ephedrine sulfate (Ephedsol, Ectasule) Alpha$_1$, beta$_1$, and beta$_2$	A: PO: 25–50 mg t.i.d./q.i.d. SC/IM: 25–50 mg IV: 10–25 mg PRN; *max* 150 mg/24 h C >2 y: PO: 2–3 mg/kg/d or 25–100 mg/m^2/d in 4–6 divided doses	To treat hypotensive states, bronchospasm, nasal congestion, orthostatic hypotension. Effective for relief of symptoms of hay fever, sinusitis, and allergic rhinitis. Also may be used for treating mild cases of asthma. Drug resistance may occur with prolonged use of ephedrine. If this occurs, stop drug for 3–5 d and then resume. *Pregnancy category:* C; PB: UK; t½: 3–6 h
Norepinephrine bitartrate (levarterenol, Levophed) Alpha$_1$ and beta$_1$	A: IV: 4 mg in 250–500 mL of D$_5$W or NSS infused initially 8–12 µg/min, then 4 µg/min; monitor blood pressure	For shock. It is a potent vasoconstrictor. It increases blood pressure and cardiac output. The blood pressure should be closely monitored every 2–5 min during infusion. IV flow is titrated according to blood pressure. *Pregancy category:* D; PB: UK; t½: UK
Metaraminol bitartrate (Aramine) Alpha$_1$ and beta$_1$	A: IV/Inf: 15–100 mg in 500 mL of D$_5$W. C: IV/Inf: 0.04 mg/kg (each 1 mg diluted in 25 mL of D$_5$W)	Treatment of acute hypotension. Infusion rate should be adjusted according to blood pressure. *Pregnancy category:* C; PB: UK; t½: UK
Dopamine HCl (Intropin) Alpha$_1$ and beta$_1$	A: IV/INF: 1–5 µg/kg/min initially; gradually increase 5–10 µg/kg/min; *max:* 50 µg/kg/min C: IV: usually the same	To correct hypotension. It does not decrease renal function in doses <5 µg/kg/min. *Pregnancy category:* C; PB: UK; t½: 2 min
Phenylephrine HCl 12-hour spray (oxymetazoline HCl) (Neo-Synephrine) Alpha	*Nasal decongestant:* A: Instill: 2–3 sprays or gtt of 0.25–0.5% sol C <6 y: Instill: 2–3 gtt of 0.125% sol C 6–12 y: Instill: 2–3 gtt of 0.25% sol Also available IM, IV	To treat nasal congestion; acts as a decongestant. Used for clients with common cold, sinusitis, and with allergic rhinitis. Have client blow nose before drug is administered. *Pregnancy category:* C; PB: UK; t½: 2.5 h
Pseudoephedrine HCl (Sudafed, Actifed, Co-Tylenol, PediaCare) Alpha and beta$_1$	*Nasal decongestant:* A: PO: 60 mg q.i.d./q6h PO/SR: 120 mg q12h: *max:* 240 mg/d C 2–6 y: PO: 15 mg q6h; *max:* 60 mg/d C 6–12 y: PO: 30 mg q6h; *max:* 120 mg/d	To treat nasal congestion. OTC drug. Check label for contraindications. Avoid taking with a history of hypertension, cardiac disease, diabetes mellitus, etc. *Pregnancy category:* C; PB: UK; t½: 9–16 h

TABLE 18–2 Adrenergic Drugs (Alpha, Beta$_1$, and Beta$_2$) *(continued)*

Generic (Brand)	Route and Dosage	Uses and Considerations

Phenylpropanolamine HCl
Decongestant:
  Dimetapp, Dristan,
  Contac 12 hour,
  Triaminicol, Triaminic
	Nasal decongestant:
	A: PO: 25 mg q4h PRN
	  PO/SR: 75 mg q12h PRN
	C 2–6 y: PO: 6.25 mg q4h PRN
	C 6–12 y: 12.5 mg q4h PRN
		To treat nasal congestion; acts as OTC drugs.

Anorexiant:
  Dexatrim, Dietac,
  Control
  Alpha and beta$_1$
	Appetite suppressant:
	A: PO/SR: 75 mg q.d. (before breakfast)
	  PO: 25 mg t.i.d. a.c.
		To control weight gain. OTC drug. Client should check with health care provider before taking an appetite suppressant. *Pregnancy category:* C: PB: UK; t½: 3–4 h

Isoproterenol HCl
  (Isuprel)
  Beta$_1$ and beta$_2$
	A: SL: 10–20 mg t.i.d.
	  max: 60 mg/d
	  Inhal: 1–2 puffs q4–6 h PRN
	  IV: 0.01–0.02 mg or 2–20 μg/min via infusion
	C: SL: 5–10 mg t.i.d.
	  Inhal: Same as adult
	  IV: 2.5 μg/min OR 0.1 μg/kg/min via infusion
		To treat cardiac decompensation, congestive heart failure (increases myocardial blood flow and cardiac output), and asthmatic attack. This drug increases heart rate and dilates bronchial tubes. *Pregnancy category:* C; PB: UK; t½: 2.5–5 min

Metaproterenol sulfate
  (Alupent, Metaprel)
  Beta$_1$ (some) and beta$_2$
	A&C: >9 y: PO: 10–20 mg t.i.d./q.i.d.
	C <6y: PO: 1–2.6 mg/kg/d in 3–4 divided doses
	C 6–9 y: PO: 10 mg t.i.d./q.i.d.
	A&C: >12 y: inhal: 2–3 puffs q3–4h; *max:* 12 puffs/d
		Treatment for bronchospasm, acute heart block (only used in atropine-refractory bradycardia). By stimulating beta$_1$, the heart rate is increased but not as strongly as isoproterenol HCl. The drug dilates the bronchial tubes. *Pregnancy category:* C: PB: UK; t½: UK

Albuterol (Proventil,
  Ventolin)
  Beta$_2$
	A: PO: 2–4 mg t.i.d./q.i.d.
	  PO/SR: 4–8 mg q12h
	  Inhal: 1–2 puffs q4–6h PRN
	  Nebulizer: 0.5 mL of 0.5% sol. in 3 mL of 0.9% NaCl in 5–15 min
	C: 2–6 y: PO: 0.1 mg/kg t.i.d.
	  6–12 y: PO: 2 mg t.i.d./q.i.d.
	C: 6–12 y: Inhal: Same as adult
		To relieve bronchospasm, due to acute and chronic obstructive airway disease such as asthma, bronchitis, emphysema. It stimulates the beta$_2$ receptors of the bronchi, thus promoting bronchodilation. *Pregnancy category:* C; PB: UK; t½: 2.5–5 h

Dobutamine HCl
  (Dobutrex)
  Beta$_1$
	A or C: IV: 2.5–20 μg/kg/min initially; increase dose gradually; *max:* 40 μg/kg/min	To treat cardiac decompensation due to depressed myocardial contractility, which may result from organic heart disease, cardiac surgery. *Pregnancy category:* C; PB: UK; t½: 2 min

Isoetharine HCl
  (Bronkosol)
  Beta$_2$
	A: IPPB: 0.5–1.0 mL of 0.5% solu OR 0.5 mL of 1% solu diluted in 3 mL of NSS
	A: inhal: 1–2 puffs
		To control asthma and chronic obstructive pulmonary disease (COPD) by dilating the bronchial tubes. *Pregnancy category:* C; PB: UK; t½: UK

Terbutaline sulfate
  (Brethine, Brethaire,
  Bricanyl)
  Beta$_2$
	Bronchodilator:
	A: PO: 2.5–5 mg t.i.d. OR q8h
	  SC: 0.25 mg initial; no more than 0.5 mg in 4h
	  Inhal: 2 puffs q4–6h
	C >12 y: PO: 2.5 mg t.i.d. OR q8h
	Premature Labor:
	A: PO: 2.5 mg q4–6h
	  IV: 10 μg/min, gradually increase; *max:* 80 μg/min
		Primary use is to correct bronchospasm. Unofficial use is during premature labor to prevent premature-term birth. *Pregnancy category:* B; PB: 25%; t½: 3–11 h

Ritodrine HCl (Yutopar) Beta$_2$ and some beta$_1$	A: PO: Initially 10 mg q2h for first 24 h; maint: 10–20 mg q4–6h; max: 120 mg/d IV: 50–100 μg/min; dose may gradually increase to 300 μg/min	Used to decrease and/or stop uterine contraction. To be effective, the heart rate must be over 100 beats per minute (bpm). Due to many side effects, the drug is not used as frequently today in controlling premature labor. *Pregnancy category:* C; PB: UK; t½: 1.6–2.6 h

KEY: A: adult; C: child; PO: by mouth; IV: intravenous; PB: protein-binding; t½: half-life; UK: unknown; SC: subcutaneous; Inf: infusion; inhal: inhalation; OTC: over-the-counter: >:greater than; <: less than.

that they regulate the release of norepinephrine by inhibiting its release. Alpha$_2$ drugs are also believed to produce a cardiovascular depression by stimulating alpha$_2$ receptors in the CNS, leading to a decrease in blood pressure (discussed in Chapter 34).

Names of adrenergic drugs, the receptors they activate, dosage information, and common uses are covered in Table 18–2.

Side Effects and Adverse Reactions

Side effects frequently result when the drug dosage is increased or the drug is nonselective (acting on several receptors). Side effects that are commonly associated with adrenergic drugs include hypertension, tachycardia, palpitations, dysrhythmias, tremors, dizziness, urinary difficulty, nausea, and vomiting.

NURSING PROCESS: ADRENERGIC AGONIST

ASSESSMENT

- Obtain vital signs (VS) for future comparison. Epinephrine stimulates the alpha$_1$ (increases blood pressure), beta$_1$ (increases heart rate), and beta$_2$ (dilates bronchial tubes) receptors. Isoproterenol (Isuprel) stimulates the beta$_1$ and beta$_2$ receptors. Albuterol (Proventil) stimulates the beta$_2$ receptor.
- Assess the drugs the client is taking and report possible drug-drug interaction. Beta blockers decrease the effect of epinephrine.
- Assess the medical history. Most adrenergic drugs are contraindicated if the client has cardiac dysrhythmias, narrow-angle glaucoma, or cardiogenic shock.
- Assess the results of laboratory values and compare with future laboratory findings.

POTENTIAL NURSING DIAGNOSES

- High risk for impaired tissue integrity
- Decreased cardiac output

PLANNING

- Client's VS will be closely monitored and will be within normal or acceptable ranges.

NURSING INTERVENTIONS

- Monitor the client's VS. Report signs of increasing blood pressure and increasing pulse rate. If the client is receiving an alpha-adrenergic drug intravenously for shock, the blood pressure should be checked every 3 to 5 min or as indicated to avoid severe hypertension.

- Report side effects of adrenergic drugs, such as tachycardia, palpitations, tremors, dizziness, and increased blood pressure.
- Check the client's urinary output and assess for bladder distention. Urinary retention can result from high drug dose or continuous use of adrenergic drugs.
- For cardiac resuscitation, administer epinephrine 1:1000 IV (1 mg/mL), which may be diluted in 10 mL of saline solution (as prescribed).
- Check IV site frequently when administering norepinephrine bitartrate (Levarterenol) or dopamine (Intropin) because infiltration of these drugs causes tissue necrosis. These drugs should be diluted sufficiently in IV fluids. An antidote for norepinephrine (Levophed) and dopamine is phentolamine mesylate (Regitine) 5 to 10 mg, diluted in 10 to 15 mL of saline infiltrated into the area.
- Offer food when giving adrenergic drugs to avoid nausea and vomiting.
- Monitor laboratory test results. Blood glucose levels may be increased.

CLIENT TEACHING

General
- Instruct the client to read labels on all over-the-counter (OTC) drugs for cold symptoms and diet pills. Many of these have properties of sympathetic (adrenergic, sympathomimetics) drugs and should not be taken if the client is hypertensive or has diabetes mellitus, cardiac dysrhythmias, or coronary artery disease.
- Instruct mothers not to take drugs containing sympathetic drugs while nursing infants. These drugs pass into the breast milk.
- Explain to the client that continuous use of nasal sprays or drops that contain adrenergics may result in nasal congestion rebound (inflamed and congested nasal tissue).

Skill

- Instruct the client and family how to administer cold medications by spray or drops in the nostrils. Spray should be used with head in upright position. The use of nasal spray lying down can cause systemic absorption. Coloration of nasal spray or drops might indicate deterioration.
- Instruct the client not to use bronchodilator sprays in excess. If the client is using a nonselective adrenergic drug that affects beta$_1$ and beta$_2$ receptors, tachycardia may occur.

Side Effects

- Instruct the client to report side effects to health care provider, i.e., rapid heart rate, palpitations, or dizziness.

EVALUATION

- Evaluate the client's response to the adrenergic drug. Continue monitoring the client's VS and report abnormal findings.

ADRENERGIC BLOCKERS (ANTAGONISTS)

Drugs that block the effects of the adrenergic neurotransmitter are called **adrenergic blockers,** adrenergic antagonists, or sympatholytics. They are antagonists to the adrenergic agonists by blocking the alpha- and beta-receptor sites. Most adrenergic blockers block either the alpha or the beta receptor. They block the effects of the neurotransmitter either directly by occupying the alpha or the beta receptors, or indirectly by inhibiting the release of the neurotransmitters, norepinephrine and epinephrine. The three sympatholytic receptors are alpha$_1$, beta$_1$, and beta$_2$. Table 18–3 lists the effects of alpha and beta blockers.

ALPHA-ADRENERGIC BLOCKERS

Drugs that block or inhibit a response at the alpha-adrenergic receptor site are called alpha-adrenergic blockers, or more commonly, **alpha blockers.** The alpha blockers promote vasodilation, thus causing a decrease in blood pressure. If the vasodilation is longstanding, orthostatic hypotension can result. Dizziness may also be a symptom of a drop in blood pressure. As the blood pressure decreases, pulse rate usually increases to compensate for the low blood pressure and inadequate blood flow. The alpha blockers can be used to treat peripheral vascular disease, such as Raynaud's disease. Vasodilation occurs, permitting more blood flow to the extremities. The alpha blockers are also discussed in Chapter 35.

BETA-ADRENERGIC BLOCKERS

Beta-adrenergic blockers, commonly referred to as **beta blockers,** decrease heart rate; a decrease in blood pressure usually follows. Some of the beta blockers are nonselective, blocking both beta$_1$ and beta$_2$ receptors. Not only does the pulse rate decrease because of beta$_1$ blocking, but bronchoconstriction also occurs. Nonselective beta blockers (beta$_1$ and beta$_2$) should be used with extreme caution in any client who has chronic obstructive pulmonary disease (COPD) or asthma. If the desired effect is to decrease pulse rate and blood pressure, then a selective beta$_1$ blocker, such as metoprolol tartrate (Lopressor), may be ordered.

Propranolol hydrochloride (Inderal) was the first beta blocker prescribed for treating angina, cardiac dysrhythmias, and hypertension. Although it is still prescribed today, it has many side effects, partly due to its nonselective response in blocking both beta$_1$ and beta$_2$ receptors. It is contraindicated for clients with asthma or second- or third-degree heart block. Propranolol is extensively metabolized by the liver, hepatic first-pass; thus, a small amount of the drug reaches the systemic circulation. Figure 18–5 describes the pharmacologic behavior of propranolol.

Pharmacokinetics

Propranolol is well absorbed from the GI tract. It crosses the blood-brain barrier and the placenta and is found in breast milk. It is metabolized by the liver and has a short half-life of 3 to 6 h.

Pharmacodynamics

By blocking both types of beta receptors, propranolol decreases heart rate and, secondarily, the blood pressure. It also causes the bronchial tubes to constrict and the uterus to contract. It is available orally in tablets and sustained-release capsules, and intravenously. The onset of action of the sustained-

TABLE 18–3 Effects of Adrenergic Blockers at Receptors

Receptor	Responses
Alpha$_1$	Vasodilation: Decreases blood pressure. Reflex tachycardia might result. Miosis: Constricts the pupil. Suppresses ejaculation.
Beta$_1$	Decreases heart rate.
Beta$_2$	Constricts bronchioles. Contracts uterus.

FIGURE 18–5. Adrenergic Blocker (Sympatholytic)

Beta₁ and Beta₂ Blocker	Dosage	**NURSING PROCESS** Assessment and Planning
Propranolol HCl (Inderal), 🍁 Apo-Propranolol, De- tensol, Novopranolol *Pregnancy Category:* C	See Antihypertension, antianginal, and antidysrhythmics A: PO: Initially: 20–40 mg, b.i.d., titrate up to 160–240 mg/d in 2–3 divided doses SR: 120–160 mg/d C: PO: 2–4 mg/kg/d in 2 divided doses	

Contraindications	Drug-Lab-Food Interactions	
Congestive heart failure, secondary heart block, cardiogenic shock, bronchial asthma, bronchospasm *Caution:* Renal or hepatic dysfunction	*Increase* atrioventricular block with digoxin, calcium channel blockers *Increase* hypotensive effect with phe- nothiazines, diuretics, antihyperten- sives *Decrease* absorption with antacids *Lab: Increase* serum potassium, uric acid, AST (SGOT), ALT (SGPT), ALP; *decrease* blood sugar	

Pharmacokinetics	Pharmacodynamics	Interventions
Absorption: PO: Well absorbed *Distribution:* PB: 93% *Metabolism:* t½: 2–4 h *Excretion:* 90% excreted in urine as metabolites	PO: Onset: 30 min Peak: 1–1.5 h (SR: 6 h) Duration: 6 h IV: Onset: Immediate Peak: 5 min Duration: UK	

	Evaluation
Therapeutic Effects/Uses: To treat cardiac dysrhythmias, hypertension, angina pectoris, myo- cardial infarction. *Mode of Action:* Blocks beta₁- (cardiac) and beta₂- (pulmonary) adrenergic receptor sites.	

Side Effects	Adverse Reactions
Bradycardia, confusion, drowsiness, fa- tigue, vertigo, pruritus, dry mouth, nasal stuffiness, brown discoloration of the tongue (rare)	Visual hallucinations, thrombocytopenia *Life-threatening:* Laryngospasm, atrioventricular heart block, agranulocytosis

KEY: A: adult; C: child; PO: by mouth; IV: intravenous; PB: protein-binding; t½: half-life; UK: unknown; SR: sustained release; 🍁: Canadian drug names.

release preparation is longer than that of the tablet; peak time and duration action are also longer for the sustained-release formulation. This form is effective for dosing once a day, especially for clients who do not comply with drug doses of several times a day.

Drug Interactions

Many drugs interact with propranolol. Phenytoin, isoproterenol, nonsteroidal antiinflammatory drugs (NSAIDs), barbiturates, and xanthines (caffeine, theophylline) decrease the drug effect of propran-

TABLE 18–4 Adrenergic Blockers

Generic (Brand)	Route and Dosage	Uses and Considerations
Tolazoline (Priscoline HCl) Alpha$_1$	A: SC/IM/IV: 10–50 mg q.i.d. *Pulmonary hypertension:* NB: IV: 1–2 mg/kg infused over 10 min, followed by 1–2 mg/kg/h, for 24–48 h	For peripheral vascular disorder and for persistent pulmonary hypertension in the newborn. Also for emergency hypertension. *Pregnancy category:* C: PB: UK; t½: 3–10 h
Phentolamine mesylate (Regitine) Alpha$_1$	A: IM/IV: 2.5–5 mg, repeat q5min until controlled, then q2–3h PRN C: IM/IV: 0.05–0.1 mg/kg, repeat if needed	Management of peripheral vascular disorder and hypertensive emergency. Antidote for dopamine infiltration. *Pregnancy category:* C: PB: UK; t½: 20 min
Doxazosin mesylate (Cardura) Alpha$_1$	A: PO: 1 mg/d, titrate dose up to *max:* 16 mg/d; maint: 4–8 mg/d	For mild to moderate hypertension and BPH. Check for orthostatic hypotension. Dizziness, headache syncope may occur. *Pregnancy category:* C; PB: 98% t½: 9–12 h
Prazosin HCl (Minipress) Alpha$_1$	A: PO: 1 mg b.i.d./t.i.d.; maint: 3–15 mg/d; max: 20 mg/d in divided doses	Management of mild to moderate hypertension. May be used in combination with other antihypertensive drugs. *Pregnancy category:* C; PB: 95%; t½: 3 h.
Terazosin HCl (Hytrin) Alpha$_1$	A: PO: 1 mg/h.s., maint: 1–5 mg in 1–2 divided doses; *max:* 20 mg/d	For hypertension. May be used in combination with diuretic or other antihypertensive drugs. May also be used for BPH. May cause dizziness, headache, edema, orthostatic hypotension. *Pregnancy category:* C; PB: UK t½: 9–12 h
Propranolol HCl (Inderal) Beta$_1$ and beta$_2$	See Prototype Drug Chart (Fig. 18–5)	Treatment of hypertension, cardiac dysrhythmias, angina pectoris, postmyocardial infarction. Contraindicated in asthma and COPD. *Pregnancy category:* C; PB: 93%; t½: 2–4 h
Nadolol (Corgard) Beta$_1$ and beta$_2$	A: PO: 40–80 mg/d; *max:* 320 mg/d	Management of hypertension and angina pectoris. Contraindicated in bronchial asthma and severe COPD because it blocks beta$_2$. *Pregnancy category:* C; PB: 30%; t½: 10–24 h
Pindolol (Visken) Beta$_1$ and beta$_2$	A: PO: 5 mg b.i.d./t.i.d.; maint: 10–30 mg in divided doses; *max:* 60 mg/d in divided doses	Management of hypertension and angina pectoris. Contraindicated in asthma, COPD, and second-third-degree heart block. *Pregnancy category:* B; PB: 40%; t½: 3–4 h
Timolol maleate (Blocadren) Beta$_1$ and beta$_2$	A: PO: Initially 10 mg b.i.d.; maint: 20–40 mg/d in 2 divided doses; *max:* 60 mg/d	Management of mild to moderate hypertension, dysrhythmias, and post-myocardial infarction. Also may be used as prophylaxis of migraine headache. For ophthalmic use to treat IOP. Use with caution for clients with asthma or COPD. *Pregnancy category:* C; PB: <10%; t½: 3–4 h
Metoprolol tartrate (Lopressor) Beta$_1$	*Hypertension:* A: PO: 50–100 mg/d in 1–2 divided doses; maint: 100–450 mg/d in divided doses; *max:* 450 mg/d in divided doses *Myocardial infarction:* A: IV: 5 mg q2min ×3 doses, then PO: 100 mg b.i.d.	Management of hypertension, angina pectoris, post-myocardial infarction. Bradycardia, dizziness, GI distress may occur. *Pregnancy category:* C; PB: 12%; t½: 3–4 h
Atenolol (Tenormin) Beta$_1$	A: PO: 25–100 mg/d	Treatment of mild to moderate hypertension and angina pectoris. May be used in combination with antihypertensive drugs. Bradycardia, dizziness, and hypotension may occur. *Pregnancy category:* C; PB: 6%–16%, t½: 6–7 h
Acebutolol HCl (Sectral) Beta$_1$	A: PO: Initially: 200–400 mg/d A: PO: maint; 200–800 mg/d in 1–2 divided doses; *max:* 1200 mg/d	Treatment for mild to moderate hypertension, angina pectoris, and supraventricular dysrhythmias. Check apical pulse; do not give if <60 bpm. *Pregnancy category:* B; PB: 26%; t½: 3–13 h

KEY: A: adult; C: child; PO: by mouth; IM: intramuscular; IV: intravenous; NB: newborn; PRN: as necessary; UK: unknown; bpm: beats per minute; COPD: chronic obstructive pulmonary disease; PB: protein-binding; t½: half-life; BPH: benign prostatic hypertrophy; IOP: intraocular pressure.

olol. When propranolol is taken with digoxin or a calcium blocker, atrioventricular (AV) heart block may occur. The blood pressure can be decreased if propranolol is taken with another antihypertensive (this may be desirable).

Beta blockers are useful in treating cardiac dysrhythmias, mild hypertension, mild tachycardia, and angina pectoris. The use of beta blockers as antihypertensives, antidysrhythmics, and drugs for angina will be discussed again in Chapters 32 and 34. Table 18–4 lists the alpha and beta blockers, their dosages, uses, and considerations.

Side Effects and Adverse Reactions

General side effects of *alpha adrenergic blockers* include dysrhythmias, flushing, hypotension, and re-

flex tachycardia. The side effects commonly associated with *beta blockers* are bradycardia, dizziness, hypotension, headaches, hyperglycemia, intensified hypoglycemia, and agranulocytosis. Usually the side effects are dose-related.

ADRENERGIC NEURON BLOCKERS

Drugs that block the release of norepinephrine from the sympathetic terminal neurons are called **adrenergic neuron blockers,** which are classified as a subdivision of the adrenergic blockers. The clinical use of neuron blockers is to decrease blood pressure. Guanethidine monosulfate (Ismelin) and guanadrel sulfate (Hylorel), examples of the adrenergic neuron blockers, are potent antihypertensive agents.

NURSING PROCESS: ADRENERGIC BLOCKERS

Adrenergic alpha and beta blockers are also presented within the antihypertensive, antianginal, and antidysrhythmia sections.

ASSESSMENT

- Obtain baseline vital signs (VS) and ECG for future comparison. Bradycardia and decrease in blood pressure are common cardiac effects of adrenergic beta blockers. Adrenergic beta blockers are frequently referred to as beta blockers, blocking beta$_1$ and beta$_2$ (nonselective) or beta$_1$ (cardiac selective).
- Assess whether the client is having respiratory problems by listening for signs of wheezing or noting dyspnea (difficulty in breathing). If the beta blocker is nonselective, not only does the pulse rate decrease but also bronchoconstriction can result. Clients with asthma should take a beta$_1$ blocker, such as metoprolol (Lopressor), and avoid nonselective beta blockers.
- Assess the drugs the client is currently taking. Report if any are phenothiazines, digoxin, calcium channel blockers, or other antihypertensives.
- Assess the client's urine output and use for future comparison.

POTENTIAL NURSING DIAGNOSES

- Decreased cardiac output
- Impaired tissue integrity

PLANNING

- The client will comply with the drug regimen.
- The client's VS will be within desired range.

NURSING INTERVENTIONS

- Monitor the client's VS. Report marked changes such as marked decrease in blood pressure and pulse rate.
- Administer IV propranolol undiluted or diluted in D$_5$W.
- Report any complaints of excessive dizziness or lightheadedness.
- Report any complaint of stuffy nose. Vasodilation results from use of alpha-adrenergic blockers, and nasal congestion can occur.
- Report if the client is a diabetic and receiving an adrenergic beta blocker; insulin dose or oral hypoglycemic may need to be adjusted.
- Clients taking beta blockers do not have normal compensatory mechanisms in shock states. To resuscitate such clients, glucagon must be given in high doses to counteract the sympatholytic effects of beta blockers.

CLIENT TEACHING

General
- Advise the client to avoid abruptly stopping a beta blocker; rebound hypertension, rebound tachycardia, or an angina attack could result.
- Instruct the client to comply with the drug regimen.
- Advise clients on insulin therapy that early warning signs of hypoglycemia (i.e., tachycardia, nervousness) may be masked by the beta blocker.
- Advise clients on insulin therapy to carefully monitor their blood sugar and follow diet orders.

Skill
- Instruct the client and family how to take pulse and blood pressure.

Side Effects
- Instruct the client to avoid orthostatic (postural) hypotension, such as by slowly rising from supine or sitting to standing positions.
- Inform the client and family of possible mood changes when taking beta blockers. Mood changes can include depression, nightmares, and suicidal tendencies.

- Advise the male client that certain beta blockers, such as propranolol, metoprolol, and pindolol, and alpha blockers, such as prazosin, may cause impotence or a decrease in libido. Usually the problem is dose related.

EVALUATION

- Evaluate the effectiveness of the adrenergic blocker. VS must be stable within desired range.

STUDY QUESTIONS

1. What are the adrenergic receptors? What are the major physiologic responses of each?
2. What is the difference between selective adrenergic drugs and nonselective drugs? Give examples of each.
3. What are the major side effects of adrenergic drugs? What are the implications for client teaching?
4. What drugs are selective and nonselective adrenergic blockers? What are the uses of alpha blockers and beta blockers?
5. What are the side effects of adrenergic blockers?
6. What are the nursing interventions associated with the use of adrenergic drugs?

Chapter 19

Cholinergics and Anticholinergics

OUTLINE

Objectives
Terms
Introduction
Cholinergics
  Direct-Acting Cholinergics
  Indirect-Acting Choliner-
    gics

Nursing Process
Anticholinergics
  Pharmacokinetics
  Pharmacodynamics
  Side Effects and Adverse
    Reactions

Antiparkinsonism-Anti-
  cholinergic Drugs
Antihistamines for Treating
  Motion Sickness
Nursing Process
Study Questions

OBJECTIVES

Name the two cholinergic receptors.

Describe the responses of cholinergic drugs and anticholinergic drugs.

Differentiate between direct-acting and indirect-acting cholinergic drugs.

List the major side effects of cholinergic and anticholinergic drugs.

Describe the uses of cholinergics and anticholinergics.

Explain the nursing process, including client teaching, associated with cholinergics and anticholinergics.

TERMS

acetylcholine
anticholinergics
anticholinesterases
cholinergic
cholinergic blocking agents

cholinesterase
direct-acting cholinergics
indirect-acting cholinergics
miosis
muscarinic receptors

mydriasis
nicotinic receptors
parasympathomimetics
parasympatholytics

INTRODUCTION

The two groups of drugs that affect the parasympathetic nervous system are (1) the cholinergics (parasympathomimetics) and (2) the anticholinergics (parasympatholytics). Drugs in these groups are discussed in this chapter. The parasympathetic nervous system (parasympathomimetics and parasympatholytics), along with the sympathetic nervous system, is discussed and compared in Chapter 17.

CHOLINERGICS

Drugs that stimulate the parasympathetic nervous system are called **cholingeric drugs,** or **parasympathomimetics,** because they mimic the parasympathetic neurotransmitter acetylcholine. Cholinergic drugs are also called cholinomimetics, cholinergic stimulants, or cholinergic agonists. **Acetylcholine (ACh)** is the neurotransmitter located at the ganglions and the parasympathetic terminal nerve endings and innervates the receptors in organs, tissues, and glands. There are two types of cholinergic receptors: (1) **muscarinic receptors** that stimulate smooth muscle and slow the heart rate and (2) **nicotinic receptors** (neuromuscular) that affect the skeletal muscles. Many cholinergic drugs are nonselective because they can affect both the muscarinic and the nicotinic receptors. However, there are selective cholinergic drugs for the muscarinic receptors that do not have an effect on the nicotinic receptors. Figure 19–1 illustrates the effects of parasympathetic or cholinergic stimulation.

There are direct-acting cholingeric drugs and indirect-acting cholinergic drugs. **Direct-acting** cholinergic drugs act on the receptors to activate a tissue response (Fig. 19–2A). **Indirect-acting** cholinergic drugs inhibit the action of the enzyme **cholinesterase** (acetylcholinesterase) by forming a chemical complex, thus permitting acetylcholine to persist and attach to the receptor (see Fig. 19–2B). A drug that inhibits cholinesterase is called a **cholinesterase inhibitor,** or an **anticholinesterase drug.** Cholinesterase may destroy acetylcholine before it reaches the receptor or after it has attached to the site. By inhibiting or destroying the enzyme cholinesterase, more acetylcholine is available to stimulate the receptor and remain in contact with it longer.

The cholinesterase inhibitors (anticholinesterases) can be separated into reversible inhibitors and irre-

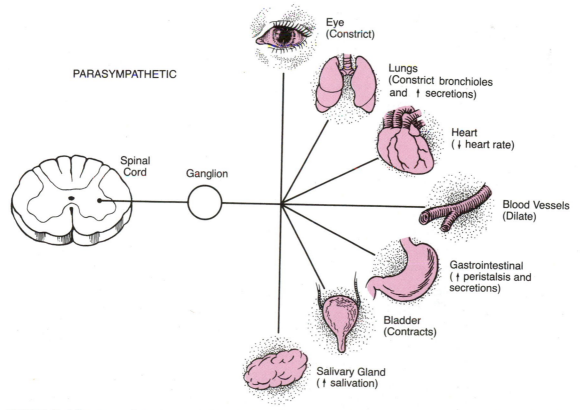

FIGURE 19–1 Parasympathetic responses. Stimulation of the parasympathetic nervous system or use of parasympathomimetic drugs causes the pupils to constrict, the bronchioles to constrict and increase bronchial secretions, heart rate to decrease, blood vessels to dilate, peristalsis and gastric secretions to increase, the bladder muscle to contract, and salivation to increase.

A Direct-Acting Parasympathomimetic
(Cholinergic Drug)

B Indirect-Acting Parasympathomimetic
(Cholinesterase Inhibitors)

FIGURE 19–2 (A) Direct-acting parasympathomimetic (cholinergic drugs). Cholinergic drugs resemble acetylcholine and act directly on the receptor. (B) Indirect-acting parasympathomimetic drug (choline-sterase inhibitors). Cholinesterase inhibitors inactivate the enzyme acetylcholinesterase (cholinesterase), thus permitting acetylcholine to react to the receptor. (Key: D: cholinergic drug; DD: cholinesterase inhibitor (anticholinesterase); AChE: acetylcholinesterase or cholinesterase; ACh: acetylcholine.)

versible inhibitors. The reversible inhibitors bind the enzyme, cholinesterase, for several minutes to hours, and the irreversible inhibitors bind the enzyme permanently. The resulting effects vary with the amount of time the cholinesterase is bound.

The major responses of cholinergic drugs are to stimulate bladder and gastrointestinal (GI) tone, constrict pupils of the eyes **(miosis),** and increase neuromuscular transmission. Other effects of cholinergic drugs include decreased heart rate and blood pressure and increased salivary, GI, and bronchial glandular secretions. Table 19–1 lists the functions of direct- and indirect-acting cholinergic drugs.

DIRECT-ACTING CHOLINERGICS

Many drugs in this category are primarily selective to the muscarinic receptors but are nonspecific because the muscarinic receptors are located in the smooth muscles of the GI and genitourinary tracts, glands, and heart. Bethanechol chloride (Urecholine), a direct-acting cholinergic drug, acts on the muscarinic (cholinergic) receptor and is used primarily to increase urination. Figure 19–3 details the pharmacologic behavior of bethanechol.

Pharmacokinetics

Bethanechol chloride (Urecholine) is poorly absorbed from the GI tract. The percentage of protein-binding and the half-life are unknown. The drug is most likely to be excreted in the urine.

Pharmacodynamics

The principal use of bethanechol is to promote micturition (urination) by stimulating the muscarinic cholinergic receptors to increase urine output. The client voids approximately 30 min to 1.5 h after taking an oral dose of bethanechol because of the increased tone of the detausor urinae muscle.

TABLE 19–1 Effects of Cholinergic Drugs

Body Tissue	Response
Cardiovascular*	Decreases heart rate, lowers blood pressure due to vasodilation, and slows conduction of atrioventricular node.
Gastrointestinal†	Increases the tone and motility of the smooth muscles of the stomach and intestine. Peristalsis is increased and the sphincter muscles are relaxed.
Genitourinary	Contracts the muscles of the urinary bladder, increases tone of the ureters, and relaxes the bladder's sphincter muscles. Stimulates urination.
Eye†	Increases pupillary constriction, or miosis (pupil becomes smaller), and increases accommodation (flattening or thickening of eye lens for distant or near vision).
Glandular*	Increases salivation, perspiration, and tears.
Bronchi (lung)*	Stimulates bronchial smooth muscle contraction and increases bronchial secretions.
Striated muscle†	Increases neuromuscular transmission and maintains muscle strength and tone.

* Tissue responses to large doses of cholinergic drugs.
† Major tissue responses to normal doses of cholinergic drugs.

FIGURE 19–3. Cholinergic

Cholinergic/Parasympathomimetic	Dosage	NURSING PROCESS
Bethanechol Chloride (Urecholine), 🍁 Duvoid, Urecholine *Pregnancy Category:* C	A: PO: 10–50 mg b.i.d./t.i.d./q.i.d.; *max:* 120 mg/d SC: 2.5–5 mg, repeat at 15–30 min intervals; PRN Do *NOT* give IM or IV	**Assessment and Planning**

Contraindications	Drug-Lab-Food Interactions	
Severe bradycardia or hypotension, chronic obstructive pulmonary disease, asthma, peptic ulcer, parkinsonism, hyperthyroidism	*Decrease* bethanechol effect with antidysrhythmics *Lab: Increase* AST, bilirubin, amylase, lipase	

Pharmacokinetics	Pharmacodynamics	Interventions
Absorption: PO: Poorly absorbed *Distribution:* PB: UK *Metabolism:* t½: UK *Excretion:* In urine	PO: Onset: 0.5–1.5 h Peak: 1–2 h Duration: 4–6 h SC: Onset: 5–15 min Peak: 0.5 h Duration: 2 h	

Therapeutic Effects/Uses: To treat urinary retention, abdominal distention.

Mode of Action: Stimulation of the cholinergic (muscarinic) receptor. Promote contraction of the bladder; increase GI peristalsis, GI secretion, pupillary constriction, and bronchoconstriction.

Evaluation

Side Effects	Adverse Reactions
Nausea, vomiting, diarrhea, salivation, sweating, flushing, frequent urination, rash, miosis, blurred vision, abdominal discomfort	Orthostatic hypotension, bradycardia, muscle weakness *Life-threatening:* Acute asthmatic attack, heart block, circulatory collapse, cardiac arrest

KEY: A: adult; C: child; PO: by mouth; SC: subcutaneous; PB: protein-binding; t½: half-life; UK: unknown; 🍁 : Canadian drug names.

Bethanechol also increases peristalsis in the GI tract. The drug should be taken on an empty stomach, and it should not be administered intramuscularly or intravenously. Bethanechol can be given subcutaneously, and micturition usually occurs within 15 min. Duration of action for oral administration is 4 to 6 h; for the subcutaneous route it is 2 h.

Direct-Acting Cholinergic: Eye

Pilocarpine is a direct-acting cholinergic drug that constricts the pupils of the eyes, thus opening the canal of Schlemm to promote drainage of aqueous humor (fluid). This drug is used to treat glaucoma by relieving fluid (intraocular) pressure in the eye. Pilocarpine also acts on the nicotinic receptor. Carbachol acts on the nicotinic receptors. These agents are discussed in more detail in Chapter 38.

INDIRECT-ACTING CHOLINERGICS

The indirect-acting cholinergic drugs do not act on receptors; instead they inhibit or inactivate the en-

TABLE 19–2 Cholinergics

Generic (Brand)	Route and Dosage	Uses and Considerations
Direct-Acting Cholinergics		
Bethanechol (Urecholine)	See Prototype Drug Chart (Fig. 19–3)	To increase urination; can stimulate gastric motility. Contraindicated in bronchial asthma, mechanical GI and urinary obstruction, and pronounced bradycardia. *Pregnancy category:* C; PB: UK; t½: UK
Carbachol (Miostat)	Ophthalmic: 0.75%–3%, 1–2 gtt, t.i.d.	To reduce intraocular pressure, miosis. See Chapter 38.
Pilocarpine HCl (Pilocar)	Ophthalmic: 0.5%–4%, 1 drop	To reduce intraocular pressure, miosis. See Chapter 38.
Cholinesterase Inhibitor		
Tacrine HCl (Cognex)	*For Alzheimer's Disease:* A: PO: 10 mg, q.i.d., increase dose at 6-wk intervals. A: PO: 40–160 mg/d pc; *max:* 160 mg/d	To improve memory in mild to moderate Alzheimer's dementia. Drug enhances cholinergic function. *Pregnancy category:* C; PB: 55%; t½: 1.5–3.5 h
Velnacrine (Mentane)	A: PO: 150–225 mg/d in divided doses	To treat Alzheimer's disease. Clinical trial drug. *Pregnancy category:* C; PB: UK; t½: 2–3 h
Indirect-Acting Cholinergics or Cholinesterase Inhibitors for the Eye		
Demecarium bromide (Humorsol)	0.125%–0.25%, 1 gt q12–48h	To reduce intraocular pressure in glaucoma, long-acting miotic. See Chapter 38.
Echothiophate iodide (Phospholine Iodide)	0.03%–0.25%, 1 gt daily or b.i.d.	To reduce intraocular pressure, long-acting miotic. See Chapter 38.
Isoflurophate (Floropryl)	0.25%, ointment q8–72h	To treat glaucoma. Apply to the conjunctival sac. See Chapter 38.
Reversible Cholinesterase Inhibitors: Myasthenia Gravis		
Ambenonium Cl (Mytelase)	A: PO: 2.5–5.0 mg t.i.d./q.i.d.; dose may be increased; maint: 5–25 mg t.i.d./q.i.d.	To increase muscle strength in myasthenia gravis; long-acting. May be used with glucocorticoids. *Pregnancy category:* C; PB: UK; t½: UK
Edrophonium Cl (Tensilon)	A: IV: 2 mg; then 8 mg if no response IM: 10 mg; may repeat with 2 mg in 30 min C <34 kg: IV: 1 mg; repeat in 30–45 sec if no response; *max:* 5 mg C >34 kg: IV: 2 mg; repeat with 1 mg if no response; *max:* 10 mg	To diagnose myasthenia gravis; very short-acting. *Pregnancy category:* C; PB: UK; t½: 1.2–2 h
Neostigmine (Prostigmin) Neostigmine methylsulfate (injectable form)	A: PO: Initially 15 mg t.i.d.; maint: 150 mg/d in divided doses; range: 15–375 mg/d IM/IV: 0.5–2.5 mg as needed C: PO: 2 mg/kg/d in 6 divided doses	To increase muscle strength in myasthenia gravis; short-acting. Used also to prevent or treat postoperative urinary retention. *Pregnancy category:* C; PB: 15–25%; t½: 1–1.5 h
Physostigmine salicylate (Eserine salicylate)	0.25%–0.5%, 1 gt daily or q.i.d.	To reduce intraocular pressure, miosis, short-acting.
Pyridostigmine bromide (Mestinon)	A: PO: 60–120 mg t.i.d./q.i.d.; maint: 600 mg/d in 3–4 divided doses; *max:* 1.5 g/d SR: 180–540 mg daily or b.i.d. IM/IV: 2 mg q2–3h C: PO: 7 mg/kg/d in 5–6 divided doses	To increase muscle strength in myasthenia gravis; moderate-acting. Prevents the destruction of the neurotransmitter acetylcholine. *Pregnancy category:* C; PB: <10%; t½: 3–4 h

KEY: A: adult; C: child; PO: by mouth; IM: intramuscular; IV: intravenous; gt: drop; gtt: drops; UK: unknown; SR: sustained-release; >: greater than; IOP: intraocular pressure; PB: protein-binding; t½: half-life; maint: maintenance; <: less than.

zyme cholinesterase, thus permitting acetylcholine to accumulate at the receptor sites (see Fig. 19–2B). This action gives them the name **cholinesterase inhibitors,** or **anticholinesterases,** of which there are two types: reversible and irreversible.

Reversible Cholinesterase Inhibitors

These inhibitors are used (1) to produce pupillary constriction in the treatment of glaucoma, and (2) to increase muscle strength in clients with myasthenia gravis (a neuromuscular disorder). Drug effects persist for several hours. Drugs used to increase muscular strength in myasthenia gravis include neostigmine (Prostigmin: short-acting), pyridostigmine bromide (Mestinon: moderate-acting), ambenonium chloride (Mytelase: long-acting), and edrophonium chloride (Tensilon: short-acting for diagnostic purposes). These drugs are discussed in more detail in Chapter 20. A reversible ophthalmic anticholinesterase drug is physostigmine (Eserine). Ophthalmic agents are discussed more thoroughly in Chapter 38.

Irreversible Cholinesterase Inhibitors

Irreversible inhibitors are potent agents because of their long-lasting effect. The enzyme cholinesterase must be regenerated before the drug effect diminishes, a process that may take days or weeks. These drugs are used to produce pupillary constriction and for manufacture of organophosphate insecticides. Examples of all types of cholinergic drugs, their standard dosages, and common uses are found in Table 19–2.

NURSING PROCESS: CHOLINERGIC DIRECT ACTING: Bethanechol (Urecholine)

ASSESSMENT

- Obtain baseline vital signs (VS) for future comparison.
- Assess urine output that should be >600 mL/d. Report decrease in urine output.
- Obtain a history from the client of health problems, such as peptic ulcer, urinary obstruction, or asthma. Cholinergics can aggravate symptoms of these conditions.

POTENTIAL NURSING DIAGNOSES

- Urinary retention
- Anxiety

PLANNING

- Client will have increased bladder and GI tone after taking cholinergics.
- Client will have increased neuromuscular strength.

NURSING INTERVENTIONS

Direct Acting
- Monitor the client's VS. Pulse rate and blood pressure decrease when large doses of cholinergics are taken. Orthostatic hypotension is a side effect of a cholinergic such as bethanechol.
- Monitor fluid intake and output. Decreased urinary output should be reported for it may be related to urinary obstruction.
- Give cholinergics 1 h before or 2 h after meals. If the client complains of gastric pain, the drug may be given with meals.
- Check serum enzyme values for amylase and lipase, as well as AST (SGOT) and bilirubin levels.

These laboratory values may increase slightly when taking cholinergics.
- Observe the client for side effects, such as gastric pain or cramping, diarrhea, increased salivary or bronchial secretions, bradycardia, and orthostatic hypotension.
- Auscultate for bowel sounds. Report decreased or hyperactive bowel sounds.
- Auscultate breath sounds for rales (cracking sounds from fluid congestion in lung tissue) or rhonchi (rough sounds due to mucus secretions in lung tissue). Cholinergic drugs can increase bronchial secretions.
- Have IV atropine sulfate (0.6 mg) available as an antidote for overdosing of cholinergics. Early signs of overdosing include salivation, sweating, abdominal cramps, and flushing.
- Note that diaphoresis (excessive perspiration) may occur; linens should be changed as needed.

Indirect Acting
- Beware of the possibility of cholinergic crisis (overdose); symptoms include muscular weakness and increased salivation.

CLIENT TEACHING

Direct Acting
General
- Instruct the client to take the cholinergic as prescribed. Compliance with the drug regimen is essential.

Side Effects
- Instruct the client to report severe side effects, such as profound dizziness or a drop in pulse rate below 60.
- Instruct the client to arise from a lying position

slowly to avoid dizziness; this is most likely due to orthostatic hypotension.
• Encourage the client to maintain effective oral hygiene if excess salivation occurs.
• Advise the client to report any difficulty in breathing due to respiratory distress.

Indirect Acting: See Drugs for Myasthenia Gravis
• Instruct the client to take the drug on time to avoid respiratory muscle weakness.

• Instruct the client to assess changes in muscle strength. Cholinesterase inhibitors (anticholinesterases) increase muscle strength.

EVALUATION

• Evaluate the effectiveness of the cholinergic or anticholinesterase drug.
• Evaluate the stability of the client's VS, and note the presence of side effects or adverse reactions.

ANTICHOLINERGICS

Drugs that inhibit the actions of acetylcholine by occupying the acetylcholine receptors are called anticholinergics or parasympatholytics. Other names for anticholinergics are **cholinergic blocking agents,** cholinergic or muscarinic antagonists, antiparasympathetic agents, antimuscarinic agents, or antispasmodics. The major body tissues and organs affected by the anticholinergic group of drugs are the heart, respiratory tract, GI tract, urinary bladder, eye, and the exocrine glands. By blocking the parasympathetic nerves, the sympathetic (adrenergic) nervous system is allowed to dominate. Anticholinergic and adrenergic drugs produce many of the same responses.

Anticholinergic and cholinergic drugs have opposite effects. The major responses to anticholinergics are a decrease in GI motility, a decrease in salivation, dilation of the pupils of the eyes **(mydriasis),** and an increase in pulse rate. Other effects of anticholinergics include decreased bladder contraction, which can result in urinary retention, and decreased rigidity and tremors related to neuromuscular excitement. Anticholinergics can act as an an-

tidote to the toxicity caused by cholinesterase inhibitors and organophosphate ingestion. The various effects of anticholinergics are described in Table 19–3.

Muscarinic receptors, which are cholinergic receptors, are involved in tissue and organ responses to anticholinergics, because anticholinergics inhibit the actions of acetylcholine by occupying these receptor sites. Figure 19–4 illustrates this action of anticholinergic drugs. Anticholinergic drugs may block the effect of direct-acting parasympathomimetics, such as bethanechol and pilocarpine, and of indirect-acting parasympathomimetics, such as physostigmine and neostigmine.

Atropine sulfate, first derived from the belladonna plant (*Atropa belladonna*) and purified in 1831, is a classic anticholinergic drug. Scopolamine was the second belladonna alkaloid produced. Atropine and scopolamine act on the muscarinic receptor, but they have little effect on the nicotinic receptor. Atropine is useful as a preoperative medication to decrease salivary secretions, as an antispasmodic drug for treating peptic ulcers because it relaxes the smooth muscles of the GI tract and decreases peristalsis, and for increasing heart rate

TABLE 19–3 Effects of Anticholinergic Drugs

Body Tissues	Responses
Cardiovascular	Increases heart rate with large doses. Small doses can decrease heart rate.
Gastrointestinal	Relaxes smooth muscle tone of GI tract, decreasing GI motility and peristalsis. Decreases gastric and intestinal secretions.
Urinary tract	Relaxes the bladder's detrusor muscle and increases constriction of the internal sphincter. Urinary retention can result.
Eye	Dilates pupils of the eye (mydriasis) and paralyzes ciliary muscle (cycloplegia), causing a decrease in accommodation.
Glandular	Decreases salivation, sweating, and bronchial secretions.
Lung	Dilates the bronchi and decreases bronchial secretions.
Central nervous system	Decreases tremors and rigidity of muscles. Drowsiness, disorientation, and hallucination can result from large doses.

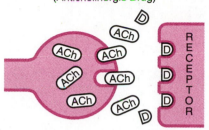

Direct-Acting Parasympatholytic
(Anticholinergic Drug)

FIGURE 19–4 Anticholinergic response. The anticholinergic drug is occupying the receptor sites, thus blocking acetylcholine. (Key: D: anticholinergic drug; ACh: acetylcholine.)

when bradycardia is present. However, if a client is on atropine or an atropine-like drug (antihistamine) for any long period, side effects can occur. Figure 19–5 details the pharmacologic behavior of atropine.

Synthetic anticholinergic drugs are also used as antispasmodics to treat peptic ulcers and intestinal spasticity. One example of such a drug is propantheline bromide (Pro-Banthine), which has been available for several decades. It decreases gastric secretions and GI spasms. Since the introduction of the histamine blockers (H_2), anticholinergic agents such as propantheline are not used as frequently to decrease gastric secretions.

PHARMACOKINETICS

Atropine sulfate is well absorbed orally and parenterally. It crosses the blood–brain barrier and exerts its effect on the central nervous system (CNS). The protein-binding is unknown; it crosses the placenta. Atropine has a short half-life; therefore, there is little cumulative effect. Most of absorbed atropine is excreted in the urine (75% to 95%).

PHARMACODYNAMICS

Atropine sulfate blocks acetylcholine by occupying the muscarinic receptor. It increases heart rate by blocking vagus stimulation, and promotes dilation of the pupil by paralyzing the iris sphincter. The two most frequent uses of atropine are preopera-

FIGURE 19–5. Anticholinergic

Anticholinergic/Parasympatholytic	Dosage	**NURSING PROCESS** Assessment and Planning
Atropine SO$_4$ (Atropine), 🍁 Atropair Atropisol (Optic) *Pregnancy Category:* C	A: PO/IM/IV: 0.4–0.6 mg q4–6h PRN C: PO/IM/IV: 0.01 mg/kg/dose; max: 0.4 mg/dose, q4–6h, PRN	
Contraindications	**Drug-Lab-Food Interactions**	
Narrow-angle glaucoma, obstructive GI disorders, paralytic ileus, ulcerative colitis, tachycardia, benign prostatic hypertrophy, myasthenia gravis, myocardial ischemia *Caution:* Renal or hepatic disorders, chronic obstructive pulmonary disease (COPD), congestive heart failure	*Increase* anticholinergic effect with phenothiazines, antidepressants, MAOIs, amantadine; may *increase* effects of atenolol	
Pharmacokinetics	**Pharmacodynamics**	Interventions
Absorption: PO/IM: Well absorbed *Distribution:* PB: UK; crosses the placenta *Metabolism:* t½: 2–3 h *Excretion:* >75% excreted in urine	PO: Onset: 0.5–1 h Peak: 1–2 h Duration: 4 h IM: Onset: 10–30 min Peak: 0.5 h Duration: 4 h IV: Onset: Immediate Peak: 5 min Duration: UK Instill: Onset: 20–30 min Peak: 30–40 min Duration: days	

Figure continues on following page

FIGURE 19–5. *Continued*

Evaluation

Therapeutic Effects/Uses: Preoperative medication to reduce salivation, increase heart rate, dilate pupils of the eye.

Mode of Action: Inhibition of acetylcholine by occupying the receptors; increase heart rate by blocking vagus stimulation; promote dilation of the pupil by blocking iris sphincter muscle.

Side Effects	Adverse Reactions
Dry mouth, nausea, headache, constipation, rash, dry skin, flushing, blurred vision, photophobia	Tachycardia, hypotension, pupillary dilatation, abdominal distention palpitations, nasal congestion *Life-threatening:* Paralytic ileus, coma

KEY: A: adult; C: child; PO: by mouth; IM: intramuscular; IV: intravenous; PB: protein-binding; t½: half-life; UK: unknown; instill: instillation: MAOIs: monoamine oxidase inhibitors; >: greater than; PRN: as necessary; ✚: Canadian drug names.

tively to decrease salivation and respiratory secretions, and to treat sinus bradycardia by increasing the heart rate. Atropine also is used ophthalmically for mydriasis and cycloplegia prior to eye refraction and to treat inflammation of the iris (iritis) and uveal tract.

Its onset of action orally is between 0.5 to 1 h and peaks at 2 to 4 h. For the intramuscular route, the onset of action is 10 to 30 min and peaks at 30 min. Duration time for both oral and intramuscular routes is 4 h. Intravenously, the onset of action is immediate and peak action is at 5 min.

SIDE EFFECTS AND ADVERSE REACTIONS

Anticholinergic drugs have many side effects. The common side effects of atropine and atropine-like drugs include dry mouth, decreased perspiration, blurred vision, tachycardia, constipation, and urinary retention. Other side effects and adverse reactions are nausea, headache, dry skin, abdominal distention, hypotension or hypertension, impotence, photophobia, and coma.

ANTIPARKINSONISM-ANTICHOLINERGIC DRUGS

At one time atropine was given to clients with Parkinson's disease to decrease salivation and drooling. It was also found to have some effect on the motor manifestation of this disease by decreasing tremors and rigidity. Additional studies indicated that anticholinergic (antimuscarinic) agents affect the central nervous system (CNS) as well as

the parasympathetic nervous system. These anticholinergic drugs affect the CNS by suppressing the tremors and muscular rigidity of parkinsonism, but they have little effect on mobility and muscle weakness. As the result of these findings, several anticholinergic drugs were developed, such as trihexyphenidyl hydrochloride (Artane), procyclidine (Kemadrin), biperiden (Akineton), and benztropine (Cogentin), for the treatment of Parkinson's disease. These drugs can be used alone in early stages of parkinsonism. Today these drugs may be used in combination with levodopa for controlling parkinsonism or used singly to treat pseudoparkinsonism resulting from the side effects of the phenothiazines in antipsychotic drugs. Drugs for parkinsonism are described in more detail in Chapter 20. Figure 19–6 lists the drug data related to trihexyphenidyl, which is used for pseudoparkinsonism.

Pharmacokinetics

Trihexyphenidyl is well absorbed from the GI tract. Its protein-binding percentage and half-life are unknown. It is excreted in the urine.

Pharmacodynamics

Trihexyphenidyl decreases involuntary movement and diminishes the signs and symptoms of tremors and muscle rigidity that occur with Parkinson's disease and pseudoparkinsonism. It is available in tablet, elixir, and sustained-release capsule. The duration of action of the sustained-release preparation is twice as long as that for the oral and elixir forms. Alcohol, narcotics, amantadine, phenothiazines,

FIGURE 19–6. Antiparkinsonism: Anticholinergic

Antiparkinsonism Anticholinergic	Dosage	NURSING PROCESS
		Assessment and Planning
Trihexyphenidyl HCl (Artane, Aphen, Hexaphen, Trihexane, Trihexy), 🍁 Aparkane, Apo-Trihex, Novohexidyl *Pregnancy Category:* C	*Parkinsonism:* A: PO: Initially 1–2 mg/d; increase to 6–10 mg/d in divided doses *Extrapyramidal symptoms: Drug induced:* A: PO: 1 mg/d; increase to 5–15 mg/d in divided doses	
Contraindications	**Drug-Lab-Food Interactions**	
Narrow-angle glaucoma, GI obstruction, urinary retention, severe angina pectoris, myasthenia gravis *Caution:* Tachycardia, benign prostatic hypertrophy, children, elderly, during lactation	*Increase* anticholinergic effect with phenothiazines, antihistamines, tricyclic antidepressants, amantadine, quinidine *Decrease* trihexyphenidyl absorption with antacids	
Pharmacokinetics	**Pharmacodynamics**	Interventions
Absorption: PO: Well absorbed *Distribution:* PB: UK *Metabolism:* t½: 5–10 h *Excretion:* In urine	PO: Onset: 1 h Peak: 2–3 h Duration: 6–12 h SR/PO: Onset: UK Peak: UK Duration: 12–24 h	

	Evaluation
Therapeutic Effects/Uses: To decrease involuntary symptoms of parkinsonism or drug-induced parkinsonism by inhibiting acetylcholine. *Mode of Action:* Blocks cholinergic (muscarinic) receptors: thus decreases involuntary movements.	

Side Effects	Adverse Reactions
Nausea, vomiting, dry mouth, constipation, anxiety, restlessness, headache, dizziness, blurred vision, photophobia, pupil dilation, dysphagia	Tachycardia, palpitations, urticaria, postural hypotension, urinary retention *Life-threatening:* Paralytic ileus

KEY: A: adult; PO: by mouth; PB: protein-binding; SR: sustained-release; t½: half-life; UK: unknown; 🍁: Canadian drug names.

and antihistamines may increase the effect of trihexyphenidyl. The side effects are similar to other anticholinergic drugs.

ANTIHISTAMINES FOR TREATING MOTION SICKNESS

The effects of anticholinergics on the CNS benefits clients prone to motion sickness. An example of such an anticholinergic, classified as an antihistamine for motion sickness, is scopolamine. It is available topically as a skin patch (Transderm Scop) to be placed behind the ear. The transdermal scopolamine is delivered over a period of 3 days and is frequently prescribed for activities that include flying, cruising on the water, and for bus or automobile trips. Other drugs classified as antihistamines for motion sickness are dimenhydrinate

(Dramamine), cyclizine (Marezine), and meclizine hydrochloride (Bonine). Most of these drugs can be purchased over-the-counter (OTC), with the exception of Transderm Scop.

Examples of anticholinergic drugs and their dosages and common uses are found in Table 19–4. Dosages may vary according to age, sex, and weight. Because anticholinergic drugs can increase intraocular pressure, they should *not* be administered to clients diagnosed with glaucoma.

Side Effects and Adverse Reactions

The side effects include dry mouth, visual disturbances (especially blurred vision due to pupillary dilation), constipation secondary to decreased GI peristalsis, urinary retention related to decreased bladder tone, tachycardia (large doses), hypotension, skin rash, muscle weakness, and flushing.

TABLE 19–4 Anticholinergics

Generic (Brand)	Route and Dosage	Uses and Considerations
Anticholinergics: GI or Cholinergic Blockers		
Atropine sulfate	See Prototype Drug Chart (Fig. 19–5)	Presurgery to decrease salivary and bronchial secretions. Increases heart rate with doses ≥0.5 mg. *Pregnancy category:* C; PB: UK; t½: 2–3 h
Dicyclomine HCl (Bentyl, Antispas, Di-Spaz)	A: PO: 10–20 mg t.i.d./q.i.d. IM: 20 mg q 6h C >2 y: PO: 10 mg t.i.d./q.i.d.	For irritable bowel syndrome. Avoid taking drug for those with narrow-angle glaucoma, severe ulcerative colitis, paralytic ileus. *Pregnancy category:* B; PB: UK; t½: 9–10 h
Glycopyrrolate (Robinul)	*GI disorders:* A: PO: 1–2 mg b.i.d./t.i.d. IM/IV: 0.1–0.2 mg t.i.d./q.i.d. *Preoperative:* A: IM: 4.4 µg/kg 30 min–1 h before surgery	Presurgery to reduce secretions and for peptic ulcer. Contraindicated in narrow-angle glaucoma, obstructive GI tract, and ulcerative colitis. *Pregnancy category:* B; PB: UK; t½: 1–4.5 h
Hyoscyamine SO₄ (Cystospaz, Anaspaz, Levsin)	A: PO/SL: 0.125–0.25 mg t.i.d./q.i.d. ac & h.s. SR: 0.375–0.75 mg/q 12h SC/IM/IV: 0.25–0.5 mg b.i.d./q.i.d. C: 2–10 y: one-half of the adult dose or individualized	Treatment of peptic ulcer and irritable bowel syndrome. Controls gastric secretion and spastic bladder. Contraindicated in narrow-angle glaucoma and severe ulcerative colitis. *Pregnancy category:* C; PB: 50%–60%; t½: 3.5 h
Isopropamide iodide (Darbid)	A: PO: 5 mg b.i.d. or q12h; may increase to 10 mg b.i.d.	To treat peptic ulcer and irritable bowel syndrome. Not for use in children under 12 y. *Pregnancy category:* C; PB: UK; t½: UK
Mepenzolate bromide (Cantil)	A: PO: 25–50 mg t.i.d. with meals and h.s.	To treat peptic ulcer, irritable bowel syndrome. Efficacy not established in children. *Pregnancy category:* C; PB: UK; t½: UK
Methscopolamine bromide (Pamine)	A: PO: 2.5 mg a.c., and 2.5–5.0 mg, h.s. C: PO: 0.2 mg/kg q.i.d.	Treatment of peptic ulcer and irritable bowel syndrome. Avoid use with prostatic hypertrophy and intestinal atony. *Pregnancy category:* C; PB: UK; t½: UK
Oxyphencyclimine HCl (Daricon)	A: PO: 5–10 mg b.i.d., t.i.d.	For peptic ulcer and irritable bowel syndrome. Not for use in children under 12 y. *Pregnancy category:* C; PB: UK; t½: UK
Propantheline bromide (Pro-Banthine)	A: PO: 15 mg a.c. t.i.d; 30 mg h.s.; max: 120 mg/d Elderly: 7.5 mg a.c. t.i.d.	Antispasmodic for peptic ulcer and irritable bowel syndrome. Also used for pancreatitis and urinary bladder spasm. *Pregnancy category:* C; PB: UK; t½: 9 h
Scopolamine hydrobromide (also hyoscine hydrobromide)	*Preoperative:* A: PO: 0.5–1.0 mg SC/IM/IV: 0.3–0.6 mg C: SC: 0.006 mg/kg or 0.2 mg/m²; max: 0.3 mg *Motion sickness:* A: PO: 0.3–0.6 mg; transderm patch: 1 patch behind ear q72h	For preanesthetic drug, irritable bowel syndrome, motion sickness, and to treat delirium. Contraindicated in narrow-angle glaucoma, obstructive GI disease, severe ulcerative colitis, and paralytic ileus. *Pregnancy category:* C; PB: <30%; t½: 8 h

TABLE 19–4 *Continued*

Generic (Brand)	Route and Dosage	Uses and Considerations
Cholinergic Antagonists: **Eye**		
Cyclopentolate HCl (Cyclogyl)	0.5%–2%, sol, 1–2 gtt	For mydriasis and cycloplegic for eye examination. See Chapter 38.
Homatropine (Isopto Homatropine)	2%–5% sol, 1–2 gtt	For mydriasis and cycloplegia (paralysis of ciliary muscle resulting in loss of accommodation) for eye examination. See Chapter 38.
Tropicamide (Mydriacyl Ophthalmic)	0.5%–1% sol, 1–2 gtt	For mydriasis and cycloplegia for eye examination. See Chapter 38.
Anticholinergic-Antiparkin- **sonism Drugs**		
Benztropine mesylate (Cogentin)	*Parkinsonism:* A: PO: IV: Initially 0.5–1.0 mg/d in 1–2 divided doses (larger dose at h.s.); maint: 0.5–6 mg/d in 1–2 divided doses	Treatment of parkinsonism and drug-induced extrapyramidal syndrome (EPS). See Chapter 20.
Biperiden lactate (Akineton)	*Parkinsonism:* A: PO: 2 mg t.i.d./q.i.d. IM/IV: 2 mg q30min for 4 doses	Same as benztropine mesylate. See Chapter 20.
Procyclidine HCl (Kemadrin)	*Parkinsonism:* A: PO: 2.5–5 mg pc t.i.d.; maint: 10–20 mg/d	Same as benztropine mesylate. See Chapter 20.
Trihexyphenidyl HCl (Artane, Trihexy)	*Parkinsonism:* A: PO: Initially 1–2 mg/d, increase to 6–10 mg/d in divided doses	Same as benztropine mesylate. See Chapter 20.

KEY: *A: adult; C: child; PO: by mouth; IM: intramuscular; IV: intravenous; PB: protein-binding; t½: half-life; ac: before meals; UK: unknown; sol: solution; <: less than; >: more than.*

NURSING PROCESS: ANTICHOLINERGIC DRUGS: Atropine

ASSESSMENT

- Obtain baseline vital signs (VS) for future comparison. Tachycardia is a side effect that occurs with large doses of anticholinergics such as atropine sulfate.
- Assess urine output. Urinary retention may occur.
- Check the client's medical history. Atropine and atropine-like drugs are contraindicated if the client has narrow-angle glaucoma, obstructive GI disorder, paralytic ileus, ulcerative colitis, benign prostatic hypertrophy (BPH), or myasthenia gravis.
- Obtain a history of the drugs the client is taking. Phenothiazines and antidepressants increase the effect of anticholinergics.

POTENTIAL NURSING DIAGNOSES

- Urinary retention
- Altered oral mucous membrane
- Constipation

PLANNING

- The client's secretions will be decreased before surgery.
- Client will not have side effects that may become a health problem.

NURSING INTERVENTIONS

- Monitor the client's VS. Report if tachycardia occurs.
- Check intake and output. Encourage the client to void before taking the medication. Report decreased urine output. Anticholinergics can cause urinary retention. Maintain adequate fluid intake.
- Check bowel sounds. Absence of bowel sounds may indicate paralytic ileus due to decrease in GI motility (peristalsis).
- Check for constipation due to the decrease in GI motility. Encourage the client to ingest foods that are high in fiber, to drink adequate amounts of fluids, and to exercise if able.

- Raise bedside rails for clients who are confused, debilitated, or elderly. Atropine could cause CNS stimulation (excitement, confusion) or drowsiness.
- Administer mouth care. Atropine decreases oral secretions and can cause dryness of the mouth.
- Administer IV atropine undiluted or diluted in 10 mL of sterile water. Rate of administration is 0.6 mg/min.

CLIENT TEACHING

General
- Instruct the client with glaucoma to avoid atropine-like drugs. Anticholinergics cause mydriasis and increase the intraocular pressure. Clients should be alerted to check labels on OTC drugs to determine if they are contraindicated for glaucoma.
- Instruct the client not to drive a motor vehicle or participate in activities that require alertness. Drowsiness is common.
- Advise the client to avoid alcohol, cigarette smoking, caffeine, and aspirin at bedtime to decrease gastric acidity.
- Instruct the client with mydriasis from an eye examination to use sunglasses in bright light because of photophobia (intolerance of bright light).

Anticholinergic
- Instruct the client to avoid hot environments and excess physical exertion. Elevations in body temperature can result from diminished sweat gland activity.

Diet
- Suggest that the client's diet include foods high in fiber and increased water intake to prevent constipation.

Side Effects
- Advise the client of common side effects from long-term use of anticholinergics, such as dry mouth, decrease in urination, and constipation.
- Instruct the client to increase fluid intake to prevent constipation when taking anticholinergics for a prolonged period of time.
- Instruct the client to urinate before taking the anticholinergic. Urinary retention can be a problem. The client should report a marked decrease in urine output.
- Suggest that the client use hard candy, ice chips, or chewing gum and maintain effective oral hygiene if the client's mouth is dry. Anticholinergics decrease salivation.
- Encourage the client to use Artificial Tears (eye drops) for dry eyes due to decreased lacrimation (tearing).

EVALUATION

- Evaluate the client's response to the anticholinergic.
- Determine if constipation, urine retention, or increased pulse rate is or remains a problem.

STUDY QUESTIONS

1. What are the actions of cholinergic drugs and anticholinergic drugs? Differentiate between direct-acting and indirect-acting cholinergic drugs.
2. What are the major side effects of cholinergic and anticholinergic drugs? What are the implications for client teaching for each of these classes of drugs?
3. What are the general uses and indications for cholinergic and anticholinergic drugs?
4. What are the nursing implications associated with the use of cholinergic and anticholinergic drugs?
5. Your client has glaucoma. What should you instruct the client regarding OTC drugs? The same client is to have surgery and atropine has been ordered. What are your nursing responsibilities?

Chapter 20

Drugs for Neuromuscular Disorders: Parkinsonism, Myasthenia Gravis, Multiple Sclerosis, and Muscle Spasms

OUTLINE

Objectives
Terms
Introduction
Parkinsonism
    Anticholinergics
    Nursing Process
    Dopaminergics
    Dopamine Agonists

Nursing Process
Myasthenia Gravis
    Acetylcholinesterase
      Inhibitors
    Nursing Process
Multiple Sclerosis
Skeletal Muscle Relaxants

Centrally Acting Muscle
    Relaxants
Peripherally Acting Muscle
    Relaxants
    Nursing Process
Case Study
Study Questions

OBJECTIVES

Define parkinsonism, myasthenia gravis, and multiple sclerosis.

Describe the actions of anticholinergic drugs and dopaminergic drugs in the treatment of parkinsonism.

Describe the side effects of antiparkinsonism drugs.

Identify the drug group for the treatment of myasthenia gravis.

Differentiate between centrally acting and peripherally acting muscle relaxants. Give an example of a drug from each group.

Describe the nursing interventions, including client teaching, of drugs used in the treatment of parkinsonism, myasthenia gravis, and muscle spasms.

Explain the treatment strategies for Multiple Sclerosis (MS).

TERMS

acetylcholinesterase inhibitor
bradykinesia
cholinergic crisis
dyskinesia

dystonic movement
multiple sclerosis
muscle relaxants
myasthenia crisis

myasthenia gravis
parkinsonism
pseudoparkinsonism

INTRODUCTION

Four types of neuromuscular disorders, and the drugs used to treat them are discussed in this chapter: parkinsonism, myasthenia gravis, multiple sclerosis, and muscle spasms. **Parkinsonism** (Parkinson's disease), a chronic neurologic disorder that affects the extrapyramidal motor tract (which controls posture, balance, and locomotion), is considered a syndrome (combination of symptoms) because of its three major features: rigidity, **bradykinesia** (slow movement), and tremors. Rigidity (abnormally increased muscle tone) increases with movement. Postural changes due to rigidity and bradykinesia include the chest and head thrust forward with the knees and hips flexed, a shuffling gait, and the absence of arm swing. Other characteristic symptoms are masked facies (no facial expression), involuntary tremors of the head and neck, and pill-rolling motions of the hands. The tremors may be more prevalent at rest.

Myasthenia gravis, a lack of nerve impulses and muscle responses at the myoneural (nerves in muscle endings) junction, causes fatigue and muscular weakness of the respiratory system, facial muscles, and extremities. Because of cranial nerve involvement, ptosis (drooping eyelid) and difficulty in chewing and swallowing occur. Respiratory arrest may result due to respiratory muscle paralysis. Myasthenia gravis is caused by an inadequate secretion of acetylcholine or a loss of acetylcholine because of an increase of the enzyme acetylcholinesterase which destroys acetylcholine at the myoneural junction.

Multiple Sclerosis (MS) treatment strategies for acute, remissions and exacerbations, and chronic progressive phases of MS are described in table form. This neuromuscular disorder is difficult to diagnose; therefore, pharmacologic treatment is necessary to control the symptoms of this disorder.

Muscle spasms have various causes, including injury or motor neuron disorders, resulting in conditions such as cerebral palsy, multiple sclerosis, spinal cord injuries (paraplegia—paralysis of the legs), and cerebral vascular accident (stroke) or hemiplegia (paralysis of one side of the body). Spasticity of muscles can be reduced with the use of skeletal muscle relaxants.

PARKINSONISM

Parkinsonism is caused by an imbalance of the neurotransmitters dopamine and acetylcholine. It seems that those with parkinsonism lack sufficient dopamine and have too much acetylcholine at the basal ganglia of the extrapyramidal motortract.

There are two neurotransmitters within neurons of the striatum of the brain: dopamine, an inhibitory neurotransmitter; and acetylcholine, an excitatory neurotransmitter. Dopamine is released from the dopaminergic neurons; acetylcholine is released from the cholinergic neurons. Dopamine normally maintains control of acetylcholine and inhibits its excitatory response. With Parkinson's disease (parkinsonism), there is a degeneration of the dopaminergic neurons (cause unknown); thus, an imbalance between dopamine and acetylcholine occurs. With less dopamine production, acetylcholine is released, thereby causing the excitation and movement disorders seen in Parkinsonism.

By the time early symptoms of Parkinson's disease appear, 80% of the striatal dopamine has been depleted. The remaining striatal neurons synthesize the dopamine from levodopa and release dopamine as needed. Before the next dose of levodopa, symptoms (slow walking, loss of dexterity) return or worsen; 30 to 60 minutes after the dose, the client's functioning is much improved.

The drugs used to treat parkinsonism by reducing the symptoms or replacing the dopamine deficit fall into two categories: (1) anticholinergics, which block the cholinergic receptors, and (2) dopaminergics, which stimulate the dopamine receptors.

ANTICHOLINERGICS

Anticholinergic drugs reduce the rigidity and some of the tremors characteristic of parkinsonism but have minimal effect on the bradykinesia. The anticholinergics are parasympatholytics that inhibit the release of acetylcholine. Anticholinergics are still used to treat drug-induced parkinsonism **(pseudoparkinsonism),** a side effect of the antipsychotic drug group phenothiazines. Examples of anticholinergics used for parkinsonism include trihexyphenidyl (Artane), benztropine (Cogentin), biperiden (Akineton), procyclidine (Kemadrin), ethopropazine (Parsidol), and orphenadrine (Norflex). The latter two drugs are the newer anticholinergics.

Table 20–1 lists the anticholinergics, their dosages, uses, and considerations. Nursing process for anticholinergics for antiparkinsonism is presented according to assessment, potential nursing diagnoses, planning, nursing interventions, and evaluation. Anticholinergics used to treat parkinsonism are also discussed in Chapter 19.

TABLE 20–1 Antiparkinsonism Drugs: Anticholinergics

Generic (Brand)	Route and Dosage	Uses and Considerations
Benztropine mesylate (Cogentin)	*Parkinsonism:* A: PO: Initially 0.5–1.0 mg/d in 1–2 divided doses (larger dose at h.s.); maint: 0.5–6 mg/d in 1–2 divided doses *Extrapyramidal syndrome:* A: PO: 1–4 mg/d in 1–2 divided doses IM/IV: 1–2 mg/d	For parkinsonism and drug-induced parkinsonism to reduce dystonia. May be taken with other antiparkinsonism drugs. Contraindicated in glaucoma, GI obstruction, severe ulcerative colitis, prostatic hypertrophy, myasthenia gravis. *Pregnancy category:* C; PB: UK; t½: UK
Biperiden HCl (Akineton)	*Parkinsonism:* A: PO: 2 mg t.i.d./q.i.d. IM/IV: 2 mg every 30 min to 4 doses; *max:* 8 mg/d C: IM/IV: 0.04 mg/kg or 1.2 mg/m², repeat if necessary	For parkinsonism and drug-induced parkinsonism (extrapyramidal symptoms [EPS]). With prolonged use, drug tolerance may occur. Similar contraindications as benztropine. Avoid taking drug with alcohol or CNS depressants. Dry mouth, blurred vision, drowsiness, muscle weakness and constipation may occur. *Pregnancy category:* C; PB: UK; t½: UK
Ethopropazine HCl (Parsidol)	*Parkinsonism:* A: PO: Initially 50 mg daily/b.i.d.; maint: 100–400 mg/d in divided doses; *max:* 600 mg/d in divided doses	For all types of parkinsonism. A phenothiazine derivative with anticholinergic and antihistamine effects. Common side effects include: dry mouth, drowsiness, dizziness, confusion, urinary retention, constipation. Contraindications: glaucoma, GU obstruction, prostatic hypertrophy. *Pregnancy category:* C; PB: UK; t½: UK
Orphenadrine HCl or citrate (Disipal, Norflex, Banflex)	A: PO: 50 mg t.i.d. or 100 mg b.i.d.	For parkinsonism. It is an antihistamine with some anticholinergic effects. Has slight CNS stimulation and can cause euphoria. *Pregnancy category:* C; PB: UK; t½: 14 h
Procyclidine HCl (Kemadrin)	*Parkinsonism:* A: PO: 2.5 mg p.c. t.i.d. *Extrapyramidal syndrome:* A: PO: Initially 2.5 mg p.c. t.i.d; maint: 2.5–5 mg p.c. t.i.d	For parkinsonism and drug-induced parkinsonism. Relieves rigidity more than tremors. May be taken with other antiparkinsonism drugs. Contraindicated in glaucoma. *Pregnancy category:* C; PB: UK; t½: UK
Trihexyphenidyl HCl (Artane)	See Prototype Drug Chart (Fig. 19–6)	For all types of parkinsonism. Most widely used antiparkinsonism drug. Contraindicated in narrow-angle glaucoma. Common side effects include nausea, dry mouth, nervousness, dizziness, blurred vision, constipation, urinary hesitancy. *Pregnancy category:* C; PB: UK; t½: 5 to 10 h

KEY: *A: adult; C: child; IM: intramuscular; IV: intravenous; PB: protein-binding; PO: by mouth: t½: half-life; UK: unknown.*

NURSING PROCESS: ANTIPARKINSONISM: Anticholinergic

ASSESSMENT

- Obtain a medical history. Report if the client has a history of glaucoma, gastrointestinal (GI) dysfunction, urinary retention, angina pectoris, or myasthenia gravis. All anticholinergics are contraindicated if the client has glaucoma.
- Obtain a drug history. Report if a drug-drug interaction is probable. Phenothiazines, tricyclic antidepressants, and antihistamines increase the effect of trihexyphenidyl.
- Assess baseline vital signs (VS) for future comparisons. Pulse rate may increase.
- Determine usual urinary output as a baseline for comparison. Urinary retention may occur with continuous use of anticholinergics.

POTENTIAL NURSING DIAGNOSES

- Impaired physical mobility
- High risk for activity intolerance

PLANNING

- Client will have decreased involuntary symptoms due to parkinsonism or drug-induced parkinsonism.

NURSING INTERVENTIONS

- Monitor VS, urine output, and bowel sounds. Increased pulse rate, urinary retention, and constipation are side effects of anticholinergics.
- Observe for involuntary movements.

General

- Advise the client to avoid alcohol, cigarette smoking, caffeine, and aspirin to decrease gastric acidity.

Diet

- Encourage the client to ingest foods that are high in fiber and to increase fluid intake to prevent constipation.

Side Effects

- Suggest that the client relieve dry mouth with hard candy, ice chips, or sugarless chewing gum. Anticholinergics decrease salivation.
- Suggest that the client use sunglasses in direct sun because of possible photophobia.

- Advise the client to void before taking the drug to minimize urinary retention. This is especially important if urine retention is present.
- Advise the client taking an anticholinergic to control symptoms of parkinsonism to have routine eye examinations to determine the presence of increased intraocular pressure, which indicates glaucoma. Clients who have glaucoma should *not* take anticholinergics.

EVALUATION

- Evaluate the client's response to trihexyphenidyl to determine if parkinsonism symptoms are controlled.

DOPAMINERGICS

Levodopa

The first dopaminergic drug was levodopa (L-dopa), introduced in 1961. Levodopa is the most effective drug for diminishing the symptoms of Parkinson's disease. Because dopamine cannot cross the blood–brain barrier, levodopa, a precursor of dopamine that can cross the blood–brain barrier, was developed. The enzyme dopa decarboxylase converts levodopa to dopamine in the brain. However, this enzyme is also found in the peripheral nervous system, thereby allowing 99% of levodopa to be converted to dopamine before it reaches the brain. Because only about 1% of levodopa is converted to dopamine in the brain, large doses of the drug are needed to achieve a pharmacologic response. Many side effects occur because of these high doses, including nausea, vomiting, dyskinesia, orthostatic hypotension, cardiac dysrhythmias, and psychosis. Levodopa has a short half-life (1 to 2 h), so the drug is taken three to four times a day. The drug is initially administered in low doses for a week and gradually increased over a period of weeks. It usually takes 2 to 4 months to achieve the maximum effect of the drug. Table 20–2 lists the purposes for drugs used to treat parkinsonism.

Carbidopa and Levodopa

Because of levodopa's side effects and the fact that so much of the levodopa is metabolized before it reaches the brain, an alternative drug, carbidopa, was developed that inhibits the enzyme dopa de-

carboxylase. By inhibiting the enzyme in the periphery, more levodopa reaches the brain. The carbidopa is combined with levodopa in a ratio of 1 part carbidopa to 10 parts levodopa. Figure 20–1 outlines the comparative action of levodopa and carbidopa-levodopa.

The advantages of combining levodopa with carbidopa are:

1. More dopamine reaches the basal ganglia.
2. A single dose per day is administered instead of multiple doses.
3. Smaller doses of levodopa are required to achieve the desired effect.

The disadvantage of the carbidopa-levodopa combination is that with more available levodopa, more side effects may be noted, including nausea, vomiting, **dystonic movements** (involuntary abnormal movements), and psychotic behavior. The drug is usually not prescribed for drug-related parkinsonism. The peripheral side effects of levodopa are not as prevalent; however, cardiac dysrhythmia, palpitations, and orthostatic hypotension may occur. Figure 20–2 lists the pharmacologic behavior of carbidopa-levodopa.

DOPAMINE AGONISTS

Other dopamine agonists stimulate the dopamine receptors. For example, amantadine hydrochloride (Symmetrel) is an antiviral drug and acts on the dopamine receptors. It may be taken as the only drug for parkinsonism or taken in combination with levodopa or an anticholinergic drug. Amantadine can be used for drug-induced parkinsonism.

TABLE 20–2 Comparison of Drugs to Treat Parkinson's Disease

Drug	Purpose
Dopaminergics Levodopa Carbidopa-levodopa	Decrease symptoms of parkinsonism. Carbidopa, a decarboxylase inhibitor, permits more levodopa to reach the striatum nerve terminals (where levodopa is converted to dopamine). With the use of carbidopa, less levodopa is needed.
Dopamine Agonists Amantadine	Amantadine was first used as an antiviral drug for influenza A. It decreases symptoms of parkinsonism. It can be given as an early treatment for Parkinson's disease, which could delay the use of levodopa. Amantadine is effective in treating drug-induced parkinsonism and has fewer side effects than anticholinergics.
Bromocriptine	A D_2 dopamine receptor agonist. Bromocriptine may be used for early treatment of Parkinson's disease. With increasing motor symptoms, bromocriptine can be given with levodopa therapy.
Pergolide	A D_1 and D_2 dopamine receptor agonist. It is more potent than bromocriptine and may be used for early treatment of Parkinson's disease. Pergolide can be used with levodopa.
MAO-B Inhibitor Selegiline	Inhibits the catabolic enzymes of dopamine. MAO-B inhibitor extends the action of dopamine. It can be given in the early diagnosed phase of Parkinson's disease. If the drug is given with levodopa, the dosage of levodopa is usually decreased.
Anticholinergics; **Antiparkinsonism**	Anticholinergics were the first group of drugs used to treat Parkinson's disease before levodopa and dopamine agonists were introduced. Anticholinergics are useful in decreasing tremors related to Parkinson's disease. Today, the major use of these agents is to treat drug-induced parkinsonism. Treatment should start with low dosages and then the dose should gradually be increased. The elderly are more susceptible to the many side effects of anticholinergics. Those clients with memory loss or dementia should *not* be on anticholinergic therapy.

Bromocriptine mesylate (Parlodel) acts directly on the dopamine receptors in the central nervous system (CNS), cardiovascular system, and GI tract. Bromocriptine is more effective than amantadine and the anticholinergics; however, it is not as effective as levodopa in alleviating parkinsonian symptoms. Clients who do not tolerate levodopa are frequently given bromocriptine. It is thought that dopamine receptors affected by bromocriptine are different from those affected by levodopa. Bromocriptine may be given with levodopa or carbidopa-levodopa.

The enzyme monoamine oxidase-B (MAO-B) causes catabolism (breakdown) of dopamine. Selegiline inhibits MAO-B, thus prolonging the action of levodopa. It may be ordered for newly diagnosed clients with Parkinson's disease. This drug could delay levodopa therapy by a year. Table 20–2

FIGURE 20–1. Levodopa and carbidopa-levodopa. *(A)* Levodopa. Ninety-nine percent of levodopa has been converted to dopamine in the periphery, and 1% of levodopa reaches the brain. *(B)* Carbidopa–levodopa. Carbidopa in this combination of carbidopa–levodopa inhibits the enzyme decarboxylase in the periphery. Thus, more levodopa reaches the brain.

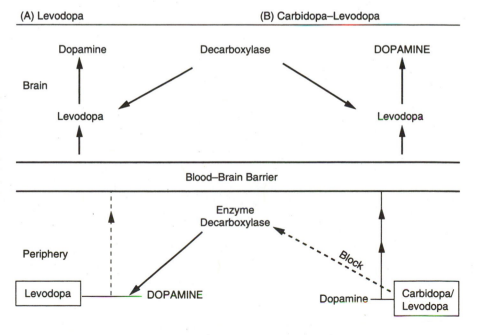

FIGURE 20–2. Antiparkinsonism: Dopaminergic

Carbidopa-Levodopa	Dosage	NURSING PROCESS Assessment and Planning
Carbidopa-Levodopa (Sinemet) Pregnancy Category: C	A: PO: 1:10 ratio; initially 10 carbidopa/100 levodopa t.i.d.; maint: 25/250 mg t.i.d.	

Contraindications	Drug-Lab-Food Interactions	
Narrow-angle glaucoma; severe cardiac, renal, or hepatic disease Caution: peptic ulcer, psychiatric disorders	Increase hypertensive crisis with MAOIs Decrease levodopa effect with anticholinergics, phenytoin, tricyclic antidepressants, pyridoxine Lab: May increase BUN, AST, ALT, ALP, LDH Food: Avoid foods containing pyridoxine (vitamin B_6)	

Pharmacokinetics	Pharmacodynamics	Interventions
Absorption: PO: Well absorbed Distribution: PB: Carbidopa: 36%; levodopa: UK Metabolism: t½: 1–2 h Excretion: In urine as metabolites	PO: Onset: 15 min Peak: 1–3 h Duration: 5–12 h	

Therapeutic Effects/Uses: To treat parkinsonism, to relieve tremors and rigidity. Mode of Action: Transmission of levodopa to brain cells for conversion to dopamine; carbidopa blocks the conversion of levodopa to dopamine in the periphery.	Evaluation

Side Effects	Adverse Reactions
Anorexia, nausea, vomiting, dysphagia, fatigue, dizziness, headache, dry mouth, bitter taste, twitching, blurred vision, insomnia	Involuntary choreiform movements, palpitations, orthostatic hypotension, urinary retention, psychosis, severe depression, hallucinations Life-threatening: Agranulocytosis, hemolytic anemia, cardiac dysrhythmias, leukopenia

KEY: A: adult; PO: by mouth; PB: protein-binding; t½: half-life; MAOIs: monoamine oxidase inhibitors; UK: unknown.

gives a comparison of the drugs used to control parkinsonism. Table 20–3 lists dopaminergics, dopamine agonists, and MAO-B inhibitors, their dosages, and uses and considerations.

Side Effects and Adverse Reactions

The common side effects of anticholinergics include dry mouth and dry secretions, urinary retention, constipation, blurred vision, and an increase in pulse rate. Mental effects, such as restlessness and confusion, may occur in the older adult.

The side effects of levodopa are numerous. GI disturbances are common since dopamine stimulates the chemoreceptor trigger zone (CTZ) in the medulla, which stimulates the vomiting center. Nausea and vomiting can be decreased by taking the drug with food or at mealtime; however, food

TABLE 20–3 Antiparkinsonism: Dopaminergics

Generic (Brand)	Route and Dosage	Uses and Considerations
Dopaminergics Carbidopa-Levodopa (Sinemet)	See Prototype Drug Chart (Fig. 20–2)	For parkinsonism. More levodopa reaches the brain; carbidopa blocks dopa decarboxylase in the periphery. Lower doses of levodopa are needed; thus fewer side effects. *Pregnancy category:* C; PB: 36% (carbidopa); t½: 1–2 h
Levodopa (or L-dopa) (Dopar, Larodopa)	A: PO: 0.5–1.0 g/d in 2–4 divided doses; increase dose gradually; average maint: 3–6 g/d with food, in divided doses; *max:* 8 mg/d	For parkinsonism. *Not* for drug-induced parkinsonism. Can cause GI upset; drug should be taken with food. Has many side effects, such as nausea, vomiting, orthostatic hypotension, cardiac dysrhythmias, and psychosis. *Pregnancy category:* C; PB: UK; t½: 1–3 h
Dopamine Agonists Amantadine HCl; (Symmetrel)	*Parkinsonism:* A: PO: 100 mg b.i.d.; may increase dose; *max:* 400 mg/d	For early onset parkinsonism, drug-induced parkinsonism, and influenza A respiratory virus. Effective for rigidity and bradykinesia; less effective for decreasing tremors. May be used alone or in combination. Has fewer side effects than anticholinergic drugs. *Pregnancy category:* C; PB: 60–70%; t½: 12–24 h
Bromocriptine mesylate (Parlodel)	A: PO: Initially 1.25–2.5 mg/d; may gradually increase dose; maint: 30–60 mg/d in 3 divided doses; *max:* 100 mg/d	For parkinsonism. Response is better than amantadine. Can be taken in adjunct with levodopa or carbidopa-levodopa. Hypotension, lightheadedness, and syncope are major side effects. Initially, small doses are given and then gradually increased over several weeks. *Pregnancy category:* C; PB: 90–96%; t½: 6–8 h: terminal phase: 50 h
Pergolide mesylate (Permax)	A: PO: Initially 0.05 mg/d × 2d; increase by 0.1–0.15 mg q3d × 12d; *max:* 5 mg/d	For parkinsonism. Usually used as adjunct with levodopa or carbidopa-levodopa. It is more potent than bromocriptine. Same side effects as bromocriptine. *Pregnancy category:* B; PB: 90%; t½: UK
MAO-B Inhibitor Selegiline HCl (Eldepryl)	A: PO: 10 mg/d in 2 divided doses	For early onset parkinsonism. May delay the use of levodopa therapy by 1 year. It can be given with levodopa preparations; dose of levodopa would need to be decreased. *Pregnancy category:* C; PB: >90%; t½: 2–20 h

KEY: *A: adult; PB: protein-binding; PO: by mouth; t½: half-life; UK: unknown; ×: times.*

will slow the absorption rate. **Dyskinesia** (impaired voluntary movement) may occur with high levodopa dosages. Cardiovascular side effects include orthostatic hypotension and increased heart rate during early use of levodopa. Cardiac dysrhythmias may occur as the levodopa dosages are increased. Psychosis (paranoia) and increased libido are additional side effects of increased levodopa dosages.

Amantadine has few side effects, but they can intensify when the drug is combined with other antiparkinsonism drugs. Orthostatic hypotension, confusion, urinary retention, and constipation are common side effects of amantadine. Side effects from bromocriptine are more common than from amantadine and include GI disturbances (nausea), orthostatic hypotension, palpitations, chest pain, edema in the lower extremities, nightmares, delusions, and confusion. If bromocriptine is taken with levodopa, usually the drug dosages are reduced and side effects and drug intolerance decrease.

Contraindications

Anticholinergics or any drugs that have anticholinergic effects are contraindicated for persons with glaucoma. Persons with severe cardiac, renal, or psychiatric health problems should avoid levodopa drugs because of adverse reactions. Clients with chronic obstructive lung diseases, such as emphysema, can have dry, thick mucous secretions due to large doses of anticholinergic drugs.

Drug-Drug Interactions

Pyridoxine (vitamin B₆) increases dopa decarboxylase action, which metabolizes levodopa in the peripheral nervous system to dopamine. Foods rich in pyridoxine such as beans (lima, navy, and kidney) and certain cereals should therefore be avoided. Antipsychotic drugs block the receptors for dopamine. Levodopa taken with a MAO inhibitor antidepressant can cause a hypertensive crisis.

NURSING PROCESS: ANTIPARKINSONISM: DOPAMINERGIC AGENT:
Carbidopa-Levodopa

ASSESSMENT

- Obtain the client's VS to use for future comparison.
- Assess the client for signs and symptoms of parkinsonism, including stooped forward posture; shuffling gait; masked facies; and resting tremors.
- Obtain a history from the client of glaucoma, heart disease, peptic ulcers, kidney or liver disease, and psychosis.
- Report if drug-drug interaction is probable. Drugs that should be avoided or closely monitored are levodopa, bromocriptine, and anticholinergics.
- Obtain a drug history.

POTENTIAL NURSING DIAGNOSES

- Impaired physical mobility
- High risk for activity intolerance

PLANNING

- Symptoms of parkinsonism will be decreased or absent after 1 to 4 wk of drug therapy.

NURSING INTERVENTIONS

- Monitor the client's VS and electrocardiogram (ECG). Orthostatic hypotension may occur during early use of levodopa and bromocriptine. Have the client rise slowly to avoid faintness.
- Check for weakness, dizziness, or syncope, which are symptoms of orthostatic hypotension.
- Administer carbidopa-levodopa (Sinemet) with low-protein foods. High-protein diets interfere with drug transport to the CNS.
- Observe for parkinsonism symptoms.

CLIENT TEACHING

General
- Advise the client not to abruptly discontinue the medication. Rebound parkinsonism (increased symptoms of parkinsonism) can occur.
- Inform the client that urine may be discolored and will darken with exposure to air. Perspiration also may be dark. Explain that both are harmless but that clothes may be stained.

- Advise the diabetic client that the blood sugar should be checked with an over-the-counter (OTC) reagent strip (Hemastix or Chemstrip bG) and not done through urine testing. With Clinitest, a false-positive test result can occur; with Tes-Tape or Clinistix, a false-negative test result can occur.

Diet
- Suggest to the client that taking levodopa with food may decrease GI upset; however, food will slow the drug absorption rate.
- Advise the client to avoid vitamins that contain vitamin B_6 (pyridoxine) and foods rich in vitamin B_6, such as beans (lima, navy, kidney) and cereals that contain the vitamin.

Side Effects
- Instruct the client to report side effects and symptoms of dyskinesia. Explain to the client that it may take weeks or months before the symptoms are controlled.

Amantadine and Bromocriptine
- Suggest that the client taking amantadine report any signs of skin lesions, seizures, or depression. A history of these health problems should have been reported to the health care provider.
- Advise the client taking bromocriptine to report symptoms of lightheadedness when changing positions (a symptom of orthostatic hypotension).
- Advise the client to avoid alcohol when taking bromocriptine.
- Teach the client to check heart rate and to report changes in rate or irregularity. The client should know baseline heart rate.
- Instruct the client not to abruptly stop the drug without first notifying the health care provider. Any adverse reactions should be reported immediately.

EVALUATION

- Evaluate the effectiveness of the drug therapy in controlling the symptoms of parkinsonism.
- Determine that there is an absence of side effects.

MYASTHENIA GRAVIS

Myasthenia gravis results from a lack of acetylcholine reaching the cholinergic receptors. This health problem is characterized by weakness and fatigue of the skeletal muscles. A possible cause of the decrease in acetylcholine (ACh) is that the enzyme acetylcholinesterase (AChE) destroys the ACh. The group of drugs for controlling myasthenia gravis is the AChE inhibitors, also known as cholinesterase inhibitors and anticholinesterase, that inhibit the action of the enzyme. As the result of this action, more ACh activates the cholinergic receptors and promotes muscle contraction. The **AChE inhibitors** are classified as parasympathomimetics.

ACETYLCHOLINESTERASE INHIBITORS

The first drug used to manage myasthenia gravis was neostigmine (Prostigmin). It is a short-acting AChE inhibitor with a half-life of 0.5 to 1 h. The drug is given every 2 to 4 h and must be given on time to prevent muscle weakness. The AChE inhibitor, pyridostigmine bromide (Mestinon), has an intermediate action and is given every 3 to 6 h. Ambenonium chloride (Mytelase) is a long-acting AChE inhibitor and is usually prescribed when the client does not respond to neostigmine or pyridostigmine. Figure 20–3 lists the drug data related to pyridostigmine. The cholinesterase (AChE) inhibitors are also discussed in Chapter 19.

Pharmacokinetics

Pyridostigmine is poorly absorbed from the GI tract. Fifty percent of the sustained-release capsule is absorbed readily and the balance is poorly absorbed. The half-life of oral pyridostigmine is 3.5 to 4 h, and intravenously it is 2 h. Because of its short half-life, it must be administered several times a day. The drug is metabolized by the liver and excreted in the urine.

Pharmacodynamics

Pyridostigmine increases muscle strength of clients with muscular weakness due to myasthenia gravis. The onset of action of oral preparations is 0.5 to 1 h. The duration of action is longer with the sustained-release drug capsule. One-thirtieth (1/30th) of the oral dose of pyridostigmine can be administered intravenously. Overdosing of pyridostigmine can result in signs and symptoms of **cholinergic crisis** (increased salivation, tears, sweating, and miosis); thus, the antidote, atropine sulfate, should be available. This crisis requires emergency medical intervention.

Edrophonium chloride (Tensilon) is a drug used in diagnosing myasthenia gravis. It is a very short-acting AChE inhibitor that increases muscle strength during its duration of action (5 to 20 min). If ptosis (droopy eyelid) is immediately corrected after administration of this drug, the diagnosis is most likely myasthenia gravis. Table 20–4 lists the acetylcholinesterase inhibitors.

TABLE 20–4 Acetylcholinesterase (AChE) Inhibitors: Myasthenia

Generic (Brand)	Route and Dosage	Uses and Considerations
Ambenonium (Mytelase)	A: PO: 2.5–5.0 mg t.i.d./q.i.d.; dose may be increased; maint: 5–40 mg t.i.d./q.i.d.	For myasthenia gravis. A long-acting acetylcholinesterase (AChE) inhibitor. It is 6 times more potent than neostigmine. Frequently used when client cannot take neostigmine or pyridostigmine because of the bromide component. It can be taken in adjunct with glucocorticoid drug. *Pregnancy category:* C; PB: UK; t½: UK
Edrophonium Cl (Tensilon)	A: IV 2 mg; then 8 mg if no response IM: 10 mg, may repeat with 2 mg in 30 min C <34 kg: IV: 1 mg, repeat in 30–45 sec if no response; *max:* 5 mg C >34 kg: IV: 2 mg, repeat with 1 mg if no response; *max:* 10 mg	For diagnosing myasthenia gravis. Ptosis should be absent in 1–5 min. Very short-acting drug. *Pregnancy category:* C; PB: UK; t½: 1.2–2 h
Neostigmine bromide (Prostigmin)	A: PO: 150 mg/d in divided doses; *range:*	For controlling myasthenia gravis. Must be given on time to prevent myasthenia crisis. Parenteral route is used if chewing, swallow-

Table continues on following page

TABLE 20–4 Acetylcholinesterase (AChE) Inhibitors: Myasthenia (*Continued*)

Generic (Brand)	Route and Dosage	Uses and Considerations
Neostigmine methylsulfate (injectable form)	15–375 mg/d IM/IV: 0.5–2.5 mg as needed C: PO: 2 mg/kg/d in divided doses or 10 mg/m² q4h	ing, and breathing are affected. Due to its short half-life, dose is usually given in 3 to 6 divided doses. Overdose can cause cholinergic reaction; nausea, abdominal cramps, excessive salivation, sweating. *Pregnancy category:* C; PB: 15%–25%; t½: 1–1.5 h
Pyridostigmine bromide (Mestinon)	See Prototype Drug Chart (Fig. 20–3).	For myasthenia gravis. Also used to reverse postoperative muscle paralysis due to a neuromuscular blocker. *Pregnancy category:* C; PB: UK; t½: 3.5–4 h

KEY: A: adult; C: child; PO: by mouth; IM: intramuscular; IV: intravenous; PB: protein-binding; t½: half-life; UK: unknown; <: less than; >: greater than.

FIGURE 20–3. Myasthenia Gravis (Drugs for)

		NURSING PROCESS

Cholinesterase inhibitor
 	
Pyridostigmine Bromide (Mestinon)
Pregnancy Category: C
	Dosage
	
	A: PO: 60–120 mg t.i.d./q.i.d.; max: 1.5 g/d
	  SR: 180–540 mg q.d. or b.i.d.
	  IM/IV: 2 mg q2–3h
	C: PO: 7 mg/kg/d in 5–6 divided doses
		NURSING PROCESS
		Assessment and Planning

Contraindications GI and GU obstruction, severe renal disease *Caution:* Asthma, bradycardia, peptic ulcer, cardiac dysrhythmias, pregnancy	**Drug-Lab-Food Interactions** *Decrease* pyridostigmine effect with atropine, muscle relaxants, antidysrhythmics, magnesium	

Pharmacokinetics
 	
Absorption: PO: Poorly absorbed; SR: 50% absorbed
Distribution: PB: UK
Metabolism: t½: PO: 3.5–4 h; IV: 2 h
Excretion: In urine and by liver
	Pharmacodynamics
	
	PO: Onset: 30–45 min
	    Peak: UK
	    Duration: 3–6 h
	PO SR: Onset: 0.5–1 h
	    Peak: UK
	    Duration: 6–12 h
	IM: Onset: 15 min
	    Peak: UK
	    Duration: 2–4 h
	IV: Onset: 2–5 min
	    Peak: UK
	    Duration: 2–3 h
		Interventions

Therapeutic Effects/Uses: To control and treat myasthenia gravis. *Mode of Action:* Transmission of neuromuscular impulses by preventing the destruction of acetylcholine.		Evaluation

Side Effects	**Adverse Reactions**
Nausea, vomiting, diarrhea, headache, dizziness, abdominal cramps, sweating, rash, miosis	Hypotension, urticaria *Life-threatening:* Respiratory depression, bronchospasm, cardiac dysrhythmias, seizures

KEY: A: adult; C: child; PO: by mouth; SR: sustained-release; IM: intramuscular; IV: intravenous; max: maximum; PB: protein-binding; t½: half-life; UK: unknown.

Overdosing and underdosing of AChE inhibitors have similar symptoms, such as muscle weakness, dyspnea (difficulty breathing), and dysphagia (difficulty swallowing). Additional symptoms that may be present with overdosing are increased salivation (drooling), bradycardia, abdominal cramping, and increased tearing and sweating. All doses of AChE inhibitors should be administered *on time* because late administration of the drug could result in muscle weakness.

Side Effects and Adverse Reactions

Side effects and adverse reactions of AChE inhibitors include GI disturbances (nausea, vomiting, diarrhea, abdominal cramps), increased salivation and tearing, miosis (constricted pupil of the eye), and possible hypertension.

NURSING PROCESS: MYASTHENIA GRAVIS (DRUGS FOR):
Pyridostigmine (Mestinon)

ASSESSMENT

- Obtain a drug history of drugs that the client is currently taking. Report if a drug-drug interaction is likely. Client should avoid atropine, atropine-like drugs, and muscle relaxants.
- Obtain baseline VS for future comparison.
- Assess the client for signs and symptoms of **myasthenia crisis,** such as muscle weakness with difficulty breathing and swallowing.

POTENTIAL NURSING DIAGNOSES

- Inability to sustain spontaneous ventilation
- High risk for activity intolerance
- Anxiety related to possible recurrence of myasthenia crisis

PLANNING

- The client's symptoms of muscle weakness and difficulty breathing and swallowing due to myasthenia gravis will be eliminated or reduced in 2 to 3 d.

NURSING INTERVENTIONS

- Monitor the effectiveness of drug therapy (acetylcholinesterase [AChE] inhibitors). Muscle strength should be increased. Both depth and rate of respirations should be assessed and maintained within normal range.

- Administer IV pyridostigmine undiluted at rate of 0.5 mg/min. Do *not* add the drug to IV fluids.
- Observe the client for signs and symptoms of cholinergic crisis due to overdosing, including muscle weakness, increased salivation, sweating, tearing, and miosis.
- Have readily available an antidote for cholinergic crisis (atropine sulfate).

CLIENT TEACHING

General
- Instruct the client to take the drugs as prescribed to avoid recurrence of symptoms.
- Encourage the client to wear a medical ID bracelet or necklace (e.g., Medic Alert) indicating the health problem and the drug(s) taken.

Diet
- Instruct the client to take the drug before meals for best drug absorption. If gastric irritation occurs, take the drug with food.

Side Effects
- Advise the client to report to the health care provider recurrence of symptoms of myasthenia gravis. Drug therapy may need to be modified.

EVALUATION

- Evaluate the effectiveness of the drug therapy. Muscle strength should be maintained.
- Determine the absence of respiratory distress.

MULTIPLE SCLEROSIS

Multiple sclerosis (MS) is characterized by multiple lesions of the myelin sheath called plaques. It is a condition in which there are remissions and exacerbations of multiple symptoms (sensory and cerebellar) such as motor weakness, spasticity, or diplopia.

MS is difficult to diagnose because there is no specific diagnostic test. Available laboratory tests that may suggest MS include elevated IgG in the cerebrospinal fluid, increased IgG/albumin ratio, and multiple lesions on magnetic resonance imaging (MRI). A study, cited by Noronha and Arnason, of monthly MRI scans of clients with MS indicated that the MRI scans identified four times the frequency of new lesions, suggestive of MS attacks, without clients having clinical symptoms. Having a scheduled treatment protocol to avoid clinical MS attacks is not recommended because of the side effects of the drugs used, such as glucocorticoids.

There are treatment strategies for three types or phases of MS: the acute attack, remission-exacerbation, and chronic progressive MS. Table 20–5 describes these three phases of MS. Goals for treatment strategies are to decrease the inflammatory process of nerve fibers and to improve conduction of demyelinating axons.

Drugs that the client with MS should avoid include histamine (H_2) blockers such as cimetidine and ranitidine, indomethacin (an NSAID), and beta blockers such as propranolol. Various drug regimens for treating MS are currently in research and development.

SKELETAL MUSCLE RELAXANTS

Muscle relaxants relieve muscular spasms and pain associated with traumatic injuries and chronic debilitating disorders, such as multiple sclerosis, strokes (cerebrovascular accident [CVA]), cerebral palsy, and spinal cord injuries. Spasticity results from increased muscle tone from hyperexcitable neurons due to increased stimulation from the cerebral neurons or lack of inhibition in the spinal cord or at the skeletal muscles. Muscle relaxants are divided into two major groups: the centrally acting

and peripherally acting. The centrally acting muscle relaxants depress neuron activity in the spinal cord or brain, and the peripherally acting muscle relaxants act directly on the skeletal muscles.

CENTRALLY ACTING MUSCLE RELAXANTS

The centrally acting muscle relaxants are used to treat acute spasms from muscle trauma. This group of muscle relaxants is not as effective against chronic neurologic disorders as the peripherally acting muscle relaxants, with the exceptions of diazepam (Valium) and baclofen (Lioresal). Examples of centrally acting muscle relaxants include carisoprodol (Soma), chlorphenesin carbamate (Maolate), chlorzoxazone (Paraflex), cyclobenzaprine (Flexeril), metaxalone (Skelaxin), methocarbamol (Robaxin), orphenadrine citrate (Norflex), and baclofen (Lioresal). Baclofen is a new agent that acts on the spinal cord. These drugs are similar in their action, side effects, and adverse reactions. The choice of drug is usually personal.

The centrally acting muscle relaxants decrease pain and increase range of motion. They have a sedative effect and should not be taken concurrently with CNS depressants, such as barbiturates, narcotics, and alcohol. The centrally acting muscle relaxants are described in Table 20–6.

Two anxiolytics, diazepam (Valium) and meprobamate (Equanil), may be effective in decreasing muscle spasms resulting from acute traumatic in-

---

TABLE 20–5 Treatment Strategies for the Three Phases of Multiple Sclerosis

Phases of Multiple Sclerosis	Characteristics	Treatment Strategies

Acute Attack	Fatigue, motor weakness, optic neuritis	• Tapering course of glucocorticoids (Prednisone)
		• Adrenocorticotropic hormone (ACTH) stimulates the adrenal cortex to secrete cortisol.
		• ACTH can be given IM or IV.
		  (1) Aqueous ACTH, 80 units in 500 mL of D_5W for 1–5 d
		  (2) Tapering doses of ACTH gel, IM for 25–30 d, starting with 40 units, b.i.d.
		• 6-alpha methylprednisolone sodium succinate (MP)
		  (1) MP 1 g/d, IV, for 5–7 d
		  (2) Tapering doses of oral glucocorticoid

Remission-Exacerbation	Recurrence of clinical MS symptoms; spasticity	• Biologic (immune) response modifiers (BRM); see Chapter 29. Betaseron, an interferon-B (IFN-B), 0.25 mg (8 mIU) every other day. It reduces spasticity and improves muscle movement. • Immunosuppressant drug azathioprine (Imuran). Reduces exacerbation (relapses). Used for MS to decrease steroid use.

Chronic Progressive	Progressive MS symptoms (wheelchair bound)	• Immunosuppressant cyclophosphamide (Cytoxan)
		Possible Treatment Protocol
		  (1) Cytoxan 600 mg/m^2 in 250 mL of D_5W, every other day × 5 doses. Monitor WBC values.
		  (2) ACTH, tapering doses for 14 d. Starting with 40 units, IM, b.i.d.

KEY: IM: intramuscular; IV: intravenous; m^2: square meter (body surface area); WBC: white blood count.

TABLE 20–6 Muscle Relaxants (Skeletal)

Generic (Brand)	Route and Dosage	Uses and Considerations
Anxiolytics		
Diazepam (Valium) CSS IV	A: PO: 2–10 mg b.i.d./q.i.d. IM/IV: 5–10 mg; may repeat	Diazepam has many uses, one of which is to relieve muscle spasms associated with paraplegia and cerebral palsy. Contraindicated in narrow-angle glaucoma. *Pregnancy category:* D; PB: 98%; t½: 20–50 h
Meprobamate (Equanil, Miltown) CSS IV	A: PO: 400 mg–1.2 g/d in divided doses	This anxiolytic has a muscle relaxant effect. *Pregnancy category:* D; PB: UK; t½: 10–12 h
Centrally Acting Muscle Relaxants		
Baclofen (Lioresal)	A: PO: Initially 5 mg t.i.d.; may increase dose; *maint:* 10–20 mg t.i.d./q.i.d.; *max:* 80 mg/d	For muscle spasms due to multiple sclerosis and spinal cord injury. Overdose may cause CNS depression. Drowsiness, dizziness, nausea, hypotension may occur. *Pregnancy category:* C; PB: 30%; t½: 3–4 h
Carisoprodol (Soma)	See Prototype Drug Chart (Fig. 20–4)	For muscle spasms and other painful musculoskeletal disorders. It is available in compound form with aspirin and aspirin with codeine. Same side effects as baclofen. *Pregnancy category:* C; PB: UK; t½: 8 h
Chlorphenesin carbamate (Maolate)	A: PO: Initially 800 mg t.i.d.; maint: 400 mg q.i.d.	For muscle spasm. For short-term treatment of acute spasm. *Pregnancy category:* C; PB: UK; t½: 3–4 h
Chlorzoxazone (Paraflex, Parafon Forte)	A: PO: 250–750 mg t.i.d./ q.i.d.; *max:* 3 g/d C: PO: 20 mg/kg/d or 600 mg m²/d in 3–4 divided doses	For acute or severe muscle spasms. Not effective for cerebral palsy. Take with food to decrease GI upset. *Pregnancy category:* C; PB: UK; t½: 1 h
Cyclobenzaprine HCl (Flexeril, Cycoflex)	A: PO: 10 mg t.i.d.; may increase dose; *max:* 60 mg/d	For short-term treatment of muscle spasms. Not effective for relieving cerebral or spinal cord disease. Take with food or milk to decrease GI upset. *Pregnancy category:* B; PB: 93%; t½: 1–3 d
Methocarbamol (Robaxin, Delaxin, Marbaxin)	A: PO: Initially 1.5 g q.i.d.; maint: 1 g q.i.d. IM/IV: 0.5–1 g q8h; *max:* 3 g/d	For acute muscle spasms; drug used for treatment of tetanus. Has CNS depressant effects (sedation). Avoid taking alcohol or CNS depressants. Urine may be green, brown, or black. Drowsiness that may occur usually decreases with continued drug use. *Pregnancy category:* C; PB: UK; t½: 1–2 h
Orphenadrine citrate (Norflex, Flexon)	A: PO: 100 mg b.i.d. IM/IV: 60 mg daily/b.i.d.	For acute muscle spasm. It can be toxic with a mild overdose. Used in combination with aspirin and caffeine (Norgesic). *Pregnancy category:* C; PB: <20%; t½: 14 h
Depolarizing Muscle Relaxants (adjunct to anesthesia) Pancuronium bromide (Pavulon)	A: IV: 0.04–0.1 mg/kg; then 0.01 mg/kg every 30–60 min as needed C>10 y: same as for adult.	Used in surgery for relaxation of skeletal muscle (e.g., abdominal wall). It is considered to be 5 times as potent as tubocurarine chloride. It does not cause hypotension or bronchospasm. *Pregnancy category:* C; PB: <10%; t½: 2 h
Succinylcholine Cl (Anectine Cl, Quelicin, Sucostrin)	A: IM: 2.5–4 mg/kg; *max:* 150 mg IV: 0.3–1.1 mg/kg; *max:* 150 mg C: IM/IV: 1–2mg/kg; *max:* IM: 150 mg	Used in surgery with anesthesia for skeletal muscle relaxation, Also used in endoscopy and intubation. *Pregnancy category:* C; PB: UK; t½: UK
Vecuronium bromide (Norcuron)	A or C >9 y: IV: Initially 0.08–0.1 mg/kg/dose; maint: 0.05–0.1 mg/kg/h as needed	Use is similar as succinylcholine chloride. It can be used for clients having asthma, renal disease or with limited cardiac reserve. Given after general anesthesia has been started. *Pregnancy category:* C; PB: 60%–80%; t½: 1–1.5 h
Recuronium bromide	*Anesthesia intubation:* A: IV: Initially: 0.45–0.6 mg/kg C: IV: 0.6 mg/kg *During surgery:* A: IV bolus: 0.9–1.2 mg/kg *Postoperative:* A: IV: 0.01–0.012 mg/kg/min	Similar to vecuronium. *Pregnancy category:* B; PB: 30%; t½: 2–18 min

Table continues on following page

TABLE 20–6 Muscle Relaxants (Skeletal) *(Continued)*

Generic (Brand)	Route and Dosage	Uses and Considerations
Peripherally Acting Muscle Relaxant Dantrolene sodium (Dantrium)	A: PO: Initially 25 mg/d; increase gradually; maint: 100 mg b.i.d.–q.i.d. C: PO: Initially 0.5 mg/kg b.i.d.; increase dose gradually by 0.5 mg/kg t.i.d./q.i.d.; *max*: 100 mg q.i.d.	For chronic neurologic disorders causing spasms such as spinal cord injuries, stroke, multiple sclerosis. Start with low doses and increase every 4 to 7 d. Avoid taking with alcohol and CNS depressants. *Pregnancy category*: C; PB: 95%; t½: 8 h

KEY: *A: adult; C: child; CSS: Controlled Substance Schedule; PO: by mouth; IM: intramuscular; IV: intravenous; PB: protein-binding; t½: half-life; UK: unknown; >: greater than.*

jury or chronic neurologic disorders. Diazepam may also be used as an adjunctive agent in the relief of muscle spasms.

PERIPHERALLY ACTING MUSCLE RELAXANTS

Dantrolene sodium (Dantrium), a peripherally acting muscle relaxant, acts on the muscles directly and has minimal effect on the CNS. This drug is most effective for spasticity or muscle contractions of neurologic origin (multiple sclerosis, CVA). The new centrally acting muscle relaxant baclofen is also effective in treating muscle spasms due to multiple sclerosis. However, high doses of dantrolene may cause hepatotoxicity, so liver enzyme blood tests should be monitored. Figure 20–4 compares the drug data of the centrally acting muscle relaxant carisoprodol and the peripherally acting muscle relaxant dantrolene.

Pharmacokinetics

Carisoprodol is well absorbed from the GI tract, but only 35% of dantrolene is absorbed. Both carisoprodol and dantrolene have moderate half-lives. The half-life for intravenous dantrolene is shorter than that for the oral preparation. The protein-binding percentage for carisoprodol is unknown; that for dantrolene is 90%. Signs and symptoms of drug accumulation of dantrolene should be assessed. Both drugs are metabolized in the liver and excreted in the urine.

FIGURE 20–4. Muscle Relaxants

Muscle Relaxants	Dosage	NURSING PROCESS Assessment and Planning
Centrally Acting Muscle Relaxant Carisoprodol *(C)* (Soma, Soprodol) *Pregnancy Category:* C *Peripherally Acting Muscle Relaxant* Dantrolene *(D)* (Dantrium) *Pregnancy Category:* C	*(C):* A: PO: 350 mg, t.i.d., h.s. C >5 y: PO 25 mg/kg/d in 4 divided doses. *(D):* A: PO: Initially: 25 mg/d; increase to 25 mg, b.i.d. to q.i.d. and in increments of 25 mg up to 100 mg, b.i.d.–q.i.d. IV: 2.5 mg/kg before surgery C >5 y: Initially: 0.5 mg/kg, b.i.d.; increase to 0.5 mg/kg t.i.d. or q.i.d. max: 100 mg. q.i.d.	
Contraindications	**Drug-Lab-Food Interactions**	Interventions
(C & D): Severe liver or renal disease *(D):* Severe heart disease	*(C & D):* Increase CNS depression with alcohol, narcotics, sedative-hypnotics, antihistamines, tricyclic antidepressants. May increase risk of ventricular fibrillation with calcium channel blockers	

FIGURE 20–4. Muscle Relaxants *Continued*

Pharmacokinetics	**Pharmacodynamics**
Absorption: PO: *(C):* well absorbed; *(D):* 35% absorbed *Distribution:* PB: *(C):* UK; *(D):* 90% *Metabolism:* t½: *(C):* 8 h; *(D):* 8–9 h; IV: 4–8 h *Excretion:* *(C & D):* in the urine	*(C):* PO: Onset: 30 min 　　Peak: 3–4 h 　　Duration: 4–6 h *(D):* PO: Onset: 1 h 　　Peak: 5 h 　　Duration: 8 h IV: Onset: rapid 　　Peak: rapid 　　Duration: 6–8 h

Therapeutic Effects/Uses: *(C):* To relax skeletal muscles; *(D):* To treat spasticity associated with stroke, spinal cord injury, multiple sclerosis, cerebral palsy

Mode of Action: *(C):* Blocks interneuronal activity. *(D):* Produces direct relaxation of the spastic muscle by interfering with the release of the calcium ion.

Evaluation

Side Effects	**Adverse Reactions**
(C): Nausea, vomiting, dizziness, weakness, insomnia *(D):* Muscle weakness, anorexia, vomiting, drowsiness, dizziness, diarrhea, sweating, photosensitivity, insomnia	*(C):* Asthmatic attack, tachycardia, hypotension, diplopia *(D):* Pleural effusions, tachycardia, hypotension, palpitations

KEY: PO: by mouth; IV: intravenous; UK: unknown; PB: protein-binding; t½: half-life; >: greater than.

Pharmacodynamics

Carisoprodol alleviates muscle spasm associated with acute painful musculoskeletal conditions. Dantrolene acts directly on the skeletal muscles and decreases the release of calcium, thereby aiding in the reduction of muscle spasticity. Both drugs have similar drug interactions. When these drugs are taken with alcohol, sedative-hypnotics, barbiturates, or tricylic antidepressants, increased CNS depression occurs.

The onset of action, peak concentration time, and duration of action for carisoprodol are shorter than they are for dantrolene. Dantrolene can be administered intravenously as well as orally, and the onset of action and peak time occur rapidly.

Table 20–6 lists the muscle relaxants, their dosages, uses, and considerations.

Side Effects and Adverse Reactions

The side effects from centrally acting muscle relaxants include drowsiness, dizziness, lightheadedness, headaches, and occasional nausea, vomiting, diarrhea, and abdominal distress. Cyclobenzaprine and orphenadrine have anticholinergic effects.

The side effects from peripherally acting muscle relaxants include liver toxicity (increased liver enzymes), drowsiness, photosensitivity, and occasional anorexia, nausea, and vomiting. Avoid use if the client has a history of breast cancer, because mammary malignancy could recur.

NURSING PROCESS: MUSCLE RELAXANT: Carisoprodol

ASSESSMENT

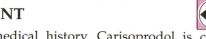

- Obtain a medical history. Carisoprodol is contraindicated if the client has severe renal or liver disease.

- Obtain baseline VS for future comparison.
- Obtain the client's history to identify the cause of muscle spasm and to determine if it is acute or chronic.

- Obtain a drug history. Report if a drug-drug interaction is probable.
- Note if there is a history of narrow-angle glaucoma or myasthenia gravis. Cyclobenzaprine and orphenadrine are contraindicated with these health problems.

POTENTIAL NURSING DIAGNOSES

- Impaired physical mobility
- Activity intolerance

PLANNING

- Client will be free of muscular pain within 1 wk.

NURSING INTERVENTIONS

- Monitor serum liver enzyme levels of clients taking dantrolene and carisoprodol. Report elevated liver enzymes, such as ALP, ALT, and GGPT.
- Monitor VS. Report abnormal results.
- Observe for CNS side effects; e.g., dizziness.

CLIENT TEACHING

General

- Inform the client that the muscle relaxant should not be abruptly stopped. Drug should be tapered over 1 wk to avoid rebound spasms.

- Advise the client not to drive or operate dangerous machinery when taking muscle relaxants. These drugs have a sedative effect and can cause drowsiness.
- Inform the client that most of the centrally acting muscle relaxants for acute spasms are usually taken for no longer than 3 wk.
- Advise the client to avoid alcohol and CNS depressants. If muscle relaxants are taken with these drugs, CNS depression may be intensified.
- Inform the client that these drugs are contraindicated during pregnancy or by lactating mothers. Check with the health care provider.

Diet

- Advise the client to take muscle relaxants with food to decrease GI upset.

Side Effects

- Instruct the client to report side effects of the muscle relaxant, such as nausea, vomiting, dizziness, faintness, headache, and diplopia. Dizziness and faintness are most likely due to orthostatic (postural) hypotension.

EVALUATION

- Evaluate the effectiveness of the muscle relaxant to determine if the client's muscular pain has decreased or disappeared.

■ CASE STUDY
Client with Parkinsonism

T. R., age 79 years, was diagnosed as having parkinsonism 10 years ago. During early treatment of parkinsonism, he was taking levodopa (L-dopa). The drug dosage had to be increased in order to alleviate symptoms.

1. What is the purpose and the action of levodopa?
2. Why does the dosage of levodopa need to be increased for treating parkinsonism?
3. What are the side effects of levodopa? Why does the drug have to be administered several times a day?

Because T. R. developed numerous side effects and adverse reactions to levodopa, the health care provider changed the drug to carbidopa-levodopa (Sinemet). The client asks the nurse why the drug was changed.

4. What would be an appropriate response to the question about changing the drug for parkinsonism?
5. How does the dose for carbidopa-levodopa differ from that for levodopa? What are the advantages of carbidopa-levodopa?

The family of T. R. say that they know a person with parkinsonism taking the antiviral drug amantadine (Symmetrel). The family asks if Symmetrel is the same as Sinemet and, if so, shouldn't the client take that drug instead of a drug containing levodopa.

6. What is the effect of amantadine on parkinsonism symptoms?
7. What would be an appropriate response to the family's question concerning the use of Symmetrel for T. R.?
8. Certain anticholinergic drugs may be used for controlling parkinsonism symptoms. What is the action of these drugs and what are their side ef-

fects? These anticholinergic drugs are usually prescribed for parkinsonism symptoms resulting from what?

STUDY QUESTIONS

1. A 66-year-old man was recently diagnosed with parkinsonism. What are four physical characteristics associated with parkinsonism?
2. This gentleman was instructed to take 250 mg of levodopa three times a day. At what time of the day should the drug be taken? What are three side effects of the drug? Why should vitamin B_6 (pyridoxine) be avoided in foods and vitamin supplements?
3. Because of the side effects, the drug therapy was changed to bromocriptine. How do these two drugs differ? Explain.
4. Selected anticholinergics are prescribed for parkinsonism. What are their effects on parkinsonism symptoms? What are the side effects of anticholinergics?
5. An AChE inhibitor is used in the treatment of myasthenia gravis. What is its action?
6. What teaching should be included concerning drug compliance and drug dose intervals?
7. Centrally acting muscle relaxants are used for what type of muscle spasms? What is the major side effect of this group of drugs?
8. The client with multiple sclerosis has muscle spasms. What are two muscle relaxants that are used to reduce this spasticity?

Unit V

Antiinflammatory and Antiinfective Agents

INTRODUCTION

Unit V discusses agents prescribed for alleviating an inflammatory process and combating disease-producing microorganisms (pathogens). Included in this unit are antiinflammatory drugs; antibacterials-antibiotics; sulfonamides; peptides; antitubercular, antifungal, antiviral, anthelmintics, and antimalarial drugs; and urinary antiseptics. Drugs for dermatologic disorders, many of which are prescribed for skin infections, are also described.

INFLAMMATION

Inflammation is a reaction to tissue injury due to the release of chemical mediators that cause both a vascular response and fluid and cells (leukocytes, or WBC) to migrate to the injured site. The chemical mediators are (1) histamines, (2) kinins, and (3) prostaglandins. Histamine, the first mediator in the inflammatory process, causes dilation of the arterioles and increases capillary permeability, allowing fluid to leave the capillaries and flow into the injured area. The kinins, such as bradykinin, also increase capillary permeability and the sensation of pain. Prostaglandins are released, causing an increase in vasodilation, capillary permeability, pain, and fever. The antiinflammatory drugs, such as nonsteroidal antiinflammatory drugs (NSAIDs) and steroids (cortisone preparations), inhibit chemical mediators, thus decreasing the inflammatory process. Figure V–1 illustrates the process of chemical mediators acting on the injured tissues. The five responses to tissue injury are referred to as the cardinal signs of inflammation: redness, swelling, pain, heat, and loss of function.

Inflammation may or may not be the result of an infection. Only a small percentage of inflammations are due to infections; other causes include trauma, surgical interventions, extreme heat or cold, and caustic chemical agents. Antiinflammatory drugs reduce fluid migration and pain, thus lessening loss of function and increasing the client's mobility and comfort.

INFECTION

Disease-producing organisms may be gram-positive or gram-negative bacteria, viruses, or fungi. The degree to which they are pathogenic depends on the microorganism and its virulence. The cell walls of bacteria differ in their structure: bacilli are elongated, cocci are spherical, and spirilla are helical.

Viruses are very small organisms that do not have an organized cellular structure. There are numerous families of virus, including herpesviruses, cytomegalovirus, adenovirus, papovavirus, and the human immunodeficiency virus (HIV). Today, an increasing number of an-

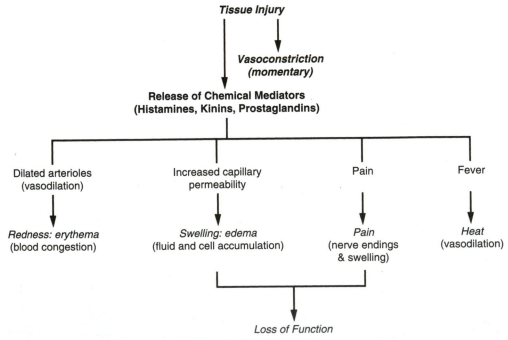

FIGURE V–1 Chemical mediator's response to tissue injury.

tiviral drugs seek to inhibit viral replication to control the virus. This pharmacologic effort has been thrust forward as we search for effective treatment and cure for acquired immunodeficiency syndrome (AIDS).

The fungi are divided into yeasts and molds. The few fungi that produce disease usually affect the skin and subcutaneous tissues in such conditions as athlete's foot and ringworm. Serious fungal infections are systemic and usually need aggressive drug therapy. Opportunistic fungal infections commonly result from prolonged antibiotic and steroidal therapies and debilitating diseases, such as cancer. The yeast *Candida albicans* is a cause of common infections of the mucous membranes of the mouth, gastrointestinal tract, vagina, and skin. *Candida,* like most fungi, is resistant to penicillin-type antibiotics because of its rigid cell wall structure. Chapter 25 describes the variety of topical and systemic drugs used in treating yeast and mold infections.

Chapter 21

Antiinflammatory Drugs

OUTLINE

Objectives
Terms
Introduction
Cardinal Signs of Inflammation
Nonsteroidal Antiinflammatory
  Drugs
    Salicylates
    Nursing Process
    Para-chlorobenzoic Acid
    Pyrazolone Derivatives
    Proprionic Acid Derivatives

Fenamates
Oxicams
Phenylacetic Acid Deriva-
  tives
Other
Nursing Process
Corticosteroids
Disease-Modifying Antirheu-
  matic Drugs
  Gold
  Nursing Process

Immunosuppressive Agents
  Antimalarials
Antigout Drugs
  Antiinflammatory Gout
    Drug: Colchicine
  Uric Acid Inhibitor
  Uricosurics
  Nursing Process
Study Questions

OBJECTIVES

Describe the action of nonsteroidal antiinflammatory drugs (NSAIDs).

List the major side effects of NSAIDs.

Explain the use of disease-modifying antirheumatic drugs (DMARDs).

Identify several side effects and adverse reactions of DMARDs.

Give nursing process, including client teaching, associated with NSAIDs and DMARDs.

Discuss the use of antigout drugs.

TERMS

chrysotherapy
DMARDs
gout

immunosuppressives
infection
inflammation

NSAIDs
prostaglandins
uricosuric

INTRODUCTION

Inflammation is a response to tissue injury and infection. When the inflammatory process occurs, a vascular reaction takes place in which fluid, elements of blood, white blood cells (leukocytes), and chemical mediators accumulate at the injured tissue or infection site. The process of inflammation is a protective mechanism in which the body attempts to neutralize and destroy harmful agents at the site of injury and to establish conditions for tissue repair.

Although there is a relationship between inflammation and infection, these terms should *not* be used interchangeably. **Infection** is caused by microorganisms and results in inflammation, but *not* all inflammations are caused by infections.

CARDINAL SIGNS OF INFLAMMATION

The five characteristics of inflammation, referred to as the cardinal signs of inflammation, are redness, heat, swelling (edema), pain, and loss of function (see Table 21–1 for the explanation of these signs). The two phases of inflammation are the vascular phase that occurs 10 to 15 min following an injury and the delayed phase. The vascular phase is associated with vasodilation and increased capillary permeability, during which blood substances and fluid leave the plasma and go to the injured site. The delayed phase occurs when leukocytes infiltrate the inflamed tissue.

Various chemical mediators are released during the inflammation process. Prostaglandins that have been isolated from the exudate at inflammatory sites are among them. **Prostaglandins** (chemical mediators) have many effects, including vasodilation, relaxation of smooth muscle, increased capillary permeability, and sensitization of nerve cells to pain. Drugs, such as aspirin, inhibit the biosynthesis of prostaglandins and therefore are referred to as prostaglandin inhibitors. Because prostaglandin inhibitors affect the inflammatory process, they are also referred to as antiinflammatory agents.

Antiinflammatory agents have additional properties, such as relief of pain (analgesic), reduction of an elevated body temperature (antipyretic), and inhibition of platelet aggregation (anticoagulant). Aspirin is the oldest antiinflammatory drug, but was first used for its analgesic and antipyretic properties. As a result of searching for a more effective drug with fewer side effects, many other antiinflammatory agents or prostaglandin inhibitors have been discovered. Although these drugs have potent antiinflammatory effects that mimic the effects of corticosteroids (cortisone), they are *not* chemically related and therefore are referred to as **nonsteroidal antiinflammatory drugs,** or **NSAIDs.**

NONSTEROIDAL ANTIINFLAMMATORY DRUGS

NSAIDs are aspirin and "aspirin-like" drugs that inhibit the synthesis of prostaglandins. These drugs, also called prostaglandin inhibitors, have varying degrees of analgesic and antipyretic effects, but are used primarily as antiinflammatory agents for relieving inflammation and pain. When administering NSAIDs for pain relief, the dosage is usually higher than for treatment of inflammation. Their antipyretic effect is less than their antiinflammatory effect. With the exceptions of aspirin and ibuprofen, NSAID preparations are not suggested for use in alleviating mild headaches and mild elevated temperature. The choice of drugs for headaches and fever are aspirin, acetaminophen, and ibuprofen (given to children and adults with high fever). NSAIDs are more appropriate for reducing swelling, pain, and stiffness in joints.

NSAIDs cost more than aspirin. Other than aspirin, the only NSAIDs that can be purchased over-the-counter (OTC) are ibuprofen (Motrin, Nuprin,

TABLE 21–1 Cardinal Signs of Inflammation

Signs	Description and Explanation
Erythema (Redness)	Redness occurs in the first phase of inflammation. Blood accumulates in the area of tissue injury due to release of the body's chemical mediators (kinins, prostaglandins, and histamine). Histamine dilates the arterioles.
Edema (Swelling)	Swelling is the second phase of inflammation. Plasma leaks into the interstitial tissue at the injury site. Kinins dilate the arterioles, increasing capillary permeability.
Heat	Heat at the inflammatory site can be due to increased blood accumulation and may result from pyrogens (substances that produce fever) that interfere with the temperature-regulating center in the hypothalamus.
Pain	Pain is due to tissue swelling and the release of chemical mediators.
Loss of function	Function is lost due to the accumulation of fluid at the tissue injury site and to pain, which decreases mobility at the affected area.

Advil, Medipren) and naproxen (Aleve). All other NSAIDs must be ordered with a prescription. If a client can take aspirin for the inflammatory process without gastrointestinal (GI) upset, then the salicylate products are usually recommended.

There are seven groups of NSAIDs:

1. Salicylates related to aspirin (see Chapter 14 for detailed effects)
2. *Para*-chlorobenzoic acid derivatives, or indoles
3. Pyrazolone derivatives
4. Proprionic acid derivatives
5. Fenamates
6. Oxicams
7. Phenylacetic acids

These agents will be discussed separately. The half-lives of NSAIDs differ greatly—some have a short half-life, others have a moderate to long half-life with a general range of 8 to 24 h. Aspirin and an NSAID should *not* be taken together because of the side effects. Also, combined therapy does not increase effectiveness.

SALICYLATES

Aspirin is the oldest antiinflammatory agent. A prostaglandin inhibitor that decreases the inflammatory process, aspirin was the most frequently used antiinflammatory agent before the introduction of ibuprofen. Because high doses of aspirin are generally needed to relieve inflammation, gastric distress is a common problem. In such cases, enteric-coated tablets may be used. Aspirin should

not be taken with other NSAIDs because it decreases the blood level and the effectiveness of the NSAID. Aspirin is also considered an antiplatelet drug for clients having cardiac or cerebrovascular disorders. Figure 21–1 gives the pharmacokinetic data of aspirin.

Pharmacokinetics

Aspirin is well-absorbed from the GI tract. It can cause GI upset; therefore, it is suggested that aspirin should be taken with water, milk, or food. The enteric-coated (EC) or buffered form can decrease gastric distress. The EC tablet should not be crushed or broken.

Aspirin has a short half-life. It should not be taken during the last trimester of pregnancy because it could cause premature closure of ductus arteriosus in the fetus. Aspirin should not be taken by children with flu symptoms because it may cause the potentially fatal Reye's syndrome.

Pharmacodynamics

Aspirin, like other NSAIDs, inhibits prostaglandin synthesis; thus, it decreases inflammation and pain. The onset of action for aspirin is within 30 min. It peaks in 1 to 2 h, and the duration of action is an average of 4 to 6 h. The action for the rectal preparation of aspirin can be erratic because of blood supply and fecal material in the rectum; it may take a week or more for a therapeutic antiinflammatory effect.

FIGURE 21–1. Analgesic and Antiinflammatory Drug: Aspirin

Salicylate	Dosage	**NURSING PROCESS** Assessment and Planning
Aspirin (A.S.A., Bayer, Astrin, Ecotrin, Alka Seltzer [in some], Empirin) 🍁 Ancasal, Astrin, Entrophen, Novasen *Pregnancy Category:* D	*Analgesic:* A: PO: 325–650 mg q4h PRN; max: 4 g/d C: PO: 40–65 mg/d in 4–6 divided doses; max: 3.5 g/d *TIA and thromboembolic condition:* A: PO: 325–650 mg/d or b.i.d. *Arthritis:* A: PO: 3.6–5.4 g/d in divided doses *TDM:* 15–30 mg/dL; 150–300 µg/mL	
Contraindications	**Drug-Lab-Food Interactions**	
Hypersensitivity to salicylates or NSAIDs, flu or virus symptoms in children, third trimester of pregnancy *Caution:* Renal or hepatic disorders	*Increase* risk of bleeding with anticoagulants; *increase* risk of hypoglycemia with oral hypoglycemic drugs; *increase* ulcerogenic effect with glucocorticoids *Lab: Decrease* cholesterol and potassium, T_3, T_4 levels; *increase* PT, bleeding time, uric acid	

FIGURE 21–1. *Continued*

Pharmacokinetics	Pharmacodynamics	Interventions

Absorption: PO: 80–100%
Distribution: PB: 59–90%, crosses placenta
Metabolism: t½: 2–3 h (low dose); 2–20 h (high dose)
Excretion: 50% in urine
	PO: Onset: 15–30 min
	     Peak: 1–2 h
	     Duration: 4–6 h
	Rectal: Onset: 1–2 h
	     Peak: 3–5 h
	     Duration: 4–7 h	

	Evaluation
Therapeutic Effects/Uses: To reduce pain and inflammatory symptoms; to decrease body temperature; to inhibit platelet aggregation. *Mode of Action:* Inhibition of prostaglandin synthesis, inhibition of hypothalamic heat-regulator center.	

Side Effects	Adverse Reactions
Anorexia, nausea, vomiting, diarrhea, dizziness, confusion, hearing loss, heartburn, rash, stomach pains, drowsiness	Tinnitus, urticaria, ulceration *Life-threatening:* Agranulocytosis, hemolytic anemia, bronchospasm, anaphylaxis, thrombocytopenia, hepatotoxicity, leukopenia

KEY: A: adult; C: child; PO: by mouth; TDM: therapeutic drug monitoring; UK; unknown: PB: protein-binding; t½: half-life; PRN: as necessary; 🍁 : Canadian drug names.

NURSING PROCESS: ANALGESIC AND ANTIINFLAMMATORY DRUG: Aspirin

ASSESSMENT

- Obtain a medical history. Determine if there is any history of gastric upset, gastric bleeding, or liver disease. Aspirin can cause gastric irritation. It prolongs bleeding time by inhibiting platelet aggregation.
- Obtain a drug history. Report if a drug-drug interaction is probable.

POTENTIAL NURSING DIAGNOSES

- High risk for injury
- Pain

PLANNING

- Client will be free of mild pain in 12 to 24 hours and mild inflammation within 1 week. Aspirin may be ordered for mild to severe arthritic condition, pain relief, antiinflammatory effects, fever reduction, and inhibition of platelet aggregation.

NURSING INTERVENTIONS

- Monitor serum salicylate (aspirin) level when the client is taking high doses of aspirin for chronic conditions such as arthritis. The normal therapeutic range is 15 to 30 mg/dL. Mild toxicity occurs at serum level of >30 mg/dL, and severe toxicity occurs at >50 mg/dL.
- Observe the client for signs of bleeding, such as dark (tarry) stools, bleeding gums, petechiae (round red spots), ecchymosis (excessive bruising), and purpura (large red spots) when the client is taking high doses of aspirin.

CLIENT TEACHING

General
- Advise the client not to take aspirin with alcohol or drugs that are highly protein-bound, such as the anticoagulant warfarin (Coumadin). Aspirin displaces drugs like warfarin from the protein-binding site, causing more free anticoagulant.
- Suggest that the client inform the dentist before

a dental visit if the client is taking high doses of aspirin.

- With the health care provider's approval, instruct the client to discontinue aspirin 3 to 7 d before surgery to reduce the risk of bleeding.
- Keep aspirin bottle out of reach of small children.
- Instruct the parent to call the poison control center immediately if a child has taken a large or unknown amount of aspirin (also acetaminophen).
- Instruct the client *not* to administer aspirin for virus or flu symptoms in children. Reye's syndrome (vomiting, lethargy, delirium, and coma) has been linked with aspirin and viral infections. Acetaminophen is usually prescribed for cold and flu symptoms.
- Inform the client that old aspirin tablets can cause GI distress.
- Inform the client with dysmenorrhea to take acetaminophen instead of aspirin 2 d before and 2 d during the menstrual period.

Diet

- Instruct the client to take aspirin (also ibuprofen) with food, at mealtime, or with plenty of fluids. Enteric-coated aspirin avoids GI disturbance.

Side Effects

- Instruct the client to report side effects such as drowsiness, tinnitus (ringing in the ears), headaches, flushing, dizziness, GI symptoms (bleeding, heartburn), visual changes, and seizures.

EVALUATION

- Evaluate the effectiveness of aspirin in relieving pain. If pain persists, another analgesic such as ibuprofen may be prescribed.
- Determine if the client is having any side effects to aspirin.

PARA-*CHLOROBENZOIC ACID*

One of the first NSAIDs introduced was indomethacin (Indocin). It is used for rheumatoid, gouty, and osteoarthritis and is a potent prostaglandin inhibitor. It is a highly protein-bound drug (90%) and displaces other protein-bound drugs, resulting in potential toxicity. It has a moderate half-life (4 to 11 h). Indomethacin is very irritating to the stomach and should be taken with meals or food.

Two other *para*-chlorobenzoic acid derivatives, sulindac (Clinoril) and tolmetin (Tolectin), produce less severe adverse reactions than indomethacin. Tolmetin is not as highly protein-bound as indomethacin and sulindac and has a short half-life. This group of NSAIDs may decrease blood pressure and cause sodium and water retention.

PYRAZOLONE DERIVATIVES

The pyrazolone group of NSAIDs, like the *para*-chlorobenzoic acid group, is highly protein-bound. Phenylbutazone (Butazolidin), 96% protein-bound, has been used for years to treat rheumatoid arthritis and acute gout. It has a very long half-life, 50 to 65 h, so adverse reactions are common and drug accumulation may occur. Gastric irritation occurs in 10% to 45% of clients.

The most dangerous adverse reactions to this group of drugs are blood dyscrasias, such as agranulocytosis and aplastic anemia. Phenylbutazone should be reserved for the treatment of arthritis and other severe inflammatory conditions when other less toxic NSAIDs have been used without success.

PROPRIONIC ACID DERIVATIVES

The proprionic acid group represents a relatively new group of NSAIDs. These drugs are aspirin-like but have stronger effects and create less GI irritation. Drugs in this group are highly protein-bound, so drug interactions might occur, especially when given with another highly protein-bound drug. Ibuprofen (Motrin) is the most widely used NSAID today, and in lower doses (200 mg) it may be purchased OTC. These NSAIDs are better tolerated than other NSAIDs. Gastric upset occurs but it is not as severe as it is with aspirin, indomethacin, and phenylbutazone. Severe adverse reactions, such as blood dyscrasias, are *not* frequently seen. Figure 21–2 details the pharmacologic behavior of ibuprofens. Five other proprionic acid agents are fenoprofen calcium (Nalfon), naproxen (Naprosyn), suprofen (Profenal); ketoprofen (Orudis), and flurbiprofen (Ansaid).

Pharmacokinetics

Ibuprofens are well absorbed from the GI tract. These drugs have a short half-life, but are highly protein-bound. If ibuprofen is taken with another highly protein-bound drug, severe side effects may occur. The drug is metabolized in the liver to inactivate metabolites and excreted as inactive metabolites in the urine.

Pharmacodynamics

Ibuprofens inhibit prostaglandin synthesis and are therefore effective in alleviating inflammation and pain. They have a short onset of action, peak concentration time, and duration of action. It may take several days for the antiinflammatory effect to be evident.

There are many drug interactions associated with ibuprofen. It can increase the effects of coumadin, sulfonamides, many of the cephalosporins, and phenytoin. When taken with aspirin, its effect can be decreased. Hypoglycemia may result when taking ibuprofen with insulin or an oral hypoglycemic drug. There is high risk of toxicity when ibuprofen is taken concurrently with calcium blockers.

FIGURE 21–2. Antiinflammatory: Nonsteroidal Antiinflammatory Drug (NSAID)

NSAID	Dosage	**NURSING PROCESS** Assessment and Planning
Ibuprofen (Motrin, Advil, Nuprin, Medipren, Rufen) Amersol Proprionic acid derivative *Pregnancy Category:* B	A: PO: 200–800 mg t.i.d./q.i.d.; max: <3.2 g/d (<3,200 mg/d) C: PO: Average: 5–10 mg/kg/d; max: 40 mg/kg/d 1–4 y: 400 mg/d in divided doses 5–7 y: 600 mg/d in divided doses >8 y: 800 mg/d in divided doses	
Contraindications	**Drug-Lab-Food Interactions**	
Severe renal or hepatic disease, asthma, peptic ulcer *Caution:* Bleeding disorders, early pregnancy, lactation, systemic lupus erythematosus (SLE)	*Increase* bleeding time with oral anticoagulants; *increase* effects of phenytoin, sulfonamides, warfarin *Decrease* effect with aspirin; may *increase* severe side effect of lithium	
Pharmacokinetics	**Pharmacodynamics**	Interventions
Absorption: PO: Well absorbed *Distribution:* PB: 98% *Metabolism:* t½: 2–4 h *Excretion:* In urine, mostly as inactive metabolites; some in bile	PO: Onset: 0.5 h Peak: 1–2 h Duration: 4–6 h	

Therapeutic Effects/Uses: To reduce inflammatory process; to relieve pain; anti-inflammatory effect for arthritic conditions and reduce fever.

Mode of Action: Inhibition of prostaglandin synthesis, thus relieving pain and inflammation.

Evaluation

Side Effects	Adverse Reactions
Anorexia, nausea, vomiting, diarrhea, edema, rash, purpura, tinnitus, fatigue, dizziness, lightheadedness, anxiety, confusion	GI bleeding *Life-threatening:* Blood dyscrasias, cardiac dysrhythmias, nephrotoxicity, anaphylaxis

KEY: A: adult; C: child; PO: by mouth; PB: protein-binding; t½: half-life; <: less than; >: greater than; : Canadian drug name.

FENAMATES

The fenamate group includes potent NSAIDs used for acute and chronic arthritic conditions. Like most NSAIDs, gastric irritation is a common side effect of fenamates, and clients with a history of peptic ulcer should avoid taking this group of drugs. Other side effects include edema, dizziness, tinnitus, and pruritus. Two fenamates are meclofenamate sodium monohydrate (Meclomen) and mefenamic acid (Ponstel).

OXICAMS

Piroxicam (Feldene) is a relatively new NSAID and, like the others, is indicated for long-term arthritic conditions, such as rheumatoid and osteoarthritis. It is well tolerated, and its major advantage over the others is its long half-life, which allows it to be dosed only once daily. It also can cause gastric problems, such as ulceration and epigastric distress, but the incidence is lower than for some of the other NSAIDs.

Full clinical response to piroxicam may take a week or two. This drug is also highly protein-bound and may interact with another highly protein-bound drug if taken together. Piroxicam should not be taken with aspirin or other NSAIDs.

PHENYLACETIC ACID DERIVATIVES

Diclofenac sodium (Voltaren), the newest NSAID, has a plasma half-life of 8 to 12 h. Its analgesic and antiinflammatory effects are similar to aspirin's, but it has minimal to no antipyretic effect. It is indicated for rheumatoid arthritis, osteoarthritis, and ankylosing spondylitis. Adverse reactions are similar to those of other NSAIDs.

OTHER

Ketorolac (Toradol) is the first injectable nonsteroidal antiinflammatory agent. Like other NSAIDs, it inhibits prostaglandin synthesis, but it has greater analgesic properties than other antiinflammatory agents. Ketorolac is recommended for short-term management of pain. For postsurgical pain it has shown analgesic efficacy equal or superior to that of opioid analgesics. It is administered intramuscularly in doses of 30 to 60 mg q6h for adults.

Table 21-2 lists the frequently used NSAIDs, their dosages, and considerations for use.

General Side Effects and Adverse Reactions

Most NSAIDs tend to have fewer side effects than aspirin when taken at antiinflammatory doses, but gastric irritation is still a common problem when taking NSAIDs without food. Also, sodium and water retention may occur when taking phenylbutazone. Alcoholic beverages consumed with NSAIDs may increase gastric irritation and should be avoided.

TABLE 21-2 Antiinflammatory: Nonsteroidal Antiinflammatory

Generic (Brand)	Route and Dosage	Uses and Considerations
Salicylates Aspirin (ASA, Bayer, Ecotrin)	A: PO: 325–650 mg PRN See Prototype Drug Chart (Fig. 21–1)	Requires large dose for inflammation, rheumatoid arthritis. GI upset and ulceration can occur. Alcohol can increase GI effects. *Pregnancy category:* D; PB: 59%–90%; t½: 2–3 h (low doses), 2–20 h (high doses)
Diflunisal (Dolobid)	A: PO: Initially: 1 g (1,000 mg); maint: 500 mg q8–12 h	Relief of mild to moderate pain; used to treat osteoarthritis and rheumatoid arthritis. Acts by inhibiting prostaglandin synthesis. Avoid if hypersensitive to aspirin. Do not use during third trimester of pregnancy. *Pregnancy category:* C; PB: 99%; t½: 1 h
Para-Chlorobenzoic Acid (Indoles) Indomethacin (Indocin)	A: PO: 25–50 mg b.i.d./t.i.d. with food SR: 75 mg q.d./b.i.d.; *max:* 200 mg/d C: PO: 1–2 mg/kg/d in 2–4 divided doses; may increase to 4 mg/kg/d; *max:* 150–200 mg/d	For moderate to severe arthritic conditions. Potent drug. GI upset and ulceration are common. Take drug with food. Avoid indomethacin if allergic to aspirin. *Pregnancy category:* B (D near term); PB: 90%–99%; t½: 3–120 h
Sulindac (Clinoril)	A: PO: 150–200 mg b.i.d.	For acute and chronic arthritis, bursitis, and tendinitis. Not as potent as indomethacin. Give with food. *Pregnancy category:* C; PB: 93%; t½: 7–18 h

TABLE 21–2 Antiinflammatory: Nonsteroidal Antiinflammatory (Continued)

Generic (Brand)	Route and Dosage	Uses and Considerations
Tolmetin (Tolectin)	A: PO: Initially: 400 mg t.i.d.; maint: 600–1800 mg/d in divided doses; *max:* 2 g/d C >2 y: PO: 20 mg/kg/d in divided doses; *max:* 30 mg/kg/d	For acute and chronic arthritis, including juvenile rheumatoid arthritis. Less potent than indomethacin; more effective than aspirin. Take drug with food. *Pregnancy category:* B (D near term); PB: 99%; t½: 1–1.5 h
Pyrazolone Phenylbutazone (Butazolidin)	A: PO: 100–400 mg/d in divided doses; *max:* 600 mg/d	For acute rheumatoid arthritis, osteoarthritis, and gouty arthritis. Potent drug. Severe side effects can occur. Take with food. Very long half-life. *Pregnancy category:* C; PB: 98%; t½: 50–100 h
Proprionic Acid Fenoprofen calcium (Nalfon)	A: PO: 300–600 mg t.i.d./q.i.d.; *max:* 3.2 g/d	Treatment of mild to moderate pain. Also for arthritic conditions. Most effective after 2–3 weeks of therapy. Take with food. *Pregnancy category:* B (D at term); PB: 90%; t½: 3 h
Flurbiprofen sodium (Ansaid, Ocufen)	A: PO: 50–300 mg/d in 2–4 divided doses; *max:* 300 mg/d *Ophthalmic use:* 0.03% sol	Treatment of acute and chronic arthritis. Take drug with food. *Pregnancy category:* C; PB: UK; t½: 5 h
Ibuprofen (Motrin, Advil, Nuprin, Medipren)	See Prototype Drug Chart (Fig. 21–2)	Relief of mild to moderate pain; used to reduce fever (adult and children) and also for arthritic conditions. Similar effect as aspirin. Can increase bleeding time. GI upset can occur. Take with food, milk, or antacids if GI discomfort occurs. *Pregnancy category:* B; PB: 98%; t½: 2–4 h
Ketoprofen (Orudis)	*Inflammatory:* A: PO: 150–300 mg/d in 3–4 divided doses *Mild-moderate pain:* A: PO: 25–50 mg q6–8h PRN; *max:* 300 mg/d	Relief of mild to moderate pain and acute and chronic arthritis. Take with food or 8 ounces of water to avoid GI upset. *Pregnancy category:* B (D at term); PB: 99%; t½: 3–4 h
Naproxen (Naprosyn)	A: PO: 250–500 mg b.i.d. C: PO: 5–10 mg/kg/d in 2 divided doses	Relief of mild to moderate pain. Also for arthritic, gout, bursitis conditions. Similar OTC drug: Aleve. Take with food or with a full glass of water. *Pregnancy category:* B; PB: 99%; t½: 10–15 h
Oxaprozin (Daypro)	A: PO: Initially: 1,200 mg/d; maint: 600 mg/d; *max:* 1800 mg/d in divided doses	Treatment of acute and chronic arthritis. Take with food for GI discomfort. *Pregnancy category:* C; PB: 99%; t½: 40 h
Anthranylic Acids (Fenamates) Meclofenamate (Meclomen)	A: PO: 200–400 mg in 3–4 divided doses	For acute and chronic arthritis. GI symptoms can be severe. Used when other NSAIDs are not effective. Take with food to avoid GI upset. *Pregnancy category:* B (D at term); PB: 99%; t½: 3 h
Mefenamic acid (Ponstel)	A: PO: Initially: 500 mg; then 250 mg q6h PRN; *max:* 1 g/d	For acute and chronic arthritis. Diarrhea is common problem. Usually discontinued after 7 days. *Pregnancy category:* C; PB: 90%; t½: 2–4 h
Oxicams Piroxicam (Feldene)	A: PO: 10 mg b.i.d. or 20 mg q.d.	For arthritic conditions. Long half-life; effective at 2 weeks. GI upset may occur. *Pregnancy category:* C; PB: 99%; t½: 30–86 h
Phenylacetic Acid Diclofenac sodium (Voltaren)	A: PO: 25–50 mg t.i.d./q.i.d. or 75 mg b.i.d.	For rheumatoid arthritis, osteoarthritis, and spondylitis. Also for acute gout, juvenile rheumatoid arthritis, bursitis, and tendinitis. If GI distress occurs, take with food. *Pregnancy category:* B; PB: 90%–99%; t½: 2 h
Etodolac (Lodine)	A: PO: 200–400 mg q6–8h PRN; *max:* 1,200 mg/d	Used for acute pain, rheumatoid arthritis, and osteoarthritis. Take with food or antacid to avoid GI distress. *Pregnancy category:* C; PR: 99%; t½: 6–7 h
Ketorolac tromethamine (Toradol)	A: <50 kg: IM: LD: 30 mg; maint: 15 mg q6h A: >50 kg: IM: LD: 30–60 mg; maint: 15–30 mg PRN	First injectable NSAID. For short-term management of pain. Also available for ophthalmic use to relieve itching due to allergic conjunctivitis. *Pregnancy category:* B; PB: 99%; t½: 5–6 h

KEY: A: adult; C: child; PO: by mouth; IM: intramuscular; IV: intravenous; >: greater than; <: less than; LD: loading dose; PRN: as necessary; PB: protein-binding; t½: half-life; sol: solution; SR: sustained-release; maint: maintenance.

NURSING PROCESS: ANTIINFLAMMATORY: Nonsteroidal Antiinflammatory Drug

ASSESSMENT

- Check the client's history of allergy to NSAIDs, including aspirin. If an allergy is present, notify the health care provider.
- Obtain a drug history and report any possible drug-drug interaction. NSAIDs can increase the effects of phenytoin (Dilantin), sulfonamides, and warfarin. Most NSAIDs are highly protein-bound and can displace other highly protein-bound drugs, like warfarin (Coumadin).
- Obtain a medical history. NSAIDs are contraindicated if the client has a severe renal or liver disease, peptic ulcer, or bleeding disorder.
- Assess the client for GI upset and peripheral edema, which are common side effects of NSAIDs.

POTENTIAL NURSING DIAGNOSES

- Impaired tissue integrity
- High risk for activity intolerance

PLANNING

- The inflammatory process will subside in 1 to 3 wk.

NURSING INTERVENTIONS

- Observe the client for bleeding gums, petechiae, ecchymoses, or black (tarry) stools. Bleeding time can be prolonged when taking NSAIDs, especially with a highly protein-bound drug such as warfarin (anticoagulant).
- Report if the client is having GI discomfort. Administer the NSAIDs at mealtime or with food to prevent GI upset.
- Monitor vital signs (VS) and check for peripheral edema, especially in the morning.

CLIENT TEACHING

General

- Instruct the client not to take aspirin and acetaminophen with NSAIDs. Taking an NSAID with aspirin could cause GI upset and possible GI bleeding.
- Instruct the client to avoid alcohol when taking NSAIDs. GI upset or gastric ulcer may result.
- Advise the client to inform the dentist or surgeon before a procedure when taking ibuprofen or other NSAIDs for a continuous period of time.
- Advise women not to take NSAIDs 1 to 2 d before menstruation to avoid heavy menstrual flow. If discomfort occurs, acetaminophen is usually prescribed.
- Advise women in the third trimester of pregnancy to avoid NSAIDs. If delivery occurs, excess bleeding might occur with NSAIDs.
- Inform the client that it may take several weeks to experience the desired drug effect of some NSAIDs and disease-modifying antirheumatic drugs (DMARDs).

Diet

- Instruct the client to take NSAIDs with meals or food to reduce GI upset.

Side Effects

- Advise the client of the common side effects of NSAIDs. Nausea, vomiting, peripheral edema, GI upset, purpura or petechiae, and/or dizziness might occur. Report occurrences of side effects.

EVALUATION

- Evaluate the effectiveness of the drug therapy, such as a decrease in pain and in swollen joints and an increase in mobility.

CORTICOSTEROIDS

Corticosteroids, such as prednisone, prednisolone, and dexamethasone, are frequently used as antiinflammatory agents. This group of drugs can control inflammation by suppressing or preventing many of the components of the inflammatory process at the injured site. Corticosteroids have been widely prescribed for arthritic conditions, and although they are not the drug of choice for arthritis because of their numerous side effects, they are frequently used to control arthritic flare-ups.

The half-life of corticosteroids is long, greater than 24 h, and with a large prescribed dose, the steroid is administered once a day. When discontinuing steroid therapy, the dosage should be tapered over a period of 5 to 10 days. Steroids are discussed in more detail in Chapter 40.

DISEASE-MODIFYING ANTIRHEUMATIC DRUGS

When NSAIDs do not control immune-mediated arthritic disease sufficiently, other drugs, though more toxic, can be prescribed to alter the disease process. The **disease-modifying antirheumatic drug (DMARD) group** includes gold drug therapy, immunosuppressive agents, and antimalarials.

GOLD

Gold drug therapy, referred to as **chrysotherapy** or heavy metal therapy, is the most frequently used DMARD. It is used to arrest progression of rheumatoid arthritis and to prevent deformities caused by the disease. It depresses migration of leukocytes and also suppresses prostaglandin activity. Gold is not used in early arthritis unless the illness is progressing rapidly and unresponsive to other therapy, nor is it used in far-advanced arthritis. It is used for palliative (relief of symptoms) and not for curative reasons. Response in alleviating symptoms is slow; with injectable gold, it could take up to 2 months and, for oral dosage of gold, it could take 3 to 6 months for clinical response. The half-life of gold is 7 to 25 days, and gold drugs are highly protein-bound. Blood should be monitored for blood dyscrasia before and during parenteral or oral gold therapy.

The newest gold salt is auranofin (Ridaura). It is the only gold preparation that can be administered orally. The two parenteral gold salts are aurothioglucose (Solganal) and gold sodium thiomalate (Myochrysine). Oral gold may be absorbed erratically; thus parenteral gold may be advised. Switching from parenteral to oral gold preparations may be necessary for long-term use. Figure 21–3 presents the drug data for the gold preparation auranofin (Ridaura).

Pharmacokinetics

Twenty-five percent of auranofin is absorbed from the GI tract. It is moderately highly protein-bound. Its half-life is long, both in the blood, 26 days, and in the body tissues, 40 to 120 days. Sixty percent of auranofin is excreted in the urine, and the drug may be present in the urine up to 15 months after it has been discontinued.

Pharmacodynamics

Auranofin is prescribed to relieve inflammation and pain from rheumatoid arthritis when NSAIDs and other measures are ineffective. The therapeutic effect may take 3 to 6 months; steady state (the average therapeutic effect that is maintained) of the drug is achieved after 2 to 4 months. Side effects and adverse reactions need to be closely monitored.

Table 21–3 details the dosages and considerations for the three gold drugs used as antiinflammatory agents for rheumatoid arthritis.

Side Effects and Adverse Reactions

Approximately 25% to 45% of clients receiving gold therapy experience side effects. The side effects may occur anytime during or several months after therapy. The numerous possible side effects include dermatitis, urticaria (hives), erythema, alopecia (loss of hair), stomatitis (mouth ulcers), pharyngitis, gastritis, colitis, hepatitis, severe blood dyscrasias (agranulocytosis, aplastic anemia), or even anaphylactic shock.

Contraindications

Gold therapy is contraindicated for clients with eczema, urticaria, colitis, hemorrhagic conditions, and systemic lupus erythematosus.

TABLE 21–3 Antiinflammatory Drugs: Gold Preparations

Generic (Brand)	Route and Dosage	Uses and Considerations
Auranofin (Ridaura)	See Prototype Drug Chart (Fig. 21–3)	For rheumatoid arthritis when unresponsive to NSAIDs. Start with low dose. Check laboratory values, especially white blood cell count, hemoglobin, and hematocrit. Check renal and liver function. *Pregnancy category:* C; PB: 60%; t½: 26 d
Aurothioglucose (Solganal)	Increase dose weekly: A: IM: 10, 25, 50 mg (sol in oil)	Same considerations as auranofin. *Pregnancy category:* C; PB: 95%; t½: 3–27 d
Gold sodium thiomalate (Myochrysine)	Increase dose weekly: A: IM: 10, 25, 50 mg (aqueous sol) until 1 g cumulative: maint: 25–50 mg q2–3wk C: TD: 10 mg, followed by 1 mg/kg/wk × 20 wk; maint: 1 mg/kg/dose every 2–4 wk	Same considerations as auranofin. Contains 50% gold. *Pregnancy category:* C; PB: 95%; t½: 3–27 d

KEY: *A: adult; C: child; IM: intramuscular; TD: test dose; PB: protein-binding; t½: half-life; sol: solution; maint: maintenance.*

FIGURE 21–3. Antiinflammatory Agent: Gold

Gold Preparation	Dosage	NURSING PROCESS
		Assessment and Planning

Gold Preparation

Auranofin
  (Ridaura)
Pregnancy Category: C

Dosage

A: PO: 6 mg/d in single or divided
  doses; may increase dose to 9 mg/d
C: Initial: 0.1 mg/kg/d in 1–2 divided
  doses; *maint:* 0.15 mg/kg/d in 1–2
  divided doses; *max:* 0.2 mg/kg/d in
  1–2 divided doses

Contraindications

Severe renal or hepatic disease, colitis,
  systemic lupus erythematosus (SLE),
  pregnancy, blood dyscrasias
Caution: Diabetes mellitus, CHF

Drug-Lab-Food Interactions

With anticancer drugs, may cause bone
  marrow depression
Lab: Slightly *increase* liver enzyme tests

Pharmacokinetics

Absorption: PO: 25% absorbed
Distribution: PB: 60%
Metabolism: t½: 26 d in blood; 40–120 d
  in tissue
Excretion: >60% in urine (may appear
  for 15 mon); in feces

Pharmacodynamics

PO: Onset: UK
  Peak: 1–2 h
  Duration: Months

Interventions

Therapeutic Effects/Uses: To alleviate inflammation and pain of rheumatoid arthritis.

Mode of Action: Inhibition of prostaglandin synthesis and decreased phagocytosis.

Evaluation

Side Effects

Anorexia, nausea, vomiting, diarrhea,
  stomatitis, abdominal cramps,
  pruritus, dizziness, headache,
  metallic taste, rash, dermatitis,
  photosensitivity

Adverse Reactions

Corneal gold deposits, urticaria,
  hematuria, proteinuria, bradycardia
Life-threatening: Nephrotoxicity,
  agranulocytosis, thrombocytopenia,
  interstitial pneumonitis

KEY: A: adult; C: child; PO: by mouth; PB: protein-binding; t½: half-life; UK: unknown; >: greater than.

NURSING PROCESS: ANTIINFLAMMATORY DRUGS: Gold

ASSESSMENT

- Obtain the client's health history. Usually, gold drugs such as auranofin are contraindicated if there is renal or hepatic dysfunction, marked hypertension, congestive heart failure, systemic lupus erythematosus (SLE), or uncontrolled diabetes mellitus.
- Check for proteinuria and hematuria before giving initial gold dose and during gold therapy.
- Observe the client for 30 min after gold injection for possible allergic reaction after the first and second injections. It takes approximately 10 to 15 min for a serious allergic reaction (anaphylaxis) to occur.
- Obtain baseline vital signs (VS) and hematology laboratory findings for future comparisons.

POTENTIAL NURSING DIAGNOSES

- Impaired physical mobility
- Pain
- High risk for impaired skin integrity

PLANNING

- The client will be free of inflammation and pain while taking the gold treatment without adverse drug reaction.

NURSING INTERVENTIONS

- Monitor the client's VS. Report abnormal findings.
- Monitor laboratory tests, e.g., complete blood count (CBC). Report abnormal findings.
- Check periodically for signs of side effects and adverse reactions to gold therapy. Side effects may include anorexia, nausea, vomiting, diarrhea, gingivitis, stomatitis, rash, itching, and decreased urine output. Most gold drugs have a long half-life; thus, a cumulative effect can result. Auranofin causes less severe adverse reactions than other gold preparations.

CLIENT TEACHING

General

- Instruct the client to perform frequent dental hygiene, including brushing the teeth with a soft toothbrush and flossing to prevent or control gingivitis and stomatitis. Use of diluted hydrogen peroxide can be helpful with mild stomatitis.
- Instruct the client to adhere to scheduled laboratory blood tests and appointments with the health care provider so any adverse reactions can be monitored.

- Inform the client that the desired therapeutic effect may take as long as 3 to 4 mon to occur.

Diet

- Suggest high-fiber diet or antidiarrheal drugs to control diarrhea. If diarrhea is continuous or severe for a prolonged time, the gold drug is usually discontinued.

Side Effects

- Explain to the client to report early symptoms of possible gold toxicity such as a metallic taste or pruritus. A rash may occur. These symptoms should be reported to the health care provider.
- Teach the client the side effects and to report them immediately. (See list of side effects and adverse reactions.)
- Instruct the client to avoid direct sunlight because the gold drug may cause photosensitivity. Use of sunblock is necessary.
- Instruct the client to report skin conditions such as dermatitis, bruising, and petechiae. Bleeding gums and blood in the stools should be reported to the health care provider.

EVALUATION

- Evaluate the effectiveness of the gold therapy by determining if the client has less pain and inflammation.
- Evaluate the client for present or repeated side effects. The gold therapy regimen may need to be changed or discontinued.

IMMUNOSUPPRESSIVE AGENTS

Immunosuppressives are used to treat refractory rheumatoid arthritis; that is, arthritis that does not respond to antiinflammatory drugs. Drugs such as azathioprine (Imuran), cyclophosphamide (Cytoxan), and methotrexate (Mexate) are used primarily to suppress cancer growth and proliferation. These drugs might be used in suppressing the inflammatory process of rheumatoid arthritis when other treatments fail.

ANTIMALARIALS

Antimalarial drugs may be used in treatment of rheumatoid arthritis when other methods of treat-

ment fail. The mechanism of action of antimalarials in suppression of rheumatoid arthritis is unclear. The effect may take 4 to 12 weeks to become apparent, and antimalarials are usually used in combination with NSAIDs in clients whose arthritis is not under control.

ANTIGOUT DRUGS

Gout is an inflammatory condition that attacks joints, tendons, and other tissues. The most common site of acute gouty inflammation is at the joint of the big toe. Gout is characterized by a defect in purine (products of certain proteins) metabolism, resulting in an increase in urates (uric acid salts) and an accumulation of uric acid (hyperuricemia) or an ineffective clearance of uric acid by the kidneys. Uric acid solubility is poor in acid urine and urate crystals may form, causing urate calculi. Fluid intake should be increased while taking antigout drugs, and the urine should be alkaline. Acetaminophen should be taken for discomfort instead of aspirin (salicylic acid) to reduce acidity. Foods rich in purine, including wine, alcohol, organ meats, sardines, salmon, and gravy, should be avoided.

ANTIINFLAMMATORY GOUT DRUG: COLCHICINE

The antiinflammatory drug colchicine inhibits the migration of leukocytes to the inflamed site. It does not inhibit uric acid synthesis and does not promote uric acid excretion. It should not be used if the client has a severe renal, cardiac, or GI problem. Gastric irritation is a common problem; therefore, colchicine should be taken with food.

Colchicine is well absorbed in the GI tract, and its peak concentration time is within 2 h. Most of the drug is excreted in the feces, but 10% to 20% is excreted in the urine.

URIC ACID INHIBITOR

Allopurinol (Zyloprim) is not an antiinflammatory drug; instead, it inhibits the final steps of uric acid biosynthesis and therefore lowers serum uric acid levels, preventing the precipitation of an attack. This drug is frequently used today for prevention (prophylaxis) of gout. Allopurinol is also indicated

for gout clients with renal impairment. Figure 21–4 lists the pharmacologic behavior of allopurinol.

Pharmacokinetics

Eighty percent of allopurinol is absorbed from the GI tract. Biosynthesis of uric acid occurs in the liver in pure form and active metabolites. The half-life of the drug itself is 2 to 3 h, and of its active metabolites is 20 to 24 h. The protein-binding percentage is unknown. Most of the drug and its metabolite are excreted in feces and some in urine.

Pharmacodynamics

Allopurinol inhibits the production of uric acid by inhibiting the enzyme xanthine oxidase, which is needed in the synthesis of uric acid. Allopurinol also improves the solubility of uric acid. Its onset of action occurs within 30 to 60 min; its peak time is average, 2 to 4 h; and it has a long duration of action.

Alcohol, caffeine, and thiazide diuretics increase the uric acid level. Use of ampicillin or amoxicillin with allopurinol increases the risk of rash formation. Allopurinol can increase the effect of coumadin and oral hypoglycemic drugs.

URICOSURICS

Uricosurics increase the rate of uric acid excretion by inhibiting its reabsorption. This group of drugs is effective in alleviating chronic gout, but they should *not* be used during acute attacks. Probenecid (Benemid) is a uricosuric that has been available since 1945. It blocks the reabsorption of uric

TABLE 21–4 Antigout Drugs

Generic (Brand)	Route and Dosage	Uses and Considerations
Antiinflammatory Gout Drug		
Colchicine (Novocolchine Colsalide)	A: PO: Initially: 0.5–1.2 mg; then 0.5–0.6 mg q1–2h for pain relief; max: 4 mg/d IV: Initially: 2 mg; then 0.5 mg q6h PRN; *max:* 4 mg/d	Treatment of acute gout and prophylaxis of recurrent gouty arthritis. Not for clients with renal or gastric disorders. Take with food. *Pregnancy category:* C; PB: 10%–30%, t½: 20–30 min
Uric Acid Biosynthesis Inhibitor		
Allopurinol (Zyloprim)	See Prototype Drug Chart (Fig. 21–4)	Treatment for hyperuricemia by preventing uric acid synthesis. Prevents acute gouty attack. Keep urine alkaline; increase fluid intake. *Pregnancy category:* C; PB: UK; t½: 2–3 h
Uricosurics		
Probenecid (Benemid)	A: PO: First week: 250 mg b.i.d.; maint: 500 mg b.i.d.; *max:* 2 g/d C < 50 kg: PO: 25–40 mg/kg/d in 4 divided doses	Treatment for hyperuricemia; promotes urinary excretion of uric acid. For gout and gouty arthritis. Alkaline urine helps to prevent renal stones. Increase fluid intake. *Pregnancy category:* B; PB: 90%; t½: 4–10 h
Sulfinpyrazone (Anturane)	A: PO: First week: 100–200 mg b.i.d.; maint: 200–400 mg b.i.d.; *max:* 800 mg/d	Used in the management of hyperuricemia; decreases gouty attacks. Can cause GI distress. Take with food. *Pregnancy category:* C; PB: 90%; t½: 3 h

KEY: *A: adult; C: child; PO: by mouth; IV: intravenous; UK: unknown; <: less than; PRN: as necessary; PB: protein-binding; t½: half-life; maint: maintenance.*

acid and promotes its excretion. Probenecid can be taken with colchicine. If gastric irritation occurs, probenecid should be taken with meals. It has an average half-life of 8 to 10 h and is 85% to 95% protein-bound. Caution should be taken when administering this drug with other highly protein-bound drugs.

Another uricosuric is sulfinpyrazone (Anturane). This drug is a metabolite of phenylbutazone and is more potent than probenecid. Sulfinpyrazone should be taken with meals or with antacids to prevent gastric irritation. Severe blood dyscrasias

might occur, especially with a history of blood dyscrasia. Table 21–4 gives the commonly used antigout drugs, their dosages, and uses and considerations.

Side Effects and Adverse Reactions

Side effects may include flushed skin, sore gums, and headache. Kidney stones, resulting from the uric acid, could be prevented by increasing water intake and maintaining a urine pH above 6.0. Blood dyscrasias occur rarely. Aspirin use should be avoided because it causes uric acid retention.

FIGURE 21–4. Antigout

Uric Acid Biosynthesis Inhibitor	Dosage	NURSING PROCESS Assessment and Planning
Allopurinol (Zyloprim) 🍁 Alloprin, Apo-Allopurinol, Novopurinol *Pregnancy Category:* C	A: PO: 200–300 mg/d (for mild gout) 400–600 mg/d (for severe gout) C: PO: 10 mg/kg/d in 2–3 divided doses <6 y: 150 mg/d in 3 divided doses	
Contraindications	**Drug-Lab-Food Interactions**	
Hypersensitivity, severe renal disease *Caution:* Hepatic disorder	*Increase* effect of warfin, phenytoin, theophylline, anticancer drugs, ACE inhibitors; *increase* rash with ampicillin, amoxicillin; *increase* toxicity with thiazide diuretics *Decrease* allopurinol effect with antacids *Lab: Increase* AST, ALT, BUN	
Pharmacokinetics	**Pharmacodynamics**	Interventions
Absorption: PO: 80% absorbed *Distribution:* PB: UK *Metabolism:* t½: Drug: 2–3 h Metabolite: 20–24 h *Excretion:* 10–20% in urine; 80–90% in feces	PO: Onset: 0.5–1 h Peak: 2–4 h Duration: 18–30 h	

Therapeutic Effects/Uses: To treat gout and hyperuricemia; prevent urate calculi.

Mode of Action: Reduction of uric acid synthesis.

Evaluation

Side Effects	Adverse Reactions
Anorexia, nausea, vomiting, diarrhea, stomatitis, dizziness, headache, rash, pruritus, malaise, metallic taste	Cataracts, retinopathy *Life-threatening:* Bone marrow depression, aplastic anemia, thrombocytopenia, agranulocytosis, leukopenia

KEY: A: adult; C: child; PO: by mouth; UK: unknown; PB: protein-binding; t½: half-life; <: less than; 🍁: Canadian drug names.

NURSING PROCESS: ANTIGOUT

ASSESSMENT

- Obtain a medical history from the client of any gastric, renal, cardiac, or liver disorders. Antigout drugs are excreted via kidneys, so sufficient renal function is needed. Drug dosage and drug selection might need to be changed.
- Obtain a drug history. Report possible drug-drug interactions. (See drug-laboratory-food interaction list.)
- Assess the serum uric acid value to be used for future comparisons.
- Assess the urine output. Use the initial urine output for future comparison.
- Obtain laboratory tests (BUN, serum creatinine, ALP, AST, ALT, LDH) and compare with future laboratory test results.

POTENTIAL NURSING DIAGNOSES

- Impaired tissue integrity
- Pain

PLANNING

- Client's "gouty pain" is absent or controlled without side effects.

NURSING INTERVENTIONS

- Report GI symptoms, gastric pain, nausea, vomiting, or diarrhea when taking antigout drugs. Take these drugs with food to alleviate gastric distress.
- Monitor the client's urine output. Because the drugs and uric acid are excreted through the urine, kidney stones might occur, so both water intake and urine output should be increased.
- Monitor laboratory tests for renal and liver function; i.e., BUN, serum creatinine, ALP, AST, and ALT.

General

- Encourage the client to keep medical appointments and to have regular scheduled laboratory tests for renal, liver, and blood cell (CBC) functions. Some antigout drugs may cause blood dyscrasias; blood tests should be monitored.
- Instruct the client to increase fluid intake; it will increase drug and uric acid excretion.

Diet

- Advise the client to avoid alcohol and caffeine because they can increase uric acid levels.
- Suggest to the client not to take large doses of vitamin C while taking allopurinol; kidney stones may occur.
- Instruct the client not to ingest foods that are high in purine content, such as organ meats, salmon and sardines, gravies, and legumes. Purine foods increase the uric acid levels.
- Instruct the client to report any gastric distress. Encourage the client to take antigout drugs with food or at mealtime.

Side Effects

- Instruct the client to report side effects of antigout drugs, such as anorexia, nausea, vomiting, diarrhea, stomatitis, dizziness, rash, pruritus, and metallic taste, to the health care provider.
- Advise the client to have a yearly eye examination because visual changes can result from prolonged use of allopurinol.

EVALUATION

- Evaluate the client's response to the antigout drug. If pain persists, the drug regimen may need modification.
- Determine the presence of adverse reactions. Drug therapy for gout pain may need to be changed.

STUDY QUESTIONS

1. What is the action of nonsteroidal antiinflammatory drugs (NSAIDs)? Give examples of common NSAIDs.
2. What are the major side effects of NSAIDs?
3. What are the uses of disease-modifying antirheumatic drugs (DMARDs)?

4. What are the side effects and adverse reactions of DMARDs?
5. What are the nursing interventions associated with the use of NSAIDs and DMARDs?
6. What drugs are used to treat gout? What are the nursing considerations?

Chapter 22

Antibacterials: Penicillins and Cephalosporins

OUTLINE

Objectives
Terms
Introduction
Antibacterial Drugs
    Mechanisms of Antibacterial Action
    Resistance to Antibacterials
    General Adverse Reactions to Antibacterials

Narrow-Spectrum and Broad-Spectrum Antibiotics
Penicillins
    Broad-Spectrum Penicillins
    Penicillinase-Resistant Penicillins
    Antipseudomonal Penicillins

Nursing Process
Cephalosporins
    First-, Second-, and Third-Generation Cephalosporins
    Nursing Process
Case Study
Study Questions

OBJECTIVES

Explain the mechanisms of action of antibacterial drugs.

Differentiate between bacteria that are naturally resistant and those that have acquired resistance to an antibiotic.

Identify several adverse effects associated with antibacterial drugs.

Differentiate between narrow-spectrum and broad-spectrum antibiotics.

Give an example each of natural, broad-spectrum (extended), penicillinase-resistant, and antipseudomonal penicillins.

Explain the expected effects of the first, second, and third generations of cephalosporins.

Describe specific nursing interventions and the client teaching that relate to the administration of penicillins and cephalosporins.

TERMS

acquired resistance
antibacterials
antimicrobials
bactericidal
bacteriostatic

broad-spectrum antibiotic
cross-resistance
immunoglobulins
inherent resistance
microorganisms

narrow-spectrum antibiotic
nephrotoxicity
nosocomial infection
superinfection

INTRODUCTION

Although the terms *antibacterial, antimicrobial,* and *antibiotic* are frequently used interchangeably, there are some subtle differences in meaning. **Antibacterial** and **antimicrobial drugs** are substances that inhibit the growth of or kill bacteria or other microorganisms (microscopic organisms including bacteria, viruses, fungi, protozoa, and rickettsiae). Technically, the term *antibiotic* refers to chemicals that are produced by one kind of microorganism that inhibit the growth of or kill another. For practical purposes, however, these terms may be used interchangeably. Several drugs, including antiinfective and chemotherapeutic agents, have actions similar to those of the antibacterial and antimicrobial agents. Antibacterial drugs do not act alone in destroying bacteria. Natural body defenses, surgical procedures to excise infected tissues, and dressing changes may be needed along with antibacterial drugs to eliminate the infecting bacteria.

Antibacterial drugs are obtained from natural sources or are manufactured. The use of moldy bread on wounds to fight infection dates back 3500 years. In 1928, Alexander Fleming, a British bacteriologist, noted that "mold" was contaminating the bacterial cultures and inhibiting the bacterial growth. Fleming called the mold *Penicillium notatum.* In 1939, Howard Florey continued with Fleming's findings and purified the penicillin so that it could be used commercially. Penicillin was used during World War II and became widely marketed in 1945. Sulfonamide, a synthetic antibacterial, was introduced in 1935. Sulfonamides are discussed in greater detail in Chapter 24.

Bacteriostatic drugs inhibit the growth of bacteria, whereas **bactericidal** drugs kill bacteria. Some antibacterial drugs, such as tetracycline and sulfonamides, have a bacteriostatic effect, whereas other antibacterials, such as penicillins and cephalosporins, have a bactericidal effect. Depending on the drug dose and serum level, certain drugs can have both bacteriostatic and bactericidal effects. Drug serum levels should be monitored.

Peaks and troughs of serum antibiotic levels are monitored for drugs with a narrow therapeutic index, such as aminoglycosides, to determine if the drug is within the therapeutic range for its desired effect. If the serum peak level is too high, drug toxicity could occur. If the serum trough level, drawn minutes before the next drug dose, is below the therapeutic range, the client is not receiving an adequate antibiotic dose to kill the microorganism.

ANTIBACTERIAL DRUGS

Antibacterial drugs are currently grouped into ten categories: penicillins, cephalosporins, macrolides, tetracyclines, lincosamides, vancomycin, aminoglycosides, chloramphenicol, fluoroquinolones, and peptides. Penicillins and cephalosporins are discussed in this chapter. Antibacterials and antibiotics II (macrolides, tetracyclines, aminoglycosides, and fluoroquinolones) are described in Chapter 23. Sulfonamides are presented in Chapter 24. Antitubercular drugs, antifungal drugs, and peptides are covered in Chapter 25. Antivirals, antimalarials, and anthelmintics are discussed in Chapter 26. Today most antibiotics are produced semisynthetically or synthetically.

TABLE 22–1 Mechanisms of Actions of Antibacterial Drugs

Action	Effect	Drugs
Inhibitions of cell wall synthesis	Bactericidal effect. a. Enzyme breakdown of the cell wall b. Inhibition of the enzyme in the synthesis of the cell wall	Penicillin Cephalosporins Bacitracin Vancomycin
Alteration in membrane permeability	Bacteriostatic or bactericidal effect. Membrane permeability is increased. The loss of cellular substances causes lysis of the cell.	Amphotericin B Nystatin Polymyxin Colistin
Inhibition of protein synthesis	Bacteriostatic or bactericidal effect. Interferes with protein synthesis without affecting normal cell. Inhibits the steps of protein synthesis.	Aminoglycosides Tetracyclines Erythromycin Lincomycins
Interference with cellular metabolism	Bacteriostatic effect. Interferes with steps of metabolism within the cells.	Sulfonamides Trimethoprim Isoniazid (INH) Naldixic acid Rifampin

MECHANISMS OF ANTIBACTERIAL ACTION

Four mechanisms of antibacterial action are responsible for the inhibition of growth or destruction of microorganisms: (1) inhibition of bacterial cell wall synthesis, (2) alteration of membrane permeability, (3) inhibition of protein synthesis, and (4) interference with metabolism within the cell. Table 22–1 discusses the four mechanisms of action and gives antibacterial drug examples.

Antibacterial drugs must not only penetrate the bacterial cell wall in sufficient concentration, but the drug must have an affinity to the binding sites on the bacterial cell. The time the drug remains at the binding sites increases the effect of the antibacterial action. The time is controlled by the pharmacokinetics (distribution, half-life, and elimination) of the drug. Antibacterials that have a longer half-life usually maintain a greater concentration at the binding site and frequent dosing is not required. Most antibacterials are not highly protein-bound, with the exception of a few, i.e., oxacillin, ceftriaxone, cefoperazone, cefonicid, cefprozil, cloxacillin, nafcillin, and clindamycin. Thus, protein-binding does not have a major influence regarding the effectiveness of the drug dose. The steady state of the antibacterial drug occurs after the fourth to fifth half-lives, and the drug is eliminated from the body after the seventh half-life.

Antibacterial drugs are used to achieve the minimum effective concentration (MEC) necessary to halt the growth of a microorganism—a concentration that depends upon the drug's pharmacokinetics (absorption, distribution, metabolism and excretion). However, when minimum bactericidal concentration (MBC) is desired, a considerably greater concentration of drug is usually needed, so

the client should be monitored and assessed for drug toxicity.

Pharmacodynamics of Antibacterials

The drug concentration at the site or the exposure time for the drug plays an important role in bacteria eradication. Many antibacterials have a bactericidal effect against the pathogen when the drug concentration remains constantly above the MEC during the dosing interval. Duration of time for use of the antibacterial varies according to the type of pathogen, site of infection, and immunocompetence of the host. With some severe infections, a continuous infusion regimen is more effective than an intermittent dosing because of constant drug concentration and time exposure. Once-daily antibacterial dosing (e.g., aminoglycosides) has been effective in eradicating pathogens and in most of those cases has not caused severe adverse reactions (ototoxicity, nephrotoxicity). In addition, once- or twice-daily drug dosing increases the client's adherence to the drug regimen.

Figure 22–1 displays the effect of three methods of drug dosing. The drug dose is effective while it remains above the MEC.

Body defenses and antibacterial drugs work together to stop the infectious process. The effect antibacterial drugs have on an infection depends not only on the drug, but also on the host's defense mechanisms. Factors such as age, nutrition, immunoglobulins, white blood cells, organ function, and circulation influence the body's ability to fight infection. If the host's natural body defense mechanisms are inadequate, drug therapy might not be as effective. As a result, drug therapy may need to be closely monitored or revised. When circulation is impeded, an antibacterial drug may not be distrib-

FIGURE 22–1 Effects of concentrated drug dosing.

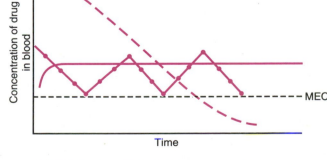

uted properly to the infected area. In addition, **immunoglobulins,** e.g., IgG, IgM, (a protein with antibody activity; part of the immune response system), and white blood cells needed to combat infections may be depleted in individuals with poor nutritional status.

RESISTANCE TO ANTIBACTERIALS

Bacteria may be sensitive or resistant to certain antibacterials. When a bacteria is sensitive to the drug, the organism is inhibited or destroyed. If a bacteria is resistant to an antibacterial, the organism continues to grow despite administration of that antibacterial drug.

Bacterial resistance may result naturally (inherent), or it may be acquired. A **natural,** or **inherent, resistance** occurs without previous exposure to the antibacterial drug. For example, the gram-negative (non-Gram-staining) bacterium *Pseudomonas aeruginosa* is resistant to penicillin G. An **acquired resistance** is caused by prior exposure to the antibacterial. For example, although *Staphylococcus aureus* was once sensitive to penicillin G, previous exposures have caused this organism to become resistant to penicillin G. Penicillinase, an enzyme produced by the microorganism, is responsible for causing penicillin resistance. This enzyme metabolizes penicillin G, causing the drug to be ineffective. Available today are penicillinase-resistant penicillins that are effective against *Staphylococcus aureus*.

In large health care institutions, there is a tendency toward drug resistance to bacteria. Mutant strains of organisms have developed, thus increasing the resistance to the antibiotics that were once effective. Infections that are acquired while clients are hospitalized are called **nosocomial infections.**

Many of these infections are caused by drug-resistant bacteria and can prolong hospitalization, which is costly to the client.

Cross-resistance can also occur between antibacterial drugs that have similar actions, such as the penicillins and cephalosporins. The organism causing the infection can be determined by culture, and the antibiotics sensitive to the organism are determined by culture and sensitivity (C & S). To determine the effect antibacterial drugs have on a specific microorganism, C & S or antibiotic susceptibility testing is performed. The susceptibility or resistance of one microorganism to several antibacterials can be determined by this method. Multi-antibiotic therapy (daily use of several antibacterials) delays the development of microorganism resistance.

GENERAL ADVERSE REACTIONS TO ANTIBACTERIALS

Three major adverse reactions associated with the administration of antibacterial drugs are allergic (hypersensitivity) reactions, superinfection, and organ toxicity. Table 22–2 describes these adverse reactions, all of which require close monitoring of the client.

NARROW-SPECTRUM AND BROAD-SPECTRUM ANTIBIOTICS

Antibacterial drugs are either narrow spectrum or broad spectrum. The **narrow-spectrum antibiotics** are primarily effective against one type of organism. For example, penicillin and erythromycin are used to treat infections caused by gram-positive bacteria. **Broad-spectrum antibiotics,** such as tetra-

TABLE 22–2 General Adverse Reactions to Antibacterial Drugs

Type	Considerations
Allergy or hypersensitivity effect	Allergic reactions to drugs may be mild or severe. Examples of mild reactions are rash, pruritus, and hives. An example of a severe response is anaphylactic shock. Anaphylaxis results in vascular collapse, laryngeal edema, bronchospasm, and cardiac arrest. Shortness of breath is frequently the first symptom of anaphylaxis. Severe allergic reaction generally occurs within 20 min. Mild allergic reaction is treated with an antihistamine; anaphylaxis requires treatment with epinephrine, bronchodilators, and antihistamines.
Superinfection	Superinfection is a secondary infection that occurs when the normal microbial flora of the body are disturbed during antibiotic therapy. Superinfections can occur in the mouth, respiratory tract, intestine, genitourinary tract, or skin. Fungus infections frequently result in superinfections, although bacterial organisms, such as *Proteus, Pseudomonas,* and staphylococci may be the offending microorganisms.
	Superinfections rarely develop when the drug is administered for less than a week. They occur more commonly with the use of broad-spectrum antibiotics. For fungal infection of the mouth, nystatin is frequently used
Organ toxicity	Organs, such as the liver and kidney, are involved in drug metabolism and excretion. Antibacterials may result in damage to these organs. For example, aminoglycosides can be ototoxic and nephrotoxic.

cycline and the cephalosporins, are effective against both gram-positive and gram-negative organisms. Because narrow-spectrum antibiotics are selective, they are more active against those single organisms than the broad-spectrum antibiotics. Broad-spectrum antibiotics are frequently used to treat infections when the offending microorganism has not been identified by culture and sensitivity.

PENICILLINS

Penicillin, a natural antibacterial agent obtained from the mold genus *Penicillium*, was introduced to the military during World War II and is considered to have saved many soldiers' lives. It became widely used in 1945 and was labeled the "miracle" drug. With the advent of penicillin, many clients survived who would have died from wound and severe respiratory infections.

Penicillin's beta lactam structure interferes with bacterial cell wall synthesis by inhibiting the bacterial enzyme that is necessary for cell division and cellular synthesis. The bacteria dies due to cell lysis (cell breakdown). The penicillins can be both bacteriostatic and bactericidal depending on the drug and dosage. Penicillin G is primarily bactericidal.

Penicillin G was the first penicillin administered orally and by injection. With oral administration, only about one-third of the dose is absorbed. Because of its poor absorption, penicillin G given by injection (intramuscular and intravenous) is more effective in achieving a therapeutic serum penicillin level. Aqueous penicillin G has a short duration of action, and the intramuscular injection is very painful due to the aqueous drug solution. Therefore, a longer-acting form of penicillin, procaine penicillin (milky color) was produced to extend the drug's activity. Procaine in the penicillin decreases the pain related to injection of this medication.

Penicillin V was the next type of penicillin produced. Although two-thirds of the oral dose is absorbed by the gastrointestinal (GI) tract, it is a less potent antibacterial drug than penicillin G. Penicillin V is effective against mild to moderate infections.

Initially, penicillin was overused. It was first introduced for the treatment of staphylococcus infections, but after a few years, mutant strains of staphylococcus developed that were resistant to penicillins G and V. In addition, staphylococcus secretes a bacterial enzyme, penicillinase, that destroys penicillin, rendering it ineffective. This led to the development of new broad-spectrum antibiotics with structures similar to penicillin to combat infections that are resistant to penicillins G and V.

BROAD-SPECTRUM PENICILLINS

The broad-spectrum penicillins are used to treat both gram-positive and gram-negative bacterias. They are not, however, as "broadly" effective against all microorganisms as they were once considered to be. This group of drugs is costlier than penicillin and therefore should not be used when ordinary penicillins, such as penicillin G are effective. The broad-spectrum penicillins are effective against some gram-negative organisms, such as *Escherichia coli, Haemophilus influenzae, Shigella dysenteriae, Proteus mirabilis,* and *Salmonella;* however, these drugs are not penicillinase-resistant. Examples of this group are ampicillin, amoxicillin, bacampicillin, and cyclacillin (Table 22–3). Amoxicillin is the most prescribed penicillin derivative for adults and children.

PENICILLINASE-RESISTANT PENICILLINS

The penicillinase-resistant penicillins (antistaphylococcal penicillins) are used for treating penicillinase-producing *Staphylococcus aureus.* Cloxacillin and dicloxacillin are oral preparations of these antibiotics; methicillin, nafcillin, and oxacillin are intramuscular and intravenous preparations. This group of drugs is not effective against gram-negative organisms, and they are less effective than penicillin G against gram-positive organisms. Figure 22–2 compares the similarities and differences of the broad-spectrum penicillin amoxicillin and the penicillinase-resistant penicillin cloxacillin.

Pharmacokinetics

Amoxicillin is well absorbed from the GI tract, whereas cloxacillin is only partially absorbed. Protein-binding power differs between the two drugs—amoxicillin is 25% protein-bound, and cloxacillin is highly protein-bound (>90%). Drug toxicity may result when other highly protein-bound drugs are used with cloxacillin. Both of these drugs have short half-lives. Seventy percent of amoxicillin is excreted in the urine; cloxacillin is excreted in the bile and urine.

Pharmacodynamics

Both amoxicillin and cloxacillin are penicillin derivatives and are bactericidal. These drugs interfere with bacterial cell wall synthesis, causing cell lysis. Amoxicillin may be produced with or without clavulanic acid, an agent that prevents the breakdown of amoxicillin by decreasing resistance to the

FIGURE 22–2. Penicillin Derivations: Amoxicillin and Cloxacillin

Penicillins	Dosage	NURSING PROCESS
		Assessment and Planning
Broad-Spectrum Penicillins Amoxicillin trihydrate (A), (Amoxil), 🍁 Apo-Amoxi Amoxicillin-clavulanate (Augmentin), 🍁 Clavulin *Pregnancy Category:* B *Penicillinase-Resistant Penicillin* Cloxacillin sodium (C) (Tegopen), 🍁 Apo-Cloxi, Novocloxin *Pregnancy Category:* B	(A) A: PO: 250–500 mg, q8h C: PO: 20–40 mg/kg/d; in 3 divided doses (C) A: PO: 250–500 mg, q6h C: PO: 12.5–25 mg/kg/d in 4 di- vided doses	

Contraindications	Drug-Lab-Food Interactions	
(A&C) Allergic to penicillin (A) Severe renal disorder *Caution:* (A&C) Hypersensitivity to cephalosporins	(A&C) *Increase* effect with aspirin, probenecid *Decrease* effect with tetracycline, erythromycin *Lab: Increase* serum AST, ALT	

Pharmacokinetics	Pharmacodynamics	Interventions
Absorption: PO: (A) >80% in intestine (C) 40–60% GI tract *Distribution:* PB: (A) 20% (C) 90–95% *Metabolism:* t½: (A) 1–1.5 h (C) 0.5–1 h *Excretion:* (A) 70% in urine; clavulanate: 30–40% in urine (C) Excreted in bile and urine	(A) PO: Onset: 0.5 h Peak: 1–2 h Duration: 6–8 h (C) PO: Onset: 0.5 h Peak: 1–2 h Duration: 6 h	

	Evaluation
Therapeutic Effects/Uses: (A) To treat respiratory tract infection, urinary tract infection, otitis media, sinusitis. (C) To treat *Staphylococcus aureus* infection. *Mode of Action:* (A&C) Inhibition of the enzyme in cell wall synthesis. Bactericidal effect.	

Side Effects	Adverse Reactions
(A&C) Nausea, vomiting, diarrhea, rash (A) Edema, stomatitis (C) Lethargy, twitching, depression, increased bleeding time	(A&C) Superinfections (vaginitis) *Life-threatening:* (A&C) Blood dyscrasias, hemolytic anemia, bone marrow depression (A) Respiratory distress (C) Agranulocytosis

KEY: A: adult; C: child; PO: by mouth; PB: protein-binding; t½: half-life; 🍁: Canadian drug names.

antibacterial drug. The addition of clavulanic acid intensifies the effect of amoxicillin. The amoxicillin-clavulanic acid preparation (Augmentin) and amoxicillin trihydrate (Amoxil) have similar pharmacokinetics and pharmacodynamics, as well as similar side effects and adverse reactions.

When aspirin and probenecid are taken with amoxicillin or cloxacillin, the serum antibacterial

TABLE 22–3 Antibacterials: Penicillins

Generic (Brand)	Route and Dosage	Uses and Considerations
Basic Penicillins		
Penicillin G procaine (Crysticillin, Wycillin)	A: IM: 600,000–1.2 million U/d in 1–2 divided doses C: IM: 300,00–600,000 U/d in 1–2 divided doses NB: IM: 50,000 U/kg/d	For moderately serious infections. Slow IM absorption with prolonged action. The solution is milky. *Pregnancy category:* B; PB: 65%; t½: 0.5 h
Penicillin G benzathine (Bicillin)	A: IM: 1.2 million U as a single dose C: IM: >27 kg: 900,00 U/dose IM: <27 kg: 50,000 U/kg/dose or 300,000–600,000 U/dose	Long- acting penicillin when given by injection. Used as a prophylaxis for rheumatic fever. *Pregnancy category:* B; PB: 65%; t½: 1 h
Penicillin G sodium/potassium (Pentids, Pfizerpen)	A: PO: 200,000–500,000 U q6h IM: 500,000–5 million U/d in divided doses IV: 4–20 million U/d in divided doses, diluted in IV fluids C: PO: 25,000–90,000 U/d in divided doses IV: 50,000–100,000 U/kg/d in divided doses	Poorly absorbed orally due to gastric acidity and food. Take before or after meals. Penicillin G is available in salts (potassium [K] and sodium [Na]). With high doses, electrolyte levels should be monitored. Injectable solution is clear. *Pregnancy category:* B; PB: 60%; t½: 0.5–1 h
Penicillin V potassium (V-Cillin K, Veetids, Betapen VK)	A: PO: 125–500 mg q6h C: PO: 15–50 mg/kg/d in 3–4 divided doses	Acid-stable and less active than penicillin G against some bacteria. Not recommended in renal failure. Take drug after meals. *Pregnancy category:* B; PB: 80%; t½: 0.5 h
Broad-Spectrum Penicillins Amoxicillin (Amoxil)	See Prototype Drug Chart (Fig. 22–2)	Effective against throat, nose, ear, skin, and genitourinary infections. Eighty percent is absorbed from the GI tract. Food does not prevent absorption.
Amoxicillin-clavulanate (Augmentin)	See Prototype Drug Chart (Fig. 22–2)	Same as amoxicillin. Clavulanic acid prevents amoxicillin breakdown. *Pregnancy category:* B; PB: 25%; t½: 1–1.5 h
Ampicillin (Polycillin, Omnipen)	A: PO: 250–500 mg q6h IM/IV: 2–8 g/d in divided doses C: PO: 50–100 mg/kg/d in divided doses IM/IV: 50–200 mg/kg/d in divided doses	First broad-spectrum penicillin. Fifty percent of drug is absorbed by GI tract. Effective against gram-negative and gram-positive bacteria. Individuals with penicillin allergies may also be allergic to ampicillin. *Pregnancy category:* B; PB: 15%–28% t½: 1–2 h
Ampicillin-sulbactam (Unasyn)	A: IV: 1.5–3.0 g q6h C: IV: 100–200 mg/kg/d, divided q6h	Same as ampicillin. Sulbactam inhibits beta lactamase, thus extending the spectrum. *Pregnancy category:* B; PB: 28%–38%; t½: 1–2 h
Bacampicillin HCl (Spectrobid)	A: PO: 400–800 mg q12h C: PO: 25–50 mg/kg/d in divided doses	Same as ampicillin. Ninety percent is absorbed. It is hydrolyzed to ampicillin during absorption from the GI tract. *Pregnancy category:* B; PB: 17%–20%; t½: 1 h
Penicillinase-Resistant Penicillins Cloxacillin (Tegopen)	A: PO: 250–500 mg q6h C: PO: 50–100 mg/kg/d in 4 divided doses	For penicillin-resistant staphylococci. Take before or after meals. *Pregnancy category:* B; PB: 90%; t½: 0.5–1 h
Dicloxacillin sodium (Dynapen)	A: PO: 125–500 mg q6h C: PO: 12.5–25 mg/kg/d in 4 divided doses	For systemic infection. Used against penicillin-resistant staphylococci. Has bactericidal effect. *Pregnancy category:* B; PB: 95%; t½: 0.5–1 h
Methicillin (Staphcillin)	A: IM: 1 g q6h IV: 1–2 g q6h diluted in NSS C: IM/IV: 100–300 mg/kg/d in 4–6 divided doses	First penicillinase-resistant penicillin. Used to treat staphylococcal infection. *Pregnancy category:* B; PB: 25%–40%; t½: 0.5–1 h

Table continued on following page

TABLE 22-3 Antibacterials: Penicillins (Continued)

Generic (Brand)	Route and Dosage	Uses and Considerations
Nafcillin (Nafcin, (Unipen)	A: PO: 250 mg–1 g q4–6h IM: 250–500 mg q6h IV: 500 mg–1g q4–6h C: PO: 25–100 mg/kg/d in 4 divided doses IM: 25 mg/kg b.i.d. IV: 50–200 mg/kg/d in divided doses	Highly effective against penicillin G-resistant *Staphylococcus aureus*. Not recommended for oral use due to its instability in gastric juices. *Pregnancy category:* B; PB: 90%; t½: 0.5–1.5 h
Oxacillin sodium (Prostaphlin, Bactocill)	A: PO: 250–1 g q4–6h IM/IV: 500 mg–2 g q4h; *max:* IM/IV: 12 g C: PO/IM/IV: 50–100 mg/kg/d in divided doses; *max:* IM/IV: 300 mg/kg/d	For penicillin-resistant staphylococci. As effective as methicillin. *Pregnancy category:* B; PB: 95%; t½: 0.5–1 h
Carbenicillin disodium (Geocillin, Geopen)	A: PO: 1.5–3.0 g/d in divided doses IM: 1–2 g q6h or 200 mg/kg/d in 4 divided doses IV: 4–6 g q4–6h C: PO: 30–50 mg/kg/d in divided doses; *max:* 2–3 g/d IM: 50–200 mg/kg/d in divided doses IV: 50–500 mg/kg/d in divided doses	The first penicillin-like drug developed to treat infections due to *Pseudomonas aeruginosa* and *Proteus* spp. It contains large amounts of sodium. Use with caution when administering to clients with hypertension or congestive heart failure. *Pregnancy category:* B; PB: 50%; t½: 1–1.5 h
Mezlocillin sodium (Mezlin)	A: IM/IV: 3–4 g q6h or 100–300 mg/kg/d in 4 divided doses; *max:* 24 g/d C: IM/IV: 50 mg/kg q4h	For serious infections, especially due to *Pseudomonas aeruginosa*. It can be given in combination with aminoglycosides and cephalosporins to obtain synergistic effect. *Pregnancy category:* B; PB: 30%–40%; t½: 1 h
Piperacillin sodium (Pipracil)	A: IM/IV: 2–4 g q6h or 100–300 mg/kg/d in divided doses; *max:* 24 g/d C: >12 y: IM/IV: 100–300 mg/kg/d in 4–6 divided doses	For serious infections. Can be given prior to and following surgery. Primarily used for gram-negative organisms. Treatment for septicemia; bone, joint, respiratory, and urinary tract infections. *Pregnancy category:* B; PB: 16%–22%; t½: 0.6–1.5 h
Ticarcillin disodium (Ticar)	A: IM/IV: 1–2 g q6h C: IM/IV: 50–200 mg/kg/d in 4 divided doses *Systemic infections:* Dose is increased	Effective against gram-positive and gram-negative bacilli. Used to treat respiratory, urinary, reproductive, skin, and soft tissue infections. It can be given in combination with aminoglycosides for synergistic effect. *Pregnancy category:* C; PB: 45%–65%; t½: 1–1.5 h
Ticarcillin-clavulanate (Timentin)	A: IV: 3.1 g q6h C: >12 y: IV: 200–300 mg/kg/d in 4–6 divided doses	Clavulanic acid protects ticarcillin from degradation by beta-lacta-

KEY: *A: adult; C: child; PO: by mouth; IM: intramuscularly; IV: intravenously; NB: newborn; PB: Protein-binding; t½: half-life; >: greater than; <: less than.*

levels may be increased. The effects of amoxicillin and cloxacillin are decreased when taken with erythromycin and tetracycline. The onset of action, serum peak concentration time, and duration of action for amoxicillin and cloxacillin are very similar.

ANTIPSEUDOMONAL PENICILLINS

The antipseudomonal penicillins are the new group of broad-spectrum penicillins. This group of drugs is effective against *Pseudomonas aeruginosa*, a gram-negative bacillus that is difficult to eradicate. These drugs are also useful against many gram-negative organisms such as *Proteus* spp., *Serratia* spp., *Klebsiella pneumoniae,* and *Acinetobacter* spp. The antipseudomonal penicillins are not penicillinase-resistant. Their pharmacologic action is similar to aminoglycosides, but they are less toxic than the aminoglycosides.

Each group of penicillins is described in Table 22–3, including drug group, drug names, dosages, uses, and considerations.

Side Effects and Adverse Reactions

Common adverse reactions to penicillin administration are hypersensitivity and **superinfection** (occurrence of a secondary infection when the flora of the body is disturbed) (see Table 22–2). Nausea, vomiting, and diarrhea are common GI disturbances.

Rash is an indicator of a mild to moderate allergic reaction. Severe allergic reaction leads to anaphylactic shock. Allergic effects occur in 5% to 10% of persons receiving penicillin compounds; therefore, close monitoring during the first dose and subsequent doses of penicillin is essential.

NURSING PROCESS: ANTIBACTERIALS: Penicillins

ASSESSMENT

- Assess for allergy to penicillin or cephalosporins. The client who is hypersensitive to amoxicillin should not take any type of penicillin products. Severe allergic reaction could occur. A small percentage of clients who are allergic to penicillin could also be allergic to a cephalosporin product.
- Check laboratory results, especially liver enzymes. Report elevated ALP, ALT, or AST.
- Assess urine output. If the amount is inadequate (<30 mL/h or <600 mL/d), drug and/or drug dosage may need to be changed.

POTENTIAL NURSING DIAGNOSES

- High risk for infection
- High risk for impaired tissue integrity
- Noncompliance with drug regimen

PLANNING

- Client's infection will be controlled and later eliminated.

NURSING INTERVENTIONS

- Send a sample of material from the infectious area to the laboratory for culture to determine antibiotic susceptibility (also known as C & S) before antibiotic therapy is started.
- Check for signs and symptoms of superinfection, especially for clients taking high doses of the antibiotic for a prolonged time. Signs and symptoms include stomatitis (mouth ulcers), genital discharge (vaginitis), and anal or genital itching.
- Check the client for allergic reaction to the penicillin product, especially after the first and second doses. This may be a mild reaction, such as a rash, or a severe reaction, such as respiratory distress or anaphylaxis.
- Have epinephrine available to counteract a severe allergic reaction.

- Check the client for bleeding if high doses of penicillin are being given; a decrease in platelet aggregation (clotting) may result.
- Monitor body temperature and infectious area.
- Dilute the antibiotic for IV use in an appropriate amount of solution as indicated in the drug circular.

CLIENT TEACHING

General

- Instruct the client to take all of the prescribed penicillin product such as amoxicillin until the bottle is empty. If only a portion of the penicillin is taken, drug resistance to that antibacterial agent may develop in the future.
- Advise the client who is allergic to penicillin to wear a medical alert (Medic-Alert) bracelet or necklace and carry a card that indicates the allergy. The client should notify the health care provider during history taking of his or her allergy to penicillin.
- Keep drugs out of reach of small children. Request child safety cap bottle.
- Inform the client to report any side effects or adverse reaction that may occur while taking the drug.
- Encourage the client to increase fluid intake; it will aid in decreasing the body temperature and in excreting the drug.
- Instruct the client or child's parent that chewable tablets must be chewed or crushed before swallowing.

Diet

- Advise the client to take medication with food if gastric irritation occurs. Take oral penicillin 1 h before or 2 h after meals to avoid delay in drug absorption.

EVALUATION

- Evaluate the effectiveness of the antibacterial agent by determining if the infection has ceased and no side effects, including superinfection, have occurred.

CEPHALOSPORINS

In 1948, a fungus called *Cephalosporium acremonium* was discovered from seawater at a sewer outlet off the coast of Sardinia. This fungus was found to be active against gram-positive and gram-negative bacteria and resistant to beta lactamase (enzyme that acts against beta lactam structure of penicillin). In the early 1960s, cephalosporins were used with clinical effectiveness. For the cephalosporins to be effective against numerous organisms, their molecules were chemically altered and semisynthetic cephalosporins were produced. Like penicillin, the cephalosporins have a beta lactam structure and act by inhibiting the bacterial enzyme that is necessary for cell wall synthesis. Lysis to the cell occurs, and the bacterial cell dies.

FIRST-, SECOND-, AND THIRD-GENERATION CEPHALOSPORINS

Three groups of cephalosporins have been developed, and they have been identified as generations. Each generation is effective against a broader spectrum of bacteria. The actions of the three generations of cephalosporins are discussed in Table 22–4.

Approximately 10% of persons allergic to penicillin are also allergic to cephalosporins because both groups of antibacterials have similar molecular structures. If a client is allergic to penicillin and taking a cephalosporin, the nurse should watch for a possible allergic reaction to the cephalosporin, even though the likelihood of a reaction is small.

Only a few cephalosporins are administered orally. These include cephalexin (Keflex), cefadroxil (Duricef), cephradine (Velosef), cefaclor (Ceclor), ce-furoxime acetoxyethyl ester (Ceftin), cefuroxime sodium (Zinacef), and cefixime (Suprax). The rest of the cephalosporins are administered intramuscularly and intravenously. Figure 22–3 compares the similarities of and differences between a first-generation cephalosporin, cefazolin sodium (Ancef, Kefzol), and a second-generation cephalosporin, cefaclor (Ceclor).

Pharmacokinetics

Cefazolin is administered intramuscularly and intravenously, and cefaclor is given orally. The protein-binding power of cefazolin is greater than that of cefaclor. The half-life of each drug is short, and the drugs are excreted 60% to 80% unchanged in the urine.

Pharmacodynamics

Cefazolin and cefaclor inhibit bacterial cell wall synthesis and produce a bactericidal action. For intramuscular and intravenous use of cefazolin, the onset of action is almost immediate, and the peak concentration time is 5 to 15 minutes for intravenous use. The peak concentration time for an oral dose of cefaclor is 30 to 60 minutes.

When probenecid is administered with either of these drugs, the urine excretion of cefazolin or cefaclor is decreased, which increases the drug's action. The effects of cefazolin and cefaclor can be decreased if the drug is given with tetracyclines or erythromycin. These drugs can cause false-positive laboratory results for proteinuria and glucosuria, especially when they are taken in large doses.

Table 22–5 lists the drugs in their designated generation, dosages, and considerations.

Side Effects and Adverse Reactions

The side effects and adverse reactions to cephalosporins include GI disturbances (nausea, vomiting, and diarrhea), alteration in blood clotting time (increased bleeding) with administration of large doses, and **nephrotoxicity** (toxicity to the kidney) in individuals with a preexisting renal disorder.

Drug Interactions

Drug interactions can occur with certain cephalosporins and ingestion of alcohol. For example, consuming alcohol while taking cefamandole, cefoperazone, or moxalactam may cause flushing, dizziness, headache, nausea and vomiting, and muscular cramps. Uricosuric drugs taken concurrently can decrease the excretion of cephalosporins, greatly increasing serum levels.

TABLE 22–4 Activity of the Three Generations of Cephalosporins

Generation	Activity
First	Effective against gram-positive bacteria, such as streptococci and most staphylococci. Effective against most gram-negative bacteria, such as *Escherichia coli* and species of *Klebsiella, Proteus, Salmonella,* and *Shigella.*
Second	Same effectiveness as the first generation. These antibiotics possess a broader spectrum against other gram-negative bacteria, such as *Haemophilus influenzae, Neisseria gonorrhoeae, Neisseria meningitidis, Enterobacter* spp., and several anaerobic organisms.
Third	Same effectiveness as the first and second generations. Also effective against gram-negative bacteria, such as *Pseudomonas aeruginosa, Serratia* spp., and *Acinetobacter* spp. Less effective against gram-positive bacteria.

FIGURE 22–3. Cephalosporins

Cephalosporins	Dosage	NURSING PROCESS Assessment and Planning

First-Generation Cephalosporin
Cefazolin (A)
  (Ancef, Kefzol)
Pregnancy Category: B
 	
Second-Generation Cephalosporin
Cefaclor (C)
  (Ceclor)
Pregnancy Category: B
	(A)
	A: IM/IV: 250 mg–2 g, q6–8h;
	  max: 12 g/d
	C: IM/IV: 25–100 mg/kg/d in 3
	  divided doses;
	  max: 4 g/d
	(C)
	A: PO: 250–500 mg, q8h
	  max: 4 g/d
	C: PO: 20–40 mg/kg/d in 3 divided
	  doses
	  max: 1 g/d	

Contraindications	Drug-Lab-Food Interactions	
(A&C) Hypersensitivity to cephalo-sporins *Caution* (A&C) Hypersensitivity to penicillins; renal disease, lactation	(A&C) *Increase* effect with probenecid; *increase* toxicity with loop diuretics, aminoglycosides, colistin, vancomycin (A&C) *Decrease* effect with tetracyclines, erythromycin (A&C) *Lab:* May *increase* BUN, serum creatinine, AST, ALT, ALP, LDH, bilirubin	

Pharmacokinetics	Pharmacodynamics	Interventions

Absorption:
(A) IM, IV
(C) PO: well absorbed
Distribution: PB:
(A) 75–85%
(C) 25%
Metabolism: t½:
(A) 1.5–2.5 h
(C) 0.5–1 h
Excretion:
(A) 70% excreted unchanged in urine
(C) 60–80% excreted unchanged in urine
	(A)
	IM: Onset: rapid
	  Peak: 0.5–2 h
	  Duration: UK
	IV: Onset: immediate
	  Peak: 5–15 min
	  Duration: UK
	(C)
	PO: Onset: rapid
	  Peak: 0.5–1 h
	  Duration: UK	

Evaluation

Therapeutic Effects/Uses: (A&C) To treat respiratory, urinary, and skin infections.
(A) To treat bone and joint infection, genital infections, and endocarditis.
(C) To treat ear infection, ampicillin-resistant strains, and certain gram-negative organisms, *E. coli, Proteus, H. influenzae,* and gram-positive strains, *Streptococcus pneumoniae, S. pyogenes,* and *Staphylococcus aureus.*

Mode of Action: Inhibition of cell wall synthesis, causing cell death; bactericidal effect.

Side Effects	Adverse Reactions
(A&C) Anorexia, nausea, vomiting, diarrhea, rash (A) Abdominal cramps, fever (C) Pruritus, headaches, vertigo, weakness	(A&C) Superinfections, urticaria *Life-threatening:* (A) Seizures (high doses), anaphylaxis (C) Renal failure

KEY: A: adult; C: child; PO: by mouth; IM: intramuscular; IV: intravenous; PB: protein-binding; t½: half-life; UK: unknown.

TABLE 22–5 Antibacterials: Cephalosporins

Generic (Brand)	Route and Dosage	Uses and Considerations
First Generation Cefadroxil (Duricef)	A: PO: 500 mg–2 g/d in 1–2 divided doses C: PO: 30 mg/kg/d in 2 divided doses	To treat urinary tract infections, beta-hemolytic streptococcal infections, and staphylococcal skin infection. It is well absorbed by the GI tract and is not affected by food. *Pregnancy category:* B; PB: 20%; t½: 1–2 h
Cefazolin sodium (Ancef, Kefzol)	A: IM/IV: 250 mg–1 g q6–8h; *max:* 12 g/d C: IM/IV: 25–100 mg/kg/d in 3 divided doses; *max:* 6 g/d	Similar to cephalothin but more effective against *E. coli* and *Klebsiella*. *Pregnancy category:* B; PB: 75%–85%; t½: 1.5–2.5 h
Cephalexin (Keflex)	*Infection:* A: PO: 250–500 mg q6h C: PO: 25–50 mg/kg/d in 3–4 divided doses *Otitis media:* C: PO: 25–100 mg/kg/d in 4 divided doses	First acid-stable cephalosporin sufficiently absorbed from the GI tract. Useful for treating urinary tract infections. *Pregnancy category:* B; PB: 10%–15%; t½: 0.5–1.2 h
Cephalothin (Keflin)	A: IM/IV: 500 mg–1 g q4–6h C: IM/IV: 20–40 mg/kg q6h	Cephalothin is the first cephalosporin used clinically. To treat respiratory, GI, genitourinary, bone, joint, skin, soft tissue infections; septicemia; endocarditis; meningitis. It is usually given IV. *Pregnancy category:* B; PB: 65%–80%; t½: 0.5–1 h
Cephapirin sodium (Cefadyl)	A: IM/IV: 500 mg–1 g q4–6h C: IM/IV: 40–80 mg/kg/d in 4 divided doses	Treatment is the same as for cephalothin. *Pregnancy category:* B; PB: 40%–50%; t½: 0.5–1 h
Cephradine (Velosef)	A: PO: 250–500 mg q6h or 500 mg–1 g q12h IM/IV: 500 mg–1 g q6–12 h C: PO: 25–50 mg/kg/d in 4 divided doses IM/IV: 50–100 mg/kg/d in 4 divided doses	Treatment is the same as for cephalothin. The oral drug is similar to cephalexin. Well absorbed from GI tract. *Pregnancy category:* B; PB: 20%; t½: 1–2 h
Second Generation Cefaclor (Ceclor)	See Prototype Drug Chart (Fig. 22–3)	Used to treat respiratory infections and otitis media, especially in children. Also effective for urinary tract and skin infections. Well absorbed by GI tract. *Pregnancy category:* B; PB: 25%; t½: 0.5–1 h
Cefamandole (Mandol)	A: IM/IV: 500 mg–1 g q4–8h	Used to treat infections of the bone, joint, and respiratory tract, as well as septicemia. *Pregnancy category:* B; PB: 60%–75%; t½: 1 h
Cefmetazole sodium (Zefazone)	A: IV: 2 g q6–12h	For treatment of lower respiratory and urinary tract infections. Also used for preoperative prophylaxis for surgery. *Pregnancy category:* B; PB: 68%; t½: 1.5–3 h
Cefonicid sodium (Monocid)	A: IM/IV: 500mg–2 g/d single dose or b.i.d.	Similar to cefamandole. Also used for surgical prophylaxis. *Pregnancy category:* B; PB: 98%; t½: 4.5 h
Ceforanide (Precef)	A: IM/IV: 500 mg–1 g q12h C: IM/IV: 20–40 mg/kg/d in 2 divided doses	For treatment of respiratory, urinary, skin, bone, and joint infections. Also used to treat septicemia, endocarditis, cardiovascular surgery, and prosthetic arthroplasty. *Pregnancy category:* B; PB: 80%; t½: 3 h
Cefoxitin sodium (Mefoxin)	A: IM/IV 1–2 g q6–8h; *max:* 12 g/d C: IM/IV: 80–160 mg/kg/d in divided doses	Used to treat severe infections and septicemia. *Pregnancy category:* B; PB: 70%; t½ 45 min–1 h
Cefpodoxime (Proxetil, Vantin)	A: PO: 100–400 mg q12h × 1–2 wk C: 6 mo–12 y: PO: 10 mg/kg/d in 2 divided doses	To treat respiratory and urinary tract infection, and otitis media. Food enhances drug absorption. *Pregnancy category:* B; PB: 20%–40%; t½: 2–3 h
Cefprozil monohydrate (Cefzil)	A: PO: 250–500 mg daily or q12h C: PO: 15 mg/kg q12h × 10 d	Effective against gram-positive bacilli including *Staphylococcus aureus*. With impaired renal function, dose is usually decreased by 50%. *Pregnancy category:* B; PB: 99%; t½: 1–2 h

Table continued on following page

TABLE 22–5 Antibacterials: Cephalosporins *(Continued)*

Generic (Brand)	Route and Dosage	Uses and Considerations
Cefuroxime (Ceftin, Zinacef)	A: PO: 250–500 mg q12h IM/IV: 750 mg–1.5 g q8h C: PO: 125–250 mg q12h IM/IV: 50–100 mg/kg/d in divided doses	Similar to cefamandole. Effective in treating meningitis and septicemia and for cardiothoracic procedures and surgical prophylaxis. *Pregnancy category:* B; PB: 50%; t½: 1.5–2 h
Loracarbef (Lorabid)	A: PO: 200 mg qd × 7 d C: PO: 15 mg/kg q12h × 7 d	For treatment of respiratory, urinary, and skin infections. If creatinine clearance is <50 mL/min, drug dose is reduced by 50%. *Pregnancy category:* B; PB: UK; t½: 1 h
Third Generation Cefixime (Suprax)	A: PO: 400 mg/d in 1–2 divided doses C: <12 y: PO: 8 mg/kg/d in 1–2 divided doses	Effective against most gram-positive and gram-negative bacilli: minimal effect against staphylococci and ineffective against *Pseudomonas aeruginosa*. Food does not affect drug dose. *Pregnancy category:* B; PB: 65%; t½ 2.5–4 h
Cefoperazone (Cefobid)	A: IM/IV: 2–4 g/d in 2 divided doses C: IV: 25–100 mg/kg q12h	To treat respiratory, urinary tract, and female genital tract infections. *Pregnancy category:* B; PB: 70%–80%; t½: 2.5 h
Cefotaxime (Claforan)	A: IM/IV: 1–2 g q8–12h C: IM/IV: 50–200 mg/kg/d in 4–6 divided doses *Life-threatening infection:* 2 g q4h	First of the third generation. Effective against *Pseudomonas aeruginosa*. Also used in treating gram-negative meningitis. *Pregnancy category:* B; PB: 30%–40%; t½: 1–1.5 h
Cefotetan (Cefotan)	A: IM/IV: 500 mg–2g q12h	Effective against some gram-negative organisms, except *Pseudomonas aeruginosa*. *Pregnancy category:* B; PB: 85%; t½: 3–5 h
Ceftazidime (Fortaz, Tazicef)	A: IM/IV: 500 mg–2 g q8–12h C: IV: 50 mg/kg q8h; *max:* 6 g/d	Most effective against *Pseudomonas* spp. *Pregnancy category:* B; PB: 10%–17%; t½: 1–2 h
Ceftriaxone (Rocephin)	A: IM/IV: 500 mg–2 g in single dose or q12h C: IM/IV: 50–75 mg/kg/d in 2 divided doses	Similar to ceftizoxime and cefotaxime. It has a very long half-life, so is given once or twice a day. It is used against neisseria and gonococcal infections and in the treatment of Lyme disease. *Pregnancy category:* B; PB: 85%–95%; t½: 8 h
Ceftizoxime sodium (Cefizox)	A: IM/IV: 500 mg–2 g q8–12h C: IV: 50 mg/kg q6–8h; *max:* 200 mg/kg/d	For treatment of respiratory, urinary tract, skin, bone, and joint infections. For surgical prophylaxis. *Pregnancy category:* B; PB: 30%–60%; t½: 2 h

KEY: A: adult; C: child; PO: by mouth; IM: intramuscularly; IV: intravenously; PB: protein-binding; t½: half-life; <: less than.

NURSING PROCESS: ANTIBACTERIALS: Cephalosporins

ASSESSMENT

- Assess for allergy to cephalosporins. If allergic to one type or class of cephalosporin, the client should not receive any other type of cephalosporin.
- Assess vital signs (VS) and urine output. Report abnormal findings, which may include an elevated temperature or a decrease in urine output.
- Check laboratory results, especially those that indicate renal and liver function, such as BUN, serum creatinine, AST, ALT, ALP, and bilirubin. Report abnormal findings. Use these laboratory results for baseline values.

POTENTIAL DRUG DIAGNOSES

- High risk for infection
- Noncompliance with drug regimen

PLANNING

- Client's infection will be controlled and later eliminated.

NURSING INTERVENTIONS

- Culture the infectious area before cephalosporin therapy is started. The organism causing the infection can be determined by culture, and the antibiotics sensitive to the organism are determined by C & S. (Antibiotic therapy may be started before culture result is reported. The antibiotic may need to be changed after C & S test result.)

- Check for signs and symptoms of a superinfection, especially if the client is taking high doses of a cephalosporin product for a prolonged period of time. Superinfection is usually caused by the fungal organism *Candida* in the mouth (mouth ulcers) or in the genital area, such as the vagina (vaginitis).
- Refrigerate oral suspensions. For IV cephalosporins, dilute in an appropriate amount of IV fluids (50–100 mL) according to the drug circular.
- Administer IV cephalosporins over 30–45 min 2–4 times a day.
- Monitor VS, urine output, and laboratory results. Report abnormal findings.

CLIENT TEACHING

General
- Keep drugs out of reach of small children. Request child safety cap bottle.
- Instruct the client to report signs of superinfection, such as mouth ulcers or discharge from the anal or genital area.

- Advise the client to ingest buttermilk or yogurt to prevent superinfection of the intestinal flora with long-term use of a cephalosporin.
- Instruct the diabetic client not to use Clinitest tablets for urine glucose testing since false test results may occur. Tes-Tape or Clinistix may be used for urine testing, or Chemstrip bG may be used for blood glucose testing.
- Instruct the client to take the complete course of medication even when symptoms of infection have ended.

Diet
- Advise the client to take medication with food if gastric irritation occurs.

Side Effects
- Instruct the client to report any side effects from use of oral cephalosporin drug; they may include anorexia, nausea, vomiting, headache, dizziness, itching, and rash.

EVALUATION

- Evaluate the effectiveness of the cephalosporin by determining if the infection has ceased and no side effects, including superinfection, have occurred.

■ CASE STUDY
Client Requiring an Antibacterial Agent

S. A., who is 6 years old, has otitis media. The health care provider ordered amoxicillin 250 mg q8h. The nurse asks S. A.'s mother if S. A. is allergic to any drugs, and her mother says she is allergic to penicillin.

1. What type of drug is amoxicillin? Is it similar to penicillin? Explain.
2. What nursing action should the nurse take? Why?

The health care provider changed the amoxicillin order to cefaclor (Ceclor) 250 mg q8h. The therapeutic dosage for children is 20–40 mg/kg/day in three divided doses. S. A. weighs 40 lb.

3. What type of drug is cefaclor?
4. Is the prescribed cefaclor dosage for S. A. within safe parameters? Explain.
5. Could S. A. be allergic to cefaclor? Explain.

STUDY QUESTIONS

1. What is the action of a bacteriostatic drug? Of a bactericidal drug?
2. What is a nosocomial infection?
3. What is meant by cross-resistance? Give an example of how it can occur.
4. When do superinfections occur? What is the nurse's role?
5. Your client is taking ampicillin. What type/category is ampicillin? Explain the drug effect against pathogen(s).
6. What is the severe adverse reaction associated with penicillin? What is an early symptom of such an adverse reaction? What emergency intervention is required?
7. Your client is taking cephalexin (Keflex) for a urinary tract infection. What generation of cephalosporin is cephalexin? What is its route of administration?
8. What antibiotics are used as penicillin substitutes?

Chapter 23

Antibacterials: Macrolides, Tetracyclines, Aminoglycosides, Fluoroquinolones

OUTLINE

Objectives
Terms
Introduction
Macrolides, Lincosamides, and
  Vancomycin
    Macrolides: Erythromycin
    Nursing Process
    Lincosamides
    Vancomycin

Tetracyclines
  Side Effects and Adverse
    Reactions
  Nursing Process
Aminoglycosides
  Pharmacokinetics
  Pharmacodynamics
  Side Effects and Adverse
    Reactions

Nursing Process
Fluoroquinolones (Quinolones)
  Pharmacokinetics
  Pharmacodynamics
  Nursing Process
Unclassified Antibacterial Drugs
Case Study
Study Questions

OBJECTIVES

Describe the pharmacokinetics and pharmacodynamics of erythromycin.

Differentiate between bacteriostatic and bactericidal drugs. Give examples of each.

Explain the nursing process for tetracyclines including the adverse reactions.

Describe the nurse's role in detecting ototoxicity and nephrotoxicity associated with the administration of aminoglycosides.

Discuss the reasons for ordering serum aminoglycosides for peak and trough concentration levels.

Explain the mechanism of action of fluoroquinolones (quinolones).

Describe the nursing interventions, including client teaching, for each of the drug categories.

TERMS

bactericidal
bacteriostatic
nephrotoxicity

ototoxicity
pathogen
photosensitivity

superinfection

INTRODUCTION

The groups of antibacterials discussed in this chapter include macrolides (erythromycin), lincosamides, vancomycin, tetracyclines, aminoglycosides, and fluoroquinolones (quinolones). The macrolides, lincosamides, and tetracyclines are primarily bacteriostatic drugs and may be bactericidal, depending on drug dose or pathogen. Vancomycin, aminoglycosides, and fluoroquinolones are bactericidal drugs.

MACROLIDES, LINCOSAMIDES, AND VANCOMYCIN

These three groups of drugs are discussed together, because although they differ in structure, they have similar spectrums of antibiotic effectiveness to penicillin. Drugs from these groups are used as penicillin substitutes, especially with individuals who are allergic to penicillin. Erythromycin is the drug frequently prescribed if the client has a hypersensitivity to penicillin.

MACROLIDES: ERYTHROMYCIN

Erythromycin, derived from the fungus-like bacterium, *Streptomyces erythraeus*, was first introduced in the early 1950s. Erythromycin inhibits protein synthesis. At low to moderate drug doses, it has a bacteriostatic effect, and with high drug doses, the effect is bactericidal. Erythromycin can be administered orally or intravenously. Because gastric acid destroys the drug, various salts of erythromycin (e.g., ethylsuccinate, stearate, and estolate) are used to decrease dissolution (breakdown in small particles) in the stomach and to allow absorption in the intestine. For intravenous use, the compounds, erythromycin lactobionate and erythromycin gluceptate, are used to increase drug absorption. Table 23–1 lists the erythromycins.

Erythromycin is active against most gram-positive bacteria, with the exception of *Staphylococcus aureus,* and it is moderately active against some gram-negative bacteria. Resistant organisms may emerge during treatment. It is often prescribed as a penicillin substitute. It is a drug of choice for mycoplasmal pneumonia and legionnaires' disease. Figure 23–1 details the pharmacologic behavior of erythromycin-based antibiotics.

Pharmacokinetics

Erythromycin oral preparations are well absorbed from the gastrointestinal (GI) tract. The drug is available intravenously, but should be diluted in 100 mL of saline or 5% dextrose in water solution to prevent phlebitis or burning sensations at the injection site. It has a short half-life and a moderate protein-binding effect. The drug is excreted in bile, feces, and to some degree, in the urine. Because a small amount is excreted in the urine, renal insufficiency is not a contraindication for erythromycin use.

Pharmacodynamics

Erythromycin suppresses bacterial protein synthesis. The onset of action of the oral preparation is 1 h, peak concentration time is 4 h, and the duration of action is 6 h.

Side Effects and Adverse Reactions

Side effects and adverse reactions to erythromycin include GI disturbances such as nausea, vomiting, diarrhea, and abdominal cramping. Allergic reactions to erythromycin are rare. Hepatotoxicity (liver toxicity) can occur if the drug is taken in high doses with other hepatotoxic drugs, such as acetaminophen (high doses), phenothiazines, and sulfonamides. Erythromycin estolate (Ilosone) appears to have more toxic effects on the liver than the other erythromycins. Liver damage is usually reversible when the drug is discontinued. Erythromycin should not be taken with clindamycin or lincomycin because they compete for receptor sites.

FIGURE 23–1. Antibacterials: Erythromycin

Macrolide	Dosage	NURSING PROCESS

Erythromycin
  (E-Mycin, Erythrocin, Erythrocin Lac-
  tobionate [IV]), ❦ Novorythro, Ery-
  thromid, Apo-Erythro-S
Pregnancy Category: B
	A: PO: 250–500 mg q6h
	  IV: 1–4 g/d in divided doses
	C: PO: 30–50 mg/kg/d in 4 divided
	  doses
	  IV: 20–50 mg/kg/d in 4–6 divided
	  doses
		Assessment and Planning

Contraindications	Drug-Lab-Food Interactions	

Severe hepatic disease
Caution: Hepatic dysfunction, lactation
	Increase effect of digoxin,
	  carbamazepine, theophylline,
	  cyclosporine, warfarin, triazolam
	Decrease effect of penicillins,
	  clindamycin	

Pharmacokinetics	Pharmacodynamics	

Absorption: PO: Well absorbed
Distribution: PB: 65%
Metabolism: t½: PO: 1–2 h
  IV: 3–5 h
Excretion: In bile, feces, and small
  amount in urine
	PO: Onset: 1 h
	  Peak: 4 h
	  Duration: 6 h
	IV: Onset: UK
	  Peak: UK
	  Duration: UK
		Interventions

Therapeutic Effects/Uses: To treat gram-positive and some gram-negative organisms; for clients who are allergic to penicillin. To treat respiratory infections, legionnaires' disease, and prevent recurrence of rheumatic fever.

Mode of Action: Inhibition of the steps of protein synthesis, bacteriostatic or bactericidal effect.

Evaluation

Side Effects	Adverse Reactions

Anorexia, nausea, vomiting, diarrhea,
  tinnitus, abdominal cramps, pruritus,
  rash
	Superinfections, vaginitis, urticaria,
	  stomatitis, hearing loss
	Life-threatening: Hepatotoxicity,
	  anaphylaxis

KEY: A: adult; C: child; PO: by mouth; IV: intravenous; PB: protein-binding; t½: half-life; UK: unknown; ❦: Canadian drug names.

TABLE 23–1 Antibacterials: Macrolides, Lincosamides, and Vancomycin

Generic (Brand)	Route and Dosage	Uses and Considerations
Macrolides		
Azithromycin (Zithromax)	A: PO: Initially: 500 mg × 1 dose; maint: 250 mg/d; *max:* 1.5 g	For treatment of mild to moderate streptococcccal infections, lower respiratory tract infections. *Pregnancy category:* C; PB: 50%, t½ 11–55 h
Clarithromycin (Biaxin)	A: PO: 250–500 mg q12h × 7–14 d C: PO: 15 mg/kg/d in 2 divided doses	For treatment of upper and lower respiratory infections, skin and soft tissue infections, and gram-positive and negative organisms. Report persistent diarrhea. *Pregnancy category:* C; PB: 65–75%; t½: 3–6 h
Erythromycin base (E-Mycin, Ilotycin) Erythromycin estolate (Ilosone)	See Prototype Drug Chart (Fig. 23–1)	Enteric-coated tablet to prevent gastric acid from destroying the drug. Higher doses are needed for severe infections. Available in liquid, chewable tablet, tablet, and capsule forms. Hepatotoxicity is associated with the estolate salt.

Generic (Brand)	Route and Dosage	Uses and Considerations
Macrolides		
Erythromycin ethylsuccinate (E.E.S., E-Mycin E, Pediamycin)		Not affected by food. Available in liquid form, chewable tablets, and coated tablets.
Erythromycin lactobionate (Erythrocin Lactobionate IV)		For intravenous administration.
Erythromycin stearate (Erythrocin)		Acid-stable. It should not be taken with food. It comes in coated tablet form. *Pregnancy category:* B; PB: 65%; t½: PO: 1–2 h, IV: 3–5 h
Lincosamides		
Clindamycin HCl (Cleocin)	A: PO: 150–450 mg q6–8h; *max:* 1,800 mg/d	For serious infections. Available in capsule form. Taken with a full glass of water. Not affected by food. *Pregnancy category:* B; PB: 94%; t½: 2–3 h
Clindamycin palmitate (Cleocin Pediatric)	C: PO: 25–40 mg/kg/d in 3–4 divided doses	Available in suspension for children and elderly.
Clindamycin phosphate (Cleocin Phosphate)	A: IM/IV: 300–900 mg q6–8h; *max:* 2,700 mg/d C: IM/IV: 20–30 mg/kg/d in 3–4 divided doses	For treatment of serious infections, such as septicemia caused by gram-negative organism. *Not* to be given as a bolus. *Pregnancy category:* B; PB: 94%; t½: 2–3 h
Lincomycin (Lincorex)	A: PO: 500 mg q6–8h; *max:* 8 g/d IM: 600 mg daily–q12h IV: 600 mg–1 g q8–12h; dilute in 100 mL of IV fluids C: PO: 30–60 mg/kg/d in 3–4 divided doses IV: 10–20 mg/kg/d in 2–3 divided doses, dilute in IV fluids	In most situations, this drug has been replaced by clindamycin. *Pregnancy category:* B; PB: 70–75%; t½: 4–6 h
Vancomycin		
Vancomycin HCl (Vancocin)	A: IV: 500 mg q6h or 1 g q12h C: IV: 40 mg/kg/d in 4 divided doses; dilute in IV fluids; run for 1–1.5 h	For *Staphylococcus aureus*-resistant infections and cardiac surgical prophylaxis in clients with penicillin allergy. Adverse reactions include possible ototoxicity, nephrotoxicity, vascular collapse. *Pregnancy category:* C; PB: 10%; t½: 5–11 h

KEY: A: adult; C: child; PO: by mouth; IM: intramuscular; IV: intravenous; PB: protein-binding; t½: half-life.

NURSING PROCESS: ANTIBACTERIALS: MACROLIDES: Erythromycin

ASSESSMENT

- Assess vital signs (VS) and urine output. Report abnormal findings.
- Check lab tests for liver enzyme values to determine liver function. Liver enzyme tests should be periodically ordered for clients taking large doses of erythromycin for a continuous period.
- Obtain a history of drugs the client is currently taking. Erythromycin can increase the effects of digoxin, oral anticoagulants, theophylline, carbamazepine, and cyclosporine. Dosing for these drugs may need to be decreased.

POTENTIAL NURSING DIAGNOSES

- High risk for infection
- High risk for impaired tissue integrity

PLANNING

- Client's infection will be controlled and later eliminated.

NURSING INTERVENTIONS

- Obtain a sample from the infected area and send to the lab for culture and sensitivity (C & S) test *before* starting erythromycin therapy. Antibiotic can be initiated after obtaining culture sample.
- Monitor VS, urine output, and laboratory values, especially liver enzymes: ALP, ALT, AST, and also bilirubin.
- Monitor the client for liver damage due to prolonged use and high dosage of macrolides, such as erythromycin. Signs of liver dysfunction include elevated liver enzyme levels and jaundice.
- Monitor bleeding times if the client is receiving an oral anticoagulant.

- Administer oral erythromycin 1 h before meals or 2 h after meals. Take with a full glass of water and not fruit juice. Take the drug with food if GI upset occurs. Chewable tablets should be chewed and not swallowed whole.
- For IV erythromycin, dilute in an appropriate amount of solution as indicated in the drug circular.

General
- Instruct the client to take the full course of antibacterial agent as prescribed. Drug compliance is most important for all antibacterials (antibiotics).

Side Effects
- Instruct the client to report side effects, including adverse reactions. Encourage the client to report nausea, vomiting, diarrhea, abdominal cramps, and itching. Superinfection, a secondary infection due to drug therapy, such as stomatitis or vaginitis may occur.
- Instruct the client to report any symptoms of hearing impairment, such as tinnitus, vertigo, or roaring noises.

EVALUATION

- Evaluate the effectiveness of erythromycin by determining if the infection has been controlled or has ceased and no side effects, including superinfection, have occurred.

LINCOSAMIDES

Clindamycin and lincomycin are examples of lincosamides. Like erythromycin, they inhibit bacterial protein synthesis and have both bacteriostatic and bactericidal actions, depending on drug dosage. Clindamycin is more widely prescribed than lincomycin because it is active against most gram-positive organisms, including *Staphylococcus aureus* and anaerobic organisms. It is not effective against the gram-negative bacteria, such as *Escherichia coli, Proteus,* and *Pseudomonas.* Clindamycin is absorbed better than lincomycin through the GI tract and maintains a higher serum drug concentration. Clindamycin is considered to be more effective than lincomycin and has fewer toxic effects. Table 23–1 lists the lincosamides.

Side Effects and Adverse Reactions

Side effects and adverse reactions to clindamycin and lincomycin include GI irritation, such as nausea, vomiting, and stomatitis. Also, rash may occur. Severe adverse reactions include colitis and anaphylactic shock.

Drug Interaction

Clindamycin and lincomycin are incompatible with aminophylline, phenytoin (Dilantin), barbiturates, and ampicillin.

VANCOMYCIN

Vancomycin, a glycopeptide bactericidal antibiotic, was widely used in the 1950s to treat staphylococcal infections. The use of the drug was almost abandoned due to the many reports of nephrotoxicity and ototoxicity. **Ototoxicity** results in damage to the auditory or vestibular branch of the eighth cranial nerve. Such damage can result in permanent hearing loss (auditory branch) or temporary or permanent loss of balance (vestibular branch). Vancomycin is still being used against drug-resistant *Staphylococcus aureus* and in cardiac surgical prophylaxis for individuals with penicillin allergies. Serum vancomycin levels are usually drawn on clients receiving this drug so that toxic effects can be minimized.

TETRACYCLINES

The tetracyclines, isolated from *Streptomyces aureofaciens* in 1948, were the first broad-spectrum antibiotics effective against gram-positive and gram-negative bacteria and many other organisms, such as mycobacteria, rickettsiae, spirochetes, and chlamydiae. Tetracyclines act by inhibiting bacterial protein synthesis and have a bacteriostatic effect. Tetracyclines are not effective against *Staphylococcus aureus* (except for the newer tetracyclines), *Pseudomonas,* or *Proteus.* They can be used against *Mycoplasma pneumoniae.*

The tetracyclines are frequently prescribed for oral use although they are also available for intramuscular and intravenous use (Fig. 23–2). Because intramuscular administration of tetracycline causes pain on injection and tissue irritation, this route of administration is seldom used. The intravenous route is used to treat severe infections. The newer oral preparations of tetracyclines, doxycycline and minocycline, are more rapidly and completely absorbed. Tetracyclines should not be taken with magnesium and aluminum preparations (antacids), milk products containing calcium, or iron-containing drugs because all of these substances bind with tetracycline and prevent absorption of the drug. It is suggested that tetracyclines, except for doxycycline and minocycline, be taken on an empty stomach 1 h before or 2 h after meals. Table 23–2 describes the tetracycline preparations, their dosages, uses, and considerations.

Although tetracyclines are widely used, they have numerous side effects, adverse reactions, toxicities, and drug interactions.

Side Effects and Adverse Reactions

GI disturbances such as nausea, vomiting, and diarrhea are side effects of tetracyclines. **Photosensi-**tivity (sunburn reaction) may occur in persons taking tetracyclines, especially demeclocycline. Pregnant women should not take tetracycline during the first trimester of pregnancy because of possible teratogenic effects. Women in the last trimester of pregnancy and children younger than 8 should *not* take tetracycline because it irreversibly discolors the permanent teeth. Minocycline can cause damage to the vestibular part of the inner ear, which may result in difficulty maintaining balance. Tetracyclines should be taken 1 h before or 2 h after meals because food, especially milk products, impairs absorption. Outdated tetracyclines should always be discarded because the drug breaks down into a toxic byproduct. Nephrotoxicity results when the tetracycline is given in high doses with other nephrotoxic drugs. **Superinfection** is another problem that might result because tetracycline can disrupt the microbial flora of the body.

TABLE 23–2 Antibacterials: Tetracyclines

Generic (Brand)	Route and Dosage	Uses and Considerations
Tetracycline (Achromycin, Tetracyn, Sumycin, Panmycin)	See Prototype Drug Chart (Fig. 23–2)	Used for respiratory and urinary tract infections. For acne the usual dose is 250 mg, b.i.d. Milk products and antacids should not be taken with tetracyclines. Should *not* be taken in the last trimester of pregnancy or before a child is 8 years old to prevent discoloration of the teeth. Also used to treat stage I of Lyme disease. Photosensitivity is a problem; wear protective clothing or sunscreen when in sunlight. *Pregnancy category:* D, PB: 20–60; t½: 6–12 h
Demeclocycline HCl (Declomycin)	A: PO: 150 mg q6h or 300 mg q12h C: >8 y: PO 6–12 mg/kg/d in 2–4 divided doses	Used for gram-positive and gram-negative bacteria. Photosensitivity may occur. *Pregnancy category:* D; PB: 35%–90%; t½: 10–17 h
Doxycycline hyclate (Vibramycin)	A: PO: 100 mg q12–24h IV: 100–200 mg/d C >8 y: PO/IV: 2–4 mg/kg/d in 1–2 divided doses	Smaller doses are effective against bacteria and microorganisms. Also used for legionella syndrome. *Pregnancy category:* D; PB: 25%–92%; t½: 20 h
Minocycline HCl (Minocin)	A: PO/IV: 100 mg q12h or 50 mg q6h C: >8 y: PO/IV: 4 mg/kg/d in 2 divided doses	Should not be administered to clients with renal insufficiency. *Pregnancy category:* D; PB: 55%–88%; t½: 11–20 h
Oxytetracycline HCl (Terramycin)	A: PO: 250–500 mg q6–12h IM: 200–300 mg/d in 2–3 divided doses IV: 250–500 mg in 2 divided doses C >8 y: PO: 25–50 mg/kg/d in 4 divided doses IM: 15–25 mg/kg/d in 2–3 divided doses; *max:* 250 mg/dose IV: 10–20 mg/kg/d in 2 divided doses	Used for urinary tract infections. Adminsistered primarily by the oral route. *Pregnancy category:* D; PB: 20%–40%; t½: 6–10 h

KEY: *A:* adult; *C:* child; *PO:* by mouth; *IV:* intravenous; *PB:* protein-binding; *t½: half-life;* >: greater than.

FIGURE 23–2. Antibacterials: Tetracyclines

Tetracycline	Dosage	NURSING PROCESS
Tetracycline (Achromycin, Tetracyn, Panmycin, Sumycin), ❧ Novotetra *Pregnancy Category:* D (includes child <8 y)	*Systemic infection:* A: PO: 250–500 mg q6h–12 h IM: 250 mg/d; 300 mg/d in 2–3 divided doses C: >8 y: PO: 25–50 mg/kg/d in 4 divided doses IM: 15–25 mg/kg/d in 2–3 divided doses; max: 250 mg/dose	**Assessment and Planning**
Contraindications	**Drug-Lab-Food Interactions**	
Hypersensitivity, pregnancy, severe hepatic or renal disease *Caution:* History of allergies, renal and hepatic dysfunction, myasthenia gravis	May *increase* or *decrease* effects of anticoagulants *Decrease* tetracycline absorption with antacids, iron, and zinc; *decrease* effects of oral contraceptives *Food:* Dairy products (milk, cheese) *decrease* effect *Lab:* Decrease serum potassium level	
Pharmacokinetics	**Pharmacodynamics**	Interventions
Absorption: PO: 75–80% absorbed *Distribution:* PB: 20–60 h *Metabolism:* t½: 6–12 h *Excretion:* Unchanged in the urine	PO: Onset: 1–2 h Peak: 2–4 h Duration: 6 h IV: Onset: Rapid Peak: 0.5–1 h Duration: UK	

Therapeutic Effects/Uses: To treat infections due to uncommon gram-positive and gram-negative organisms, skin infections or disorders, chlamydial infection, gonorrhea, syphilis, rickettsial infection.

Mode of Action: Inhibition of the steps of protein synthesis. Bacteriostatic or bactericidal

Evaluation

Side Effects	Adverse Reactions
Nausea, vomiting, diarrhea, rash, flatulence, abdominal discomfort, headache, photosensitivity, pruritus, epigastric distress, heartburn	Superinfections, (candidiasis) *Life-threatening:* Blood dyscrasias, hepatotoxicity, nephrotoxicity, exfoliative dermatitis, intracranial hypertension

KEY: A: adult; C: child; PO: by mouth; IM: intramuscular; IV: intravenous; PB: protein-binding; t½: half-life; UK: unknown; >: greater than; ❧ : Canadian drug name.

NURSING PROCESS: ANTIBACTERIALS: Tetracyclines

ASSESSMENT

- Assess VS and urine output. Report abnormal findings.
- Check laboratory results, especially those that indicate renal and liver function, such as BUN, serum creatinine, AST, ALT, APT, and bilirubin.
- Obtain a history of dietary intake and drugs the client is currently taking. Dairy products and antacids decrease drug absorption.

POTENTIAL NURSING DIAGNOSES

- High risk for infection
- Noncompliance with drug regimen
- High risk for impaired skin integrity

PLANNING

- Client's infection will be controlled and later eliminated.

NURSING INTERVENTIONS

- Obtain a sample for culture from the infected area and send to the laboratory for C & S test. Antibiotic therapy can be started after the culture sample has been taken.
- Administer tetracycline 1 h before meals or 2 h after meals for absorption.
- Monitor laboratory values for liver and kidney functions; these include liver enzymes, BUN, and serum creatinine.
- Monitor VS and urine output.

CLIENT TEACHING

General
- Instruct the client to store tetracycline out of the light and extreme heat. Tetracycline decomposes in light and heat, causing the drug to become toxic.
- Advise the client to check the expiration date on the bottle of tetracycline; out-of-date tetracycline can be toxic.
- Advise a woman who is contemplating pregnancy who has an infection to inform her health care provider and to avoid taking tetracycline because of possible teratogenic effect.
- Inform parents that children less than 8 years old should not take tetracycline because it can cause discoloration of permanent teeth.
- Instruct the client to take the complete course of tetracycline as prescribed.

Diet
- Instruct the client to avoid milk products, iron, and antacids. Tetracycline should be taken 1 h before meals or 2 h after meals with a full glass of water. If GI upset occurs, drug can be taken with nondairy foods.

Side Effects
- Instruct the client to use sunblock/protecting clothing during sun exposure. Photosensitivity is associated with tetracycline.
- Instruct the client to report signs of a superinfection (mouth ulcers, anal or genital discharge).
- Advise client to use additional contraceptive techniques and not to rely on oral contraceptives when taking drug because effectiveness may decrease.
- Advise the client to use effective oral hygiene several times a day to prevent or alleviate mouth ulcers (stomatitis).

EVALUATION

- Evaluate the effectiveness of tetracycline by determining if the infection has been controlled or has ceased and there are no side effects.

AMINOGLYCOSIDES

Aminoglycosides act by inhibiting bacterial protein synthesis. The aminoglycoside antibiotics are used against gram-negative bacteria, such as *Escherichia coli*, *Proteus* spp., and *Pseudomonas* spp. Some gram-positive cocci are resistant to aminoglycosides, so penicillins or cephalosporins may be used.

Streptomycin sulfate, derived from the bacterium *Streptomyces griseus* in 1944, was the first aminoglycoside available for clinical use and was used in the treatment of tuberculosis. Due to its ototoxicity and the bacterial resistance that can develop, it is infrequently used today. The aminoglycosides that are currently used to treat *Pseudomonas aeruginosa* infection include gentamicin (1963), tobramycin (1970), amikacin (1970s), and netilmicin (1980s). Netilmicin is one of the latest aminoglycosides, and the occurrence of toxicities from this drug is not as frequent or as intense as those from other aminoglycosides. Figure 23–3 lists the drug data related to the aminoglycosides gentamicin (Garamycin) and netilmicin (Netromycin).

Pharmacokinetics

Gentamicin and netilmicin are administered intramuscularly and intravenously. Both drugs have a short half-life, and drug dose can be given 3 to 4 times a day. Netilmicin has a low protein-binding power. Excretion of these drugs is primarily unchanged in the urine.

Pharmacodynamics

Gentamicin and netilmicin inhibit bacterial protein synthesis and both have a bactericidal effect. Although netilmicin is the newer aminoglycoside,

FIGURE 23–3. Antibacterials: Aminoglycosides

Aminoglycosides	**Dosage**	**NURSING PROCESS** Assessment and Planning

Gentamicin sulfate *(G)*
  (Garamycin)
Pregnancy Category: C
 	
Netilmicin sulfate *(N)*
  (Netromycin)
Pregnancy Category: D
	(G)
	A: IM: 3 mg/kg/d in 3–4 divided
	     doses
	  IV: 3–5 mg/kg/d in 3–4 divided
	     doses
	C: IM:/IV: 2–2.5 mg/kg, q8–12 h
	TDM: 5–10 μg/mL; peak: 10–12
	  μg/mL; trough: 0.5–2 μg/mL
	(N)
	A: IM/IV: 3–6 mg/kg/d in 3 divided
	     doses
	C: IM/1V: 5–8 mg/kg/d in 3 divided
	     doses
	TDM: Peak: 0.5–10 μg/mL; trough: <4
	  μg/mL	

Contraindications	**Drug-Lab-Food Interactions**	

(G & N)
Hypersensitivity, severe renal disease,
  pregnancy, and breast feeding
Caution: (G & N) Renal disease, neuro-
  muscular disorders (myasthenia
  gravis, parkinsonism), heart failure,
  elderly, neonates
	(G & N)
	Increase risk of ototoxicity with loop
	  diuretics, methoxyflurane; *increase*
	  risk of nephrotoxicity with
	  amphotericin B, polymyxin,
	  cisplatin, furosemide, vancomycin
	Lab: *Increase* BUN, serum AST, ALT,
	  LDH, bilirubin, creatinine
	Decrease serum potassium and
	  magnesium	

Pharmacokinetics	**Pharmacodynamics**	Interventions

Absorption: Both: IM, IV
Distribution: PB:
  (G) UK, *(N)* 10%
Metabolism: t½:
  (G) 2 h, *(N)* 2–3 h
Excretion: (G) unchanged in urine, *(N)*
  90% excreted unchanged in urine
	(G)
	IM/IV: Onset: rapid
	          Peak: 1–2 h
	          Duration: 6–8 h
	(N)
	IM: Onset: rapid
	          Peak: 0.5–1.5 h
	          Duration: UK
	IV: Onset: immediate
	          Peak: 0.5–1 h
	          Duration: UK	

	Evaluation
Therapeutic Effects/Uses: (G & N) To treat serious infections caused by gram-negative or- ganisms, such as *Pseudomonas aeruginosa, Proteus;* to treat pelvic inflammatory disease (PID). *(G)* Effective against methicillin-resistant *Staphylococcus aureus* infections. *(N)* Effec- tive against gentamicin-resistant bacteria. *Mode of Action:* Inhibition of bacterial protein synthesis. Bactericidal effect.	

Side Effects	**Adverse Reactions**

(G & N) Anorexia, nausea, vomiting,
  rash, numbness, visual disturbances,
  tremors, tinnitus, pruritus, muscle
  cramps or weakness, photosensitivity
	(G & N) Oliguria, urticaria, palpitation,
	  superinfection
	Life-threatening: (G & N) Ototoxicity,
	  nephrotoxicity, thrombocytopenia,
	  agranulocytosis, neuromuscular
	  blockade, liver damage

KEY: G: gentamicin sulfate; N: netilmicin sulfate; A: adult; C: child; IM: intramuscular; IV: intravenous; PB: protein-binding; t½: half-life; UK: unknown; TDM: therapeutic drug monitoring; <:
less than; >: more than.

its pregnancy category is D, whereas gentamicin has a pregnancy category of C. The onset of action for both drugs is similar (rapid or immediate). The peak action for netilmicin is 30 minutes faster than gentamicin.

Aminoglycosides are not readily absorbed through the GI tract; thus, they are administered intramuscularly and intravenously. To ensure a desired blood level, the drug is usually administered intravenously. The aminoglycosides can be given with penicillins and cephalosporins, but should not be mixed together in the same administered container. When combinations of antibiotics are given intravenously, the IV line is flushed after each an-

tibiotic has been administered to ensure that the antibiotic is completely delivered.

Side Effects and Adverse Reactions

The serious adverse reactions to aminoglycosides include ototoxicity and nephrotoxicity. Nephrotoxicity might occur, depending on renal function, drug dose, and age (young and elderly). Careful drug dosing is especially important with young and old clients. The nurse must assess changes in clients' hearing, balance, and urinary output. Prolonged use of aminoglycosides could result in a superinfection. Table 23–3 lists the aminoglycosides, their dosages, uses, and considerations.

TABLE 23–3 Antibacterials: Aminoglycosides

Generic (Brand)	Route and Dosage	Uses and Considerations
Amikacin SO$_4$ (Amikin)	A&C: IM/IV: 15 mg/kg/d in 2–3 divided doses; *max:* 1.5 g/d NB: IV: 7.5 mg/kg q12h TDM: Peak: 15–30 mg/mL; trough: 5–10 mg/mL	Synthetic derivative of kanamycin. Effective against *Pseudomonas* spp. Hearing changes should be monitored. *Pregnancy category:* C; PB: 4%–11%; t½: 2–3 h
Gentamicin SO$_4$ (Garamycin)	See Prototype Drug Chart (Fig. 23–3)	Effective against gram-negative bacteria, including *Pseudomonas* spp. Urinary output should be monitored. *Pregnancy category:* C; PB: UK: t½: 2 h
Kanamycin SO$_4$ (Kantrex)	A: PO: 1 g q6h *Hepatic coma:* 8–12 g/d in divided doses IM/IV: 15 mg/kg/d in 2 divided doses C: IV: Same as adult	Used orally for hepatic coma. Effective against gram-negative bacteria with the exception of *Pseudomonas aeruginosa.* Monitor for hearing loss and urinary output. *Pregnancy category:* D; PB: 10%; t½: 2–3 h
Neomycin SO$_4$ (Mycifradin)	A: PO: GI surgery: 1 g qh for 4 doses; then 1 g q4h For 24 h or other regimens *Hepatic coma:* 4–12 g/d in divided doses IM: 15 mg/kg/d in 4 divided doses; *max:* 1 g/d C: PO: 10 mg/kg in q4–6h for 3 d	Decreases bacteria in the bowel and is used as a preoperative bowel antiseptic. It is also available as a topical antibiotic ointment. *Pregnancy category:* C; PB: 10%; t½: 2–3 h
Netilmicin (Netromycin)	A: IM/IV: 3–6 mg/kg/d in 3 divided doses C: IM/IV: 5–8 mg/kg/d in 3 divided doses TDM: Peak: 0.5–10 μg/mL; trough: <4 μg/mL	This newer aminoglycoside is effective against gram-negative bacteria and has fewer side effects. Similar to gentamicin and tobramycin. *Pregnancy category:* D; PB: 10%; t½: 2–3 h
Paromomycin (Humatin)	*Intestinal amebiasis:* A&C: PO: 25–35 mg/kg/d in 3 divided doses for 5–10 d	Used in treating hepatic coma and parasitic infections. Hearing changes and urinary output should be monitored. Is not systemically absorbed. *Pregnancy category:* C; PB: UK; t½: UK
Streptomycin SO$_4$	*Tuberculosis:* A: IM: 1 g daily for 2–3 mo; then 1 g 3 × wk *Endocarditis:* A: IM: 1 g q12h for 1 wk; dose may be decreased	First aminoglycoside. Used with antituberculosis drugs in treatment of tuberculosis. Ototoxicity is a major problem. *Pregnancy category:* C; PB: 30%; t½: 2–3 h

TABLE 23–3 Antibacterials: Aminoglycosides *(Continued)*

Generic (Brand)	Route and Dosage	Uses and Considerations
Tobramycin SO$_4$ (Nebcin)	A: IM/IV: 3–5 mg/kg/d in 3 divided doses C: IM/IV: 6–7.5 mg/kg/d in 3–4 divided doses TDM: Peak: 10–12 μg/mL; trough: 0.5–2 μg/mL	Very effective against *Pseudomonas aeruginosa*. Hearing changes and urinary output should be monitored. Toxic effects are less than for other aminoglycosides. *Pregnancy category:* D; PB: 10%; t½: 2–3 h

KEY: A: adult; C: child; PO: by mouth; IM: intramuscular; IV: intravenous; NB: newborn; PB: protein-binding; t½: half-life; TDM: therapeutic drug monitoring; UK: unknown; <: less than.

NURSING PROCESS: ANTIBACTERIALS: Aminoglycosides

ASSESSMENT

- Assess VS and urine output. Compare these results with future VS and urine output. An adverse reaction to most aminoglycosides is nephrotoxicity.
- Assess laboratory results to determine renal and liver functions, including BUN, serum creatinine, ALP, ALT, AST, and bilirubin. Serum electrolytes should also be checked. Aminoglycosides may decrease the serum potassium and magnesium levels.
- Obtain a medical history related to renal or hearing disorders. Large doses of aminoglycosides could cause nephrotoxicity or ototoxicity.

POTENTIAL NURSING DIAGNOSES

- High risk for infection
- High risk for impaired tissue integrity
- High risk for altered tissue perfusion: renal

PLANNING

- Client's infection will be controlled and later eliminated.

NURSING INTERVENTIONS

- Send a sample from the infected area to the laboratory for culture to determine organism and antibiotic sensitivity (C & S) before aminoglycoside is started.
- Monitor intake and output. Urine output should be at least 600 mL/d. Immediately report if urine output is decreased. Urinalysis may be ordered daily. Check results for proteinuria, casts, blood cells, or appearance.
- Check for hearing loss. Aminoglycosides can cause ototoxicity.

- Check laboratory results and compare with baseline values. Report abnormal results.
- Monitor VS. Note if body temperature has decreased.
- For IV use, dilute the aminoglycoside in 50–200 mL of normal saline solution (NSS) or D$_5$W solution and administer in 30–60 min.
- Check that therapeutic drug monitoring (TDM) has been ordered for peak and trough drug levels. The TDM for gentamicin is 5–10 μg/mL. Blood should be drawn 45–60 min after drug has been administered for peak levels and minutes before the next drug dosing for trough levels. Drug peak values should be 10–12 μg/mL, and trough values should be 0.5–2 μg/mL.
- Monitor for signs and symptoms of superinfection, such as stomatitis (mouth ulcers), genital discharge (vaginitis), and anal or genital itching.

General
- Unless fluids are restricted, encourage the client to increase fluid intake.
- Instruct the client never to take leftover antibiotics.

Side Effects
- Instruct the client to report side effects resulting from the aminoglycosides, including nausea, vomiting, tremors, tinnitus, pruritus, and muscle cramps.
- Instruct the client to use sunblock lotion and protective clothing during sun exposure. Photosensitivity can be caused by aminoglycosides.

EVALUATION

- Evaluate the effectiveness of the aminoglycoside by determining if the infection has ceased and no side effects have occurred.

FLUOROQUINOLONES (QUINOLONES)

The mechanism of action of fluoroquinolones is to interfere with the enzyme DNA gyrase, which is needed for the synthesis of bacterial DNA. Their antibacterial spectrum includes both gram-positive and gram-negative organisms. They are bactericidal. Nalidixic acid and cinoxacin are the earliest derivatives of the fluoroquinolone group, which is prescribed primarily for urinary tract infection caused by common gram-negative organisms, such as *Escherichia coli* (Table 23–4).

Ciprofloxacin and norfloxacin are synthetic antibacterials related to nalidixic acid. These two fluoroquinolones have a broad spectrum of action on gram-positive and gram-negative organisms, including *Pseudomonas aeruginosa*. Norfloxacin is indi-

FIGURE 23–4. Antibacterials: Fluoroquinolones (Quinolones)

Fluoroquinolone	Dosage	NURSING PROCESS Assessment and Planning
Ciprofloxacin (Cipro) Quinolone, fluoroquinoline *Pregnancy Category:* C (X at term), breast feeding	A: PO: 250–500 mg q12h *Severe infections:* A: PO: 500–750 mg q12h IV: 200 mg q12h *Mild to moderate infections:* A: IV: 400 mg q12h	

Contraindications	Drug-Lab-Food Interactions	
Severe renal disease, hypersensitivity to other quinolones, pregnancy and breast feeding *Caution:* Seizure disorders, renal disorders, children <14 y, elderly, clients receiving theophylline	*Increase* effect with probenecid; *increase* effect of theophylline, caffeine *Decrease* drug absorption with antacids, iron *Lab: Increase* AST, ALT	

Pharmacokinetics	Pharmacodynamics	Interventions
Absorption: PO: 70% absorbed *Distribution:* PB: 20% *Metabolism:* $t\frac{1}{2}$: 3–4 h *Excretion:* 50% unchanged in urine	PO: Onset: 0.5–1 h Peak: 1–2 h Duration: UK	

Therapeutic Effects/Uses: To treat lower respiratory tract, renal, bone, and joint infections.

Mode of Action: Interference with the enzyme DNA gyrase, which is needed for bacterial DNA synthesis. Bactericidal effect.

Evaluation

Side Effects	Adverse Reactions
Nausea, vomiting, diarrhea, abdominal cramps, flatulence, headache, dizziness, fatigue, restlessness, insomnia, rash, flushing, tinnitus, photosensitivity	Urticaria, oral candidiasis, crystalluria, hematuria, seizures

KEY: A: adult; PB: protein-binding; $t\frac{1}{2}$: half-life; PO: by mouth; IV: intravenous; <: less than; UK: unknown.

cated for urinary tract infections, and ciprofloxacin has FDA approval for urinary tract infections; lower respiratory tract infections; and skin, soft tissue, bone, and joint infections.

The use of fluoroquinolones as urinary antibiotics is discussed in Chapter 27. Figure 23–4 lists the drug data related to ciprofloxacin. Ciprofloxacin's use is not limited to urinary tract infections but is equally effective for treating bone, joint, and soft tissue infections.

Pharmacokinetics

Approximately 70% of ciprofloxacin hydrochloride (Cipro) is absorbed from the GI tract. It has a low protein-binding effect and a moderately short half-

life of 3 to 4 h. About one-half of the drug is excreted unchanged in the urine.

Pharmacodynamics

Ciprofloxacin inhibits bacterial DNA synthesis by inhibiting the enzyme DNA gyrase. The drug has a high tissue distribution. If possible, it should be taken before meals since food slows the absorption rate. Antacids also decrease absorption rate. When taking probenecid with ciprofloxacin, the drug action of ciprofloxacin is increased. Ciprofloxacin prolongs the drug action of theophylline.

Ciprofloxacin has an average onset of action of 0.5 to 1.0 h, and the peak concentration time is 1 to 2 h. The duration of action is unknown.

TABLE 23–4 Antibacterials: Fluoroquinolones (Quinolones) and Unclassified

Generic (Brand)	Route and Dosage	Uses and Considerations
Fluoroquinolones		
Cinoxacin (Cinobac)	A: PO: 1 g/d 2–4 divided doses for 1–2 wk C >12 y: Same as adult	For acute and chronic urinary tract infections (UTIs). Effective against gram-negative organisms except for *Pseudomonas*. Absorbed in prostatic tissue. More effective than nalidixic acid. *Pregnancy category:* B; PB: 60%–80%; t½: 1.5 h
Ciprofloxacin HCl (Cipro)	See Prototype Drug Chart (Fig. 23–4)	Has a broad-sprectrum antibacterial effect. For UTI, skin and soft tissue infections, and bone and joint infections. Antacid inhibits drug absorption. *Pregnancy category:* C (X at term); PB: 20%; t½: 3–4 h
Enoxacin (Penetrex)	A: PO: 200–400 mg b.i.d. 7–14 d	To treat UTI including those caused by *E. coli, Proteus, Pseudomonas.* *Pregnancy category:* C; PB: 40%; t½: 3–6 h
Lomefloxacin HCl (Maxaquin)	A: PO: 200–400 mg/d × 7–14 d	For complicated and uncomplicated UTIs, transurethral surgery, lower respiratory infections. Drug dose is reduced for clients with a low creatinine clearance. *Pregnancy category:* C; PB: UK; t½: 6–8 h
Nalidixic acid (NegGram)	A: PO: 1 g q.i.d. for 1–2 wk; 1 g b.i.d. for long-term use C: PO: 55 mg/kg/d in 4 divided doses for 1–2 wk; 33 mg/kg/d for long-term use	For acute and chronic UTIs. Drug resistance may occur. Is not distributed in prostatic fluid. *Pregnancy category:* B; PB: 95%; t½: 2–6 h
Norfloxacin (Noroxin)	A: PO: 400 mg b.i.d., a.c. or p.c. for 1–3 wk	For acute and chronic UTIs. Most potent drug of the fluoroquinolone group. Food may inhibit drug absorption. *Pregnancy category:* C; PB: 10%–15%; t½: 3–4 h
Ofloxacin (Floxin)	A: PO: 200–400 mg q12h × 10 d	For respiratory and UTIs, prostatitis, and skin infections. Not to be given with meals. Superinfection may result. Avoid excessive sunlight. *Pregnancy category:* C; PB: 20%; t½: 5–8 h
Unclassified		
Aztreonam (Azactam)	*Urinary tract infections:* A: IM/IV: 0.5–1.0 g q8–12h *Severe infections:* A: IM/IV: 1.0–2.0 g q6–8h; *max:* 8 g/d	For treatment of gram-negative infections of the lower respiratory tract, UTIs, and skin and gynecologic infections. May be used in combination with other antibacterials. *Pregnancy category:* B; PB: 56%; t½: 1.7–2.1 h
Chloramphenicol (Chloromycetin)	A&C: PO/IV: 50 mg/kg/d in 4 divided doses (q6h) NB: 25 mg/kg/d in 4 divided doses (q6h)	For treatment of severe infections. Drug can be toxic. *Pregnancy category:* C; PB: 50%–60%; t½: 1.5–4.0 h

Generic (Brand)	Route and Dosage	Uses and Considerations
Imipenem-cilastatin (Primaxin)	A: IM: 500–750 mg q12h IV: 250 mg–1 g q6–8h C: IV: 15–25 mg/kg q6h	For treatment of severe infections of the lower respiratory tract, UTIs, skin, bones, joints, and septicemia. *Pregnancy category: C; PB: 20%; t½: 1 h*
Spectinomycin HCl (Trobicin)	A: IM: 2–4 g as single dose	Has a bacteriostatic effect. Effective against *Neisseria gonorrhoeae*. Ineffective against syphilis. *Pregnancy category: B; PB: 10% t½: 1–3 h*

KEY: *A: adult; C: child; PO: by mouth; IM: intramuscular; IV: intravenous; NB: newborn; PB: protein-binding; t½: half-life; UTI: urinary tract infection.*

NURSING PROCESS: ANTIBACTERIALS: Fluoroquinolones

ASSESSMENT

- Assess VS and intake and urine output. Compare these results with future VS and urine output. Fluid intake should be at least 2,000 mL/d.
- Assess laboratory results to determine renal function: BUN and serum creatinine.
- Obtain a drug and diet history. Antacids and iron preparations decrease absorption of fluoroquinolones such as ciprofloxacin (Cipro). Ciprofloxacin can increase the effects of theophylline and caffeine.

POTENTIAL NURSING DIAGNOSES

- High risk for infection
- High risk for impaired tissue integrity
- Noncompliance with drug regimen

PLANNING

- Client's infection will be controlled and later eliminated.

NURSING INTERVENTIONS

- Obtain specimen from the infected site and send to the laboratory for C & S before initiating antibacterial drug therapy.
- Monitor intake and output. Urine output should be at least 750 mL/d. Client should be well hydrated, and fluid intake should be >2,000 mL/d to prevent crystalluria. Urine pH should be <6.7.
- Monitor VS. Report abnormal findings.
- Check laboratory results, especially BUN and serum creatinine. Elevated values may indicate renal dysfunction.
- Administer ciprofloxacin 1 h before or 2 h after

meals or 2 h before or after antacids and iron products for absorption. Take with a full glass of water. If GI distress occurs, drug may be taken with food.
- For IV ciprofloxacin, dilute the antibiotic in an appropriate amount of solution as indicated in the drug circular. Infuse over 60 min.
- Check for signs and symptoms of superinfection such as stomatitis (mouth ulcers), furry black tongue, anal or genital discharge, and itching.
- Monitor serum theophylline levels. Ciprofloxacin can increase theophylline levels. Check for symptoms of CNS stimulation: nervousness, insomnia, anxiety, and tachycardia.

CLIENT TEACHING

General
- Instruct the client to drink at least 6 to 8 glassfuls (8 oz) of fluid daily.
- Instruct the client to avoid caffeinated products.

Side Effects
- Advise the client to avoid operating hazardous machinery or operating a motor vehicle while taking the drug or until drug stability has occurred due to possible drug-related dizziness.
- Advise the client that photosensitivity is a side effect of most fluoroquinolones. The client should use sunglasses, sunblock, and protective clothing when in the sun.
- Instruct the client to report side effects, such as dizziness, nausea, vomiting, diarrhea, flatulence, abdominal cramps, tinnitus, and rash. Older adults are more likely to develop side effects.

EVALUATION

- Evaluate the effectiveness of the fluoroquinolone by determining if the infection has ceased and the body temperature has returned within normal range.

UNCLASSIFIED ANTIBACTERIAL DRUGS

Several antibacterials, such as chloramphenicol, spectinomycin, imipenem-cilastatin, and aztreonam, do not belong to any major drug group. Chloramphenicol (Chloromycetin) was discovered in 1947 and has a bacteriostatic action by inhibiting bacterial protein synthesis. Because of the toxic effects of chloramphenicol, including blood dyscrasias related to bone marrow suppression, it is used only for treatment of serious infections. It is effective against gram-negative and gram-positive bacteria, and many other microorganisms, such as rickettsiae, mycoplasmas, and *Haemophilus influenzae*.

Spectinomycin hydrochloride (Trobicin), introduced in 1971, is used against *Neisseria gonorrhoeae*, the microbe that causes gonorrhea. It is also prescribed for persons allergic to penicillins, cephalosporins, or tetracyclines. It is administered intramuscularly as a single dose.

Imipenem with cilastatin sodium (Primaxin) is a new antibacterial introduced in 1986. It is effective against gram-positive bacteria, including *Staphylococcus aureus* and *Pseudomonas aeruginosa*.

Aztreonam (Azactam) is a monobactam antibacterial. Though aztreonam has the same beta lactam structure as penicillin and cephalosporins, it has a different spectrum of activity. It is not effective against gram-positive bacteria but is effective against the gram-negative bacteria *Neisseria gonorrhoeae* and *Haemophilus influenzae*.

■ CASE STUDY:
Client with a Pseudomonal Infection

A. J. N., 46 years old, has a wound infection. The culture report stated that the infection was due to *Pseudomonas aeruginosa*. A. J. N.'s temperature was 104°F (40°C). Amikacin sulfate (Amikin) is to be administered intravenously in 100 mL of D$_5$W over 45 min, every 8 h. Dosage is 15 mg/kg/day in three divided doses. A. J. N. weighs 165 lb.

1. What is the drug classification of amikacin? How many milligrams of amikacin should A. J. N. receive every 8 h?
2. What type of intravenous infusion should be used? What would be the IV flow rate?
3. Why should a wound culture be taken before determining the antibacterial agent?

The nurse assessed A. J. N. for hearing and urinary function before and during amikacin therapy.

4. What should a hearing assessment include?
5. A. J. N.'s urine output in the last 8 h was 125 mL. Explain the possible cause for the amount of urine output. What nursing action should be taken?
6. What laboratory tests monitor renal function?
7. The health care provider requests peak and trough serum amikacin levels. When should the blood samples to determine peak serum level and trough serum level be drawn?

STUDY QUESTIONS

1. Name two groups of drugs that are classified as bacteriostatic drugs.
2. What antibacterial drugs are used as penicillin substitutes?
3. Give an example of a macrolide.
4. What is the nurse's role in client teaching about tetracycline?
5. What type of antibacterial drug are aminoglycosides?
6. What two types of toxicities are related to aminoglycosides? What signs and symptoms should the nurse assess?
7. Fluoroquinolones are used to treat what health problems?
8. Name four GI problems associated with a fluoroquinolone such as ciprofloxacin.

Chapter 24

Antibacterials: Sulfonamides

OUTLINE

Objectives
Terms
Introduction
Sulfonamides
    Pharmacokinetics

Pharmacodynamics
Side Effects and Adverse
    Reactions
Topical and Ophthalmic
    Sulfonamides

Nursing Process
Case Study
Study Questions

OBJECTIVES

Differentiate between short-acting and intermediate-acting sulfonamides.

Describe the uses, side effects, and adverse reactions to all the sulfonamides.

Explain the nursing interventions, including client teaching, related to sulfonamides.

TERMS

bacteriostatic
cross-sensitivity
crystalluria

erythema multiforme
exfoliative dermatitis
photosensitivity

synergistic effect

INTRODUCTION

Sulfonamides are one of the oldest antibacterial agents used to combat infection. When penicillin was marketed initially, the sulfonamide drugs were not widely prescribed because penicillin was considered the "miracle drug." Today, however, new sulfonamides, and the combination drug of sulfonamide with an antibacterial agent in such preparations as trimethoprim-sulfamethoxazole (Bactrim, Septra) have increased the usage of sulfonamides.

SULFONAMIDES

Sulfonamides were first isolated from the coal tar analine compound in the early 1900s and were produced for clinical use against coccal infections in 1935. It was the first group of drugs used against bacteria. Sulfonamides are not classified as an antibiotic because they were not obtained from biologic substances. The sulfonamides are bacteriostatic, acting by inhibiting bacterial synthesis of folic acid. The clinical usefulness of sulfonamides has decreased due to the availability and effectiveness of penicillin and other antibiotics and the development of bacterial resistance to some sulfonamides. However, they are still used in treating urinary tract and ear infections and may be used in newborn eye prophylaxis. Sulfonamides are not effective against viruses and fungi.

Trimethoprim is a new antibacterial agent that interferes with bacterial folic acid synthesis. It is effective in preventing bacterial resistance to sulfonamide agents. This drug is effective against the gram-negative bacteria *Proteus* spp., *Klebsiella* spp., and *Escherichia coli*. Trimethoprim is used in combination with the sulfonamide, sulfamethoxazole (Bactrim, Septra) to obtain a better response against many organisms. The two drugs have a synergistic effect, increasing the desired drug response. Figure 24–1 describes the pharmacologic behavior of trimethoprim-sulfamethoxazole (co-trimoxazole).

PHARMACOKINETICS

Co-trimoxazole (Bactrim, Septra) is well absorbed from the gastrointestinal (GI) tract and is moderately protein-bound. Its half-life is 8 to 12 h; thus, it is administered twice a day. It is excreted as unchanged metabolites in the urine.

PHARMACODYNAMICS

Co-trimoxazole is a combination of trimethoprim and sulfamethoxazole. Trimethoprim, a nonsulfonamide antibiotic, enhances the activity of the drug combination. Co-trimoxazole blocks steps in bacterial synthesis of protein and nucleic acid, producing a bactericidal effect.

Co-trimoxazole can be administered orally or intravenously. Orally, the drug has a moderately rapid onset of action, and intravenously the drug action is immediate. Serum peak concentration time for oral use is 2 to 4 h and shorter for intravenous use, 0.5 to 1.0 h. Co-trimoxazole, when taken with an oral hypoglycemic agent sulfonylurea, increases the hypoglycemic response. Also, it can increase the activity of oral anticoagulants.

Many of the sulfonamides are for oral use because they are absorbed readily by the GI tract. They also are available in solution and ointment for ophthalmic use and in cream form, silver sulfadiazine (Silvadene) and mafenide acetate (Sulfamylon), for burns. Sulfonamide drugs are well distributed to body tissues and the brain. The liver metabolizes the sulfonamide drug, and the kidneys excrete it.

Most of the early sulfonamides are highly protein-bound and displace other drugs by competing for protein sites. There are three categories of sulfonamides, classified according to their duration of action:

1. Short-acting sulfonamides (rapid absorption and excretion rate)
2. Intermediate-acting sulfonamides (moderate to slow absorption and a slow excretion rate)
3. Long-acting sulfonamides (sulfamethoxypyridazine and sulfameter are no longer prescribed); this group is excreted slowly and can cause toxicity

Sulfonamides are described in Table 24–1.

SIDE EFFECTS AND ADVERSE REACTIONS

The side effects of sulfonamides may include an allergic response, such as skin rash and itching. Anaphylaxis is not common. Blood disorders, such as hemolytic anemia, aplastic anemia, and low white blood cell and platelet counts, could result from prolonged use and high dosages. GI disturbances (anorexia, nausea, and vomiting) may also occur. The early sulfonamides were insoluble in acid urine; thus, **crystalluria** (crystals in urine) and hematuria were common problems. Crystalluria occurs less commonly with sulfisoxazole (Gantrisin) than it does with sulfadiazine and sulfamethoxazole. Increasing fluid intake dilutes the drug, which helps to prevent crystalluria from occurring. **Photosensitivity** can occur, so the client should avoid sunbathing and excess ultraviolet light. **Cross-sen-**

TABLE 24–1 Antibacterials: Sulfonamides

Generic (Brand)	Route and Dosage	Uses and Considerations
Short-Acting Sulfadiazine (Microsulfon)	A: PO: LD: 2–4 g; then 2–4 g/d in 4 divided doses C: PO: LD: 75 mg/kg or 2 g/m²; then 150 mg/kg/d in 4–6 divided doses	For treatment of systemic infections. This drug could be classified as a short–immediate-acting sulfonamide. When taking this drug, increase the fluid intake to >2000 mL/d. *Pregnancy category:* C; PB: 20%–30%; t½: 8–12 h
Sulfamethizole (Sulfasol, Thiosulfil Forte)	A: PO: 0.5–1 g in 3–4 divided doses C: PO: 30–45 mg/kg/d in 4 divided doses	For treatment of urinary tract infections. It is highly soluble. Fluid intake should be at least 2000 mL/d. *Pregnancy category:* C; PB: 90%; t½: 1.5 h
Sulfisoxazole (Gantrisin)	A: PO: LD: 2–4 g; then 4–8 g/d in 4–6 divided doses C: PO: LD: 75 mg/kg or 2 g/m²; then 150 mg/kg/d in 4–6 divided doses	Popular drug for treating urinary tract infections because it is more soluble in urine. Rapidly absorbed from GI tract. Used for treatment and prophylaxis of otitis media. Often ordered with a one-time initial loading dose. Fluid intake ≥2000 mL/d. *Pregnancy category:* C; PB: 85%–95%; t½: 4.5–7.5 h
Intermediate-Acting Sulfamethoxazole (Gantanol)	A: PO: LD: 2 g; then 2–3 g/d in 2–3 divided doses for 7–10 d C: PO: LD: 50–60 mg/kg; then 25–30 mg/kg q12h; *max:* 75 mg/kg/d	For urinary tract infections, otitis media, and meningococcal A strain meningitis prophylaxis. Similar to Gantrisin, except it is absorbed and excreted slowly. Fluid intake should be at least 2000 mL/d. *Pregnancy category:* C; PB: 60%–70%; t½: 7–12 h
Sulfasalazine (Azulfidine, Salazoprine)	A: PO: Initially: 1 g q6–8h; maint: 2 g q6h C: >2 y: PO: Initially: 40–60 mg/kg/d in 4–6 divided doses; maint: 20–30 mg/kg/d in 4 divided doses; max: 2 g/d	For treatment of ulcerative colitis, Crohn's disease, rheumatoid arthritis (some cases). Take after eating. Side effects include nausea, vomiting, bloody diarrhea. *Pregnancy category:* C (near term: D); PB: 99%; t½: 5.5 h
Trimethoprim-sulfamethoxazole: co-trimoxazole (Bactrim, Septra)	See Prototype Drug Chart (Fig. 24–1)	For urinary tract and ear infections. Single-strength tablet contains 80 mg of trimethoprim (T) and 400 mg of sulfamethoxazole (S). Drug of choice for treating *Pneumocystis carinii* pneumonia. Most frequently used as a sulfonamide. *Pregnancy category:* C (near term: D); PB: 50%–65%; t½: 8–12 h
Long-Acting Sulfamethoxypyridazine (Kynex, Midicel)		No longer used owing to very slow excretion rate and toxicity.
Sulfameter (Sulla)		Same as for sulfamethoxypyridazine

KEY: A: adult; C: child; LD: loading dose; PB: protein-binding; PO: by mouth; (S): sulfamethoxazole; (T): trimethoprim; t½: half-life; >: greater than.

sitivity might occur with the different sulfonamides, but does not occur with other antibacterial drugs. Sulfonamides should be avoided during the third trimester of pregnancy.

TOPICAL AND OPHTHALMIC SULFONAMIDES

Sulfonamides can be administered for topical and ophthalmic uses. Topical use of sulfonamides can cause hypersensitivity reactions; therefore, they are not frequently used. Mafenide acetate (Sulfamylon) is a sulfonamide derivative prescribed for second- and third-degree burns to prevent sepsis. Silver sulfadiazine (Silvadene) is another topical sulfonamide

used in treatment of burns. Both of these drugs are discussed in more detail in Chapter 39.

Sulfacetamide sodium (AK-Sulf, Cetamide, Isopto Cetamide, Sodium Sulamyd, Sulf-10) is a sulfonamide for ophthalmic and topical uses. For the ophthalmic preparations (liquid/drop and ointment), sulfacetamide sodium is used to treat conjunctivitis, corneal ulcers, and prophylactic treatment after eye injury or removal of a foreign body. Do *not* use ointment for the eye unless it has "ophthalmic" printed on the drug label. This drug is discussed in more detail in Chapter 38.

Topical sulfacetamide sodium for the skin is an ointment, and is used to treat seborrheic dermatitis and secondary bacterial skin infections. This form is *not* used for the eye.

FIGURE 24–1. Antibacterials: Sulfonamides (Trimethoprim-Sulfamethoxazole)

		NURSING PROCESS Assessment and Planning
Co-trimoxazole *Co-trimoxazole* (Bactrim, Septra) Sulfonamide: trimethoprim (TMP)– sulfamethoxazole (SMZ) *Pregnancy Category:* C	**Dosage** A: PO: 160/800 mg q12h (160 mg [TMP]/800 mg [SMZ]) C: PO: 8/40 mg q12h (8 mg [TMP]/40 mg [SMZ]) Dosing is based on trimethoprim component	
Contraindications Severe renal or hepatic disease, hyper- sensitivity to sulfonamides	**Drug-Lab-Food Interactions** *Increase* anticoagulant effect with warfarin; *increase* hypoglycemic effect with an oral hypoglycemic drug *Lab:* May *increase* BUN, serum creati- nine, AST, ALT, ALP	
Pharmacokinetics *Absorption:* PO: Well absorbed *Distribution:* PB: 50–65%; crosses placenta *Metabolism:* t½: 8–12 h *Excretion:* In urine as metabolites	**Pharmacodynamics** PO: Onset: 0.5–1 h Peak: 2–4 h Duration: UK IV: Onset: Immediate Peak: 0.5–1 h Duration: UK	Interventions

Therapeutic Effects/Uses: To treat urinary tract infection, otitis media, bronchitis, pneumonia, *Pneumocystis carinii* infection, rheumatic fever, burns.

Mode of Action: Inhibition of protein synthesis of nucleic acids. Bactericidal effect.

Evaluation

Side Effects Anorexia, nausea, vomiting, diarrhea, rash, stomatitis, fatigue, depression, headache, vertigo, photosensitivity	**Adverse Reactions** *Life-threatening:* Leukopenia, thrombocytopenia, increased bone marrow depression, hemolytic anemia, aplastic anemia, agranulocy- tosis, Stevens-Johnson syndrome, renal failure

Note: Sulfa drugs should NOT be used in infants <2 mo.
KEY: TMP: trimethoprim; SMZ: sulfamethoxazole; A: adult; C: child; PO: by mouth; UK: unknown; IV: intravenous; PB: protein-binding; t½: half-life.

NURSING PROCESS: ANTIBACTERIALS: Sulfonamides

ASSESSMENT

- Assess the client's renal function by checking urinary output (>600 mL/d), BUN (normal, 8 to 25 mg/dL), and serum creatinine (normal, 0.5 to 1.5 mg/dL).
- Obtain a medical history from the client. Sulfonamides such as co-trimoxazole (trimethoprim-

sulfamethoxazole [Bactrim, Septra]) are contraindicated for clients with severe renal or liver disease.
- Assess if the client is hypertensive to sulfonamides. An allergic reaction can include rash, skin eruptions, and itching. A severe hypersensitivity reaction includes erythema multiforme (erythematous macular, papular, or vesicular

eruption; if severe, can cover the entire body) or exfoliative dermatitis (desquamation, scaling, and itching of skin).

- Obtain a drug history of drugs the client is currently taking. Oral antidiabetic drugs (sulfonylureas) with sulfonamides increase the hypoglycemic effect; the use of warfarin with sulfonamides increases the anticoagulant effect.
- Assess baseline laboratory results, especially CBC. Blood dyscrasias may occur due to high doses of sulfonamides over a continuous period of time, causing life-threatening conditions.

POTENTIAL NURSING DIAGNOSES

- High risk for infection
- High risk for impaired tissue integrity
- Altered patterns of urinary elimination

PLANNING

- Client's infection will be controlled and later alleviated.

NURSING INTERVENTIONS

- Administer sulfonamides with a full glass of water. Extra fluid intake can prevent crystalluria and kidney stone formation.
- Monitor the client's intake and output. Urine output should be at least 1,200 mL/d to decrease the risk of crystalluria. The sulfonamides sulfadiazine and sulfamethoxazole are more likely to cause crystalluria than are sulfisoxazole (Gantrisin) and combination drugs. Fluid intake should be at least 2000 mL/d.
- Monitor vital signs (VS). Note if the temperature has decreased.
- Observe the client for hematologic reaction that may lead to life-threatening anemias. Early signs are sore throat, purpura, and decreasing white blood cell and platelet counts. Check the client's CBC and compare with baseline findings.

- Check for signs and symptoms of superinfection (secondary infection caused by a different organism than the primary infection). Symptoms include stomatitis (mouth ulcers), furry black tongue, anal or genital discharge, and itching.

General

- Instruct the client to drink several quarts of fluid daily while taking sulfonamides to avoid the complication of crystalluria.
- Advise the pregnant woman to avoid sulfonamides during the last 3 mo of pregnancy.
- Instruct the client not to take antacids with sulfonamides because antacids decrease the absorption rate.
- Advise the client who has an allergy to one sulfonamide that all sulfonamide preparations should be avoided, with the health care provider's approval, due to the possibility of cross-sensitivity. Observe the client for rash or any skin eruptions.

Skill

- Instruct the client to take the sulfonamide 1 h before or 2 h after meals with a full glass of water.

Side Effects

- Instruct the client to report bruising or bleeding that could be caused from drug-induced blood disorder. Advise the client to have blood cell count monitored on a regular basis.
- Advise the client to avoid direct sunlight and to use sunblock and protective clothing to decrease the risk of photosensitive reactions.

EVALUATION

- Evaluate the effectiveness of the sulfonamide by determining if the infection has been alleviated and the blood cell count is within normal range.

■ CASE STUDY
Client Taking a Sulfonamide Drug

R. M., age 46 years, has a severe urinary tract infection (UTI). She is taking co-trimoxazole 160 mg/800 mg, every 6 hours.

1. Is the drug dose within recommended drug dose and dosing interval? What is the nurse's responsibility?

2. What are the side effects of trimethoprim-sulfamethoxazole or co-trimoxazole? What is stomatitis?
3. What are the adverse reactions of co-trimoxazole?
4. What would be a sign of thrombocytopenia? Of hemolytic anemia?

Client teaching is an important part of nursing implications and interventions. Explain the nurse's role in regard to client teaching concerning the following:

5. The required amount of daily fluid intake which should be taken
6. Cross-sensitive effects if allergic to other sulfonamide preparations; allergic reaction may include _____.
7. The time of day for taking the sulfonamide
8. Reporting bruising, bleeding; why?
9. Protective measures to take to prevent effects from possible photosensitive reaction

R. M. is taking the anticoagulant Coumadin 7.5 mg daily.

10. What effect does co-trimoxazole have on warfarin? Should R.M.'s Coumadin dose be increased or decreased? What is the nurse's responsibility?

STUDY QUESTIONS

1. Why would a nurse instruct a client taking a sulfonamide to increase fluid intake? Why is the use of sunblock lotion indicated for sun exposure for a client taking a sulfonamide drug?
2. If your client is allergic to a sulfonamide drug, what should you advise the client about the use of other sulfonamides?
3. What is the generic name for Gantrisin? What is its main clinical use? Is it classified as a short-acting, intermediate-acting, or long-acting sulfonamide?
4. What is the purpose of the drug trimethoprim-sulfamethoxazole/co-trimoxazole (Bactrim, Septra)?
5. Your client is taking a sulfonylurea (oral hypoglycemic to promote insulin production). What effect may co-trimoxazole have on the sulfonylurea? What is the nurse's responsibility if the client is receiving both drugs?
6. What effects can co-trimoxazole have on the following laboratory tests: AST, ALT, ALP, BUN, serum creatinine?
7. What hematologic conditions can occur because of excessive or long-term use of sulfonamides such as co-trimoxazole?

Chapter 25

Antitubercular Drugs, Antifungal Drugs, Peptides

OUTLINE

Objectives
Terms
Antitubercular Drugs
    Pharmacokinetics
    Pharmacodynamics
    Side Effects and Adverse
      Reactions

Nursing Process
Antifungal Drugs
    Polyenes
    Imidazole Group
    Antimetabolite
    Nursing Process

Peptides
    Side Effects and Adverse
      Reactions
Case Study
Study Questions

OBJECTIVES

Differentiate between first-line and second-line antitubercular drugs and give examples of each.

Name the three classes of antifungal drugs.

Identify examples of polyenes and explain their uses.

Describe the adverse reactions of antitubercular, antifungal, and peptide drugs.

Describe the nursing interventions, including client teaching, for clients taking antitubercular drugs, antifungal drugs, and peptides.

TERMS

AIDS
antifungal drugs
antimycotic
antitubercular drugs
first-line drugs

hepatoxicity
HIV infection
neurotoxicity
opportunistic infection
paresthesias

peptides
prophylaxis
second-line drugs

INTRODUCTION

Antitubercular, antifungal, and peptide drugs are presented in this chapter. Although these categories of drugs differ from each other, these drugs inhibit or kill organisms that cause diseases.

This chapter includes a drug table and nursing process for each of the three categories of drugs. Prototype drugs for antitubercular drugs and antifungal drugs are included.

ANTITUBERCULAR DRUGS

Tuberculosis (TB) is caused by the bacillus *Mycobacterium tuberculosis*. It is transmitted from one person to another by droplets dispersed in the air through coughing and sneezing. The organisms are inhaled into the alveoli (air sacs) of the lung. Prior to 1944, many people died from this disease because of the absence of drug therapy. Streptomycin, a parenteral antibiotic, was the first drug used for treating TB. Isoniazid (INH) was discovered in 1952 and was the first oral drug preparation effective against the tubercle bacillus. Group names for drugs used in treating tuberculosis include antimycobacterial agents and antitubercular drugs.

The occurrence of TB decreased until the 1980s. The rising incidence is partly due to clients whose immune responses are compromised (immunocompromised) and the increasingly crowded living conditions in urban cities. Clients susceptible to TB in-

FIGURE 25–1. Antitubercular Drugs

Isoniazid	Dosage	NURSING PROCESS Assessment and Planning
Isoniazid (INH, Nydrazid, Laniazid), 🍁 Isotamine, PMS, Isoniazid *Pregnancy Category:* C	A: PO/IM: 5–10 mg/kg/d in a single dose; max: 300 mg/d *Prophylaxis:* 300 mg/d C: PO/IM: 10–20 mg/kg/d in a single dose; max: 300 mg/d *Prophylaxis:* 10 mg/kg/d in a single dose	
Contraindications	**Drug-Lab-Food Interactions**	
Severe renal or hepatic disease, alcoholism, diabetic retinopathy	*Increase* effect with alcohol, rifampin, cycloserine *Lab:* Increase AST, ALT, bilirubin	
Pharmacokinetics	**Pharmacodynamics**	Interventions
Absorption: PO: Well absorbed *Distribution:* PB: 10% *Metabolism:* t½: 1–4 h *Excretion:* 50% unchanged in urine	PO: Onset: 0.5 h Peak: 1–2 h Duration: PO: 6–8 h IM: 6 h	

Therapeutic Effects/Uses: To treat tuberculosis; prophylactic measure against tuberculosis. *Mode of Action:* Inhibition of bacterial cell wall synthesis.	Evaluation

Side Effects	Adverse Reactions
Drowsiness, tremors, rash, blurred vision, photosensitivity	Psychotic behavior, peripheral neuropathy, vitamin B_6 deficiency *Life-threatening:* Blood dyscrasias, thrombocytopenia, seizures, agranulocytosis, hepatotoxicity

KEY: A: adult; C: child; PO: by mouth; IM: intramuscular; PB: protein-binding; t½: half-life; max: maximum; 🍁: Canadian drug name.

TABLE 25–1 Antitubercular Drugs

Generic (Brand)	Route and Dosage	Uses and Considerations
Aminosalicylate sodium, P.A.S. sodium	A: PO: 14–16 g/d in 2–3 divided doses C: PO: 275–420 mg/kg/d in 3–4 divided doses; take with food	Second-line antitubercular drug. To treat pulmonary and extrapulmonary tuberculosis. Used in combination with other antitubercular drugs. Take after meals to reduce gastric irritation. *Pregnancy category:* C; PB: 15%; t½: 1 h
Ethambutol HCl (Myambutol)	A: PO: 15 mg/kg as a single dose *Retreatment* A: PO: 25 mg/kg as a single dose for 2 mo; then decrease to 15 mg/kg/d C: >12 y: same as adult	Used as a combination drug for active tuberculosis. Decrease dose if renal insufficiency is present. *Pregnancy category:* C; PB: 10%–20%; t½: 3–4 h (8 h with renal dysfunction)
Isoniazid (INH, Nydrazid)	See Prototype Drug Chart (Fig. 25–1)	Used in combination drug therapy against active tuberculosis. For prophylactic use against tuberculosis, vitamin B_6 frequently given to prevent peripheral neuropathy and when isoniazid is given on an extended basis. *Pregnancy category:* C; PB: 10%; t½: 1–4 h
Pyrazinamide (Tebrazid; Canadian drug)	A: PO: 20–35 mg/kg/d in 3–4 divided doses; *max:* 3 g/d	Second-line antitubercular drug. Used in combination with other antitubercular drugs for short-term and initial phase of therapy. Promote fluid intake. *Pregnancy category:* C; PB: 10%–20%; t½: 9.5 h
Rifabutin (Mycobutin)	A: PO: 300 mg/d in 1 or 2 divided doses	To treat *Mycobacterium tuberculosis* infection; to prevent disseminated *Mycobacterium avium* complex (MAC) disease in clients with advanced HIV infection. *Pregnancy category:* B; PB: 85%; t½: 16–69 h
Rifampin (Rifadin, Rimactane)	A: PO: 600 mg/d as a single dose C: PO: 10–20 mg/kg/d as a single dose; *max:* 600 mg/d	Used as a combination drug for active tuberculosis. For selective gram-positive and gram-negative bacteria, including *Neisseria meningitidis.* Liver enzymes should be monitored. *Pregnancy category:* C; PB: 85%–90%; t½: 3 h
Streptomycin SO_4	A: IM: 1 g daily or 7–15 mg/kg/d for 2–3 mo, then 2–3× wk C: IMP: 20–40 mg/kg/d in divided doses	Used against tuberculosis as the third drug with isoniazid and rifampin or with isoniazid and ethambutol. First drug use to treat tuberculosis. *Pregnancy category:* C; PB: 30%; t½: 2–3 h

KEY: *A: adult; C: child; PO: by mouth; IM: intramuscular; PB: protein-binding; t½: half-life; >: greater than.*

clude those with alcohol addiction, acquired immunodeficiency syndrome (AIDS), and debilitated persons. Prophylactic antitubercular therapy is suggested for persons who have been in close contact with those with TB and human immunodeficiency virus (HIV)-positive persons who have a positive TB skin test or close contact with a person with TB. Prophylactic therapy is contraindicated for those persons with liver disease. Isoniazid is the primary drug used and may cause isoniazid-induced liver damage. Other antitubercular drugs may also cause liver damage if given in high doses over an extended period of time.

Single-drug therapy with isoniazid proved to be ineffective in treating tuberculosis because resistance to the drug developed in a short time. It was discovered that by using a combination of antitubercular drugs, bacterial resistance did not occur. In fact, the duration of treatment was reduced from 2 years to 6 to 9 months. Different combinations of drugs can be used, for example, isoniazid and rifampin, or isoniazid, rifampin, and ethambutol, or

isoniazid, rifampin, and pyrazinamide. Rifampin and ethambutol were discovered in the early 1960s and either drug given alone is not effective against the tubercle bacillus. Isoniazid can be prescribed alone as a prophylaxis measure against tuberculosis. When a person is diagnosed with tuberculosis, the family members are given prophylactic doses of isoniazid for 6 months to a year. Figure 25–1 lists the drug data for isoniazid.

PHARMACOKINETICS

Isoniazid is well absorbed from the gastrointestinal (GI) tract. It can also be administered intramuscularly and intravenously. It has a very low protein-binding rate (10%), and its half-life is 1 to 4 h. Isoniazid is metabolized by the liver, and 75%–95% of the drug is excreted in the urine.

PHARMACODYNAMICS

Isoniazid inhibits cell wall synthesis of the tubercle bacillus. It is usually prescribed with other antitubercular agents. The onset of action and peak concentration time for oral and intramuscular routes of isoniazid are the same. Peripheral neuropathy is an adverse reaction to isoniazid; thus pyridoxine, vitamin B₆, is usually taken with isoniazid to decrease the probability of neuropathy. Alcohol ingestion with the drug can increase the incidence of peripheral neuropathy. If phenytoin is taken with isoniazid, the effect of phenytoin may be decreased. Antacids decrease isoniazid absorption.

Antitubercular drugs in the treatment of TB are divided into two categories, first-line and second-line drugs. **First-line drugs** (isoniazid, rifampin, ethambutol, and streptomycin) are considered to be more effective and less toxic than second-line drugs in treating TB. **Second-line drugs** (*para*-aminosalicylic acid, kanamycin, cycloserine, ethionamide, capreomycin and pyrazinamide) are not as effective as first-line drugs and some can be more toxic. Second-line drugs may be used in combination with first-line drugs, especially to treat disseminated TB. First-line drugs and some second-line drugs are described in Table 25–1.

SIDE EFFECTS AND ADVERSE REACTIONS

Side effects and adverse reactions differ according to the drug prescribed. For isoniazid, peripheral neuropathy can be a problem, especially to the malnourished, those with diabetes mellitus, and alcoholics. Peripheral neuropathy can be prevented by giving pyridoxine (vitamin B₆). Hepatotoxicity is an adverse reaction to isoniazid, from which hepatitis can result. Clients with liver disorders should not take isoniazid or isoniazid and rifampin unless liver enzymes are closely monitored. Rifampin can increase liver enzyme levels.

NURSING PROCESS: ANTITUBERCULAR DRUGS

ASSESSMENT

- Obtain a history from the client of any past instances of tuberculosis, last purified protein derivative (PPD) tuberculin test and reaction, last chest x-ray and result, and allergy to any of the antitubercular drugs if taken previously.
- Obtain a medical history from the client. Most antitubercular drugs are contraindicated if the client has a severe hepatic disease.
- Check laboratory tests for liver enzyme values, bilirubin, BUN, and serum creatinine. These baseline values can be compared with future laboratory test results.
- Assess the client for signs and symptoms of peripheral neuropathy, such as numbness or tingling of the extremities.
- Check the client for hearing changes if the antitubercular drug regimen includes streptomycin. Ototoxicity is an adverse reaction to streptomycin.

POTENTIAL NURSING DIAGNOSES

- High risk for infection
- High risk for impaired tissue integrity

PLANNING

- Client's sputum test for acid-fast bacilli will be negative in 2 to 3 mo after the prescribed antitubercular therapy.

NURSING INTERVENTIONS

- Administer the commonly ordered antitubercular drug isoniazid (INH) 1 h before or 2 h after meals. Food decreases absorption rate.
- Administer pyridoxine (vitamin B₆) as prescribed with isoniazid to prevent peripheral neuropathy.
- Monitor serum liver enzyme levels, especially if the client is taking isoniazid or rifampin. Elevated levels may indicate liver toxicity.
- Collect sputum specimens for acid-fast bacilli early in the morning. Usually three consecutive morning sputum specimens are sent to the laboratory, and the routine is repeated several weeks later.
- Have eye examinations performed on clients taking isoniazid and ethambutol. Visual disturbances may result in clients taking these antitubercular drugs.
- Emphasize the importance of complying with drug regimen.

CLIENT TEACHING

General
- Instruct the client to take the antitubercular drug such as isoniazid 1 h before meals or 2 h after meals for better absorption.
- Instruct the client to take the antitubercular drugs as prescribed. Ineffective treatment of tuberculosis might occur if the drugs are taken intermittently or discontinued when symptoms are

decreased or when the client is feeling better. Compliance with the drug regimen is a must.

- Instruct the client not to take antacids while taking antitubercular drug(s) because they decrease the drug absorption. The client should also avoid alcohol because it may increase the risk of hepatotoxicity.
- Advise the client to keep medical appointments and to participate in sputum testing. Sputum testing is important to determine the effectiveness of the drug regimen.
- Advise the woman contemplating pregnancy to first check with her health care provider about taking the antitubercular drugs ethambutol and rifampin.

Side Effects

- Instruct the client to report any numbness, tingling, or burning of the hands and feet. Peripheral neuritis is a common side effect of isoniazid. Vitamin B$_6$ prevents peripheral neuropathy. Neu-

ritis may not occur if the client eats a balanced diet daily.

- Advise the client to avoid direct sunlight to decrease the risk of photosensitivity. Client should use sunblock while in the sun.
- Inform the client taking rifampin that urine, feces, saliva, sputum, sweat, and tears may be a harmless red-orange color. Soft contact lenses may be permanently stained.
- Advise the client receiving ethambutol to take daily single doses to avoid visual problems. Divided doses of ethambutol may cause visual disturbances.

EVALUATION

- Evaluate the effectiveness of the antitubercular drug(s). Sputum specimen for acid-fast bacilli should be negative after taking antitubercular drugs for several weeks to months.

ANTIFUNGAL DRUGS

Antifungal drugs, also called **antimycotic drugs,** are used to treat two types of fungal infections: superficial fungal infections of the skin or mucous membrane and systemic fungal infections of the lung or central nervous system. Fungal infections may be mild, such as tinea pedis (athlete's foot), or severe, as in pulmonary conditions or meningitis. Fungi, such as *Candida* spp. (yeast), are part of the normal flora of the mouth, skin, intestine, and vagina. Candidiasis might occur as an opportunistic infection when the body's defense mechanisms are impaired, allowing for overgrowth of the fungus. Drugs such as antibiotics, oral contraceptives, and immunosuppressives may also alter the body's defense mechanisms. Opportunistic fungal infections can be mild (yeast infection in the vagina) or severe (systemic fungal infection).

The antifungal drugs are classified into four groups:

1. Polyenes, including amphotericin B and nystatin
2. Imidazoles, which include ketoconazole, miconazole, and clotrimazole
3. The antimetabolic antifungal flucytosine
4. Topical antifungals for superficial infections

POLYENES

The polyene antifungal drug of choice for treating severe systemic infection is amphotericin B. Introduced in 1956 and used today with close supervision because of its toxicity, amphotericin B is effective against numerous fungal diseases, including

histoplasmosis, cryptococcosis, coccidioidomycosis, aspergillosis, blastomycosis, and candidiasis (systemic infection). Amphotericin B is not absorbed from the GI tract; therefore, it is administered intravenously in low doses for treating systemic fungal infections.

Amphotericin B is highly protein-bound and has a long half-life, and only 5% of the drug is excreted in the urine. Renal disease does not affect the excretion of amphotericin B.

Side Effects and Adverse Reactions

Side effects of and adverse reactions to amphotericin B include flushing, fever, chills, nausea, vomiting, hypotension, paresthesias, and thrombophlebitis. Amphotericin B is considered *highly toxic* and can cause nephrotoxicity and electrolyte imbalance, especially hypokalemia and hypomagnesemia (low serum potassium and magnesium levels). Urinary output, BUN, and serum creatinine levels need to be closely monitored.

Nystatin (Mycostatin), a polyene antifungal drug, is administered orally or topically to treat candida infection. It is available in suspensions, cream, ointment, and vaginal tablets. Nystatin is poorly absorbed via the GI tract; however, the oral tablet form is used for intestinal candidiasis. The more common use of nystatin is in oral suspension for candida infection in the mouth. The client is instructed to swish the liquid within the mouth to have contact with the mucous membrane, and then to swallow the liquid after a few minutes. If the throat area is involved, instruct the client to gargle with nystatin after swishing and before swallowing. Figure 25–2 describes the pharmacologic behavior of nystatin.

Pharmacokinetics

Nystatin is poorly absorbed. Its protein-binding power and half-life are unknown. The drug is excreted unchanged in feces.

Pharmacodynamics

Nystatin increases permeability of the fungal cell membrane, thus causing the fungal cell to become unstable and to discharge the content. This drug has a fungistatic and fungicidal action. The onset of action for both suspension and tablet is rapid. The onset of action for vaginal tablet or cream is approximately 24 or more hours.

IMIDAZOLE GROUP

The imidazole group is effective against candidiasis (superficial and systemic), coccidioidomycosis, cryptococcosis, histoplasmosis, and paracoccidioidomycosis. Ketaconazole is the first effective antifungal drug that is orally absorbed. Fluconazole and itraconazole are two new imidazole drugs for systemic fungal infection. These two antifungals can be taken orally, unlike amphotericin B, which is only administered intravenously.

FIGURE 25–2. Antifungals

Nystatin	Dosage	NURSING PROCESS
		Assessment and Planning
Nystatin (Mycostatin), ★Nadostine, Nyaderm *Antifungal* *Pregnancy Category:* C	A: Topical use as directed *Intestinal infections:* A: PO: 500,000–1,000,000 U t.i.d. or q8h *Oral candidiasis:* A: PO: 400,000–600,000 U q6–8h Neonate (<7 d): PO: 100,000 U q.i.d. C: PO: 250,000–500,000 U q.i.d.	
Contraindications	**Drug-Lab-Food Interactions**	
Hypersensitivity Vag: Pregnancy	None significant known	
Pharmacokinetics	**Pharmacodynamics**	Interventions
Absorption: PO: Poorly absorbed *Distribution:* PB: UK *Metabolism:* t½: UK *Excretion:* In feces unchanged	PO: Onset: Rapid Peak: UK Duration: 6–12 h Vaginally: Onset: 24–72 h Peak: UK Duration: UK	

	Evaluation
Therapeutic Effects/Uses: To treat *Candida* infections. *Mode of Action:* Increase permeability of the fungal cell membrane.	

Side Effects	Adverse Reactions
PO: Anorexia, nausea, vomiting, diarrea (large doses), stomach cramps, rash Vag: Rash, burning sensation	None known

KEY: A: adult; **C:** child; **PO:** by mouth; **<:** less than; **Vag:** Vaginal; **UK:** unknown; **PB:** protein-binding; **t½:** half-life; ★: Canadian drug names.

Three of the imidazoles, clotrimazole (Lotrimin, Mycelex), butoconazole nitrate (Femstat), and econazole nitrate (Spectazole), are for topical use only. The last imidazole is miconazole (Monistat), and is for intravenous and topical use. Topically, it is frequently used in the treatment of vaginitis. Intravenously, it is used to treat bladder infections and meningitis.

ANTIMETABOLITE

The antimetabolite flucytosine has antifungal action. It is well absorbed from the GI tract. Flucytosine is used in combination with other antifungal drugs, such as amphotericin B. Table 25–2 lists the commonly used antifungal drugs, their dosages, uses, and considerations.

TABLE 25–2 Antifungal Drugs

Generic (Brand)	Route and Dosage	Uses and Considerations
Polyenes		
Amphotericin B (Fungizone)	*Test dose:* A: IV: 0.25–1.0 mg in 20 mL of D_5W infused over 20–30 min A: IV: 0.25–1.0 mg/kg/d in D_5W or 1.5 mg/kg q.o.d.: *max:* 1.5 mg/kg/d C: IV: Same as adult, except dilution and infuse time differ	For treatment of a variety of systemic fungal (mycotic) infections, such as aspergillosis, blastomycosis, coccidioidomycosis, cryptococcosis, histoplasmosis. Nephrotoxicity may occur when given in high doses. Hypokalemia might occur. *Pregnancy category:* B; PB: 95%; t½: 24 h
Nystatin (Mycostatin)	See Prototype Drug Chart (Fig. 25–2)	For oral and intestinal candidiasis. Absorption is poor. Oral tablets are for intestinal candidiasis. Liquid form is for oral candidiasis; use by swish and swallow or expectorate. *Pregnancy category:* C; PB: UK; t½: UK
Imidazoles		
Fluconazole (Diflucan)	A: PO/IV: 50–400 mg/d; maint: 100–200 mg/d C: PO/IV: 3–6 mg/kg/d	For a variety of fungal infections. Highly selective inhibitor of fungal cytochrome P-450. Used to treat cryptococcal meningitis in AIDS clients and oropharyngeal and systemic candidiasis. *Pregnancy category:* C; PB: 12%; t½: 20–40 h
Itraconazole (Sporanox)	A: PO: Loading dose: 200 mg q8h × 3 d: maint: 200 mg/d: *max:* 400 mg/d in 2 divided doses	Effective against various systemic fungal infections, particularly blastomycosis and histoplasmosis. *Pregnancy category:* C; PB: 99%; t½: 21–42 h
Ketoconazole (Nizoral)	A: PO: 200–400 mg/d as a single dose C: PO: 3.3–6.6 mg/kg/d as single dose C: <20 kg: PO: 50 mg daily	For infections by *Candida* spp., histoplasmosis, blastomycosis, and others. Treatment could last 1–6 months for systemic infections. Take with food to avoid GI discomfort. *Pregnancy category:* C; PB: 95%; t½: 2–8 h
Miconazole nitrate (Monistat, Micatin)	A: IV: 200–3,600 mg/d in D_5W in 3 divided doses; infuse IV over 30–60 min C: IV: 20–40 mg/kg/d in divided doses; *max:* 15 mg/kg/inf A: Supp: 100 mg vag h.s. for 7 d Available: Vaginal cream 2%; lotion	For fungal meningitis and fungal bladder infections. Also for vaginal fungal infections. *Pregnancy category:* B; PB: 92%; t½: 2–24 h
Terbinafine HCl (Lamisil)	A & C: Topical: Cream 1%, apply 1–2 × per day	For treatment of superficial mycosis; i.e., tinea pedis, tinea cruris, and tinea corporis. *Pregnancy category:* B; PB: NA; t½: NA
Antimetabolites		
Flucytosine (Ancobon)	A: PO: 50–150 mg/kg/d in 4 divided doses C: <50 kg: PO: 1.5–4.5 g/m²/d in 4 divided doses	Use with amphotericin B may increase therapeutic action as well as toxicity. Fungal resistance occurs if the drug is given alone. *Pregnancy category:* C; PB: UK; t½: 3–6 h
Antiprotozoal		
Atovaquone (Mepron)	A: PO: 750 mg t.i.d. with food × 21 d	For treatment of mild to moderate *Pneumocystis carinii* pneumonia. *Pregnancy category:* C; PB: 99%; t½: 2–3 d

KEY: *A: adult; C: child; PO: by mouth; IV: intravenous; PB: protein-binding; Supp: suppository; t½: half-life; UK: unknown; Vag: vaginal; >: greater than; <: less than.*

NURSING PROCESS: ANTIFUNGALS

ASSESSMENT

- Obtain a medical history from the client of any serious renal or hepatic disorder. Antifungal agents such as amphotericin B, fluconazole (Diflucan), flucytosine (Ancobon), and ketoconazole (Nizoral) are contraindicated if the client has a serious renal or liver disease.
- Check laboratory tests for liver enzyme values (ALP, ALT, AST, GGT), BUN, bilirubin, and serum creatinine. Elevated levels can indicate liver or renal dysfunction. These test results may be used for future comparisons.
- Obtain baseline vital signs (VS) for future comparison.

POTENTIAL NURSING DIAGNOSES

- High risk for infection
- High risk for impaired tissue integrity

PLANNING

- Client's fungal infection will be resolved.

NURSING INTERVENTIONS

- Obtain a culture to determine the fungus; e.g., *Candida.*
- Monitor the client's urinary output; many of the antifungal drugs may cause nephrotoxicity.
- Monitor the laboratory results and compare with baseline findings; i.e., BUN, serum creatinine, ALP, ALT, AST, bilirubin, and electrolytes. Certain antifungals could cause hepatotoxicity as well as nephrotoxicity when taking high doses over a prolonged period of time.
- Monitor VS. Compare with baseline findings.
- Observe for side effects and adverse reactions to antifungal drugs (antimycotics), such as nausea, vomiting, headache, phlebitis, and signs and symptoms of electrolyte imbalance (hypokalemia with amphotericin B).

CLIENT TEACHING

General
- Instruct the client to take the drug as prescribed. Compliance is of utmost importance since discontinuing the drug too soon may result in a relapse.
- Advise the client to obtain laboratory testing as indicated. Serum liver enzymes, BUN, creatinine, and electrolytes should be monitored.
- Advise the client taking ketoconazole not to consume alcohol.

Skill
- Instruct the client on the administration of nystatin (Mycostatin) suspension. Place the nystatin dose, usually 1 to 2 teaspoons, in the mouth. Swish the solution in the mouth and swallow (swish and swallow), or after swishing, have the client expectorate the solution (check with health care provider).

Side Effects
- Advise the client to avoid operating hazardous equipment or a motor vehicle when taking amphotericin B, ketoconazole, or flucytosine because these drugs may cause visual changes, sleepiness, dizziness, or lethargy.
- Instruct the client to report side effects, such as nausea, vomiting, diarrhea, dermatitis, rash, dizziness, tinnitus, edema, and flatulence. These symptoms may occur when taking certain antifungal drugs.

EVALUATION

- Evaluate the effectiveness of the antifungal (antimycotic) drug by noting the absence of the fungal infection, e.g., decreased itching, redness, and rawness.

PEPTIDES

The two groups of **peptides** used as antibiotics are the polymyxins and bacitracin. Polymyxins were one of the early groups of antibacterials, but many of the early drugs were discontinued due to nephrotoxicity. Today two polymyxins, colistin and polymyxin B, are approved for pharmaceutical use. Polymyxins produce a bactericidal effect by inter-fering with the cellular membrane of the bacterium, thereby causing cell death. They affect most gram-negative bacteria, such as *Pseudomonas aeruginosa*, *Escherichia coli*, *Klebsiella* spp., and *Shigella* spp.

Except for colistin, which exerts action on the colon and is excreted in the feces, the polymyxins are not absorbed through the oral route. Intramuscular injection of polymyxins produces marked pain at the injection site. Intravenous administra-

TABLE 25–3 Antibacterials: Peptides

Generic (Brand)	Route and Dosage	Uses and Considerations
Bacitracin (Bactrin USP)	C <2.5 kg: IM: <900 U/kg/d in 2–3 divided doses C >2.5 kg: IM: <1000 U/kg/d in 2–3 divided doses. Available in topical and ophthalmic ointment	It is seldom used parenterally except for children. Topical ointment for skin infection and ophthalmic ointment for infections of the eye. *Pregnancy category:* C; PB: <20%; t½: UK
Colistin (PO) (Coly-Mycin S, Polymyxin E)	A & C: PO: 5–15 mg/kg/d in 3 divided doses	For treating *Pseudomonas aeruginosa* infection. For gastroenteritis due to Shigella spp. *Pregnancy category:* C; PB: UK; t½: 2–3 h
Colistimethate sodium (IM/IV) (Coly-Mycin M)	IM/IV: 2.5–5 mg/kg/d in divided doses	For treating *Pseudomonas aeruginosa* infection. *Pregnancy category:* C; PB: UK; t½: 2–3 h
Polymyxin B SO$_4$ (Aerosporin)	A: IM: 25,000 U/kg/d in divided doses IV: 15,000–25,000 U/kg/d in 2 divided doses (q12h) C >2 y: Same as adult	For systemic use; also available in ointment form. May cause nephrotoxicity if given with aminoglycosides or amphotericin. *Pregnancy category:* B; PB: UK; t½: 4.5–6 h

KEY: *A: adult; C: child; IM: intramuscular; IV: intravenous; PB: protein-binding; t½: half-life; UK: unknown; >: greater than; <: less than.*

tion of polymyxins at a slow infusion rate is, therefore, the suggested method. Table 25–3 lists the polymyxins, their dosage, and uses.

High serum levels of polymyxins can cause nephrotoxicity and neurotoxicity. With nephrotoxicity, the blood urea nitrogen (BUN) and serum creatinine levels are elevated; however, when the serum drug level decreases, renal toxicity is usually reversed. Signs and symptoms of **neurotoxicity** are numbness and tingling of the extremities, paresthesias (abnormal sensation), and dizziness. Neurotoxicity is usually reversible when the drug is discontinued.

Bacitracin has a polypeptide structure and acts by inhibiting bacterial cell wall synthesis and damaging the cell wall membrane. The drug action can be bacteriostatic or bactericidal. Bacitracin is not absorbed by the GI tract and if given orally is excreted in the feces. It is, therefore, given intravenously or intramuscularly. It crosses the blood–brain barrier and, thus, is effective in treating meningitis. Bacitracin is effective against most gram-positive bacteria and some gram-negative bacteria. Over-the-counter (OTC) bacitracin ointment is available for application to the skin.

SIDE EFFECTS AND ADVERSE REACTIONS

The side effects of bacitracin include nausea and vomiting. Severe adverse reactions are renal damage, respiratory paralysis, blood dyscrasias (life-threatening anemias), and mild to severe allergic reactions, ranging from hives to anaphylaxis.

■ CASE STUDY
Client with Tuberculosis

C.J., 41 years old, has had a constant cough and night sweats for several months. He consumes 1 pint of whiskey per day. Sputum taken revealed that it was positive for acid-fast (tubercle) bacillus. The physician ordered 6- to 9-month antitubercular drug regimen (time of therapy to be determined according to sputum and x-ray test results). For 2 months, C.J. was prescribed isoniazid, rifampin and pyrazinamide daily. The next 4 to 7 months, C.J. would receive isoniazid and rifampin biweekly.

1. What do you think are the contributing causes for C.J.'s contacting tuberculosis?
2. Which of the drug(s) are first-line and second-line antitubercular drugs? Why are these drugs used in combination?
3. What is the nurse's role in client teaching concerning the drug regimen?
4. Name at least two serious adverse reactions that can occur when antitubercular drugs are given over an extended period of time.
5. What laboratory tests should be monitored while C.J. is taking isoniazid and rifampin? Why?

The health care provider ordered pyridoxine to be given daily.

6. What type of drug is pyridoxine?
7. For what reason would this drug be given?
8. What health agencies may the nurse suggest that could be helpful to C.J. during and after therapy?

STUDY QUESTIONS

1. What is the purpose of combination drug therapy in the treatment of tuberculosis?
2. What is a common side effect of isoniazid? Why should some clients receive pyridoxine (vitamin B$_6$) while taking isoniazid? What are the signs and symptoms of peripheral neuropathy?
3. What is a potential adverse reaction to the use of isoniazid and rifampin? Would the problem be intensified if the drugs were taken by an alcoholic or a client with a liver disorder? Explain.
4. Your client is to receive nystatin or an oral fungal infection. How would you instruct the client to use the oral suspension of nystatin?
5. What is the type of electrolyte imbalance associated with the use of amphotericin B? What other adverse effect might result from the use of amphotericin B?
6. Two new oral antifungal drugs that may be taken for systemic fungal infections are _____ and _____. How do these drugs differ from one another according to their protein-binding and half-life? What are the advantages of these drugs over amphotericin B?
7. Why should kidney function be assessed with polymyxin administration? Against what bacteria are polymyxins and colistin effective?

Chapter 26

Antiviral, Antimalarial, and Anthelmintic Drugs

OUTLINE

Objectives
Terms
Antiviral Drugs
    Antiviral Antimetabolites
    Nursing Process

Antimalarial Drugs
    Pharmacokinetics
    Pharmacodynamics
    Side Effects and Adverse
        Reactions
    Nursing Process

Anthelmintic Drugs
    Side Effects and Adverse
        Reactions
    Nursing Process
Study Questions

OBJECTIVES

Name several antiviral and antimalarial drugs and explain their uses.

Identify the various helminths and the human body sites for their infestation.

Describe the action of anthelmintics.

Explain the side effects of and adverse reactions to antiviral, antimalarial, and anthelmintic drugs.

Identify several nursing interventions, including client teaching, for antiviral, antimalarial, and anthelmintic drug therapy.

TERMS

AIDS
anthelmintic drugs
antimalarial drugs
antiviral drugs

ARC
erythrocytic phase
helminths
helminthiasis

opportunistic infection
prophylaxis
tissue phase
trichinosis

ANTIVIRAL DRUGS

Viruses are more difficult to eradicate than most bacterias. Viruses depend on the biochemical processes of the host cells for viral reproduction. The growth cycle of viruses depends on the host cell enzymes and cell substrates for viral replication. Antiviral drug development has been slower than the prolific antibacterial drug production. This may be partly because of the toxic effects of some antivirals to the body cells, related to their inability to differentiate viral from host cells.

Today, the **antiviral drugs** are used to destroy, prevent, or delay the spread of a viral infection. A virus replicates itself in several steps. The purpose of antiviral drugs is to prevent the replication of the virus by inhibiting one of these steps, thus preventing it from reproducing. This group of drugs is effective against influenza, herpes species, and human immunodeficiency virus (HIV).

Amantadine hydrochloride (Symmetrel) has been used to treat parkinsonism and has also been found to be effective against the virus that causes influenza A. The drug is used prophylactically during epidemics and in minimizing influenza symptoms following early diagnosis. However, amantadine is *not* effective against influenza B. The drug is excreted unchanged in the urine, so adequate urinary output and renal function are essential. Dosages of amantadine might need to be decreased if renal function is impaired. Rimantadine HCl is a new antiviral drug to treat influenza A. As with amantadine HCl, the client's renal and hepatic function should be monitored.

ANTIVIRAL ANTIMETABOLITES

Before 1994, there were four antiviral antimetabolites. Today there are eight approved antiviral antimetabolites and many more that are in the experimental stages. Those that are marketed include acyclovir (Zovirax), didanosine (Videx), famciclovir (Famvir), ganciclovir (Cytovene), ribavirin (Virazole), vidarabine monohydrate (Vira-A), zalcitabine (Hivid), and zidovudine (AZT, Retrovir). The topical drugs are idoxuridine (Herplex) and trifluridine (Viroptic) and are available in ophthalmic solution and ointment.

Vidarabine was first introduced as an antineoplastic drug for the treatment of leukemia. In 1964, it was discovered that vidarabine exerts an antiviral effect against herpes simplex type I, herpes zoster, varicella zoster, and cytomegalovirus. Although it is not effective against genital herpes simplex II, vidarabine has been used effectively in treating herpes simplex viral encephalitis.

Acyclovir was introduced as an antineoplastic drug and later found to be effective against herpesvirus, especially genital herpes simplex II, but also against herpes simplex I, herpes zoster (shingles), and cytomegalovirus (which can cause congenital defects). There has been reported resistance to acyclovir due to the lack of viral-producing enzyme (thymidine kinase) needed to convert the drug to an effective antiviral compound. Figure 26–1 lists the drug data for acyclovir.

Pharmacokinetics

Acyclovir is slowly absorbed, depending on the dose, and is widely distributed to body and organ tissues. Fifty percent passes into the cerebrospinal fluid. Ten to thirty percent of the drug is protein-bound. The half-life is 2 to 3 h with normal renal function. Acyclovir is excreted unchanged in the urine.

Pharmacodynamics

Acyclovir interferes with the virus's synthesis of DNA, thereby short-circuiting its replication. The onset of action for the oral preparation is unknown and for the intravenous route is rapid. The peak concentration time is within 2 h for both routes of administration, and the duration of action for both is similar.

Probenecid can increase the effect of acyclovir. If aminoglycoside or amphotericin B is taken with acyclovir, the incidence of nephrotoxicity is increased.

The antiviral drug ribavirin was marketed in 1986. It is being used to treat respiratory syncytial virus (RSV) in children and respiratory infections caused by the influenza A and B viruses in the aged. Ribavirin is administered by aerosol.

Zidovudine, didanosine, and zalcitabine are Food and Drug Administration (FDA)–approved antiviral drugs for treating persons with acquired immunodeficiency syndrome **(AIDS)** and AIDS-related complex **(ARC)**. Zidovudine is thought to suppress the replication of the HIV virus by inhibiting the action of viral reverse transcriptase, preventing the synthesis of DNA, and allowing the T4 (helper) lymphocytes to increase initially to destroy any free virus in the system. As the disease progresses, however, these lymphocytes decrease. If zidovudine is given within 20 h after exposure to the virus, it usually prevents the lymphocytes from being infected with the virus. It is usually given to prolong the life of the person with AIDS by preventing opportunistic infections.

Didanosine (Videx) is a new approved drug prescribed for clients with advanced HIV infection and those clients who cannot tolerate zidovudine. It also can be substituted for zidovudine following 4 months of HIV treatment. Zalcitabine is administered in combination with zidovudine for treating advanced HIV infection. Table 26–1 lists the commonly used antiviral drugs, their dosages, uses, and considerations.

Side Effects and Adverse Reactions
Amantadine and Rimantadine

The side effects of and adverse reactions to amantadine include central nervous system (CNS) effects, such as insomnia, depression, anxiety, confusion, and ataxia; orthostatic hypotension; neurologic problems, such as weakness, dizziness, slurred speech; and gastrointestinal (GI) disturbances, including anorexia, nausea, vomiting, and diarrhea. Rimantadine's CNS side effects occur less often than with amantadine.

FIGURE 26–1. Antivirals

Acyclovir sodium	Dosage	NURSING PROCESS
		Assessment and Planning
Acyclovir sodium (Zovirax) Antiviral Pregnancy Category: C	A: PO: 200 mg q4h, 3–5×/d IV: 5 mg/kg q8h × 5d (diluted in D₅W) C <12 y: IV: 250 mg/m² q8h × 5d; infuse over 1 h	

Contraindications	Drug-Lab-Food Interactions	
Hypersensitivity, severe renal or hepatic disease Caution: Electrolyte imbalance, lactation	Increase nephro-neurotoxicity with aminoglycosides, probenecid, interferon Lab: May increase AST, ALT, BUN	

Pharmacokinetics	Pharmacodynamics	Interventions
Absorption: PO: Slowly absorbed Distribution: PB: 10–30% Metabolism: t½: PO: 2–3 h Excretion: 95% unchanged in urine	PO: Onset: UK Peak: 1.5–2 h Duration: 4–8 h IV: Onset: Rapid Peak: 1–2 h Duration: 4–8 h	

Therapeutic Effects/Uses: To treat herpes simplex I, genital herpes II.

Mode of Action: Interference with viral synthesis of DNA.

Evaluation

Side Effects	Adverse Reactions
Nausea, vomiting, diarrhea, headache, tremors, lethargy, rash, pruritus, increased bleeding time, phlebitis at IV site	Urticaria, anemia, gingival, hyperplasia Life-threatening: Nephrotoxicity (large doses), neuropathy, bone marrow depression, granulocytopenia, thrombocytopenia, leukopenia, seizure, acute renal failure

KEY: A: adult; C: child; PO: by mouth; IV: intravenous; <: less than; PB: protein-binding; t½: half-life.

Vidarabine, Acyclovir, and Ganciclovir

The side effects of and adverse reactions to vidarabine, ganciclovir, and acyclovir include GI disturbances (nausea, vomiting, diarrhea). With vidarabine, there might be CNS disturbances, such as weakness, malaise, tremors, and confusion. Adverse reactions can include a decrease in hemoglobin, white blood cells, and platelets; liver involvement (transient); and thrombophlebitis. With acyclovir, there might be headache, dizziness, and hematuria. Insomnia, depression, and hypotension, although infrequent, can also occur. Elevated BUN and serum creatinine levels can result from renal involvement; such involvement is usually transient.

Ganciclovir can cause thrombocytopenia and granulocytopenia. Because of the possible serious adverse reactions, this drug should be prescribed primarily for severe systemic cytomegalovirus infections for immunocompromised clients.

TABLE 26–1 Antivirals

Generic (Brand)	Route and Dosage	Uses and Considerations
General		
Amantadine HCl (Symmetrel)	*Influenza A:* A: PO: 200 mg/d in 1–2 divided doses; C 1–8 y: PO: 4.4–8.8 mg/kg/d in 2–3 divided doses; C 9–12 y: PO: 100–200 mg/d in 1–2 divided doses	Primary use is prophylaxis against influenza A. Well absorbed by the GI tract. *Pregnancy category:* C; PB: UK; t½: 24 h
Rimantadine HCl (Flumadine)	A: PO: 200 mg/d in 1 or 2 divided doses; C: PO: 5–7 mg/kg/d	For prophylaxis and treatment against influenza A virus. Drug dose is usually reduced for clients with severe hepatic or renal impairment. *Pregnancy category:* C; PB: 40%; t½: 33 h
Antimetabolites		
Acyclovir (Zovirax)	See Prototype Drug Chart (Fig. 26–1)	For treatment of herpes simplex viruses (HSV–1, HSV–2). Food does not affect oral absorption. Renal function should be monitored. *Pregnancy category:* C; PB: 10%–30%; t½: 2–3 h
Didanosine (Videx)	*HIV infections:* A >75 kg: PO: 300 mg q12h; 50–75 kg: 200 mg q12h; 35–50 kg: 125 mg q12h; C: PO: tab: 1.1–1.4 m². 100 mg b.i.d. Pedi Powder: 0.8–1 m²: 75 mg q12h; 0.5–0.7 m²: 50 mg q12h; <0.4 m²: 25 mg q12h	Used for advanced HIV infection especially if intolerant to zidovudine (AZT). Take with water 30 min to 1 h before meals. *Pregnancy category:* B; PB: UK; t½: 1.5 h
Famiciclovir (Famvir)	*Herpes zoster:* A: PO: 500 mg q8h × 7 d	For treatment of herpes zoster. *Pregnancy category:* C; PB: UK; t½: UK
Ganciclovir sodium (Cytovene)	A&C: IV: Initially: 5 mg/kg q12h × 14–21 d; maint: 5 mg/kg/d × 7d or 6 mg/kg/d × 5 d	For treatment of cytomegalovirus (CMV) systemic infection in immunocompromised clients. *Pregnancy category:* C; PB: 1%–2%; t½: 2.5–6 h
Ribavirin (Virazole)	A&C: By aerosol inhalation administration	For respiratory syncytial viral infection in infants and children. *Pregnancy category:* X; PB: NA; t½: 24 h
Vidarabine monohydrate (Vira-A)	A: IV: 10–15 mg/kg/d infused over 12–24 h	Effective against serious herpes simplex 1 (HSV–1), herpes zoster, and varicella zoster. *Pregnancy category:* C; PB; 20%–30%; t½: 1.5–3 h
Zalcitabine (Hivid)	*HIV infections:* A: PO: 0.75 mg q8h given with zidovudine 200 mg q8h	To treat advanced HIV infection. May be used in combination with zidovudine. Dose is reduced if creatinine clearance is <40 mL/min. *Pregnancy category:* C; PB: <4%; t½: 1.2–2 h
Zidovudine (Retrovir)	A: PO: 100–200 mg q4h; IV: 1–2 mg/kg q4h; max: 1,200 mg/d; C: PO: 90–180 mg/m² q6h; max: 200 mg q6h	For AIDS and ARC treatment. Blood count should be monitored for leukopenia and anemia. *Pregnancy category:* C; PB: 25%–38%; t½: 1 h

KEY: A: adult; C: child; IV: intravenous; m²: body surface area; PB: protein-binding; PO: by mouth; t½: half-life; <: less than; >: more than.

NURSING PROCESS: ANTIVIRALS

ASSESSMENT

- Obtain a medical history of any serious renal or hepatic disease.
- Obtain baseline vital signs (VS) and a complete blood count. Use these findings for comparison with future results.
- Assess baseline laboratory results, particularly BUN, serum creatinine, liver enzymes, bilirubin, and electrolytes. Use these results for future comparisons.
- Assess baseline VS and urine output. Report abnormal findings.

POTENTIAL NURSING DIAGNOSES

- High risk of infection
- High risk for impaired tissue integrity

PLANNING

- Symptoms of viral infections will be eliminated or diminished.

NURSING INTERVENTIONS

- Monitor the client's complete blood count (CBC). Report abnormal results, such as leukopenia, thrombocytopenia, and low hemoglobin and hematocrit.
- Monitor other laboratory tests, such as BUN, serum creatinine, and liver enzymes, and compare with baseline values.
- Monitor the client's urinary output. An antiviral drug such as acyclovir can affect renal function.
- Monitor VS, especially blood pressure. Acyclovir and amantadine may cause orthostatic hypotension.
- Observe for signs and symptoms of side effects. Most antiviral drugs have many side effects; see Prototype Drug Chart (Fig. 26–1).
- Check for superimposed infection (superinfection) due to high dose and prolonged use of an antiviral drug such as acyclovir.

- Administer oral acyclovir as prescribed. Oral dose can be taken at mealtime.
- For IV use, dilute the antiviral drug in an appropriate amount of solution as indicated in the drug circular. Administer the IV drug over 60 min. *Never* give acyclovir as a bolus (IV push).

CLIENT TEACHING

General

- Advise the client to maintain an adequate fluid intake to ensure sufficient hydration for drug therapy and to increase urine output.
- Instruct the client with genital herpes to avoid spreading the infection by sexual abstinence or the use of a condom. Advise these women to have a Pap test done every 6 mon or as indicated by the health care provider. Cervical cancer is more prevalent in women with genital herpes simplex.
- Instruct clients taking zidovudine to have blood cell count monitored.

Side Effects

- Instruct the client to perform oral hygiene several times a day. Gingival hyperplasia (red, swollen gums) can occur with prolonged use of antiviral drugs.
- Instruct the client to report adverse reactions, including decrease in urine output and CNS changes such as dizziness, anxiety, or confusion.
- Advise the client with dizziness due to orthostatic hypotension to arise slowly from a sitting to a standing position.
- Instruct the client to report any side effects associated with the antiviral drug, such as nausea, vomiting, diarrhea, increased bleeding time, rash, urticaria, or menstrual abnormalities.

EVALUATION

- Evaluate the effectiveness of the antiviral drug in eliminating the virus or in decreasing symptoms.
- Determine if side effects are absent.

ANTIMALARIAL DRUGS

Malaria, caused by the protozoan parasites *Plasmodium* spp. that is carried by an infected *Anopheles* mosquito, is still one of the most prevalent protozoan diseases. After the infected mosquito bites the human, the protozoan parasite passes through two phases, the tissue phase and the erythrocytic phase. The **tissue phase** produces no clinical symptoms in the human, but the **erythrocytic phase** (invasion of the red blood cells) causes symptoms of chills, fever, and sweating.

Treatment of malaria depends on the type of Plasmodium and the organism's life cycle. Quinine was the only antimalarial drug available from 1820 until the early 1940s. Synthetic **antimalarial drugs** have since been developed that are as effective as quinine and cause fewer toxic effects. When drug-resistant malaria occurs, combinations of antimalarials are used to facilitate effective treatment. Many of the synthetic antimalarials, such as chloroquine, primaquine, and pyrimethamine-sulfadoxine are used prophylactically. The prototype drug (chloroquine HCl) of the antimalarial drug group is displayed in Figure 26–2.

PHARMACOKINETICS

Chloroquine HCl is well absorbed from the GI tract. It is moderately protein-binding, and the drug has a long half-life. The first two doses have a loading dose effect. Because of the long half-life, the next dose is given on the second day, and the fourth dose is given on the third day. Chloroquine is metabolized in the liver to active metabolites and excreted in the urine.

PHARMACODYNAMICS

Chloroquine HCl inhibits the malaria parasite's growth by interferring with its protein synthesis. Whether the drug is taken orally or given intramuscularly, the onset of action is rapid. The peak effect is slower when given orally. The duration of effect of the drug is very long—days to weeks.

Table 26–2 lists commonly ordered antimalarial drugs, their dosage, uses, and considerations. (*Note:* Quinine and quinidine are *not* the same drug. Quinine is an antimalarial drug and quinidine is an antidysrhythmic drug).

SIDE EFFECTS AND ADVERSE REACTIONS

General side effects of and adverse reactions to antimalarials include GI upset, eighth cranial nerve involvement (quinine and chloroquine), renal impairment (quinine), and cardiovascular effects (quinine).

TABLE 26–2 Antimalarials

Generic (Brand)	Route and Dosage	Uses and Considerations
Chloroquine HCl (Aralen HCl)	*Acute malaria:* A: PO: 600 mg base/dose; then 6 h later: 300 mg/dose; then at 24 and 48 h: 300 mg/dose IM: 200 mg/base q6h PRN C: PO: 10 mg base/kg/dose, then 6 h later: 5 mg base/kg/dose; 24–48 h later: 5 mg base/kg/dose. IM: 5 mg base/kg q12h *Prophylaxis:* 2 wk before and 6–8 wk after exposure A&C: PO: 5 mg/kg/wk; *max:* 300 mg base/wk	Treatment of acute malaria. For prophylactic use, the drug should be taken 2 weeks prior to possible exposure and after the return visit. Chloroquine is considered to be the drug of choice; however, it can be combined with primaquine. *Pregnancy category:* C; PB: 50%–65%; t½: 2.5–5 d
Hydroxychloroquine SO₄ (Plaquenil SO₄)	*Acute malaria:* A: PO: 800 mg/dose; 6 h later: 400 mg; then 400 mg daily for 2 d C: PO: 10 mg base/kg/dose, 6 h: 5 mg base/kg; 5 mg base/kg daily for 2 d *Prophylaxis:* 1 wk before and 6–8 wk after exposure A&C: PO: 5 mg base/kg/wk; max: 300 mg base/wk	Alternative to chloroquine. Dosage varies for treating malaria. Can be used adjunctively with primaquine. Give drug with meals to reduce the occurrence of GI distress. *Pregnancy category:* C; PB: 55% t½: 2.5–5 d

Table continued on page 393

FIGURE 26–2. Antimalarials: Chloroquine HCl

Antimalarial	Dosage	NURSING PROCESS
		Assessment and Planning

Antimalarial

Chloroquine HCl
  (Aralen HCl)
Pregnancy Category: C

Dosage

Acute Malaria:
A: PO: 600 mg base/dose; then 6 h
  later: 300 mg/dose; then at 24 and
  48 h: 300 mg/dose
  IM: 200 mg/base q6h, PRN
C: PO: 10 mg base/kg/dose, then 6 h
  later: 5 mg base/kg/dose; then 5 mg
  base/kg/d for 2 d
IM: 5 mg base/kg q12h
Prophylaxis:
2 wk before and 6–8 wk after exposure
A&C: PO: 5 mg/kg/wk; max: 300 mg
  base/wk

NURSING PROCESS
Assessment and Planning

Contraindications

Hypersensitivity to 4-aminoquinolones,
  renal disease, psoriasis, retinal
  changes
Caution: Alcoholism; liver dysfunction;
  G-6-PD deficiency; GI, neurologic,
  and hematologic disorders

Drug-Lab-Food Interactions

Increase effects of digoxin, anticoagulants, neuromuscular blocker
Decrease absorption with antacids and
  laxatives
Lab: *Decrease* red blood cell (RBC)
  count, hemoglobin, hematocrit

Pharmacokinetics

Absorption: well absorbed from GI tract
Distribution: PB: 50–65%
Metabolism: t½: 1–2 months
Excretion: excreted slowly in urine

Pharmacodynamics

PO: Onset: rapid
  Peak: 3.5 h
  Duration: days to weeks
IM: Onset: Rapid
  Peak: 0.5 h
  Duration: days to weeks

Interventions

Therapeutic Effects/Uses: To treat acute malaria and for prophylaxis.

Mode of Action: Increased pH in the malaria parasite inhibits parasitic growth.

Evaluation

Side Effects

Anorexia, nausea, vomiting, diarrhea,
  abdominal cramps, fatigue, pruritus,
  nervousness, visual disturbances
  (blurred vision)

Adverse Reactions

ECG changes, hypotension, psychosis
Life-threatening: Agranulocytosis, aplastic anemia, thrombocytopenia, ototoxicity, cardiovascular collapse

KEY: A: adult; C: child; PO: by mouth; IM: intramuscular; PB: protein-binding; t½: half-life.

TABLE 26–2 Antimalarials *(Continued)*

Generic (Brand)	Route and Dosage	Uses and Considerations
Mefloquine HCl (Lariam)	A: PO: Single dose: 1,250 mg; then 250 mg qwk × 4 wk	New antimalarial drug. Action is similar to chloroquine HCl. *Pregnancy category:* C; PB: 98%; t½: 21 d
Primaquine phosphate	*Malaria prophylaxis:* A: PO: 15 mg/d for 14 d (single doses) C: PO: 0.3 mg/kg/d for 14 d (single doses)	Prophylaxis against certain *Plasmodium* spp. (*P. vivax* and *P. ovale*) and for relapse. Can affect white blood cell production (granulocytopenia). *Pregnancy category:* C; PB: UK; t½: 3.7–9.6 h
Pyrimethamine (Daraprim)	*Malaria prophylaxis:* A&C: > 10 y: PO: 25 mg/wk C <4 y: PO: 6.25 mg/wk C 4–10 y: PO: 12.5 mg/wk	Prophylaxis use for malaria. For treatment of chloroquine-resistant *Plasmodium falciparum* infections. May be used with quinacrine, quinine, or chloroquine. *Pregnancy category:* C; PB: 80%; t½: 1.5–2 d
Quinacrine HCl (Atabrine HCl)	*Malaria supression:* A: PO: 100 mg/d C: PO: 50 mg/d	For treating *Plasmodium malariae* and *Plasmodium vivax* infections. *Pregnancy category:* C; PB: UK; t½: UK
Quinine SO₄ (Quin-260, Quiphile)	*Acute malaria:* A: PO: 650 mg q8h for 3–7 d C: PO: 25 mg/kg/d in 3 divided doses (q8h) for 3–7 d	Used in combination drug therapy or for chloroquine-resistant malaria. Used to treat nocturnal leg cramps. *Pregnancy category:* X; PB: 70%–95%; t½: 6–14 h

KEY: *A: adult; C: child; PB: protein-binding; PO: by mouth; IM: intramuscular; t½: half-life; UK: unknown; >: greater than; <: less than.*

NURSING PROCESS: ANTIMALARIAL DRUGS

ASSESSMENT

- Assess the client's hearing, especially if taking quinine or chloroquine. These drugs may affect the eighth cranial nerve.
- Assess the client for visual changes. Clients on chloroquine and hydroxychloroquine should have frequent ophthalmic examinations.

POTENTIAL NURSING DIAGNOSES

- High risk of infection
- High risk for impaired tissue integrity

PLANNING

- Client will be free of malarial symptoms.

NURSING INTERVENTIONS

- Monitor the client's urinary output and liver function by checking the urine output (>600 mL/day) and the liver enzymes. Antimalarial drugs concentrate first in the liver; serum liver enzyme levels should be checked especially if the person drinks considerable amounts of alcohol or has a liver disorder.
- Report if the client's serum liver enzymes are elevated.

CLIENT TEACHING

- Advise clients traveling to malaria-infested countries to receive prophylactic doses of antimalarial drug prior to leaving, during the visit, and upon return.
- Instruct the client to take oral antimalarial drugs with food or at mealtime if GI upset occurs.
- Monitor the client returning from a malaria-infested area for malarial symptoms.
- Instruct the client on chloroquine or hydroxychloroquine to report vision changes immediately.
- Avoid consuming large quantities of alcohol.

EVALUATION

- Evaluate the effectiveness of the antimalarial drug by determining that the client is free of symptoms.

TABLE 26–3 Anthelmintic Drugs

Drug	Dosage	Uses and Considerations
Diethylcarbamazine (Hetrazan)	A: PO: 2–3 mg/kg/t.i.d.	Treatment for nematode–filariae
Mebendazole (Vermox)	A: PO: 100 mg b.i.d. × 3 d Repeat in 2–3 wks if necessary C >2y: PO: same as adult	Treatment for giant roundworm, hookworm, pinworm, whipworm. *Pregnancy category:* C
Niclosamide (Niclocide)	A: PO: 2 g, single dose C >34 kg: PO: 1.5 g, single dose C 11–34 kg: PO: 1 g, single dose A: PO: 2 g/d × 1 wk C >34 kg: PO: 1.5 g, single dose, then 1 g/d × 6 days	Treatment for beef and fish tapeworms. *Pregnancy category:* B Treatment of dwarf tapeworms.
Oxamniquine (Vansil)	A: PO: 15 mg/kg/b.i.d. for 1–2 d C: PO: 10–15 mg/kg/b.i.d. for 1–2 d	Treatment against mature and immature worms. *Pregnancy category:* C

Piperazine citrate (Antepar, Vermizine)	*Roundworm:*
	A: PO: 3.5 g/d × 2 d
	C: PO: 75 mg/kg/d × 2 d
	  max: 3.5 g/d
	Pinworms:
	A&C: 65 mg/kg/d × 7 d
	  max: 2.5 g/d
		Treatment of roundworms and pinworms. *Pregnancy category:* B

Praziquantel (Biltricide)	A&C: PO: 10–20 mg/kg single dose A&C: PO: 20 mg/kg, t.i.d., × 1 d A&C: 25 mg/kg, t.i.d., 1–2 d	Treatment for beef, pork, fish tapeworms. Treatment for blood flukes. Treatment for liver, lung, and intestinal flukes. *Pregnancy category:* B; PB: UK; t½: 0.8–1.5 h
Pyrantel pamoate (Antiminth)	A&C: PO: 11 mg/kg single dose Repeat in 2 wks if necessary	Treatment of giant roundworm, hookworm, pinworm. *Pregnancy category:* C
Thiabendazole (Mintezol, Minzolum)	A&C: PO: 25 mg/kg, for 2–5 d Repeat in 2 d if necessary	Treatment of threadworm and pork worm. *Pregnancy category:* C

KEY: A: adult; C: child; PB: protein-binding; PO: by mouth; t½: half-life; UK: unknown; >: greater than; <: less than.

ANTHELMINTIC DRUGS

Helminths are large organisms (parasitic worms) that feed on host tissue. The most common site for **helminthiasis** (worm infestation) is the intestine. Other sites for parasitic infestation are the lymphatic system, blood vessels, and liver.

There are four groups of helminths: (1) cestodes (tapeworms), (2) trematodes (flukes), (3) nematodes intestine (roundworms), and (4) nematodes tissue invading (tissue roundworms and filariae). The cestodes (tapeworms) are segmented and enter the intestine via contaminated food. There are four species of cestodes: *Taenia solium* (pork tapeworm), *Taenia saginata* (beef tapeworm), *Diphyllobothrium latum* (fish tapeworm), and *Hymenolepis nana* (dwarf tapeworm). The segmented cestodes have heads and have hooks or suckers that attach to the tissue.

The trematodes (flukes) are flat, nonsegmented parasites that feed on the host. Four types of trematodes exist: *Fasciola hepatica* (liver fluke), *Fasciolopsis buski* (intestinal fluke), *Paragonimus wester-* *mani* (lung fluke), and *Schistosoma* species (blood fluke). Five types of nematodes may feed on the intestinal tissue; these include *Ascaris lumbricoides* (giant roundworm), *Necator americanus* (hookworm), *Enterobius vermicularis* (pinworm), *Stronglyloides stercolaris* (threadworm), and *Trichuris trichiura* (whipworm). Two types of nematodes that are tissue invading include *Trichinella spiralis* (pork roundworm), and *Wuchereria bancrofti* (filariae). The pork roundworm or *Trichinella spiralis* can cause **trichinosis,** which can be diagnosed by a muscle biopsy. By thoroughly cooking pork, the roundworm, if present, is destroyed.

Table 26–3 lists eight anthelmintic drugs that are prescribed to treat various types of parasitic worms.

SIDE EFFECTS AND ADVERSE REACTIONS

The common side effects of anthelmintics include GI upset such as anorexia, nausea, vomiting, and occasionally diarrhea and stomach cramps. The neurologic problems associated with anthelmintics are dizziness, weakness, headache, and drowsiness. Adverse reactions do not occur frequently because the drugs are usually given only for a short period of time (1 to 3 days), except for niclosamide for treatment of dwarf tapeworms, piperazine for treatment of pinworms, and thiabendazole for treatment of threadworms and pork worms. Thiabendazole should be avoided if the client has liver disease.

NURSING PROCESS: ANTHELMINTICS

ASSESSMENT

- Obtain a history of foods the client has eaten, especially meat and fish, and how the food was prepared.
- Note if any other person in the household has been checked for helminths (worms).
- Assess baseline vital signs (VS) and collect a stool specimen.

POTENTIAL NURSING DIAGNOSES

- Altered comfort related to GI symptoms
- Activity intolerance related to dizziness, headache, drowsiness

PLANNING

- The client will be free of helminths.
- The client will understand how to prepare foods properly to avoid reoccurrence of helminths.

NURSING INTERVENTIONS

- Collect a stool specimen in a clean container. Avoid having the stool come in contact with water, urine, or chemicals, which could destroy the presence of parasitic worms.
- Administer the prescribed anthelmintics after meals to prevent or minimize the occurrence of GI distress.

- Report to the health care provider if the client is having any side effects.

- Explain to the client the importance of washing hands before eating and after going to the toilet. The parasite can be transferred within the family due to poor hygiene.
- Instruct the client to take daily showers and *not* baths.
- Instruct the client to change sheets, bedclothes, towels, and underwear daily.
- Explain to the client that if the problem persists after therapy, a second course of anthelmintics may be necessary.
- Emphasize the importance of taking the prescribed drug at designated times and to keep health care appointments.
- Alert the client that drowsiness may occur and that he or she should avoid operating a car or machinery if drowsiness occurs.
- Instruct the client to report any side effects to the health care provider.

EVALUATION

- Evaluate the effect of the anthelmintics and the absence of side effects.
- Determine if the client is using proper hygiene to avoid spread of parasitic worms.

STUDY QUESTIONS

1. Amantadine is an antiviral drug. For what other disease is this drug used? What are some side effects of and adverse reactions to amantadine?
2. Vidarabine and acyclovir are antiviral antimetabolites. How are these drugs similar and how do they differ in their uses?
3. What three antiviral drugs may be prescribed for advanced HIV infection?
4. Your client is to receive chloroquine as a prophylactic against malaria. How does chloroquine act to prevent malaria? What is the schedule for administration when it is used prophylactically? Discuss the significance of chloroquine HCl's protein-binding and half-life.

5. The client's hematology tests should be monitored while the client is taking chloroquine HCl. Why?
6. Concerning the use of antimalarials, what should be included in client teaching?
7. What are helminths? Most types of helminths are concentrated in what part of the body?
8. Trichinosis is caused by what organism? How can this health problem be prevented? How is it diagnosed?
9. What client teaching instructions should be included for a client diagnosed as having helminths?

Chapter 27

Drugs for Urinary Tract Disorders

OUTLINE

Objectives
Terms
Introduction
Urinary Antiseptics/Antiinfec-
  tives and Antibiotics
    Nitrofurantoin

Methenamine
Trimethoprim
Fluoroquinolones
  (Quinolones)
    Nursing Process
Urinary Analgesics

Phenazopyridine
  Nursing Process
Urinary Stimulants
Urinary Antispasmodics
Study Questions

OBJECTIVES

Identify the groups of drugs that are urinary antiseptics and antiinfectives.

Describe the side effects of and adverse reactions to urinary antiseptics and antiinfectives.

Give uses for a urinary analgesic, a urinary stimulant, and a urinary antispasmodic.

Describe the nursing process, including client teaching, regarding urinary antiseptic/antiinfective drugs and urinary analgesics.

TERMS

bacteriostatic
bactericidal
micturition

urinary analgesics
urinary antiseptics/antiin-
  fectives

urinary antispasmodics
urinary stimulants
urinary tract infection (UTI)

INTRODUCTION

The largest number of urinary tract disorders are due to **urinary tract infections (UTIs).** UTIs may result from an upper urinary tract infection, such as pyelonephritis, or from a lower urinary tract infection, such as cystitis or prostatitis. A group of drugs called **urinary antiseptics/antiinfectives** prevent bacterial growth in the kidneys and bladder but are not effective for systemic infections. Urinary antiseptics/antiinfectives have a bacteriostatic effect when given in lower dosages. They also have a bactericidal effect when given in higher dosages.

Urinary antiseptics/antiinfectives, urinary stimulants, urinary antispasmodics, and urinary analgesics are presented in this chapter. Antibacterials/antibiotics and sulfonamides that are used in treating urinary tract infections are discussed in Chapters 22, 23, and 24. Diuretics are discussed in Chapter 33.

Cystitis, a lower UTI frequently occurring in females because of their shorter (compared with the male) urethra, is commonly caused by *Escherichia coli (E. coli).* Symptoms include pain and burning on urination, and urinary frequency and urgency. A urine culture is taken prior to the start of any antiinfective/antibiotic drug therapy. In males, a lower UTI is most likely to be prostatitis with symptoms similar to cystitis.

URINARY ANTISEPTICS/ ANTIINFECTIVES AND ANTIBIOTICS

Urinary antiseptics/antiinfectives are limited to the treatment of UTIs. The drug action occurs in the renal tubule and bladder, and thus is effective in reducing bacterial growth. A urinalysis and culture and sensitivity test are usually performed prior to the initiation of drug therapy. The groups of urinary antiseptics/antiinfectives are nitrofurantoin, methenamine, trimethoprim, and the fluoroquinolones.

NITROFURANTOIN

Nitrofurantoin (Furolan, Macrodantin) was first prescribed for UTI in 1953. Nitrofurantoin is bacteriostatic or bactericidal, depending on drug dosage, and is effective against many gram-positive and gram-negative organisms, especially *E. coli.* It is used in the treatment of acute and chronic UTIs. The drug data for nitrofurantoin are given in Figure 27–1.

Pharmacokinetics

Nitrofurantoin is well absorbed from the gastrointestinal (GI) tract. The drug is usually taken with food to decrease GI distress. Decreased absorption occurs when the drug is taken with antacids. Nitrofurantoin is moderately protein-bound. With normal renal function, the drug is rapidly eliminated because of a short half-life of 20 minutes; however, it accumulates in the serum with urinary dysfunction.

Pharmacodynamics

When nitrofurantoin is given in low doses for prophylactic use, the drug has a bacteriostatic effect. High concentration of nitrofurantoin causes a bactericidal effect. Nitrofurantoin is effective against many gram-positive and gram-negative organisms such as *E. Coli, Neisseria,* streptococci, *Staphylococcus aureus,* and others. It is not as effective against *Pseudomonas aeruginosa, Proteus* species, and some species of *Klebsiella.* The onset and duration of action are unknown. Peak action occurs one-half hour after absorption. If the client develops sudden onset of dyspnea, chest pain, cough, fever, and chills, the client should contact the health care provider. Symptoms resolve after discontinuing the drug.

METHENAMINE

Methenamine (Mandelamine, Hiprex) produces a bactericidal effect when the urine pH is less than 5.5. It is available as mandelate salt (short-acting) and as hippurate salt. Methenamine is effective against gram-positive and gram-negative organisms, especially *E. coli* and *P. aeruginosa.* It is used for chronic UTIs. Methenamine should not be taken with sulfonamides because crystalluria would likely occur. It is absorbed readily from the GI tract, and approximately 90% of the drug is excreted unchanged. Methenamine forms ammonia and formaldehyde in acid urine; therefore, the urine needs to be acidified to exert a bactericidal action. Cranberry juice (several eight-ounce glasses per day), ascorbic acid, and ammonium chloride can be taken to decrease the urine pH.

TRIMETHOPRIM

Trimethoprim (Proloprim, Trimpex) can be used alone (although frequently it is not) for the treatment of UTIs or in combination with a sulfonamide, sulfamethoxazole (the combined preparation is generically referred to as co-trimoxazole), to prevent the occurrence of trimethoprim-resistant organisms. It produces slow-acting bactericidal effects against most gram-positive and gram-negative

FIGURE 27–1. Urinary Antiinfectives

Antiinfective	Dosage	NURSING PROCESS Assessment and Planning
Nitrofurantoin (Furalan, Furan, Macrodantin), 🍁 Apo-nitrofurantoin, Novofuran *Pregnancy Category:* B	*Initial/Recurrent UTI:* A: PO: 50–100 mg q.i.d. with meals and h.s.; take with food C: PO: >1 mo: 5–7 mg/kg in 4 divided doses *Long-term Prophylaxis:* A: PO: 50–100 mg h.s. A: PO: 1–2 mg/kg in 1–2 divided doses	

Contraindications	Drug-Lab-Food Interactions	
Hypersensitivity moderate to severe renal impairment, oliguria, anuria, $Cl_{cr} < 40$ mL/min, infants <1 mo, term pregnancy, lactation with infant suspected of having G-6-PD deficiency *Caution:* Vitamin B deficiency, electrolyte imbalance, diabetes mellitus	*Decrease* effect with probenecid; *decrease* absorption with antacids	

Pharmacokinetics	Pharmacodynamics	Interventions
Absorption: Well absorbed from GI tract; enhanced with food *Distribution:* PB: 60%, crosses placenta and enters breast milk *Metabolism:* t½: 20–60 min *Excretion:* In urine; small amounts in bile	PO: Onset: UK Peak: 30 min Duration: UK	

	Evaluation
Therapeutic Effects/Uses: To treat acute and chronic UTIs. *Mode of Action:* Inhibits bacterial enzymes and metabolism.	

Side Effects	Adverse Reactions
Anorexia, nausea, vomiting, rust/brown discoloration of urine, diarrhea, rash, pruritus, dizziness, headache, drowsiness	Superinfection, peripheral neuropathy, hemolytic anemia, agranulocytosis *Life-threatening:* Anaphylaxis, hepatotoxicity, Stevens-Johnson syndrome

KEY: A: adult; C: child; PO: by mouth; UK: unknown; PB: protein-binding; t½: half-life; >: greater than; <: less than; Cl_{cr}: creatinine clearance; 🍁: Canadian drug names.

TABLE 27–1 Antiseptics and Urinary Antiinfectives

Generic (Brand)	Route and Dosage	Uses and Considerations
Methenamine mandelate (Mandelamine, Mandameth)	A: PO: 1 g q.i.d. p.c. C 6–12 y: PO: 0.5 g q.i.d. p.c. C <6 y: PO: 50 mg/kg in 4 divided doses p.c.	For chronic UTIs. Urine pH should be acidic (<5.5). It should not be used with sulfonamides. May cause crystalluria, so push fluids. It can cause GI irritation, so take the drug with meals. *Pregnancy category:* C; PB: UK; t½: 3–6 h
Methenamine hippurate (Hiprex, Urex)	A: PO: 1 g b.i.d. C 6–12 y: 0.5–1 g b.i.d.	Same as above
Nitrofurantoin (Furalan, Macrodantin, Nitrofan)	See Prototype Drug Chart (Fig. 27–1)	For acute and chronic UTIs. A normal creatinine clearance assures the effectiveness of the drug. Peripheral neuropathy is an adverse effect. It may cause GI irritation. Taking with food decreases GI upset. *Pregnancy category:* B; PB: 40%; t½: 20–60 min
Trimethoprim (Proloprim, Trimpex)	A: PO: 100 mg q12h or 200 mg q24h; if Cl_{cr} (CrCl) is 15–30 mL/min: 50 mg q12h; if Cl_{cr} <15 mL/min: do not use	For prevention and treatment of acute and chronic UTIs in both males and females. High doses can cause GI upset. Drug can be combined with sulfamethoxazole (Bactrim). *Pregnancy category:* C; PB:
Quinolones (Fluoro-quinolones) Cinoxacin (Cinobac)	A: PO: 1 g/d in 2–4 doses for 1–2 wk; *Renal dysfunction:* Initially: 500 mg; if Cl_{cr} is >80 mL/min: 500 mg b.i.d.; 80–50 mL/min: 250 mg t.i.d.; 50–20 mL/min: 250 mg b.i.d.; <20 mL/min: 250 mg q.d. Not recommended for infants or prepubertal children	For acute and chronic UTIs. More effective than nalidixic acid. Absorbed in prostatic tissue. Can cause dizziness and photosensitivity. Avoid excessive exposure to sunlight. *Pregnancy category:* C; PB: 60%–80%; t½: 1.5 h
Ciprofloxacin (Cipro)	A: PO: mild to moderate: 250 mg q12h; severe/complicated: 250–500 mg q12h *Renal dysfunction:* If Cl_{cr} >50 mL/min (PO), >30 mL/min (IV): Usual dose 30–50 mL/min: 250–500 mg q12h 5–29 mL/min: 250–500 mg q18h (PO); 200–400 mg q18–24h (IV) *Hemo or peritoneal dialysis:* 250–500 mg q24h after dialysis	Has a broad-spectrum antibacterial effect. For UTI, skin and soft tissue infections, and bone and joint infections. Antacid inhibits drug absorption. Use with caution in clients with seizure disorders. Can be taken without food. Photosensitivity can occur. Avoid excessive exposure to sunlight. *Pregnancy category:* C; PB: 20%–40%; t½: 4–6 h
Enoxacin (Penetrex)	*Uncomplicated UTI:* A: PO: 200 mg q12h for 7 d *Complicated or severe UTI:* A: PO: 400 mg q12h for 14 d If Cl_{cr} <30 mL/min, reduce dose by 50%	Effective against complicated and uncomplicated UTIs. Fluid intake should be increased. Take before or after meals. Phototoxicity may occur. *Pregnancy category:* C (pregnant: X); PB: UK; t½: 3–6 h
Lomefloxacin (Maxaquin)	A: PO: 400 mg/d × 10 d	For UTIs and transurethral surgery prophylaxis. *Pregnancy category:* C; PB: UK; t½: 6.25–7.75 h
Nalidixic acid (NegGram)	A: PO: 1 g q.i.d. for 1–2 wk; 1 g b.i.d. for long-term use C: PO: 55 mg/kg/d in 4 divided doses for 1–2 wk; 33 mg/kg/d for long-term use C: <3 mo: Do not use	For acute and chronic UTIs. Resistance to drug may occur. Highly protein-bound. Not distributed in prostatic fluid. Take with food to avoid GI upset. Photosensitivity can occur. Avoid excessive exposure to sunlight. Contact health care provider if seizures or severe headaches occur. *Pregnancy category:* B; PB: 93%; t½: 1–2 h (elderly: 12 h)
Norfloxacin (Noroxin)	A: PO: 400 mg b.i.d. for 1–2 wk on empty stomach *Uncomplicated cystitis due to* E. coli, K. pneumoniae, P. mirabilis: 400 mg b.i.d. × 3d *Uncomplicated due to any other organism:* 400 mg b.i.d. × 7–10d *Complicated:* 400 mg b.i.d. × 10–21d *Renal impairment (Cl_{cr} <30 mL/min):* 400 mg q.d.	For acute and chronic UTIs. Most potent drug of the quinolone group. Food may inhibit drug absorption. *Pregnancy category:* C; PB: 10%–15%; t½: 3–4 h

Table continued on following page

TABLE 27–1 Antiseptics and Urinary Antiinfectives *(Continued)*

Generic (Brand)	Route and Dosage	Uses and Considerations
Ofloxacin (Floxin)	A: PO: IV: 200 mg q12h × 10 d	For UTIs, respiratory tract and skin infections. May cause headaches, dizziness, insomnia. *Pregnancy category:* C; PB: 20%–32%; t½: 5–7.5 h
Other Aztreonam (Azactam)	A: IM/IV: 500 mg–1 g q8–12h	Treatment of UTIs caused by gram-negative organisms. Also useful for low respiratory infection, septicemia. *Pregnancy category:* B; PB: 56%–60%; t½: 1.5–2 h
Imipenem/cilastatin sodium (Primaxin)	A: IV: 250 mg–1 g q6h max: 4 g/d or 50 mg/kg/d, whichever is the lesser amount C: Safety and efficacy not established Dosing adjustment with renal impairment	Treatment of serious UTIs. Also useful for lower respiratory, bone, and joint infections; and septicemia and endocarditis. *Pregnancy category:* C; PB: 20%–40%; t½: 1 h
Methylene blue (Urolene Blue)	*Cystitis, urethritis:* A: PO: 60–125 mg b.i.d./t.i.d. p.c. with glass of water	For urinary calculi. Urine, sweat, and/or stool may be blue-green due to the dye in the drug. *Pregnancy category:* C; PB: UK; t½: UK
Co-trimoxazole or sulfamethoxazole-trimethoprim (Bactrim, Septra)	See sulfonamides, Chapter 24 (Fig. 24–1)	Effective for serious UTIs. Useful for otitis media. See Chapter 24. *Pregnancy category:* C; PB: 60%–70%; t½: 9 h
Polymyxin B SO₄ (Aerosporin)	A&C: IV: 15,000–25,000 U/kg/d in divided doses q12h	Effective for UTIs and to prevent bacteruria occurring from indwelling catheter. Can cause nephrotoxicity. Monitor renal function (BUN, serum creatinine). *Pregnancy category:* B; PB: UK; t½: 4–6 h

KEY: *A: adult; C: child; PO: by mouth; IM: intramuscular; IV: intravenous; UK: unknown, Cl_{cr}: creatinine clearance; >: greater than; <: less than; PB: protein-binding; t½: half-life.*

organisms. Trimethoprim is used in the treatment and prevention of acute and chronic UTIs. The amount of trimethoprim in the prostatic fluid is about two to three times greater than the amount in the vascular fluid. The half-life of trimethoprim is normally 9 to 11 h; the half-life is longer with renal dysfunction.

FLUOROQUINOLONES (QUINOLONES)

Fluoroquinolones are one of the newest groups of urinary antiseptics and are effective against lower UTIs. Nalidixic acid (NegGram) was developed in 1964, and cinoxacin (Cinobac), norfloxacin (Noroxin), and ciprofloxacin hydrochloride (Cipro) were marketed in the 1980s. Enoxacin was marketed in the late 1980s or early 1990s; ofloxacin in 1990; and lomefloxacin in 1992. The newer fluoroquinolones (norfloxacin, ciprofloxacin, enoxacin, ofloxacin, and lomefloxacin) are effective against a wide variety of UTIs. Drug dosage should be decreased when renal dysfunction is present. The half-lives of these drugs are 2 to 4 h but are prolonged with renal dysfunction. Table 27–1 lists the urinary antiseptics/antiinfectives, their dosages, uses, and considerations.

Side Effects and Adverse Reactions

The side effects of and adverse reactions to urinary antiseptics are listed below by category.

Nitrofurantoin

Side effects of nitrofurantoin use include GI disturbances such as anorexia, nausea, vomiting, diarrhea, and abdominal pain, and pulmonary reactions such as dyspnea, chest pain, fever, and cough.

Methenamine

Methenamine use also has GI side effects, including nausea, vomiting, and diarrhea. There are some allergic reactions to the dye in Hiprex. Bladder irritation and crystalluria (with large doses) may occur.

Trimethoprim

GI symptoms, including nausea and vomiting and skin problems, such as rash and pruritus, can accompany trimethoprim use.

Fluoroquinolones

Nalidixic acid use can have the following side effects: headaches, dizziness, syncope (fainting), peripheral neuritis, visual disturbances, and rash. Nausea, vomiting, diarrhea, headaches, and visual disturbances can occur with cinoxacin and norfloxacin use. Photosensitivity is a common side effect associated with fluoroquinolones.

Drug-Drug Interactions

The following drug-drug interactions can occur.

1. Nalidixic acid enhances the effects of warfarin

2. Antacids decrease nitrofurantoin absorption.
3. Most urinary antiseptics cause false-positive Clinitest results.
4. Sodium bicarbonate inhibits the action of methenamine.
5. Methenamine taken with sulfonamides increases the risk of crystalluria.

The nursing process for nitrofurantoin is applicable for other urinary antiseptics/antiinfectives.

NURSING PROCESS: URINARY ANTIINFECTIVES: Nitrofurantoin

ASSESSMENT

- Obtain a history from the client of clinical problems with urinary tract infection (UTI) or other urinary tract disorders.
- Assess the client for signs and symptoms of UTI, such as pain or burning sensation on urination and frequency and urgency of urination.
- Assess CBC on clients with long-term therapy; monitor regularly.
- Assess renal and hepatic function.
- Assess urine pH; 5.5 is desired; however, alkalinization of the urine is *not* recommended.

POTENTIAL NURSING DIAGNOSIS

- Altered; comfort, pain
- High risk for infection

PLANNING

- Client will be free of signs and symptoms of UTI within 10 d.

NURSING INTERVENTIONS

- Monitor the client's output. Careful attention to output is required when administering urinary antiseptics to clients with anuria and oliguria. Report promptly any decrease in urine output.
- Before the start of drug therapy, obtain a urine culture to determine the organism causing the UTI.
- Observe the client for side effects of and ad-

verse reactions to urinary antiseptic drugs. Peripheral neuropathy (tingling, numbness of extremities) may result from renal insufficiency (inability to excrete drug) or long-term use of nitrofurantoin. Peripheral neuropathy may be irreversible.
- Dilute IV nitrofurantoin in 500 mL of IV solution before administering; reconstitute in sterile water without preservative.

CLIENT TEACHING

General
- Advise the client not to crush tablets or open capsules.
- Advise the client to rinse mouth thoroughly after taking oral nitrofurantoin. This drug can stain the teeth.
- Avoid antacids because they interfere with drug absorption.
- Instruct client to shake suspension well before taking and protect it from freezing.
- Advise client not to drive a motor vehicle or operate dangerous machinery; drug may cause drowsiness.
- Advise the diabetic client not to use Clinitest to test for glucose because a false-positive may result.

Diet
- Instruct the client to increase fluids and take the drug with food; this minimizes GI upset.

Side Effects
- Advise the client that urine may turn a harmless brown.

- Advise the client to report any signs of secondary fungal or bacterial infection (superinfection), such as stomatitis or anogenital discharge or itching.

Methenamine

- Advise the client to drink cranberry juice or take vitamin C with approval of the health care provider in order to keep the urine acidic. Foods that are alkaline, such as milk and some vegetables, may increase the urine pH. The urine pH should be less than 5.5 for the antiseptic to be effective.

Fluoroquinolones

- Advise the client to avoid operating hazardous machinery or driving a car while taking the drug, especially if dizziness is present.

- Instruct the client to take the drug with food and to avoid antacids because they interfere with drug absorption.
- Advise the client that the urine may turn a harmless brown because of the drug.
- Advise the client to report any signs of superinfection or a secondary fungal or bacterial infection.
- Avoid excessive exposure to sunlight.

EVALUATION

- Evaluate the effectiveness of the urinary antiinfectives in alleviating the UTI. Client is free of side effects and adverse reactions to drug.

URINARY ANALGESICS
PHENAZOPYRIDINE

Phenazopyridine hydrochloride (Pyridium), an azo dye, is a **urinary analgesic** that has been available for almost 40 years. It is used to relieve pain, burning sensation, and the frequency and urgency of urination that are symptomatic of lower UTIs. The drug can cause GI disturbances, hemolytic anemia, nephrotoxicity, and hepatotoxicity. The urine becomes a harmless reddish orange color because of the dye. Phenazopyridine can alter the glucose urine test (Clinitest), so a blood test should be used to monitor sugar levels. Figure 27–2 describes the pharmacologic behavior of phenazopyridine.

Pharmacokinetics

Phenazopyridine is well absorbed from the GI tract. Its protein-binding percentage and half-life are unknown. Phenazopyridine is metabolized by the liver and excreted in the urine, which is colored a reddish orange because of the harmless dye in the drug.

Pharmacodynamics

Phenazopyridine has been available for decades for decreasing urinary pain and discomfort. It has an anesthetic effect on the urinary tract mucosa; exact action is unknown. The serum peak concentration time for this drug is 5 h, and its duration of action is 6 to 8 h. Phenazopyridine is usually administered several times a day. With severe liver or renal diseases, hepatotoxicity or nephrotoxicity, respectively, may occur.

NURSING PROCESS: URINARY ANALGESIC: Phenazopyridine (Pyridium)

ASSESSMENT

- Obtain a history from the client of clinical problems with the urinary tract.
- Obtain a drug history; report probable drug-drug interactions.
- Assess the client for signs and symptoms of UTI such as pain or burning sensation on urination and frequency and urgency of urination.
- Assess hepatic function studies, especially serum liver enzymes, with long-term therapy.

POTENTIAL NURSING DIAGNOSES

- Altered patterns of urinary elimination
- Pain due to renal problem

PLANNING

- The client will be free of urinary tract pain within 3 d.

NURSING INTERVENTIONS

- Administer drug with food or milk to decrease gastric distress. Chewable tablets should be chewed.
- Observe client for side effects of and adverse reaction to urinary analgesic.

CLIENT TEACHING

General

- Instruct client to take medication exactly as ordered; recommended dosage should not be exceeded. Advise to take with food or milk.

Side Effects

- Advise the client that urine will be harmless reddish orange but does permanently stain clothing and tears will stain contact lenses.

- Instruct client to report signs of hepatotoxicity, including yellowing of skin or sclera, clay-colored stools, abdominal pain, diarrhea, dark urine, or fever.

Bethanechol

- Instruct the client to report abdominal discomfort, diarrhea, nausea, vomiting, increased salivation, urgency, flushing, or sweating.

EVALUATION

- Evaluate the effectiveness of the drug in alleviating the urinary tract pain. Client is free of side effects and adverse reactions to drug.

FIGURE 27–2. Urinary Analgesic

Antipruritic, local anesthetic	Dosage	**NURSING PROCESS** Assessment and Planning
Phenazopyridine (Pyridium, Urodine); ✤ Phenazo, Pyronium *Pregnancy Category:* B	A: PO: 100–200 mg t.i.d. p.c. × 2 d C: PO: 12 mg/kg in 3 divided doses	
Contraindications	**Drug-Lab-Food Interactions**	
Severe liver or renal disease, pregnancy or breast feeding	May interfere with urinalysis color reactions, urinary glucose, ketones, proteins, steroids	
Pharmacokinetics	**Pharmacodynamics**	Interventions
Absorption: PO: Well absorbed *Distribution:* PB: UK *Metabolism:* t½: UK *Excretion:* In urine	PO: Onset: UK Peak: 5–6 h Duration: 6–8 h	

Evaluation

Therapeutic Effects/Uses: For relief of UTI from infection, trauma, and surgery (use with urinary antiseptic).

Mode of Action: Produces analgesia/local anesthesia on urinary tract mucosa. Exact mechanism of action unknown.

Side Effects	Adverse Reactions
Anorexia, nausea, vomiting, diarrhea, heartburn, red-orange discoloration of urine, rash, pruritus, headache, vertigo	*Life-threatening:* Agranulocytosis, hepatotoxicity, nephrotoxicity, thrombocytopenia, leukopenia, hemolytic anemia

KEY: A: adult; C: child; PO: by mouth; UK: unknown; PB: protein-binding; t½: half-life; ✤: Canadian drug names.

TABLE 27–2 Urinary Analgesic, Stimulant, and Antispasmodics

Generic (Brand)	Route and Dosage	Uses and Considerations
Urinary Analgesic Phenazopyridine HCl (Pyridium, Urodine)	See Prototype Drug Chart (Fig. 27–2)	For chronic cystitis to alleviate pain and burning sensation during urination. Urine will be reddish orange. Can be taken concurrently with an antibiotic. It treats only symptoms, not the underlying cause of the pain; therefore, do not use long term for undiagnosed urinary tract pain. *Pregnancy category:* B; PB: UK; t½: UK
Urinary Stimulant Bethanechol Cl (Urecholine, Duvoid, Urabeth)	A: PO: 10–50 mg t.i.d./q.i.d. 1 h a.c. or 2 h p.c. SC: 2.5–10 mg t.i.d./q.i.d. PRN C: PO: 0.6 mg/kg/d in 3–4 divided doses	For hypotonic or atonic bladder. Should not be taken if peptic ulcer is present. Can cause epigastric distress, abdominal cramps, nausea, vomiting, diarrhea, and flatulence. Can cause dizziness, lightheadedness, and fainting, especially when standing up from lying or sitting position. *Pregnancy category:* C; PB: UK; t½: UK
Urinary Antispasmodics Dimethyl sulfoxide (DMSO, Rimso-50)	*Bladder instillation:* 50 mL of 50% sol retained for 15 min; repeat q2wk until relief	For cystitis. Administered into the bladder to remain for 15 min. Additional effects are antiinflammatory, anesthetic, and bacteriostatic. Can cause a garlic-like taste and odor on breath/skin for up to 72 hours. *Pregnancy category:* C; PB: UK; t½: UK
Flavoxate HCl (Urispas)	A: PO: 100–200 mg t.i.d. or q.i.d.	For urinary tract spasms. To be avoided by persons with glaucoma. Cautious use by the elderly. Side effects include nausea, vomiting, dry mouth, drowsiness, blurred vision. *Pregnancy category:* B; PB: UK; t½: UK
Oxybutynin Cl (Ditropan)	A: PO: 5 mg b.i.d. or t.i.d. C: >5 y: PO: 5 mg b.i.d. C 1–5 y: PO: 0.2 mg/kg b.i.d.-q.i.d.	For urinary tract spasms. Contraindicated for persons with cardiac, renal, hepatic, and prostate problems. Side effects include drowsiness, blurred vision, dry mouth. *Pregnancy category:* B; PB: UK; t½: 1–3 h
Propantheline bromide (Pro-Banthine)	A: PO: 15 mg t.i.d. 30 min a.c. and 30 mg h.s.; max: 120 mg/d Elderly: 7.5 mg t.i.d./q.i.d. C: PO: 2–3 mg/kg/d in divided doses	Effective for ureteral and urinary bladder spasm. Frequent dosing may cause urinary hesitancy or retention. Have client void before each dose. *Pregnancy category:* C; PB: UK; t½: 1.5 h

KEY: *A: adult; C: child; PO: by mouth; S.C.: subcutaneous; >: greater than; <: less than; a.c.: before meals; p.c.: after meals; UK: unknown; PB: protein-binding; t½: half-life; sol: solution.*

URINARY STIMULANTS

When bladder function is decreased or lost due to a neurogenic bladder (a dysfunction due to a lesion of the nervous system) as a result of a spinal cord injury (paraplegia, hemiplegia) or severe head injury, a parasympathomimetic may be used to stimulate **micturition** (urination). The drug of choice, bethanechol chloride (Urecholine), is a **urinary stimulant,** also known as a direct-acting parasympathomimetic (cholinomimetic). The drug action is to increase bladder tone by increasing tone of the detrusor urinal muscle, which produces a contraction strong enough to stimulate urination. Bethanechol is discussed in detail in Chapter 19.

URINARY ANTISPASMODICS

Urinary tract spasms due to infection or injury can be relieved with **antispasmodics** that have a direct action on the smooth muscles of the urinary tract. This group of drugs (dimethyl sulfoxide [also called DMSO], oxybutynin, and flavoxate) is contraindicated for use if urinary or GI obstruction is present or if the client has glaucoma. Antispasmodics have the same effects as antimuscarinics, parasympatholytics, and anticholinergics (discussed in Chapter 19). Side effects include dry mouth, increased heart rate, dizziness, intestinal distention, and constipation. Table 27–2 lists drugs that are urinary analgesics, stimulants, and antispasmodics.

STUDY QUESTIONS

1. What are the symptoms of UTIs? What group of drugs is used to alleviate these symptoms?
2. What is the major group of side effects associated with most urinary antiseptics/antiinfectives. How can they be prevented?
3. What type of drug is phenazopyridine and what is its purpose? What are two nursing interventions related to this drug?
4. What are the side effects of urinary antispasmodics? Why? Why should a person with glaucoma avoid taking a drug from this group?

Unit VI

Antineoplastic Agents

Cancer continues to be a major health problem in our society. Causes of some cancers may be attributed to the environment (chemicals, radiation, and infections) and to genetic background. Cancer (malignant) cells are characterized by (1) fast growth, (2) undifferentiated tissue mass, and (3) spread, or metastasis, to other body cells and organs. Cancer cells that divide rapidly respond more effectively to anticancer therapy than the slow-growing cells or solid tumors.

In the last two decades, more advances have been made to control and eradicate cancer through the use of numerous anticancer drugs, research, and treatment protocols that include select combinations of anticancer drugs. Nurses are taking an active role in various health facilities and in the home care of clients receiving anticancer therapy. To be a resourceful participant in the care of clients with cancer, the nurse first needs to understand the type of drug therapy the client is receiving, contraindications, drug interactions, therapeutic effects, side effects, and adverse reactions.

Chapter 28 discusses the cell cycle, the phases of cell duplication, and how certain anticancer drugs inhibit or prevent cell reproduction. The anticancer drugs are grouped as cell-cycle specific and cell-cycle nonspecific. Drugs in these groups are presented according to their effects on the cell cycle. Alkylating compounds, antimetabolites, antitumor antibiotics, vinca alkaloids, and steroids are anticancer drug categories discussed.

Chapter 29 describes the evolving state of biologic response modifiers, which have the following functions: (1) enhance host immunologic function, (2) destroy or interfere with tumor activities, and (3) promote differentiation of stem cells.

The nursing process is used throughout these two chapters to illustrate the importance of the role of the nurse in drug therapy.

Chapter 28

Anticancer Drugs

OUTLINE

Objectives
Terms
Introduction
   The Cell Cycle and Its
     Phases
Alkylating Drugs
   Cyclophosphamide
     Nursing Process

Antimetabolites
   Fluorouracil
     Nursing Process
Antitumor Antibiotics
   Pharmacokinetics
   Pharmacodynamics
   Side Effects and Adverse
     Reactions

Vinca Alkaloids
Hormones and Hormone Antag-
   onists
Miscellaneous Antineoplastics
Summary
Case Study
Study Questions

OBJECTIVES

Differentiate between cell-cycle specific and cell-cycle nonspecific drugs.

Identify general side effects of and adverse reactions to anticancer drugs.

Describe the uses and considerations for the following types of drugs: alkylating compounds, antimetabolites, antitumor antibiotics, vinca alkaloids, and hormones.

Explain the nursing implications of anticancer drugs.

TERMS

alopecia
androgens
anticancer drugs
antiestrogens
antineoplastic drugs
body surface area
cell-cycle nonspecific

cell-cycle specific
chemotherapeutic agents
corticosteroids
DNA
doubling time
growth fraction
irritants

nonvesicants
progestins
RNA
stomatitis
tumoricidal
vesicants
vinca alkaloids

INTRODUCTION

Anticancer drugs, also called cancer **chemotherapeutic agents** or **antineoplastic drugs,** were introduced in the treatment of cancer in the 1940s. These first antineoplastic drugs included estrogen for prostatic cancer and the nitrogen mustard drug mechlorethamine hydrochloride (Mustargen). Many of the early anticancer drugs, such as methotrexate, 5-fluorouracil, 6-mercaptopurine, and cyclophosphamide, are still in use today. Since the beginning of the 1970s more anticancer drugs have been marketed, and drug protocols (detailed plans) using combinations of drugs have been proven effective in curing specific leukemias and Hodgkin's disease. Today anticancer drugs are given for several reasons, including cure, control, and palliation. Chemotherapy may be used as the sole treatment of cancer or in conjunction with radiation and surgery.

THE CELL CYCLE AND ITS PHASES

Some anticancer drugs act at certain phases of the cell cycle. To understand the action of these drugs, the nurse needs to know the cell cycle. There are five phases in cell replication:

1. G_1: enzyme production needed for **DNA** (deoxyribonucleic acid)
2. S, or synthesis: DNA synthesis and replication
3. G_2: **RNA** (ribonucleic acid) and protein synthesis
4. M, or mitosis: cell division
5. G_0: resting phase

Cancer cells move more quickly through the phases than normal cells. Figure 28–1 demonstrates the phases of the cell cycle and gives an explanation of each.

Anticancer drugs interfere with either all phases or a specific phase of the cell cycle. There are two types of anticancer drugs: **cell-cycle nonspecific** (CCNS) drugs, which act on any phase during the cell cycle; and **cell-cycle specific** (CCS) drugs, which act on a specific phase of the cell cycle. CCNS drugs (also called cell-cycle independent) kill the cell during the dividing and resting phase. CCS drugs (also called cell-cycle dependent) are effective against rapidly growing cancer cells. In general, the groups of CCNS drugs (some alkylating agents are CCS) are the alkylating drugs, antitumor antibiotics, and hormones. The CCS drugs are the antimetabolites and the vinca alkaloids. Table 28–1 identifies the types, group, and the phase of the cell cycle that they affect.

Growth fraction and doubling time are two factors that play a major role in the cancer cell response to the anticancer drug. **Growth fraction** is the percentage of the cancer cell that is actively dividing. A high growth fraction occurs when the cell is *rapidly* dividing, and a low growth fraction occurs when the cell divides *slowly*. In general, anticancer drugs are more effective against the cancer cells that have a high growth fraction. Leukemias and some lymphomas have high growth fractions and, thus, respond well to anticancer drug therapy. Carcinomas of the breast and colon and melanomas have a low growth fraction, so they respond poorly to antineoplastics. Small and early forming cancer cells and fast-growing tumors respond well to anticancer drugs. Drug therapy for cancer diagnosed in its early stage is more effective and has a higher cure rate than cancer diagnosed in the advanced stages. Solid tumors have a large percentage of the cell mass in the G_0 phase, so these tumors have a low growth fraction and are less sensitive to anticancer drugs. Higher doses of drugs result in better **tumoricidal** (tumor-killing) effects.

Doubling time, which is related to the growth fraction, is the time required for a number of cancer cells to double their mass. When the tumor ages and enlarges, its growth fraction decreases

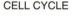

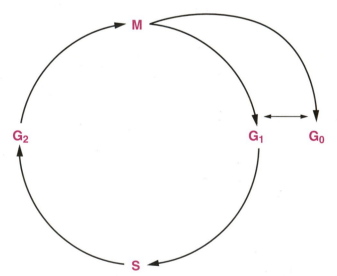

FIGURE 28–1 Cell cycle. *G_1 phase (Postmitotic gap):* Production of enzyme for DNA synthesis. Time of G_1 phase is 15–18 h. *S phase (Synthesis):* The DNA is doubled. Time of S phase is 10–20 h. *G_2 phase (Premitotic gap):* RNA synthesis for later mitosis. Time of G_2 phase is 3 h. *M phase (Mitosis):* Cell division, producing two identical cells. Time of M phase is 1 h. *G_0 phase (Resting phase):* remain in this phase or return to the cell cycle for cell replication. Cells in this phase are not as sensitive to many antineoplastic drugs.

TABLE 28–1 Groups of Cell-Cycle Nonspecific (CCNS) and Cell-Cycle Specific (CCS) Drugs

Drug Type	Drug Group	Cell-Cycle Effect
CCNS	Alkylating drugs	All phases. Act more effectively in G_1 and S phases.
	Antitumor antibiotics	All phases. Bleomycin more effective at the G_2 phase; daunorubicin and doxorubicin more effective at the S phase, and mitomycin more effective at the G_1 and S phases.
	Nitrosoureas	All phases
	Steroids (corticosteroids, estrogen, androgens)	All phases. Act more effectively at the S and M phases.
CCS	Antimetabolites	Effective at the S phase
	Vinca alkaloids	Effective at the M phase
	Antitumor antibiotics	See CCNS antitumor antibiotics.

and its doubling time increases. Compare, for example, breast cancer, whose growth fraction is 1% and whose doubling time is 55 days, and lymphocytic leukemia, whose growth fraction is 50% and whose doubling time is 4 days.

Cancer Chemotherapy

Tumor cells are similar to normal cells in that it is difficult for anticancer drugs to be selective in killing tumor cells and not normal cells. If large anticancer doses are given to kill malignant cells, normal cells also usually are killed; thus, the death of the client could result.

Antibacterials (antibiotics) differ from anticancer drugs because they are selective in killing bacterial cells. Antibacterials do not harm normal-functioning cells. Many of the antibacterials, such as penicillin, attack and destroy the bacterial cell walls. The bacterial cell dies and the normal cells remain. Malignant cells do not have definite cell walls. Anticancer drug research is directed toward developing a drug that will be selective in killing cancer cells only.

With antibacterial drugs, the client's immune defense mechanism aids in destroying the bacterially infected cells, whereas the anticancer drugs compromise the immune system and the drug fails to attack only cancer cells.

There are various drug protocols for successful chemotherapy. If the chemotherapy is extended too long or the doses are too high, toxicity is likely to occur. To eliminate every cancer cell can be difficult. When symptoms disappear, it had once been thought that malignant cells were eradiated. Unfortunately, this generally is not true, because 1 million cancer cells could still remain when there are

no symptoms. It is still not fully known how long cancer therapy should be continued. With continuous research and protocol drug therapy, an answer is anticipated in the near future.

Drug Resistance

Tumor resistance can develop against an anticancer drug because the drug is used too infrequently or the tumor's location limits the drug's effectiveness. Brain tumors respond poorly to anticancer drugs because most drugs do not cross the blood–brain barrier. Nitrosoureas, however, do cross the blood–brain barrier. Intraarterial infusion of the drugs at the site may be necessary.

Changes in DNA are a major cause of drug resistance, and mutation of cancer cells is also a factor in drug resistance. As the tumor ages, cancer cells mutate as they multiply; thus, the cancer cells are no longer identical. The mutated cells may differ in response to drug therapy.

Combination Chemotherapy

Single-agent drug therapy is seldom used; instead, combinations of drugs are used to enhance tumoricidal effects. CCS and CCNS drugs are often combined to maximize cell death. Use of combination drugs has the following advantages: (1) decreased drug resistance and, in general, shortened and intensified drug therapeutic effect; (2) increased destruction of cancer cells by effectiveness against the various mutated cells; and (3) reduced drug toxicity because of the use of several anticancer drugs at lower doses and with less injury to normal cells.

General Side Effects and Adverse Reactions

Anticancer drugs cause adverse reactions on rapidly growing normal cells, such as those in blood and hair. These drugs can also cause disturbances of the gastrointestinal (GI) tract, mucous membrane, and reproductive system. Table 28–2 lists the general adverse reactions to anticancer drugs on the fast-growing cells of the body. Selected nursing measures and considerations are included.

ALKYLATING DRUGS

One of the largest groups of anticancer drugs are the alkylating compounds. Drugs in this group belong to the CCNS category and affect all phases of the cell cycle. Thus, they are effective against many types of cancer: acute and chronic leukemias, lymphomas, multiple myeloma, and solid tumors (in the breast, ovaries, uterus, lungs, bladder, and stomach). Drugs in this category are divided into four groups: (1) nitrogen mustards (mechlorethamine, cyclophosphamide, chlorambucil, ifosfamide, and melphlan), (2) nitrosoureas (lomustine, carmustine, semustine, streptozocin), (3) alkyl sulfonate (busulfan), and (4) alkylating-like drugs (cisplatin, carboplatin). Adverse reactions to these drugs are the same as those shown in Table 28–2.

CYCLOPHOSPHAMIDE

Nitrogen mustard was the first alkylating drug that became available for clinical use during World War II. It is marketed as mechlorethamine and is used to treat Hodgkin's disease and solid tumors. An analog of nitrogen mustard commonly prescribed orally and intravenously is cyclophosphamide (Cytoxan). The client should be well hydrated while taking this drug in order to prevent hemorrhagic cystitis (bleeding due to severe bladder inflammation). Bone marrow suppression and alopecia are common side effects. Figure 28–2 details the pharmacologic behavior of cyclophosphamide.

Pharmacokinetics

Cyclophosphamide (Cytoxan) is well absorbed from the GI tract. Its half-life is moderate and it is moderately protein-bound. The drug is metabolized by the liver, and less than 50% is excreted unchanged in the urine.

TABLE 28–2 General Adverse Reactions to Anticancer Drugs

Adverse Reactions	Nursing Measures and Considerations
Bone Marrow Suppression	
Low white blood cell (WBC) count (neutropenia)	Susceptibility to infections is probable with a decreased WBC. Friends and family with colds or infections should take precautions (i.e., wear mask) or avoid visiting the client. Fever, chills, or sore throat should be reported. Neutrophils are the primary WBCs that fight infections.
Low platelet count (thrombocytopenia)	Petechiae, ecchymoses, bleeding of gums, and nosebleeds are signs of a low platelet count and should be reported.
Gastrointestinal Disturbances	
Anorexia	Loss of appetite may be due to the bitter taste in the mouth from drugs or the nausea caused by drugs.
Nausea and vomiting	Antineoplastic drugs stimulate the vomiting centers. Antiemetics are given several hours before the chemotherapy and for 12–48 h after the treatment.
Diarrhea	Hydration should be maintained. Hot foods (increase peristalsis) and high-fiber foods should be avoided.
Other	
Stomatitis	Good mouth care is necessary to minimize mouth ulcers. Saline or sodium bicarbonate mouth rinses may be used. If superinfection occurs, an antifungal medication may be used.
Alopecia	Varying degrees of hair loss occur after the first or second treatment. A wig should be purchased before treatment starts. After final treatment, some hair growth is apparent in several months.
Infertility	If infertility occurs, it could be irreversible. Pretreatment counseling is advised.

FIGURE 28–2. Antineoplastic: Alkylating Drug

Alkylating Drug	Dosage	NURSING PROCESS
Cyclophosphamide (Cytoxan), 🍁 Procytox *Pregnancy Category:* D	A: PO: Initially: 1–5 mg/kg over 2–5 d; maint: 1–5 mg/kg/d IV: Initially: 40–50 mg/kg in divided doses over 2–5 d C: PO/IV: Initially: 2–5 mg/kg in divided doses for 6 d; maint: 10–15 mg/kg every 7–10 d If bone marrow depression occurs, dosage adjustment is necessary	Assessment and Planning
Contraindications	**Drug-Lab-Food Interactions**	
Hypersensitivity, severe bone marrow depression *Caution:* Pregnancy, liver or kidney disease	Thiazides, anticoagulants, digoxin, phenobarbital, rifampin *Lab:* Uric acid, Pap test, purified protein derivative (PPD), mumps, candida	
Pharmacokinetics	**Pharmacodynamics**	Interventions
Absorption: PO: Well absorbed *Distribution:* PB: 50% *Metabolism:* t½: 3–12 h *Excretion:* 25–40% in urine unchanged; 5–20% in feces	*Effects on blood count:* PO/IV: Onset: 7 d Peak: 10–14 d Duration: 21 d	

Therapeutic Effects/Uses: To treat breast, lung, ovarian cancers; Hodgkin's disease; leukemias; and lymphomas; an immunosuppressant agent.

Mode of Action: Inhibition of protein synthesis through interference with DNA replication by alkylation of DNA.

Evaluation

Side Effects	Adverse Reactions
Nausea, vomiting, diarrhea, weight loss, hematuria, alopecia, impotence, sterility, ovarian fibrosis, headache, dizziness, dermatitis	Hemorrhagic cystitis, secondary neoplasm *Life-threatening:* Leukopenia, thrombocytopenia, cardiotoxicity (very high doses), hepatotoxicity (long term)

KEY: A: adult; C: child; PO: by mouth; IV: intravenous; PB: protein-binding; t½: half-life; 🍁 : Canadian drug name.

Pharmacodynamics

Cyclophosphamide is an early anticancer drug and is frequently used today as one of the drugs for the anticancer protocols. The onset of action begins within hours; however, the desired effect may take several days. It is one of the anticancer drugs that can be administered orally.

Several drug interactions may occur with cyclophosphamide: thiazides and allopurinol can increase bone marrow depression, the effect of digoxin decreases, and the effect of insulin increases, causing hypoglycemia. Phenobarbital and rifampin may increase cyclophosphamide toxicity. Adverse reactions should be observed and reported.

Table 28–3 lists some of the alkylating drugs, their dosages, uses, and considerations.

TABLE 28–3 Antineoplastics: Alkylating Drugs

Generic (Brand)	Route and Dosage*	Uses and Considerations
Nitrogen Mustards		
Chlorambucil (Leukeran)	A: PO: 0.1–0.2 mg/kg/d	For treating lymphocytic leukemia, lymphomas, and cancer of the breast and ovaries. Side effects include nausea, vomiting, anorexia, diarrhea, abdominal upset, and leukopenia. *Pregnancy category:* D; PB: 99%; t½: 1.5 h
Cyclophosphamide (Cytoxan)	See Prototype Drug Chart (Fig. 28–2)	For treating lymphocytic leukemia, Hodgkin's disease, certain solid tumors. One of the major drugs for combination drug therapy. Fluids should be forced to prevent hemorrhagic cystitis. Orally, it is taken without food or with meals. *Pregnancy category:* D; PB: 50%; t½: 3–12 h
Estramustine phosphate sodium (Emcyt)	*Palliation prostate cancer:* A: PO: 10–16 mg/kg/d in 3–4 divided doses for 28–90 d; determine if response occurred	For treatment of progressive carcinoma of prostate. Consists of estrogen and nitrogen mustard. Common side effects: nausea, peripheral edema, thrombophlebitis, breast tenderness. *Pregnancy category:* C; PB: UK; t½: 20 h
Ifosfamide (Iflex)	A: IV: 1–2 g/m²/d for 5 d q21–28 d C: IV: 1800 mg/m²/d for 3–5 d q21–28 d	For treating testicular cancer, lymphoma, lung cancer, and sarcomas. Mesna, a uroprotective agent, is added to prevent hemorrhagic cystitis. *Pregnancy category:* D; PB: UK; t½: 12–15 h (high dose)
Mechlorethamine HCl (Mustargen)	A: IV: 0.4 mg/kg/dose or 6–10 mg/m² as single dose or in divided doses	For treating Hodgkin's disease, solid tumors, and pleural effusion due to cancer of lung. Similar side effects as chlorambucil. *Pregnancy category:* D; PB: UK; t½: <1 min
Melphalan (Alkeran)	A: PO: 6 mg/d	For treating multiple myeloma, melanoma, and cancer of the breast, ovary, and testes. *Pregnancy category:* D; PB: <30%; t½: 1.5 h
Uracil mustard	*Palliation chronic lymphocytic leukemia, non-Hodgkin's lymphoma:* A: PO: 0.15 mg/kg/wk for 4 wk C: PO: 0.30 mg/kg/wk for 4 wk	For chronic lymphocytic and myelocytic leukemia; non-Hodgkin's disease of the cervix, ovary, and lung. GI distress may occur. *Pregnancy category:* X; PB: UK; t½: UK
Nitrosoureas		
Carmustine (BiCNU)	A: IV: 75–100 mg/m²/d for 2 d or 200 mg/m² q6 wk as single dose or divided into 2 doses on successive days; next course is dependent on blood count	For treating Hodgkin's disease, multiple myeloma, melanoma, and central nervous system (CNS) tumors, such as brain tumors. May be used for cancer of the breast and lung. Nausea, vomiting, and stomatitis may occur. *Pregnancy category:* D; PB: UK; t½: 15–30 min
Lomustine (CeeNu)	A: PO: 130 mg/m²/d as single dose	For treating advanced Hodgkin's disease and CNS tumors. *Pregnancy category:* D; PB: 50%; t½: 1–2 d
Streptozocin (Zanosar)	A: IV: 500 mg/m²/d for 5 d or 1 g/m²/wk	For treating pancreatic islet cell tumor and cancer of the lung. May also be used for Hodgkin's disease, colorectal cancer. Nausea, vomiting, diarrhea, and leukopenia may occur. *Pregnancy category:* C; PB: UK; t½: 30–45 min
Alkyl Sulfonates		
Busulfan (Myleran)	A: PO: 4–8 mg/d; *max:* 12 mg/d C: PO: 0.06–0.12 mg/kg/d	For treating myelocytic leukemia. WBC should be closely monitored. May be used as preparation agent in bone marrow transplant. *Pregnancy category:* D; PB: UK; t½: UK
Alkylating-like Drugs		
Altretamine (Hexalen)	A: PO: 4–12 mg/kg/d in 3–4 divided doses for 28–90 d	Primarily for ovarian cancer. Also used for breast, cervix, colon, endometrium, head/neck, and lung cancers; lymphomas. Nausea and vomiting and peripheral neuropathy may occur. *Pregnancy category:* D; PB: 6%; t½: 13 h
Carboplatin (Paraplatin)	A: IV: 360 mg/m² q4 wk *Solid tumors:* C: 560 mg/m² once every 4 wk *Brain tumor:* C: 175 mg/m² once weekly for 4 wk	For treatment of recurrent ovarian cancer. May be used as preparation agent in bone marrow transplant. *Pregnancy category:* D; PB: 0%; t½: 2–6 h

Table continued on following page

TABLE 28–3 Antineoplastics: Alkylating Drugs (Continued)

Generic (Brand)	Route and Dosage*	Uses and Considerations
Cisplatin (Platinol)	A: IV: 20 mg/m² / d for 5 d; then 50–70 mg/m² q3wk or 100 mg/m² q4wk	For treating ovarian and testicular cancer. Used as adjunctive treatment. Has been used for cancer of the bladder, head and neck, and endometrium. Nausea, vomiting, peripheral neuropathy, stomatitis, tinnitus, and blurred vision may occur. Ototoxicity occurs in 30% of clients. *Pregnancy category:* D; PB: >90%; t½: 1–60 h
Dacarbazine (DTIC)	*Hodgkin's disease:* A: IV: 150 mg/m² daily for 5 d; repeat course q28d or 375 mg/m² on day 1 of combination therapy: repeat course q15d *Metastatic malignant melanoma:* A: IV: 2–4.5 mg/kg daily for 10 d; repeat q28d	For metastatic malignant melanoma, sarcomas, neuroblastoma, and refractory Hodgkin's disease. May be given as an IV bolus (push) injection or by infusion. Common side effects are anorexia, nausea, and vomiting. *Pregnancy category:* C; PB: 5%–10%; t½: 5 h
Pipobroman (Vercyte)	*Chronic myelocytic leukemia:* A: PO: Initially: 1.5–2.5 mg/kg/d for 30 d; maint: 10–175 mg/d	Treatment for polycythemia and chronic myelocytic leukemia. *Pregnancy category:* D; PB: UK; t½: UK
Triethylenethiophosphoramide (thiotepa)	A: IV: 0.2 mg/kg/d for 4–5 d; then 0.3–0.4 mg/kg at 2 to 4 wk intervals	For palliation of neoplastic diseases, especially breast and ovary. *Pregnancy category:* D; PB: UK; t½: 1.5–2 h

KEY: A: adult; C: child; PO: by mouth; m²: body surface area; IV: intravenous; PB: protein-binding; t½: half-life; UK: unknown.
* For full discussion of body surface area in dosage calculation, see Chapter 4.

NURSING PROCESS: ALKYLATING DRUGS: Cyclophosphamide

ASSESSMENT

- Assess CBC, differential, and platelet count weekly. Withhold drug if platelets <75,000 cells/mm³ or WBC <4,000 cells/mm³; notify health care provider.
- Assess results of pulmonary function tests, chest x-rays, and renal and liver function studies during therapy.
- Assess temperature; fever may be early sign of infection.

POTENTIAL NURSING DIAGNOSES

- High risk for infection
- Body image disturbance

PLANNING

- Client will experience improved blood count status indicative of improvement/remission of the specific cancer growth.

NURSING INTERVENTIONS

- Hydrate client with IV and/or oral fluids before chemotherapy starts.
- Administer antacid before oral drug.
- Administer antiemetic 30 to 60 min before giving drug.
- Monitor IV site frequently for irritation and phlebitis.
- Increase fluids to 2 to 3 L/d to reduce risk of hemorrhagic cystitis, urate deposition, or calculus formation.
- Store drug in airtight container at room temperature.

CLIENT TEACHING

General

- Advise women who are contemplating pregnancy while taking antineoplastics to first seek medical advice. There may be teratogenic effects to the fetus. Pregnancy should be avoided for 3 to 4 mo after completing antineoplastic therapy in most situations. Some sources recommend

that both men and women avoid conception for 2 y after completing treatment.
- Remind client to consult health care provider before administration of any vaccination.

Diet
- Advise client to follow diet low in purines (organ meats, beans, and peas) to alkalize urine.
- Advise client to avoid citric acid.

Side Effects
- Instruct client about good oral hygiene with soft toothbrush for stomatitis; do not use toothbrush when platelet count is < 50,000 cells / mm³.
- Emphasize with client protective isolation precautions. Advise the client not to visit anyone with any type of respiratory infection. A de-

creased WBC puts the client at high risk for acquiring an infection.
- Instruct client to report promptly signs of infection (fever, sore throat), bleeding (bleeding gums, petechiae, bruises, hematuria, blood in the stool), and anemia (increased fatigue, dyspnea, orthostatic hypotension).
- Remind female client that she may experience amenorrhea, menstrual irregularities, or sterility and remind male client that he may experience impotence.
- Advise client of possible hair loss; recommend considerations of wig or hairpiece.

EVALUATION

- Client will be free of cancer as indicated by improved blood counts and free of side effects of drug.

ANTIMETABOLITES

Antimetabolites are the oldest group of anticancer drugs, except for the original nitrogen mustard. They are classified as cell-cycle specific and affect the S phase (DNA synthesis and me-tabolism). 5-Fluorouracil and floxuridine could be classified as CCNS as well as CCS. This group is subdivided into folic acid (folate) antagonists (methotrexate), pyrimidine analogs (5-fluorouracil, floxuridine, and cytarabine), and purine analogs (6-mercaptopurine and thioguanine). Other miscellaneous groups of anticancer drugs include ribonucleotide reductase inhibitor, antimicrotubule, enzyme inhibitor, and podophyllotoxin derivative.

Methotrexate was discovered in 1948 and is used for noncancer conditions, such as immunosuppression following organ transplant. Methotrexate, a folic acid antagonist, acts by substituting for folic acid, which is needed for the synthesis of proteins and DNA. Since its discovery in 1957, 5-fluorouracil (abbreviated as 5-FU) is commonly used as a single drug or in combination to cure or alleviate the symptoms of cancer.

The types of cancer that respond to antimetabolites are lymphomas, acute leukemias, cancer within the gastrointestinal tract, and breast cancer. Figure 28–3 presents the pharmacologic data of fluorouracil.

FLUOROURACIL

Pharmacokinetics

Fluorouracil is administered intravenously for carcinoma and topically for superficial basal cell carci-

noma. Protein-binding is less than 10%, and the half-life for the intravenous route is short (10 to 20 min). A small amount of the drug is excreted in the urine and up to 80% is excreted by lungs as carbon dioxide (CO_2).

Pharmacodynamics

Fluorouracil, a CCS drug, blocks the enzyme action necessary for DNA and RNA synthesis. The drug has a low therapeutic index. Fluorouracil can be used alone or in combination with other anticancer drugs.

Fluorouracil can cross the blood–brain barrier. The duration of action is 30 d.

Side Effects and Adverse Reactions

Side effects for fluorouracil are similar to other anticancer drugs, which include anorexia, nausea, vomiting, diarrhea, stomatitis, alopecia, photosensitivity, increased pigmentation, rash, and erythema. Adverse reactions may occur 4 to 8 days after the beginning of drug therapy. These include hematologic toxic effects such as leukopenia, thrombocytopenia, and agranulocytosis.

The general side effects for antimetabolite drugs include bone marrow suppression (leukopenia, thrombocytopenia), **stomatitis** (inflammation of the oral [mouth] mucosa), and alopecia. Table 28–4 lists the antimetabolite drugs, their dosages, uses, and considerations.

FIGURE 28–3. Antineoplastic: Antimetabolite

Antimetabolite	Dosage	**NURSING PROCESS** Assessment and Planning
Fluorouracil (Adrucil, 5-FU, Efudex) *Pregnancy Category:* D	A: IV: 12 mg/kg/d × 4 d; max: 800 mg/d; repeat with 6 mg/kg on day 6, 8, 10, and 12 Maint: 10–15 mg/kg/wk as single dose; max: 1 g/wk Topical: 1–2% sol/cream b.i.d. to head/neck lesions; 5% to other body areas Refer to specific protocol.	
Contraindications	**Drug-Lab-Food Interactions**	
Hypersensitivity, pregnancy, severe infection, myelosuppression, marginal nutritional status	Bone marrow depressants, live virus vaccines, cimetidine, calcium *Lab:* Liver function studies, albumin, AST, ALT	
Pharmacokinetics	**Pharmacodynamics**	Interventions
Absorption: IV and topical: 5–10% *Distribution:* PB: UK *Metabolism:* t½: 10–20 min *Excretion:* In urine and expired carbon dioxide	*Effects on blood count:* IV: Onset: 1–9 d Peak: 9–21 d Duration: 30 d Topical: Onset: 2–3 d Peak: 2–6 wk Duration: 4–8 wk	

Therapeutic Effects/Uses: To treat cancer of breast, cervix, colon, liver, ovary, pancreas, stomach, and rectum. In combination with levamisole after surgical resection in clients with Duke's Stage C colon cancer.

Mode of Action: Prevention of thymidine production, thereby inhibiting DNA and RNA synthesis. Not phase specific.

Evaluation

Side Effects	Adverse Reactions
Nausea, vomiting, diarrhea, stomatitis, alopecia, rash	Anemia *Life-threatening:* Thrombocytopenia, myelosuppression, hemorrhage, renal failure

KEY: A: adult; IV: intravenous; UK: unknown; PB: protein-binding; t½: half-life.

TABLE 28–4 Antineoplastics: Antimetabolites

Generic (Brand)	Route and Dosage*	Uses and Considerations
Folic Acid Antagonist Methotrexate (Amethopterin, MTX)	A: PO/IM: Induction: 3.3 mg/m²/d for 4–6 wk; maint: 30 mg/m²/wk in divided doses (2 × wk) C: Pediatric dosing varies with protocol and indication	For treating solid tumors, sarcomas, choriocarcinoma, leukemia. At higher doses, clients should be hydrated and keep urine pH 7.0 for drug solubility for excretion. Higher doses require use of Leucovorin as a rescue for normal cells. *Pregnancy category:* D; PB: 50%; t½: 8–16 h
Pyrimidine Analogs Cytarabine HCl (Cytosar-U, ARA-C)	A: IV: 100–200 mg/m²/d or 3 mg/kg/d as continuous 12- or 24-h infusion	For treating acute leukemias and lymphomas. Also used as an immunosuppressive drug after organ transplant. May be used in combination with other anticancer drugs. Nausea, vomiting, leukopenia, and thrombocytopenia are common side effects. *Pregnancy category:* D; PB: 15%; t½: 1–3 h
Floxuridine (FUDR)	A: Intraarterial: 0.1–0.6 mg/kg/d for 14 d IV: 0.5–1 mg/kg/d for 7–15 d	For treating metastatic colon cancer and hepatomas. *Pregnancy category:* D; PB: UK; t½: 20 h
5-Fluorouracil (Adrucil, 5-FU)	See Prototype Drug Chart (Fig. 28–3)	For treating solid tumors in the breast, bladder, ovaries, cervix, and GI tract. WBC should be monitored. Can be administered by IV push or in continuous IV fluids. Common side effects are anorexia, nausea, vomiting, diarrhea, stomatitis. *Pregnancy category:* D; PB: <10%; t½: 10–20 min
Procarbazine HCl (Matulane)	A: PO: Initially: 2–4 mg/kg/d in divided doses for 7 d; then increase to 4–6 mg/kg/d until desired leukocyte/platelet counts	Palliative treatment of advanced Hodgkin's disease and for solid tumor. May be used with other anticancer drugs. *Pregnancy category:* D; PB: UK; t½: 10 min
Purine Analogs 6-Mercaptopurine (Purinethol)	A&C: PO: 1.5–2.5 mg/kg/d; max: 5 mg/kg/d	First used in 1952 for treating acute lymphatic leukemia. Also used as an immunosuppressive drug. Adverse reactions may include hepatoxicity, bone marrow depression, hyperuricemia. *Pregnancy category:* D; PB: 19%; t½: 45 min
Thioguanine	A&C: PO: 2–3 mg/kg/d	For treating acute and chronic myelogenous leukemia. Long duration of action. *Pregnancy category:* D; PB: UK; t½: 2–11 h
Miscellaneous **Ribonucleotide Reductase Inhibitor** Hydroxyurea (Hydrea)	*Palliation:* A: PO: 20–30 mg/kg/d or 80 mg/kg q3d C: No dosage regimens established	For treating melanoma, resistant chronic myelocytic leukemia, and ovarian cancer. Has a long duration of action. *Pregnancy category:* D; PB: UK; t½: 3–4 h
Trimetrexate glucuronate (NeuTrexin)	A: IV: 45 mg/m²/d by infusion over 1–1.5 h with Leucovorin 20 mg/m², q6h (PO or IV)	Alternative drug therapy for *Pneumocystis carinii* pneumonia; treatment for clients with AIDS. May be used for colorectal cancer. CBC should be monitored. *Pregnancy category:* D; PB: 86%–94%; t½: 11–13 h
Antimicrotubule Paclitaxel (Taxol)	*Ovarian cancer:* A: IV: 135 mg/m² for 24 h q3wk; shortened infusions approved for refractory breast cancer	For treating metastatic ovarian and breast cancer. Monitor vital signs and electrocardiogram. Has a long duration of action (3 wk). Peak action is 11 d. *Pregnancy category:* D; PB: 80%–90%; t½: 5–17 h
Enzyme Inhibitor Pentostatin (Nipent)	*Hairy cell leukemia:* A: IV: 4 mg/m² every other wk	For treating hairy cell leukemia refractory to alpha-interferon. Causes DNA death. Has a very long duration of action. *Pregnancy category:* D; PB: UK; t½: 6 h
Podophyllotoxin Derivative Etoposide (VePesid, VP-16)	A: IV: 50–100 mg/m²/d on days 1–5, q3–4wk for 3–4 treatment therapy	For treating refractory testicular tumors, small cell lung carcinoma, Hodgkin's and non-Hodgkin's lymphomas, and acute myelogenous leukemia. Has standard chemotherapy side effects. Has a long duration of action. *Pregnancy category:* D; PB: 97%; t½: 4–11 h
Teniposide (Vumon, VM-26)	*Leukemia:* C: IV: over ≥30–60 min: 165 mg/m² and cytarabine 300 mg/m² 2 × wk for 8–9 doses	For treating acute lymphoblastic leukemia (ALL) in children. Used in combination with other anticancer drugs. Severe adverse reactions include bone marrow depression and anaphylaxis. *Pregnancy category:* D; PB: 99%; t½: 5 h

Table continued on following page

TABLE 28-4 Antineoplastics: Antimetabolites *(Continued)*

Generic (Brand)	Route and Dosage*	Uses and Considerations
Others		
Cladribine (Leustatin)	*Hairy cell leukemia:* A: IV: 0.09–0.1 mg/kg/d continuous infusion for 7 d	For treatment of hairy cell leukemia and chronic lymphocytic leukemia. Adverse reactions: bone marrow suppression, fever, nausea, vomiting, diaphoresis. *Pregnancy category:* D; PB: 20%; t½: 5.4 h
Fludarabine (Fludara)	*Chronic lymphocytic leukemia; acute leukemia:* A: IV: 25 mg/m²/d for 5 consecutive d/q28d	For treatment of chronic lymphocytic leukemia in clients who have not responded to other alkylating drugs; low-grade non-Hodgkin's lymphoma. Anorexia, nausea, diarrhea, fever, and peripheral edema may occur. *Pregnancy category:* D; PB: UK; t½: 9 h

KEY: *A: adult; C: child; PO: by mouth; IV: intravenous; >: greater than; <: less than; PB: protein-binding; t½: half-life; m²: square meter of body surface area; UK: unknown.*
* For full discussion of body surface area in dosage calculation, see Chapter 4.

NURSING PROCESS: ANTIMETABOLITES: Fluorouracil

ASSESSMENT

- Assess the client's vital signs (VS) and use for future comparison.
- Assess CBC and platelet count weekly. Notify health care provider and withhold drug if WBC is <3500/mm³ or platelet count is <100,000 cells/mm³.
- Assess renal function studies before and during drug therapy.
- Assess temperature every 4 to 6h; fever may be early sign of infection.

POTENTIAL NURSING DIAGNOSES

- High risk for infection
- Altered nutrition; less than body requirements
- Body image disturbance

PLANNING

- Client will have blood tests with values in the desired range.
- Client will be free of adverse reactions to drug therapy.
- Client's neoplasm will decrease in size.

NURSING INTERVENTIONS

- Handle drug with care during preparation; avoid direct skin contact with anticancer drugs. Follow protocols. Solution is colorless to light yellow.
- Administer IV dose over 1 to 2 min. Apply firm prolonged pressure to injection site if thrombocytopenia is present.
- Monitor IV site frequently. Extravasation produces severe pain. If this occurs, apply ice pack and notify health care provider.

- Administer antiemetic 30 to 60 min before drug to prevent vomiting.
- Offer the client food and fluids that may decrease nausea, such as cola, crackers, or ginger ale.
- Administer antibiotics prophylactically for infection, analgesics for pain, and antispasmodics for diarrhea, as ordered.
- Maintain strict medical asepsis.
- Encourage fluid intake of 2 to 3 L/d, unless contraindicated, to prevent dehydration.
- Support good oral hygiene; brush teeth with soft toothbrush and use waxed dental floss.
- Monitor fluid intake and output and nutritional intake. GI effects are common on the fourth day of treatment.

CLIENT TEACHING

General

- Emphasize protective precautions, as necessary.
- Teach the client to examine mouth daily and report stomatitis (ulceration in mouth). Good oral hygiene several times a day is essential. If stomatitis occurs, rinse mouth with baking soda or saline. Do not use a toothbrush when the platelet count is <50,000/mm³.
- Advise women who are contemplating pregnancy while taking antineoplastics to first seek medical advice. Teratogenic effects to the fetus can occur from antineoplastics. Pregnancy should be avoided for 3 to 4 mo after completing antineoplastic therapy in most situations. Some sources recommend that both men and women avoid conception for 2 y after completion of treatment.
- Advise the client not to visit anyone with any type of respiratory infection. A decreased WBC count puts the client at high risk for acquiring an infection.

Side Effects

- Advise the client to promptly report signs of bleeding, anemia, and infection to the health care provider.

EVALUATION

- The client's tumor size will be decreased.
- Evaluate the client's blood tests results.
- Evaluate for side effects or adverse reactions to drug therapy.

ANTITUMOR ANTIBIOTICS

Antitumor antibiotics (bleomycin, dactinomycin, daunorubicin, doxorubicin, mitomycin, and plicamycin) inhibit protein and RNA synthesis and bind DNA, causing fragmentation. Except for bleomycin, which has its major effect on the G_2 phase, they are classified as CCNS drugs. Dactinomycin was the first antibiotic used in the treatment of tumors in animals in the early 1940s. Bleomycin and plicamycin were introduced in 1962. These antitumor antibiotics differ from one another and are used for various cancers.

Figure 28–4 compares the similarities of and differences between doxorubicin and plicamycin.

PHARMACOKINETICS

Doxorubicin and plicamycin are administered intravenously. Doxorubicin is metabolized in the liver to active and inactive metabolites. The various metabolites affect the half-life, with the initial phase being 12 min, the intermediate phase 3.5 h, and the final phase 30 h.

PHARMACODYNAMICS

The primary effects of doxorubicin and plicamycin differ although they are classified as antitumor antibiotics. Doxorubicin is prescribed in combination with other anticancer agents for treatment of cancer of the breast, ovaries, lung, and bladder, and for leukemias and lymphomas. Plicamycin may be used in combination with other anticancer agents for the treatment of testicular carcinoma. Its primary use is for correction of hypercalcemia.

Because plicamycin affects bleeding time, use of aspirin, anticoagulants, and thrombolytic agents should be avoided. The use of cyclophosphamide with doxorubicin can increase the chance of occurrence of hemorrhagic cystitis.

Table 28–5 lists the antitumor antibiotics, their dosages, uses, and considerations.

NURSING PROCESS
Assessment and Planning

FIGURE 28–4. Antitumor Antibiotics

Antibiotics: Anticancer	Dosage
Doxorubicin (Adriamycin): (D) *Pregnancy Category:* D Plicamycin (Mithracin): (P) *Pregnancy Category:* X	*(D): Solid tumors:* A: IV: 60–75 mg/m²; repeat q21d, OR 30 mg/m²/d for 2–3 successive d, q4wk *(P) Testicular tumor:* A: IV: 25–30 μg/kg/d for 8–10 d Hypercalcemia: A: IV: 15–25 μg/kg/d for 3–4 d Reduce dose with renal impairment

Contraindications	Drug-Lab-Food Interactions
(D) Pregnancy, severe cardiac disease *Caution:* Hepatic and renal impairment (P) Hypocalcemia, bleeding disorders, myelosuppression *Caution:* Hepatic and renal impairment	(D): *Increase* hypercalcemia with Vitamin D *Increase* cardiotoxicity with daunorubicin *Lab:* ECG changes, *increase* uric acid (P) *Increase* hemorrhaging with aspirin, NSAIDs, anticoagulants, thrombolytic drugs, dipyridamole, sulfinpyrazone, valproic acid; *increase* serum calcium level with calcium drugs and Vitamin D *Lab: Decrease* calcium and phosphorus; *increase* BUN and creatinine, ALP

FIGURE 28–4. Antitumor Antibiotics (*Continued*)

Pharmacokinetics	Pharmacodynamics	Intervention

Absorption: IV
Distribution: PB: (D) 80–90%, (P) UK
Metabolism: t½: (D) 3–30 h; (P) 2–8 h
Excretion: (D) 50% in bile and 5% in urine; (P) urine
	(D)
	IV: Onset: 7–10 d
	    Peak: 14 d
	    Duration: 21 d
	(P)
	IV: Onset: 24 h
	    Peak: 48–72 h
	    Duration: 5–15 d	

	Evaluation
Therapeutic Effects/Uses: (D) To treat breast, bladder, ovarian, lung cancers, leukemias, lymphomas. (P) To correct hypercalcemia, hypercalciuria, and to treat testicular carcinoma. *Mode of Action:* (D) Inhibits DNA and RNA synthesis. Has immunosuppressant activity. (P) Inhibits hypercalcemic action of vitamin D and action by the parathyroid hormone. Inhibits DNA and RNA synthesis.	

Side Effects	Adverse Reactions
(D) and (P): Stomatitis, anorexia, nausea, vomiting, diarrhea, rash (D): Alopecia (P): Dizziness, weakness, headache, mental depression	(D): Esophagitis, anemia, hyperpigmentation of nails, tongue, and oral mucosa, especially in blacks (P): Nose bleeds, purpura, ecchymoses *Life-threatening:* (D) and (P): thrombocytopenia, leukopenia (D) Cardiotoxicity, CHF, ECG severe changes, severe myelosuppression, anaphylaxis (P) Hemorrhage

KEY: A: adult; IV: intravenous; PB: protein-binding; t½: half-life; CHF: congestive heart failure.

SIDE EFFECTS AND ADVERSE REACTIONS

The adverse reactions to the antitumor antibiotics are similar to the general adverse reactions to antineoplastics, which include alopecia, nausea, vomiting, stomatitis, leukopenia, and thrombocytopenia. Most antitumor antibiotics, except bleomycin and plicamycin, are capable of causing **vesication** (blistering of tissue). Some antitumor antibiotics can cause organ toxicities: bleomycin causes pulmonary toxicity, and daunorubicin, doxorubicin, and idarubicin cause cardiac toxicity.

VINCA ALKALOIDS

The **vinca alkaloids,** vincristine, vinblastine, and vinorelbine tartrate are classified as cell-cycle spe-

cific and act on the M phase (blocking cell division). These drugs can be used as single drugs or in combination drug therapy. Adverse reactions include leukopenia, partial to complete alopecia, stomatitis, nausea, vomiting, and neurotoxicity with vincristine and occasionally with vinblastine. Signs and symptoms of neurotoxicity might include decrease in muscular strength (numbness, tingling of fingers and toes), constipation, ptosis (drooping of the upper eyelid), hoarseness, and motor instability. Table 28–5 lists the vinca alkaloids, their dosages, uses, and considerations.

HORMONES AND HORMONE ANTAGONISTS

Hormones (steroids) are used in combination therapy for treating various cancers. The anticancer hormones have two major actions: (1) as agonists

TABLE 28-5 Antitumor Antibiotics and Vinca Alkaloids

Generic (Brand)	Route and Dosage*	Uses and Considerations
Antitumor Antibiotics Bleomycin SO$_4$ (Blenoxane)	A: IM/IV: 10–20 U/m^2/wk or 0.25–0.5 U/kg/wk Reduce dose with renal impairment	For treating squamous-cell carcinomas, testicular tumor (when used with vinblastine and cisplatin), and lymphomas. Low incidence of bone marrow suppression. Total lifetime dose is 450 U. A serious adverse reaction is anaphylaxis. Has a long duration of action. *Pregnancy category:* D; PB: 1%; t½: 2 h
Dactinomycin (Actinomycin D, Cosmegen)	A: IV: 500 μg/m^2/d for 5 d; may repeat at 2–4 wk C: IV: 15 μg/kg/d for 5 d; may repeat at 2–4 wk; *max:* 500μg	For treating testicular tumors. Wilms' tumor, choriocarcinoma, and rhabdomyosarcoma. Nausea and vomiting may occur during the first 24 hours. Has a long duration of action. *Pregnancy category:* C; PB: 80%–90%; t½: 36 h
Daunorubicin HCl (Cerubidine)	*Leukemias:* A: IV: 30–60 mg/m^2/d for 2–3 d; repeat dose in 3–4 wk Reduce dose with hepatic/renal impairment	For treating leukemias, Ewing's sarcoma, Wilms' tumor, neuroblastoma, and non-Hodgkin's lymphoma. Has a long duration of action. *Pregnancy category:* D; PB: 80%; t½: 19 h
Doxorubicin (Adriamycin)	*Solid tumors:* A: IV: 60–75 mg/m^2; repeat q21d Reduce dose with hepatic impairment	For treating breast, lung, and genitourinary cancers, leukemias, lymphomas, and ovarian tumors. Lower dose required when used in combinations. Total lifetime dose is 550 mg/m^2. *Pregnancy category:* D; PB: 80%–90%; t½: 3–22 h
Idarubicin (Idamycin)	*Solid tumor:* A: IV: 12–15 mg/m^2/d for 3 d *Leukemia:* A: IV: 10–12 mg/m^2/d for 3–4 d; repeat q3 wk Reduce dose with hepatic/renal impairment	For treating acute monocytic leukemia and solid tumors. More potent than daunorubicin or doxorubicin. Vesicant, monitor CBC. Urine may be red. *Pregnancy category:* D; PB: 97%; t½: 22 h
Mitomycin (Mutamycin)	A: IV: 10–20 mg/m^2 q6–8wk Reduce dose with renal impairment	For treating disseminated adenocarcinoma of breast, stomach, and pancreas. Also used for cancer of the head, neck, cervix, and lung. Monitor temperature and CBC. *Pregnancy category:* D; PB: UK; t½: 12 min
Plicamycin (Mithracin)	*Testicular tumor:* A: IV: 25–30 μg/kg/d for 8–10 d *Hypercalcemia:* A: IV: 15–25 μg/kg/d for 3–4 d Reduce dose with renal impairment	For treating hypercalcemia due to metastatic cancer. High doses may cause liver and renal damage. Monitor serum calcium levels. Has standard chemotherapy drug's side effects. *Pregnancy category:* D; PB: 0%; t½: 2–8 h
Mitoxantrone (Novantrone)	*Solid tumor:* A: IV: 12 mg/m^2/d × 3. Dilute with 50 mL NSS or D$_5$W over 15–30 min	For treating acute nonlymphocytic leukemia; may be used for breast cancer. Rash, dyspnea, hypotension, facial swelling, blue urine, sclera, skin hue change may occur. Severe hepatic dysfunction with decreased total body clearance. *Pregnancy category:* D; PB: 95%; t½: 1.5–13 d
Vinca Alkaloids Vinblastine SO$_4$ (Velban)	A: IV: Initial: 3.7 mg/m^2; after 7 d, increase dose weekly; *max:* 18.5 mg/m^2 C: IV: Initial: 2.5 mg/m^2; increase dose weekly; *max:* 12.5 mg/m^2	For treating cancer of the testes, breast, and kidney and for treatment of lymphomas, lymphosarcomas, and neuroblastomas. Nausea, vomiting, and alopecia are common side effects. Check CBC before dosing. *Pregnancy category:* D; PB: 75%; t½: 25 h
Vincristine SO$_4$ (Oncovin)	A: IV: 0.4–1.4 mg/m^2/wk; *max:* 2 mg/dose C: IV: 1–2 mg/m^2/wk; *max:* 2 mg/dose	For treating cancer of the breast, lungs, and cervix; multiple myelomas, sarcomas, lymphomas, Wilms' tumor. Neurologic difficulties should be assessed. Used for treating Hodgkin's disease in combination therapy, MOPP: mechlorethamine, vincristine, procarbazine, and prednisone. *Never* should be given intrathecally. *Pregnancy category:* D; PB: 75%; t½: triphasic 2–85 h
Vinorelbine (Navelbine)	A: IV: 30 mg/m^2 weekly as a 6- to 10-min IV infusion	For use as a first-line treatment for ambulatory clients with advanced, unresectable non-small cell lung cancer (NSCLC). May be used alone or in combination with cisplatin for stage IV NSCLC and in combination with cisplatin for stage III NSCLC. *Pregnancy category:* D; PB: UK; t½: UK

KEY: *A: adult; C: child; PO: by mouth; IM: intramuscular; IV: intravenous; CBC: complete blood count; m^2: square meter of body surface area; UK: unknown; PB: protein-binding; t½: half-life.*
* *For full discussion of body surface area in dosage calculation, see Chapter 4.*

that inhibit tumor cell growth, and (2) as antagonists that compete with endogenous hormone. Examples of agonists are estrogen, progestins, androgens, and adrenocorticosteroids. Examples of antagonists are aminoglutethimide, flutamide, goserelin acetate, and tamoxifen. Table 28–6 lists the hormones, hormone antagonists, and miscellaneous anticancer drugs.

Groups of hormones are the corticosteroids (cortisone), estrogens, progestins, and androgens. **Cor-**

TABLE 28–6 Antineoplastic: Androgens and Miscellaneous

Generic (Brand)	Route and Dosage*	Uses and Considerations
Androgens		
Testolactone (Teslac) CSS III	*Palliation breast carcinoma:* A: PO (females): 250 mg q.i.d.	For palliative treatment of breast carcinoma in postmenopausal women. Serum calcium levels should periodically be checked. Voice may deepen and facial hair may occur. *Pregnancy category:* D; PB: UK; t½: UK
Progesterone (Gesterol 50)	*Endometrial and breast cancer* A: IM: 5–10 mg/d for 6–8 d	For palliative treatment of endometrial and breast carcinoma. *Pregnancy category:* X; PB: UK; t½: 5 min
Miscellaneous: Hormonal Antagonists, Enzymes		
Aminoglutethimide (Cytadren)	A: PO: 250 mg q6h; increased q2 wk to 2 g/d in 2–3 divided doses to decrease nausea and vomiting	For treating adrenal carcinoma, ectopic adrenocorticotropic hormone (ACTH)-producing tumors. Drug suppresses adrenal activity. May be used in breast cancer therapy. Treatment usually used for 3 mo. *Pregnancy category:* D; PB: 20%–25%; t½: 7–15 h
Asparaginase (Elspar)	Start with intradermal skin test A: IV/IM: 6,000 U/m² q.o.d. for 3–4 wk or 1000–20,000 U/m² for 10–20 d or 200 IU/kg/d for 28 d	For treating acute lymphocytic leukemia. Used in combination with another anticancer drugs. Common side effects include nausea, vomiting, anorexia, leukopenia, and impaired pancreatic function. *Pregnancy category:* C; PB: 30%; t½: 8–30 h (IV)
Flutamide (Eulexin)	A: PO: 250 mg q8h *Note:* Give simultaneously with luteinizing hormone–releasing hormone (LHRH) analog therapy, e.g., leuprolide acetate, 7.5 mg IM/mo	For treating metastatic prostatic carcinoma, usually in combination with other anticancer drugs. *Pregnancy category:* D; PB: 95%; t½: 5–10 h
Goserelin acetate (Zoladex)	*Palliation prostate cancer:* A: SC: 3.6 mg into upper abdomen q28d	For treating metastatic prostatic carcinoma. It is a synthetic luteinizing hormone-releasing analog. May also be used in breast cancer and endometriosis. Gynecomastia, breast swelling, and hot flashes may occur. *Pregnancy category:* X; PB: UK; t½: 4–6 h
Megestrol acetate	*Breast cancer:* A: PO: 40 mg q.i.d. *Endometrial cancer:* A: PO: 40–320 mg/d in divided doses; *max:* 800 mg/d	For palliative treatment of advanced carcinoma of the breast and endometrium. May promote weight gain by increasing appetite. *Pregnancy category:* X; PB: UK; t½: 15–20 h
Mitotane (Lysodren)	*Palliation adrenal cortical carcinoma:* A: PO: 1–6 g/d in divided doses; increasing to 8–10 g/d in 3–4 divided doses; *max:* 18 g/d	For palliative treatment of inoperable adrenal cortical carcinoma. Adverse reactions include hemorrhagic cystitis, hypouricemia, and hypercholesterolemia. Monitor vital signs. *Pregnancy category:* C; PB: UK; t½: 20–160 d
Polyestradiol PO₄ (Estradurin)	*Palliation prostate cancer:* A: IM: 40 mg q2–4 wk; *max:* 80 mg	For palliative treatment of inoperable prostatic carcinoma. Estrogen derivative. Side effects may include fluid retention, nausea, vomiting, hypertension, weight change, and thromboembolic disorders. *Pregnancy category:* X; PB: UK; t½: UK
Tamoxifen citrate (Nolvadex)	*Palliation/adjunctive, treatment of breast carcinoma:* A: PO: 10–20 mg b.i.d.	For palliative treatment of advanced breast carcinoma with positive lymph nodes in postmenopausal women. Competes with estradiol at estrogen receptor sites. It decreases DNA synthesis. *Pregnancy category:* D; PB: UK; t½: 7 d

KEY: A: adult; C: child; PO: by mouth; IM: intramuscular; IV: intravenous; UK: unknown; PB: protein-binding; t½: half-life; CSS: Controlled Substance Schedule.

* *For full discussion of body surface area in dosage calculation, see Chapter 4.*

ticosteroids (glucocorticoids) are classified as anti-inflammatory agents, suppressing the inflammatory process that occurs with tissue involvement. This hormone also suppresses leukocytes and is effective in controlling leukemia and lymphoma. It is used in conjunction with other drugs as part of an antineoplastic regimen, an example of which is the MOPP regimen (mechlorethamine, Oncovin [vincristine], procarbazine, and prednisone), which is used for Hodgkin's disease. Prednisone is a frequently prescribed, inexpensive cortisone derivative. Dexamethasone and hydrocortisone can be administered intramuscularly and intravenously. These drugs can decrease cerebral edema caused by a brain tumor (neoplasm). Cortisone drugs give the client a sense of well-being and varying degrees of euphoria.

Cortisone derivatives that are taken internally produce many side effects, such as fluid retention, potassium loss, a risk of infection, increase in blood sugar, increase in fat distribution, muscle weakness, increased bleeding tendency, and euphoria.

Estrogen therapy is a palliative treatment used in men to decrease the progression of prostatic cancer and in postmenopausal women to decrease the progression of breast cancer. Estrogen preparations suppress tumor growth, and the drug promotes remission of the cancer for 6 months to a year. Examples of this group of drugs are diethylstilbestrol (Estrobene), ethinyl estradiol (Estinyl), chlorotrianisene (Tace), and conjugated estrogens (Premarin).

Two **antiestrogens** used to treat advanced breast cancer are tamoxifen citrate (Nolvadex) and an investigative agent, nafoxidine, which act by suppressing the growth of estrogen-dependent tumors.

Progestins are prescribed for breast cancer, endometrial carcinoma, and renal cancer. These drugs—hydroxyprogesterone caproate (Duralutin), medroxyprogesterone acetate (Depo-Provera), and megestrol acetate (Megace)—act by shrinking the cancer tissues. Adverse reactions include fluid retention and thrombotic (clot) disorders.

Androgens are given to treat advanced breast cancer in premenopausal women. This male hormone promotes regression of the tumor. If androgen therapy is used for a long time, masculine secondary sexual characteristics, such as body hair growth, lowering of the voice, and muscle growth, will occur. Flutamide (Eulexin) and leuprolide acetate (Lupron) are two other androgens used in the treatment of advanced prostatic cancer.

MISCELLANEOUS ANTINEOPLASTICS

There are a number of antineoplastic drugs whose mechanism of action or chemical configuration does not allow them to be categorized as an alkylator, antimetabolite, antitumor antibiotic, vinca alkaloid, or hormone. These agents include paclitaxel (Taxol), pentostatin (Nipent), etoposide (VP-16), and others. The miscellaneous antineoplastics are used in combination with other cancer chemotherapeutics to treat a variety of solid tumors and hematologic malignancies.

SUMMARY

The anticancer drugs act by blocking phases of the G_1, S, G_2, and M cancer cell-cycle phases. The groups of antineoplastic drugs (alkylating compounds, antimetabolites, antitumor antibiotics, vinca alkaloids, and hormones) can have either a palliative or a curative effect with single or combination drug therapy. These groups of anticancer drugs are classified as either cell-cycle specific (CCS) or cell-cycle nonspecific (CCNS). Figure 28–5 shows the phases of the cell cycle and the groups of antineoplastics that affect the different phases.

The nursing implications are to report the adverse effects and to participate as a health professional in alleviating these effects. The nurse instructs the client to use good oral hygiene for stomatitis, encourages the client to purchase a wig or use scarfs for alopecia, and instructs family and friends with upper or lower respiratory infections to minimize their visits with the client or use precautions, such as wearing a mask.

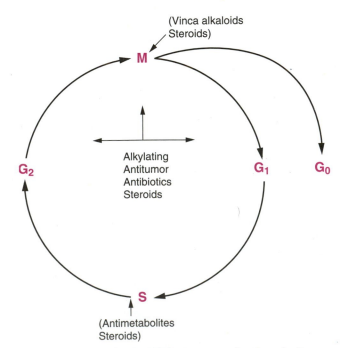

FIGURE 28–5 Phases and drug groups of antineoplastics.

■ CASE STUDY
Client with Breast Cancer

A.B., age 55 years, has recently been diagnosed as having breast cancer. Cancer chemotherapy was prescribed. A.B. received 5-fluorouracil intravenously for 4 days. Also, A.B. received doxorubicin (Adriamycin) intravenously, 60 mg/m², and this dosage is to be repeated in 21 days.

1. Fluorouracil is in what group of anticancer drugs? What is the action of this group of drugs?
2. Is fluorouracil in the CCS or CCNS category? Explain.
3. What are the side effects and adverse reactions of fluorouracil?
4. What nursing interventions and client teaching should be included in A.B.'s care?
5. Doxorubicin is classified in what group of drugs? What is the action of this group of drugs?
6. Why is a combination of antineoplastics/anticancer drugs desirable? Explain.

After several months, A.B.'s serum calcium was 12.3 mEq/L. Doxorubicin and fluorouracil were discontinued. Plicamycin and cyclophosphamide (Cytoxan) were prescribed.

7. Why was plicamycin ordered? From what group of drugs is plicamycin? What is its action?
8. What laboratory test(s) should be monitored while A.B. is taking plicamycin?

9. What group of drugs does cyclophosphamide belong to? Explain.
10. Is cyclophosphamide a CCS or CCNS drug? Explain.
11. What are the common side effects and the adverse reactions of cyclophosphamide?
12. What nursing interventions and client teaching should be included in A.B.'s care?

STUDY QUESTIONS

1. What are the five phases of the cell cycle? Name the groups of drugs that are cell-cycle specific and cell-cycle nonspecific.
2. Your client is receiving cyclophosphamide, methotrexate, and 5-fluorouracil for the treatment of breast cancer. What information would you include when teaching about self-care activities after receiving this drug?
3. What are the adverse reactions to most antineoplastic drugs? Explain.
4. What is combination drug therapy? What are its advantages?
5. What type of drug is plicamycin (Mithracin)? How is it used to correct electrolyte imbalances in clients with advanced cancer?
6. What is the action of corticosteroids, such as prednisone, in the treatment of cancer?
7. What is the definition of vesicant? List the anticancer drugs with vesicant properties.
8. What special safe handling precautions should be taken during the preparation, administration, and disposal of cancer chemotherapeutic drugs?

Chapter 29

Biologic Response Modifiers

Anne E. Lara

OUTLINE

Objectives
Terms
Introduction
Interferons
    Pharmacokinetics
    Side Effects and Adverse
      Reactions

Colony-Stimulating Factors
Erythropoietin
Granulocyte Colony-Stimulating
    Factor
Granulocyte Macrophage
    Colony-Stimulating Factor

Interleukins
    Pharmacokinetics
    Side Effects and Adverse
      Reactions
    Nursing Process
Summary
Case Study
Study Questions

OBJECTIVES

Discuss the actions of the biologic response modifiers.

Identify two client populations who may benefit from biologic response modifiers.

List three common side effects of interferons, colony-stimulating factors, and interleukin-2.

Describe the nursing process, including client teaching, needed to care for clients receiving biologic response modifiers.

TERMS

absolute neutrophil count
biologic response modifiers
colony-stimulating factors
erythropoietin
granulocyte
granulocyte colony-stimulating factor

granulocyte macrophage-colony-stimulating factor
hybridoma technology
interferons
interleukins
lymphokines
macrophage

nadir
neutrophil
recombinant DNA

INTRODUCTION

Biologic response modifiers (BRMs) are a class of agents used to enhance the body's immune system. Advances in biochemical technology have led to the discovery of BRMs and the identification of their clinical activities. **Recombinant DNA** (genetic engineering process to produce mass quantities of human proteins) and **hybridoma** (process to mass produce monoclonal antibodies using mice) **technology** (Figs. 29–1 and 29–2) are two advances that have led to commercial mass production of BRM.

Interleukins, colony-stimulating factors, interferons (α, β, γ), tumor necrosis factor, and monoclonal antibodies are some currently known BRMs. With the exception of the monoclonal antibodies, BRMs are complex proteins produced by the cells of the immune system (Fig. 29–3).

To date, three BRM functions have been identified:

1. Enhance host immunologic function (immunomodulation)
2. Destroy or interfere with tumor activities (cytotoxic/cytostatic effects)
3. Promote differentiation of stem cells (other biologic effects) (Table 29–1)

The indications for BRMs are currently being investigated in clinical trials. Erythropoietin, granulocyte colony-stimulating factors, granulocyte macrophage colony-stimulating factor, and interferon alpha are Food and Drug Administration (FDA) approved and commercially available. The interleukins, tu-

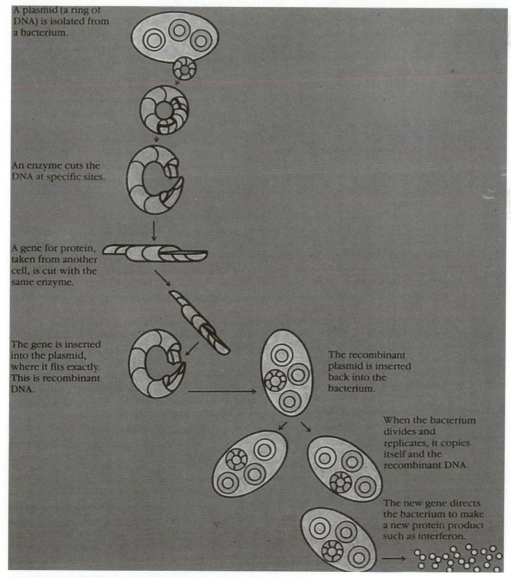

FIGURE 29–1 Recombinant DNA. (*Source:* From NIH Publication No. 88-529 [1991]: *Understanding the Immune System,* p. 29.)

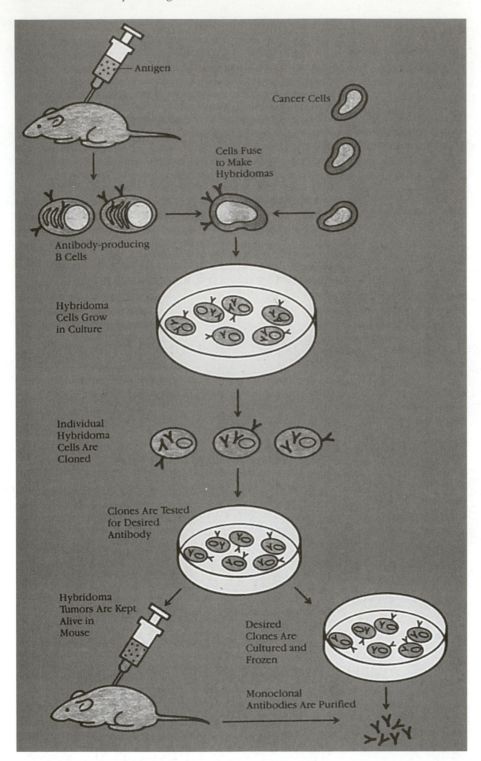

FIGURE 29–2 Hybridoma therapy. (*Source:* From NIH Publication No. 88-529 [1991]: *Understanding the Immune System*, p. 28.)

mor necrosis factor, and monoclonal antibodies continue to be studied in clinical trials. Interferons, interleukins, and colony-stimulating factors will be discussed in this chapter.

INTERFERONS

Interferons (IFNs) are a family of naturally occurring proteins that were first discovered in the 1950s. Three major types of IFNs have been identified: alpha (α) IFN, beta (β) IFN, and gamma (γ) IFN. Each type is produced by a different cell within the immune system. All three types can be manufactured using recombinant DNA technology; only IFN-α, however, is FDA approved for commercial use.

Interferon alpha is produced by B cells, T cells, macrophages, and null cells in response to the

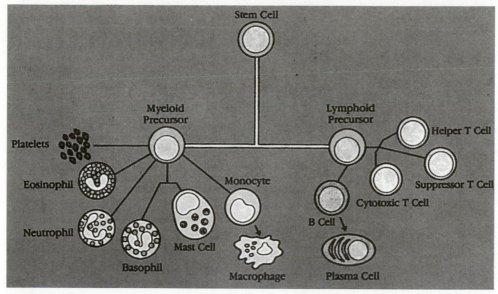

FIGURE 29–3 Cells of the immune system. (*Source:* From NIH Publication No. 88-529 [1991]: *Understanding the Immune System,* p. 5.)

presence of viruses or tumor cells. Interferon alpha has been shown to have antiviral, antiproliferative, and immunomodulatory effects, which means that IFN-α inhibits intracellular replication of viral DNA, interferes with tumor cell growth, and enhances natural killer cell (antitumor) activity. Recombinant IFN-α is manufactured as Roferon-A and as Intron A.

In 1986, IFN-α was approved by the FDA for use in treating hairy-cell leukemia, and in 1989 it was approved for use in acquired immunodeficiency syndrome (AIDS)-related Kaposi's sarcoma. Clinically, alpha IFN has been used in the treatment of non-Hodgkin's lymphoma, multiple myeloma, chronic myelogenous leukemia, renal cell carcinoma, malignant melanoma, bladder cancer, and carcinoid (type of cancer-like disease). Intravesical administration of IFN-α has proved successful for low-grade bladder tumors, intraperitoneal administration of IFN-α has been used for ovarian cancer clients, and intralesional application of IFN-α has been used to treat melanoma and basal cell carci-

noma. Benign conditions such as laryngeal papillomata and condyloma acuminata have also been treated with alpha IFN. IFN is currently being investigated in clinical trials as a chemotherapy-enhancing agent in clients with colon cancer.

PHARMACOKINETICS

Interferon is metabolized by the liver and filtered by the kidney. Approximately 80% of the dose, however, is absorbed by the body. Peak serum concentrations are reached 4 to 8 h after administration. Interferon can be administered subcutaneously, intramuscularly, and intravenously, although subcutaneous or intramuscular administration is preferred. Subcutaneous administration is recommended for clients with platelet counts below 50,000.

Roferon-A is available in both liquid and powder forms. The liquid is supplied in 3 million IU/mL vials and 18 million IU/mL vials. At a concentration of 3 million IU/0.5 mL, the powder is available as 18 million IU/vial. When mixed with 3 mL of bacteriostatic water diluent, the vial concentration is 6 million IU/mL, or 3 million IU/0.5 mL. Both the liquid and the powder should be refrigerated at 2 to 8°C, and used within 1 month. The vials should not be frozen or shaken.

Intron A is supplied as a lyophilized powder in 3, 5, 10, and 25 million IU. The powder is reconstituted with bacteriostatic water diluent. Final vial concentrations are 3 million IU/vial (3 million IU/vial with 1 mL of diluent), 5 million IU/mL (5 million IU/vial with 2 mL of diluent), and 5 million IU/mL (25 million IU/vial with 5 mL of dilu-

TABLE 29–1 Action of Biologic Response Modifiers (BRMs)

BRMs	Action
Interleukins	I
Interferons	I, C
Monoclonal antibodies	C
Tumor necrosis factor	C
Colony-stimulating factors	O

KEY: I: immunomodulation; C: cytotoxic/cytostatic; O: other biologic activity.

ent). The vials can be shaken to hasten powder dissolution. The final solution is stable for 30 days when stored at 2 to 8°C. The IFN alphas are listed in Table 29–2 with their dosages, uses, and considerations.

SIDE EFFECTS AND ADVERSE REACTIONS

The major side effect of IFN-α is a flu-like syndrome. Other effects are seen in the gastrointestinal (GI), neurologic, cardiopulmonary, renal, hepatic, hematologic, and dermatologic systems.

The flu-like syndrome is characterized by fever, chills, fatigue, malaise, and myalgias. Chills can occur 3 to 6 h after IFN-α administration and may progress to rigors. A fever as high as 39 to 40°C may occur within 30 to 90 min after the onset of chills and last for 24 h. Fatigue, malaise, and myalgias are cumulative side effects; fatigue is the dose-limiting toxicity (the side effect that would result in decrease in dose or discontinuation of drug).

GI side effects include nausea, diarrhea, vomiting, anorexia, taste alterations, and xerostomia (dry mouth). These side effects are mild, with anorexia considered to be the dose-limiting toxicity for this system.

Neurologic side effects are reversible (after the drug is stopped) and occur in 70% of clients who receive IFN-α. These effects are manifested by mild confusion, somnolence (sleepiness), irritability, poor concentration, seizures, transient aphasia (temporary loss of ability to speak), hallucinations, paranoia, and psychoses.

Cardiopulmonary side effects are dose-related and occur more frequently in the elderly and in those clients with an underlying cardiac disease. The effects include tachycardia, pallor, cyanosis, tachypnea, nonspecific electrocardiographic changes, rare myocardial infarction, and orthostatic hypotension.

Renal and hepatic effects are dose-dependent and usually result in few or no symptoms. The effects are manifested by increased blood urea nitrogen (BUN) and creatinine levels, proteinuria, and elevated transaminases.

Hematologic effects are reversible and dose-limiting. Neutropenia (decreased number of neutrophils in the blood) and thrombocytopenia are manifestations of such effects. Neutropenia is usually rare and does not predispose the client to infection. Thrombocytopenia is more common in clients with hematopoietic (affecting the formation of blood cells) diseases than in those with solid tumors.

TABLE 29–2 Biologic Response Modifiers: Interferons

Generic (Brand)	Route and Dosage	Uses and Considerations
Interferon alfa-2a (Roferon-A)	*Hairy-cell leukemia, condylomata acuminata:* A: SC/IM: 3 million IU daily for 16–24 wk	For treating hairy-cell leukemia, condyloma acuminata and AIDS-related Kaposi's sarcoma. Flu-like symptoms such as fatigue, aches, pain, fever, chills, headaches may occur. *Pregnancy category:* C; PB: UK; t½: 2–3 h
Interferon alfa-2b (Intron A)	A: SC: 2 million IU/m² × 3 wk *Kaposi's sarcoma:* A: IM/SC/IV: Initially: 36 million IU daily for 10–12 wk; maint: 36 million IU 3 × wk	For treating hairy-cell leukemia, condyloma acuminata, AIDS-related Kaposi's sarcoma, and chronic hepatitis B and non-A hepatitis. Flu-like symptoms may occur. Monitor CBC, AST, ALT, ALP, LDH. *Pregnancy category:* C; PB: UK; t½: 2 h
Interferon gamma-1b (Actimmune)	*Body surface area >0.5 m²:* A: SC: 50 μg/m² 3 × wk *Body surface area <0.5 m²:* A&C >1 y: SC: 1.5 μg/kg 3 × wk	For treating chronic granulomatous disease. Flu-like symptoms may occur. *Pregnancy category:* C; PB: UK; t½: 0.5–6 h
Interferon alfa-n3 (Alferon N)	*Condylomata acuminata:* A: Inject into wart: 250,000 U (0.05 mL) twice weekly; max: 8 wk Do *not* repeat for >3 mo after end of therapy	For treating recurring condylomata acuminata (genital, venereal warts). Flu-like symptoms may occur. Monitor CBC, AST, ALT, ALP, LDH. *Pregnancy category:* C; PB: UK; t½: 6–8 h
Interferon beta-1b (Betaseron)	*Reduce number of clinical exacerbations of multiple sclerosis:* A: >18 y: SC: 8 million U q.o.d. C: Not recommended	For treating multiple sclerosis (MS). Flu-like symptoms may occur. *Pregnancy category:* C; PB: UK; t½: 8 min–4.3 h

KEY: *A: adult; C: child; SC: subcutaneous; IM: intramuscular; IV: intravenous; UK: unknown; CBC: complete blood count; >: greater than; <: less than; PB: protein-binding; t½: half-life.*

Maculopapular rashes of the trunk and extremities, pruritis, irritation at the injection site, desquamation (shedding of epithelial cells of the skin), and alopecia are dermatologic effects of IFN-α. Alopecia can occur after more than 4 months of therapy.

The administration of IFN-α is contraindicated in clients with known hypersensitivity to IFN-α, mouse immunoglobulin, or any component of the product. It should be used cautiously in clients with severe cardiac, renal, or hepatic disease, or those with seizure disorders or central nervous system dysfunction. Manufacturers recommend administering the agent to persons 18 years or older only under the supervision of a qualified physician. There have been no studies demonstrating the safety and effectiveness of IFN-α in pregnant women, nursing mothers, or children. Women of child-bearing age should use contraceptives while receiving IFN-α due to the agent's effects on serum estradiol and progesterone concentrations. Studies have demonstrated no fertility or teratogenic effects in males.

It is recommended that baseline and periodic complete blood counts (CBCs) and liver function tests be performed during the course of IFN therapy. Manufacturers suggest that clients be treated for at least 6 months before a decision is made to continue treatment in those who respond or discontinue treatment in those who do not; optimal treatment duration has not been determined. Dose reductions of 50% or drug discontinuation should be considered if adverse reactions occur. Concurrent or prior treatment with chemotherapeutic agents or radiation therapy may increase the effectiveness and the toxicity of IFN-α.

COLONY-STIMULATING FACTORS

Hematopoietic **colony-stimulating factors** (CSFs) are proteins that stimulate or regulate the growth, maturation, and differentiation of bone marrow stem cells (Fig. 29–4). The CSFs are manufactured through recombinant DNA techniques.

Although CSFs are not directly tumoricidal, they are useful in cancer treatment because they

1. Decrease the length of posttreatment neutropenia (the length of time the neutrophils [a type of white blood cell] are decreased secondary to chemotherapy), thereby reducing the incidence and duration of infection.
2. Permit the delivery of higher doses of drugs. Myelosuppression (suppression of bone marrow activity) is often a dose-limiting toxicity of chemotherapy. Higher, possibly tumoricidal doses of drugs cannot be administered because

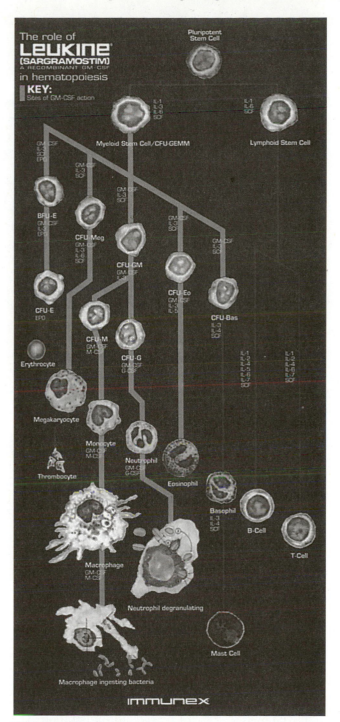

FIGURE 29–4 The role of Leukine (sargramostim) in hematopoiesis. (*Source:* From Immunex Corp.)

of potentially life-threatening side effects. CSFs can minimize the myelosuppression toxicity, thus allowing the delivery of higher doses of drugs.
3. Reduce bone marrow recovery time after bone marrow transplantation.
4. Enhance macrophage or granulocyte tumor-, virus-, and fungus-destroying ability.

Colony-stimulating factors have been used to treat clients with neutropenia secondary to disease or treatment and can be administered both intravenously and subcutaneously. Three CSFs are FDA approved for clinical use: erythropoietin, granulocyte colony-stimulating factor (G-CSF), and granulocyte macrophage colony-stimulating factors (GM-CSF).

ERYTHROPOIETIN

Erythropoietin (EPO) is a glycoprotein produced by the kidney that stimulates red blood cell production in response to hypoxia (decreased oxygen to body tissues). Specifically, EPO stimulates the division and differentiation of committed red blood cell progenitors (parent cells destined to become circulating red blood cells) in the bone marrow. EPO is currently FDA approved for use in clients with anemia secondary to chronic renal failure or AZT (zidovudine)-treated human immunodeficiency virus (HIV) infections. Its use in clients with anemia secondary to cancer or its treatment remain under investigation. The use of EPO in these anemic clients may decrease the need for and frequency of red cell transfusion. Erythropoietin is marketed under the brand name Epogen.

Pharmacokinetics

Erythropoietin can be administered both intravenously (IV push) or subcutaneously. According to the manufacturer, intravenously administered EPO is eliminated at a rate consistent with first-order kinetics (process by which the drug is eliminated in part by hepatic and renal blood flow), with a circulating half-life ranging from approximately 4 to 13 h in clients with chronic renal failure (CRF). Plasma levels of EPO have been detected for at least 24 h. After subcutaneous administration of EPO to CRF clients, peak serum levels were achieved within 5 to 24 h after administration. The half-life of intravenously administered EPO is approximately 20% shorter in normal volunteers than in CRF clients. Pharmacokinetic studies have not been done with HIV-infected clients. See Figure 29–5.

Erythropoietin should be administered at starting doses of 50 to 100 U/kg three times a week. The dose of EPO should be reduced when the hematocrit reaches the 30% to 33% range or increases by more than four points in any 2-week period. The dosage needs to be individualized to maintain the hematocrit within the target range. Dose changes

should be made in the range of 25 U/kg three times a week.

According to the manufacturer, if a client does not respond to or maintain a response, the following situations must be considered and evaluated:

1. Iron deficiency
2. Underlying infections, inflammatory or malignant processes
3. Occult blood loss
4. Underlying hematologic disease
5. Folic acid or vitamin B_{12} deficiency
6. Hemolysis
7. Aluminum intoxication
8. Osteitis fibrosa cystica (fibrous degeneration with formation of cysts and nodules secondary to hyperparathyroidism)

Side Effects and Adverse Reactions

The side effects of erythropoietin include hypertension, headache, arthralgias (joint pain), nausea, edema, fatigue, diarrhea, vomiting, chest pain, injection site skin reaction, asthenia (weakness), dizziness, seizures, thromboses (clots), and allergic reactions. Studies demonstrate that EPO administration was well tolerated with no reports of serious allergic reactions or anaphylaxis. Rare transient skin reactions have been reported. Blood pressure may rise in CRF clients receiving EPO during the early phase of treatment when the hematocrit (Hct) is rising. About 25% of CRF clients receiving dialysis may require initiation of or increase in antihypertensive therapy. It is postulated that increases in blood pressure may relate to increases in Hct; therefore, it is recommended that the dose of EPO be decreased if the Hct increase exceeds four points in any 2-week period. Similarly, a rise in Hct may cause increased vascular access clotting (clots in blood vessel at connection site with artificial kidney) in hemodialysis clients. Clients may require increased heparinization during EPO therapy to prevent clotting of the artificial kidney. Seizures occurred in CRF clients receiving EPO during clinical trials; activity was particularly evident during the first 90 days of therapy.

EPO administration is contraindicated in clients with (1) uncontrolled hypertension, (2) known hypersensitivity to mammalian cell-derived products, and (3) known hypersensitivity to human albumin. Evaluation of iron stores should occur during EPO therapy. Transferrin saturation should be at least 20% and ferritin should be at least 100 ng/mL. Iron supplements may be needed to increase and maintain transferrin saturation to support EPO-stimulated erythropoiesis.

The safety and effectiveness of EPO therapy in

FIGURE 29–5. Biologic Response Modifiers: Erythropoietin

Epoetin Alfa (Erythropoietin [EPO])	Dosage	**NURSING PROCESS** Assessment and Planning
Epoetin Alfa (Erythropoietin [EPO]) (Epogen, Procit), 🍁 Eprex *Pregnancy Category:* C	A: 50–100 U/kg 3 × wk IV: Dialysis clients IV/SC: Nondialysis, CRF clients IV/SC: 100 U/kg 3 × wk for 8 wk in AZT-treated HIV-infected clients Initial dose to those with EPO levels <500 mU/mL and receiving <4,200 mg of AZT/wk. Clients with EPO level >500 mU/mL are unlikely to respond to EPO therapy .	
Contraindications	**Drug-Lab-Food Interactions**	
Uncontrolled hypertension, hypersensitivity to mammalian cell–derived products or human albumin *Caution:* Pregnancy, lactation, porphyria; safety in children not known	*Drug:* None known *Lab:* Increase hematocrit, decreased plasma volume	
Pharmacokinetics	**Pharmacodynamics**	Interventions
Absorption: SC, IV *Distribution:* PB: UK *Metabolism:* t½: 4–13 h in clients with CRF; 20% less in those with normal renal function *Excretion:* In urine	IV: Onset: 7 to 10 d Peak: 2–4 wk Duration: UK SC: Onset: 7 to 10 d Peak: 5–24 h Duration: UK	

Therapeutic Effects/Uses: To treat anemia secondary to CRF or AZT (zidovudine) treatment of HIV infections. Use in clients with anemia secondary to cancer or its treatment is under investigation.

Mode of Action: Increased production of RBCs, triggered by hypoxia or anemia.

Evaluation

Side Effects	Adverse Reactions
Sense of well-being, hypertension, arthralgias, nausea, edema, fatigue, injection site reaction, rash, diarrhea, shortness of breath	Seizures, hyperkalemia *Life-threatening:* Cerebrovascular accident, myocardial infarction

KEY: A: adult; SC: subcutaneous; IV: intravenous; <: lesser than; >: greater than; UK: unknown; PB: protein-binding; t½: half-life. 🍁 : Canadian drug name.

pregnant women, nursing mothers, and children have not been established. There are no known EPO drug interactions.

The manufacturers' preparation and administration recommendations for EPO are

1. Do not shake, because shaking may denature the glycoprotein, rendering it biologically inactive.
2. Use only one dose per vial. Do not reenter the vial. Discard any unused portion because the vial contains no preservatives.
3. Store the 2000-, 3000-, 4000-, 10,000-, or 20,000-unit vials at 2 to 8°C. Do not freeze.
4. Warm the vial to room temperature before subcutaneous (SC) administration.
5. Use the smallest volume of EPO per injection (1 mL or less per injection) to decrease injection site discomfort.

6. Use ice to numb the injection site.
7. Do not use the same needle to draw medication into the syringe and to inject the medication. Use a new needle to inject medication.

GRANULOCYTE COLONY-STIMULATING FACTOR

Granulocyte colony-stimulating factor (G-CSF), marketed as filgrastim (Neupogen), is a human **granulocyte** (type of WBC responsible for fighting infection) colony-stimulating factor produced by recombinant DNA technology. G-CSF, which is a glycoprotein produced by monocytes (a type of WBC), fibroblasts (immature fiber-producing cells), and endothelial (cells that line the heart cavity, and blood and lymph vessels) cells, regulates the production of **neutrophils** (granular leukocytes, WBCs) within the bone marrow. G-CSF is FDA approved and commercially available to decrease the incidence of infections in clients receiving myelosuppressive chemotherapeutic agents. G-CSF has been evaluated as an adjunct to chemotherapy for both solid tumor and hematologic malignancies and in studies employing a number of different chemotherapy regimens. Figure 29–6 gives the drug data for filgrastim.

FIGURE 29–6. Granulocyte Colony-Stimulating Factor

Filgrastim	Dosage	NURSING PROCESS
		Assessment and Planning
Filgrastim (Neupogen) Granulocyte colony-stimulating factor (G-CSF) *Pregnancy Category:* C	A: IV inf/SC: 5 μg/kg/d C: 5–10 μg/kg/d Refer to specific protocols.	
Contraindications	**Drug-Lab-Food Interactions**	
Hypersensitivity to *E. coli*–derived proteins; 24 h before or after cytotoxic chemotherapy *Caution:* Pregnancy, lactation; safety in children not known	*Drug:* None known *Lab: Increase* lactic acid, LDH, alkaline phosphatase: transient *increase* in neutrophils	
Pharmacokinetics	**Pharmacodynamics**	Interventions
Absorption: SC: Well absorbed *Distribution:* PB: UK *Metabolism:* t½: 2–3.5 h *Excretion:* Probably in urine	IV/SC: Onset: 24 h Peak: 3–5 d Duration: 4–7 d	

Therapeutic Effects/Uses: To decrease incidence of infection in clients receiving myelosuppressive chemotherapeutic agents; adjunct to chemotherapy for both solid tumor and hematologic malignancies.

Mode of Action: Increases production of neutrophils and enhances their phagocytosis

Evaluation

Side Effects	Adverse Reactions
Nausea, vomiting, skeletal pain, alopecia, diarrhea, fever, skin rash, anorexia, headache, cough, chest pain, sore throat, constipation	Neutropenia, dyspnea, splenomegaly, psoriasis, hematuria *Life-threatening:* Thrombocytopenia, myocardial infarction, adult respiratory distress syndrome in clients with sepsis

KEY: A: adult; C: child; IV: intravenous; UK: unknown; SC: subcutaneous; PB: protein-binding; t½: half-life.

Pharmacokinetics

Filgrastim administration results in a two-phase neutrophil response. An early response is seen within 24 h of administration. Following the chemotherapy-induced **nadir** (low point), a second peak in circulating neutrophils is observed. The proliferation-induced increase in neutrophils usually commences 4 to 5 days after administration is initiated, but timing may vary based on the type and dose of the myelosuppressive therapy and the client's underlying disease and prior treatment history. The elimination half-life of G-CSF in both normal and cancer clients is 3.5 h. Clearance rates are approximately 0.5 to 0.7 mL/min/kg.

G-CSF can be administered subcutaneously and by intravenous infusion. Administration of G-CSF by intravenous bolus is currently being investigated. The recommended starting dose of G-CSF is 5 μg/kg/day SC or IV infusion daily. The maximum tolerated dose has not been established. Doses may be increased in 5 μg/kg increments for each chemotherapy cycle, according to the duration and severity of the absolute neutrophil count nadir. The **absolute neutrophil count** (ANC) is determined by

Total white blood count (WBC) × percentage of neutrophils + percentage of bands

G-CSF should not be administered 24 h before or 24 h after the administration of therapeutic agents because of the potential sensitivity of rapidly dividing myeloid cells to chemotherapy. G-CSF may stimulate the proliferation of rapidly dividing cells, which may be destroyed by chemotherapy drugs.

G-CSF causes a transient increase in neutrophil counts 1 to 2 days after initiation of therapy. To achieve a sustained therapeutic response, however, G-CSF therapy should be continued until postchemotherapy nadir ANC is 10,000/mm^3. Premature discontinuation of G-CSF therapy before expected ANC recovery is not recommended.

Side Effects and Adverse Reactions

The side effects of filgrastim therapy include nausea, vomiting, skeletal pain, alopecia, diarrhea, neutropenia, fever, mucositis, fatigue, anorexia, dyspnea, headache, cough, skin rash, chest pain, generalized weakness, sore throat, stomatitis, constipation, and pain of unspecified origin. Of these reactions, bone pain was the only consistently observed reaction attributed to G-CSF therapy. The bone pain was of mild to moderate severity and well controlled with nonnarcotic analgesia. It was more frequently seen in clients receiving higher (20 to 100 μg/kg/day) intravenous doses than in clients receiving lower (3 to 10 μg/kg/day) subcutaneous doses.

G-CSF administration has no demonstrable effects on fertility in male and female rats. Its carcinogenic potential is not known. Caution should be used when G-CSF is given to pregnant women and nursing mothers. The manufacturer recommends that the benefits justify the potential risks.

Filgrastim's efficacy has not been demonstrated in children, although safety data indicate that it does not cause any greater toxicity in children than adults.

There has been no evidence of other drug interaction with filgrastim, but its administration is contraindicated in clients with known hypersensitivity to *Escherichia coli* derivant proteins.

Neupogen is supplied as 1-mL vials containing 300 μg of filgrastim or as 1.6-mL vials containing 480 μg of filgrastim. Both vials are preservative-free, and, therefore, the manufacturer recommends the vials be used one time only and that any vial left at room temperature for longer than 6 h should be discarded. Filgrastim should be stored in a refrigerator at 2 to 8°C. Freezing and shaking of the vials should be avoided.

GRANULOCYTE MACROPHAGE COLONY-STIMULATING FACTOR

Granulocyte macrophage colony-stimulating factor (GM-CSF) belongs to a group of growth factors that support survival, clonal expression, and differentiation (maturation) of hematopoietic progenitor cells. GM-CSF induces partially committed progenitor (parent) cells to divide and differentiate in the granulocyte macrophage (a type of WBC responsible for recognizing and destroying bacteria through phagocytosis) pathway. GM-CSF, unlike G-CSF, is a multilineage factor, promoting proliferation of myelomonocytic, megakaryocytic, and erythroid progenitors. Activated T cells, endothelial cells, and fibroblasts produce GM-CSF in vivo. Commercial production of GM-CSF is accomplished through recombinant DNA technology. GM-CSF is FDA approved for commercial use to induce and support myeloid reconstitution after autologous bone marrow transplant (BMT). Figure 29–7 presents the drug data for sargramostim.

Pharmacokinetics

GM-CSF has been found to effectively accelerate myeloid engraftment (growth and development of bone marrow and subsequent circulating blood cell activity) in autologous BMT. After autologous BMT in clients with non-Hodgkin's lymphoma, acute

FIGURE 29–7. Granulocyte Macrophage Colony-Stimulating Factor

Sargramostim	Dosage	**NURSING PROCESS** Assessment and Planning
Sargramostim (Leukine) Granulocyte macrophage colony-stimulating factor (GM-CSF) *Pregnancy Category:* C	A: IV 250 μg/m^2/d as a 2-h inf for 21 d after autologous BMT; a maximum tolerated dose has not been determined Some protocols use SC administration.	
Contraindications	**Drug-Lab-Food Interactions**	
Within 24 h of chemotherapy administration or within 12 h after last dose of radiation therapy, excessive leukemia myeloid blast cells in bone marrow, hypersensitivity to GM-CSF, yeast-derived products *Caution:* Pregnancy, lactation, congestive heart failure; safety in children not established; not FDA approved for children	Lithium and steroids may *increase* effect *Lab: Increase* in WBC and platelet counts	
Pharmacokinetics	**Pharmacodynamics**	Interventions
Absorption: IV: Essentially complete *Distribution:* PB: UK *Metabolism:* t½: 2 h *Excretion:* Probably in urine	IV: Onset: 7–14 d Peak: UK Duration: Baseline WBC by 1 wk after administration	

	Evaluation
Therapeutic Effects/Uses: To accelerate growth and development of bone marrow and circulating blood cell activity in autologous BMT. *Mode of Action:* Increased production and functional activity of eosinophils, macrophages, monocytes, and neutrophils	

Side Effects	Adverse Reactions
Generally well tolerated; diarrhea, fatigue, chills, weakness, local irritation at injection site, peripheral edema, rash	Pleural/pericardial effusion, rigors, GI hemorrhage, dyspnea

KEY: A: adult; IV: intravenous; UK: unknown; PB: protein-binding; t½: half-life; GI: gastrointestinal; BMT: bone marrow transplant; SC: subcutaneous.

lymphoblastic leukemia, or Hodgkin's disease, GM-CSF administration resulted in accelerated myeloid engraftment, decreased duration of antibiotic use, reduced duration of infectious episodes, and shortened hospitalizations.

A GM-CSF product is commercially available as sargramostim: Leukine.

The recommended dose of GM-CSF is 250 μg/m^2/day for 21 days as a 2-h infusion beginning 2 to 4 h after autologous bone marrow infusion.

GM-CSF should not be administered within 24 h of chemotherapy administration or within 12 h after the last dose of radiation therapy. Manufacturers recommend dose reduction or discontinuation in the presence of a severe adverse reaction, blast cell (immature, possibly malignant cell) appearance, or underlying disease progression. GM-CSF therapy should be stopped if ANC is greater than 20,000 cells/mm^3 to avoid potential complications associated with leukocytosis.

Side Effects and Adverse Reactions

Side effects of GM-CSF administration include fever, mucous membrane disorder, asthenia, malaise, sepsis, nausea, diarrhea, vomiting, anorexia, liver damage, alopecia, rash, peripheral edema, dyspnea, blood dyscracias, renal dysfunction, and central nervous system disorder. GM-CSF should be administered with caution to clients with preexisting pleural or precardial effusions because it may increase fluid retention. Sequestration of granulocytes in the pulmonary circulation has been seen with GM-CSF administration. The phenomenon has resulted in dyspnea and suggests that special attention be given to respiratory symptoms during or immediately following GM-CSF infusions, a caution that is especially important for clients with underlying pulmonary disease. If dyspnea occurs, the GM-CSF infusion should be reduced by half or discontinued.

Supraventricular dysrhythmia has been observed during GM-CSF infusion, suggesting cautious administration in clients with preexisting cardiac disease. Renal and hepatic dysfunction, as indicated by elevated serum creatinine, bilirubin, and liver function tests, have occurred with GM-CSF administration. If these values become elevated, GM-CSF dosage should be reduced or therapy interrupted.

GM-CSF therapy is contraindicated in clients with excessive leukemia myeloid blast cells in the bone marrow or peripheral blood (>10%), or in clients with known hypersensitivity to GM-CSF, yeast-derived products, or any component of the product. Because of the sensitivity of rapidly dividing hematopoietic progenitor cells to cytotoxic chemotherapy or radiologic therapy, GM-CSF should not be administered within 24 h preceding or following chemotherapy or within 12 h preceding or following radiation therapy.

GM-CSF should be administered to pregnant women or nursing mothers only if clearly indicated; that is, if the benefits outweigh the risks. Efficacy in the pediatric population has not been established.

Carcinogenic, mutagenic, or fertility effects have not been determined. Full evaluation of drug interactions have not been conducted; however, drugs that may potentiate the myeloproliferative effects of GM-CSF, such as lithium and corticosteroids, should be used with caution.

Leukine is supplied as a sterile, white, preservative-free lyophilized powder (powder that goes into solution quickly) in vials containing 250 μg or 500 μg of sargramostim. The powder is reconstituted with 1 mL of sterile water for injection. During reconstitution the diluent should be directed at the side of the vial and contents gently swirled but not shaken. Further dilution with 0.9% sodium chloride only is performed in preparation for the 2-h intravenous infusion. The final concentration of solution should be greater than 10 μg/mL. The infusion should be completed within 6 h of preparation to ensure stability and potency. Sargramostim powder, reconstituted vials, and diluted solution should be refrigerated at 2 to 8°C.

INTERLEUKINS

Interleukins are a group of proteins that are produced by the body's white blood cells—the lymphocytes. Because interleukins are hormone-like glycoproteins manufactured by the lymphocytes, they are sometimes referred to as **lymphokines.** One of the most widely studied interleukins is interleukin-2 (IL-2).

This substance, first defined in 1976, has been found to have antitumor activities. The greatest antitumor effect has been identified in clients with renal cell cancer or malignant melanoma.

IL-2 is produced commercially through recombinant DNA technology. It is marketed as aldesleukin (Proleukin) for use in the treatment of clients with metastatic renal cell carcinoma.

PHARMACOKINETICS

IL-2, administered either by IV infusion or subcutaneous injection, is rapidly distributed to the extravascular, extracellular space and eliminated from the body by metabolism in the kidney. The serum half-life of IL-2 is short. Because of this rapid clearance, IL-2 is administered in frequent, short infusions.

Proleukin is supplied in single-use vials, each of which contains 22×10^6 units of Proleukin. Unreconstituted vials should be stored in a refrigerator at 2 to 8°C (36 to 46°F). When reconstituted aseptically with 1.2 mL of sterile water for injection, each vial contains 18 million IU (1.1 mg) of Proleukin. Bacteriostatic water should not be used. The sterile water should be injected into the vial. The contents should be gently swirled, not shaken. The resulting solution should be a clear, colorless to pale yellow liquid. Any unused portion of the liquid should be discarded. The indicated dose of Proleukin should be withdrawn from the vial and diluted into a 50-mL 5% dextrose IV bag. The IV bag, if not used immediately, can be stored for 48 hours in a refrigerator. The Proleukin should be infused over a 15-min period through nonfiltered IV tubing. See Table 29–3 for dosage and administration information.

TABLE 29–3 Interleukin

Drug	Dosage	Uses and Considerations
Interleukin-2 (Proleukin)	*Metastatic renal cancer:* A: IV: 600,000 IU/kg (0.037 mg/kg) by a 15-min IV infusion q8h for a total of 14 doses. Following 9 days of rest, the schedule is repeated for another 14 doses, for a maximum of 28 doses per course	For treating metastatic renal cancer.
	Renal cancer studies: 18 million IU/m²/d for 5 days, followed by 2 days rest, then 9 million or 18 million IU/m²/d, 5 d/wk, for 5 wks	This dosage schedule and route have also been used in renal cancer studies.
	PATIENTS RECEIVING IL-2 BY ANY ROUTE, IN ANY DOSE, AND IN ANY SETTING—INPATIENT AND/OR OUTPATIENT—SHOULD BE MONITORED CLOSELY FOR SIGNS OF TOXICITY.	

KEY: A: adult; IV: intravenous; m²: square meter of body surface area.

TABLE 29–5 Organ System Toxicities with Interleukin-2 (IL-2)

Organ System	Permanently Discontinue Treatment for the Following Toxicities
Cardiovascular	Sustained ventricular tachycardia (≥ 5 beats)
	Cardiac rhythm disturbances not controlled or unresponsive to management
	Recurrent chest pain with electrocardiographic changes, documented angina or myocardial infarction
	Pericardial tamponade
Pulmonary	Intubation required > 72 hours
Renal	Renal dysfunction requiring dialysis > 72 hours
Central nervous system	Coma or toxic psychosis lasting > 48 hours
	Repetitive or difficult to control seizures
Gastrointestinal	Bowel ischemia/perforation/GI bleeding requiring surgery

Source: Proleukin: Aldesleukin for Injection. Cetus/Chiron Corp., Emeryville, CA. Printed with permission.

SIDE EFFECTS AND ADVERSE REACTIONS

The side effects most frequently reported as a result of IL-2 include hypotension, nausea, vomiting, diarrhea, mental status changes, oliguria/anuria, anemia, thrombocytopenia, fever, chills, sinus tachycardia, pulmonary congestion, dyspnea, pain at injection site, fatigue, weakness, malaise, and elevated liver function tests. See Table 29–4 for additional side effects. According to the manufacturer, Proleukin should be permanently discontinued for certain organ system toxicities (Table 29–5) and held and restarted under specific parameters for other toxicities (Table 29–6).

TABLE 29–4 Incidence of Adverse Events to Interleukin-2

Events by Body System	% of Patients	Events by Body System	% of Patients
Cardiovascular		**Gastrointestinal**	
Hypotension	85	Nausea and Vomiting	87
(requiring pressors)	71	Diarrhea	76
Sinus Tachycardia	70	Stomatitis	32
Arrhythmias	22	Anorexia	27
Atrial	8	GI Bleeding	13
Supraventricular	5	(requiring surgery)	2
Ventricular	3	Dyspepsia	7
Junctional	1	Constipation	5
Bradycardia	7	Intestinal Perforation/Ileus	2
Premature Ventricular Contractions	5	Pancreatitis	< 1
Premature Atrial Contractions	4		
Myocardial Ischemia	3	**Neurologic**	
Myocardial Infarction	2	Mental Status Changes	73
Cardiac arrest	2	Dizziness	17
Congestive heart failure	1	Sensory Dysfunction	10
Myocarditis	1	Special Sensory Disorders (vision, speech, taste)	7
Stroke	1	Syncope	3
Gangrene	1	Motor Dysfunction	2
Pericardial Effusion	1	Coma	1
Endocarditis	1	Seizure (grand mal)	1
Thrombosis	1		

Source: Proleukin: Aldesleukin for Injection. Cetus/Chiron Corp., Emeryville, CA. Printed with permission.

TABLE 29–6 Interleukin-2 Dose Held and Given, Listed According to Organ System

Organ System	Hold Dose For	Subsequent Doses May Be Given If
Cardiovascular	Atrial fibrillation, supraventricular tachycardia, or bradycardia that requires treatment or is recurrent or persistent Systolic bp < 90 mmHg with increasing requirements for pressors Any ECG change consistent with MI or ischemia with or without chest pain; suspicion of cardiac ischemia	Client is asymptomatic with full recovery to normal sinus rhythm Systolic bp ≥ 90 mmHg and stable or improving requirements for pressors Client is asymptomatic, MI has been ruled out, clinical suspicion of angina is low
Pulmonary	O_2 saturation < 94% on room air or < 90% with 2 L O_2 by nasal prongs	O_2 saturation ≥ 94% on room air or ≥ 90% with 2 L O_2 by nasal prongs
Central Nervous System	Mental status changes, including moderate confusion or agitation	Mental status changes completely resolved
Systemic	Sepsis syndrome, client is clinically unstable	Sepsis syndrome has resolved, client is clinically stable, infection is under treatment
Renal	Serum creatinine ≥ 4.5 mg/dL or a serum creatinine of 4 mg/dL in the presence of severe volume overload, acidosis, or hyperkalemia Persistent oliguria, urine output of ≤ 10 mL/hour for 16 to 24 hours with rising serum creatinine	Serum creatinine < 4 mg/dL and fluid and electrolyte status is stable Urine output > 10 mL/hour with a decrease of serum creatinine ≥ 1.5 mg/dL or normalization of serum creatinine
Hepatic	Signs of hepatic failure including encephalopathy, increasing ascites, liver pain, hypoglycemia	All signs of hepatic failure have resolved*
Gastrointestinal	Stool guaiac repeatedly > 3–4 +	Stool guaiac negative
Skin	Bullous dermatitis or marked worsening of preexisting skin condition (avoid topical steroid therapy)	Resolution of all signs of bullous dermatitis

KEY: *bp: blood pressure; ECG: electrocardiographic; MI: myocardial infarction.*
* *Discontinue all further treatment for that course. Consider starting a new course of treatment at least 7 weeks after cessation of adverse event and hospital discharge.*
Source: Proleukin: Aldesleukin for Injection. Cetus/Chiron Corp., Emeryville, CA. Printed with permission.

NURSING PROCESS: BIOLOGIC RESPONSE MODIFIERS

ASSESSMENT

- Obtain baseline information about the client's physical status, including height, weight, vital signs (VS), laboratory values (CBC, uric acid, electrolytes, BUN, creatinine, and liver function tests), cardiopulmonary assessment, intake and output, skin assessment, daily activities status (ability to perform activities of daily living, sleep-rest cycle), nutritional status, presence or absence of underlying symptoms of disease, and the use of current or past medication and treatment.
- Assess CBC and platelet count (with filgrastim and sargramostim) before therapy and biweekly throughout therapy to avoid leukocytosis. Assess renal and hepatic function tests in clients with dysfunction (liver enzymes, BUN, serum creatinine). With erythropoietin, assess blood pressure before start and especially early in therapy. Most clients will need supplemental iron. Desired levels are > 100 ng/mL for serum ferritin and > 20% for serum iron transferrin saturation.
- Obtain baseline data regarding the client's psychosocial status, including educational level, ability and desire to learn, support systems, past coping strategies, presence or absence of emotional difficulties, and self-care abilities.
- Assess the client for signs and symptoms of biologic response modifiers (BRM), such as fatigue, chills, diarrhea, and weakness. With filgrastim, be alert to changes in clients with preexisting cardiac conditions.
- Assess the client's and family's ability to administer subcutaneous BRM.
- Determine the client's and family's understanding of BRM and related side effects.

POTENTIAL NURSING DIAGNOSES

- Altered nutrition; less than body requirements
- High risk for infection
- High risk for fluid volume deficit
- Altered oral mucous membrane
- Fatigue
- Body image disturbance
- Anxiety
- Fear
- High risk for caregiver role strain

PLANNING

- Client and family will verbalize an understanding of the importance of reporting BRM-related side effects.
- Client and family will demonstrate correct and safe BRM administration.
- Client and family will identify strategies to deal with BRM-related side effects.
- Client will remain free of infection (filgrastim and sargramostim).

NURSING INTERVENTIONS

- Monitor the client's temperature at the onset of chills.
- Administer prescribed meperidine 25 to 50 mg IV to decrease rigors.
- Premedicate the client with acetaminophen to reduce chills and fever and with diphenhydramine to reduce nausea.
- Cover the client with blankets to promote warmth during chills.
- Encourage the client to rest when tired and to notify health care provider if profound fatigue or anorexia occurs.
- Encourage the client to drink at least 2 L of fluid a day to promote excretion of cellular breakdown products.
- Administer antiemetic as necessary. Premedicate the client with antiemetic and administer antiemetic around the clock for 24 h after BRM administration to further delay nausea or vomiting.
- Consult the dietitian, social worker, and physical or occupational therapist as necessary.
- Provide the client and family the opportunity to discuss the effect of BRM therapy on the quality of life.
- Refer the client and family to a financial counselor if reimbursement of BRM therapy is problematic.
- Administer BRM at bedtime to decrease the consequences of fatigue.
- Continue with the same brand of BRM, and no-

tify the health care provider if you are considering changing the brand.

- Remember, with sargramostim, use only one dose per vial; be alert for expiration date. Avoid shaking vial. Reconstituted solutions are clear; use within 6 h and discard unused portion. Recall that albumin may be added, depending on drug concentration, to prevent adsorption of drug to components of the drug delivery system.
- Remember, with filgrastim, drug vials are for one-time use; any vial left at room temperature for more than 6 h should be discarded. Drug vials are preservative free. Store in refrigerator at 2 to 8°C. Avoid shaking vials.

CLIENT TEACHING

General
- Explain to the client and family the rationale for BRM therapy.
- Explain the frequency and rationale for studies and procedures during BRM therapy.
- Inform the client and family that most BRM side effects disappear within 72 to 96 h after discontinuation of therapy.
- Instruct clients of childbearing age to use contraceptives during BRM therapy and for 2 y after completion of therapy.
- Provide the client with information regarding the effect on sexuality of BRM-related fatigue.

Side Effects
- Advise the client to report episodes of difficulty in concentration, confusion, or somnolence.
- Report weight loss.
- Report dyspnea, palpitations, and signs of infection or bleeding.

Skill
- Demonstrate correct drug administration techniques.
- Provide the client and family with written or video instructions regarding BRM self-administration.

EVALUATION

- Evaluate the client's and family's education strategies by asking them to discuss the potential effect of BRM therapy on the quality of life.
- Evaluate the client's and family's BRM self-administration technique.
- Evaluate periodically the client's and family's management of BRM-related side effects.
- There will be a decreased incidence of infection in clients after autologous bone marrow transplant.

SUMMARY

BRM therapy is in its infancy. As clinical trial results yield more information about BRM activity and clinical efficacy, the indications for the use of BRMs will expand. As more is learned about the effect of BRMs on the quality of client life, attention will be directed toward side effect management and symptom prevention. Nurses play a key role in both the identification and management of BRM-related toxicities. Through assessment of clients receiving BRMs and a knowledge of BRM activity, nurses can develop a plan of care that will result in clients receiving BRM therapy in a safe and comfortable manner.

■ CASE STUDY
Client's Treatment for Cancer

J.W. is a 55-year-old man with metastatic nonsmall-cell cancer of the lung. His past treatment regimen included external-beam chest irradiation and combination chemotherapy. Two weeks prior to hospitalization, J.W. received a course of carboplatin, Velban, and methotrexate as an outpatient. He was admitted to the hospital with neutropenia and anemia. Upon assessment J.W. was cachectic, weak, and able to perform activities of daily living only with assistance. Admitting laboratory data were Hgb (hemoglobin) 7.4; Hct 21.9; platelets 116,000; and WBC 600 with ANC of 96. J.W. was started on Neupogen 480 μg, SC, daily and EPO 10,000 U, SC, every other day. Parenteral antibiotic therapy was also initiated. Nursing diagnoses for J.W. included a potential for infection related to neutropenia, fatigue related to anemia, and anxiety related to hospitalization.

Nursing interventions included

1. Good handwashing before and after client contact
2. No one with cold or infection to enter client's room
3. Vital signs and pulmonary assessment every 4 h
4. Inspection of all sites associated with a high risk for infection (venipuncture sites, oral cavity, perirectal area) every shift
5. No rectal temps, suppositories, enemas, or urinary catheters
6. Daily laboratory monitoring
7. Masks worn at all times during client contact
8. Bedside physical therapy
9. Emotional support of client and family
10. Client and family instruction in giving subcutaneous injections and about the signs and symptoms of infection.

J.W. was continued on filgrastim (Neupogen) and erythropoietin (EPO). The following laboratory data were obtained:

Lab Tests	Day 1	Day 2	Day 3	Day 4	Day 5
Hgb	6.9	6.5	7.1	7.8	7.9
Hct	20.6	19.4	21.6	22.9	22.9
Platelets	107.000	115,000	125,000	142,000	159,000
WBC/ANC	600/0	1000/0	1200/168	9400/4700	31500/18270

Neupogen was discontinued on day 5, and antibiotics were discontinued on day 4, but EPO was continued. J.W.'s physical therapy was continued in the physical therapy department. Because J.W. refused red blood cell transfusion on the basis of religious beliefs, he was discharged to home (day 5) on EPO 10,000 U, SC, every other day.

STUDY QUESTIONS

1. Identify the three functions of BRMs.
2. Describe how colony-stimulating factors exert their effect in the body.
3. List the side effects of interferon alpha, G-CSF; GM-CSF, and interleukin-2.
4. Discuss client and family teaching strategies for clients receiving erythropoietin.
5. Explain how to administer EPO, G-CSF, and GM-CSF.
6. Describe the nursing assessment for clients receiving IL-2 (discussion should include preadministration, administration, and post administration assessments).

Unit VII

Respiratory Agents

RESPIRATORY SYSTEM

The respiratory tract is divided into two major parts: (1) the upper respiratory tract, which consists of the nares, nasal cavity, pharynx, and larynx, and (2) the lower respiratory tract, which comprises the trachea, bronchi, bronchioles, alveoli, and alveolar-capillary membrane. Air enters through the upper respiratory tract and travels to the lower respiratory tract where gas exchanges take place. Figure VII–1 illustrates these components.

Ventilation and *respiration* are distinct terms and should not be used interchangeably. **Ventilation** is the movement of air from the atmosphere through the upper and lower airways to the alveoli. **Respiration** is the process whereby gas exchange occurs at the alveolar-capillary membrane.

Respiration has three phases: (1) ventilation, in which oxygen passes through the airways; (2) perfusion, in which blood from the pulmonary circulation is adequate at the alveolar-capillary bed; and (3) diffusion (molecules move from higher concentration to lower concentration) of gases, in which oxygen passes into the capillary bed to be circulated and carbon dioxide leaves the capillary bed and diffuses into the alveoli for ventilatory excretion.

Perfusion is influenced by alveolar pressure. For gas exchange, the perfusion of each alveolus must be matched by adequate ventilation. Factors such as mucosal edema, secretions, and bronchospasm increase the resistance to airflow and decrease ventilation and diffusion of gases.

The chest cavity is a closed compartment bounded by 12 ribs, the diaphragm, thoracic vertebrae, sternum, neck muscles, and intercostal muscles between the ribs. The pleura is a membrane that encases the lungs. The lungs are divided into lobes: the right lung has three lobes and the left lung has two lobes. The heart, which is not attached to the lungs, lies on the midleft side in the chest cavity.

LUNG COMPLIANCE

Lung compliance (lung volume based on the unit of pressure in the alveoli) determines the lung's ability to stretch; i.e., its tissue elasticity. Lung compliance is determined by (1) connec-

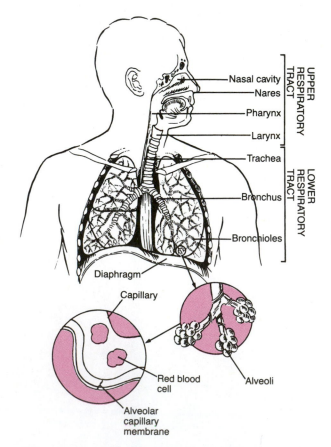

FIGURE VII–1 Basic structures of the respiratory tract.

tive tissue (collagen and elastin) and (2) surface tension in the alveoli that is controlled by surfactant. Surfactant lowers the surface tension in the alveoli and prevents interstitial fluid from entering. Increased (high) lung compliance is present with chronic obstructive pulmonary disease (COPD), and decreased (low) lung compliance occurs with restrictive pulmonary disease. With low compliance, there is decreased lung volume, due to increased connective tissue or increased surface tension; the lungs become "stiff," and it takes greater than normal pressure to expand lung tissue.

CONTROL OF RESPIRATION

Oxygen (O_2), carbon dioxide (CO_2), and hydrogen (H^+) ion concentration in the blood influence respiration. Chemoreceptors are sensors that are stimulated by changes in these gases and ion. The central chemoreceptors, located in the medulla near the respiratory center and cerebrospinal fluid, respond to an increase in CO_2 and a decrease in pH by increasing ventilation. However, if the CO_2 level remains elevated, the stimulus to increase ventilation is lost.

Peripheral chemoreceptors located in the carotid and aortic bodies respond to changes in oxygen (Po_2) levels. A low blood O_2 level ($Po_2 < 60$ mmHg) stimulates the peripheral chemoreceptors, which in turn stimulate the respiratory center in the medulla, and ventilation is increased. If O_2 therapy increases the oxygen level in the blood, the Po_2 may be too high to stimulate the peripheral chemoreceptors, and ventilation will be depressed.

BRONCHIAL SMOOTH MUSCLE

The tracheobronchial tube is composed of smooth muscle whose fibers spiral around the tracheobronchial tube, becoming more closely spaced as they near the terminal bronchioles (Fig. VII–2). Contraction of these muscles constricts the airway. The sympathetic and parasympathetic nervous systems affect the bronchial smooth muscle in opposite ways. The vagus nerve (parasympathetic nervous system) releases acetylcholine, which causes bronchoconstriction. The sympathetic nervous system releases epinephrine, which stimulates the beta$_2$ receptor in the bronchial smooth muscle, resulting in bronchodilation. These two nervous systems counterbalance each other to maintain homeostasis.

Cyclic adenosine monophosphate (cyclic AMP) in the cytoplasm of bronchial cells increases bronchodilation by relaxing the bronchial smooth muscles. The pulmonary enzyme phosphodiesterase can inactivate cyclic AMP. Drugs of the methylxanthine group (theophylline) inactivate phosphodiesterase, thus permitting cyclic AMP to function.

This unit includes Chapter 30, Drugs for Common Upper Respiratory Infections, and Chapter 31, Drugs for Acute and Chronic Lower Respiratory Disorders. Chapter 30 discusses drugs that are used to relieve cold symptoms, such as antihistamines, decongestants, antitussives, and expectorants. Drugs that are used to alleviate and control airway obstruction are presented in Chapter 31. These include the sympathomimetics (adrenergics), particularly the beta$_2$ adrenergics; the methylxanthines, such as theophylline; glucocorticoids; cromolyn sodium; and mucolytics. Use of the aerosol inhaler is described. Drug charts are included in each chapter, and the nursing process with client teaching is emphasized.

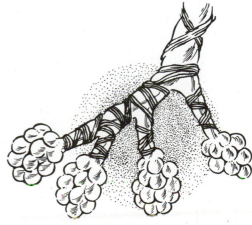

FIGURE VII–2 The bronchial smooth muscle fibers become more closely spaced as they near the alveoli.

Chapter 30

Drugs for Common Upper Respiratory Infections

OUTLINE

Objectives
Terms
Introduction
Common Cold and Acute
  Rhinitis
    Antihistamines

Nursing Process
Nasal and Systemic
  Decongestants
Antitussives
Expectorants
Sinusitis

Acute Pharyngitis
Acute Tonsillitis
Acute Laryngitis
Nursing Process: Common Cold
Study Questions

OBJECTIVES

Define antihistamine, decongestant, antitussive, and expectorant.

Define rhinitis, sinusitis, pharyngitis, and laryngitis.

Identify the side effects of nasal decongestants and explain how they can be avoided.

Describe the nursing process, including client teaching, for drugs used to treat the common cold.

TERMS

acute rhinitis
allergic rhinitis
antihistamine
antitussive
common cold

decongestant
expectorant
laryngitis
pharyngitis
rebound nasal congestion

rhinorrhea
sinusitis
tonsillitis

INTRODUCTION

Upper respiratory infections (URIs) include the common cold, acute rhinitis, sinusitis, acute tonsillitis, and acute laryngitis. The common cold is the most prevalent type of URI. Adults have an average of two to four colds per year, and children have an average of four to twelve colds per year. Incidence is seasonally variable, with approximately 50% of the population having a winter cold and 25% having a summer cold. Normally, a cold is not considered to be a life-threatening illness; however, it causes physical and mental discomfort and loss of time at work and school. The common cold is a very expensive illness in the United States: over $500 million is spent each year on over-the-counter (OTC) cold and cough preparations.

COMMON COLD AND ACUTE RHINITIS

The **common cold** is caused by the rhinovirus and affects primarily the nasopharyngeal tract. **Acute rhinitis** (acute inflammation of the mucous membranes of the nose) usually accompanies the common cold. Acute rhinitis is not the same as **allergic rhinitis,** often referred to as "hay fever," which is caused by pollen or a foreign substance such as animal dander. There are increased nasal secretions in both acute rhinitis and allergic rhinitis.

A cold is most contagious 1 to 4 days prior to the onset of symptoms (the incubation period) and during the first 3 days of the cold. Transmission occurs more frequently from touching contaminated surfaces and then touching the nose or mouth than from viral droplets from sneezing.

There is an old saying, "Curing a cold takes 1 week with treatment or 7 days without treatment." Home remedies include rest, chicken noodle soup, hot toddy (sugar, alcohol, and tea), vitamin C (debatable), and megadoses of vitamins (controversial). The four groups of drugs used to manage cold symptoms are antihistamines (H_1 blocker), decongestants (sympathomimetic amines), antitussives, and expectorants. These drugs can be used singly or in combination preparations.

Symptoms of the common cold include **rhinorrhea** (watery nasal discharge), nasal congestion, cough, and increased mucosal secretions. If a bacterial infection secondary to the cold occurs, infectious rhinitis may result and the nasal discharge becomes tenacious, mucoid, and yellow or yellowgreen in color. The nasal secretions are discolored by white blood cells and cellular debris that are byproducts of the fight against the bacterial infection.

ANTIHISTAMINES

Antihistamines, or H_1 blockers, compete with histamine for receptor sites, thus preventing a histamine response. H_1 blockers are also called histamine antagonists. The two types of histamine receptors, H_1 and H_2, cause different responses. When the H_1 receptor is stimulated, the extravascular smooth muscles, including those lining the nasal cavity, are constricted. With stimulation of the H_2 receptor, an increase in gastric secretions occurs, which is a cause of peptic ulcer (see Chapter 37). These two types of histamine receptors should not be confused. Antihistamines decrease nasopharyngeal secretions by blocking the H_1 receptor.

The anticholinergic properties of most antihistamines cause dryness of the mouth and decreased secretions, making them useful in treating rhinitis caused by the common cold. Antihistamines also decrease the nasal itching and tickling that cause sneezing. Many OTC cold remedies contain an antihistamine, which can cause drowsiness. Clients should be alerted not to drive or operate dangerous machinery if they are taking a medication that contains an antihistamine.

The antihistamines are not useful in an emergency situation such as anaphylaxis. Most antihistamines are rapidly absorbed in 15 minutes, but they are not potent enough to combat anaphylaxis. The antihistamine diphenhydramine (Benadryl) has been available for years, and it is frequently combined with other ingredients in cold remedy preparations. Its primary use is to treat rhinitis. Figure 30–1 lists the pharmacologic behavior of diphenhydramine.

Pharmacokinetics

Diphenhydramine can be administered orally, intramuscularly, or intravenously. It is well absorbed from the gastrointestinal (GI) tract, but systemic absorption from topical use is minimal. It is highly protein-bound (98% to 99%) and has an average half-life of 2 to 7 h. Diphenhydramine is metabolized by the liver and excreted as metabolites in the urine.

Pharmacodynamics

Diphenhydramine blocks the effects of histamine by competing for and occupying H_1 receptor sites. It has anticholinergic effects and should be avoided

FIGURE 30–1. Antihistamine

Antihistamine	**Dosage**	**NURSING PROCESS** Assessment and Planning
Diphenhydramine HCl (Benadryl), 🍁 Allerdryl *Pregnancy Category:* B	A: PO: 25–50 mg q6–8h A: IM/IV: 10–50 mg as single dose, q4–6h; max; 400 mg/d C: PO/IM/IV 5 mg/kg/d in 4 divided doses; max: 300 mg/d	
Contraindications	**Drug-Lab-Food Interactions**	
Acute asthmatic attack, severe liver disease, lower respiratory disease, neonate; MAOIs *Caution:* Narrow-angle glaucoma, benign prostatic hypertrophy, pregnancy, newborn or premature infant, breast feeding, urinary retention	*Increase* CNS depression with alcohol, narcotics, hypnotics, barbiturates; avoid use of MAOIs	
Pharmacokinetics	**Pharmacodynamics**	Interventions
Absorption: PO: Well absorbed *Distribution:* PB: 82% *Metabolism:* t½: 2–7 h *Excretion:* In urine as metabolites	PO: Onset: 15–45 min Peak: 1–4 h Duration: 4–8 h IM: Onset: 15–30 min Peak: 1–4 h Duration: 4–7 h IV: Onset: Immediate Peak: 0.5–1 h Duration: 4–7 h	

	Evaluation
Therapeutic Effects/Uses: To treat allergic rhinitis, itching; to prevent motion sickness; sleep aid; antitussive. *Mode of Action:* Blocks histamine, thereby decreasing allergic response. Affects respiratory system, blood vessels, and GI system.	

Side Effects	**Adverse Reactions**
Drowsiness, dizziness, fatigue, nausea, vomiting, urinary retention, constipation, blurred vision, dry mouth and throat, reduced secretions, hypotension, epigastric distress, blurred vision, hearing disturbances; excitation in children; photosensitivity	*Life-threatening:* Agranulocytosis, hemolytic anemia, thrombocytopenia

KEY: A: adult; C: child; PO: by mouth; IM: intramuscular; IV: intravenous; PB: protein-binding; MAOIs: monoamine oxidase inhibitors; t½: half-life; 🍁 : Canadian drug names.

by clients with narrow-angle glaucoma. Drowsiness is a major side effect of the drug, and in fact it has been used as an ingredient in "sleep aid" products. This drug is also used as an antitussive (for cough). Its onset of action can occur in as few as 15 minutes when taken orally and intramuscularly. The onset of action is immediate with intravenous use. The duration of action is 4 to 8 h.

Diphenhydramine can cause central nervous system depression if taken with alcohol, narcotics, hypnotics, or barbiturates.

Table 30–1 lists selected antihistamines or antihistamine-like agents that are useful for treating rhinitis.

Side Effects and Adverse Reactions

The most common side effects are drowsiness, dizziness, fatigue, and disturbed coordination. Skin rashes and anticholinergic symptoms, such as dry mouth, urine retention, blurred vision, and wheezing, may be seen.

NURSING PROCESS: ANTIHISTAMINE: Diphenhydramine

ASSESSMENT

- Obtain baseline vital signs (VS).
- Obtain drug history; report if drug-drug interaction is probable.
- Assess for signs and symptoms of urinary dysfunction, including retention, dysuria, and frequency.
- Assess CBC during drug therapy.
- Assess cardiac and respiratory status.
- If allergic reaction, obtain history of environmental exposures, drugs, recent foods, and stress.

POTENTIAL NURSING DIAGNOSES

- Fluid volume deficit, potential
- Sleep pattern disturbance

PLANNING

- Client will have improvement of histamine-associated (allergy) effects.
- Client will have improved sleep, if used as a sleep aid.

NURSING INTERVENTIONS

- Give with food to decrease gastric distress.
- Administer IM in large muscle. Avoid SC injection.

CLIENT TEACHING

General

- Instruct client to avoid driving a motor vehicle and other dangerous activities if drowsiness occurs or until stabilized on drug.

- Avoid alcohol and other CNS depressants.
- Instruct client to take drug as prescribed. Notify health care provider if confusion or hypotension occurs.
- For prophylaxis of motion sickness, take drug at least 30 min before offending event and then before meals and h.s. during the event.
- Inform the breast-feeding mother that small amounts of drug pass into the breast milk. Because children are more susceptible to the side effects of antihistamines, such as unusual excitement or irritability, breast feeding is not recommended while on these drugs.

Side Effects

- Instruct family member(s) or parent(s) that children are more sensitive to the effects of antihistamines; nightmares, nervousness, and irritability are more likely to occur.
- Inform older adults that they are more sensitive to the effects of antihistamines. Confusion, difficult or painful urination, dizziness, drowsiness, feeling faint, and dryness of the mouth, nose, or throat are more likely to occur in the older client.
- For temporary relief of mouth dryness, suggest using sugarless candy or gum, ice chips, or using a saliva substitute.

EVALUATION

- Evaluate effectiveness of drug in relieving allergic symptoms or as a sleep aid.

TABLE 30–1 Antihistamines for Treatment of Allergic Rhinitis

Generic (Brand)	Route and Dosage	Uses and Considerations
Antihistamines		
Chlorpheniramine maleate (Chlor-Trimeton, Kloromin, Phenetron, Telechlor, Teldrin)	A: PO: 2–4 mg q4–6h; max: 24 mg/24 h SR: 8–12 mg q8–12 h C: 6–12 y: PO: 2 mg q4–6h	For allergies including allergic rhinitis. May be in combination with nasal decongestant. *Pregnancy category:* C; PB: 72%; t½: 20–24 h
Diphenhydramine (Benadryl)	See Prototype Drug Chart (Fig. 30–1)	For allergic rhinitis, urticaria, nausea, and vomiting due to motion sickness. May be used as a nighttime sleep aid and as an antitussive drug. *Pregnancy category:* B; PB: 82%; t½: 2–7 h
Phenothiazines (Antihistamine Action)		
Promethazine HCl (Phenergan, Prometh, Prorex, V-Gan)	A: PO/IM: 12.5–25 mg q4–6h PRN a.c. & h.s.; *max:* 150 mg/d C: PO/IM: 0.5 mg/kg q4–6h Tab & suppository not recommended <2 y; *max:* 18.75 mg/d	For allergies, rhinitis, nausea, vomiting, motion sickness, and adjunct to analgesics for pain. Has a pronounced sedative effect. Avoid alcohol and CNS depressants. *Pregnancy category:* C; PB: UK; t½: UK
Trimeprazine tartrate (Temaril)	*Non-SR:* A: PO: 2.5 mg q.i.d. C 3–12 y: PO: 2.5 mg t.i.d. C 0.5–3 y: 1.25 mg t.i.d. *SR:* A: PO: 5 mg q12h C >6 y: PO: 5 mg/d	For allergies, rhinitis, and relief of pruritic symptoms. *Pregnancy category:* C; PB: UK; t½: UK
Piperazine Derivative		
Hydroxyzine (Atarax, Vistaril)	A: PO: 25–100 mg t.i.d./q.i.d. C >6 y: 50–100 mg/d in divided doses; *For pruritus:* C: <6 y: PO: 50 mg/d in divided doses	For allergies, relief of tension and anxiety, and to prevent nausea and vomiting. Has a pronounced sedative effect. Avoid alcohol and CNS depressants. *Pregnancy category:* C; PB: UK; t½: 3 h
Butyrophenone Derivative		
Terfenadine (Seldane)	A: PO: 60 mg b.i.d. C >6 y: PO: 30 mg b.i.d. C 3–6 y: PO: 15 mg b.i.d.	Relief of allergic rhinitis (sneezing, red itching eyes, tearing). Give with food. *Pregnancy category:* C; PB: 97%; t½: 20 h
Ethanolamine Derivative		
Carbinoxamine and pseudoephedrine (Carbiset, Carbodec, Rondec)	A: PO: 5 mL q.i.d. or 1 tab q.i.d. C <18 mo: PO: 0.25–1 mL q.i.d. C 1.5–6 y: PO: 2.5 mL t.i.d./q.i.d. C >6 y: PO: 5 mL b.i.d./q.i.d.	For allergy control. Combination of an antihistamine and decongestant. *Pregnancy category:* C; PB: UK; t½: 10–20 h
Clemastine fumarate (Tavist)	A: PO: 1.34–2.68 mg, b.i.d., t.i.d.; *max:* 8 mg/d C <12 y: PO: 0.67–1.34 mg, b.i.d.	For relief of allergic rhinitis and urticaria. *Pregnancy category:* C; PB: UK; t½: UK
Ethylenediamine Derivative		
Tripelennamine HCl (Pelamine)	A: PO: 25–50 mg q4–6h or SR: 100 mg q8–12h; *max:* 600 mg/d C: PO: 5 mg/kg/d q 4–6 h in divided doses; *max:* 300 mg/d	For allergies. Has a mild CNS depressant effect. Take with food to decrease GI upset. *Pregnancy category:* B; PB: UK; t½: UK
Piperidine Derivatives		
Azatadine maleate (Optimine)	A: PO: 1–2 mg b.i.d., t.i.d. C <12 y: PO: not recommended	Relief of allergic rhinitis and chronic urticaria. Drowsiness, dizziness, and hypotension may occur. *Pregnancy category:* B; PB: UK; t½: 9–12 h
Cyproheptadine HCl (Periactin)	A: PO: 4–20 mg/d divided q8h; *max:* 0.5 mg/kg/d C >6 y: PO: 4 mg q8–12h; *max:* 16 mg/d C (2–6 y): PO: 2 mg, q8–12 h	For allergies (rhinitis, conjunctivitis, pruritus). Common side effects include drowsiness, dry mouth, dizziness, epigastric distress. *Pregnancy category:* B; PB: UK; t½: UK
Propylamine Derivatives		
Brompheniramine maleate (Bromphen, Dimetane, Histaject, Nasahist B, Oraminic II)	A: PO: 4 mg q4–6h or SR: 8 mg q8–12h; *max:* 24 mg/d IM/IV/SC: 10 mg q8–12h; *max:* 40 mg/d C 6–12 y: PO: 2 mg q4–6h; *max:* 12–16 mg/d	For allergies. Also present in various cough and decongestant formulas. *Pregnancy category:* C; PB: UK; t½: 25–36 h
Dexchlorpheniramine maleate (Dexchlor, Poladex, Polaramine)	A: PO: 2 mg q4–6h or SR: 4–6 mg q8–12h or h.s. C >6 y: PO: 1 mg q4–6h or SR: 4 mg h.s.	Relief of allergic rhinitis. May be used with epinephrine to treat anaphylactic reaction. *Pregnancy category:* B; PB: UK; t½: UK

TABLE 30–1 Antihistamines for Treatment of Allergic Rhinitis (*Continued*)

Generic (Brand)	Route and Dosage	Uses and Considerations
Triprolidine and pseu-doephedrine (Actifed)	A: PO: 1 tab, q4–6h; *max:* 4 tab/d C >6 y: PO: ½ tab q6–8h; *max:* 2 tab/d	For rhinitis. A combination of an antihistamine and decongestant. *Pregnancy category:* B; PB: UK; t½: 3 h
Triprolidine HCl (Alleract, Myidyl)	A: PO: 2.5 mg q6–8h; *max:* 10 mg/d C 6–12 y: PO: 1.25 mg q6–8h; *max:* 5 mg/d C 2–5 y: PO: 0.6 mg t.i.d./q.i.d.; *max:* 2.5 mg/d C 4 mo–2 y: PO: 0.3 mg t.i.d./q.i.d.; *max:* 1.25 mg/d	For allergies. Similar effects as other antihistamines. *Pregnancy category:* C; PB: UK; t½: UK
Other Cromolyn sodium (Intal)	*Prophylaxis bronchial asthma:* A&C >5 y: Inhal: 2 metered sprays or PO: 20 mg ≤ 1 h before exercise *Allergic rhinitis:* A&C >5 y: 1 spray per nostril t.i.d./q.i.d.; *max:* 6 per day	For treatment of allergic rhinitis, bronchial asthma, and prevention of bronchospasm. It is *not* an antihistamine. *Pregnancy category:* B; PB: UK; t½: 1.5 h
Miscellaneous Astemizole (Hismanal)	A: PO: 30 mg on day 1; 20 mg on day 2, 10 mg on day 3 and thereafter; take on empty stomach C 6–12 y: PO: 5 mg/d C <6 y: PO: 0.2 mg/kg/d	Treatment of allergic rhinitis and urticaria. Has less anticholinergic effect than diphenhydramine. *Pregnancy category:* C; PB: 96%; t½: 2.5 d
Cetirizine	A: 5–10 mg/d	For allergies. *Pregnancy category:* C; PB: 93%; t½: 8 h
Loratadine (Claritin)	A: PO: 10 mg daily	Relief of allergic rhinitis. Long-acting H$_1$ blocking effect. *Pregnancy category:* B; PB: UK; t½: 8–11 h
Methdilazine HCl (Tacaryl)	A: PO: 8 mg b.i.d./q.i.d. C >3 y: PO: 4 mg b.i.d./q.i.d.	For allergies and pruritus. *Pregnancy category:* B; PB: UK; t½: UK

KEY: A: adult; C: child; PO: by mouth; SC: subcutaneous; IM: intramuscular; IV: intravenous; >: greater than; <: less than; UK: unknown; PB: protein-binding; t½: half-life; SR: sustained-release; tab: tablet; CNS: central nervous system; inhal: inhaler.

NASAL AND SYSTEMIC DECONGESTANTS

Nasal congestion results from dilation of nasal blood vessels due to infection, inflammation, or allergy. With this dilation, there is a transudation of fluid into the tissue spaces, resulting in swelling of the nasal cavity. Nasal **decongestants** (sympathomimetic amines) stimulate the alpha-adrenergic receptors, thus producing vascular constriction (vasoconstriction) of the capillaries within the nasal mucosa. The result is shrinking of the nasal mucous membranes and a reduction in fluid secretion (runny nose).

Nasal decongestants are administered by nasal spray or drops or in tablet, capsule, or liquid form. Frequent use of decongestants, especially nasal spray or drops, can result in tolerance and **rebound nasal congestion** (rebound vasodilation instead of vasoconstriction). The rebound nasal congestion is caused by irritation of the nasal mucosa.

The systemic decongestants (alpha-adrenergic agonists) are available in tablet, capsule, and liquid forms and are primarily used for allergic rhinitis, including hay fever, and acute coryza (profuse nasal discharge). Examples of systemic decongestants are ephedrine, phenylpropanolamine, phenylephrine, and pseudoephedrine. These agents are frequently combined with an antihistamine, analgesic, or antitussive in oral cold remedies. The advantage of systemic decongestants is that they relieve nasal congestion for a longer period of time than the nasal decongestants; however, today there are long-acting nasal decongestants. The nasal decongestants usually act promptly and cause fewer side effects than the systemic decongestants. Table 30–2 provides drugs, dosages, and uses and considerations of systemic and nasal decongestants.

Side Effects and Adverse Reactions

The incidence of side effects is low with use of topical preparations such as nose drops. Decongestants

TABLE 30–2 Systemic and Nasal Decongestants (Sympathomimetic Amines)

Generic (Brand)	Route and Dosage	Uses and Considerations
Ephedrine SO$_4$ (Ectasule, Ephedsol, Vatronol)	A: PO: 25–50 mg t.i.d./q.i.d. PRN SC/IM/IV: 25–50 mg; may repeat q10min; max: 150 mg/24 h	Relief of allergic rhinitis, nasal congestion, sinusitis, mild acute and chronic asthma; improves narcotic-impaired respiration; corrects hypotension. It is an alpha- and beta-adrenergic agonist. OTC drug used alone or in combination. *Pregnancy category:* C; PB: UK; t½: 3–6 h
Naphazoline HCl (Allerest, Albalon)	A&C >12 y: 2 gtt or 0.05% spray in each nostril; q3–6h ≤ 5 d C (6–12 y): 0.025%, 1–2 gtt in each nostril	Relief of nasal congestion, allergic rhinitis. Can cause rebound congestion, transient hypertension, bradycardia, cardiac dysrhythmias. Use only 3–5 d. *Pregnancy category:* C; PB: UK; t½: UK
Oxymetazoline HCl (Afrin)	A&C >6 y: 0.05% gtt or spray; 2–3 gtt or 1–2 sprays q nostril b.i.d. C 2–5 y (0.025% gtt only): 2–3 gtt b.i.d. (q10–12h)	Long-acting decongestant. Taken twice a day, morning and evening. Can cause rebound congestion. Use only 3–5 d. *Pregnancy category:* C; PB: UK; t½: UK
Phenylephrine HCl (Neo-Synephrine, Sinex)	A: Sol (0.25–1%): 2–3 gtt or 1–2 sprays in each nostril q4h C 6–12 y: Sol (0.25%): 2–3 gtt or sprays in each nostril q4h C 6 mo–5 y: Sol (0.125–0.16%): 1–2 gtt in each nostril q4h	For rhinitis. Less potent than epinephrine. Can cause transient hypertension and headaches. Do not use for longer than 3–5 d. *Pregnancy category:* C; PB: UK; t½: 2.5 d
Phenylpropanolamine HCl (Allerest, Dimetapp)	A: PO: 25–50 mg t.i.d./q.i.d.; *max:* 150 mg/d C 6–12 y: 12.5 mg q4h; *max:* 75 mg/d C 2–5 y: 6.25 mg q4h; *max:* 37.5 mg/d	For rhinitis, may be used to treat obesity. Various combinations. Has less CNS stimulation than ephedrine. *Pregnancy category:* B; PB: UK; t½: 3–4 h
Pseudoephedrine (Actifed, Novafed, Sudafed)	A: PO: 60 mg q4–6h; 120 mg SR q12h; *max:* 240 mg/d C 6–12 y: 30 mg q4–6h; *max:* 120 mg/d C 2–5 y: 15 mg q4–6h; *max:* 60 mg/d	For rhinitis. Less CNS stimulation and hypertension than ephedrine. *Pregnancy category:* C; PB: UK; t½: 9–15 h
Tetrahydrozoline HCl (Tyzine)	A&C >6 y: 2–4 gtt (0.1%) or spray q4–6h PRN C 2–6 y: 2–3 gtt (0.05%) q4–6h PRN Direct medical supervision for use >3–5 d	Relief of nasal congestion, rhinitis, sinusitis. *Pregnancy category:* C; PB: UK; t½: UK
Xylometazoline HCl (Otrivin)	A&C >12 y: 1–2 gtt (0.1%) or 1–2 sprays q8–10h; *max:* 3 × in 24 h C <12 y: 2–3 gtt (0.05%) or 1 spray q8–10h; *max:* 3 × in 24 h	Relief of nasal congestion, rhinitis, sinusitis. Excessive use can cause rebound nasal congestion. *Pregnancy category:* C; PB: UK; t½: UK

KEY: *A: adult; C: child; PO: by mouth; SC: subcutaneous; IM: intramuscular; IV: intravenous; PRN: as necessary; gtt: drops; >: greater than; PB: protein-binding; t½: half-life; OTC: over-the-counter; sol: solution; SR: sustained release; CNS: central nervous system; <: less than.*

can make a client jittery, nervous, or restless. These side effects decrease or disappear as the body adjusts to the drug.

Usage of nasal decongestants longer than 5 days could result in **rebound nasal congestion.** Instead of the nasal membranes constricting, vasodilation occurs, causing increased stuffy nose and nasal congestion. The nurse should emphasize the importance of limiting the use of nasal sprays and drops.

As with any alpha-adrenergic drug (e.g., decongestants), blood pressure and blood glucose levels can increase. These drugs are contraindicated or to be used with extreme caution for clients having hypertension, cardiac disease, hyperthyroidism, and diabetes mellitus.

Drug Interactions

When using decongestants with other drugs, drug interactions can occur. Pseudoephedrine may decrease the effect of beta blockers. Taking monoamine oxidase (MAO) inhibitors may increase the possibility of hypertension or cardiac dysrhythmias. The client should also stay away from caffeine (coffee, tea) in large amounts because it can increase the restlessness and palpitations caused by decongestants.

ANTITUSSIVES

Antitussives act on the cough control center in the medulla to suppress the cough reflex. The cough is a protective way to clear the airway of secretions or any collected material. A sore throat may cause coughing that increases throat irritation. If the cough is nonproductive and irritating, an antitussive may be taken. Hard candy may decrease the constant, irritating cough. Dextromethorphan, a nonnarcotic antitussive, is widely used in OTC cold remedies. Figure 30–2 lists the drug data related to dextromethorphan.

Pharmacokinetics

Dextromethorphan is available in syrup or liquid form, chewable capsules, and lozenges in numer-ous cold and cough remedy preparations. Brand name formulations include Robitussin DM, Romi-lar, PediaCare, Contac Cold Formula, Sucrets cough formulas, and many others. The drug is rapidly absorbed and exerts its effects 15 to 30 min after oral administration. The protein-binding percentage and half-life are unknown. Dextromethorphan is metabolized by the liver.

Pharmacodynamics

Dextromethorphan is a nonnarcotic antitussive that suppresses the cough center in the medulla. If the cough lasts longer than 1 week and a fever or rash

FIGURE 30–2. Antitussive

Antitussive	Dosage	NURSING PROCESS
		Assessment and Planning
Dextromethorphan hydrobromide (Robitussin DM, Romilar, Sucrets Cough Control, PediaCare, Benylin DM, and others); 🍁 Balminil DM, Neo-DM; Ornex DM	A: PO: 10–30 mg q4–8h; max: 120 mg/24 h	
OTC preparation	C 6–12 y: PO: 5–10 mg q4–6h; max: 60 mg/d	
Pregnancy Category: C	C 2–5 y: PO: 2.5–7.5 mg q4–8h; max: 30 mg/d	
	Sustained Action Liquid (Delsym): A: 60 mg q12h	
	C 6–12 y: 30 mg q12h	
	C 2–5 y: 15 mg q12h	

Contraindications	Drug-Lab-Food Interactions	
Chronic obstructive pulmonary disease, chronic productive cough, hypersensitivity, clients taking MAOIs	*Increase* effect/toxicity with MAOIs, narcotics, sedative-hypnotics, barbiturates, antidepressants, alcohol	

Pharmacokinetics	Pharmacodynamics	Interventions
Absorption: PO: Rapidly absorbed	PO: Onset: 15–30 min	
Distribution: PB: UK	Peak: UK	
Metabolism: t½: UK	Duration: 3–6 h	
Excretion: In urine, UK		

	Evaluation
Therapeutic Effects/Uses: To provide temporary suppression of a nonproductive cough; to reduce viscosity of tenacious secretions.	
Mode of Action: Inhibition of the cough center in the medulla.	

Side Effects	Adverse Reactions
Nausea, dizziness, drowsiness, sedation	Hallucinations at high doses
	Life-threatening: None known

KEY: A: adult; C: child; PO: by mouth; PB: protein-binding; t½: half-life; UK: unknown; 🍁: Canadian drug names.

is present, medical care should be sought. Clients with underlying medical conditions should seek prompt medical attention.

The onset of action for dextromethorphan is rela- tively fast and the duration is 3 to 6 h. Usually preparations containing dextromethorphan can be used several times a day. Central nervous system depression can increase if the drug is used with al-

TABLE 30–3 Antitussives and Expectorants

Generic (Brand)	Route and Dosage	Uses and Considerations
Narcotic Antitussives		
Codeine CSS II	A: PO: 10–20 mg q4–6h; *max*: 120 mg/d C 6–12 y: PO: 5–10 mg q4–6h; *max*: 60 mg/d C 2–5 y: PO: 2.5–4.5 mg q4–6h; *max*: 18 mg/d	Schedule II drug. Can be a Schedule V drug when combined in cough syrup. Usually mixed with an antihistamine, decongestant, and/or expectorant. Can cause drowsiness, dizziness, nausea, constipation, respiratory depression. *Pregnancy category*: C; PB: 7%; t½: 2.5–4 h
Guaifenesin and codeine (Cheracol, Robitussin A-C) CSS V	*Temporary relief of cough due to minor irritation:* A: PO: 5–10 mL of q6–8h C 2–6 y: PO: 2.5 mL q6–8h, PRN	An expectorant that is combined with a narcotic antitussive. Also to control a cough due to the common cold or bronchitis. *Pregnancy category*: C; PB: UK; t½: UK
Hydrocodone bitartrate (Hycodan) CSS III	A: PO: 5–10 mg q4–6h, *max*: 15 mg/d C: PO: 0.6 mg/kg/d in 3–4 divided doses, not to exceed 10 mg/single dose	Relief of cough and pain. Has similar side effects as codeine. *Pregnancy category*: C; PB: UK; t½: 3–4 h
Nonnarcotic Antitussives		
Benzonatate (Tessalon)	*Relief of nonproductive cough:* A: PO: 100 mg t.i.d. or q4h; *max*: 600 mg/d C (<10 y): PO: 8 mg/kg/d in 3–6 divided doses	Relief of cough. It does not decrease the respiratory center. Has few side effects. *Pregnancy category*: C; PB: UK; t½: UK
Dextromethorphan hydrobromide (Benylin, Romilar, Sucrets Cough Control, and others)	See Prototype Drug Chart (Fig. 30–2)	Suppresses cough due to common cold or inhaled irritants. Nonprescription cough medication. Does not depress respiration. Does not cause physical dependence, and tolerance does not develop. *Pregnancy category*: C; PB: UK; t½: UK
Diphenhydramine (Benadryl)	See Prototype Drug Chart (Fig. 30–1)	Used as a cough suppressant. Has antihistamine properties. Can cause drowsiness and dry mouth. *Pregnancy category*: B; PB: 82%; t½: 2–7 h
Promethazine with dextromethorphan	A: PO: 5 mL q4–6h; *max*: 30 mL/d C 6–12 y: PO: 2.5–5 mL q4–6h; *max*: 20 mL/d C 2–6 y: PO: 1.25–5 mL, q4–6h	For cough. A combination of a phenothiazine and a nonnarcotic antitussive. *Pregnancy category*: C; PB: UK; t½: UK
Expectorants		
Guaifenesin (Robitussin, Anti-Tuss, Glyco-Tuss)	A: PO: 200–400 mg q4h; *max*: 2.4 g/d C 6–12 y: PO: 100–200 mg q4h; *max*: 1.2 g/d C 2–5 y: PO: 50–100 mg q4h; *max*: 600 mg/d	For dry, unproductive cough. Can cause nausea, vomiting. Can be combined with other cold remedies. Take with glass of water to loosen mucus. *Pregnancy category*: C; PB: UK; t½: UK
Iodinated glycerol (Iophen)	A: PO: 60 mg q.i.d.; sol: 20 gtt q.i.d.; elix: 5 mL q.i.d. C: PO: Up to half adult dose according to weight	Same as potassium iodide. *Pregnancy category*: X; PB: UK; t½: UK
Potassium iodide (SSKI)	A: PO: 300–650 mg b.i.d., t.i.d. C: PO: 60–250 mg q8–12h	Stimulates bronchial secretions and fluids. Avoid if hyperkalemia is present. Can cause nausea and vomiting. *Pregnancy category*: D; PB: UK; t½: UK
Antitussive/Expectorant		
Guaifenesin and dextromethorphan (Robitussin-DM)	A: PO: 10 mL q6–8h C 6–12 y: PO: 5 mL q6–8h C 2–5 y: PO: 2.5 mL q6–8h	For nonproductive cough. *Pregnancy category*: C; PB: UK; t½: UK

KEY: *A: adult; C: child; PO: by mouth; UK: unknown; max: maximum; PB: protein-binding; t½: half-life; CSS: Controlled Substance Schedule; PRN: as necessary; elix: elixir; <: less than.*

cohol, narcotics, sedative-hypnotics, barbiturates, or antidepressants.

Antitussives are of three types: nonnarcotic, narcotic, or combination preparations. Usually these drugs are used in combination with other agents (Table 30–3).

EXPECTORANTS

Expectorants loosen bronchial secretions so they can be eliminated with coughing. They can be used with or without other pharmacologic agents. Expectorants are found in many OTC cold remedies along with analgesics, antihistamines, decongestants, and antitussives. The most common expectorant in such preparations is guaifenesin. Table 30–3 lists the drug data for antitussives and expectorants. Hydration is the best expectorant.

SINUSITIS

Sinusitis is an inflammation of the mucous membranes of one or more of the maxillary, frontal, ethmoid, or sphenoid sinuses. A systemic or nasal decongestant may be indicated. Acetaminophen, fluids, and rest may also be helpful. For acute or severe sinusitis, an antibiotic may be prescribed.

ACUTE PHARYNGITIS

Acute pharyngitis (inflammation of the throat, or "sore throat") can be caused by a virus or by beta-hemolytic streptococci (strep throat) or other bacteria. It can occur alone or with the common cold and rhinitis or acute sinusitis. Symptoms include elevated temperature and cough. A throat culture should be taken to rule out beta-hemolytic streptococcal infection. Saline gargles, lozenges, and increased fluid intake are usually indicated. Acetaminophen may be taken for the elevated temperature. A 10-day course of antibiotics is often prescribed if the throat culture is positive for beta-hemolytic streptococci. Antibiotics are not effective for viral pharyngitis.

ACUTE TONSILLITIS

Acute tonsillitis is inflammation of the tonsils. *Streptococcus* is the usual causative microorganism. Symptoms include sore throat, pain on swallowing, chills, fever, and aching muscles. A throat culture should be taken to determine whether the causative organism is beta-hemolytic streptococcus. Saline gargle, increased fluid intake, and antibiotics are normal treatment modalities.

ACUTE LARYNGITIS

In acute **laryngitis,** edema of the vocal cords causes the voice to be weak or husky. It may be due to stress, overuse of the vocal cords, or a respiratory infection. Drug therapy has minimal value. Voice rest is usually necessary, and smoking should be avoided.

NURSING PROCESS: COMMON COLD

ASSESSMENT

- Determine if there is a history of hypertension, especially if a decongestant is one of the ingredients of the cold remedy.
- Obtain baseline vital signs (VS). An elevated temperature of 99°F (37.2°C) to 101°F (38.3°C) may indicate a viral infection caused by a cold.

POTENTIAL NURSING DIAGNOSES

- Fatigue
- Sleep deprivation due to chronic coughing
- High risk for infection

PLANNING

- Client will be free of nonproductive cough. A secondary bacterial infection does not occur.

NURSING INTERVENTIONS

- Monitor vital signs. Blood pressure can become elevated when a decongestant is taken. Dysrhythmias can also occur.
- Observe color of bronchial secretions. Yellow or green mucus is indicative of a bronchial infection. Antibiotics may be needed.
- Be aware that codeine preparations for cough suppression can lead to tolerance and physical dependence.

CLIENT TEACHING

- Instruct the client on proper use of a nasal spray. With a puff or squeeze, inhale. Do not use more than one or two puffs, 4 to 6 times a day for 5 to 7 days. Rebound congestion can occur with overuse.
- Advise the client to read the label on OTC drugs

and check with the health care provider before taking cold remedies. This is especially important when taking other drugs or when the client has a major health problem such as hypertension or hyperthyroidism.

- Inform the client that antibiotics are not helpful in treating the common cold viruses. They may be prescribed if a secondary infection occurs.
- Advise the older client with heart disease, asthma, emphysema, diabetes mellitus, or hypertension to contact the health care provider concerning the selection of drug, including OTC drugs.
- Advise the client not to drive when starting on a cold remedy containing an antihistamine because drowsiness is common.
- Instruct the client to maintain adequate fluid intake. Fluids liquify bronchial secretions to ease elimination by coughing.
- Instruct the client not to take a cold remedy near or at bedtime. Insomnia may occur if it contains a decongestant.
- Instruct the client to drink the diluted liquid form of saturated solution of potassium iodide (SSKI) through a straw to avoid discoloration of tooth enamel.
- Encourage the client to get adequate rest.
- Instruct the client that common cold and flu viruses are transmitted frequently by hand-to-hand contact or touching a contaminated surface. Cold viruses can live on the skin for several hours, and on hard surfaces for several days.
- Instruct the client to avoid environmental pollutants, smoking, and dust.
- Instruct the client/parents to have child perform three effective coughs before bedtime to promote uninterrupted sleep.
- Instruct the client/parents to keep the drug stored out of reach of small children; request child safety caps.
- Advise the client to contact the health care provider if cough persists for >1 wk or is combined with chest pain, fever, or headache.

Skill
- Instruct the client to cough effectively, to take deep breaths before coughing and to be in the upright position.

EVALUATION
- Evaluate the effectiveness of the drug therapy. Determine that the client is free of a nonproductive cough, has adequate fluid intake and rest, and is afebrile.

STUDY QUESTIONS

1. Antihistamines can be used for the common cold. What are the desired and undesired effects of antihistamines?
2. What are antitussives and expectorants? How are they administered?
3. Your client has a cold and is complaining of nasal congestion. He has been using a nasal decongestant every 3 hours for several days. He says that the nasal congestion is as bad as it had been before he started the nasal decongestant. What nursing interventions, including client teaching, should be given?
4. Your client is complaining of a "sore throat." The pharynx appears red. What nursing action should be taken?
5. P.T. states she has had a cold for 5 days and now has "lost her voice." What client teaching instructions should be included?
6. M.P. says she was with Tom the day before he "got a head cold." She asks whether she can avoid the cold by staying away from Tom. What would your response be? What client teaching is recommended?

Chapter 31

Drugs for Acute and Chronic Lower Respiratory Disorders

OUTLINE

Objectives
Terms
Introduction
Chronic Obstructive Pulmonary
   Disease (COPD)
     Bronchial Asthma
Sympathomimetics: Alpha- and
   Beta-Adrenergic Agonists

Metaproterenol
Use of Aerosol Inhaler
   Nursing Process
Methylxanthine (Xanthine)
   Derivatives
     Theophylline
Glucocorticoids (Steroids)
   Side Effects and Adverse
     Reactions

Cromolyn Sodium
Anticholinergics
Mucolytics
Antimicrobials
   Nursing Process
Case Study
Study Questions

OBJECTIVES

Define chronic obstructive pulmonary disease (COPD) and restrictive lung disease.

List the drug groups that are used for COPD and asthma and the desired effects of each.

Describe the side effects of beta$_2$-adrenergic agonists and methylxanthines.

State the therapeutic serum or plasma theophylline level and the toxic level.

Explain the therapeutic effects of glucocorticoids, cromolyn, antihistamines, and mucolytics for asthma and COPD.

Describe the nursing process, including client teaching, related to drugs commonly used for COPD, including asthma, and restrictive lung disease.

TERMS

bronchial asthma
bronchiectasis
bronchodilator
bronchospasm

chronic bronchitis
chronic obstructive pul-
   monary disease (COPD)
emphysema

glucocorticoids
mucolytic
restrictive lung disease

INTRODUCTION

Chronic obstructive pulmonary disease (COPD) and restrictive pulmonary disease are the two major categories of lower respiratory tract disease. COPD is caused by airway obstruction with increased airway resistance to airflow to lung tissues. In **restrictive lung disease** there is a decrease in total lung capacity due to fluid accumulation or loss of elasticity of the lung. Pulmonary edema, pulmonary fibrosis, pneumonitis, lung tumors, thoracic deformities (scoliosis), and disorders affecting the thoracic muscular wall such as myasthenia gravis are among the types and causes of restrictive pulmonary disease.

Drugs discussed in this chapter are used primarily to treat COPD, particularly asthma. These drugs include bronchodilators (sympathomimetics [primarily beta$_2$-adrenergic agonists], methylxanthines [xanthines]), glucocorticoids, cromolyn, anticholinergics, and mucolytics. Some of these drugs may also be used for the treatment of restrictive pulmonary diseases.

CHRONIC OBSTRUCTIVE PULMONARY DISEASE

COPD includes four main lung diseases: (1) asthma, (2) chronic bronchitis, (3) emphysema, and (4) bronchiectasis. Bronchial asthma is characterized by bronchospasm (constricted bronchioles), wheezing, and dyspnea. There is resistance to airflow due to obstruction of the airway. In acute and chronic asthma, minimal to no changes are seen in the structure and function of lung tissues when the disease process is in remission. In chronic bronchitis, emphysema, and bronchiectasis there is permanent, irreversible damage to the physical structure of the lung tissue. Frequently, there is steady deterioration over a period of years.

Chronic bronchitis is a progressive lung disease caused by smoking or chronic lung infections. Bronchial inflammation and excessive mucus secretion result in airway obstruction. Productive coughing is a response to excess mucus production and chronic bronchial irritation. Inspiratory and expiratory rhonchi may be heard on auscultation. Hypercapnia (increased carbon dioxide retention) and hypoxemia (decreased blood oxygen) lead to respiratory acidosis.

In **bronchiectasis** there is abnormal dilatation of the bronchi and bronchioles secondary to frequent infection and inflammation. The bronchioles become obstructed due to the breakdown of the epithelium of the bronchial mucosa. Tissue fibrosis may result.

Emphysema is a progressive lung disease caused by cigarette smoking, atmospheric contaminants, or lack of the alpha$_1$-antitrypsin protein that inhibits proteolytic enzymes that destroy alveoli (air sacs). The proteolytic enzymes are released in the lung by bacteria or phagocytic cells. The terminal bronchioles become plugged with mucus, causing a loss of fiber and elastin network in the alveoli. The alveoli enlarge as many of the alveolar walls are destroyed. Air becomes trapped in the overexpanded alveoli, leading to inadequate gas (O_2 and CO_2) exchange.

BRONCHIAL ASTHMA

Bronchial asthma is a chronic obstructive pulmonary disease characterized by periods of bronchospasm resulting in wheezing and difficulty in breathing. **Bronchospasm,** or bronchoconstriction, results when the lung tissue is exposed to extrinsic or intrinsic factors that stimulate a bronchoconstrictive response. Factors that can trigger an asthmatic attack (bronchospasm) include humidity, air pressure changes, temperature changes, smoke, fumes (exhaust, perfume), stress, emotional upset, and allergies to animal dander, food, and drugs such as aspirin, indomethacin, and ibuprofen. Reactive airway disease (RAD) is a cause of asthma due to sensitivity stimulation from allergens, dust, temperature changes, and cigarette smoking.

Mast cells, found in connective tissue throughout the body, are directly involved in the asthmatic response, particularly to extrinsic factors. Mast cells stimulate the release of chemical mediators such as histamine, serotonin, ECF-A (eosinophil chemotactic factor of anaphylaxis), and leukotrienes. Histamine and ECF-A are strong bronchoconstrictors. Bronchial smooth muscles are wrapped spirally around the bronchioles, and the bronchioles contract as they are stimulated by these mediators.

Cyclic adenosine monophosphate (cyclic AMP, or cAMP), a cellular substance, is involved in many cellular activities and is responsible for maintaining bronchodilation. When histamine, ECF-A, and leukotrienes inhibit the action of cAMP, bronchoconstriction results. The sympathomimetic (adrenergic) **bronchodilators** and methylxanthines increase the amount of cAMP in bronchial tissue cells. Figure 31–1 shows the factors contributing to bronchoconstriction.

In an acute asthmatic attack, the sympathomimetics (beta-adrenergic agonists) are the first line of defense. They promote cAMP production and enhance bronchodilation. Sympathomimetics (adrenergics) are also discussed in Chapter 18.

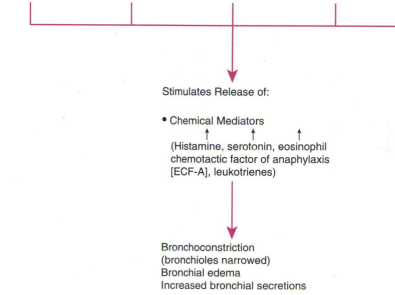

	ENVIRONMENT		POLLUTANTS	ALLERGIC SUBSTANCE	DRUGS
	External	*Internal*			
	Humidity	Emotion	Smoke	Food	Aspirin
	Air pressure changes	Stress	Air pollution (cars, industry)	Animal dander	NSAIDs (Ibuprofen)
	Temperature changes		Perfume	Plants, trees	
	Work			Flowers	
	Exercise				

Stimulates Release of:

• Chemical Mediators

(Histamine, serotonin, eosinophil chemotactic factor of anaphylaxis [ECF-A], leukotrienes)

Bronchoconstriction (bronchioles narrowed)
Bronchial edema
Increased bronchial secretions

FIGURE 31–1 Factors contributing to bronchoconstriction.

SYMPATHOMIMETICS: ALPHA- AND BETA₂-ADRENERGIC AGONISTS

Sympathomimetics increase cyclic AMP, causing dilation of the bronchioles. In an acute bronchospasm due to anaphylaxis from an allergic reaction, the nonselective sympathomimetic epinephrine (Adrenalin), which is an $alpha_1$ $beta_1$, and $beta_2$ agonist, is given subcutaneously to promote bronchodilation and elevate the blood pressure. Epinephrine is administered in emergency situations to restore circulation and increase airway patency (see Chapter 47).

For bronchospasm associated with chronic asthma or COPD, selective $beta_2$-adrenergic agonists are given by aerosol or as a tablet. These drugs act primarily on the $beta_2$ receptors; therefore, the side effects are *less severe* than those of epinephrine, which acts on alpha, $beta_1$, and $beta_2$ receptors.

The first beta-adrenergic agent used for bronchospasm was isoproterenol (Isuprel), which was introduced in 1941. It has no alpha agonist properties, but it is a nonselective beta agonist because it stimulates both $beta_1$ and $beta_2$ receptors. Because the $beta_1$ receptors are stimulated, the heart rate increases and tachycardia may result. $Beta_2$ stimulation promotes bronchodilation. Isoproterenol cannot be given orally because it is metabolized in the gastrointestinal (GI) tract. It may be administered sublingually, by inhalation using an aerosol inhaler or nebulizer, or intravenously for severe asthmatic attacks. Its duration of action is short.

METAPROTERENOL

The second beta-adrenergic agent is metaproterenol (Alupent, Metaprel), which was first marketed in 1961. It has some $beta_1$ effect, but it is primarily used as a $beta_2$ agent. It may be administered orally or by inhalation with a metered-dose inhaler or a nebulizer.

For long-term asthma treatment, $beta_2$-adrenergic agonists are frequently administered by inhalation. Usually more drug is delivered by inhalation directly to the constricted bronchial site. The effective inhalation drug dose is less than it would be by the oral route; there are also fewer side effects in using this route.

The onset of action of the drug is more rapid (1 to 15 min) by inhalation than orally. If the client does not receive effective relief from the inhaler, either the client's technique is faulty or the cannister is empty (see Chapter 3 on determining the amount of drug left in the cannister). A spacer device may be attached to the inhaler to improve drug delivery to the lung with less deposition in the mouth. If the client does not use the inhaler properly to deliver the drug dose, the medication may be trapped in the upper airways. Because of drug inhalation, mouth dryness and throat irritation could result. Figure 31–2 lists the pharmacologic behavior for metaproterenol.

Pharmacokinetics

Metaproterenol is well absorbed from the GI tract. Its protein-binding percent and half-life are unknown. It is metabolized by the liver and excreted in the urine.

FIGURE 31–2. Bronchodilator: Adrenergic

Adrenergic Bronchodilator	Dosage	NURSING PROCESS Assessment and Planning
Metaproterenol SO$_4$ (Alupent, Metaprel) *Pregnancy Category:* C	A&C >9 y and >27 kg: PO: 20 mg, q6–8 h C 6–9 y or <27 kg: PO: 10 mg, q6–8 h A&C >12 y: MDI 2–3 inhalations as single dose; wait 2 min before second dose, if necessary; use only q3–4 h to maximum of 12 inhalations/d	
Contraindications	**Drug-Lab-Food Interactions**	
Hypersensitivity, cardiac dysrhythmias *Caution:* Narrow-angle glaucoma, cardiac disease, hypertension	*Increase* action of both with sympathomimetics *Decrease* with beta blockers *Lab:* Decreased serum potassium	
Pharmacokinetics	**Pharmacodynamics**	Interventions
Absorption: PO: Well absorbed *Distribution:* PB: UK *Metabolism:* t½: UK *Excretion:* In urine as metabolites	PO: Onset: 15–30 min Peak: 1 h Duration: 4 h SC: Onset: 1–5 min Peak: 1 h Duration: 3–4 h	

	Evaluation
Therapeutic Effects/Uses: To treat bronchospasm, asthma; to promote bronchodilation. *Mode of Action:* Relaxation of smooth muscle of bronchi.	

Side Effects	Adverse Reactions
Nervousness, tremors, restlessness, insomnia, headache, nausea, vomiting, hyperglycemia, muscle cramping in extremities	Tachycardia, palpitations, hypertension *Life-threatening:* Cardiac dysrhythmias, cardiac arrest, paradoxical bronchoconstriction

KEY: A: adult; C: child; PO: by mouth; >: greater than; <: less than; UK: unknown; MDI: metered-dose inhaler; PB: protein-binding; t½: half-life.

Pharmacodynamics

Metaproterenol reverses bronchospasm by relaxing the bronchial smooth muscle. The drug acts on the beta$_2$ receptor, promoting bronchodilation, and increases cyclic AMP.

The onset of action for oral and inhalational metaproterenol is fast and its duration is short. Excessive use of the drug by inhalation may cause tolerance and paradoxic bronchoconstriction. Because it has some beta$_1$ properties, it can cause tremor, nervousness, heart palpitations, and increased heart rate when taken in large doses. There are a few drug interactions that need to be considered. When metaproterenol is taken with a beta-adrenergic blocker, its effects are decreased. Other sympathomimetic agents increase the effects of metaproterenol.

The newer beta-adrenergic drugs for asthma are more selective for beta$_2$ receptors. High doses or overuse of the beta$_2$-adrenergic agents for asthma may cause some degree of beta$_1$ response such as nervousness, tremor, and increased pulse rate. The ideal beta$_2$ agonist is one that has a rapid onset of action, longer duration of action, and very few side effects. Albuterol (Proventil, Ventolin) is a selective beta$_2$ drug that is effective for treatment and control of asthma by causing bronchodilation.

USE OF AN AEROSOL INHALER*

If the beta$_2$ agonist is given by a metered-dose inhaler, correct use of the inhaler and dosage intervals need to be explained to the client. The correct method of using the inhaler is as follows (Fig. 31–3):

1. Insert the medication canister into the plastic holder.
2. Shake the inhaler well *before using*. Remove cap from mouthpiece.
3. Breathe *out* through the mouth, expelling air. Place mouthpiece into the mouth or in front of the open mouth, holding the inhaler upright.
4. If a spacer is used, attach the spacer to the inhaler, and place the end of the spacer in the mouth, passing the teeth and above the tongue.

* See Chapter 3.

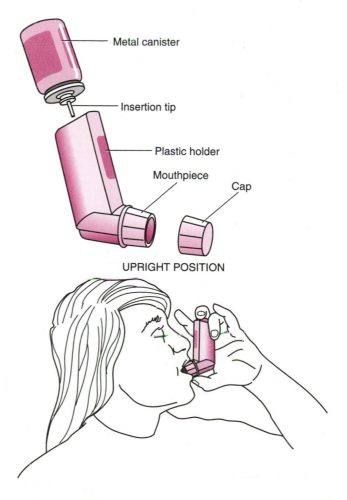

FIGURE 31–3 Technique for using the aerosol inhaler.

5. Keep the lips securely around the mouthpiece and *inhale. While inhaling, push the top of the medication canister* once.

6. Hold your breath for a few seconds, remove the mouthpiece and take your finger off the canister, and *exhale slowly.*

7. If a second dose is required, wait 2 minutes and repeat the procedure by first shaking the canister in the plastic holder with the cap on.

8. Cleanse the mouthpiece. If the inhaler has not been used recently or when it is first used, "test spray" before administering the metered dose.

9. If a glucocorticoid inhalant is to be used with a bronchodilator, wait 5 minutes before using the inhaler containing the steroid to allow time for the bronchodilator to take effect.

Excessive use of the aerosol drug can lead to tolerance and loss of drug effectiveness. Occasionally, clients have developed severe paradoxic airway resistance (bronchoconstriction) with repeated, excessive use of sympathomimetic oral inhalation, especially isoproterenol. Frequent dosing can cause tremors, nervousness, and increased heart rate. Table 31–1 lists the sympathomimetics used as bronchodilators.

Side Effects and Adverse Reactions

Epinephrine

The side effects and adverse reactions of epinephrine include tremors, dizziness, hypertension, tachycardia, heart palpitations, dysrhythmias, and angina. The client needs to be closely monitored when epinephrine is administered.

Beta$_2$ Adrenergics

The side effects associated with beta$_2$ drugs (albuterol, terbutaline) include tremors, headaches, nervousness, increased pulse rate, palpitations (high doses), and minimal lowering of the blood pressure. The beta$_2$ agonists may increase blood glucose levels; diabetics who take beta$_2$ agonists should be taught to closely monitor their serum glucose levels. Side effects of the beta$_2$ agonists may diminish after a week or longer. The bronchodilating effects may decrease with continued use. It is believed that tolerance to these drugs can develop; if this occurs, the dose may need to be increased. Failure to respond to a previously effective dose may indicate worsening asthma that requires reevaluation prior to increasing the dose.

TABLE 31–1 Sympathomimetics: Adrenergic Bronchodilators and Anticholinergics

Generic (Brand)	Route and Dosage	Uses and Considerations
Alpha- and Beta-adrenergic Ephedrine SO$_4$ (Ephedsol) Alpha$_1$, beta$_1$, beta$_2$	A: PO: 25–50 mg q3–4h; *max:* 150 mg/d PRN; SC/IM/IV: 12.5–25 mg PRN C >2 y: PO: 2–3 mg/kg/d in 4–6 divided doses C 6–12 y: PO: 6.25–12.5 mg q4h; *max:* 75 mg	Relief of allergic rhinitis and sinusitis; improves respiration due to narcotic excess; corrects hypotensive state. Nervousness, tachycardia, and insomnia could occur. *Pregnancy category:* C; PB: UK; t½: 3–6 h
Epinephrine (Adrenalin, Primatene Mist, Bronkaid Mist) Alpha$_1$, beta$_1$, beta$_2$	A: SC: 0.1–0.5 mg or mL of 1:1,000 sol; may repeat q10–15 min C: SC: 0.01 mg or mL of 1:1,000 sol; may repeat q20min–4h Inhal: 1–2 puffs of 1:100 q15 min × 2 doses then q3h	For acute bronchoconstriction and to combat anaphylactic reaction. It is a nonselective (alpha, beta$_1$, and beta$_2$) adrenergic drug. Used frequently by nebulizer. Side effects include nervousness, tremors, dizziness, palpitations, tachycardia, and other cardiac dysrhythmias. *Pregnancy category:* C; PB: UK; t½: UK
Beta-Adrenergic Albuterol (Proventil, Ventolin) Beta$_2$	A&C >6 y: Inhal: 1–2 puffs q4–6h or 2 puffs 15 min before exercise A: PO: 2–4 mg t.i.d. or q.i.d.; *max:* 8 mg q.i.d. SR: 4–8 mg q12h C 6–12 y: PO: 2 mg t.i.d./q.i.d. C 2–6 y: PO: 0.1 mg/kg t.i.d.	Treatment of acute and chronic asthma, bronchitis, and exercise-induced bronchospasm. Onset of action orally is 30 min and duration of action is 4–6 h; SR: 8–12 h. *Pregnancy category:* C; PB: UK; t½: 4–5 h
Bitolterol mesylate (Tornalate) Beta$_1$ (some), beta$_2$	A: Inhal: 2 (1–3 min apart), q4–6h; *max:* 12 inhal/d	Treatment of asthma and acute bronchitis. It can be used as a single-treatment therapy or in combination with theophylline or corticosteroid. Tremors, nervousness may occur. Has a longer duration of action than many other adrenergics (5–8 h) by inhalation. *Pregnancy category:* C; PB: UK; t½: 3 h
Isoetharine HCl (Bronkosol) Beta$_1$ (some), beta$_2$	Inhal: 1–2 puffs A: IPPB: 0.5–1.0 mL of 5% sol or 0.5 mL of 1% sol diluted in 3 mL of NSS	For bronchoconstriction and reversible obstructive pulmonary disease. Rapid onset (1–5 min); short duration of action (1–4 h). *Pregnancy category:* C; PB: UK; t½: UK

TABLE 31–1 Sympathomimetics: Adrenergic Bronchodilators and Anticholinergics (*Continued*)

Generic (Brand)	Route and Dosage	Uses and Considerations
Isoproterenol (Isuprel) Beta$_1$ and beta$_2$	A&C: Inhal: 1–2 puffs q4–6h A: SL: 10–20 mg q6–8h C: SL: 5–10 mg q6–8h	For bronchoconstriction. Nonselective (beta$_1$ and beta$_2$). Beta$_1$ effect causes heart rate to increase. Monitor heart rate and blood pressure. The absorption of the sublingual drug can be variable and unpredictable. *Pregnancy category:* C; PB: UK; t½: 2–5 min
Metaproterenol sulfate (Alupent, Metaprel) Beta$_1$ (some) and beta$_2$	See Prototype Drug Chart (Fig. 31–2)	Relief of bronchospasm due to asthma, bronchitis, and emphysema. Nervousness, tremors, tachycardia, and palpitations may occur. *Pregnancy category:* C; PB: UK; t½: UK
Pirbuterol acetate (Maxair) Beta$_2$	*Prevention:* A&C > 12 y: Inhal: 2 puffs q4–6h *Bronchospasm:* A&C > 12 y: Inhal: 2 puffs (1–3 min apart) followed by 1 puff; not to exceed 12 inhalations/d	Treatment of asthma. Moderate duration of action (5 h). *Pregnancy category:* C; PB: UK; t½: 2–3 h
Salmeterol (Serevent) Beta$_2$	*Maintenance bronchodilation:* A&C > 12 y: Inhal: 2 puffs q12h *Prevention exercise-induced bronchospasm* A&C > 12 y: Inhal: 2 puffs ≥ 30–60 min before exercise	Treatment for chronic asthma and exercise-induced bronchospasm. Not effective for treating acute bronchospasms. Has a long duration of action (12 h). *Pregnancy category:* C; PB: 94%–98%; t½: 5.5 h
Terbutaline SO$_4$ (Brethine, Bricanyl) Beta$_2$	Inhal: 1–2 puffs q4–6h A: PO: 2.5–5 mg t.i.d. 　SC: 0.25–0.5 mg q8h 　IV: 10 μg/min, gradually increase; *max:* 80 μg/min C > 12 y: PO: 2.5 mg t.i.d.	To treat reversible airway obstruction due to asthma, bronchitis, and emphysema. May cause nervousness, tremors, lightheadedness, palpitations, tachycardia if taken in excess. Slow to moderate onset (15–30 min); long oral duration (4–8 h) and moderate inhaled duration (3–6 h). *Pregnancy category:* B; PB: 25%; t½: 3–11 h
Anticholinergics Ipratropium bromide (Atrovent)	*COPD:* A: Inhal: 2 puffs t.i.d., q.i.d. > 4 h intervals; *max:* 12 inhal/d	To treat bronchospasm associated with COPD, including asthma. Use with caution in clients with narrow-angle glaucoma. *Pregnancy category:* B; PB: UK; t½: 1.5–2h

KEY: A: adult; C: child; PO: by mouth; SR: sustained-release; SL: sublingual; IV: intravenous; COPD: chronic obstructive pulmonary disease; >: greater than; PB: protein-binding; t½: half-life; IPPB: intermittent positive-pressure breathing; sol: solution; NSS: normal saline solution; inhal: inhalation.

NURSING PROCESS: BRONCHODILATOR: Adrenergic

ASSESSMENT

- Obtain a medical and drug history; report probable drug-drug interactions.
- Obtain baseline vital signs (VS) for abnormalities and for future comparisons.
- Assess for wheezing, decreased breath sounds, cough, and sputum production.
- Assess sensorium levels for confusion and restlessness due to hypoxia and hypercapnia.
- Assess hydration; diuresis may result in dehydration in the elderly and children.

POTENTIAL NURSING DIAGNOSES

- Airway clearance, ineffective
- Noncompliance with drug therapy

PLANNING

- Client will be free of wheezing and lung fields will be clear within 2 to 5 d.
- Client is taking oral drug(s) and using inhaler as prescribed.

NURSING INTERVENTIONS

- Monitor VS. Blood pressure and heart rate can increase greatly. Check for cardiac dysrhythmias.
- Provide adequate hydration. Fluids aid in loosening secretions. Monitor drug therapy. Observe for side effects.
- Administer medication after meals to decrease GI distress.

Skill

• Instruct to correctly use the inhaler or nebulizer. Caution against overuse since side effects and tolerance may result.

Correct use of metered-dose inhaler to deliver beta$_2$ agonist:

1. Insert the medication canister into the plastic holder.
2. Shake the inhaler well *before* using. Remove cap from mouthpiece.
3. Breathe *out* through the mouth. Open mouth wide and hold mouthpiece 1 to 2 inches from mouth or place inhaler mouthpiece in mouth. A spacer may be used. Discuss technique with health care provider.
4. With mouth open, take *slow deep* breath through mouth and at same time push the top of the medication canister once.
5. Hold breath for a few seconds; exhale slowly through pursed lips.
6. If a second dose is required, wait 2 min and repeat the procedure by first shaking the canister in the plastic holder with the cap on.

7. If the inhaler has not been used recently or when it is first used, "test spray" before administering the metered dose.
8. If a glucocorticoid inhalant is to be used with a bronchodilator, wait 5 min before using the inhaler containing the steroid for the bronchodilator effect.
• Teach client to monitor pulse rate.
• Teach client to monitor amount of medication remaining in the canister.
• Advise client not to take over-the-counter (OTC) preparations without first checking with the health care provider. Some OTC products may have an additive effect.
• Instruct the client to avoid smoking. Smoking increases drug elimination.
• Discuss ways to alleviate anxiety such as relaxation techniques and music.
• Advise client having asthma attacks to wear an ID bracelet or tags.

EVALUATION

• Evaluate the effectiveness of the bronchodilator. The client is breathing without wheezing and without side effects of the drug.

METHYLXANTHINE (XANTHINE) DERIVATIVES

The second group of bronchodilators used for asthma are the methylxanthine (xanthine) derivatives, which include aminophylline, theophylline, and caffeine. Xanthines also stimulate the central nervous system (CNS) and respiration, dilate coronary and pulmonary vessels, and cause diuresis. Because of their effect on respiration and pulmonary vessels, the xanthines are used in the treatment of asthma.

THEOPHYLLINE

The first theophylline preparation produced was aminophylline in 1936. Aminophylline is still the treatment of choice for acute asthma when it is administered as an intravenous solution. The solution contains 85% theophylline. Theophylline relaxes the smooth muscles of the bronchi, bronchioles, and pulmonary blood vessels by inhibiting the enzyme phosphodiesterase, resulting in an increase in cyclic AMP, which promotes bronchodilation.

Theophylline has a low therapeutic index and a narrow therapeutic range of 10 to 20 μg/mL. The serum or plasma theophylline concentration level

should be monitored frequently to avoid severe side effects. Toxicity is likely to occur when the serum level is greater than 20 μg/mL. Certain theophylline preparations can be given with sympathomimetic (adrenergic) drug agents, but the dose may need to be adjusted.

Figure 31–4 presents the drug data related to theophylline preparations.

Pharmacokinetics

Theophylline is usually well absorbed after oral administration, but absorption may vary according to the specific dosage form. Theophylline is also well absorbed from oral liquids and uncoated plain tablets. Sustained-release dosage forms are slowly absorbed. Food and antacids may decrease the rate, but not the extent, of absorption; large volumes of fluid and high-protein meals may increase the rate of absorption. The rate of absorption also can be affected by the size of the dose: larger doses are absorbed more slowly. Theophylline can be administered intravenously in IV fluids.

The theophylline drugs are metabolized by liver enzymes, and 90% of the drug is excreted by the kidneys. Tobacco smoking increases metabolism of theophylline drugs, thereby decreasing the drug's

FIGURE 31–4. Bronchodilator; Methylxanthine

Methylxanthine	Dosage	**NURSING PROCESS** Assessment and Planning
Theophylline (Theo-Dur, Theophyllin KI, Elixophyllin-KI, Somophyllin, Slophyllin, Slo-bid, Quibron), 🍁 PMS Theophylline, Pulmophylline Respiratory smooth muscle relaxant *Pregnancy Category:* C	*Bronchospasm, Bronchial Asthma:* A: PO: 250–500 mg q8–12h C: PO: 50–100 mg q6h; max: 12 mg/kg/d Dosing is highly individualized and is based on therapeutic serum levels 10 and 20 μg/mL. Monitor levels and client response.	

Contraindications	Drug-Lab-Food Interactions	
Severe cardiac dysrhythmias, hyperthyroidism, hypersensitivity to xanthines, peptic ulcer disease, uncontrolled seizure disorder *Caution:* With young children and elderly	*Increase* effect with allopurinol, oral contraceptives, ciprofloxacin, cimetidine, ranitidine, calcium blockers, erythromycin *Decrease* effects of neuromuscular blockers, phenytoin, lithium; *decrease* effect with smoking, rifampin, phenobarbital, corticosteroids, and others *Food: Increase* metabolism with low-carbohydrate, high-protein diet *Decrease* elimination with high-carbohyrate diet (*increase* t½) *Lab:* Interaction with laboratory result is not common; however, check with each laboratory	

Pharmacokinetics	Pharmacodynamics	Interventions
Absorption: PO: Well absorbed; SR: slowly absorbed *Distribution:* PB: Approx 60% *Metabolism:* t½: 7–9 h nonsmokers; 4–5 h smokers *Excretion:* In urine	PO: Onset: 30 min Peak: 1–2 h Duration: 6 h PO-SR: Onset: 1–3 h Peak: 4–8 h Duration: 8–24 h PO: Onset: Rapid Peak: UK Duration: 6–8 h	

	Evaluation
Therapeutic Effects/Uses: To promote bronchodilation; to treat asthma and chronic obstructive pulmonary disease. *Mode of Action:* Increased cyclic AMP results in bronchodilation; diuresis; cardiac, CNS, and gastric acid stimulaton.	

Side Effects	Adverse Reactions
Anorexia, nausea, vomiting, restlessness, dizziness, insomnia, flushing, rash, headache	Irritability, tremors, tachycardia, palpitations, urticaria *Life-threatening:* Seizures, cardiac dysrhythmias, convulsions

KEY: A: adult; C: child; PO: by mouth; SR: sustained release; IV: intravenous; PB: protein-binding; t½: half-life; UK: unknown; 🍁: Canadian drug names.

half-life. The half-life is shortened in smokers and in children. With a short drug half-life, theophylline is readily excreted by the kidneys, and the drug dose may need to be increased to maintain the therapeutic serum or plasma range. In non-smokers and older adults, the average half-life of theophylline is 7 to 9 hours, and the dose requirements may be decreased. In smokers and children, the half-life is 4 to 5 hours and the dose requirement may be increased. In premature infants, the half-life is 15 to 55 h. In clients who have congestive heart failure (CHF), cor pulmonale, COPD, or liver disease, the half-life is 12 h. Creatinine clearance may be decreased in older adults, so caution should be taken related to theophylline dosage in order to avoid drug toxicity.

Pharmacodynamics

Theophylline increases the level of cyclic AMP, resulting in bronchodilation. The average time of onset of action for oral theophylline preparations is 30 minutes; for sustained-release capsules it is 1 to 2 hours. The duration of action for the sustained-release form is 8 to 24 hours, and for other oral and intravenous theophylline preparations, approximately 6 hours.

Table 31–2 lists the theophylline preparations, their dosages, and uses and considerations.

Side Effects and Adverse Reactions

Side effects and adverse reactions include anorexia, nausea and vomiting, gastric pain due to increased gastric acid secretion, intestinal bleeding, nervousness, dizziness, headache, irritability, cardiac dysrhythmias, tachycardia, palpitations, marked hypotension, hyperreflexia, and seizures.

Clients should not take other xanthines while taking theophylline in order to decrease the potential for side effects. Adverse CNS reactions are often more severe in children than in adults; i.e., headaches, irritability, restlessness, nervousness, insomnia, dizziness, and seizures.

Theophylline toxicity is most likely to occur when serum concentrations exceed 20 μg/mL. Theophylline can cause hyperglycemia, decreased clotting time and, rarely, increased white blood cell count (leukocytosis). Because of the diuretic effect of xanthines, including theophylline, clients should be advised to avoid caffeine products such as coffee, tea, cola drinks, and chocolate and to increase their fluid intake.

Rapid intravenous administration of aminoph-

TABLE 31–2 Theophylline Preparations

Generic (Brand)	Route and Dosage	Uses and Considerations
Aminophylline—theophylline ethylenediamine (Somophyllin)	A: PO: LD 500 mg; then 250–500 mg q6–8h IV: LD 6 mg/kg over 30 min; then 0.2–0.9 mg/kg/h C: PO: LD: 7.5 mg/kg; then 3–6 mg/kg q6–8h IV: LD 5.6 mg/kg then 1 mg/kg/h *Caution:* Need to stress that individual titration is based on serum theophylline levels.	IV for acute asthmatic attack. For IV use, drug must be diluted. Oral preparations are tablets or elixirs. For oral use, give with food to avoid GI distress. Side effects include restlessness, syncope, palpitation, tachycardia, hyperventilation, cardiac dysrhythmias. *Pregnancy category:* C; PB: UK; t½: 4–9 h
Dyphylline—dihydroxypropyl theophylline (Dyline, Dilor, Lufyllin)	A: PO: 200–800 mg q.i.d. or q6h A: IM: 250–500 mg q6h C >6 y: PO: 4–7 mg/kg/d in 4 divided doses Therapeutic serum theophylline range: 10–20 μg/mL	Treatment of asthma, chronic bronchitis, and emphysema. One-tenth as potent as theophylline. *Pregnancy category:* C; PB: UK; t½: 2 h
Oxtriphylline—choline theophyllinate (Choledyl)	A: PO: 200 mg q.i.d. or q6h C: 2–12 y: PO: 4 mg/kg q6h Therapeutic serum theophylline range: 10–20 μg/mL	Relief of asthma and COPD. Useful for long-term therapy. Drug tolerance is infrequent. *Pregnancy category:* C; PB: UK; t½: 3–13 h
Theophylline	See Prototype Drug Chart (Fig. 31–4)	Used for moderate to severe asthma. Also for bronchospasm due to bronchitis and emphysema. Drug comes in tablets, timed-release tablets, liquid, elixirs, suspension, and in combination with other drugs. Monitor serum theophylline levels (10–20 μg/mL). Has many side effects; see prototype drug. *Pregnancy category:* C; PB: 60%; t½: nonsmokers: 7–9 h; smokers: 4–5 h

KEY: A: adult; C: child; PO: by mouth; LD: loading dose; IV: intravenous; UK: unknown; >: greater than; PB: protein-binding; t½: half-life.

ylline (a theophylline product) can cause dizziness, flushing, hypotension, severe bradycardia, and palpitations. Intravenous theophylline preparation should be administered slowly or via an infusion pump in order to avoid severe side effects.

Drug Interactions

Beta blockers, cimetidine (Tagamet), propranolol (Inderal), and erythromycin decrease the liver metabolism rate and increase the half-life and effects of theophylline; barbiturate and carbamazepine decrease its effects. In both situations, the theophylline dosage would need adjustment. Theophylline increases the risk of digitalis toxicity, decreases the effects of lithium, and decreases theophylline levels with phenytoin. If theophylline and beta-adrenergic agonist are given together, a synergistic effect can occur; cardiac dysrhythmias may result.

GLUCOCORTICOIDS (STEROIDS)

Glucocorticoids, members of the corticosteroid family are used in the treatment of respiratory disorders, particularly asthma. These drugs have an antiinflammatory action and are indicated if the asthma is unresponsive to bronchodilator therapy or if the client has an asthma attack while on maximum doses of a theophylline or an adrenergic drug.

Side effects are significant with long-term oral use and include fluid retention, hyperglycemia, and impaired immune response. It is thought that glucocorticoids have a synergistic effect when given with a beta$_2$ agonist.

Glucocorticoids can be given by (1) aerosol inhaler: beclomethasone (Vanceril, Beclovent); (2) tablet: triamcinolone (Amcort, Aristocort, Azmacort), dexamethasone (Decadron), prednisone, prednisolone, and methylprednisolone; and (3) injectable form: dexamethasone (Decadron), hydrocortisone. Inhaled glucocorticoids are *not* helpful in treatment of a severe asthmatic attack. It may take 1 to 4 weeks for an inhaled steroid to reach its full effect.

Glucocorticoid preparations are discussed in detail in Chapter 40.

These drugs can be irritating to the gastric mucosa and should be taken with food to avoid ulceration. When discontinuing glucocorticoids, the dosage should be tapered slowly to prevent adrenal insufficiency. A single dose usually does not cause adrenal suppression. The use of an oral inhaler minimizes the risk of adrenal suppression that is associated with oral systemic glucocorticoid

therapy. Inhaled glucocorticoids are preferred to the oral preparations unless they fail to control the asthma.

SIDE EFFECTS AND ADVERSE REACTIONS

Side effects associated with the oral inhalers generally are local rather than systemic (e.g., throat irritation, hoarseness, dry mouth, and coughing). Oral, laryngeal, and pharyngeal fungal infections have occurred but are reversible with discontinuation and antifungal treatment. Using a spacer for the inhaler may prevent these effects.

Oral and injectable glucocorticoids have many side effects. Occasionally, short-term use does not cause significant side effects. Most adverse reactions are seen within 2 weeks of glucocorticoid therapy.

When steroids are used over a prolonged time, fluid retention (puffy eyelids, edema in the lower extremities, moon face, and weight gain), thinning of the skin, purpura, abnormal subcutaneous (fat) distribution, increased blood sugar, and impaired immune response are likely to occur.

CROMOLYN SODIUM

Cromolyn sodium (Intal) is used for prophylactic treatment of bronchial asthma and therefore must be taken on a daily basis. It is *not* used for acute asthmatic attacks. Cromolyn does not have bronchodilator or antiinflammatory properties, but acts by inhibiting the release of histamine, which can cause an asthma reaction. The most common side effects are cough and a bad taste in the mouth. These effects can be decreased by drinking a few sips of water before and after the inhalation.

The method of administration of cromolyn is by inhalation. It can be used with beta adrenergics and xanthine derivatives. Rebound bronchospasm is a serious side effect of cromolyn. The drug should not be discontinued abruptly because a rebound asthmatic attack can result.

ANTICHOLINERGICS

The beta-adrenergic agonists and methylxanthines have replaced the anticholinergic drugs in treating asthma. Recently a new anticholinergic drug, ipratropium bromide (Atrovent), was introduced to treat asthmatic conditions by dilating the bronchioles. Unlike other anticholinergics, ipratropium has few systemic effects. It is administered by aerosol.

Clients using a beta-agonist inhalant should use it 5 minutes before using ipratropium. When using the anticholinergic agent in conjunction with an inhaled glucocorticoid (steroid) or cromolyn, the ipratropium should be used 5 minutes before the steroid or cromolyn. This causes the bronchioles to dilate so that the steroid or cromolyn can be deposited in the bronchioles.

MUCOLYTICS

Mucolytics act like detergents by liquifying and loosening thick mucous secretions so they can be expectorated. Acetylcysteine (Mucomyst) is admin-

istered by nebulization. The drug should not be mixed together with other drugs. The medication should be administered with a bronchodilator for clients with asthma or hyperactive airways disease because the increased secretions may obstruct the bronchial airways. The bronchodilator should be given 5 minutes before the mucolytic. Side effects include nausea and vomiting, stomatitis (oral ulcers), and "runny nose."

ANTIMICROBIALS

Antibiotics are used only if an infection results from retained mucous secretions.

NURSING PROCESS: BRONCHODILATOR

ASSESSMENT

- Obtain a medical and drug history; report probable drug-drug interaction.
- Obtain baseline vital signs (VS) for identifying abnormalities and for future comparisons.
- Assess for wheezing, decreased breath sounds, cough, and sputum production.
- Assess sensorium levels for confusion and restlessness due to hypoxia and hypercapnia.
- Assess theophylline blood levels. Toxicity occurs at a higher frequency with levels of >20 μg/mL.
- Assess hydration; diuresis may result in dehydration in the elderly and children.

POTENTIAL NURSING DIAGNOSIS

- Airway clearance, ineffective
- Activity intolerance
- Knowledge deficit related to over-the-counter (OTC) drugs

PLANNING

- Client will be free of wheezing or significantly improved and lung fields will be clear within 2 to 5 d.
- Client is taking oral drug(s) and using inhaler as prescribed.

NURSING INTERVENTIONS

- Monitor VS. Blood pressure may decrease and heart rate may increase. Check for cardiac dysrhythmias.
- Provide adequate hydration. Fluids aid in loos-

ening secretions. Monitor drug therapy. Observe for side effects.
- Check serum plasma theophylline levels (normal level is 10 to 20 μg/mL).
- Administer medication at regular intervals around the clock to have a sustained therapeutic level.
- Administer medication after meals to decrease GI distress.
- Do *not* crush enteric-coated or sustained-release (SR) tablets or capsules.
- Provide pulmonary therapy by chest clapping and postural drainage, as appropriate.

CLIENT TEACHING

General
- Advise the client that if allergic reaction occurs (rash, urticaria), drug should be discontinued and health care provider notified.
- Advise the client not to take OTC preparations without first checking with the health care provider. Some OTC products may have an additive effect.
- Encourage the client to stop smoking under medical supervision. Avoid marked sudden changes in smoking amounts, which could affect theophylline blood levels. Smoking increases drug elimination, which may require an increase of drug dose.
- Discuss ways to alleviate anxiety such as relaxation techniques and music.
- Advise the client having frequent or severe asthma attacks to wear an ID bracelet or tags.
- Encourage the client contemplating pregnancy to seek medical advice before taking a theophylline preparation.

- Advise the client to keep drug stored out of reach of small children; request child safety caps.

Skill
- Instruct the client to correctly use the nebulizer in conjunction with theophylline.
- Teach the client to monitor pulse rate and report any irregularities in comparison to baseline to health care provider.

Diet
- Advise the client that a high-protein, low-carbohydrate diet increases theophylline elimination.

Conversely, a low-protein, high-carbohydrate diet prolongs the half-life; dosage may need adjustment.

EVALUATION

- Evaluate the effectiveness of the bronchodilators. The client is breathing without wheezing and without side effects of the drug:
- Evaluate serum theophylline levels to make sure they are within the accepted range.
- Evaluate tolerance to activity.

■ CASE STUDY
Client with Asthma

M.A., age 55 years, was recently diagnosed as having bronchial asthma. She has a family history of asthma: her mother and three brothers also have asthma. In the past year, M.A. has had three asthmatic attacks that were treated with prednisone and albuterol (Proventil) inhaler. Prednisone 10 mg was prescribed for 5 days as follows: day 1, one tablet four times that day; day 2, one tablet three times that day; day 3, one tablet two times that day; day 4, one tablet in the morning; day 5, one-half tablet in the morning.

1. What is prednisone and why is it prescribed for an asthmatic attack? Why is the prednisone dosage decreased (tapered) over a period of 5 days?
2. What type of drug is albuterol (Proventil)? What effect does it have on asthma?
3. Albuterol is administered by an inhaler. For each drug dose, M.A. is to receive two puffs. What instructions would you give her concerning the use of the inhaler?

To minimize the frequency of asthmatic attacks, the health care provider prescribed TheoDur 200 mg, b.i.d., for M.A. The albuterol inhalation is to be taken as needed. Nursing interventions include client history of asthmatic attacks and physical assessment.

4. What should the nurse include when taking the client's history concerning asthmatic attacks? What physical assessment would suggest an asthmatic attack?
5. What type of drug is TheoDur? Why should the nurse ask Mrs. M.A. if she smokes?

6. What are the side effects and adverse reactions and drug interactions related to TheoDur?
7. What nonpharmacologic measures can the nurse suggest that may decrease the frequency of asthmatic attacks?

STUDY QUESTIONS

1. Your client is using an albuterol aerosol inhaler four times a day to prevent an asthmatic attack. What type of drug is albuterol? What is its action? What client teaching would you include concerning dose administration and side effects?
2. Theophylline drugs are administered by tablets for preventing asthmatic attacks and in intravenous fluids for an acute asthmatic attack. What is the effect of theophylline? What is its serum therapeutic range? Why is the serum level monitored?
3. When is cromolyn sodium used for treating asthma? Why should cromolyn not be discontinued abruptly?
4. S. D. is to use two aerosol inhalers, one a bronchodilator (Proventil) and the second a glucocorticoid (Vanceril). What client teaching would you include on administering these drugs together?
5. E. W. was having a mild asthmatic attack. The health care provider ordered methylprednisolone 4 mg for 6 days with decreasing dosages over the 6 days (6 tablets the first day, 5 tablets the second day, 4 tablets the third day, and so forth). The questions the client asks include: What is the purpose of this drug for treating my asthma? Why am I taking fewer tablets each day? Why do I take it with food or after a meal? What are appropriate responses?
6. What are mucolytics? When are they used?

Unit VIII

Cardiovascular Agents

The cardiovascular system includes the heart, blood vessels (arteries and veins), and blood. Blood rich in oxygen, nutrients, and hormones moves through vessels called arteries, which narrow to arterioles. Capillaries transport rich nourished blood to body cells and absorb waste products such as carbon dioxide (CO_2), urea, creatinine, and ammonia. The deoxygenated blood with waste products is returned to the circulation by the venules and veins for elimination by the lungs and kidneys (Fig. VIII–1).

The pumping action of the heart is the energy source for circulation of blood to body cells. Blockage of vessels can inhibit blood flow.

HEART

The heart is composed of four chambers: the right and left atria and the right and left ventricles (Fig. VIII–2). The right atrium receives deoxygenated blood from the circulation, and the right ventricle pumps blood to the pulmonary artery to the lungs for gas exchange (CO_2 for O_2). The left atrium receives oxygenated blood, and the left ventricle pumps the blood into the aorta for systemic circulation.

The heart muscle is called the **myocardium** and surrounds the atria and ventricles. The ventricles are thick walled, especially the left ventricle, to achieve the muscular force needed to pump blood to the pulmonary and systemic circulations. The atrium is thin walled, because it serves as a receptacle for blood from the circulation and from the lungs and has no pumping action.

The heart has a fibrous covering called the **pericardium** that protects it from injury and infection. The **endocardium** is a three-layered membrane that lines the inner part of the heart chambers. Four valves, two atrioventricular (tricuspid and mitral) and two semilunar (pulmonic and aortic), control blood flow between the atria and ventricles and between the ventricles and the pulmonary artery and the aorta. Three major coronary arteries, right, left, and circumflex, provide nutrients to the myocardium. Blockage in one or more of these arteries can result in a myocardial infarction, or heart attack.

CONDUCTION OF ELECTRICAL IMPULSES

The myocardium is capable of generating and conducting its own electrical impulses. The cardiac impulse usually originates in the **sinoatrial (SA) node** located in the posterior wall of the right atrium. The SA node is frequently referred to as the *pacemaker*, because it regulates the heartbeat (firing of cardiac impulses), which is approximately 60 to 80 beats a minute. The **atrioventricular (AV) node,** located in the posterior right side of the interatrial septum, has a continuous tract of fibers called the bundle of His, or the AV bundle. These two conducting systems (SA node and AV node) can act independently of each other. The ventricle can contract independently 30 to 40 times per minute.

Drugs that affect cardiac contraction include calcium, digitalis preparations, and quinidine and related preparations. The autonomic nervous system (ANS) and the drugs that stimulate or inhibit it influence heart contractions. The sympathetic nervous system and drugs that stimulate it increase heart rate; the parasympathetic nervous system and drugs that stimulate it decrease heart rate.

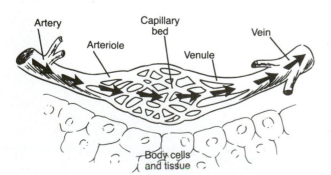

FIGURE VIII–1 Basic structures of the vascular system.

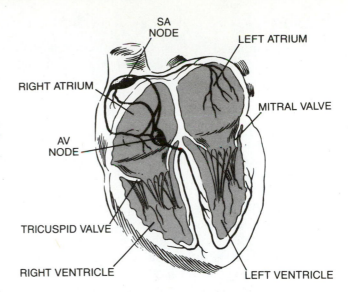

FIGURE VIII–2 Anatomy of the heart. (Key: SA node: sinoatrial node; AV node: atrioventricular node.)

Labels on figure: SA NODE, LEFT ATRIUM, RIGHT ATRIUM, MITRAL VALVE, AV NODE, TRICUSPID VALVE, RIGHT VENTRICLE, LEFT VENTRICLE

REGULATION OF HEART RATE AND BLOOD FLOW

The heart beats approximately 60 to 80 times a minute in an adult, pumping blood into the systemic circulation. As blood travels, resistance to blood flow develops and arterial pressure increases. The average systemic arterial pressure, known as blood pressure, is 120/80 mmHg. Arterial blood pressure is determined by peripheral resistance and **cardiac output,** the volume of blood expelled from the heart in 1 minute, which is calculated by multiplying the heart rate by the stroke volume. The average cardiac output is 4 to 8 L/min. **Stroke volume,** the amount of blood ejected from the left ventricle with each heart beat, is approximately 70 mL/beat.

Three factors, preload, contractility, and afterload, determine the stroke volume (Fig. VIII–3). **Preload** refers to the blood flow force that stretches the ventricle. **Contractility** is the force of ventricular contraction, and **afterload** is the resistance to ventricular ejection of blood caused by opposing pressures in the aorta and systemic circulation.

Specific drugs can increase or decrease preload and afterload, affecting both stroke volume and cardiac output. Most vasodilators decrease preload and afterload, thus decreasing arterial pressure and cardiac output.

CIRCULATION

There are two types of circulation—systemic, or peripheral, and pulmonary. With pulmonary circulation, the heart pumps deoxygenated blood from the right ventricle through the pulmonary artery to the lungs. In this situation, the artery is carrying blood that has a high concentration of CO_2. Oxygenated blood is returned to the left atrium by the pulmonary vein.

With systemic or peripheral circulation, the heart pumps blood from the left ventricle to the aorta into the general circulation. The blood is carried by arteries and arterioles to capillary beds. Nutrients in the capillary blood are transferred to cells in exchange for waste products. Blood returns to the heart through venules and veins.

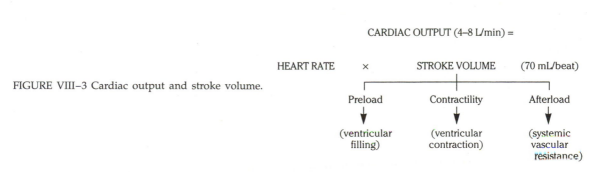

FIGURE VIII–3 Cardiac output and stroke volume.

CARDIAC OUTPUT (4–8 L/min) =

HEART RATE × STROKE VOLUME (70 mL/beat)

Preload — (ventricular filling)

Contractility — (ventricular contraction)

Afterload — (systemic vascular resistance)

471

BLOOD

Blood is composed of plasma, red blood cells (erythrocytes), white blood cells (leukocytes), and platelets. Plasma, made up of 90% water and 10% solutes, constitutes 55% of the total blood volume. The solutes in plasma include glucose, protein, lipids, amino acids, electrolytes, minerals, lactic and pyruvic acids, hormones, enzymes, oxygen, and carbon dioxide.

The major function of blood is to provide nutrients, including oxygen, to body cells. Most of the oxygen is carried in the hemoglobin of red blood cells (RBCs). The white blood cells (WBCs) are the major defense mechanism of the body and act by engulfing microorganisms. They also produce antibodies. The platelets are large cells that cause blood to coagulate. RBCs have a life span of approximately 120 days, where as the WBCs' life span is only 2 to 24 hours.

Unit VIII, Cardiovascular Agents, is composed of four chapters dealing with drugs for cardiac disorders, diuretics and antihypertensive drugs, and drugs for circulatory disorders. Cardiac glycosides, antianginals, and antidysrhythmics are described in Chapter 32. Six categories of diuretics are included in Chapter 33. Five major categories of antihypertensive agents are presented in Chapter 34. Anticoagulants, thrombolytics, antilipidemics, and peripheral vasodilators are the four drug groups discussed in Chapter 35. Two case studies and four groups of study questions are presented in this unit.

Chapter 32

Drugs for Cardiac Disorders

OUTLINE

Objectives
Terms
Introduction
Cardiac Glycosides
    Digoxin
    Nursing Process
Antianginals

Nitrates
Beta Blockers
Calcium Channel Blockers
    Nursing Process
Antidysrhythmics
    Pharmacokinetics
    Pharmacodynamics

Side Effects and Adverse
    Reactions
    Nursing Process
Case Study
Study Questions

OBJECTIVES

Explain the actions of cardiac glycosides, antianginal drugs, and antidysrhythmics.

Describe the signs and symptoms of digitalis toxicity.

Identify the side effects and adverse reactions of nitrates, beta blockers, calcium channel blockers, quinidine, and procainamide.

Explain the nursing process, including client teaching, related to cardiac glycosides, antianginal drugs, and antidysrhythmic drugs.

TERMS

afterload
angina pectoris
antianginal drugs
antiarrhythmics
antidysrhythmics
atrial fibrillation
atrial flutter
bradycardia
beta blockers

calcium channel blockers
cardiac dysrhythmias
cardiac glycosides
chronotropic
congestive heart failure
depolarization
dromotropic
heart failure
hypercapnia

hypokalemia
hypoxia
inotropic
myocardial ischemia
nitrates
preload
repolarization
tachycardia
therapeutic serum level

INTRODUCTION

Three groups of drugs, the cardiac glycosides, the antianginals, and the antidysrhythmics, are discussed in this chapter. Drugs in these groups regulate heart contraction, heart rate and rhythm, and blood flow to the myocardium (heart muscle).

CARDIAC GLYCOSIDES

Digitalis, one of the oldest drugs, used as early as 1200 A.D., is still used today in a purified form. Obtained from the purple and white foxglove plant, it can be poisonous. In 1785, William Withering of England used digitalis for alleviating "dropsy," edema of the extremities caused by kidney and cardiac insufficiency. Digitalis preparations are effective in treating congestive heart failure (CHF). (Withering did not realize that "dropsy" was the result of heart failure.) When the heart muscle (myocardium) weakens and enlarges; it loses its ability to pump blood through the heart and into the systemic circulation. This is called **heart failure,** or pump failure. When compensatory mechanisms fail and the peripheral and lung tissues are congested, the condition is **congestive heart failure.** Heart failure can be left sided or right sided. The client is in left-sided heart failure when the left ventricle does not contract sufficiently to pump the blood returned from the left atrium and lungs into the aorta, causing excessive amounts of blood to remain in the lung tissue. Right-sided heart failure occurs when the heart does not pump sufficiently for the amount of blood returning from the systemic circulation, and the blood and its constituents are pushed into peripheral tissues. One type of heart failure can lead to the other. Digitalis preparations are also used to correct **atrial fibrillation** (cardiac dysrhythmia with rapid uncoordinated contractions of atrial myocardium) and **atrial flutter** (cardiac dysrhythmia with rapid contractions of 200 to 300 beats per minute [bpm]).

Cardiac glycosides are also called digitalis glycosides. This group of drugs inhibits the sodium-potassium pump; thus, they increase intracellular calcium, which causes the cardiac muscle fibers to contract more efficiently. Digitalis preparations have three effects on the heart muscle: (1) a positive **inotropic** action (increases myocardial contraction), (2) a negative **chronotropic** action (decreases heart rate), and (3) a negative **dromotropic** action (decreases conduction of the heart cells). The increase in myocardial contractility increases cardiac, peripheral, and kidney function by increasing cardiac output, decreasing preload, improving blood flow to the periphery and kidneys, decreasing edema, and increasing fluid excretion. As a result, fluid retention in the lung and extremities is decreased.

DIGOXIN

Figure 32–1 gives the pharmacologic data for digoxin.

Pharmacokinetics

The absorption rate of digoxin in oral tablet form is >70%, and with the liquid preparation is 90%. The protein-binding power for digoxin is low; however, its half-life is 36 h, and thus drug accumulation can occur. Side effects and serum digoxin level should be closely monitored to detect digitalis toxicity.

Thirty percent of digoxin is metabolized by the liver and 65% is excreted by the kidneys mostly unchanged. Kidney dysfunction can affect the excretion of digoxin. Thyroid dysfunction can alter metabolism of cardiac glycosides. For clients with hypothyroidism, the dose of digoxin should be decreased; in hyperthyroidism, the dose may need to be increased.

Digitoxin is a potent cardiac glycoside that has a very long half-life and is highly protein-bound. Today this drug is seldom prescribed. The names of *digoxin* and *digitoxin* are very similar, and the nurse must be extremely careful to administer the correct drug. The client should consistently take the same brand-name digoxin to avoid unnecessary side effects or adverse reactions.

Pharmacodynamics

In clients with a failing heart, cardiac glycosides increase myocardial contraction, which increases cardiac output and improves circulation and tissue perfusion. Because these drugs decrease conduction through the atrioventricular node, the heart rate is decreased.

The onset and peak actions of oral and intravenous digoxin vary. The **therapeutic serum level** is 0.5 to 2.0 ng/mL for digoxin and 10 to 35 ng/mL for digitoxin. To treat CHF, the lower serum therapeutic levels should be obtained, and for atrial flutter or fibrillation, the higher therapeutic serum levels are required.

Of these two drugs, digoxin is more frequently used. It can be administered orally or intravenously. Table 32–1 lists the drug data for digitalis preparations.

Digitalis Toxicity

Overdose or accumulation of digoxin causes digitalis toxicity. Signs and symptoms include

FIGURE 32–1. Cardiac Glycosides (Inotropic Agents, Cardiotonics)

Cardiac Glycoside	Dosage	**NURSING PROCESS** Assessment and Planning
Digoxin (Lanoxin), ❦ Novodigoxin *Pregnancy Category:* C	A: PO: 0.5–1 mg initially in 2 divided doses (digitalization); maint: 0.125–0.5 mg/d; elderly: 0.125 mg/d IV: Same as PO dose given over 5 min C: PO: 1 mo–2 y: 0.01–0.02 mg/kg in 3 divided doses 2–10 y: 0.012–0.04 mg/kg in divided doses; maint: 0.012 mg/kg/d in 2 divided doses. Pediatric doses are usually ordered in μg (mcg) in elixir form. IV: Dosage varies	

Contraindications	Drug-Lab-Food Interactions	
Ventricular dysrhythmias, 2nd- or 3rd-degree heart block *Caution:* AMI, renal disease, hypothyroidism, hypokalemia	*Increase* digoxin serum level with quinidine, flecainide, verapamil *Decrease* digoxin absorption with antacids, colestipol *Increase* risk for digoxin toxicity with thiazide diuretics, loop diuretics *Lab:* hypokalemia, hypomagnesemia, hypercalcemia	

Pharmacokinetics	Pharmacodynamics	Interventions
Absorption: PO: 60–76%; liq PO: 90% *Distribution:* PB: 25% *Metabolism:* t½: 30–45 h *Excretion:* 70% in urine; 30% by liver metabolism	PO: Onset: 1–5 h Peak: 6–8 h Duration: 2–4 d IV: Onset: 5–30 min Peak: 1–5 h Duration: 2–4 d	

	Evaluation
Therapeutic Effects/Uses: To treat CHF, atrial tachycardia, flutter, or fibrillation. *Mode of Action:* It inhibits the sodium-potassium ATPase, thus promoting increased force of cardiac contraction, cardiac output, and tissue perfusion; decreases ventricular rate.	

Side Effects	Adverse Reactions
Anorexia, nausea, vomiting, headache, blurred vision (yellow-green halos), diplopia, photophobia, drowsiness, fatigue, confusion	Bradycardia, visual disturbances *Life-threatening:* Atrioventricular block, cardiac dysrhythmias

KEY: A: adult; C: child; PO: by mouth; IV: intravenous; AMI: acute myocardial infarction; CHF: congestive heart failure; PB: protein-binding; t½: half-life; ❦: Canadian drug name.

TABLE 32–1 Cardiac Glycosides

Generic (Brand)	Route and Dosage	Uses and Considerations
Rapid-Acting Digitalis		
Digoxin (Lanoxin)	See Prototype Drug Chart (Fig. 32–1)	For CHF atrial flutter, or atrial fibrillation. Low pulse rate may indicate digitalis toxicity. Serum therapeutic level is 0.5–2. *Pregnancy category:* C; PB: 25%; t½: 30–45 h
Long-Acting Digitalis		
Digitoxin (Crystodigin)	A: PO/IV: LD: 0.8–1.2 mg; maint: PO: 0.05–3 mg/d	For CHF. Serum therapeutic level is 15–30 ng/mL. Due to its long half-life, this drug is seldom given. *Pregnancy category:* C; PB: 97%; t½: 1–3 wk
Positive Inotropic Bipyridines		
Amrinone lactate (Inocor)	A: IV: LD: 0.75 mg/kg within 2–3 min; maint: 5–10 µg/kg/min; *max:* 10 mg/kg/d	For CHF, amrinone may be prescribed when digoxin and diuretics have not been effective. It may be used in conjunction with diuretic. Drug is for short-term use. *Pregnancy category:* C; PB: 10%–50%; t½: 3.5–7 h
Milrinone lactate (Primacor)	A: IV: Initially: 50 µg/kg/over 10 min *Continuous infusion:* 0.375–0.75 µg/kg/min with 0.45–0.9% saline	For short-term treatment of CHF. May be given prior to heart transplantation. Heart rate and blood pressure should be monitored. *Pregnancy category:* C; PB: 70%; t½: 1.5–2.5 h

KEY: *A: adult; PO: by mouth; IV: intravenous; LD: loading dose; PB: protein-binding; t½: half-life; CHF: congestive heart failure.*

anorexia, diarrhea, nausea and vomiting, **bradycardia** (pulse rate below 60 beats per minute [bpm]), premature ventricular contractions, cardiac dysrhythmias, headaches, malaise, blurred vision, visual illusions (white, green, yellow halos around objects), confusion, and delirium. Older adults are more prone to toxicity.

Cardiotoxicity is a serious adverse reaction to digoxin; ventricular dysrhythmias result. There are three cardiac altered functions that contribute to digoxin-induced ventricular dysrhythmias: (1) suppression of atrioventricular (AV) conduction, (2) increased automaticity, and (3) decreased refractory period in ventricular muscle. The antidysrhythmics phenytoin and lidocaine are effective in treating digoxin-induced ventricular dysrhythmias.

Drug Interactions

Drug interaction with digitalis preparations can cause digitalis toxicity. Many of the potent diuretics such as furosemide (Lasix) and hydrochlorothiazide (HydroDIURIL) promote the loss of potassium from the body. The resultant **hypokalemia** (low serum potassium level) increases the effect of the digitalis preparation, and digitalis toxicity results. Cortisone preparations taken systemically promote sodium retention and potassium excretion or loss, and can also cause hypokalemia. Clients taking digoxin along with a potassium-wasting diuretic or a cortisone drug should consume foods rich in potassium or take potassium supplements to avoid hypokalemia and digitalis toxicity. Antacids can decrease digitalis absorption if taken at the same time. Staggering doses avoids this problem.

NURSING PROCESS: CARDIAC GLYCOSIDES

ASSESSMENT

- Obtain a drug history. Report if a drug-drug interaction is probable. If the client is taking digoxin and a potassium-wasting diuretic or cortisone drug, hypokalemia might result, causing digitalis toxicity. A low serum potassium level enhances the action of digoxin. A client taking a thiazide and/or cortisone along with digoxin should be taking a potassium supplement.
- Obtain a baseline-pulse rate for future comparisons. Apical pulse should be taken for a full minute and should be >60 bpm.

- Assess for signs and symptoms of digitalis toxicity. Common symptoms include anorexia, nausea, vomiting, bradycardia, cardiac dysrhythmias, and visual disturbances. Report symptoms immediately to the health care provider.

POTENTIAL NURSING DIAGNOSES

- Decreased cardiac output
- Altered tissue perfusion (cardiopulmonary, cerebral)
- Anxiety related to cardiac problem

PLANNING

- Client checks pulse rate daily before taking digoxin. Client will report pulse rate of <60 bpm or a marked decline in pulse rate.
- Client eats foods rich in potassium to maintain a desired serum potassium level (see Client Teaching, Diet).

NURSING INTERVENTIONS

- Do *not* confuse **digoxin** with **digitoxin.** Read the drug labels carefully. Digoxin has a long half-life but has a shorter half-life than digitoxin.
- Check the apical pulse rate before administering digoxin. Do *not* administer if pulse rate is <60 bpm.
- Check the signs of peripheral and pulmonary edema, which indicate CHF.
- Check the serum digoxin level. The normal therapeutic drug range for digoxin is 0.5 to 2.0 ng/mL. A serum digoxin level of >2.0 ng/mL is indicative of digitalis toxicity. Check serum potassium level (normal range, 3.5 to 5.3 mEq/L) and report if hypokalemia (<3.5 mEq/L) is present.

CLIENT TEACHING

General
- Explain to the client the importance of compliance with the drug therapy. A visiting nurse may ensure that the medications are properly taken.

- Advise the client not to take over-the-counter (OTC) drugs without first consulting the health care provider to avoid adverse drug interactions.
- Keep drugs out of reach of small children. Request child safety cap bottle.
- Instruct the parent to check child's pulse rate before administering the drug.

Skill
- Instruct the client how to check the pulse rate before taking digoxin and to call the health care provider for pulse rate <60 bpm or irregular pulse.

Diet
- Advise the client to eat foods rich in potassium such as fresh and dried fruits, fruit juices, and vegetables, including potatoes.

Side Effects
- Instruct the client to report side effects such as a pulse rate of <60 bpm, nausea, vomiting, headache, and visual disturbances, including diplopia.

EVALUATION

- Evaluate the effectiveness of digoxin by noting the client's response to the drug (decreased heart rate, decreased chest rales), and the absence of side effects. Continue monitoring the pulse rate.

ANTIANGINAL DRUGS

Antianginal drugs are used to treat **angina pectoris** (acute cardiac pain from inadequate blood flow due to plaque occlusion in the coronary arteries of the myocardium or due to spasms of the coronary arteries). With decreased blood flow, there is a decrease in oxygen to the myocardium that causes pain. Anginal pain is frequently described by the client as tightness, pressure in the center of the chest, and pain radiating down the left arm. Referred pain felt in the neck and left arm commonly occurs with severe angina pectoris. Anginal attacks may lead to myocardial infarction (heart attack). Anginal pain usually lasts for only a few minutes.

The frequency of anginal pain depends on many factors, including the type of angina, which includes (1) classic (stable), which occurs with stress or exertion; (2) unstable (preinfarction), which occurs frequently over the course of a day with progressive severity, and (3) variant (Prinzmetal),

which occurs during rest. The first two types are caused by a narrowing or partial occlusion of the coronary arteries; variant angina is due to vessel spasm (vasospasm). It is not uncommon for the client to have both classic and variant angina. Unstable angina often indicates an impending myocardial infarction (MI).

Antianginal drugs increase blood flow either by increasing oxygen supply or by decreasing oxygen demand by the myocardium. Three types of antianginals are the nitrates, beta blockers, and calcium channel blockers. The major systemic effect of nitrates is a reduction of venous tone, which decreases the workload of the heart and promotes vasodilation. Beta blockers and calcium channel blockers decrease the workload of the heart and decrease oxygen demands.

Nonpharmacologic ways of decreasing anginal attacks are to avoid heavy meals, smoking, extremes in weather changes, strenuous exercise, and emotional upset. Proper nutrition, moderate exercise (only after consulting with a health care provider if the client already has angina), adequate rest, and relaxation techniques should be employed as preventive measures.

Stress tests, cardiac profile laboratory tests, and cardiac catheterization may be needed to determine the degree of blockage in the coronary arteries. A combination of pharmacologic and nonpharmacologic measures is usually necessary to control and prevent anginal attacks.

NITRATES

Nitrates, developed in the 1840s, were the first agents used to relieve angina. Nitroglycerin is not swallowed because it undergoes first-pass metabolism by the liver, which decreases its effectiveness; instead it is given sublingually (under the tongue) and is absorbed readily into the circulation through the sublingual vessels. The sublingual tablet comes in various dosages, but the average dose prescribed is 0.4 mg or gr 1/150 following cardiac pain, repeated every 5 min for a total of three doses. The client may experience dizziness, faintness, or headache due to the peripheral vasodilation. If pain persists, the client should immediately call for medical assistance. Nitroglycerin is also available in topical (ointment, transdermal patch) and intravenous forms. Figure 32–2 summarizes the action of the nitroglycerin (nitrates).

Pharmacokinetics

Nitroglycerin, taken sublingually, is absorbed rapidly and directly into the internal jugular vein and the right atrium. Approximately 40% to 50% of nitrates absorbed through the gastrointestinal (GI) tract are inactivated by liver metabolism (first-pass metabolism of the liver). The nitroglycerin in Nitro-Bid ointment and in the Transderm-Nitro patch is absorbed slowly through the skin. It is excreted primarily in the urine.

Pharmacodynamics

Nitroglycerin acts directly on the smooth muscle of blood vessels, causing relaxation and dilation. It decreases cardiac **preload** (the amount of blood in the ventricle at the end of diastole) and **afterload** (peripheral vascular resistance) and reduces myocardial oxygen demand. With dilation of the veins, there is less blood return to the heart, and with dilation of the arteries, there is less vasoconstriction and resistance.

The onset of action of nitroglycerin depends on the method of administration. With sublingual and intravenous use, the onset of action is rapid (1 to 3 min); it is slower with the transdermal method (30 to 60 min). The duration of action of the Transderm-Nitro patch is approximately 24 h. Because Nitro-Bid ointment is effective for only 6 to 8 h, it must be reapplied three to four times a day. The use of Nitro-Bid ointment has declined since the advent of the Transderm-Nitro patch, which needs to be applied only once a day. Table 32–2 lists drug data for the nitrates.

Side Effects and Adverse Reactions

Headaches are one of the most common side effects of nitroglycerin, but they may become less frequent with continued use. Otherwise, acetaminophen may provide some relief. Other side effects include hypotension, dizziness, weakness, and faintness. When nitroglycerin ointment or transdermal patches are discontinued, the dose should be tapered over several weeks to prevent the rebound effect of severe pain due to **myocardial ischemia** (lack of blood supply to the heart muscle). Nitrate tolerance can occur with a continual increase in dosage or with prolonged use.

BETA BLOCKERS

Beta-adrenergic blockers block the beta$_1$ receptor site. Beta blockers decrease the effects of the sympathetic nervous system by blocking the release of the catecholamines epinephrine and norepinephrine, thereby decreasing the heart rate and blood pressure. They are used as antianginal, antidysrhythmic, and antihypertensive drugs. Beta blockers are effective as antianginals because by decreasing the heart rate and myocardial contractility, they reduce the need for oxygen consumption and, consequently, the pain of angina. These drugs are more useful for classic angina.

Beta blockers, which are discussed in detail in Chapter 18, are subdivided into nonselective beta blockers (blocking beta$_1$ and beta$_2$) and selective (cardiac) beta blockers (blocking beta$_1$). Examples of nonselective beta blockers are propranolol (Inderal), nadolol (Corgard), and pindolol (Visken). These drugs decrease the pulse rate and can cause bronchoconstriction. The selective (cardioselective) beta blockers act more strongly on the beta$_1$ receptor, thus decreasing the pulse rate. Examples are atenolol (Tenormin) and metoprolol (Lopressor). This latter group is the choice for controlling

FIGURE 32–2. Antianginals: Nitroglycerin

Nitrate	Dosage	NURSING PROCESS
Nitroglycerin (Nitrostat, Nitro-Bid, Transderm-Nitro patch, NTG), 🍁 Nitrogard SR, Nitrol *Nitrate* *Pregnancy Category:* C	A: PO/SL: 0.3, 0.4, 0.6 mg; repeat q5min ×3 as needed. SR: 2.5 mg q8–12 h IV: Initially: 5 μg/min; dose may be increased Oint: 2% 1–2 inch to chest or thigh area Patch: 2.5–15 mg/d to chest or thigh area	Assessment and Planning

Contraindications	Drug-Lab-Food Interactions	
Marked hypotension, AMI, increased intracranial pressure (ICP), severe anemia *Caution:* Severe renal or hepatic disease, early MI	*Increase* effect with alcohol, beta blockers, calcium blockers, antihypertensives *Decrease* effects of heparin	

Pharmacokinetics	Pharmacodynamics	
Absorption: SL: >75% absorbed; oint and patch: slow absorption *Distribution:* PB: 60% *Metabolism:* t½: 1–4 min *Excretion:* Liver and urine	SL: Onset: 1–3 min Peak: 4 min Duration: 20–30 min SR: Cap: Onset: 20–45 min Duration: 3–8 h Oint: Onset: 20–60 min Peak: 1–2 h Duration: 3–8 h Patch: Onset: 30–60 min Peak: 1–2 h Duration: 20–24 h IV: Onset: 1–3 min Duration: 0.5–2 h	Interventions

Therapeutic Effects/Uses: To control angina pectoris (anginal pain). *Mode of Action:* Decrease myocardial demand for oxygen; decrease preload by dilating veins, thus indirectly decreasing afterload.	Evaluation

Side Effects	Adverse Reactions
Nausea, vomiting, headache, dizziness, syncope, weakness, flushing, confusion, pallor, rash, dry mouth	Hypotension, reflex tachycardia, paradoxical bradycardia *Life-threatening:* Circulatory collapse

KEY: A: adult; C: child; PO: by mouth; SL: sublingual; SR: sustained-release; IV: intravenous; PB: protein-binding; t½: half-life; NTG: nitroglycerin; AMI: acute myocardial infarction; MI: myocardial infarction; 🍁: Canadian drug names.

angina pectoris. Table 32–2 lists the beta blockers most frequently used for angina.

Pharmacokinetics

Orally, the beta blockers are well absorbed. Absorption of sustained-release capsules is slow. The half-life of propranolol (Inderal) is 3 to 6 h. Of the selective beta blockers, atenolol (Tenormin) has a half-life of 6 to 7 h and metoprolol (Lopressor), 3 to 7 h. Propranolol and metoprolol are metabolized and excreted by the liver. Fifty percent of atenolol is excreted unchanged by the kidneys, and 50% is excreted unabsorbed in the feces.

TABLE 32–2 Antianginals

Generic (Brand)	Route and Dosage	Uses and Considerations
Nitrates		
Amyl nitrite	A: Inhal: 0.18–0.3 mL amp PRN	For acute anginal attack. Rarely used. *Pregnancy category:* C; PB: UK; t½: 1–4 min
Isosorbide dinitrate (Isordil, Sorbitrate)	A: SL: 2.5–10 mg q.i.d. Chewable: 5–10 mg PRN PO: 2.5–30 mg q.i.d. a.c. and h.s. SR: 40 mg, q6–12h	To prevent anginal attacks. Drug can lower blood pressure. Tolerance builds up over time. Headaches, dizziness, lightheadedness, and flushing may occur. *Pregnancy category:* C; PB: UK; t½: 1–4 h
Isosorbide mononitrate (Imdur)	A: PO: SR: 30–60 mg q morning: *max:* 240 mg/d	To prevent anginal attacks. Sustained-release form provides controlled delivery and a 6-h drug-free period. By allowing a drug-free period, tolerance to nitrates is reduced; effectiveness is increased. *Pregnancy category:* C; PB: 5%; t½: 6.6 h
Nitroglycerin (Nitrostat, Nitro-Bid, Transderm-Nitro)	See Prototype Drug Chart (Fig. 32–2)	To control angina pectoris. IV used for treating severe angina and hypertension. Headaches occur approximately 50% when first used. *Pregnancy category:* C; PB: 60%; t½: 1–4 min (IV)
Pentaerythritol tetranitrate (Peritrate)	A: PO: 10–40 mg t.i.d./q.i.d. SR: 20–80 mg q12h	To prevent anginal attacks. Tolerance builds up over time. *Pregnancy category:* C; PB: UK; t½: 10 min
Beta-Adrenergic Blockers		
Atenolol (Tenormin) (Beta₁)	A: PO: 50–100 mg/d; *max:* 200 mg/d	To control angina pectoris. Also effective in managing hypertension. Blood pressure and heart rate should be monitored. Cardioselective drug, blocking beta₁. Can be used by asthmatic clients. *Pregnancy category:* C; PB: 5%–15%; t½: 6–7 h
Metoprolol tartrate (Lopressor)(Beta₁)	A: PO: Initially: 50–100 mg/d in 1–2 divided doses; maint: 100–400 mg/d SR: 100 mg, daily; *max:* 400 mg/d	Same as atenolol. Monitor heart rate and blood pressure. *Pregnancy category:* C; PB: 12%; t½: 3–7 h
Propranolol HCl (Inderal) (Beta₁ and beta₂)	A: PO: Initially: 10–20 mg t.i.d./q.i.d.; maint: 20–60 mg t.i.d./q.i.d.; *max:* 320 mg/d SR: 80–160 mg/d	First beta blocker, blocking beta₁ and beta₂. It is no longer the drug of choice to prevent angina because of the risk of bronchospasm. Heart rate, blood pressure, and respiratory status should be monitored. *Pregnancy category:* C; PB: 90%; t½: 3–6 h

Pharmacodynamics

Because beta blockers decrease the force of myocardial contraction, the oxygen demand by the myocardium is reduced, and the client can tolerate increased exercise with less oxygen need. Beta blockers tend to be more effective for classic angina than for variant angina.

The onset of action of the nonselective beta blocker propranolol is 30 min, its peak action is reached in 1 to 1.5 h, and its duration is 4 to 12 h. For the selective beta blockers, the onset of action of atenolol is 60 min, the peak action occurs in 2 to 4 h, and the duration of action is 24 h; the onset of action of metoprolol is reached in 15 min and the duration of action is 6 to 12 h.

Side Effects and Adverse Reactions

Both nonselective and selective beta blockers cause a decrease in pulse rate and blood pressure. For the nonselective beta blockers, bronchospasm, behavioral or psychotic response, and impotence (with use of Inderal) are potential adverse reactions.

The vital signs need to be closely monitored in the early stages of beta blocker therapy. With discontinuation of use, the dosage should be tapered for a week or two to prevent a rebound effect (reflex tachycardia and vasoconstriction).

CALCIUM CHANNEL BLOCKERS

Calcium channel blockers, also known as calcium blockers, are the newest group of drugs to be marketed (1982) for the treatment of angina pectoris, certain dysrhythmias, and hypertension. Calcium activates myocardial contraction, increasing the workload of the heart and the need for more oxygen. Calcium blockers decrease cardiac contractility (negative inotropic effect by relaxing smooth muscle) and the workload of the heart, thus decreasing

TABLE 32–2 Antianginals *(Continued)*

Generic (Brand)	Route and Dosage	Uses and Considerations
Calcium Channel Blockers Amlodipine (Norvasc)	IV: See Antidysrhythmics A: PO: Initially: 10 mg; maint: 2.5–10 mg/d	Management of angina pectoris. May be given with another antianginal or antihypertensive drug. *Pregnancy category:* C; PB: 95%; t½: 30–50 h
Bepridil HCl (Vascor)	A: PO: Initially 200 mg/d × 10 d; maint: 300 mg/d; *max:* 400 mg/d	Treatment of angina pectoris. May be used as single drug or in combination with nitrates. Given as a single dose. *Pregnancy category:* C; PB: 99%; t½: 2–24 h
Diltiazem HCl (Cardizem)	A: PO: 30–60 mg q.i.d.; may increase to 360 mg/d in 4 divided doses SR: 60 mg q12h; *max:* 360 mg/d CD: 120–180 mg/d; *max:* 360 mg/d	For angina pectoris. Hypotensive effect is not as severe as with nifedipine. Kidney function should be monitored. *Pregnancy category:* C; PB: 70%–85%; t½: 3.5–9 h
Isradipine (DynaCirc)	A: PO: 2.5–7.5 mg t.i.d.	Primary use is to treat hypertension. Also can be given for angina pectoris. *Pregnancy category:* C; PB: 99%; t½: 5–11 h
Nicardipine HCl (Cardene, Cardene SR)	A: PO: 20 mg t.i.d.; maint: 20–40 mg t.i.d. SR: 30 mg b.i.d.; maint: 30–60 mg b.i.d.	Used for angina pectoris. May be used alone or in combination with other antianginals. Used also for hypertension. Peripheral edema, headache, dizziness, and lightheadedness may occur. *Pregnancy category:* C; PB: 95%; t½: 5 h
Nifedipine (Procardia, Adalat)	A: PO: 10–30 mg q6–8h; *max:* 180 mg/d	For angina pectoris. Blood pressure should be closely monitored, especially if client is taking nitrates or beta blockers. Is a potent calcium blocker. *Pregnancy category:* C; PB: 92%–98%; t½: 2–5 h
Verapamil HCl (Calan, Isoptin, Verelan)	A: PO: 40–120 mg t.i.d.; *max:* 480 mg/d IV: 5–10 mg over 2 min	Treatment of angina pectoris, cardiac dysrhythmias, and hypertension. Peripheral edema, constipation, dizziness, headache, and hypotension may occur. *Pregnancy category:* C; PB: 90%; t½: 3–8 h

KEY: *A: adult; PO: by mouth; IV: intravenous; SL: sublingual; SR: sustained-release; CD: controlled delivery; a.c.: before meals; PB: protein-binding; t½: half-life; PRN: as necessary; UK: unknown.*

the need for oxygen. They are effective in controlling variant angina by relaxing coronary arteries and for classic angina by decreasing oxygen demand.

Pharmacokinetics

Three calcium blockers, verapamil (Calan), nifedipine (Procardia), and diltiazem (Cardizem), have been effectively used in long-term treatment of angina. Eighty to ninety percent of calcium channel blockers are absorbed through the GI mucosa. However, the first-pass metabolism by the liver decreases the availability of free circulating drug, and only 20% of verapamil, 45% to 65% of diltiazem, and 35% to 40% of nifedipine are bioavailable. All three drugs are highly protein-bound (80%–90%) and their half-life is 2 to 6 h.

Several new calcium blockers are available: nicardipine HCl (Cardene), amlodipine (Norvasc), and bepridal HCl (Vascor). All three of these drugs are highly protein-bound (>95%). Nicardipine has the shortest half-life of the three drugs.

Pharmacodynamics

Bradycardia is a common problem with verapamil, the first calcium blocker. Nifedipine, the most potent of the calcium blockers, promotes vasodilation of the coronary and peripheral vessels, and hypotension can result. The onset of action is 10 min for verapamil and 30 min for nifedipine and diltiazem. Duration of action is 3 to 7 h (PO) and 2 h (IV) for verapamil and 6 to 8 h for nifedipine and diltiazem.

Table 32–2 presents the drug data for the calcium blockers used in treating angina.

Side Effects and Adverse Reactions

The side effects of calcium blockers include headache, hypotension (more common with nifedipine and less common with diltiazem), dizziness, and flushing of the skin. Reflex tachycardia can occur due to hypotension. Calcium blockers can cause changes in liver and kidney function, and serum liver enzymes should be checked periodically. Calcium blockers are frequently given with other antianginal drugs such as nitrates to prevent angina.

NURSING PROCESS: ANTIANGINALS: Nitroglycerin, Beta and Calcium Blockers

ASSESSMENT

- Obtain baseline vital signs (VS) for future comparisons.
- Obtain health and drug histories. Nitroglycerin is contraindicated for marked hypotension or acute myocardial infarction (AMI).

POTENTIAL NURSING DIAGNOSES

- Decreased cardiac output
- Anxiety related to cardiac problem(s)
- Acute pain
- Activity intolerance

PLANNING

- Client takes nitroglycerin or other antianginals and angina pain is controlled.

NURSING INTERVENTIONS

- Monitor VS. Hypotension is associated with most antianginal drugs.
- Have the client sit or lie down when taking a nitrate for the first time. After administration, check the VS while the client is lying down and then sitting up. Have the client rise slowly to a standing position.
- Offer sips of water before giving sublingual (SL) nitrates; dryness may inhibit drug absorption.
- Monitor effects of IV nitroglycerin. Report angina that persists.
- Apply Nitro-Bid ointment to the designated mark on paper. Do *not* use fingers because the drug can be absorbed; use a tongue blade or gloves. For the Transderm-Nitro patch, do not touch the medication portion.
- Do *not* apply the Nitro-Bid ointment or the Transderm-Nitro patch in any area on the chest in the vicinity of defibrillator-cardioverter paddle placement. Explosion and skin burns may result.

CLIENT TEACHING

General
- A nitroglycerin SL tablet is used if chest pain occurs. Repeat in 5 min if the pain has not sub-

sided and again in another 5 min if it persists. Do *not* give more than 3 tablets. If the chest pain persists >15 min, immediate medical help is necessary.
- Instruct the client not to ingest alcohol while taking nitroglycerin to avoid hypotension, weakness, and faintness.
- Tolerance to nitroglycerin can occur. If the client's chest pain is not completely alleviated, the client should notify the health care provider.

Beta Blockers and Calcium Blockers
- Instruct the client not to discontinue these drugs without the health care provider's approval. Withdrawal symptoms, such as reflex tachycardia and pain, may be severe.

Skill
- Instruct the client about SL nitroglycerin tablets. The tablet is placed under the tongue for quick absorption. A stinging or biting sensation may indicate the tablet is fresh. With the newer SL nitroglycerin, the biting sensation may not be present. The bottle is stored away from light and kept dry.
- Instruct the client about the Transderm-Nitro patch. Apply once a day, usually in the morning. Rotation of skin sites is necessary. Usually the patch is applied to the chest wall; however, the thighs and arms are used. Avoid hairy areas.

Side Effects
- Headaches commonly occur when first taking nitroglycerin products and last about 30 min. Acetaminophen is suggested for relief.
- If hypotension results from SL nitroglycerin, place the client in supine position with legs elevated.

Beta Blockers and Calcium Blockers
- Instruct the client how to take a pulse rate. Advise the client to call the health care provider if dizziness or faintness occurs; this may indicate hypotension.

EVALUATION

- Evaluate the nitrate product for relieving anginal pain. Note headache, dizziness, or faintness.

ANTIDYSRHYTHMICS

A **cardiac dysrhythmia (arrhythmia)** is defined as any deviation from the normal rate or pattern of the heartbeat; this includes heart rates that are too slow (bradycardia), too fast (**tachycardia**), or irregular. The terms *dysrhythmia* (disturbed heart rhythm) and *arrhythmia* (absence of rhythm) are used interchangeably, despite the slight difference in meaning.

The electrocardiogram (ECG) identifies the type of dysrhythmia. The P wave of the ECG reflects atrial activation, the QRS complex indicates the ventricular depolarization, and the T wave reflects ventricular **repolarization** (return of cell membrane potential to resting after depolarization). The PR interval indicates atrioventricular conduction time, and the QT interval reflects the ventricular action potential duration. Atrial dysrhythmias prevent proper filling of the ventricles and decrease the cardiac output by one third. Ventricular dysrhythmias are life-threatening because ineffective filling of the ventricle results in decreased or absent cardiac output. With ventricular tachycardia, ventricular fibrillation is likely to occur, followed by death. Cardiopulmonary resuscitation (CPR) is a necessity in treating these clients.

Cardiac dysrhythmias frequently follow a myocardial infarction (heart attack) or can result from **hypoxia** (lack of oxygen to body tissues), **hypercapnia** (increased carbon dioxide in the blood), excess catecholamines, or electrolyte imbalance. The desired action of antidysrhythmics is restoration of normal cardiac rhythm, which is accomplished by various mechanisms (Table 32–3).

The antidysrhythmics are grouped into four classes: (1) fast (sodium) channel blockers IA (I), IB (II), and IC (III); (2) beta blockers; (3) those that prolong repolarization; and (4) slow (calcium) channel blockers.

When sodium and calcium enter a cardiac cell, **depolarization** (myocardial contraction) occurs.

Sodium enters rapidly to start the depolarization, and calcium enters later to maintain it. These electrolytes irritate the cell and cause contraction. In the presence of myocardial ischemia, the contraction can be irregular.

Cardiac action potentials are frequent depolarization followed by repolarization of myocardial cells. Figure 32–3 illustrates the action potential of a cardiac cell to conduct impulses. There are five phases. Phase 0 is the depolarization caused by an influx of sodium ions. Phase 1 is rapid repolarization. Phase 2 is the influx of calcium ion, which prolongs the action potential and promotes atrial and ventricular muscle contraction. Phase 3 is rapid repolarization due to the potassium ion. Phase 4 is the spontaneous depolarization, or automaticity, which initiates the action potential cycle.

Fast (sodium) channel blockers decrease the fast sodium influx to the cardiac cells. The drug response is (1) decreased conduction velocity in the cardiac tissues; (2) suppression of the automaticity that decreases the likelihood of ectopic foci; and (3) increased recovery time (repolarization or refractory period). There are three subgroups of fast channel blockers: IA (I) slows conduction and prolongs repolarization (quinidine, procainamide), IB (II) slows conduction and shortens repolarization (lidocaine, mexiletine HCl), and IC (III) prolongs conduction with little to no effect on repolarization (encainide, flecainide). Figure 32–4 summarizes the action of the fast channel blocker procainamide HCl.

PHARMACOKINETICS

The IA or fast (sodium) channel blockers I, quinidine (Cardioquin, Quinidex), procainamide (Pronestyl, Procan), and disopyramide (Norpace), are absorbed rapidly from the GI mucosa. Food and pH change the absorption rate. The salt content of quinidine affects absorption: quinidine sulfate is

TABLE 32–3 Pharmacodynamics of Antidysrhythmics

Mechanisms of Action
Block adrenergic stimulation of the heart.
Depress myocardial excitability and contractility.
Decrease conduction velocity in cardiac tissue.
Increase recovery time (repolarization) of the myocardium.
Suppress automaticity (spontaneous depolarization to initiate beats).

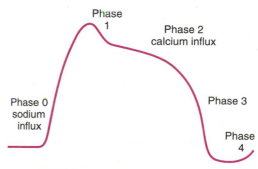

FIGURE 32–3 Cardiac action potential.

FIGURE 32–4. Antidysrhythmics: Fast Channel Blocker (IA)

Fast Channel Blocker I (IA)	Dosage	NURSING PROCESS

Fast Channel Blocker I (IA)

Procainamide HCl
  (Procan, Pronestyl)
Fast channel (sodium) blocker I
Pregnancy Category: C

Dosage

A: PO: 250–500 mg q3–4h
  SR: 250 mg–1 g q6h or 50 mg/kg/d
  in 4 divided doses
  IV: 20–30 mg/min; maint: 1–4
  mg/min; max: 17 mg/kg
C: PO: 40–60 mg/kg/d in 4 divided
  doses
  IV: 3–6 mg/kg q10–30 min; max: 100
  mg/dose
TDM: 4–8 μg/mL

NURSING PROCESS
Assessment and Planning

Contraindications

Hypersensitivity to procaine, blood
  dyscrasias, heart block, cardiogenic
  shock, myasthenia gravis
Caution: Hypotension, CHF, MI,
  renal or hepatic insufficiency

Drug-Lab-Food Interactions

Increase effects with histamine$_2$ blockers; *increase* hypotensive effects with
  antihypertensives, nitrates
Decrease effects with barbiturates
Lab: May *increase* ALP, AST, LDH,
  bilirubin

Pharmacokinetics

Absorption: PO: 75–95%
Distribution: PB: 20%
Metabolism: t½: 3–4 h
Excretion: 60% unchanged in urine (half
  as an active metabolite)

Pharmacodynamics

PO: Onset: 30 min
  Peak: 1–1.5 h
  Duration: 3–4 h (SR: 8 h)
IV: Onset: Minutes
  Peak: 25–60 min
  Duration: 3–4 h

Interventions

Therapeutic Effects/Uses: To control cardiac dysrhythmias (premature ventricular contractions [PVCs], ventricular tachycardia.

Mode of Action: Depression of myocardial excitability by slowing conduction of cardiac
tissue through the atrium, bundle of His, and ventricle to decrease cardiac dysrhythmias.

Evaluation

Side Effects

Anorexia, nausea, vomiting, diarrhea,
  headache, dizziness, weakness, flushing, rash, pruritus, lupus-like syndrome with rash

Adverse Reactions

Life-threatening: Atrioventricular block,
  pleural effusion, ventricular tachy-
  cardia/fibrillation, thrombocytopenia, agranulocytosis, cardiovascular
  collapse, torsades de pointes

KEY: A: adult; C: child; PO: by mouth; IV: intravenous; TDM: therapeutic drug monitoring; SR:
sustained-release; PB: protein-binding; t½: half-life.

absorbed more readily than quinidine gluconate or quinidine polygalacturonate.

Quinidine is highly protein-bound, whereas procainamide is 20% protein-bound, and disopyramide is moderately protein-bound. All of these antidysrhythmics are excreted by the kidneys unchanged. Procainamide has a shorter half-life than quinidine or disopyramide.

PHARMACODYNAMICS

Quinidine, procainamide, and disopyramide have similar onset-of-action times. The peak action is longer with disopyramide and the duration is shorter with procainamide.

Table 32–4 lists the drug data for the commonly administered antidysrhythmics.

TABLE 32–4 Antidysrhythmics

Generic (Brand)	Route and Dosage	Uses and Considerations
Class I **Fast (Sodium) Channel Blockers I** Disopyramide phosphate (Norpace, Napamide)	A: PO: 100–200 mg q6h CR: 300 mg q12h C 4–12 y: PO: 10–15 mg/kg/d in divided doses 13–18 y: PO: 6–15 mg/kg/d in divided doses	Prevention and suppression of unifocal and multifocal premature ventricular contractions (PVCs). For ventricular dysrhythmias. May cause anticholinergic symptoms. Serum therapeutic level: 3–8 μg/mL. *Pregnancy category:* C; PB: 50%–66%; t½: 4–10 h
Procainamide (Pronestyl, Procan)	See Prototype Drug Chart (Fig. 32–4)	For atrial and ventricular dysrhythmias. Has less hypotensive effect than quinidine. Serum therapeutic level: 4–8 μg/mL. *Pregnancy category:* C; PB: 20%; t½: 3–4 h
Quinidine sulfate, polygalactorate, gluconate (Quinidex, Cardioquin)	A: PO: 200–400 mg t.i.d./q.i.d. C: PO: 30 mg/kg or 900 mg/m^2 in 5 divided doses	For atrial, ventricular, and supraventricular dysrhythmias. Nausea, vomiting, diarrhea, abdominal pain, or cramps are common side effects. If given with digoxin, it can increase digoxin concentration. Serum therapeutic level: 2–6 μg/mL. *Pregnancy category:* C; PB: 80%; t½: 6–7 h
Fast (Sodium) Channel Blockers II Lidocaine (Xylocaine)	A: IV: 50–100 mg bolus in 2–3 min; then 20–50 μg/kg/min	For acute ventricular dysrhythmias following MI and cardiac surgery. Serum therapeutic range: 1.5–6 μg/mL. *Pregnancy category:* B; PB: 60%–80%; t½: 1.5–2 h
Mexiletine HCl (Mexitil)	A: PO: 200–400 mg q8h	Analog of lidocaine. Treatment for acute and chronic ventricular dysrhythmias. Take with food to decrease GI distress. Common side effects include nausea, vomiting, heartburn, tremor, dizziness, nervousness, lightheadedness. Serum therapeutic range: 0.5–2 μg/mL. *Pregnancy category:* C; PB: 50%–60%; t½: 10–12 h
Fast (Sodium) Channel Blockers III Encainide HCl **Available for compassionate use only**	A: PO: 25 mg q8h; may increase to 50–75 mg q8h	For ventricular dysrhythmia, but may cause new ventricular dysrhythmia. FDA approved for life-threatening situations. *Pregnancy category:* B; PB: 75%–85%; t½: 3–12 h
Flecainide (Tambocor)	A: PO: Initial: 50–100 mg q12h, increase by 50 mg q12h, q4d; *maint:* 150 mg, q12h; *max:* 300 mg/d	For life-threatening ventricular dysrhythmias; prevention of paroxysmal supraventricular tachycardia (PSVT) and paroxysmal atrial fibrillation or flutter (PAF). Avoid use in cardiogenic shock, second- or third-degree heart block, or right bundle branch block. *Pregnancy category:* C; PB: UK; t½: 12–27 h
Propafenone HCl (Rythmol)	A: PO: 150–300 mg q8h; *max:* 900 mg/d	Treatment of life-threatening ventricular dysrhythmias. Avoid use if cardiogenic shock, uncontrolled CHF, heart block, severe hypotension, bradycardia, and bronchospasms occur. *Pregnancy category:* C; PB: 97%; t½: 5–8 h
Tocainide HCl (Tonocard)	A: PO: LD: 600 mg PO: 400 mg q8h; *max:* 2.4 g/d	For ventricular dysrhythmias, especially PVC. Similar to lidocaine except in oral form. Serum therapeutic level: 4–10 μg/mL. *Pregnancy category:* C; PB: 70%–80%; t½: 10–17 h
Class II **Beta-Adrenergic Blockers** Acebutolol HCl (Sectral) Beta$_1$ blocker	A: PO: 200 mg b.i.d.; may increase dose	Management of ventricular dysrhythmias. Also used for angina pectoris and hypertension. Primarily for PVC. New beta blocker that affects the beta$_1$ receptor in the heart. Can cause bradycardia and decrease cardiac output. *Pregnancy category:* B; PB: 26%; t½: 3–13 h
Propranolol HCl (Inderal) Beta$_1$ and beta$_2$ blocker	A: PO: 10–30 mg t.i.d./q.i.d. A: IV bolus: 0.5–3 mg at 1 mg/min	For ventricular dysrhythmias, PAT, and atrial and ventricular ectopic beats. Asthmatic clients should not use drug. *Pregnancy category:* C; PB: 90%; t½: 3–6 h
Sotalol HCl (Betapace) Beta$_1$ and beta$_2$ blocker	A: PO: 80 mg b.i.d.; *max:* 240–320 mg/d Increase dose interval with renal dysfunction	For ventricular dysrhythmias. Avoid if bronchial asthma or heart block is present. *Pregnancy category:* B; PB: 0%; t½: 12 h

Table continues on following page

TABLE 32–4 Antidysrhythmics (Continued)

Generic (Brand)	Route and Dosage	Uses and Considerations
Class III **Prolong Repolarization** Adenosine (Adenocard)	A: IV: 6 mg (bolus: 1–2 sec); repeat if necessary, 12 mg bolus	Treatment of paroxysmal supraventricular tachycardia (PSVT), Wolff-Parkinson-White syndrome. Avoid if second- or third-degree AV block or atrial flutter or fibrillation is present. *Pregnancy category:* C; PB: UK; t½: <10 sec
Amiodarone HCl (Cordarone)	A: PO: LD: 400–1600 mg/d in divided doses; maint: 200–600 mg/d	For life-threatening ventricular dysrhythmias. Initially dosage is greater and then decreases over time. Therapeutic serum level: 1–2.5 µg/mL. *Pregnancy category:* C; PB: 96%; t½: 5–100 d
Bretylium tosylate (Bretylol)	A: IM: 5–10 mg/kg q6–8h IV: 5–10 mg/kg; repeat in 15–30 min, IV drip or IV bolus	For ventricular tachycardia and fibrillation (to convert to a normal sinus rhythm). Used when lidocaine and procainamide are ineffective. *Pregnancy category:* C; PB: UK; t½: 4–17 h
Class IV **Calcium Channel Blockers** Verapamil HCl (Calan)	A: PO: 240–480 mg/d in 3–4 divided doses IV: 5–10 mg IV push	For supraventricular tachydysrhythmias, prevention of PSVT. Also used for angina pectoris and hypertension. Avoid use if cardiogenic shock, second- or third-degree AV block, severe hypotension, severe CHF occur. Serum therapeutic level 80–300 ng/mL or 0.08–0.3 µg/mL. *Pregnancy category:* C; PB: 90%; t½: 3–8 h
Diltiazem (Cardizem)	A: IV: 0.25 mg/kg IV bolus over 2 min, or 5–10 mg/h in IV infusion	For PSVT and atrial flutter or fibrillation. Avoid use if second- or third-degree AV block or hypotension occurs. *Pregnancy category:* C; PB: 70%–80%; t½: 3–8 h
Others Phenytoin (Dilantin)	A: IV: 100 mg q5–10 min until dysrhythmia ceases; *max:* 1000 mg	Treatment of digitalis-induced dysrhythmias. Not approved as dysrhythmic drug by FDA. Serum level <20 µg/mL. *Pregnancy category:* D; PB: 95%; t½: 22 h
Digoxin (Lanoxin)	A: IV: LD: 0.6–1 mg/d in 24 h C >10 y: IV: LD: 8–12 µg/kg	For atrial flutter or fibrillation; to prevent recurrence of paroxysmal atrial tachycardia. *Pregnancy category:* A; PB: 20%–25%; t½: >36 h

KEY: A: adult; C: child; PO: by mouth; IV: intravenous; UK: unknown; PB: protein-binding; t½: half-life; m²: square meter of body surface area; LD: loading dose; MI: myocardial infarction; CHF: congestive heart failure; AV: atrioventricular; >: greater than; <: less than.

Lidocaine, a IB or fast (sodium) channel blocker II, was used in 1940s as a local anesthetic and is still used for that purpose. Later, it was determined that lidocaine had antidysrhythmic properties and was and still is most effective for treating acute ventricular dysrhythmias. It slows conduction velocity and decreases action potential amplitude. Onset of action (intravenously) is rapid.

SIDE EFFECTS AND ADVERSE REACTIONS

Quinidine and Procainamide

Quinidine, the first drug used to treat cardiac dysrhythmias, has many side effects, such as nausea, vomiting, diarrhea, confusion, and hypotension. It can also cause heart block and neurologic and psychiatric symptoms. Procainamide causes less cardiac depression than quinidine.

Lidocaine

High doses of lidocaine could cause cardiovascular depression, bradycardia, and hypotension. Side effects may include dizziness, lightheadedness, and confusion.

Beta Blockers

The drugs in the second class, beta blockers, decrease conduction velocity, automaticity, and recovery time (refractory period). Examples are propranolol (Inderal) and acebutolol (Sectral). Side effects of beta blockers are bradycardia and hypotension.

Prolong Repolarization

Drugs in the third class prolong repolarization and are used in emergency treatment of ventricular dysrhythmias when other antidysrhythmics are not effective. These drugs, bretylium (Bretylol) and amiodarone (Cordarone), increase the refractory period (recovery time) and prolong the action potential duration (cardiac cell activity). Bretylium and amiodarone can cause nausea, vomiting, hypotension, and neurologic problems.

Calcium Blockers

The fourth class, the calcium channel blocker Verapamil (Calan, Isoptin), a slow (calcium) channel blocker, blocks calcium influx, thus decreasing the excitability and contractility (negative inotropic) of the myocardium. It increases the refractory period of the AV node, which decreases ventricular response. Verapamil is contraindicated for clients with AV block or congestive heart failure. The side effects of calcium blockers are nausea, vomiting, hypotension, and bradycardia.

NURSING PROCESS: ANTIDYSRHYTHMICS

ASSESSMENT

- Obtain health and drug histories. The history may include shortness of breath (SOB), heart palpitations, coughing, chest pain (type, duration, and severity), previous angina or cardiac dysrhythmias, and drugs that the client is currently taking.
- Obtain baseline vital signs (VS) and ECG for future comparisons.
- Check early cardiac enzyme results (AST, LDH, CPK) to compare with future laboratory results.

POTENTIAL NURSING DIAGNOSES

- Decreased cardiac output
- Anxiety related to irregular heartbeat
- High risk for activity intolerance

PLANNING

- Client will no longer experience abnormal sinus rhythm.
- Client will comply with the antidysrhythmic drug regimen.

NURSING INTERVENTIONS

- Monitor VS. Hypotension can occur.
- When the drug is ordered IV push or bolus, administer it over a period of 2 to 3 min or as prescribed.
- Monitor ECG for abnormal patterns and report

findings, such as PVCs, increased PR and QT intervals, and/or widening of the QRS complex. Increased QT interval is a risk factor for torsade des pointes.

CLIENT TEACHING

General
- Instruct the client to take the prescribed drug as ordered. Drug compliance is essential.
- Provide specific instructions for each drug, such as photosensitivity for amiodarone.

Side Effects
- Instruct the client to report side effects and adverse reactions to the health care provider. These can include dizziness, faintness, nausea, and vomiting.
- Advise the client to avoid alcohol, caffeine, and cigarettes. Alcohol can intensify the hypotensive reaction; caffeine increases the catecholamine level; and cigarette smoking promotes vasoconstriction.

EVALUATION

- Evaluate the effectiveness of the prescribed antidysrhythmic by comparing heart rates with the baseline heart rate and assessing the client's response to the drug. Report side effects and adverse reactions. The drug regimen may need to be adjusted. A proarrhythmic effect may occur, which may require discontinuation of the drug.

■ CASE STUDY
Client with Congestive Heart Failure and Potassium Imbalance*

Mrs. S. T., age 64 years, has congestive heart failure (CHF), which has been controlled with digoxin, furosemide (Lasix), and a low-sodium diet. She is taking potassium chloride (KCl) 20 mEq orally per day. Three days ago, Mrs. S. T. had flu-like symptoms of anorexia, lethargy, and diarrhea. Her fluid and food intake were diminished. She refused to take the KCl, stating that the drug makes her "sick." She has taken the daily digoxin and furosemide.

The nurse's assessment during the home visit includes poor skin turgor, poor muscle tone, irregular pulse rate, and decreased bowel sounds. The nurse obtained a blood sample for serum electrolytes; results indicated potassium (K) 2.9 mEq/L, sodium (Na) 137 mEq/L, and chloride (Cl) 96 mEq/L.

1. What are the reference values for serum K, serum Na, and serum Cl?
2. The serum potassium level and physical findings indicate what type of electrolyte imbalance? Explain.
3. What are the reasons for the electrolyte imbalance?
4. Mrs. S. T. said she was not taking KCl because the drug makes her "sick." What information can you give her concerning the administration of potassium?
5. What type of drug is furosemide? What is its effect on digoxin when there is a potassium deficit?
6. Is it possible for digitalis toxicity to occur? Explain. What are the signs and symptoms of digitalis toxicity?

Mrs. S. T. was referred to the health care provider because of the serum potassium deficit and its effect on digoxin. A repeat serum potassium determination was taken and the result was 2.8 mEq/L. A liter of dextrose 5% in water with KCl 40 mEq/L was administered over a 4-h period.

7. How many milliequivalents of KCl per hour would Mrs. S. T. receive? Does this amount constitute an acceptable dosage?
8. Why is it important that the nurse check the rate of intravenous fluids containing potassium, the hourly urine output, and vital signs?
9. Because of the low serum potassium level, what other electrolyte value should be checked and why?

After Mrs. S. T.'s serum electrolytes returned to normal, the health care provider instructed her to continue to take the prescribed KCl dosage daily with her other medications.

10. Mrs. S. T. asked why she has to continue taking these drugs. What should your response be?
11. The nurse instructs Mrs. S. T. to eat foods rich in potassium. Which foods are the richest sources of potassium?

STUDY QUESTIONS

1. Your client is taking digoxin 0.25 mg/d. What are the nursing responsibilities for client teaching in regard to pulse monitoring and side effects? What is the serum therapeutic range?
2. Drug interactions are associated with digitalis drugs. What are the effects of potassium-wasting diuretics and cortisone with digitalis?
3. What effects do electrolytes have on digitalis toxicity?
4. How are nitroglycerin products administered? Explain. What is a common side effect (temporary) of nitrates that occurs early in the course of administration? How is this side effect treated?
5. Beta blockers are administered from which drug groups for cardiac conditions? What are two side effects of beta blockers?
6. Calcium blockers are given from what drug groups for cardiac conditions? Which calcium blockers are used for dysrhythmias?
7. How do the fast sodium channel blockers affect the heart?

*Refer to Chapter 10, Fluid and Electrolyte Replacements, for information on potassium imbalance and Chapter 33, Diuretics, and Chapter 34, Antihypertensive Drugs, for a discussion of potassium-wasting diuretics.

Chapter 33

Diuretics

OUTLINE

Objectives
Terms
Introduction
Diuretics
    Thiazides and Thiazide-
      Like Diuretics
    Nursing Process

Loop (High-Ceiling)
    Diuretics
      Nursing Process
Osmotic Diuretics
Carbonic Anhydrase
    Inhibitors

Mercurial Diuretics
    Potassium-Sparing Diur-
      etics
Nursing Process
Study Questions

OBJECTIVES

Explain the action and uses of diuretics.

Identify the various groups of diuretics.

Describe several side effects and adverse reactions related to thiazide, loop, and potassium-sparing diuretics.

Explain the nursing interventions, including client teaching, related to diuretics, especially thiazide, loop, and potassium-sparing diuretics.

TERMS

antihypertensives
diuresis
diuretics
hypercalcemia
hyperglycemia

hypertension (essential or
    secondary)
hyperuricemia
hypokalemia
natriuresis

oliguria
osmolality
potassium-sparing diuretics
potassium-wasting diuretics
saluretic

INTRODUCTION

Diuretics are used for two main purposes: (1) to lower blood pressure in hypertension, and (2) to decrease edema (peripheral and pulmonary) in congestive heart failure (CHF) and renal or liver disorders. Diuretics discussed in this chapter are used either singly or in combination to decrease blood pressure and reduce edema.

DIURETICS

Diuretics produce increased urine flow (diuresis) by inhibiting sodium and water reabsorption from the kidney tubules. Most sodium and water reabsorption occurs throughout the renal tubular segments (proximal, loop of Henle [descending loop and ascending loop], and collecting tubule). Diuretics can affect one or more segments of the renal tubules. Figure 33–1 illustrates the renal tubule along with the normal process of water and electrolyte reabsorption and diuretic effects on the tubules.

Every 1½ h, the total volume of the body's extracellular fluid (ECF) goes through the kidneys

(glomeruli) for cleansing; this is the first process for urine formation. Small particles such as electrolytes, drugs, glucose, and waste products from protein metabolism are filtered in the glomeruli. Larger products such as protein and blood are not filtered with normal renal function and they remain in the circulation. Sodium and water are the largest filtrate substances.

Normally, 99% of the filtered sodium that passes through the glomeruli is reabsorbed. Fifty to 55 percent of sodium reabsorption occurs in the proximal tubules, 35% to 40% in the loop of Henle, 5% to 10% in the distal tubules, and <3% in the collecting tubules. Diuretics that act on the tubules closest to the glomeruli have the greatest effect in causing natriuresis (sodium loss in the urine). A classic example is the osmotic diuretic mannitol. The diuretic effect is dependent on the drug reaching the kidneys and its concentration in the renal tubules.

Diuretics have an antihypertensive effect by promoting sodium and water loss by blocking sodium and chloride reabsorption. This causes a decrease in fluid volume and lowering of blood pressure.

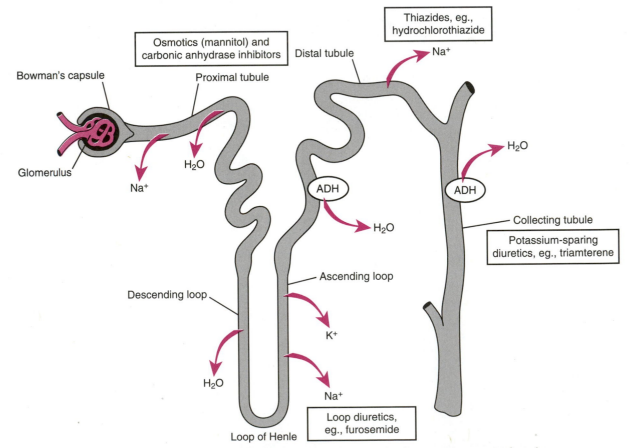

FIGURE 33–1 Diuretics act on different segments of the renal tube: osmotic, mercurial, and carbonic anhydrase inhibitor diuretics affect the proximal tubule; loop (high ceiling) diuretics affect the loop of Henle; thiazides affect the distal tubule; and potassium-sparing diuretics act primarily on the collecting tubules. (Key: ADH: antidiuretic hormone.

Also with fluid loss, edema (fluid retention in body tissues) should decrease. When sodium is retained, water is also retained in the body and the blood pressure increases.

Many diuretics cause loss of other electrolytes, including potassium, magnesium, chloride, and bicarbonate. The diuretics that promote potassium excretion are classified as **potassium-wasting diuretics,** and those that promote potassium retention are called **potassium-sparing diuretics.** In the last decade, combination diuretics have been marketed that have both potassium-wasting and potassium-sparing action.

The six categories of diuretics effective in removing water and sodium are (1) thiazide and thiazide-like, (2) loop or high-ceiling, (3) osmotic, (4) carbonic anhydrase inhibitor, (5) mercurial, and (6) potassium-sparing. The thiazide, loop or high-ceiling, and potassium-sparing diuretics are the most frequently prescribed types for hypertension and edema associated with CHF. All of these diuretics are potassium wasting, with the exception of the potassium-sparing group.

THIAZIDES AND THIAZIDE-LIKE DIURETICS

The first thiazide marketed was chlorothiazide (1957), followed 1 year later by hydrochlorothiazide. Today there are numerous thiazide and thiazide-like preparations (Table 33–1). Thiazides act on the distal convoluted renal tubule, beyond the loop of Henle, to promote sodium, chloride, and water excretion. Thiazides are used in the treatment of hypertension and peripheral edema. They are not effective for immediate diuresis.

This diuretic group is primarily used for clients with normal renal function. If the client has a renal disorder and his or her creatinine clearance test is below 30 mL/min, the effectiveness of the thiazide diuretic is greatly decreased. Thiazides cause a loss of sodium, potassium, and magnesium, but they promote calcium reabsorption. **Hypercalcemia** (calcium excess) may result, which can be a hazard to the client if he or she is digitalized or has cancer causing hypercalcemia. Thiazides affect glucose tolerance; thus, hyperglycemia can occur.

TABLE 33–1 Diuretics: Thiazides

Generic (Brand)	Route and Dosage	Uses and Considerations
Short Acting		
Chlorothiazide (Diuril, Diachlor)	*Hypertension:* A: PO: 250–500 mg q.d. or b.i.d. *Edema:* A: PO: 500–2000 mg daily or b.i.d. C >1 y: PO: 20 mg/kg/d C <6 mon: PO: 10–30 mg/kg/d in divided doses	For hypertension and peripheral edema. Adults may be given IV chlorothiazide, but it is not recommended for infants and children. *Pregnancy category:* D; PB: 20%–80%; t½: 1–2 h
Hydrochlorothiazide (HydroDIURIL, HCTZ)	See Prototype Drug Chart (Fig. 33–2)	For hypertension and edema. Hydrochlorothiazide (HCTZ) is inexpensive and is usually well tolerated by most clients. Usually HCTZ is the first thiazide prescribed. HCTZ may be used as a single antihypertensive drug or in combination with other antihypertensives. It is used in edema associated with CHF, cirrhosis of the liver, and steroids (glucocorticoids). Electrolyte imbalance can occur. *Pregnancy category:* B; PB: 65%; t½: 6–15 h
Intermediate Acting		
Bendroflumethiazide (Naturetin)	A: PO: 2.5–20 mg/d C: PO: maint: 0.05–0.1 mg/kg/d or 1.5–3 mg/m² daily or in divided doses	Treatment of hypertension and edema associated with CHF and cirrhosis. Has similar effects as the prototype drug HCTZ. Hypokalemia, hyperglycemia, and hyperuricemia may occur. *Pregnancy category:* UK; PB: 94%; t½: 3–4 h
Benzthiazide (Aquatag, Hydrex)	*Hypertension:* A: PO: 25–100 mg/daily or 25–100 mg in divided doses *Edema:* A: PO: 25–200 mg daily C: PO: 1–4 mg/kg/d in 3 divided doses	Similar to hydrochlorothiazide. *Pregnancy category:* D: PB: UK; t½: UK
Hydroflumethiazide (Saluron, Diucardin)	*Hypertension:* A: PO: 50–100 mg/d *Edema:* A: PO: 25–200 mg/d C: PO: 1 mg/kg/d	Similar to hydrochlorthiazide, its effects, side and adverse reactions, and abnormal laboratory results. *Pregnancy category:* C: PB: 74%; t½: 17 h

Table continued on following page

TABLE 33–1 Diuretics: Thiazides *(Continued)*

Generic (Brand)	Route and Dosage	Uses and Considerations
Long Acting Methyclothiazide (Aquatensen, Enduron)	*Hypertension/edema:* A: PO: 2.5–10 mg/d C: PO: 0.05–0.1 mg/kg/d	For hypertension and edema associated with CHF, renal and liver dysfunction. Side effects and drug interactions are similar to HCTZ. It has a long duration of action. *Pregnancy category:* C; PB: UK; t½: UK
Polythiazide (Renese-R)	*Hypertension:* A: PO: 2–4 mg/d *Edema:* A: PO: 1–4 mg/d C: PO: 0.02–0.08 mg/kg/d	Similar to hydrochlorothiazide. *Pregnancy category:* D; PB: 84%; t½: 25 h
Trichlormethiazide (Metahydrin, Naqua)	*Hypertension:* A: PO: 2–4 mg *Edema:* A: PO: 1–4 mg daily or b.i.d. C: PO: 0.07 mg/kg/d in divided doses	Similar to HCTZ. It has a long duration of action (24 h). *Pregnancy category:* B; PB: UK; t½: 2.5–7 h
Thiazide-Like Diuretics (This group has similar effects to but not exactly like HCTZ) Chlorthalidone (Hygroton)	*Hypertension:* A: PO: 12.5–50 mg/d *Edema:* A: PO: 25–100 mg/d C: PO: 2 mg/kg 3×wk	For hypertension and edema associated with CHF, renal and liver dysfunction. It has a very long duration of action (24–72 h). *Pregnancy category:* C; PB: 75%; t½: 40–54 h
Indapamide (Lozol)	*Hypertension and edema:* A: PO: 2.5 mg/d; may increase to 5 mg/d	For hypertension and edema. A long-acting diuretic. May be classified as a loop diuretic. *Pregnancy category:* B; PB: 75%; t½: 14–18 h
Metolazone (Zaroxolyn)	*Hypertension:* A: PO: 2.5–5.0 mg/d *Edema:* A: PO: 5–20 mg/d	For hypertension and edema. Intermediate-acting diuretic. More effective than thiazides in clients with decreased renal function. *Pregnancy category:* D; PB: 33%; t½: 8–14 h
Quinethazone (Hydromox)	A: PO: 50–100 mg/d; *max:* 200 mg/d in divided doses	For edema. Intermediate-acting diuretec. *Pregnancy category:* D; PB: UK; t½: UK

KEY: *A: adult; C: child; PO: by mouth; m²: body surface area; >: greater than; <: less than; PB: protein-binding; t½: half-life.*

Thiazides should be used with caution in clients with diabetes mellitus. Laboratory test (electrolytes and glucose) results need to be monitored. The pharmacologic data for the prototype thiazide diuretic hydrochlorothiazide are presented in Figure 33–2.

Pharmacokinetics

Thiazides are well absorbed from the gastrointestinal (GI) tract. Hydrochlorothiazide has a moderate protein-binding power, and the half-life of the thiazide drugs is longer than that of the loop diuretics. For this reason, thiazides should be administered in the morning to avoid nocturia (nighttime urination) and sleep interruption.

Pharmacodynamics

Thiazides act directly on arterioles, causing vasodilation, which can lower blood pressure. Other action is the excretion of sodium chloride and water, causing a decrease in vascular fluid and thus decreasing cardiac output and blood pressure. The onset of action of hydrochlorothiazide occurs within 2 h. The peak concentration times are long, 3–6 h. Thiazides are divided into three groups according to their duration of action: the short-acting thiazides with a duration time of less than 12 h; intermediate-acting, with a duration time of 12 to 24 h; and long-acting, with a duration time of greater than 24 h.

Table 33–1 lists the drugs, dosages, and uses and considerations for the thiazide and thiazide-like diuretics. Drug dosages for hypertension and edema are similar.

Side Effects and Adverse Reactions

Side effects and adverse reactions of thiazides include electrolyte imbalances (hypokalemia, hypercalcemia, hypomagnesemia, and bicarbonate loss), **hyperglycemia** (elevated blood sugar), **hyperuricemia** (elevated serum uric acid level), and hyperlipidemia (elevated blood lipid level). Signs and symptoms of hypokalemia should be assessed, and

FIGURE 33–2. Diuretic: Thiazides

Thiazide Diuretic	Dosage	**NURSING PROCESS** Assessment and Planning
Hydrochlorothiazide (HydroDIURIL, HCTZ, Esidrix, Oretic); 🍁 Apo-Hydro, Urozide *Pregnancy Category:* B	A: PO: Hypertension: 12.5–100 mg/d Edema: Initially: 25–200 mg in divided doses; maint: 25–100 mg/d C: PO: 1–2 mg/kg/d in divided doses C: <6 mo: PO: 1–3 mg/kg/d in divided doses	

Contraindications	Drug-Lab-Food Interactions	
Renal failure with anuria, electrolyte depletion *Caution:* Hepatic cirrhosis, renal dysfunction, diabetes mellitus, gout, systemic lupus erythematosus (SLE)	*Increase* digitalis toxicity with digitalis and hypokalemia; *increase* potassium loss with steroids; potassium loss *Decrease* antidiabetic effect; decrease thiazide effect with cholestyramine and colestipol *Lab: Increase* serum calcium, glucose, uric acid *Decrease* serum potassium, sodium, magnesium	

Pharmacokinetics	Pharmacodynamics	
Absorption: Readily absorbed from the Gi tract *Distribution:* PB: 65% *Metabolism:* t½: 6–15 h *Excretion:* In urine	PO: Onset: 2 h Peak: 3–6 h Duration: 6–12 h	Interventions

Therapeutic Effects/Uses: To increase urine output. To treat hypertension, edema from CHF, hepatic cirrhosis, renal dysfunction.

Mode of Action: Action is on the renal distal tubules by promoting sodium, potassium, and water excretion, decreasing preload and cardiac output; also edema. Acts on arterioles, causing vasodilation, thus decreasing blood pressure.

Evaluation

Side Effects	Adverse Reactions
Dizziness, vertigo, weakness, nausea, vomiting, diarrhea, hyperglycemia, constipation, rash, photosensitivity	Severe dehydration, hypotension *Life-threatening:* Severe potassium depletion, marked hypotension, uremia, aplastic anemia, hemolytic anemia, thrombocytopenia, agranulocytosis

KEY: A: adult; C: child; PO: by mouth; <: less than; PB: protein-binding; t½: half-life; CHF: congestive heart failure; 🍁: Canadian drug names.

serum potassium levels must be closely monitored. Potassium supplements are frequently needed. Serum calcium and uric acid levels should be checked because thiazides block calcium and uric acid excretion; **hypercalcemia** (elevated blood calcium levels) and hyperuricemia may result. Thiazides affect the metabolism of carbohydrates, and hyperglycemia can result, especially in clients with high to high-normal blood sugar levels. Thiazides can increase serum cholesterol, low-density lipoprotein, and triglyceride levels. A drug to lower blood lipids may be ordered. Other side effects include dizziness, headaches, nausea, vomiting, constipation, urticaria (hives) (rare), and blood dyscrasias (rare).

Table 33–2 summarizes the serum chemistry abnormalities that can occur with the use of thiazides.

Contraindications

Thiazides are contraindicated for use in renal failure. Symptoms of severe kidney impairment or shutdown include **oliguria** (marked decrease in urine output), elevated blood urea nitrogen (BUN), and elevated serum creatinine.

Drug Interactions

Of the numerous drug interactions, the most serious occurs with digoxin. Thiazides can cause hypokalemia, which enhances the action of digoxin, and digitalis toxicity can occur. Potassium supplements are frequently prescribed and serum potassium levels are monitored. Thiazides also induce hypercalcemia, which enhances the action of digoxin that may cause digitalis toxicity. Signs and symptoms of digitalis toxicity (bradycardia, nausea,

TABLE 33–2 Serum Chemistry Abnormalities Associated with Thiazides

Serum Chemistry Parameter	Abnormal Results
Electrolytes Potassium	Hypokalemia (low serum potassium) is excreted from the distal renal tubule.
Magnesium	Hypomagnesemia (low serum magnesium). Potassium and sodium loss prompt magnesium loss.
Calcium	Hypercalcemia (elevated serum calcium). Thiazides may block calcium excretion.
Chloride	Hypochloremia (low serum chloride). Sodium and potassium losses produce chloride loss.
Bicarbonate	Minimal bicarbonate loss from proximal tubule.
Uric acid	Hyperuricemia (elevated uric acid). Thiazides can block uric acid excretion.
Blood sugar	Hyperglycemia (increased blood sugar). Thiazides increase fasting blood sugar levels and those of prediabetic state.
Blood lipids	Cholesterol, low-density lipoproteins, and triglycerides can be elevated.

NURSING PROCESS: DIURETICS: Thiazides

ASSESSMENT

- Assess vital signs (VS), weight, urine output, and serum chemistry values (electrolytes, glucose, uric acid) for baseline levels.
- Check peripheral extremities for presence of edema. Note pitting edema.
- Obtain a history of drugs that are taken daily. Review for drugs that may cause drug interaction, including digoxin, corticosteroids, antidiabetics.

POTENTIAL NURSING DIAGNOSES

- High risk for fluid volume deficit
- Altered patterns of urinary elimination

PLANNING

- Client's blood pressure will be decreased and/or return to normal value.
- Client's edema will be decreased.
- Client's serum chemistry levels remain within normal ranges.

NURSING INTERVENTIONS

- Monitor VS and serum electrolytes, especially potassium, glucose, uric acid, and cholesterol levels. Report changes. If client is taking digoxin and hypokalemia occurs, digitalis toxicity frequently results.
- Observe for signs and symptoms of hypokalemia, such as muscle weakness, leg cramps, and cardiac dysrhythmias.
- Check the client's weight daily at a specified time. A weight gain of 2.2 to 2.5 lb is equivalent to an excess liter of body fluids.
- Monitor urine output to determine fluid loss or retention.

CLIENT TEACHING

General
- Emphasize the need for compliance. Client may not "feel better" for some time or may not "feel worse" if treatment is missed or discontinued.
- Suggest that the client take hydrochlorothiazide in early morning to avoid sleep disturbance due to nocturia.

- Keep drugs out of reach of small children. Request child safety cap bottle.

Skill

- Instruct the client or family member how to take and record his or her blood pressure. Record daily results.

Diet

- Instruct the client to eat foods rich in potassium, such as fruits, fruit juices, and vegetables. Potassium supplements may be ordered.
- Advise the client to take drugs with food to avoid GI upset.

Side Effects

- Instruct the client to change positions from lying to standing slowly because dizziness may occur due to orthostatic (postural) hypotension.

- Advise the client who may be prediabetic to have blood sugar checked periodically because large doses of hydrochlorothiazide increase blood glucose levels.
- Advise the client to use sunscreen when in direct sunlight.

EVALUATION

- Evaluate the effectiveness of drug therapy. Client's blood pressure and edema will be reduced and blood chemistry will remain within normal range.
- Determine the absence of side effects and adverse reactions to therapy.

---

vomiting, visual changes) should be reported. Thiazides also enhance the action of lithium, and lithium toxicity can occur. Thiazides potentiate the action of other antihypertensive drugs, which may be used in combination drug therapy for hypertension.

LOOP (HIGH-CEILING) DIURETICS

The loop, or high-ceiling, diuretics act on the ascending loop of Henle by inhibiting chloride transport of sodium into the circulation (inhibits passive reabsorption of sodium). Sodium and water are lost, together with potassium, calcium, and magnesium. They have little effect on the blood sugar; however, the uric acid level increases. The drugs in this group are potent and cause marked depletion of water and electrolytes. The effects of loop diuretics are dose related; i.e., increasing the dose increases the effect and response of the drug. This response is referred to as high-ceiling diuretics. Loop diuretics are more potent than thiazides as diuretics, inhibiting reabsorption of sodium two to three times more effectively, but are less effective as antihypertensive agents.

Loop diuretics can increase renal blood flow up to 40%. It is a common choice of diuretic for clients whose creatinine clearance results are below 30 mL/min and for those with end-stage renal disease. This group of diuretics causes excretion of calcium, unlike thiazides, which inhibit calcium loss.

Ethacrynic acid (Edecrin) (late 1950s) and furosemide (Lasix) (1960) were the first loop diuretics marketed. Bumetanide (Bumex) is more potent than furosemide per milligram-for-milligram basis.

Furosemide and bumetamide are derivatives of sulfonamides. Ethacrynic acid, a phenoxyacetic acid derivative, is a seldom-chosen loop diuretic, usually reserved for a client who is allergic to sulfa drugs. Figure 33–3 lists the drug data for the loop diuretic furosemide.

Pharmacokinetics

Loop diuretics are rapidly absorbed by the GI tract. These drugs are highly protein-bound with half-lives (t½) that vary from 30 min to 1.5 h. Loop diuretics compete for protein-binding sites with other highly protein-bound drugs.

Pharmacodynamics

Loop diuretics have a great **saluretic** (sodium-losing) effect and can cause rapid diuresis, thus decreasing vascular fluid volume and causing a decrease in cardiac output and blood pressure. Furosemide is a more potent diuretic than thiazide diuretics. It causes a vasodilatory effect, thus increasing renal blood flow before diuresis. It is used when other conservative measures fail, such as sodium restriction and use of less potent diuretics. The oral dose of furosemide is usually twice that of an intravenous dose.

The onset of action of loop diuretics occurs within 30 to 60 min. The onset of action for intravenous (IV) furosemide is 5 min. Duration of action is shorter than that of the thiazides.

Side Effects and Adverse Reactions

The most common side effects are fluid and electrolyte imbalances, such as hypokalemia, hyponatremia, hypocalcemia, hypomagnesemia, and hypochloremia. Hypochloremic metabolic alkalosis may result, which can worsen the hypokalemia. Orthostatic hypotension can occur. Thrombocytope-nia, skin disturbances, and transient deafness are seen rarely. Prolonged use of loop diuretics could cause thiamine deficiency.

FIGURE 33–3. Diuretic: Loop (High-Ceiling)

High-Ceiling (Loop) Diuretic	Dosage	**NURSING PROCESS** Assessment and Planning

Furosemide
   (Lasix, Furodide); 🍁 fumide,
   furomide
Pregnancy Category C
	A: PO: 20–80 mg single dose; repeat in
	   6–8 h max: 600 mg/d
	   IM/IV: 20–80 mg single dose; over
	   1–2 min IV; repeat 20 mg in 2 h
	C: PO: 2 mg/kg single dose; repeat in
	   6–8 h; max: 6 mg/kg/d
	   IM/IV: 1 mg/kg/ single dose; repeat
	   1 mg/kg in 2 h	

Contraindications	**Drug-Lab-Food Interactions**	

Presence of severe electrolyte
   imbalances, hypovolemia, anuria,
   hypersensitivity to sulfonamides,
   hepatic coma
	Increase orthostatic hypotension with
	   alcohol; *increase* ototoxicity with
	   aminoglycosides; *increase* bleeding
	   with anticoagulants; *increase*
	   potassium loss with steroids; *increase*
	   digitalis toxicity and cardiac
	   dysrhythmias with digitalis and
	   hypokalemia; *increase* lithium
	   toxicity; *increase* amphotericin B
	   ototoxicity and nephrotoxicity
	Lab: Increase BUN, blood/urine glucose,
	   serum uric acid, ammonia
	Decrease potassium, sodium, calcium,
	   magnesium, chloride serum levels	

Pharmacokinetics	**Pharmacodynamics**	Interventions

Absorption: PO: Readily absorbed from
   the GI tract
Distribution: PB: 95%
Metabolism: t½: 30–50 min
Excretion: In urine, some in feces;
   crosses placenta
	PO: Onset: <60 min
	   Peak: 1–4 h
	   Duration: 6–8 h
	IV: Onset: 5 min
	   Peak: 20–30 min
	   Duration: 2 h	

Therapeutic Effects/Uses: To treat fluid retention/fluid overload due to CHF, renal dysfunc-tiion, cirrhosis; hypertension; acute pulmonary edema.

Mode of Action: Inhibition of sodium and water reabsorption from the loop of Henle and distal renal tubules. Potassium, magnesium, and calcium also may be excreted.

Evaluation

Side Effects	Adverse Reactions

Nausea, diarrhea, electrolyte
   imbalances, vertigo, cramping, rash,
   headache, weakness, ECG changes,
   blurred vision, photosensitivity
	Severe dehydration; marked
	   hypotension
	Life-threatening: Renal failure,
	   thrombocytopenia, agranulocytosis

KEY: A: adult; C: child; PO: by mouth; IM: intramuscular; IV: intravenous; PB: protein-binding; <: less than; t½: half-life; CHF: congestive heart failure; 🍁: Canadian drug names.

Drug Interaction

The major drug interaction is with digitalis preparations. If the client takes digoxin with a loop diuretic, digitalis toxicity can result. The client needs potassium replacement with food or supplements. Hypokalemia enhances the action of digoxin and increases the risk of digitalis toxicity. Table 33–3 lists the data for the four loop (high-ceiling) diuretics.

OSMOTIC DIURETICS

Osmotic diuretics increase the **osmolality** (concentration) of the plasma and fluid in the renal tubules. Sodium, chloride, potassium (to a lesser degree), and water are excreted. This group of drugs is used to prevent kidney failure, to decrease intracranial pressure (ICP), e.g., cerebral edema, and to decrease intraocular pressure (IOP), e.g., glaucoma. Mannitol is a potent potassium-wasting diuretic that is used frequently in emergency situations such as for ICP and IOP. Also, mannitol can be used with cisplatin and carboplatin in cancer chemotherapy in order to induce a frank diuresis with decreased side effects of treatment.

Mannitol is the most frequently prescribed osmotic diuretic, followed by urea. Diuresis occurs within 1 to 3 h after intravenous administration. Table 33–3 describes the two osmotic diuretics.

Side Effects and Adverse Reactions

Mannitol

The side effects and adverse reactions of this osmotic diuretic include fluid and electrolyte imbalance, pulmonary edema from rapid shift of fluids, nausea, vomiting, tachycardia from rapid fluid loss, and acidosis. Crystallization of mannitol in the vial may occur when the drug is exposed to a low temperature. The vial should be warmed to dissolve the crystals. The mannitol solution should *not* be used for intravenous infusion if the crystals are present and have not been dissolved.

CARBONIC ANHYDRASE INHIBITORS

The carbonic anhydrase inhibitors acetazolamide, dichlorphenamide, ethoxzolamide, and methazolamide block the action of the enzyme carbonic an-

TABLE 33–3 Diuretics: Loop (High-Ceiling) Osmotics, Carbonic Anhydrase Inhibitors

Generic (Brand)	Route and Dosage	Uses and Considerations
Loop (High-Ceiling)		
Bumetanide (Bumex)	A: PO: 0.5–2.0 mg/d, *max:* 10 mg/d IV: 0.5–1.0 mg/dose; repeat in 2–4 h C: PO: 0.015 mg/kg/d	Treatment of hypertension and edema associated with CHF, and renal disease. Similar effects as furosemide. *Pregnancy category:* C; PB: 95%; t½: 1–1.5 h
Ethacrynic acid (Edecrin)	A: PO: 50–200 mg/d IV: 0.5–1.0 mg/kg/dose C: PO: 25 mg/d	For severe edema (pulmonary and peripheral). It is a potent diuretic and has rapid action. Also used for mild-moderate hypertension, and for hypercalcemia. *Pregnancy category:* B; PB: 95%; t½: 1–1.5 h
Furosemide (Lasix)	See Prototype Drug Chart (Fig. 33–3)	For pulmonary and peripheral edema due to CHF, hypertension, renal failure *without* anuria, and hypercalcemia. Furosemide promotes calcium excretion. Hypokalemia may result. *Pregnancy category:* C; PB: 95%; t½: 0.5–1 h
Torsemide (Demadox)	*Hypertension A:* PO/IV: Initially: 5 mg/d; maint: PO: 5–10 mg/d IV: in 2 min *CHF:* A: PO/IV: 10–20 mg/d	Similar to furosemide. *Pregnancy category:* C; PB: >97%; t½: 2–4 h
Osmotics		
Mannitol	*ICP, IOP:* A: IV: 1.5–2.0 g/kg; 15%–25% sol infused over 30–60 min *Edema, ascites, or oliguria:* A: IV: 50–100 g; 10%–20% sol infused over 90 min to 6 h	For decreasing ICP (increased intracranial pressure) and for oliguria. To prevent acute renal failure. Used in narrow-angle glaucoma for reducing intraocular pressure. Client should have effective renal function. It is a potent diuretic. *Pregnancy category:* C; PB: UK; t½: 1.5 h
Urea (Ureaphil)	A: IV: 1.0–1.5 g/kg of 30% solution C (>2 yr): IV: 0.5–1.5 g/kg of 30% solution	Same uses as mannitol. Not the drug of choice. Used during prolonged surgery to prevent acute renal failure. *Pregnancy category:* C; PB: UK; t½: 1 h

Table continued on next page

Generic (Brand)	Route and Dosage	Uses and Considerations
Carbonic Anhydrase Inhibtors		
Acetazolamide (Diamox)	A: PO/IV: 250 mg q12h; dose may vary C: PO: 10–15 mg/kg/d in divided doses C: IV: 5–10 mg/kg q6h	For edema, treating absence (petit mal) seizures, and open-angle glaucoma. May cause hyperglycemia, hyperuricemia, and hypercalcemia. Metabolic acidosis can result. *Pregnancy category:* C; PB: 90%; t½: 2.5–5.5 h
Dichlorphenamide (Daranide, Oratrol)	A: PO: 100 mg q12h; maint: 25–50 mg qd/t.i.d.	Treatment of open-angle glaucoma by reducing the intraocular pressure (IOP) and for narrow-angle glaucoma prior to surgery. *Pregnancy category:* C; PB: UK; t½: UK
Methazolamide (Neptazane)	A: PO: 50–100 mg b.i.d./t.i.d.	Similar to dichlorphenamide. *Pregnancy category:* C; PB: 50%–60%; t½: 14 h

KEY: A: adult; C: child; PO: by mouth; IV: intravenous; ICP; intracranial pressure; IOP; intraocular pressure; CHF: congestive heart failure; maint: maintenance dose; >: greater than; PB: protein-binding; t½: half-life.

NURSING PROCESS: DIURETICS: Loop (High-Ceiling)

ASSESSMENT

- Obtain a history of drugs that are taken daily. Note if client is taking a drug(s) that may cause an interaction, such as alcohol, aminoglycosides, anticoagulants, corticosteroids, lithium, amphotericin B, or digitalis. Recognize that furosemide is highly protein-bound and can displace other protein-bound drugs such as Coumadin.
- Assess vital signs (VS), serum electrolytes, weight, and urine output for baseline levels.
- Compare client's drug dose with recommended dose and report discrepancy.
- Note if client is hypersensitive to sulfonamides.

POTENTIAL NURSING DIAGNOSIS

- High risk for fluid volume deficit

PLANNING

- Client's edema and/or hypertension will be decreased.
- Client's serum chemistry levels will remain within normal ranges.

NURSING INTERVENTIONS

- Check the half-life of furosemide. With a short half-life, the drug can be repeated or given more than once a day.
- Check onset of action for furosemide, orally and intravenously. If the drug is given intravenously, the urine output should increase in 5 to 20 min. If urine output does not increase, notify the health care provider. Severe renal disorder may be present.
- Monitor urinary output to determine body fluid gain or loss. Urinary output should be at least 25 mL/h or 600 mL/24 h.
- Check the client's weight to determine fluid loss or gain. A loss of 2.2 to 2.5 lb is equivalent to a fluid loss of 1 liter.
- Monitor VS. Be alert for marked decrease in blood pressure.
- Administer IV furosemide slowly; hearing loss may occur if rapidly injected.
- Observe for signs and symptoms of hypokalemia (<3.5 mEq/L), such as muscle weakness, abdominal distention, leg cramps, and/or cardiac dysrhythmias.
- Check serum potassium levels, especially when a client is taking digoxin. Hypokalemia enhances the action of digitalis, causing digitalis toxicity.

CLIENT TEACHING

General
- Instruct the client to take furosemide early in the morning and *not* in the evening, to prevent sleep disturbance and nocturia.

Diet
- Suggest taking furosemide at mealtime or with food to avoid nausea.

Side Effects
- Instruct the client to arise slowly to prevent dizziness due to fluid loss.

EVALUATION

- Evaluate the effectiveness of drug action: decreased fluid retention or fluid overload, decreased respiratory distress, and increased cardiac output.
- Check for side effects and increase in urine output.

hydrase needed to maintain the acid-base balance (hydrogen and bicarbonate ion balance). Inhibition of this enzyme causes increased sodium, potassium, and bicarbonate excretion. With prolonged use, metabolic acidosis can occur.

This group of drugs is used primarily to decrease intraocular pressure in clients with open-angle (chronic) glaucoma. These drugs are not used in narrow-angle or acute glaucoma. Other uses include diuresis, management of epilepsy, and treatment of high-altitude or acute mountain sickness. Table 33–3 presents the drug data for carbonic anhydrase inhibitor diuretics. The drug may also be used for a client in metabolic alkalosis who needs a diuretic. Carbonic anhydrase inhibitors may be alternated with a loop diuretic.

Side Effects and Adverse Reactions

Acetazolamide

This carbonic anhydrase inhibitor can cause fluid and electrolyte imbalance, metabolic acidosis, nausea, vomiting, anorexia, confusion, orthostatic hypotension, and crystalluria. Hemolytic anemia and renal calculi can also occur. These drugs are contraindicated during the first trimester of pregnancy.

MERCURIAL DIURETICS

Mercurial diuretics are no longer available in the United States. They were discontinued in favor of safer, more effective agents. Mercury toxicity was of great concern.

Potassium-Sparing Diuretics

Potassium-sparing diuretics, weaker than thiazides and loop diuretics, are used as mild diuretics or in combination with antihypertensive drugs. These drugs act primarily in the collecting distal duct renal tubules to promote sodium and water excretion and potassium retention. The drugs interfere with the sodium-potassium pump that is controlled by the mineralocorticoid hormone aldosterone (sodium retained and potassium excreted). Potassium is reabsorbed and sodium is excreted. Among the combination potassium-sparing and potassium-wasting diuretics are triamterene hydrochlorothiazide (Dyazide) and spironolactone hydrochlorothiazide (Aldactazide), which have intensified diuretic effect and minimal potassium-wasting.

Spironolactone (Aldactone), an aldosterone antagonist discovered in 1958, was the first potassium-sparing diuretic. Aldosterone is a mineralocorticoid hormone that promotes sodium retention and potassium excretion. Aldosterone antagonists inhibit the sodium-potassium pump; i.e., potassium is retained and sodium is excreted. Amiloride and triamterene (Fig. 33–4) gives the pharmacologic data for triamterene) are two additional potassium-sparing diuretics commonly prescribed today. Table 33–4 lists the potassium-sparing diuretics and the combination potassium-wasting and potassium-sparing diuretics. When diuretic combinations are used, either combined in one tablet or as separate tablets, the dose of each is usually less than the dose of any single drug.

Side Effects and Adverse Reactions

The main side effect of these drugs is hyperkalemia. Caution must be used when giving potassium-sparing diuretics to a client with poor renal function, because 80% to 90% of the potassium is excreted by the kidneys. Urine output should be at least 600 mL per day. Clients should *not* use potassium supplements while taking potassium-sparing diuretics unless the serum potassium level is low. If a potassium-sparing diuretic is given with the antihypertensive drug angiotensin-converting enzyme (ACE) inhibitor, hyperkalemia could become severe or life-threatening because both drugs retain potassium. Monitoring serum potassium levels is necessary. GI disturbances can occur.

NURSING PROCESS: DIURETIC: Potassium-Sparing

ASSESSMENT

- Obtain a history of drugs that are taken daily. Note if the client is taking a potassium supplement or using a salt substitute.
- Assess vital signs (VS), serum electrolytes, weight, and urinary output for baseline levels.
- Compare the client's drug dose with the recommended dose and report any discrepancy.

POTENTIAL NURSING DIAGNOSIS

- High risk for fluid volume deficit

PLANNING

- Client's fluid retention and blood pressure will be decreased.
- Client's serum electrolytes remain within their normal values.

FIGURE 33–4. Diuretic: Potassium-Sparing

NURSING PROCESS
Assessment and Planning

Potassium-Sparing Diuretic	**Dosage**
Triamterene (Dyrenium) *Pregnancy Category:* B	A: PO: Edema: 100 mg q.d., b.i.d.; not to exceed 300 mg/d C: PO: 2–4 mg/kg/d in divided doses

Contraindications	**Drug-Lab-Food Interactions**
Severe kidney or hepatic disease, severe hyperkalemia *Caution:* Renal or hepatic dysfunction, diabetes mellitus	*Increase* serum potassium level with potassium supplements; *increase* effects of antihypertensives and lithium; life-threatening hyperkalemia if given with ACE inhibitor *Lab: Increase* serum potassium level; may *increase* BUN, AST, alkaline phosphatase levels *Decrease* serum sodium, chloride

Interventions

Pharmacokinetics	**Pharmacodynamics**
Absorption: PO: Rapidly absorbed from GI tract *Distribution:* PB: 67% *Metabolism:* t½: 1.5–2.5 h *Excretion:* In urine, mostly as metabolites and bile	PO: Onset: 2–4 h Peak: 6–8 h Duration: 12–16 h

Evaluation

Therapeutic Effects/Uses: To increase urine output; to treat fluid retention/overload associated with CHF, hepatic cirrhosis, or nephretic syndrome.

Mode of Action: Action on the distal renal tubules to promote sodium and water excretion and potassium retention.

Side Effects	**Adverse Reactions**
Nausea, vomiting, diarrhea, rash, dizziness, headache, weakness, dry mouth, photosensitivity	*Life-threatening:* Severe hyperkalemia, thrombocytopenia, megaloblastic anemia

KEY: A: adult; C: child; PO: by mouth; PB: protein-binding; CHF: congestive heart failure; t½: half-life.

TABLE 33–4 Diuretic: Potassium-Sparing

Generic (Brand)	Route and Dosage	Uses and Considerations
Single Agents Amiloride HCl (Midamor)	A: PO: 5 mg/d; may increase to 10–20 mg/d in 1–2 divided doses	For diuretic-induced hypokalemia; used for hypertension, CHF, and cirrhosis of the liver. Serum potassium level should be monitored to detect hyperkalemia. *Pregnancy category:* B; PB: 23%; t½: 6–9 h
Spironolactone (Aldactone)	*Hypertension:* A: PO: 25–100 mg/d *Edema:* A: PO: 25–200 mg/d in divided doses C: PO: 3.3 mg/kg/d in divided doses	For edema and hypertension. Dosage for hypertension is usually slightly lower than for edema. Has a long duration of action. *Pregnancy category:* C; PB: 98%; t½: 1.5–2 h
Triamterene	See Prototype Drug Chart (Fig. 33–4)	It blocks the luminal sodium channels. For edema due to CHF, cirrhosis, nephrosis, and steroid-induced edema. Should be taken with meals. Intermediate-acting diuretic. *Pregnancy category:* B; PB: 67%; t½: 1.5–2.5 h

Table continued on following page

TABLE 33–4 Diuretic: Potassium-Sparing *(Continued)*

Generic (Brand)	Route and Dosage	Uses and Considerations
Combinations		
Amiloride HCl and hydrochlorothiazide (Moduretic)	A: PO: 1–2 tab (amiloride 5 mg/hydrochlorothiazide 50 mg)	Combinations contain potassium-wasting and potassium-sparing diuretics. Drugs are to control hypertension and edema. They are used to prevent the occurrence of hypokalemia.
Spironolactone and hydrochlorothiazide (Aldactazide)	A: PO: 25/25 and 50/50 mg tab	Same as Moduretic
Triamterene and hydrochlorothiazide (Dyazide, Maxzide)	A: PO: 1–2 cap b.i.d., p.c. (triamterene 50 mg/hydrochlorothiazide 25 mg)	Dyazide: each tablet contains triamterene 50 mg and hydrochlorothiazide 25 mg. Maxzide comes in two strengths: triamterene 37.5 mg or 75 mg and hydrochlorothiazide 50 mg or 75 mg. *Pregnancy category:* B; PB: UK; t½: UK

KEY: *A: adult; C: child; cap: capsule; PO: by mouth; CHF: congestive heart failure; p.c.: after meals; UK: unknown; PB: protein-binding; t½: half-life.*

NURSING INTERVENTIONS

- Check the half-life of triamterene. With a long half-life, drug dose is usually administered once a day and sometimes twice a day.
- Monitor urinary output. Urine output should increase. Report if urine output is <30 mL/h, or 600 mL/day.
- Monitor VS. Report abnormal changes.
- Observe for signs and symptoms of hyperkalemia (increased serum potassium level: >5.3 mEq/L), such as nausea, diarrhea, abdominal cramps, tachycardia and later bradycardia, peaked narrow T wave (ECG), or oliguria.
- Administer triamterene in the early morning and not in the evening, to avoid nocturia.

CLIENT TEACHING

General
- Instruct the client to take triamterene with or after meals to avoid nausea.

- Do not discontinue drug without consulting the health care provider.

Diet
- Advise clients with high average serum potassium levels to avoid foods rich in potassium when taking potassium-sparing diuretics.

Side Effects
- Instruct the client to avoid exposure to direct sunlight because the drug can cause photosensitivity.
- Advise the client to report possible side effects of the drug, such as rash, dizziness, or weakness.

EVALUATION

- Evaluate the effectiveness of the potassium-sparing diuretic such as triamterene. The presence of fluid retention (edema) is decreased or absent.
- Determine if urine output has increased and the serum potassium level is within normal range.

STUDY QUESTIONS

1. The client is receiving hydrochlorothiazide (HydroDIURIL) 50 mg daily and digoxin 0.25 mg daily. Is hydrochlorothiazide a potassium-wasting or potassium-sparing diuretic? What types of electrolyte imbalances can occur? Explain.
2. Client teaching is essential when caring for a client receiving the two drugs in question 1. How would you instruct the client regarding diet and vital signs? What are the signs and symptoms of digitalis toxicity?
3. What electrolyte imbalances may occur when taking hydrochlorothiazide over a prolonged period of time?

4. Your client has diabetes mellitus and is taking hydrochlorothiazide. Why should the client's blood glucose level be closely monitored?
5. Furosemide (Lasix) is what type of diuretic? What electrolyte imbalances can be caused by this drug?
6. Your client is taking triamterene. What type of diuretic is triamterene? What effect may this have on the potassium level?
7. Why would a combination diuretic (triamterene and hydrochlorothiazide) be prescribed?
8. The client's blood pressure is 142/92. What nonpharmacologic measures would you suggest to lower the blood pressure?

Chapter 34

Antihypertensive Drugs

OUTLINE

Objectives
Terms
Introduction
Nonpharmacologic Control of
  Hypertension
Stepped-Care Approach
Antihypertensive Drugs
  Sympatholytics (Sympathetic
    Depressants)
      Beta-Adrenergic Blockers
        Nursing Process

Centrally Acting Sym-
  patholytics (Adrener-
  gic Blockers)
Alpha-Adrenergic Block-
  ers
Adrenergic Neuron
  Blockers (Peripherally
  Acting Sympatholytics)
Alpha- and Beta-Adren-
  ergic Blockers
    Nursing Process

Direct-Acting Arteriolar
  Vasodilators
Angiotensin Antagonists
  (Angiotensin-Converting
  Enzyme Inhibitors)
    Nursing Process
Calcium Channel Blockers
Case Study
Study Questions

OBJECTIVES

Identify the categories of antihypertensive drugs and the stepped-care approach to antihypertensive drugs.

Explain the pharmacologic action of the individual groups of antihypertensive drugs.

Describe the side effects and adverse reactions to sympatholytics (beta blockers, centrally acting and peripherally acting alpha blockers, alpha and beta blockers), direct-acting vasodilators, and angiotensin antagonists.

Explain the nursing interventions, including client teaching, related to antihypertensives.

TERMS

antihypertensives
hypertension (essential and
  secondary)

stepped-care hypertensive
  approach

sympatholytics

INTRODUCTION

Hypertension is an increase in blood pressure such that the systolic pressure is greater than 140 mmHg and the diastolic pressure is greater than 90 mmHg. **Essential hypertension** is the most common type, affecting 90% of persons with high blood pressure. The exact origin of essential hypertension is unknown; however, contributing factors include (1) a family history of hypertension, (2) hyperlipidemia, (3) African-American racial background, (4) diabetes, (5) obesity, (6) aging, (7) stress, and (8) excessive smoking and alcohol ingestion. Ten percent of hypertension is related to renal and endocrine disorders and is classified as **secondary hypertension.**

The kidneys and the blood vessels strive to regulate and maintain a "normal" blood pressure. The kidneys regulate blood pressure via the renin-angiotensin system. The process is illustrated in Figure 34–1. Renin (from the renal cells) stimulates production of angiotensin II (a potent vasoconstrictor), which causes the release of aldosterone (adrenal hormone that promotes sodium retention and thereby water retention). Retention of sodium and water causes fluid volume to increase, thus elevating blood pressure. The baroreceptors in the aorta and carotid sinus and the vasomotor center in the medulla assist in the regulation of blood pressure. Norepinephrine, an adrenal hormone of the sympathetic nervous system, increases blood pressure.

There are physiologic risk factors that contribute to hypertension. Diet with excess fat and carbohydrate can increase blood pressure. Carbohydrate intake can affect sympathetic nervous activity. Mild to moderate sodium restriction can decrease blood pressure. Alcohol increases renin secretions, thus causing the production of angiotensin II. Obesity affects the sympathetic and cardiovascular systems by increasing cardiac output, stroke volume, and left ventricular filling. Two-thirds of hypertensive persons are obese. Normally, weight loss can decrease hypertension.

NONPHARMACOLOGIC CONTROL OF HYPERTENSION

A sufficient decrease in blood pressure may be accomplished by nonpharmacologic methods. There are many nonpharmacologic ways to decrease blood pressure; however, if the systolic pressure is greater than 140 mmHg, antihypertensive drugs are generally ordered. Nondrug methods to decrease blood pressure include (1) stress reduction techniques, (2) exercise (increases high-density lipoproteins [HDL]), (3) salt restriction, (4) decreased alcohol ingestion, and (5) weight reduction.

When hypertension *cannot* be controlled by nonpharmacologic means, antihypertensive drugs are prescribed. However, nonpharmacologic methods should be combined with antihypertensive drugs to control hypertension. Antihypertensive drugs, used either singly or in combination with other drugs, are classified into five categories: (1) diuretics, (2) sympathetic depressants (sympatholytics), (3) direct arteriolar vasodilators, (4) angiotensin antagonists, and (5) calcium channel blockers. Hydrochlorothiazide (HydroDIURIL) is the most frequently prescribed diuretic to control mild hypertension. Hydrochlorothiazide can be used alone for recently diagnosed or mild hypertension or with other antihypertensive drugs. The various types of diuretics that are prescribed for hypertension are discussed in Chapter 33. Many antihypertensive drugs can cause fluid retention; therefore, diuretics are often administered with antihypertensive drugs.

STEPPED-CARE APPROACH

The American Heart Association's Joint National Committee on Detection, Evaluation, and Treatment of High Blood Pressure has recommended a "stepped-care approach" to pharmacologic treatment of hypertension. Severity of hypertension is classified within four stages of blood pressure range (Table 34–1). Step I drugs are used to control stage I hypertension. If the blood pressure is not controlled, then step II drugs are prescribed. Adverse effects are more prevalent with each increasing step. By using less potent drugs and combination therapy (lower dosages) for controlling high blood pressure, side effects are decreased. The stepped-care approach to management of hypertension is illustrated in Figure 34–2.

Since the publication of these guidelines, many health care providers have moved toward a more individualized approach to the treatment of hyper-

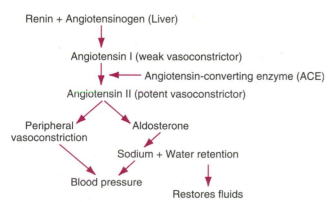

FIGURE 34–1 Renin-angiotensin system. Renin is an enzyme located in the juxtaglomerular cells of the kidney and is released when there is a decrease in blood pressure. The process of the renin-angiotensin system for restoring fluid and blood pressure is illustrated.

TABLE 34–1 Four Stages of Hypertension According to Blood Pressure

| Stages | Blood Pressure Range (mmHg) | |
	Systolic	Diastolic
Normal	<130	<85
Stage 1	140–159	90–99
Stage 2	160–179	100–109
Stage 3	180–209	110–119
Stage 4	>210	>120

tension. All drugs are considered as initial agents, and reduction of other cardiovascular risk factors and the use of fewer drugs (substituting instead of adding drugs) at the lowest effective doses are emphasized.

ANTIHYPERTENSIVE DRUGS

It has been estimated that some 20% to 30% of clients being treated with antihypertensive drugs are not truly hypertensive when hypertension is determined by 24-h ambulatory blood pressure measurement. Another large percentage are being overtreated due to a perceived inefficacy of antihypertensive drugs and the subsequent increase in dosage or numbers of antihypertensive drugs.

SYMPATHOLYTICS (SYMPATHETIC DEPRESSANTS)

The sympatholytics comprise five groups of drugs: (1) beta-adrenergic blockers, (2) centrally acting sympatholytics (adrenergic blockers), (3) alpha-adrenergic blockers, (4) adrenergic neuron blockers (peripherally acting sympatholytics), and (5) alpha- and beta-adrenergic blockers. The beta-adrenergic blockers block the beta receptors. The alpha-adrenergic blockers block the alpha receptors.

Beta-Adrenergic Blockers

Beta-adrenergic blockers, frequently referred to as *beta blockers,* are used as step I antihypertensive drugs or in combination with a diuretic in the step II approach to treating hypertension. Beta blockers are also used as antianginals and antidysrhythmics (see Chapter 32).

Beta (B_1 and B_2)-adrenergic blockers reduce cardiac output by diminishing the sympathetic nervous system response. With continued use of beta blockers, vascular resistance is diminished and blood pressure is lowered. Beta blockers also reduce renin release. There is a greater hypotensive response by clients who have higher renin levels.

Hypertensive clients who are African-Americans do not respond well to beta blockers for control of hypertension. However, with this group of people, hypertension can be controlled by combining beta blockers with diuretics.

There are numerous types of beta blockers. The nonselective beta blockers such as propranolol (Inderal) inhibit beta$_1$ (heart) and beta$_2$ (bronchial) receptors. Heart rate slows (blood pressure decreases secondary to the decrease in heart rate), and bronchoconstriction occurs. Cardioselective beta blockers are preferred because they act mainly on the beta$_1$ rather than the beta$_2$ receptors; as a result, bronchoconstriction is less likely to occur. Acebutolol (Sectral), atenolol (Tenormin), betaxolol (Ker-

STEP I

Diuretics
Beta blockers
Calcium blockers
Angiotensin-converting enzyme

STEP II

Diuretics with beta blockers
Sympatholytics

STEP III

Direct-acting vasodilators
Sympatholytic with diuretic

STEP IV

Adrenergic neuron blocker
Combinations from Step I, II, and III

FIGURE 34–2 Stepped-care approach for pharmacologic management of hypertension.

lone), bisoprolol (Zebeta), and metoprolol (Lopressor) are cardioselective beta blockers, blocking beta$_1$ receptors.

Cardioselectivity does not confer absolute protection from bronchoconstriction. In tests measuring FEV$_1$, as a measure of B$_2$ reactivity, only atenolol demonstrated true protection. Other cardioselective beta blockers were only partially effective. Studies also show that at the upper end of the dosage range, cardioselectivity is less effective. In clients with preexisting bronchospasms or other pulmonary disease beta blockers, even those considered cardioselective, should be used with caution. Some experts regard this as a relative contraindication. The real value of beta selectivity is in maintaining renal blood flow and minimizing the hypoglycemic effects of beta blockade.

Again, beta blockers tend to be more effective in lowering blood pressure in clients who have an elevated serum renin level. The cardioselective prototype drug metoprolol (Lopressor) is presented in Figure 34–3.

FIGURE 34–3. Antihypertensives: Beta Blocker

Beta Blocker	Dosage	NURSING PROCESS
Metoprolol tartrate (Lopressor), Betaloc, Apo-Metoprolol, Toprol SR Adrenergic blocker, sympatholytic, beta$_2$ blocker *Pregnancy Category:* C	*Hypertension:* A: PO: 50–100 mg/d in 1–2 divided doses; maint: 100–450 mg in divided doses; max: 450 mg/d in divided doses SR: 50–100 mg/d; max: 450 mg/d *Myocardial Infarction:* A: PO: 100 mg b.i.d. IV: 5 mg q2min × 3 doses	Assessment and Planning
Contraindications	**Drug-Lab-Food Interactions**	
Second- and third-degree heart block, cardiogenic shock, CHF, sinus bradycardia *Caution:* Hepatic, renal, or thyroid dysfunction; asthma; peripheral vascular disease, IDDM	*Increase* bradycardia with digitalis; *increase* hypotensive effect with other antihypertensives, alcohol, anesthetics	
Pharmacokinetics	**Pharmacodynamics**	Interventions
Absorption: PO: 95% *Distribution:* PB: 12% *Metabolism:* t½: 3–4 h *Excretion:* In urine	PO: Onset: 15 min Peak: 1.5 h Duration: 10–19 h IV: Onset: Immediate Peak: 20 min Duration: 5–10 h	

Therapeutic Effects/Uses: To control hypertension.

Mode of Action: Promotion of blood pressure reduction via beta$_1$-blocking effect.

Evaluation

Side Effects	Adverse Reactions
Fatigue, weakness, dizziness, nausea, vomiting, diarrhea, mental changes, nasal stuffiness, impotence, decrease libido, depression	Bradycardia, thrombocytopenia *Life-threatening:* Complete heart block, bronchospasm, agranulocytosis

KEY: A: adult; PO: by mouth; IV: intravenous; PB: protein-binding; t½: half-life; IDDM: insulin-dependent diabetes mellitus; : Canadian drug names.

Pharmacokinetics

Metoprolol is well absorbed from the GI tract. Its half-life is short. Metoprolol is highly protein-bound and will compete with other highly protein-bound drugs. Free drug will be released from the protein-binding site and can have adverse effects.

Pharmacodynamics

Beta-adrenergic blockers block sympathetic stimulation, thus decreasing heart rate and blood pressure. The nonselective beta blockers block beta$_2$ receptors, which can result in bronchial constriction. Beta blockers cross the placental barrier and can enter breast milk.

The onset of action of oral beta blockers is usually 30 min or less, and the duration of action is 6 to 12 h. When beta blockers are administered intravenously, the onset of action is immediate, peak time is 20 min intravenously (compared to 1½ h orally), and duration of action is 4 to 10 h.

Side Effects and Adverse Reactions

Side effects and adverse reactions include decreased pulse rate, markedly decreased blood pressure, and bronchospasm (nonselective beta$_2$ blockers). Beta blockers should not be abruptly discontinued because rebound hypertension, angina, dysrhythmias, and myocardial infarction can result. Other side effects are discussed in Chapter 32. Table 34–2 presents the drug data for beta blockers that are commonly used in treating hypertension.

Noncardioselective beta blockers inhibit the liver's ability to convert glycogen to glucose in response to hypoglycemia. In addition, the depression of heart rate masks the symptom (tachycardia) of hypotension. Because of this side effect, beta blockers should be used with caution in clients with diabetes mellitus.

Centrally Acting Sympatholytics (Adrenergic Blockers)

Centrally acting sympatholytics decrease the sympathetic response from the brain stem to the peripheral vessels. Centrally acting sympatholytics stimulate the alpha$_2$ receptors, which in turn decrease sympathetic activity, increase vagus activity, and decrease serum epinephrine, norepinephrine, and renin release; thus, peripheral vascular resistance is reduced.

NURSING PROCESS: ANTIHYPERTENSIVES: Beta Blockers

ASSESSMENT

- Obtain a medication history from the client. Report if a drug-drug interaction is probable.
- Obtain vital signs (VS). Report abnormal blood pressure. Compare VS with baseline finding.
- Check laboratory values related to renal and liver function. An elevated BUN and serum creatinine may be caused by metoprolol or cardiac disorder. Elevated cardiac enzymes, such as AST and LDH, could result from use of metoprolol or from a cardiac disorder.

POTENTIAL NURSING DIAGNOSES

- Decreased cardiac output
- Noncompliance with drug regimen
- Altered sexual dysfunction

PLANNING

- Client's blood pressure will be decreased and/or return to normal value.
- Client takes the medication as prescribed.

NURSING INTERVENTIONS

- Monitor VS, especially blood pressure and pulse.
- Monitor laboratory results, especially BUN, serum creatinine, AST, and LDH.

CLIENT TEACHING

General
- Instruct the client to comply with drug regimen: *abrupt discontinuation of the antihypertensive drug may cause rebound hypertension.*
- Suggest that the client avoid OTC drugs without first checking with the health care provider. Many OTC drugs carry warnings against use in the presence of hypertension.
- Suggest that the client wear a Medic Alert bracelet or carry a card indicating the health problem and prescribed drugs.
- Instruct the client in a trauma situation to inform the health care provider of drugs taken daily, such as a beta blocker. Beta blockers block the compensatory effects of the body to the shock state. Glucagon may be needed to reverse the effects so that the client can be resuscitated.

Skill

- Instruct the client or family member how to take a radial pulse and blood pressure. Advise the client to report abnormal findings to the health care provider.

Diet

- Teach the client and family members nonpharmacologic methods to decrease blood pressure, such as a low-fat and low-salt diet, weight control, relaxation techniques, exercise, smoking cessation, and decreased alcohol ingestion (1 to 2 oz/d).
- Advise the client to report constipation. Foods high in fiber, a stool softener, and increased water intake (except in clients with CHF) are usually indicated.

Side Effects

- Advise the client that antihypertensives may cause dizziness due to orthostatic hypotension and possible sexual dysfunction due to impotence. Instruct the client to remain in a sitting position for several minutes before standing.
- Instruct the client to report dizziness, slow pulse rate, changes in blood pressure, heart palpitation, confusion, or GI upset to the health care provider.
- Caution client with diabetes mellitus of possible hypoglycemic symptoms.

EVALUATION

- Evaluate the effectiveness of the drug therapy, i.e., decreased blood pressure and the absence of side effects.
- Determine that the client is adhering to the drug regimen.

This group of drugs has minimal effects on cardiac output and blood flow to the kidneys. Drugs in this group include methyldopa, clonidine, guanabenz, and guanfacine. Methyldopa (Aldomet) was one of the first drugs widely used in controlling hypertension. In high doses methyldopa and clonidine can cause sodium and water retention. Frequently, this group of drugs are administered with diuretics, vasodilators, calcium blockers, or ACE inhibitors. Beta blockers are not given with centrally acting sympatholytics that can interfere with the antihypertensive effect. Guanabenz and guanfacine are new centrally acting sympatholytics with effects similar to clonidine.

Clonidine is now available in a transdermal preparation that provides a 7-day duration of action. New transdermal patches are replaced every 7 days. Skin irritations have occurred in approximately 20% of the clients. Guanfacine has a long half-life and usually is taken once a day. Table 34–2 lists the centrally acting sympatholytics along with the beta blockers.

Side Effects and Adverse Reactions

The side effects and adverse reactions include drowsiness, dry mouth, dizziness, and slow heart rate (bradycardia). Methyldopa should not be used in clients with impaired liver function, and serum liver enzymes should be monitored periodically in all clients. This group of drugs must not be abruptly discontinued because a hypertensive crisis can result. If the drug needs to be stopped immediately, another antihypertensive drug is usually prescribed to avoid rebound hypertensive symptoms such as restlessness, tachycardia, tremors, headache, and increased blood pressure. Rebound hypertension is less likely to occur with guanabenz and guanfacine. The nurse should emphasize the need to take the medication as prescribed. This group of drugs can cause sodium and water retention, resulting in peripheral edema. A diuretic may be ordered with methyldopa or clonidine to decrease water and sodium retention (edema). Clients who are pregnant or contemplating pregnancy should avoid clonidine. Methyldopa is frequently used to treat chronic or pregnancy-induced hypertension; however, it crosses the placental barrier, and small amounts may enter breast milk in a lactating client.

Alpha-Adrenergic Blockers

This group of drugs block the alpha-adrenergic receptors, resulting in vasodilation and decreased blood pressure. They help to maintain the renal blood flow rate. The alpha blockers are useful in treating hypertensive clients with lipid abnormalities. They decrease the very low-density lipoproteins (VLDL) and the low-density lipoproteins (LDL) that are responsible for the buildup of fatty plaques in the arteries (atherosclerosis). Also, they increase high-density lipoprotein (HDL) levels ("friendly" lipoprotein). Alpha blockers are safe for

TABLE 34–2 Antihypertensives: Beta Blockers and Central Alpha$_2$ Agonists

Generic (Brand)	Route and Dosage	Uses and Considerations
Beta-Adrenergic Blockers		
Acebutolol HCl (Sectral) Cardioselective beta$_1$	A: PO: 400–800 mg/d in 1 or 2 divided doses; *max:* 1,200 mg/d	For hypertension and cardiac dysrhythmia. It may be used alone or in combination with a diuretic. Side effects include dizziness, fatigue, hypotension, bradycardia, constipation/diarrhea. Vital signs should be closely monitored. *Pregnancy category:* B; PB: 26%; t$\frac{1}{2}$: 3–13 h
Atenolol (Tenormin) Cardioselective beta$_1$	A: PO: 25–100 mg/d	For hypertension and angina. Similar side effects as acebutolol. *Pregnancy category:* C; PB: 6%–16%; t$\frac{1}{2}$: 6–7 h
Betaxolol HCl (Kerlone) Cardioselective beta$_1$	A: PO: 10–20 mg/d Also for ophthalmic use: glaucoma	For hypertension and glaucoma. Ophthalmic preparation is used to decrease intraocular pressure (IOP). *Pregnancy category:* C; PB: UK; t$\frac{1}{2}$: 14–22 h
Bisoprolol fumarate (Zebeta) Beta$_1$ blocker	A: PO: Initially: 5 mg/d; maint: 2.5–20 mg/d	For hypertension and angina pectoris. Long-acting beta$_1$ blocker. Heart rate and blood pressure may be decreased. *Pregnancy category:* C; PB: <30%; t$\frac{1}{2}$: 9–12 h
Carteolol HCl (Cartrol) Nonselective beta$_1$ and beta$_2$	A: PO: 2.5–5.0 mg/d	For hypertension and glaucoma. It should be avoided for clients who have asthma because of its beta$_2$ effect. It may be used in combination with a thiazide diuretic. *Pregnancy category:* C; PB: 23%–30%; t$\frac{1}{2}$: 4–6 h
Metoprolol (Lopressor) Cardioselective beta$_1$	See Prototype Drug Chart (Fig. 34–3)	For hypertension and angina pectoris. A commonly used drug to decrease blood pressure. *Pregnancy category:* C; PB: 12%; t$\frac{1}{2}$: 3–4 h
Nadolol (Corgard) Nonselective beta$_1$ and beta$_2$	A: PO: 40–80 mg/d; *max:* 320 mg/d	For hypertension and angina pectoris. Similar to carteolol HCl. *Pregnancy category:* C; PB: 30%; t$\frac{1}{2}$: 10–24 h
Penbutolol SO$_4$ (Levatol) Nonselective beta$_1$ and beta$_2$	A: PO: 10–20 mg/d; *max:* 80 mg/d	Treatment of stage 1 and 2 hypertension. Clients with asthma should avoid taking drug. *Pregnancy category:* C; PB: 80%–98%; t$\frac{1}{2}$: 5 h
Pindolol (Visken) Nonselective beta$_1$ and beta$_2$	A: PO: 5 mg b.i.d., t.i.d.; maint: 10–30 mg in divided doses; *max:* 60 mg/d in divided doses	For hypertension. May be used alone or in combination with thiazide diuretic. Also may be used for angina pectoris. *Pregnancy category:* B; PB: 50%; t$\frac{1}{2}$: 3–4 h
Propranolol (Inderal) Nonselective beta$_1$ and beta$_2$	A: PO: Initially: 40 mg b.i.d. SR: 80 mg/d; maint: 120–240 mg/d in divided doses C: PO: Initially 1 mg/kg/d in 2 divided doses; maint: 2 mg/kg/d	For hypertension, angina, and cardiac dysrhythmias. The first beta blocker. May cause bronchospasm, decrease in heart rate and blood pressure. *Pregnancy category:* C; PB: 90%; t$\frac{1}{2}$: 3–6 h
Timolol maleate (Blocadren) Nonselective beta$_1$ and beta$_2$	A: PO: Initially 10 mg b.i.d.; maint: 20–40 mg/d in 2 divided doses; *max:* 60 mg/d Also for ophthalmic use: glaucoma	For hypertension, angina pectoris, and glaucoma. It is used as step 1 antihypertensive, like most of the beta blockers. Similar to propranolol. *Pregnancy category:* C; PB: 60%; t$\frac{1}{2}$: 3–4 h
Central Alpha$_2$ Agonists		
Clonidine HCl (Catapres)	A: PO: Initially: 0.1 mg b.i.d.; maint: 0.2–1.2 mg/d in divided doses; *max:* 2.4 mg/d A: Transdermal patch: 100 μg (0.1 mg)/d 200 μg (0.2 mg)/d 300 μg (0.3 mg)/d	For hypertension. Long-acting. Well absorbed from GI tract. Can be taken with a diuretic. Step 2 antihypertensive drug. Decreases sympathetic effect. Drowsiness, dizziness, and dry mouth may occur. *Pregnancy category:* C; PB: 20%–40%; t$\frac{1}{2}$: 6–20 h
Guanabenz acetate (Wytensin)	A: PO: 4 mg b.i.d.; may increase to 4–8 mg/d; *max:* 32 mg b.i.d.	For hypertension and tachycardia. Can be taken with a thiazide diuretic. Intermediate-acting. May cause drowsiness, dizziness, headache, fatigue, and dry mouth. If GI distress occurs, take with food. *Pregnancy category:* C; PB: 90%; t$\frac{1}{2}$: 4–14 h
Guanfacine HCl (Tenex)	A: PO: 1 mg h.s.; may increase to 2–3 mg/d	For hypertension. Long-acting. May be taken alone or with a thiazide diuretic. *Pregnancy category:* B; PB: 70%; t$\frac{1}{2}$: >17 h
Methyldopa (Aldomet)	A: PO: 250–500 mg b.i.d.; *max:* 3 g/d IV: 250 mg–1 g q6h C: PO: 10 mg/kg/d in 2–4 divided doses	For stage 1 to 3 hypertension. May be used alone or in combination with a diuretic. Long-acting. Can be given intravenously. If GI upset occurs, take with food. *Pregnancy category:* C; PB: <15%; t$\frac{1}{2}$: 1.7 h

KEY: A: adult; C: child; PO: by mouth: IV: intravenous; PB: protein-binding; t$\frac{1}{2}$: half-life; >: greater than; <: less than.

diabetics because they do not affect glucose metabolism. They do not affect respiratory function.

The more potent alpha blockers phentolamine, phenoxybenzamine and tolazoline are used primarily for hypertensive crisis and severe hypertension resulting from tumors of the adrenal medulla (pheochromocytomas).

Prazosin, terazosin, and doxazosin (selective alpha-adrenergic blockers) are used mainly for reducing blood pressure and can be used in treatment of benign prostatic hypertrophy (BPH). Prazosin is a commonly prescribed drug. Doxazosin and terazosin have longer half-lives than prazosin, and they are normally given once a day. When prazosin is taken with alcohol or other antihypertensives, the hypotensive state can be intensified.

These drugs, like the centrally acting sympatholytics, cause sodium and water retention with edema, and diuretics are frequently given with them to decrease fluid accumulation in the extremities. Use of prazosin, terazosin, or doxazosin as a single drug is classified as step II therapy; however, if a diuretic is added to the drug regimen, then it is step III therapy.

Side Effects and Adverse Reactions
PHENTOLAMINE

Side effects include hypotension, reflex tachycardia due to the severe drop in blood pressure, nasal congestion because of the vasodilating effect, and GI disturbances.

PRAZOSIN, DOXAZOSIN, AND TERAZOSIN

The side effects include orthostatic hypotension (dizziness, faintness, light-headedness, increased heart rate), which may occur with first dose, nausea, drowsiness, nasal congestion due to vasodilation, edema, and weight gain.

Drug Interactions

Drug interactions occur when alpha-adrenergic blockers are taken with antiinflammatory drugs and nitrates (nitroglycerin) for angina. Peripheral edema is intensified when prazosin and an antiinflammatory drug are taken daily. Nitroglycerin taken for angina will lower the blood pressure. If prazosin is taken with nitroglycerin, syncope (faintness) due to a drop in blood pressure can occur. The selective alpha-adrenergic blocker prazosin is presented in Figure 34-4.

Pharmacokinetics

Prazosin is absorbed through the GI tract; however, a large portion of prazosin is lost during hepatic first-pass metabolism. The half-life is short, so the drug should be administered twice a day. Prazosin is highly protein-bound, and when it is given with other highly protein-bound drugs, the client should be assessed for adverse reactions.

Pharmacodynamics

The selective alpha-adrenergic blockers dilate the arterioles and venules, decreasing peripheral resistance and lowering the blood pressure. With prazosin, the heart rate is only slightly increased, whereas with alpha blockers such as phentolamine and tolazoline, the blood pressure is greatly reduced and reflex tachycardia can occur. Alpha blockers are more effective for treating acute hypertension, and the selective alpha blockers are more useful for long-term essential hypertension.

The onset of action of prazosin occurs between 30 min and 2 h. The duration of action of prazosin is 10 h. Table 34-2 presents the drug data for selective and nonselective alpha blockers.

Adrenergic Neuron Blockers (Peripherally Acting Sympatholytics)

Adrenergic neuron blockers are potent antihypertensive drugs that block norepinephrine from the sympathetic nerve endings, causing a decrease in norepinephrine release that results in a lowering of blood pressure. There is a decrease in both cardiac output and peripheral vascular resistance. Reserpine and guanethidine (the most potent of the two drugs) are used to control severe hypertension. Orthostatic hypotension is a common side effect: the client should be advised to rise slowly from a reclining or sitting position. The drugs in this group can cause sodium and water retention. Use of reserpine may cause vivid dreams, nightmares, and suicidal intention. They are classified as step IV drugs and can be taken alone or with a diuretic to decrease peripheral edema.

Alpha- and Beta-Adrenergic Blockers

Labetalol blocks the alpha and beta receptors (Table 34-3). Its effect on the alpha receptor is stronger than its effect on the beta receptor; therefore, it lowers the blood pressure and moderately decreases the pulse rate. Side effects include orthostatic hypotension, GI disturbances, nervousness, dry mouth, and fatigue. This drug is new and not yet classified in the stepped-care approach to drug therapy.

FIGURE 34–4. Antihypertensives: Alpha-Adrenergic Blocker

Alpha-Adrenergic Blocker	Dosage	**NURSING PROCESS** Assessment and Planning
Prazosin HCl (Minipress) Sympatholytic, selective alpha-adrenergic blocker *Pregnancy Category:* C	A: PO: 1 mg b.i.d./t.i.d.; maint: 3–15 mg/d; max: 20 mg/d in divided doses	
Contraindications	**Drug-Lab-Food Interactions**	
Renal disease	*Increase* hypotensive effect with other antihypertensives, nitrates, alcohol	
Pharmacokinetics	**Pharmacodynamics**	Interventions
Absorption: GI 60% (5% to circulation) *Distribution:* PB: 95% *Metabolism:* t½: 3 h *Excretion:* 10% in urine; in bile and feces	IV: Onset: 0.5–2 h Peak: 2–4 h Duration: 10 h	

	Evaluation
Therapeutic Effects/Uses: To control hypertension, refractory CHF, treatment of benign prostatic hypertrophy (BPH). *Mode of Action:* Dilation of peripheral blood vessels via blocking the alpha-adrenergic receptors.	

Side Effects	Adverse Reactions
Dizziness, drowsiness, headache, nausea, vomiting, diarrhea, impotence, vertigo, urinary frequency, tinnitus, dry mouth, incontinence, abdominal discomfort	Orthostatic hypotension, palpitations, tachycardia, pancreatitis

KEY: A: adult; PO: by mouth; PB: protein-binding; CHF: congestive heart failure; t½: half-life.

DIRECT-ACTING ARTERIOLAR VASODILATORS

Vasodilators are potent antihypertensive drugs. Direct-acting vasodilators are step III drugs that act by relaxing the smooth muscles of the blood vessels, mainly the arteries, causing vasodilation. Vasodilators promote an increase in blood flow to the brain and kidneys. With vasodilation, the blood pressure drops and sodium and water are retained, resulting in peripheral edema. Diuretics can be given with a direct-acting vasodilator to decrease the edema. Reflex tachycardia is caused by the vasodilation and drop in blood pressure. Beta blockers are frequently prescribed with arteriolar vasodilators to decrease the heart rate; this counter-acts the effect of reflex tachycardia. Two of the direct-acting vasodilators, hydralazine and minoxidil, are used for moderate to severe hypertension; nitroprusside and diazoxide are prescribed for acute hypertensive emergency. The latter two drugs are very potent vasodilators that rapidly decrease the blood pressure. Nitroprusside acts on the arterial and venous vessels, and diazoxide acts on the arterial vessels. Table 34–3 lists direct-acting vasodilators.

Side Effects and Adverse Reactions

The effects of hydralazine are numerous and include tachycardia, palpitations, edema, nasal con-

TABLE 34–3 Antihypertensives: Sympatholytics: Alpha-Adrenergic and Peripherally Acting Blockers and Direct-Acting Vasodilators

Generic (Brand)	Route and Dosage	Uses and Considerations
Selective Alpha-Adrenergic Blockers		
Doxazosin mesylate (Cardura)	A: PO: Initially: 1 mg/d; maint: 2–4 mg/d; *max:* 16 mg/d	For stage 1 or 2 hypertension. May be used alone or with another antihypertensive. May cause orthostatic hypotension, headache, dizziness, and GI upset. *Pregnancy category:* C; PB: 98%; t½: 22 h
Prazosin HCl (Minipress)	See Prototype Drug Chart (Fig. 34–4)	For hypertension. Intermediate-acting. May be taken with a diuretic. Commonly used antihypertensive. *Pregnancy category:* C; PB: 95%; t½: 3 h
Terazosin HCl (Hytrin)	A: PO: Initially 1 mg h.s.; maint: 1–5 mg/d; *max:* 20 mg/d	For stage 1 or 2 hypertension. May be used alone or with another antihypertensive drug. Dizziness and headache may occur. *Pregnancy category:* C; PB: 95%; t½: 9–12 h
Alpha-Adrenergic Blockers		
Phenoxybenzamine HCl (Dibenzyline)	A: PO: Initially: 10 mg/d; maint: 20–40 mg/d C: PO: 0.2 mg/kg/d in 1–2 divided doses; may increase dose by 0.2 mg	For hypertension related to adrenergic excess, pheochromocytoma. It lowers peripheral resistance. Has a long action. *Pregnancy category:* C; PB: UK; t½: 24 h
Phentolamine (Regitine)	A: IM/IV: 2.5–5 mg; repeat q5min until controlled; then q2–3h PRN C: IM/IV: 0.05–0.1 mg/kg; repeat if needed	For hypertensive crisis due to pheochromocytoma, MAO inhibitors, or clonidine withdrawal. It is a potent antihypertensive drug. In heart failure, it decreases afterload and increases cardiac output. For hypertension, it antagonizes the effects of epinephrine and norepinephrine causing vasodilation. *Pregnancy category:* C; PB: UK; t½: 20 min
Tolazoline HCl (Priscoline HCl)	NB: IV: Initially: 1–2 mg/kg; followed by 1–2 mg/kg/h for 24–48 h; expected effect within 30 min of initial dose A: IM/IV: 10–50 mg q.i.d.	For pulmonary hypertension of newborn, and for peripheral vasospastic disorders. *Pregnancy category:* C; PB: UK; t½: 3–10 h
Peripherally Acting Sympatholytics		
Guanadrel sulfate (Hylorel)	A: PO: Initially: 5 mg b.i.d.; maint: 20–75 mg/d in divided doses	For moderate to severe hypertension. Intermediate-acting duration. Rapid onset. *Pregnancy category:* B; PB: 20%; t½: 10–12 h
Guanethidine monosulfate (Ismelin sulfate)	A: PO: Initially: 10 mg/d; maint: 25–50 mg/d; *max:* 300 mg/d C: PO: 0.2 mg/kg/d; *max:* 1–1.6 mg/kg/d	For severe hypertension. Long-acting. Can be taken with a diuretic. Potent antihypertensive drug. May cause marked orthostatic hypotension, edema, weight gain, diarrhea, bradycardia. *Pregnancy category:* C; PB: UK; t½: 5 d
Reserpine (Serpasil)	A: PO: Initially: 0.25–5.0 mg daily for 1–2 wk; maint: 0.1–0.25 mg/d	One of the early antihypertensives. For hypertension. Not frequently used today. May cause nightmares, vivid dreams. *Pregnancy category:* D; PB: UK; t½: 4.5–11 h
Alpha- and Beta-Adrenergic Blocker		
Labetalol HCl (Trandate)	A: PO: Initially: 100 mg b.i.d.; maint: 200–800 mg/d in 2 divided doses A: IV: 2 mg/min in infusion; *max:* 300 mg as total dose	For stage 1 or 2 hypertension. May be used alone or with a thiazide diuretic. May cause orthostatic hypotension, palpitation, syncope. *Pregnancy category:* C; PB: 50%; t½: 4–8 h
Direct-Acting Vasodilators		
Diazoxide (Hyperstat, Proglycem)	A&C: IV: 1–3 mg/kg in bolus (30 sec); repeat in 5–15 min as needed; *max:* 150 mg	For hypertensive emergency. Dose may be repeated in 5–15 min until adequate decrease in blood pressure is achieved. Oral antihypertensive drugs may follow. *Pregnancy category:* C; PB: 90%; t½: 20–45 h
Hydralazine HCl (Apresoline HCl)	A: PO: Initially: 10 mg q.i.d.; maint: 25–50 mg q.i.d. Severe hypertension IM–IV: 10–40 mg: repeat as needed C: PO: 3–7.5 mg/kg/d in 4 divided doses	For hypertension. Short-acting duration. Can be taken with diuretic to decrease edema and beta blocker to prevent tachycardia. Dizziness, tremors, headaches, tachycardia, and palpitation may occur. Vital signs should be closely monitored. *Pregnancy category:* C; PB: 87%; t½: 2–6 h

Table continued on following page

TABLE 34–3 Antihypertensives: Sympatholytics: Alpha-Adrenergic and Peripherally Acting Blockers and Direct-Acting Vasodilators *(Continued)*

Generic (Brand)	Route and Dosage	Uses and Considerations
Minoxidil (Loniten, Rogaine, Minodyl)	A: PO: Initially: 5 mg/d; maint: 10–40 mg/d in single or divided doses; *max:* 100 mg/d C: PO: Initially: 0.2 mg/kg/d; *max:* 5 mg/d; maint: 0.25–1 mg/kg/d in divided doses; *max:* 50 mg/d *Topical for alopecia:* 2% sol b.i.d.	For hypertension. Can be taken with a diuretic to reduce edema and with a beta blocker to prevent tachycardia. Long-acting effect. When discontinuing drug, it should be slowly decreased to avoid rebound hypertension; should not be abruptly withdrawn. Vital signs should be closely monitored. *Pregnancy category:* C; PB: 0%; $t\frac{1}{2}$: 3.5–4 h
Sodium nitroprusside (Nipride, Nitropress)	A: IV: 1–3 μg/kg/min in D_5W; *max:* 10 μg/kg/min	For hypertensive crisis. A potent antihypertensive drug. Drug decomposes in light; container must be wrapped in aluminum foil. Good for 24 hours. Drug should be discarded if red or blue. Can cause cyanide toxicity. Measure cyanide and thiocyanate levels. May cause profound hypotension. *Pregnancy category:* C; PB: UK; $t\frac{1}{2}$: 2–7 d

KEY: *A: adult; C: child; PO: by mouth; IM: intramuscular; IV: intravenous; UK: unknown; PB: protein-binding; $t\frac{1}{2}$: half-life; MAO: monoamine oxidase; maint: maintenance; sec: second.*

NURSING PROCESS: ANTIHYPERTENSIVES: Alpha-Adrenergic Blockers

ASSESSMENT

- Obtain a medication history from the client, including current drugs. Report if a drug-drug interaction is probable. Prazosin is highly protein-bound and can displace other highly protein-bound drugs.
- Obtain baseline vital signs (VS) and weight for future comparisons.
- Check urinary output. Report if it is decreased (<600 mL/d), because drug is contraindicated if renal disease is present.

POTENTIAL NURSING DIAGNOSES

- High risk for activity intolerance
- Knowledge deficit related to drug regimen
- Altered sexuality patterns

PLANNING

- Client's blood pressure will decrease.
- Client will follow proper drug regimen.

NURSING INTERVENTIONS

- Monitor VS. The desired therapeutic effect of prazosin may not fully occur for 4 wk. A sudden marked decrease in blood pressure should be reported.

- Check daily for fluid retention in the extremities. Prazosin may cause sodium and water retention.

CLIENT TEACHING

General
- Instruct the client to comply with drug regimen. *Abrupt discontinuation of the antihypertensive drug may cause rebound hypertension.*
- Inform the client that orthostatic hypotension may occur. Explain that before rising, the client should dangle his or her feet.

Skill
- Instruct the client or family member how to take a blood pressure reading. A record for daily blood pressures should be kept.

Diet
- Encourage the client to decrease salt intake unless otherwise indicated by the health care provider.

Side Effects
- Caution the client that dizziness, lightheadedness, and drowsiness may occur, especially when the drug is first prescribed. If these symptoms occur, the health care provider should be notified.
- Inform the male client that impotence may occur if high doses of the drug are prescribed. This

problem should be reported to the health care provider.

- Instruct the client to report if edema is present in the morning.
- Instruct the client not to take cold, cough, or allergy over-the-counter (OTC) medications without first contacting the health care provider.

EVALUATION

- Evaluate the effectiveness of the drug in controlling blood pressure and the absence of side effects.
- Evaluate the client's adherence to medication schedule.

gestion, headache, dizziness, GI bleeding, lupus-like symptoms, and neurologic symptoms (tingling, numbness). Minoxidil has similar side effects, along with tachycardia, edema, and excess hair growth. It can precipitate an anginal attack.

Nitroprusside and diazoxide can cause reflex tachycardia, palpitations, restlessness, agitation, nausea, and confusion. Hyperglycemia can occur with diazoxide because the drug inhibits insulin release from the beta cells of the pancreas. Nitroprusside and diazoxide are discussed in greater detail in Chapter 47.

ANGIOTENSIN ANTAGONISTS (ANGIOTENSIN-CONVERTING ENZYME INHIBITORS)

Drugs in this group inhibit angiotensin-converting enzyme (ACE), which in turn inhibits the formation of angiotensin II (vasoconstrictor) and blocks the release of aldosterone. Aldosterone promotes sodium retention and potassium excretion. When aldosterone is blocked, sodium is excreted along with water. ACE inhibitors cause little change in cardiac output or heart rate, and they lower peripheral resistance. Figure 34–1 describes the renin-angiotensin system.

Benazepril, captopril, enalapril, lisinopril, and ramipril are five angiotensin antagonists presented in Table 34–4. These drugs can be used in clients who have elevated serum renin levels. These drugs are not intended for first-line antihypertensive therapy. Figure 34–5 gives the pharmacologic data related to captopril. African Americans and the elderly do not respond with effective reduction in blood pressure to ACE inhibitors, but when taken with a diuretic, the blood pressure usually will be lowered. ACE inhibitors should not be given during pregnancy because they reduce placental blood flow.

Side Effects and Adverse Reactions

The side effects of these drugs include nausea, vomiting, diarrhea, headache, dizziness, fatigue, insomnia, serum potassium excess (hyperkalemia), and tachycardia. Due to the risk of hyperkalemia, these drugs should not be taken with potassium-sparing diuretics.

CALCIUM CHANNEL BLOCKERS

Slow calcium channels are found in the myocardium (heart muscle) and smooth muscle cells. Free calcium increases muscle contractility, peripheral resistance, and blood pressure. Calcium channel blockers, also known as calcium antagonists and calcium blockers, decrease calcium levels and promote vasodilation. The large arteries are not as sensitive to calcium blockers as the coronary and cerebral arteries and the peripheral resistance vessels. Calcium blockers are highly protein-bound but have a short half-life. Slow-release preparations decrease the frequency of administering calcium blockers.

Nifedipine (Procardia) decreases blood pressure in those with low serum renin values and in the elderly. Nifedipine and verapamil are potent calcium blockers. Normally, beta blockers are not prescribed with calcium blockers because both drugs decrease myocardium contractility. Calcium blockers lower blood pressure better in African Americans than with other drug categories. Table 34–4 lists the calcium blockers along with the ACE inhibitors.

Side Effects and Adverse Reactions

The side effects and adverse reactions of calcium blockers include flushing, headache, dizziness, ankle edema, bradycardia, and atrioventricular block.

FIGURE 34–5. Antihypertensives: Angiotensin Antagonist

		NURSING PROCESS
Angiotensin-Converting Enzyme (ACE) Inhibitor *Captopril* (Capoten), 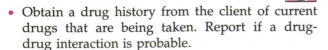 Apo-Captopril, Novo-Capto *Pregnancy Category:* C	**Dosage** A: PO: Initially: 12.5–25 mg b.i.d./t.i.d.; max: 450 mg/d; maint: 25–50 mg t.i.d.	Assessment and Planning
Contraindications Heart block *Caution:* Leukemia, chronic obstructive pulmonary disease (COPD), renal or thyroid disease	**Drug-Lab-Food Interactions** *Increase* hypotensive effect with nitrates, diuretics, adrenergic block- ers, vasodilators, other antihyperten- sives *Increase* serum potassium with potassium-sparing diuretics or with potassium supplements	

Pharmacokinetics
 	
Absorption: PO: 65% (food decreases ab-
sorption)
Distribution: PB: 25–30%
Metabolism: t½: normal kidney
function: 2–3 h
Excretion: In urine
	Pharmacodynamics
	
	PO: Onset: 15 min
	    Peak: 1 h
	    Duration: 6–12 h
		Interventions

Therapeutic Effects/Uses: To reduce blood pressure; to control CHF.

Mode of Action: Suppression of the angiotensin-converting enzyme (ACE); inhibits angiotensin I conversion to angiotensin II.

Evaluation

Side Effects Dizziness, cough, nocturia, impotence, rash, polyuria, hyperkalemia, taste disturbance	**Adverse Reactions** Oliguria, urticaria, severe hypotension *Life-threatening:* Acute renal failure, bronchospasm, angioedema, agranulocytosis

KEY: A: adult; C: child; PO: by mouth; UK: unknown; PB: protein-binding; t½: half-life; CHF: congestive heart failure; ACE: angiotensin-converting enzyme; 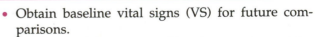: Canadian drug names.

NURSING PROCESS: ANTIHYPERTENSIVES: Angiotensin Antagonist (ACE) Inhibitor

ASSESSMENT

- Obtain a drug history from the client of current drugs that are being taken. Report if a drug-drug interaction is probable.

- Obtain baseline vital signs (VS) for future comparisons.
- Check the laboratory values for serum protein, albumin, BUN, creatinine, and WBC, and compare with future serum levels.

TABLE 34-4 Antihypertensives: Angiotensin Antagonists and Calcium Blockers

Generic (Brand)	Route and Dosage	Uses and Considerations
Angiotensin Antagonists (ACE Inhibitors)		
Benazepril HCl (Lotensin)	A: PO: Initially: 10 mg/d; maint: 20–40 mg/d in 2 divided doses	Management of stage 1 and 2 hypertension. Headache, dizziness, hypotension, nausea, diarrhea, or constipation may occur. *Pregnancy category:* D; PB: 97%; t½: 10 h
Captopril (Capoten)	See Prototype Drug Chart (Fig. 34–5)	For stage 1 or 2 hypertension and CHF. Can be taken alone or with a diuretic. Duration of action is moderate. Food can decrease absorption time. Commonly prescribed drug. Should *not* be taken with potassium-sparing diuretics to avoid hyperkalemia (potassium excess). *Pregnancy category:* C; PB: 25%–30%; t½: 2–3 h
Enalapril maleate (Vasotec)	A: PO: Initially: 5 mg/d; maint: 10–40 mg/d in 1–2 divided doses IV: 1.25 mg q6h infuse in 5 min	For hypertension and CHF. Similar to captopril and benazepril. Has a long duration of action (orally). *Pregnancy category:* D; PB: 50%–60%; t½: 1.5–2 h
Lisinopril (Prinivil, Zestril)	A: PO: Initially: 10 mg/d; maint: 20–40 mg/d; *max:* 80 mg/d	For hypertension and CHF. Usually given in combination with a diuretic. Has a long duration of action (24 h). Monitor vital signs. *Pregnancy category:* D; PB: 0%; t½: 12 h
Ramipril (Altrace)	A: PO: 2.5–5 mg/d; *max* 20 mg/d	Treatment of stage 1 and 2 hypertension and CHF. Similar to captopril. Has a long duration of action (24 h). *Pregnancy category:* D; PB: 97%; t½: 2–3 h
Calcium Channel Blockers		
Diltiazem HCl (Cardizem, Cardizem CD or SR)	A: PO SR: Initially: 60–120 mg b.i.d.; *max:* 240–360 mg/d	For hypertension (sustained-release form). Also for angina pectoris; IV form for cardiac dysrhythmias (atrial fibrillation). Headache, bradycardia, and hypotension may occur. *Pregnancy category:* C; PB: 70%–80%; t½: 3.5–9 h
Felodipine (Plendil)	A: PO: Initially: 5 mg; maint: 5–10 mg/d; *max:* 20 mg/d	Treatment for stage 1 and 2 hypertension, CHF, and angina. More potent calcium blocker. Flushing, peripheral edema, palpitations, dizziness, headache may occur. Long duration of action. *Pregnancy category:* C; PB: 99%; t½: 10–16 h
Isradipine (DynaCirc)	*Hypertension:* A: PO: 1.25–10 mg b.i.d.; *max:* 20 mg/d	Management of hypertension, CHF, and angina pectoris. For hypertension, drug may be used alone or with a diuretic. *Pregnancy category:* C; PB: 99%; t½: 5–11 h
Nifedipine (Procardia)	A: PO: 10–20 mg t.i.d. A: PO SR: 30–90 mg/d; *max:* 120 mg/d	For hypertension and angina pectoris. Potent calcium channel blocker. Common side effects include dizziness, lightheadedness, headache, flushing, peripheral edema, and nausea. Drug may be taken alone or with a diuretic. *Pregnancy category:* C; PB: 92%–98%; t½: 2–5 h
Verapamil (Calan SR, Isoptin SR)	A: PO SR: 120–240 mg/d in 2 divided doses; *max:* 480 mg/d	For hypertension (sustained release form). One of the first calcium blockers. Also used for variant angina and cardiac dysrhythmias. Common side effects: dizziness, headache, hypotension, bradycardia, and constipation. *Pregnancy category:* C; PB: 90%; t½: 3–8 h

KEY: *A:* adult; *PO:* by mouth; *SR:* sustained-release; *PB:* protein-binding; *t½:* half-life; *CHF:* congestive heart failure; *maint: maintenance.*

POTENTIAL NURSING DIAGNOSES

- Knowledge deficit related to drug regimen
- Anxiety related to hypertensive state

PLANNING

- Client's blood pressure will be within desired range.
- Client is free of moderate to severe side effects.

NURSING INTERVENTIONS

- Monitor laboratory tests related to renal function (BUN, creatinine, protein) and blood glucose levels. Caution: Watch for hypoglycemic reaction in a client with diabetes mellitus. Urine protein may be checked in the morning using a dipstick.
- Report to the health care provider occurrences of bruising, petechiae, and/or bleeding. These may indicate a severe adverse reaction to an angiotensin antagonist such as captopril.

CLIENT TEACHING

General

- Instruct the client not to abruptly discontinue use of captopril without notifying the health care provider. *Rebound hypertension could result.*
- Inform the client not to take over-the-counter (OTC) drugs (cold, allergy medications) without first contacting the health care provider.

Skill

- Teach the client how to take and record his or her blood pressure. Blood pressure chart should be established, and blood pressure changes should be reported.

Diet

- Instruct the client to take captopril 20 min to 1 h before a meal. Food decreases 35% of captopril absorption.
- Inform the client that the taste of food may be diminished during the first month of drug therapy.

Side Effects

- Explain to the client that dizziness and/or lightheadedness may occur during the first week of captopril therapy. If dizziness persists, the health care provider should be notified.
- Instruct the client to report any occurrence of bleeding.

EVALUATION

- Evaluate the effectiveness of the drug therapy: the absence of severe side effects and blood pressure return to desired range.

■ CASE STUDY

G.G., a 72-year-old African American, has congestive heart failure (CHF). She is a diabetic. Her vital signs are BP: 176/94; P: 92; R: 30. Her medications include hydrochlorothiazide 50 mg/d, atenolol 50 mg/d, and digoxin 0.25 mg/d.

1. What type of drug is hydrochlorothiazide? (Refer to Chapter 33 if necessary.)
2. Abnormal electrolytes and other laboratory test results may occur when taking hydrochlorothiazide. Indicate if the serum electrolyte and laboratory values *increase or decrease.*
   a. Sodium _____ d. Magnesium _____
   b. Potassium _____ e. Glucose _____
   c. Calcium _____ f. Uric acid _____
3. Why should G.G.'s blood glucose level be monitored when taking hydrochlorothiazide?
4. What effect may result when G.G. takes digoxin and hydrochlorothiazide? Explain.
5. Atenolol is what type of antihypertensive? Would atenolol be effective in lowering G.G.'s blood pressure if given as the only antihypertensive drug? Explain.
6. According to the stepped-care approach, atenolol is step _____. Hydrochlorothiazide is step _____. Atenolol and hydrochlorothiazide when administered together are step _____.

7. How effective is the combination of hydrochlorothiazide and atenolol for controlling G.G.'s blood pressure? Explain.
8. When using a combination drug therapy to correct hypertension, would the dosage for each drug be the same? Explain.
9. When abruptly discontinuing beta blockers for hypertension without the client taking another antihypertensive, what could occur? Explain.

G.G.'s blood glucose is 229. Her drugs for controlling hypertension are changed to prazosin 10 mg, t.i.d. Her cholesterol and low-density lipoprotein are elevated. Her serum potassium level was low, 3.2 mEq/L.

10. Why were G.G.'s drugs hydrochlorothiazide and atenolol discontinued? Explain.
11. What type of antihypertensive is prazosin? What is the physiologic action of prazosin for lowering the blood pressure?
12. What effect does prazosin have on the blood glucose level?
13. What effect could prazosin have on G.G.'s abnormal lipid levels? Explain.

G.G.'s ankles have become edematous. Hydrochlorothiazide was prescribed.

14. In the stepped-care approach for management of hypertension, what step is prazosin? When

prazosin is combined with hydrochlorothiazide, the step would be _____.

15. Why was hydrochlorothiazide added to the drug regime? Give at least two reasons.
16. Is the prazosin daily dose within the safe therapeutic prescribed range? See prototype drug chart for prazosin (Fig. 34–4). Explain.
17. What groups of antihypertensive drugs can cause sodium and water retention?

STUDY QUESTIONS

1. What nonpharmacologic methods can be practiced to decrease blood pressure?
2. What is the purpose of the stepped-care approach in the treatment of hypertension? Explain the function of diuretics in controlling hypertension.
3. A major side effect of sympatholytic drugs and direct-acting vasodilators is sodium and water retention. How would you assess this problem? What drug is given with the antihypertensives to decrease this side effect? What electrolyte imbalances might occur with the use of the additional drug?
4. What antihypertensive drug might be given for a hypertensive crisis? How would it be administered?
5. Describe the nursing process as it relates to administering beta-adrenergic blockers, alpha-adrenergic blockers, angiotensin antagonists, and calcium blockers.

Chapter 35

Drugs for Circulatory Disorders

OUTLINE

Objectives
Terms
Introduction
   Thrombus Formation
Anticoagulants
   Heparin
   Oral Anticoagulants
   Nursing Process
Thrombolytics

Pharmacokinetics
Pharmacodynamics
Side Effects and Adverse
   Reactions
Nursing Process
Antilipemics
   Pharmacokinetics
   Pharmacodynamics

Side Effects and Adverse
   Reactions
   Nursing Process
Peripheral Vasodilators
   Isoxsuprine
   Nursing Process
Case Study
Study Questions

OBJECTIVES

Describe the action of each of the four main drug groups: anticoagulants, thrombolytics, antilipemics, and peripheral vasodilators.

Identify the side effects and adverse reactions of anticoagulants, thrombolytics, antilipemics, and peripheral vasodilators.

Describe the nursing process, including client teaching, of anticoagulants, thrombolytics, antilipemics, and peripheral vasodilators.

TERMS

aggregation
activated partial thromboplastin time (APTT)
anticoagulants
antilipemics
chylomicrons
fibrinolysis
high-density lipoproteins
   (HDL)

hyperlipidemia
ischemia
lipoproteins
low-density lipoproteins
   (LDL)
myocardial infarction
necrosis
partial thromboplastin time
   (PTT)

peripheral vasodilators
prothrombin time (PT)
thromboembolism
thrombolytics
thrombosis
very low-density lipopro-
   teins (VLDL)

INTRODUCTION

Various drugs are used to maintain, preserve, or restore circulation. The four major groups are (1) anticoagulants and antiplatelets (antithrombotics), (2) thrombolytics, (3) antilipemics, and (4) peripheral vasodilators. Anticoagulants prevent the formation of clots that inhibit circulation. The antiplatelets prevent platelet aggregation (clumping together of platelets to form a clot). The thrombolytics, popularly referred to as *clot busters,* attack and dissolve blood clots that have already formed.

Antilipemics, also called *hypolipemics* or *antihyperlipemics,* decrease blood lipid concentrations. The peripheral vasodilators promote dilation of vessels narrowed by vasospasm. Each of these four drug groups are discussed separately.

THROMBUS FORMATION

A clot is a thrombus that has formed in an arterial or venous vessel. The formation of an arterial thrombus could be due to blood stasis (because of decreased circulation), platelet aggregation on the blood vessel wall, and blood coagulation. Arterial thrombus begins with platelet adhesion to the vessel wall. Adenosine diphosphate (ADP) is released from platelets, which in turn causes more platelet aggregation. As the thrombus inhibits blood flow, fibrin, platelets, and red blood cells (erythrocytes) surround the clot, building the clot's size and structure. As the clot occludes the blood vessel, tissue ischemia occurs.

The venous thrombus usually develops because of slow blood flow. The venous clot can occur rapidly. Small pieces of the venous clot can detach and travel to the pulmonary artery and then to the lung. Inadequate oxygenation and gas exchange in the lungs result.

Oral and parenteral anticoagulants (warfarin and heparin) primarily act by preventing venous thrombosis, whereas antiplatelet drugs act primarily by preventing arterial thrombosis. However, both groups of drugs suppress thrombosis.

ANTICOAGULANTS

Anticoagulants are used to inhibit clot formation. Unlike thrombolytics, they do *not* dissolve clots that have already formed but rather act prophylactically to prevent new clots. Anticoagulants are used in clients with venous and arterial vessel disorders that put them at high risk for clot formation. The venous problems include deep vein thrombosis and pulmonary embolism (ultimately an arterial problem), and the arterial problems include coro-

nary thrombosis (myocardial infarction), presence of artificial heart valves, and cerebrovascular accidents (CVA, or stroke). Antiplatelet drugs such as aspirin, dipyridamole (Persantine), and sulfinpyrazone (Anturane) are prescribed for the prevention of platelet aggregation.

HEPARIN

Anticoagulants are administered orally or parenterally (subcutaneously and intravenously). Heparin, introduced in 1938, is a natural substance in the liver that prevents clot formation. It was first used in blood transfusions to prevent clotting. Heparin is used in open heart surgery to prevent blood from clotting and in the critically ill client with disseminated intravascular coagulation (DIC). Its primary use is to prevent venous thrombosis that can lead to pulmonary embolism or stroke.

Heparin combines with antithrombin III, thus inactivating thrombin and other clotting factors. By inhibiting the action of thrombin, conversion of fibrinogen to fibrin does not occur and the formation of a fibrin clot is prevented (Fig. 35–1).

Heparin is poorly absorbed through the GI mucosa, and much is destroyed by heparinase, a liver enzyme. Because heparin is poorly absorbed orally, it is given subcutaneously for prophylaxis or intravenously to treat acute thrombosis. It can be administered as an intravenous (IV) bolus or in IV fluid for continuous infusion. Heparin prolongs clotting time, and **partial thromboplastin time (PTT)** and **activated partial thromboplastin time (APTT)** are monitored during therapy. Heparin can decrease the platelet count, causing thrombocytopenia. If hemorrhage occurs, the anticoagulant antag-

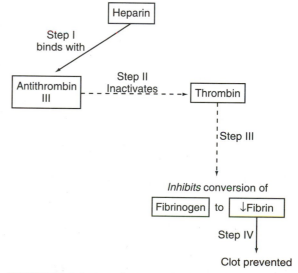

FIGURE 35–1 Action of parenteral anticoagulant: heparin.

onist protamine sulfate is given intravenously. Protamine can be an anticoagulant, but in the presence of heparin, it is an antagonist. Prior to discontinuing heparin, oral therapy with warfarin therapy is begun.

Low Molecular Weight Heparins (LMWHs)

These derivatives of standard heparin were recently introduced for the prevention of venous thromboembolism. By extracting only the low molecular weight fractions of standard heparin, studies have shown the equivalent of anticoagulation with a lower risk of bleeding. LMWHs produce more stable responses at recommended doses. As a result, frequent laboratory monitoring is not required. These newer subcutaneous heparins (dalteparin sodium and enoxaparin sodium) appear to have less effect on platelet activity. Although LMWHs have been approved for prophylactic therapy, their use for the treatment of venous thrombosis is still under study.

ORAL ANTICOAGULANTS

The coumarin group of oral anticoagulants consists of warfarin (Coumadin) and dicumarol. Warfarin is the most widely used coumarin. Oral anticoagulants inhibit hepatic synthesis of vitamin K, thus affecting the clotting factors II, VII, IX, and X. These drugs are used mainly to prevent thromboembolic conditions, such as thrombophlebitis, pulmonary embolism, and embolism formation caused by atrial fibrillation. Oral anticoagulants prolong clotting time and are monitored by the **prothrombin time (PT).** This laboratory test is usually performed before administering the next drug dose until the therapeutic level has been reached. **International normalized ratio (INR)** is a new laboratory test, introduced to account for the variability in reported PTs from different laboratories. Reagents used in the PT test are compared to an international reference standard and reported as the INR. The normal INR is 1.3 to 2.0. Clients on warfarin therapy are maintained at an INR of 2.0 to 3.0.

Monitoring at regular intervals is required for the duration of drug therapy. The coumarins have long half-lives and very long durations of action (dicumarol has a longer action than warfarin); therefore, drug accumulation can occur, which may cause internal bleeding. The nurse must observe for petechiae, ecchymosis, tarry stools, and hematemesis.

Parenteral and oral anticoagulants (heparin and warfarin) are presented in Figure 35–2.

Pharmacokinetics

Heparin is poorly absorbed through the GI mucosa, and much is destroyed by heparinase, a liver enzyme. Heparin is given parenterally, either subcutaneously for prophylactic anticoagulant therapy or intravenously (bolus or continuous infusion) for an immediate response. Warfarin, an oral anticoagulant, is well absorbed through the GI mucosa; however, food will delay but inhibit absorption.

The half-life of heparin is dose-related; high doses prolong the half-life. The half-life of warfarin is 0.5 to 3 days, in contrast to 1 to 2 h for heparin. Because warfarin has a long half-life and is highly protein-bound, the drug can have cumulative effects. Bleeding can occur, especially if another highly protein-bound drug is administered with warfarin. Kidney and liver disease prolong the half-life of both heparin and warfarin. Warfarin is metabolized to inactive metabolites that are excreted by the kidneys and in bile.

Pharmacodynamics

Heparin, administered for acute thromboembolic disorders, prevents thrombus formation and embolism. It has been effectively used in disseminated intravascular coagulation (DIC), which causes multiple thrombi in small blood vessels. Warfarin is effective for long-term anticoagulant therapy. The PT level should be 1.5 to 2 times the reference value to be therapeutic, or INR should be 2.0 to 3.0. INR has effectively replaced the use of PT, because PT can vary from laboratory to laboratory, plus reagent to reagent. Higher INR levels are usually required for clients with prosthetic heart valves, cardiac valvular disease, and recurrent emboli. Heparin does not cross the placental barrier, unlike warfarin; therefore, warfarin use is not suggested during pregnancy.

Intravenous heparin has a rapid onset, its peak time of action is reached in minutes, and its duration of action is short. After an IV heparin dose, the client's clotting time will return to normal in 2 to 6 h. Subcutaneous heparin is more slowly absorbed through the blood vessels in fatty tissue. The coumarins (warfarin and dicumarol) have long onset of action, peak concentration, and duration of action times; thus, drug accumulation may occur. Dicumarol has a longer action time than warfarin. Vitamin K counteracts the effect of warfarin, but it can take up to 24 h for it to be effective.

Table 35–1 gives the comparison summary between oral and parenteral anticoagulants, according to methods of administration, drug action, uses, contraindications, laboratory tests, side/adverse effects, and antidotes.

FIGURE 35–2. Anticoagulants

Anticoagulants	Dosage	

Anticoagulants

Heparin (H)
(Lipo-Hepin, Calciparine), ❧ Hepalean, Calcilean
Pregnancy Category: C

Warfarin sodium (W)
(Coumadin), ❧ Warfilone
Pregnancy Category: D

Dosage

H:
A: SC: 5000–7500 units, q6h or
8000–10,000 units q8h
IV: Bolus: 5000 units;
inf: 20,000–40,000 units over 24 h
C: IV: 50 units/kg bolus; 50–100
units/kg q4h or 20,000 units m²/24 h
W:
A: PO: LD: 10 mg/d for 2–3 d; maint:
2–10 mg/d
Elderly: PO: 2.5 mg/d
IV: Dose is usually titrated according
to INR

NURSING PROCESS
Assessment and Planning

Contraindications

H and W:
Bleeding disorder, peptic ulcer, severe
hepatic or renal disease, hemophilia,
CVA
W: Blood dyscrasias, eclampsia

Drug-Lab-Food Interactions

H:
Increase effect with aspirin, NSAIDs,
thrombolytics, probenecid
Decrease effect with nitroglycerin, protamine
W:
Increase effect with amiodarone, aspirin, NSAIDs, sulfonamides, thyroid
drugs, allopurinol, histamine₂ blockers, oral hypoglycemics, metronidazole, miconazole, methyldopa, diuretics, oral antibiotics, vitamin E
Decrease effect with barbiturates, laxatives, phenytoin, estrogens, vitamins
C and K, oral contraceptives, rifampin
Lab: May increase AST, ALT
Food: Decrease diet rich in vitamin K

Pharmacokinetics

Absorption: (H): SC or IV; (W): PO: well
absorbed
Distribution: PB: (H): >80%; (W): 99%
Metabolism: t½: (H): 1–2 h; (W): 0.5–3 d
Excretion: (H): slowly in urine and
reticuloendothelial system; (W): in
urine and bile

Pharmacodynamics

(H):
SC: Onset: 20–60 min
Peak: 2 h
Duration: 8–12 h
IV: Onset: immediate
Peak: 5–10 min
Duration: 2–6 h
(W):
PO: Onset: >2 d
Peak: 1–3 d
Duration: 2.5–5 d

Interventions

Therapeutic Effects/Uses: (H and W): To prevent blood clotting.

Mode of Action: (H): Inhibits thrombin, which prevents the conversion of fibrinogen to
fibrin.
(W): Depression of hepatic synthesis of vitamin K clotting factors (II [prothrombin], VII,
IX, and X).

Evaluation

Figure continued on next page

FIGURE 35–2. *Continued*

Side Effects	Adverse Reactions
(H): Itching, burning *(W):* Anorexia, nausea, vomiting, diarrhea, abdominal cramps, rash, fever	*(H and W):* Bleeding, ecchymoses *(W):* stomatitis *Life threatening: (H and W):* hemorrhage

KEY: A: Adult; C: Child; PO: by mouth; SC: subcutaneous; IV: intravenous; PB: protein-binding; t½: half-life; >: greater than; 🍁: Canadian drug names.

Drug Interactions

Because warfarin and dicumarol are highly protein-bound, they are affected by drug interactions. Aspirin, nonsteroidal antiinflammatory drugs (NSAIDs), antiinflammatory drugs, sulfonamides, phenytoin, cimetidine (Tagamet), allopurinol, and oral hypoglycemic drugs for diabetes can displace warfarin or dicumarol from the protein-bound site, causing more free circulating anticoagulant. Numerous drugs increase the action of warfarin, and bleeding is apt to occur. Acetaminophen (Tylenol) should be used instead of aspirin for clients taking warfarin or dicumarol. For frank bleeding resulting from excess free drug, parenteral vitamin K is given as a coagulant to decrease bleeding and promote clotting. However, caution must be used with this approach because the prothrombin can remain depressed for prolonged periods.

Table 35–2 lists the drug data for the anticoagulants, the antiplatelets, and the anticoagulant antagonists.

TABLE 35–1 Comparison of Oral and Parenteral Anticoagulants

Factors to Consider	Heparin	Warfarin (Coumadin)
Methods of administration	Subcutaneously Intravenously	Primarily orally
Drug action	Binds with antithrombin III, which inactivates thrombin and clotting factors, thus inhibiting fibrin formation	Inhibits hepatic synthesis of vitamin K, which decreases prothrombin and the clotting factors VII, IX, X
Uses	Treatment of venous thrombosis, pulmonary embolism, thromboembolic complications; e.g., heart surgery, disseminated intravascular coagulation (DIC)	Treatment of deep venous thrombosis, pulmonary embolism, transient ischemic attack (TIA), prophylactic for cardiac valves
Contraindication/caution	Hemophilia, peptic ulcer, severe (stage 3 or 4) hypertension, severe liver or renal disease, dissecting aneurysm	Hemophilia, peptic bleeding ulcer, blood dyscrasias, severe liver or kidney disease, acute myocardial infarction (AMI), alcoholism
Laboratory tests	PTT (partial thromboplastin time): 60–70 sec Anticoagulant: 1.5–2 × control in seconds aPTT (activated partial thromboplastin time): 40 sec Anticoagulant: PTT: 60–80 sec	PT (prothrombin time): 11–15 sec Anticoagulant: 1.25–2.5 × control in seconds INR (international normalized ratio): 1.3–2.0 Anticoagulant: INR 2.0–3.0
Side/adverse effects	Bleeding, hemorrhage, hematoma, severe hypotension	Bleeding, hemorrhage, GI bleeding, ecchymoses, hematuria
Antidote	Protamine sulfate, 1 mg per 100 units of heparin; see Table 35–2	Vitamin K_1 PO/SC/IM/IV: 2.5–10 mg, C: SC/IM: 5–10 mg Infant: 1 mg Vitamin K_4: A: PO/IM/IV: 5–15 mg/d; see Table 35–2

TABLE 35–2 Anticoagulants, Antiplatelets, and Anticoagulant Antagonists

Generic (Brand)	Route and Dosage	Uses & Considerations
Anticoagulant: LMWHs Dalteparin sodium (Fragmin)	A: SC: 2500 IU/d for 5 to 10 d starting 1–2 h before surgery	For prevention of DVT prior to surgery and for those who are at risk of thromboembolism. Similar to enoxaparin. *Pregnancy category:* B; PB: UK; t½: UK
Enoxaparin sodium (Lovenox)	A: SC: 30 mg b.i.d.	For thromboembolism. Prevents and treats DVT and pulmonary embolism. Bleeding is an adverse reaction. Monitor CBC. *Pregnancy category:* B; PB: UK; t½: 4.5 h
Heparins Heparin sodium (Lipo-Hepin)	A: SC: 5000–7500 units q6h or 8000–10,000 units q8h A: IV: Bolus: 5000 units Inf: 20,000–40,000 units over 24 h; dose varies according to aPTT level C: IV: units/kg bolus, 50–100 units/kg q4h or 20,000 units/m²/24 h	For thromboembolism as a prophylaxis against clotting. Is not given IM because of pain and hematoma. Drugs that inactivate heparin: digitalis, tetracycline, IV penicillin, phenothiazine, and quinidine. aPTT should be monitored. Protamine sulfate is the antidote for bleeding control. Dose is 1–1.5 mg for every 100 units of heparin, S.C. *Pregnancy category:* C, PB: 95%; t½: 1–1.5 h
Anticoagulants: Coumarins Dicumarol (Bishydroxycoumarin)	A: PO: LD: 200–300 mg/24 h; maint: 25–200 mg/d based on PT	For thromboembolism as long-term prophylaxis. Has a longer duration than warfarin. INR should be monitored. Oral absorption may be erratic. *Pregnancy category:* D; PB: 99%; t½: 1–2 d
Warfarin (Coumadin)	See Prototype Drug Chart (Fig. 35–2)	Used in thromboembolism for long-term prophylaxis after heparin is discontinued. Monitor PT or INR. PT should be 1.25–2.5 times the control. INR should be 2.0–3.0. Drug has many drug interactions; see text. Has a long half-life. Check for bleeding. *Pregnancy category:* D; PB: 99%; t½: 0.5–3 d
Antiplatelets Aspirin	A: PO: 325 mg/d or q.o.d.	For prevention of thrombosis prior to or after CVA or MI. Client should check with health care provider before taking aspirin for antiplatelet therapy. Aspirin should be avoided with peptic ulcer or liver dysfunction. Enteric-coated preparation decreases GI upset. *Pregnancy category:* D; PB: 55%; t½: 10–12 h
Dipyridamole (Persantine)	A: PO: 50–100 mg t.i.d./q.i.d.	For prevention of thromboembolism post-MI and associated with prosthetic devices (heart valves and hip replacement); prevention of TIA. Monitor blood pressure. *Pregnancy category:* C; PB: >91%; t½: 10–12 h
Sulfinpyrazone (Anturane)	A: PO: 200–400 mg b.i.d.; *max:* 800 mg/d	Used for treating gout. Has antiplatelet function. May be used in AV shunts for hemodialysis to prevent clotting. *Pregnancy category:* C; PB: 95%–99%; t½: 3 h
Anticoagulant Antagonists Protamine SO₄	A: IV: Initially: 1 mg/100 units heparin administered; 10–50 mg in 3–10 min slow push; *max:* 50 mg in any 10-min period	Used to stop bleeding during heparin therapy. Binds and neutralizes heparin. *Pregnancy category:* C; PB: UK; t½: UK
Vitamin K₁, phytonadione (AquaMEPHYTON, Mephyton, Konakion)	A: PO/IM/IV: 2–10 mg q12–24 h as needed C: SC/IM: 5–10 mg	For control of bleeding due to warfarin or dicumarol. If frank bleeding occurs, fresh or frozen plasma or plasmanate may be needed. Depending on form and route, vitamin K takes effect in 1–24 h. Hemorrhage is usually controlled in 3–6 h. *Pregnancy category:* C; PB: UK; t½: UK
Vitamin K₄, menadiol sodium diphosphate	A: PO/SC/IM/IV: 5–10 mg/d C: PO: 50–100 μg/d	For control of bleeding due to warfarin or dicumarol. Not effective to control bleeding due to heparin. *Pregnancy category:* C; PB: UK; t½: UK

KEY: *A: adult; C: child; PO: oral; IM: intramuscular; IV: intravenous; SC: subcutaneous; I: initially; PT: prothrombin time; aPTT: activated partial thromboplastin time; max: maximum dose; CVA: cerebrovascular accident; MI: myocardial infarction; AV: arteriovenous; UK: unknown; PB: protein-binding; t½: half-life; TIA: transient ischemic attack; DVT: deep vein thrombosis; LMWHs: low molecular weight heparins.*

NURSING PROCESS: ANTICOAGULANTS: Warfarin (Coumadin) and Heparin

ASSESSMENT

- Obtain a history of abnormal clotting or health problems that affect clotting, such as severe alcoholism or severe liver or renal disease. Warfarin is contraindicated for clients with blood dyscrasias, peptic ulcer, cerebral vascular accident (CVA), hemophilia, or severe hypertension. Caution its use in a client with acute traumatic injury.
- Obtain a drug history of current drugs the client is taking. Report if a drug-drug interaction is probable. Warfarin is highly protein-bound and can displace other highly protein-bound drugs, or warfarin could be displaced, which may result in bleeding.
- Develop a flow chart that lists PT or INR and warfarin dosages. A baseline PT or INR should be taken before warfarin is administered.

POTENTIAL NURSING DIAGNOSES

- High risk for injury (bleeding)
- Knowledge deficit

PLANNING

- Client's PT will be 1.25 to 2.5 times the control level or INR will be 2.0 to 3.0. For a client receiving heparin, the aPTT should be checked.
- Abnormal bleeding will be rapidly addressed while the client is taking an anticoagulant. The PT, INR, PTT, or aPTT level(s) will be closely monitored.

NURSING INTERVENTIONS

- Monitor vital signs (VS). An increased pulse rate followed by a decreased systolic pressure can indicate a fluid volume deficit due to external or internal bleeding.
- Check PT or INR for warfarin (Coumadin) and aPTT for heparin before administering the anticoagulant. The PT should be 1.25 to 2.5 times the control level or INR 2.0 to 3.0. The platelet count should be monitored, because anticoagulants can decrease platelet count.
- Check for bleeding from the mouth, nose (epistaxis), urine (hematuria), and skin (petechiae, purpura).

- Check stools periodically for occult blood.
- Monitor elderly clients receiving warfarin closely for bleeding. Their skin is thin and capillary beds are fragile.
- Keep anticoagulant antagonists (protamine for heparin and vitamin K or vitamin K for warfarin) available when drug dose is increased or there are indications of frank bleeding. Fresh or frozen plasma may be needed for transfusion.

CLIENT TEACHING

General

- Instruct the client to inform the dentist when taking an anticoagulant. Contacting the health care provider may be necessary.
- Instruct the client to use a soft toothbrush to avoid causing the gums to bleed.
- Instruct the client to shave with an electric razor. Bleeding from shaving cuts may be difficult to control.
- Advise the client to have laboratory tests such as PT performed as ordered by the health care provider. Warfarin dose is regulated according to the INR derived from the PT.
- Instruct the client to carry or wear a medical identification card or jewelry (Medic Alert) listing the person's name, telephone number, and drug name.
- Encourage the client *not* to smoke. Smoking increases drug metabolism; thus, the warfarin dose may need to be increased. If the person insists on smoking, notify the health care provider.
- Instruct the client to check with the health care provider before taking over-the-counter (OTC) drugs. Aspirin should *not* be taken with warfarin because aspirin intensifies its action and bleeding is apt to occur. Suggest that the client use acetaminophen.
- Teach the client to control external hemorrhage (bleeding) from accidents or injuries by applying firm, direct pressure for at least 5 to 10 min with a clean, dry absorbent material.

Diet

- Advise the client to avoid alcohol, which could contribute to increased bleeding, and large amounts of green leafy vegetables, fish, liver, coffee, or tea (caffeine), which are rich in vitamin K.

Side Effects
- Advise the client to report bleeding, such as petechiae, ecchymosis, purpura, tarry stools, bleeding gums, epistaxis, or expectoration of blood.

EVALUATION

- Evaluate the effectiveness of drug therapy. Client's PT or INR values are within the desired range, and client is free of significant side effects.

THROMBOLYTICS

Thromboembolism (occlusion of an artery or vein due to a thrombus or embolus) results in ischemia (deficient blood flow) that causes **necrosis** (death) of the tissue distal to the obstructed area. It takes approximately 1 to 2 weeks for the blood clot to disintegrate by natural fibrinolytic mechanisms. If a new thrombus or embolus could be dissolved more quickly, the necrosis would be minimized and blood flow would be reestablished faster. This is the basis for thrombolytic therapy.

Thrombolytics have been used since the early 1980s to promote the fibrinolytic mechanism (converting plasminogen to plasmin, which destroys the fibrin in the blood clot). The thrombus, or blood clot, disintegrates when a thrombolytic drug is administered within 6 h following an **acute myocardial infarction** (AMI); necrosis due to the blocked artery is prevented or minimized and hospitalization time may be decreased. The need for cardiac bypass or coronary angioplasty can be evaluated soon after thrombolytic treatment. These drugs are also used for pulmonary embolism, deep vein thrombosis, and noncoronary arterial occlusion from an acute thromboembolism.

Four commonly used thrombolytics are streptokinase, urokinase, tissue plasminogen activator (t-PA, alteplase), and anisoylated plasminogen streptokinase activator complex (APSAC, anistreplase). Streptokinase and urokinase are enzymes that act systemically and promote the conversion of plasminogen to plasmin. tPA and APSAC activate plasminogen by acting specifically on the clot. They also promote the conversion of plasminogen to plasmin. Plasmin, an enzyme, digests the fibrin in the clot. Plasmin also degrades fibrinogen, prothrombin, and other clotting factors. These four drugs induce fibrinolysis (fibrin breakdown). Figure 35–3 gives the pharmacologic data for streptokinase.

PHARMACOKINETICS

Streptokinase has a short half-life (20 min), but can persist up to 82 min. It is administered intravenously and absorbed immediately.

PHARMACODYNAMICS

Streptokinase stimulates the fibrinolytic mechanism to dissolve blood clots. Streptokinase is derived from bacterial species so that antibody formation can occur. In rare cases, anaphylaxis has been reported. Initially, a large loading dose is needed to prevent antibody resistance and to induce lysis. The onset of action and peak time are immediate and rapid. Duration of action can be extended to 12 h. After drug therapy is discontinued, the risk of bleeding can persist for 24 h.

The most expensive thrombolytic is t-PA, which costs approximately $2500 per treatment. It changes the plasminogen to plasmin in breaking down and destroying the fibrin in the clot. It has the advantage of a short half-life (5 to 7 min) and is not associated with anaphylactic reactions.

SIDE EFFECTS AND ADVERSE REACTIONS

Allergic reactions can complicate thrombolytic therapy. Anaphylaxis (vascular collapse) occurs more frequently with streptokinase than with the other thrombolytics. If the drugs are administered through an intracoronary catheter after myocardial infarction, reperfusion dysrhythmia or hemorrhagic infarction at the myocardial necrotic area can result. The major complication of thrombolytic drugs is hemorrhage. The antithrombolytic drug aminocaproic acid (Amicar) is used to stop bleeding by inhibiting plasminogen activation, which inhibits thrombolysis.

Table 35–3 lists the drug data for the thrombolytic drugs.

FIGURE 35–3. Thrombolytics

Thrombolytic Enzyme	**Dosage**	**NURSING PROCESS** Assessment and Planning
Streptokinase (Streptase, Kabikinase) *Pregnancy Category:* C	*Myocardial Infarction:* A: IV: 1,500,000 IU diluted in 45 mL; infuse over 60 min *Pulmonary Embolism (PE) and Deep Vein* *Thrombosis (DVT):* A: IV: LD: 250,000 IU Inf: 100,000 IU/h for 24–72 h (24 h for PE; 72 h for DVT)	
Contraindications	**Drug-Lab-Food Interactions**	
Recent CVA, cerebral neoplasm, active bleeding, severe hypertension, ulcerative colitis, anticoagulant therapy	*Increase* risk of bleeding with heparin, oral anticoagulants, aspirin, an- tiplatelets, NSAIDs	
Pharmacokinetics	**Pharmacodynamics**	Interventions
Absorption: IV: Directly administered *Distribution:* PB: UK *Metabolism:* t½: 20–80 min *Excretion:* In urine and bile	IV: Onset: Immediate Peak: Rapid Duration: 4–12 h	

Therapeutic Effects/Uses: To dissolve blood clots due to coronary artery thrombi, deep vein thrombosis, pulmonary embolism.

Mode of Action: Conversion of plasminogen to plasmin (fibrinolysin) for dissolving fibrin deposits.

Evaluation

Side Effects	**Adverse Reactions**
Headache, nausea, flushing, rash, fever	Bleeding, urticaria, unstable blood pressure *Life-threatening:* Hemorrhage, bronchospasm, cardiac dysrhythmias, anaphylaxis

KEY: A: adult; C: child; IV: intravenous; LD: loading dose; Inf: infusion; NSAIDs: nonsteroidal antiinflammatory drugs; UK: unknown; PB: protein-binding; t½: half-life.

TABLE 35–3 Thrombolytics

Generic (Brand)	Route and Dosage	Uses & Considerations
Thrombolytics Anistreplase (APSAC, Eminase)	A: IV: 30 units over 2–5 min	Treatment following an AMI, causing lysis of the thrombi. Decreases the infarction size. *Pregnancy category:* C; PB: UK; t½: 1.5–2 h
Streptokinase (Streptase, Kabikinase)	See Prototype Drug Chart (Fig. 35–3)	For DVT, PE, coronary thrombosis, AV cannula occlusion. Least expensive of the three drugs. May be associated with anaphylactic reactions. Anistreplase and streptokinase should not be administered for more than 5 days or within 6

Table continued on following page

TABLE 35–3 Thrombolytics *Continued*

Generic (Brand)	Route and Dosage	Uses & Considerations
		months of last dose because of possible formation of antistreptokinase antibodies, which decrease effectiveness and increase the likelihood of allergic reaction. If thrombin time is not significantly different from the normal after 4 h, discontinue due to streptokinase resistance. *Pregnancy category:* C; PB UK; t½: 20–80 min
Tissue-type plasminogen activator (t-PA, alteplase, Activase)	*Acute Myocardial Infarction (AMI)* A: IV: Total: 100 mg over 1.5 h Bolus: 15 mg (over 2 min); then 0.75 mg/kg (not to exceed 50 mg) over 30 min; then 0.5 mg/kg (not to exceed 35 mg) over 60 min	For coronary thrombosis. A clot-specific drug. Very expensive drug. Not associated with anaphylactic reactions. Also used for pulmonary thromboembolism. Adverse reactions include internal and superficial bleeding. *Pregnancy category:* C, PB: UK; t½: 30 min
Urokinase (Abbokinase)	A: IV: LD: 4400 IU/kg diluted over 10 min Inf: 4400 IU/kg over 12–24 h *Occluded coronary artery:* Dose may be increased	Same uses as streptokinase. Causes less allergic reaction and is more expensive than streptokinase. Not susceptible to antistreptokinase antibodies. May also be used for peripheral artery occlusion. *Pregnancy category:* B; PB: UK; t½: 10–20 min
Plasminogen Inactivator Aminocaproic acid (Amicar)	A: PO/IV: LD: 5 g first hour Inf: 1–1.25 g/h for 8 h; *max:* 30 g/d	Treatment for excessive bleeding that may result from heart surgery, severe trauma, abruptio placentae, and thrombolytic drugs such as streptokinase, t-PA, urokinase. Side effects include dizziness, headache, orthostatic hypotension, thrombophlebitis. *Pregnancy category:* C; PB: 0%; t½: 1–2 h

KEY: *A: adult; IV: intravenous; LD: loading dose; DVT: deep vein thrombosis; MI: myocardial infarction; PE: pulmonary embolism; AV: arteriovenous; IU: international units; UK: unknown; PB: protein-binding; t½: half-life.*

NURSING PROCESS: THROMBOLYTICS

ASSESSMENT

- Assess baseline vital signs (VS) and compare with future values.
- Check baseline CBC, PT, or INR values before administration of streptokinase.
- Obtain a medical and drug history. Contraindications for use of streptokinase include a recent CVA, active bleeding, severe hypertension, and anticoagulant therapy. It should be reported if the client is taking aspirin or NSAIDs. Thrombolytics are contraindicated for the client with a recent history of traumatic injury, especially head injury.

POTENTIAL NURSING DIAGNOSES

- Decreased cardiac output
- Anxiety related to severe health problem
- Impaired tissue integrity
- Risk for injury

PLANNING

- The blood clot will be dissolved, and the client will be closely monitored for active bleeding.
- Client's VS will be monitored for stability during and after thrombolytic therapy.
- Thrombolytic drug should be administered 4 to 6 h after MI.

NURSING INTERVENTIONS

- Monitor VS. Increased pulse rate followed by decreased blood pressure usually indicates blood loss and impending shock. Record VS and report changes.
- Observe for signs and symptoms of active bleeding from the mouth or rectum. Hemorrhage is a serious complication of thrombolytic treatment. Aminocaproic acid can be given as an intervention to stop the bleeding.
- Check for active bleeding for 24 h after thrombolytic therapy has been discontinued: q15min

for the first hour, q30min until the eighth hour, and then hourly.

- Observe for signs of allergic reaction to streptokinase, such as itching, hives, flushing, fever, dyspnea, bronchospasm, hypotension, and/or cardiovascular collapse.
- Avoid administering aspirin or NSAIDs for pain or discomfort when the client is receiving a thrombolytic.
- Monitor the ECG for the presence of reperfusion dysrhythmias as the blood clot is dissolving; antidysrhythmic therapy may be indicated.
- Avoid venipuncture/arterial sticks.

CLIENT TEACHING

General

- Explain the thrombolytic treatment to the client and family. Be supportive.

Side Effects

- Instruct the client to report any side effects, such as lightheadedness, dizziness, palpitations, nausea, pruritus, or urticaria.

EVALUATION

- Determine the effectiveness of drug therapy. The client's clot has dissolved; VS are stable; there are no signs and symptoms of active bleeding; and the client is pain free.

ANTILIPEMICS

Antilipemics lower abnormal blood lipid levels. Lipids composed of cholesterol, triglycerides, and phospholipids are transported in the body bound to protein in various amounts. These lipoproteins are classified as **chylomicrons, very low-density lipoproteins (VLDL), low-density lipoproteins (LDL),** and **high-density lipoproteins (HDL).** The HDL (friendly or good lipoproteins) have a higher percentage of protein and less lipids. Their function is to remove cholesterol from the blood stream and deliver it to the liver. The other three lipoproteins are composed mainly of cholesterol and triglycerides and contribute to atherosclerotic plaque in the blood vessels; they are "bad" lipoproteins. Table 35–4 presents the composition of the lipoproteins.

Serum cholesterol and triglyceride measurements are frequently part of a regular physical examination or readmission evaluation and are used as baseline test results. If the levels are high, a 14-hour fasting lipid profile may be ordered. When cholesterol, triglycerides, and LDL are elevated, the client is at increased risk for coronary artery disease. Table 35–5 lists the various serum lipids and their reference values (normal serum levels) according to a risk classification.

In many cases, diet alone will not lower blood lipid levels. Because 75% to 85% of serum cholesterol is endogenously (internally) derived, dietary modification alone will typically lower total cholesterol levels by only 10% to 30%. This, and the fact that adherence to dietary restrictions is often short lived, explains why many clients do not respond to diet modification alone. When hyperlipemia (hyperlipidemia) cannot be controlled by diet (avoiding saturated fats from animal sources) and exer-

TABLE 35–4 Lipoprotein Groups

Lipoprotein Subgroups	Composition of the Lipoproteins			
	Protein (%)	*Cholesterol* (%)	*Triglycerides* (%)	*Phospholipids* (%)
Chylomicrons	1–2	1–3	80–95	3–6
Very low density (VLDL)	6–10	8–20	45–65	15–20
Low density (LDL)	18–22	45–50	4–8	18–24
High density (HDL)	45–55	15–20	2–7	26–32

(*Source: Adapted from Henry:* Clinical Diagnosis and Management by Laboratory Methods, *18th ed., Philadelphia, WB Saunders, p. 189, 1991.*)

TABLE 35–5 Serum Lipid Values

Lipids	Normal Value (mg/dL)	Level of Risk for CAD		
		Low Risk (mg/dL)	Moderate Risk (mg/dL)	High Risk (mg/dL)
Cholesterol	150–240	<200	200–240	>240
Triglycerides	40–190	Values vary with age		>190
Lipoproteins:				
(LDL)	60–160	<130	130–159	>160
(HDL)	29–77	>60	35–50	<35

KEY: LDL: low-density lipoproteins; HDL: high-density lipoproteins; CAD: coronary artery disease; <: less than; >: greater than.

cise, antilipemic drugs are usually prescribed. It must be emphasized to the client that dietary changes need to be followed even after drug therapy has been initiated. The type of antilipemics ordered depends on the lipoprotein phenotype (Table 35–6).

One of the first antilipemics was cholestyramine (Questran), introduced in 1959. It is a resin that binds with bile acids in the intestine and is effective against hyperlipidemia type II. The drug comes in a gritty powder, which is mixed thoroughly in water or juice.

Colestipol (Colestid) is a new resin antilipemic similar to cholestyramine. Both of these drugs are effective in lowering cholesterol. Bile acid sequestrants should not be used as the only therapy in clients with elevated triglycerides, because they typically raise triglyceride levels.

Clofibrate (Atromid-S) and gemfibrozil (Lopid) are fibric acid derivatives that are effective in reducing triglyceride and VLDL levels. They are used primarily to reduce hyperlipidemia type IV but can also be used for type II hyperlipidemia. These

drugs are highly protein-bound and should not be taken with anticoagulants because they compete for protein sites. The anticoagulant dose should be reduced during antilipemic therapy, and the INR should be closely monitored. Clofibrate, once a popular antilipemic, is not suggested for long-term use due to its many side effects, such as cardiac dysrhythmias, angina, thromboembolism, and gallstones.

Nicotinic acid, or niacin (vitamin B$_2$), reduces VLDL and LDL. Nicotinic acid is actually very effective at lowering cholesterol levels, and its effect on the lipid profile is highly desirable. Because it has numerous side effects and large doses are required, as few as 20% of clients can tolerate niacin initially; however, with proper client counseling, careful drug titration, and concomitant use of aspirin, this number can be increased to as high as 60% to 70%.

Lovastatin is effective in lowering LDL (hyperlipidemia type II) within several weeks. GI disturbances, headaches, muscle cramps, and tiredness are early complaints. Serum liver enzymes should be monitored and an annual eye examination done because cataract formation may result from lovastatin therapy. Probucol is also useful in lowering LDL and cholesterol levels in (type II) hyperlipidemia, but GI disturbances can occur. It is contraindicated for clients with cardiac dysrhythmias.

Newer antilipemic drugs are pravastatin sodium (Pravachol), simvastatin (Zocor), and fluvastatin (Lescol). These drugs have actions that are similar to lovastatin and decrease serum cholesterol, LDL, VLDL, and triglycerides, and they slightly elevate HDL.

PHARMACOKINETICS

Thirty percent of lovastatin is absorbed, and much of the drug is lost due to extensive first-pass metabolism by the liver. When taken with food, 50%

TABLE 35–6 Hyperlipidemia: Lipoprotein Phenotype

Type	Major Lipids
I	Increased chylomicrons and increased triglycerides. Uncommon.
IIA	Increased low-density lipoprotein (LDL) and increased cholesterol.
IIB	Increased very low-density lipoprotein (VLDL), increased LDL, increased cholesterol and triglycerides. Very common.
III	Moderately increased cholesterol and triglycerides. Uncommon.
IV	Increased VLDL and markedly increased triglycerides. Very common.
V	Increased chylomicrons, VLDL, and triglycerides. Uncommon.

Types II and IV are commonly associated with coronary artery disease.

of lovastatin is absorbed. Lovastatin is highly protein-bound, and other highly protein-bound drugs such as warfarin should be avoided when taking antilipemics. Figure 35–4 gives the drug data for lovastatin.

PHARMACODYNAMICS

Lovastatin inhibits hepatic synthesis of cholesterol, thus lowering the serum cholesterol level. If the drug has not been effective in lowering the serum lipid levels after 3 months, it should be discontinued and another antilipemic started. Lovastatin should not be administered with gemfibrozil.

The onset and peak time of action of lovastatin occurs in hours; however, it takes several days for the drug to have a therapeutic effect. Duration of action may be up to 3 weeks.

Table 35–7 lists the drug data for the antilipemics.

SIDE EFFECTS AND ADVERSE REACTIONS

Cholestyramine

Side effects and adverse reactions include constipation and peptic ulcer. Constipation can be decreased or alleviated by increasing intake of fluids

FIGURE 35–4. Antilipemic

Antilipemic, Antihyperlipidemic	Dosage	**NURSING PROCESS** Assessment and Planning
Lovastatin (Mevacor) *Pregnancy Category:* X	A: PO: 20–80 mg/d in 1–2 divided doses with meals	
Contraindications	**Drug-Lab-Food Interactions**	
Hepatic disease, pregnancy *Caution:* Increase with alcohol consumption, seizure disorder, trauma	*Increase* effect with other antilipemics; *increase* effect of Coumadin *Lab:* May *increase* CPK, AST, ALT	
Pharmacokinetics	**Pharmacodynamics**	Interventions
Absorption: PO: 30% *Distribution:* PB: 95% *Metabolism:* t½: 1–2 h *Excretion:* 10% in urine, 80% in feces, bile	PO: Onset: 2–3 d Peak: UK Duration: UK	

	Evaluation
Therapeutic Effects/Uses: To control hypercholesterolemia; to decrease low-density lipoprotein (LDL); and to slightly increase high-density lipoprotein (HDL). *Mode of Action:* Reduction of HMG-CoA reductase (enzyme), which inhibits cholesterol synthesis.	

Side Effects	Adverse Reactions
Nausea, diarrhea or constipation, abdominal pain or cramps, flatulence, dizziness, headache, blurred vision, rash, pruritus	Hepatic dysfunction (elevated serum liver enzymes), myositis

KEY: A: adult; C: child; UK: unknown; PO: by mouth; PB: protein-binding; t½: half-life.

TABLE 35–7 Antilipemics

Generic (Brand)	Route and Dosage	Uses & Considerations
Cholestyramine resin (Questran)	A: PO: 4 g t.i.d. a.c. and hs; mix powder in 120–240 mL of fluid; *max:* 24 g/d	Cholestyramine resin was the first antilipemic produced. For type II hyperlipoproteinemia (LDL). Decrease in LDL is apparent in a week. Drug powder should be mixed well in fluid. It does not have any effect on VLDL and HDL, but could increase triglyceride levels. GI upset and constipation can occur. Vitamin A, D, K deficiency may occur due to decreased GI absorption. *Pregnancy category:* C; PB: UK; t½: UK
Clofibrate (Atromid-S)	A: PO: 500 mg q.i.d.	For lowering cholesterol, VLDL, and triglyceride; and for types IIB (VLDL), IV, V hyperlipidemia. Drug is more effective for higher cholesterol levels. Therapeutic effect occurs in 2–5 d. Drug should not be taken during pregnancy. Gallstones can occur with long-term use. *Pregnancy category:* C; PB: 90%–95%; t½: 12–25 h
Colestipol HCl (Colestid)	A: PO: 10–30 g/d in divided doses before meals	To reduce cholesterol and LDL levels. Same as cholestyramine. *Pregnancy category:* C; PB: UK; t½: UK
Fenofibrate (Lipidil)	A: PO: 100 mg/d	Treatment of type IV and V hyperlipidemia. Specified diet should be part of the drug therapy. *Pregnancy category:* UK; PB: UK; t½: UK
Fluvastatin (Lescol)	A: PO: Initially: 20 mg h.s.; maint: 20–40 mg/d in 1 or 2 divided doses	A recently approved antilipemic drug. Treatment of types IIA and IIB hyperlipidemia, total cholesterol, and elevated triglycerides. HDL is slightly increased. Monitor liver function (liver enzymes). *Pregnancy category:* B; PB: UK; t½: UK
Gemfibrozil (Lopid)	A: PO: 600 mg b.i.d. before meals; *max:* 1500 mg/d	For VLDL and elevated triglycerides; LDL may decrease and HDL may increase. For types II (VLDL, LDL), III, IV, V hyperlipidemia. Do not use in combination with lovastatin due to increase in CPK. *Pregnancy category:* B; PB: >90%; t½: 1.5 h
Lovastatin (Mevacor)	See Prototype Drug Chart (Fig. 35–4)	For LDL and elevated cholesterol (type II hyperlipidemia), and to increase HDL. Dose dependent on serum cholesterol level. Monitor liver function. Do not exceed 20 mg/d in clients on immunosuppressive drugs. Do not use in combination with gemfibrozil. *Pregnancy category:* X; PB: 95%; t½: 1–2 h
Nicotinic acid (Niacin)	A: PO: Initially: 100 mg t.i.d.; maint: 1–3 g/d p.c. in 3 divided doses; *max:* 6 g/d	For VLDL and LDL: types II, III, IV, V hyperlipidemia. Doses are 100 times higher than for RDA to lower VLDL. See text. *Pregnancy category:* C; PB: UK; t½: 45 min
Pravastatin sodium (Pravachol)	A: PO: 10–40 mg/d	A recently approved antilipemic drug. Decreases serum cholesterol, LDL, VLDL, and triglycerides. HDL is slightly increased. Monitor liver enzymes. *Pregnancy category:* X; PB: 55%; t½: 1.5–2.5 h
Probucol (Lorelco)	A: PO: 500 mg b.i.d. with meals	For LDL and elevated cholesterol (type II hyperlipidemia). Contraindicated in clients with cardiac dysrhythmias. *Pregnancy category:* B; PB: UK; t½: 20 d
Simvastatin (Zocor)	A: PO: Initially: 5–10 mg/d in evening; maint: 20–40 mg/d in 1 or 2 divided doses; *max:* 40 mg/d	Similar to lovastatin. Monitor liver enzymes. *Pregnancy category:* X; PB: 95%; t½: UK

KEY: A: adult; PO: by mouth; LDL: low-density lipoprotein; VLDL: very low-density lipoprotein; HDL: high-density lipoprotein; CPK: creatinine phosphokinase; RDA: recommended daily allowance; UK: unknown; PB: protein-binding; t½: half-life.

and foods high in fiber. Early signs of peptic ulcer are nausea and abdominal discomfort, followed later by abdominal pain and distention. To avoid GI discomfort, the drug must be taken with and followed by sufficient fluids.

Nicotinic Acid

The many side effects of nicotinic acid, including GI disturbances, flushing of the skin, abnormal liver function (elevated serum liver enzymes), hyperglycemia, and hyperuricemia, decrease its usefulness. However, as mentioned, aspirin and careful drug titration can reduce side effects to a manageable level in most clients.

NURSING PROCESS: ANTILIPEMICS: Lovastatin (Mevacor) and Others

ASSESSMENT

- Assess vital signs (VS) and serum chemistry values (cholesterol, triglycerides, AST, ALT, CPK) for baseline values.
- Obtain a medical history. Lovastatin is contraindicated for clients with a liver disorder. Pregnancy category is X.

POTENTIAL NURSING DIAGNOSES

- Impaired tissue integrity
- Anxiety related to elevated cholesterol level

PLANNING

- Client's cholesterol level will be <200 mg/dL in 6 to 8 wk.
- Client will be taught to choose foods low in fat, cholesterol, and complex sugars.

NURSING INTERVENTIONS

- Monitor the client's blood lipid levels (cholesterol, triglycerides, low-density lipoprotein [LDL], and high-density lipoprotein [HDL] every 6 to 8 wk for the first 6 mon after lovastatin therapy and then every 3 to 6 mon. For lipid level profile, the client should fast for 12 to 14 h. Desired cholesterol value is <200 mg/dL; triglyceride value is <150 mg/dL (can vary); LDL is <130 mg/dL; and HDL is >60 mg/dL. Cholesterol levels of >240 mg/dL, LDL levels of >160 mg/dL, and HDL levels of >35 mg/dL can lead to severe cardiovascular or cerebral vascular accident.
- Monitor laboratory tests for liver function, such as ALT, ALP, and GGTP. Antilipemic drugs may cause liver disorder.
- Observe for signs and symptoms of GI upset. Taking the drug with sufficient water or with meals may alleviate some of the GI discomfort.

CLIENT TEACHING

General
- Advise the client that if there is a family history of hyperlipidemia, his or her children should have a baseline blood lipid level obtained and monitored. Instruct the client that children should decrease fatty foods in the diet.
- Emphasize the need to comply with the drug regimen to lower the blood lipids. Side effects should be reported to the health care provider.
- Inform the client that it may take several weeks before blood lipid levels decline. Explain that laboratory tests for blood lipids (cholesterol, triglycerides, LDL, and HDL) are usually ordered every 3 to 6 mo.
- Advise the client to have serum liver enzymes monitored as indicated by the health care provider. Lovastatin, pravastatin, and simvastatin are contraindicated in acute hepatic disease and pregnancy.
- Instruct the client to have an annual eye examination and to report changes in visual acuity.

Clofibrate, Gemfibrozil, Probucol
- Advise the client taking clofibrate and probucol that decreased libido and impotence may occur and should be reported. Drug dosage can be changed or another antilipemic may be ordered.
- Instruct diabetic or prediabetic clients to monitor blood glucose levels if they are taking gemfibrozil. Dietary changes or insulin adjustment may be necessary.
- Advise the client with cardiac dysrhythmias to tell the health care provider before starting probucol. Cardiac dysrhythmias should be monitored and reported.

Skill

Cholestyramine and Cholestipol
- Instruct the client to mix the powder well in water or juice.

Diet
- Explain to the client that GI discomfort is a common problem with most antilipemics. Suggest increasing fluid intake when taking the medication.
- Instruct the client to maintain a low-fat diet by eating foods that are low in animal fat, cholesterol, and complex sugars. Lovastatin and other antilipemics are not a substitute for a diet that is low in fat.

Nicotinic Acid
- Advise the client to take the drug with meals to decrease GI discomfort.

Side Effects
Cholestyramine, Cholestipol, and
Nicotinic Acid (Niacin)
- Advise the client that constipation may occur with cholestyramine and cholestipol. Increasing fluid intake and food bulk should help in alleviating the problem.
- Explain to the client that flushing is common and should decrease with continued use of the drug. Usually, the drug is started at a low dose.
- Advise the client that large doses of nicotinic acid can cause vasodilation, producing dizziness, and faintness (syncope).

EVALUATION

- Evaluate the effectiveness of the antilipemic drug. The client's cholesterol level is within desired range.
- Determine that the client is on a low-fat, low-cholesterol diet.

PERIPHERAL VASODILATORS

Peripheral vasodilators increase blood flow to the extremities. They are used in peripheral vascular disorders of venous and arterial vessels. They are more effective for disorders resulting from vasospasm (Raynaud's disease) than from vessel occlusion or arteriosclerosis (arteriosclerosis obliterans, thromboangiitis obliterans [Buerger's disease]). In Raynaud's disease, cold exposure or emotional upset can trigger vasospasm of the toes and fingers; these clients have benefited from vasodilators.

Although the following drugs have different actions, they all promote vasodilation: tolazoline (Priscoline), an alpha-adrenergic blocker; isoxsuprine (Vasodilan) and nylidrin (Arlidin), beta-adrenergic agonists; and cyclandelate (Cyclan), nicotinyl alcohol, and papaverine (Cerespan, Genabid), direct-acting peripheral vasodilators. The alpha blocker prazosin (Minipress), and the calcium channel blocker nifedipine (Procardia) have also been used. A new drug, the hemorrheologic pentoxifylline (Trental), increases microcirculation and tissue perfusion. It does not act as a vasodilator.

ISOXSUPRINE

Pharmacokinetics

Isoxsuprine is readily absorbed from the GI tract. It has a short half-life of 1.25 to 1.5 h. Because of its half-life, the drug can be taken three to four times a day.

Pharmacodynamics

Isoxsuprine is a beta$_2$-adrenergic agonist. It causes vasodilation on arteries within the skeletal muscles. Bronchodilation also may occur. This drug has a short onset of action, peak time, and duration of action. Figure 35–5 gives the drug data for isoxsuprine.

Side Effects and Adverse Reactions

Lightheadedness, dizziness, orthostatic hypotension, tachycardia, palpitation, flushing, and GI distress may occur.

The effectiveness of these drugs in increasing blood flow by vasodilation is questionable in the presence of arteriosclerosis. These drugs may decrease some of the symptoms of cerebrovascular insufficiency. The drug data for the peripheral vasodilators are given in Table 35–8.

FIGURE 35–5. Vasodilators

Peripheral Vasodilator	Dosage	NURSING PROCESS
		Assessment and Planning
Isoxsuprine HCl (Vasodilan, Voxsuprine) Beta-adrenergic agonist *Pregnancy Category:* C	A: PO: 10–20 mg t.i.d./q.i.d.	
Contraindications	**Drug-Lab-Food Interactions**	
Arterial bleeding, severe hypotension, postpartum, tachycardia *Caution:* Bleeding disorders, tachycardia	*Decrease* blood pressure with antihypertensives	
Pharmacokinetics	**Pharmacodynamics**	Interventions
Absorption: PO: Readily absorbed *Distribution:* PB: UK *Metabolism:* t½: 1.25–1.5 h *Excretion:* In urine	PO: Onset: 0.5 h Peak: 1 h Duration: 3 h	

Evaluation

Therapeutic Effects/Uses: To increase circulation due to peripheral vascular disease (Raynaud's disease, arteriosclerosis obliterans) and cerebrovascular insufficiency.

Mode of Action: Action is directly on vascular smooth muscle.

Side Effects	Adverse Reactions
Nausea, vomiting, dizziness, syncope, weakness, tremors, rash, flushing, abdominal distention, chest pain	Hypotension, tachycardia, palpitations

KEY: A: adult; PO: by mouth; PB: protein-binding; t½: half-life; UK: unknown.

TABLE 35–8 Vasodilators (Peripheral)

Generic (Brand)	Route and Dosage	Uses & Considerations
Alpha-Adrenergic Blocker Tolazoline HCl (Priscoline HCl)	A: SC/IM/IV: 10–50 mg q.i.d. NB: IV: Initially: 1–2 mg/kg, followed by 1–2 mg/kg/h for 24–48 h; initial dose effect: 30 min	For neonatal pulmonary hypertension and in vascular occlusive diseases in adults. Causes vasodilation and decreases peripheral resistance. Improves circulation in thromboangiitis obliterans, Raynaud's disease, frostbite, and peripheral vasospastic disorders. *Pregnancy category:* C; PB: UK; t½: A: 10 h, NB: 3–10 h
Beta₂-Adrenergic Agonists Isoxsuprine HCl (Vasodilan)	See Prototype Drug Chart (Fig. 35–5)	For symptoms of TIA and peripheral vascular diseases (e.g., Raynaud's and Buerger's diseases). May cause hypotension and tachycardia. May take several weeks for therapeutic effects. *Pregnancy category:* C; PB: UK; t½: 1.25–1.5 h

Table continued on following page

TABLE 35–8 Vasodilators (Peripheral) *Continued*

Generic (Brand)	Route and Dosage	Uses & Considerations
Nylindrin HCl (Arlidin)	A: PO: 3–12 mg t.i.d./q.i.d.	For peripheral vascular disorders. May cause tachycardia and heart palpitations. *Pregnancy category:* C; PB: UK; t½: UK
Direct-Acting Peripheral Vasodilators Cyclandelate (Cyclospasmol)	A: PO: 20 mg q.i.d.; maint: 400–800 mg/d in 2–4 divided doses; dose may be reduced; *max:* 1600 mg/d	For peripheral vascular disorders. Acts on vascular smooth muscle. Has greater vasodilating effect than papaverine. Skin flushing and tachycardia can occur. Short-term use rarely of benefit; long-term treatment usually needed. *Pregnancy category:* C; PB: UK; t½: UK
Ergoloid mesylates (Hydergine)	A: PO/SL: 1 mg t.i.d.; dose may increase to 4–12 mg/d	For cerebrovascular insufficiency. To improve cognitive skills, self-care, and mood, especially in the older adult. SL tablets should be placed under the tongue. May cause GI distress, orthostatic hypotension. *Pregnancy category:* C; PB: UK; t½: 3–12 h
Nicotinyl alcohol (Ronigen [Canada only])	A: PO: 150–300 mg b.i.d.	Acts as vasodilator. Can cause flushing and orthostatic hypotension. *Pregnancy category:* UK; PB: UK; t½: UK
Papaverine (Pavabid)	A: PO: 100–300 mg, 3–5 × d SR: 150 mg q12h; *max:* 300 mg q12h IV: 30–120 mg q3h PRN	For arterial spasms. Reduces ischemia of the brain, heart, and peripheral vessels. One of the oldest vasodilators. Side effects: flushing, GI upset, headaches, increased heart rate and respiration. *Pregnancy category:* C; PB: 90%; t½: 1.5 h
Hemorrheologic Pentoxifylline (Trental)	A: PO: 400 mg t.i.d. with meals	For peripheral vascular disorders. Alleviates intermittent claudication. Also improves cerebral function for those with cerebrovascular insufficiency and may decrease stroke incidence for those having recurrent TIA. *Pregnancy category:* C; PB: UK; t½: 0.5–1 h

KEY: *A: adult; NB: newborn; PO: by mouth; SR: sustained-release tablet; SL: sublingual; TIA: transient ischemic attack; PRN: as necessary; UK: unknown; PB: protein-binding; t½: half-life.*

NURSING PROCESS: VASODILATORS: Isoxsuprine (Vasodilan)

ASSESSMENT

- Obtain baseline vital signs (VS) for future comparison.
- Assess for signs of inadequate blood flow to the extremities: pallor, coldness of extremity, and pain.

POTENTIAL NURSING DIAGNOSES

- Impaired tissue integrity
- Pain related to inadequate blood flow to extremity

PLANNING

- Client's blood flow to the extremities will improve, and the client's pain will be controlled.

NURSING INTERVENTIONS

- Monitor VS, especially blood pressure and heart rate. Tachycardia and orthostatic hypotension can be problematic with peripheral vasodilators.

CLIENT TEACHING

General

- Inform the client that a desired therapeutic response may take 1.5 to 3 mo.
- Advise the client not to smoke; smoking increases vasospasm.
- Instruct the client to use aspirin or aspirin-like compounds only with the health care provider approval. Salicylates help in preventing platelet aggregation.

Diet

- Advise the client with GI disturbances to take isoxsuprine with meals.
- Advise the client not to ingest alcohol with a vasodilator because it may cause a hypotensive reaction.

Side Effects

- Encourage the client to change position slowly but frequently to avoid orthostatic hypotension. Orthostatic hypotension is common when taking high doses of a vasodilator.
- Instruct the client to report side effects of isoxsuprine, such as flushing, headaches, and dizziness.

EVALUATION

- Evaluate the effectiveness of the isoxsuprine therapy; blood flow is increased in the extremities and pain has subsided.
- Client is experiencing no side effects from the prescribed drug.

■ CASE STUDY
Client Treated for Thrombophlebitis

T.M., 57 years old, has thrombophlebitis in the right lower leg. IV heparin, 5000 units by bolus, was given. Following the IV bolus, heparin 5000 units, SC, q6h was prescribed. Other therapeutic means to decrease pain and alleviate swelling and redness were also prescribed. An aPTT test was ordered.

1. Was T.M.'s heparin order per day within the safe daily range?
2. What does IV bolus mean? How are subcutaneous injections given? (See Chapter 3 if necessary.)
3. What is an aPTT test? Why was it ordered? Explain.

After 5 days of heparin therapy, T.M. was prescribed warfarin (Coumadin) 5 mg, PO, daily. PT and INR tests were ordered.

4. What is the pharmacologic action of warfarin?
5. Is the warfarin dose within the daily dosage range? Explain.
6. What is the half-life and protein-binding for warfarin? If a client is taking a drug that is highly protein-bound, would there be a drug interaction? Explain.
7. What are PT and INR tests? When are they ordered? Explain.
8. What serious adverse reactions could result with prolonged use and/or large doses of warfarin?
9. What client teaching interventions should the nurse include? Give three client teaching interventions.

10. Months later, T.M. had hematemesis. What nursing action should be taken?

STUDY QUESTIONS

1. In what routes can heparin be administered? When? Why? Give rationale for your explanations.
2. What drugs can enhance the action of Coumadin (drug interaction)? How is Coumadin therapy monitored? Explain.
3. Explain how protamine is used. What is its action?
4. Plan a nursing plan of care for a client with thrombocytopenia.
5. The client has had an AMI within the last 3 hours. A thrombolytic drug is given. What type of nursing assessment should be performed and for how long?
6. Name at least three client situations that would contradict the use of thrombolytic therapy.
7. Explain the difference between an anticoagulant and a thrombolytic.
8. The client has a serum cholesterol level of 265 mg/dL, a triglyceride level of 235 mg/dL, and an LDL level of 180 mg/dL. Do these serum levels indicate hypolipidemia, normolipidemia, or hyperlipidemia? What nonpharmacologic measure should the nurse suggest that can aid in decreasing blood lipids?
9. Name the "friendly" lipoprotein. Which antilipemics tend to elevate this lipoprotein?
10. What are the uses of peripheral vasodilators? What two common side effects can occur?

Unit IX

Gastrointestinal Agents

INTRODUCTION

The gastrointestinal (GI) system (tract), comprising the alimentary canal and the digestive tract, begins at the oral cavity of the mouth and ends at the anus. Major structures of the GI system are (1) the oral cavity (mouth, tongue, and pharynx), (2) the esophagus, (3) the stomach, (4) the small intestine (duodenum, jejunum, and ileum), (5) the large intestine (cecum, colon, and rectum), and (6) the anus. The accessory organs and glands that contribute to the digestive process are (1) the salivary glands, (2) the pancreas, (3) the gallbladder, and (4) the liver (Fig. IX–1). The main functions of the GI system are digestion of food particles and absorption of the digestive contents (nutrients, electrolytes, minerals, and fluids) into the circulatory system for cellular use. Absorption and digestion take place in the small intestine and, to a lesser extent, in the stomach. Undigested material passes through the lower intestinal tract with the aid of peristalsis to the rectum and anus, where it is excreted as feces, or stool.

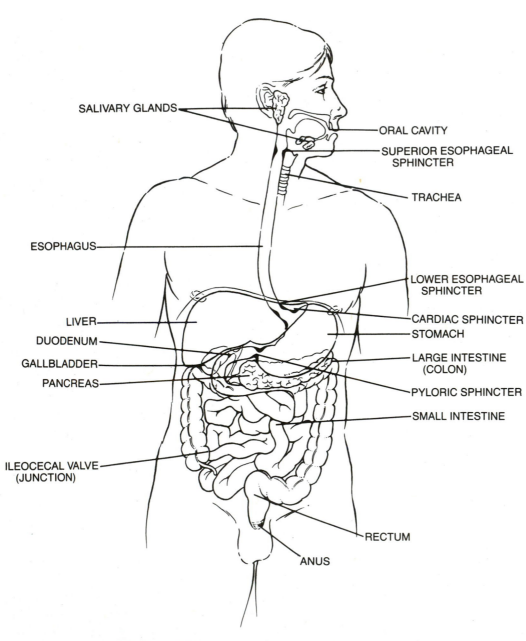

FIGURE IX–1 The gastrointestinal system and alimentary canal.

ORAL CAVITY

The oral cavity, or mouth, starts the digestive process by (1) breaking up food into smaller particles; (2) adding saliva, which contains the enzyme amylase for digesting starch (the beginning of the digestive process); and (3) swallowing, a voluntary movement of food that becomes involuntary (peristalsis) in the esophagus, stomach, and intestines. Swallowing occurs in the pharynx (throat), which connects the mouth and esophagus.

ESOPHAGUS

The esophagus, a tube that extends from the pharynx to the stomach, is composed of striated muscle in its upper portion and smooth muscle in its lower portion. The inner lining of the esophagus is a mucous membrane that secretes mucus. The peristaltic process of contraction begins in the esophagus and ends in the lower large intestine. There are two sphincters: the superior esophageal (hyperpharyngeal) sphincter and the lower esophageal sphincter. The lower esophageal sphincter prevents gastric reflux into the esophagus, a condition called *reflux esophagitis*.

STOMACH

The stomach is a hollow organ that lies between the esophagus and the intestine. The body of the stomach has lesser and greater curvatures. It can hold 1000 to 2000 mL of gastric contents, and empties in 2 to 6 h (average, 3 to 4 h), depending on gastric content and motility. Two sphincters, the cardiac sphincter, which lies at the upper opening of the stomach, and the pyloric sphincter, located at the lower portion of the stomach or the head of the duodenum, regulate the entrance of food into the stomach.

The interior lining of the stomach has mucosal folds that contain glands that secrete gastric juices. The four types of cells in the stomach mucosa that secrete these juices are (1) the chief cells, which secrete the proenzyme pepsinogen (pepsin), (2) the parietal cells, which secrete hydrochloric acid (HCl), (3) the gastrin-producing cells, which secrete gastrin, a hormone that regulates enzyme release during digestion, and (4) mucus-producing cells that release mucus to protect the stomach lining, which extends into the duodenum.

SMALL INTESTINE

The small intestine begins at the pyloric sphincter of the stomach and extends to the ileocecal valve at the cecum. Most drug absorption occurs in the duodenum, but lipid-soluble drugs and alcohol are absorbed from the stomach. The digestive process begins in the stomach, but most of the digestive contents are absorbed from the small intestine. The duodenum releases the hormone secretin, which suppresses gastric acid secretion, causing the intestinal juices to have a higher pH than the gastric juices. The intestinal cells also release the hormone cholecystokinin, which in turn stimulates the release of pancreatic enzymes and contraction of the gallbladder to release bile into the duodenum. Hormones, bile, and pancreatic enzymes (trypsin, chymotrypsin, lipase, and amylase) complete the digestion of carbohydrates, protein, and fat in preparation for absorption.

LARGE INTESTINE

The large intestine accepts undigested material from the small intestine, absorbs water, secretes mucus, and with peristaltic contractions moves the remaining intestinal contents to the rectum for elimination. Defecation completes the process.

DRUGS FOR GASTROINTESTINAL DISORDERS

Vomiting, diarrhea, and constipation are gastrointestinal problems that frequently require drug intervention. Chapter 36 describes the antiemetics used to control vomiting. Antiemetic groups include antihistamines, anticholinergics, selected phenothiazines, cannabinoids, and nonclassified antiemetics. Also discussed in the chapter are drugs that induce vomiting for elimination of ingested toxins and drugs. The antidiarrheal drugs include opiates, opiate-related drugs, and adsorbent drugs. Osmotic, contact-stimulant, bulk-forming, and emollient laxatives are discussed. The nursing process is considered in relation to each of the drug groups.

Drugs used to prevent and treat peptic ulcers (gastric and duodenal) are discussed in Chapter 37. Predisposing factors for peptic ulcers are described. Drug groups used for treating peptic ulcers include (1) selected tranquilizers, (2) anticholinergics, (3) antacids, (4) histamine$_2$ (H$_2$) blockers, (5) pepsin inhibitor (also known as mucosal protective drug), (6) gastric acid secretion inhibitor, (7) prostaglandin E$_1$ analog, and (8) GI stimulants. The nursing process is discussed in relation to these drugs.

Chapter 36

Drugs for Gastrointestinal Tract Disorders

OUTLINE

Objectives
Terms
Introduction
Vomiting
    Nonpharmacologic Measures
    Nonprescription Antiemetics
    Prescription Antiemetics

Nursing Process
Emetics
    Ipecac
    Apomorphine
    Nursing Process
Diarrhea
    Nonpharmacologic Measures
    Antidiarrheals

Nursing Process
Constipation
    Nonpharmacologic Measures
    Laxatives
Case Study
Study Questions

OBJECTIVES

Identify causes of vomiting, diarrhea, and constipation.

Explain the action and side effects of antiemetics, emetics, antidiarrheals, and laxatives.

Describe the nursing process, including client teaching, of antiemetics, emetics, antidiarrheals, and laxatives.

Identify contraindications to use of antiemetics, emetics, antidiarrheals, and laxatives.

TERMS

adsorbents
antidiarrheals
antiemetics
cannabinoids
cathartics
chemoreceptor trigger zone (CTZ)

constipation
diarrhea
emetics
emollients
laxatives
opiates
osmotics

purgatives
vomiting center

INTRODUCTION

Drug groups used to correct or control vomiting, diarrhea, and constipation are antiemetics, emetics, antidiarrheals, and laxatives. Each of these drug groups will be discussed separately. Drugs used to treat peptic ulcers are discussed in Chapter 37.

VOMITING

Vomiting (emesis), the expulsion of gastric contents, has a multitude of causes, such as motion sickness, viral and bacterial infection, food intolerance, surgery, pregnancy, pain, shock, selected drugs including antineoplastics, radiation, and disturbances of the middle ear affecting equilibrium. The cause of the vomiting needs to be identified. Nausea, a queasy sensation, may or may not precede the act of vomiting. Antiemetics can mask the underlying cause of vomiting and should not be used until it has been determined, unless the vomiting is so severe as to cause dehydration and electrolyte imbalance.

Two major cerebral centers, the **chemoreceptor trigger zone (CTZ)** that lies near the medulla and the **vomiting center** in the medulla, cause vomiting when stimulated (Fig. 36–1). The CTZ receives most of the impulses from drugs, toxins, and the vestibular center in the ear and transmits them to the vomiting center. The neurotransmitter dopamine stimulates the CTZ, which in turn stimulates

the vomiting center. Levodopa, a drug with dopamine-like properties, can cause vomiting by stimulating the CTZ. Some sensory impulses are transmitted directly to the vomiting center, such as odor, smell, taste, and gastric mucosal irritation. The neurotransmitter acetylcholine is also a vomiting stimulant. When the vomiting center is stimulated, the motor neuron responds by causing contraction of the diaphragm, the anterior abdominal muscles, and the stomach. The glottis closes, the abdominal wall moves upward, and vomiting occurs.

Nonpharmacologic measures should be used first when nausea and vomiting occur. If the nonpharmacologic measures are not effective, then antiemetics are combined with nonpharmacologic measures. There are two major groups of antiemetics: nonprescription (antihistamines, bismuth subsalicylate, phosphorated carbohydrate solution) and prescription (antihistamines, phenothiazine, benzodiazepines, cannabinoids, and miscellaneous antiemetics).

NONPHARMACOLOGIC MEASURES

The nonpharmacologic methods of decreasing nausea and vomiting include administration of weak tea, flattened carbonated beverage, gelatin, Gatorade, and Pedialyte (children). Crackers and dry toast may be helpful. When dehydration becomes severe, intravenous fluids are needed to restore body fluid balance.

NONPRESCRIPTION ANTIEMETICS

Nonprescription **antiemetics** (antivomiting agents) can be purchased as over-the-counter (OTC) drugs. These drugs are frequently used to prevent motion sickness and have minimal effect on controlling severe vomiting due to anticancer agents (antineoplastics), radiation, and toxins. To prevent motion sickness, the antiemetic should be taken 30 min prior to travel. These drugs are not effective in relieving motion sickness if taken after vomiting has occurred.

Selected antihistamine antiemetics such as dimenhydrinate (Dramamine), cyclizine hydrochloride (Marezine), meclizine hydrochloride (Antivert), and diphenhydramine hydrochloride (Benadryl) can be purchased OTC to prevent nausea, vomiting, and dizziness (vertigo) due to motion by inhibiting vestibular stimulation in the middle ear. Benadryl is also used to prevent or alleviate allergic reactions to drugs, insects, and food by acting as an antagonist to the histamine$_1$ (H$_1$) receptors.

The side effects of these drugs are similar to those of anticholinergics: drowsiness, dryness of

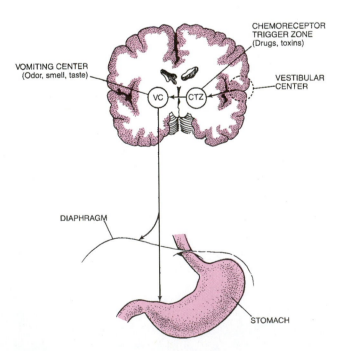

FIGURE 36–1 The chemoreceptor trigger zone and vomiting center.

TABLE 36–1 Nonprescription Antiemetics: Antihistamine

Generic (Brand)	Route and Dosage	Uses & Considerations
Motion Sickness		
Buclizine HCl (Bucladin-S [Softab])	*Prophylaxis:* A: PO: 50 mg 0.5 h before travel; may repeat in 4–6 h	Prevention of motion sickness that may cause nausea and vomiting. Drowsiness and dry mouth can occur. Avoid taking alcohol and central nervous system (CNS) depressants. *Pregnancy category:* C; PB: UK; t½: UK
Cyclizine HCl (Marezine)	A: PO: 50 mg 0.5 h before travel; may repeat in 4–6 h; *max: 200 mg/d* IM: 50 mg q4–6h PRN C 6–12 y: PO: 25 mg q.d./t.i.d. *Postoperative vomiting:* A: IM: 50 mg 0.5 h before surgery ends; may repeat q4–6h PRN	Similar to buclizine. Has been used for postoperative nausea and vomiting. *Pregnancy category:* B; PB: UK; t½: UK
Dimenhydrinate (Calm-X, Dimetabs, Dramamine)	A: PO: 50–100 mg q4–6h; *max: 400 mg/d;* IM/IV: 50 mg PRN C 6–12 y: PO: 25–50 mg q6–8h; *max: 150 mg/d* C < 2 y: Not recommended	Primarily used to prevent motion sickness. Drowsiness, dizziness, dry mouth, and hypotension may occur. *Pregnancy category:* B; PB: UK; t½: UK
Meclizine HCl (Antivert, Antrizine, Bonine)	A&C > 12 y: PO: 25–50 mg 1 h before travel, after meal; may repeat q24h *Vertigo:* A: PO: 25–100 mg/d in divided doses	Prevention of nausea, vomiting, and dizziness. Drowsiness and dry mouth may occur. *Pregnancy category:* B; PB: UK; t½: UK

KEY: A: adult; C: child; PO: by mouth; >: greater than; <: less than; UK: unknown; PB: protein-binding; t½: half-life; max: maximum; PRN: as necessary.

the mouth, and constipation. Table 36–1 lists the nonprescription antihistamines used for vomiting associated with motion sickness.

Several nonprescription drugs such as bismuth subsalicylate (Pepto-Bismol) act directly on the gastric mucosa to suppress vomiting. They are marketed in liquid and chewable tablet forms and can be taken for gastric discomfort or diarrhea. Phosphorated carbohydrate solution (Emetrol), a hyperosmolar carbohydrate, decreases nausea and vomiting by changing the gastric pH; it may also decrease smooth muscle contraction of the stomach. Its effectiveness as an antiemetic has not been verified. Clients with diabetes mellitus should avoid this drug due to its high sugar content.

Antiemetics were once used frequently for the treatment of nausea and vomiting during the first trimester of pregnancy, but today they are not recommended due to possible harm to the fetus. Nonpharmacologic methods should be used to alleviate nausea and vomiting and OTC antiemetics should be avoided. If the vomiting becomes severe and threatens the well-being of the mother and fetus, an antiemetic such as trimethobenzamide (Tigan) can be administered.

PRESCRIPTION ANTIEMETICS

Prescription antiemetics are classified into five groups: (1) antihistamines, (2) anticholinergics, (3) phenothiazines, (4) cannabinoids (for cancer clients), and (5) miscellaneous. Many of these drugs act as antagonists to dopamine, histamine, and acetylcholine, which are associated with vomiting. Antihistamines and anticholinergics act primarily on the vomiting center; they also act by decreasing stimulation of the CTZ and vestibular pathways. Phenothiazines and the miscellaneous antiemetics such as benzquinamide, diphenidol, metoclopramide, and trimethobenzamide act on the CTZ center. The cannabinoids act on the cerebral cortex.

Antihistamines and Anticholinergics

Only a few prescription antihistamines and anticholinergics are used in the treatment of nausea and vomiting; Table 36–2 lists these drugs, dosages, and uses and considerations.

Side Effects and Adverse Reactions

Side effects include drowsiness, which can be a major problem, dry mouth, blurred vision due to pupillary dilation, tachycardia (with use of anticholinergics), and constipation. These drugs should *not* be used in clients with glaucoma due to dilation of the pupils (mydriasis).

Phenothiazine Antiemetics

The largest group of drugs used for nausea and vomiting are the phenothiazines, primarily the piperazine phenothiazines.* These drugs are used to treat severe nausea and vomiting due to surgery, anesthetics, chemotherapy, and radiation sickness. They act by inhibiting the CTZ. When used in cancer clients, these drugs are commonly given the night before treatment, the day of the treatment, and for 24 h after treatment. Not all phenothiazines are effective antiemetic agents. When prescribed for vomiting, the drug dosage is usually smaller than when used for psychiatric disorders. Promethazine (Phenergan), a phenothiazine introduced as an antihistamine in the 1940s, has a sedative effect and can be used for motion sickness.

Chlorpromazine (Thorazine) and prochlorperazine edisylate (Compazine) were the first tranquilizers used for both psychosis and vomiting. Prochlorperazine, a piperazine phenothiazine, is the most frequently prescribed antiemetic drug. It is administered orally, intramuscularly, and rectally. Among the newer phenothiazines are perphenazine (Trilafon), fluphenazine (Prolixin), thiethylperazine (Torecan), and triflupromazine (Vesprin).

Figure 36–2 describes the action and effects of perphenazine (Trilafon), a phenothiazine antiemetic that is frequently used with anticancer therapy.

Pharmacokinetics

Absorption of the oral solid form of perphenazine is erratic; however, the liquid form is more stable with a faster absorption rate. It has a long protein-binding power and its half-life is moderate. Perphenazine is metabolized by the liver and gastrointestinal (GI) mucosa, and most of the drug is excreted in the urine.

Pharmacodynamics

Perphenazine inhibits dopamine in the CTZ, thus decreasing CTZ stimulation of the vomiting center. This drug is also used as an antipsychotic. The onset of action of oral perphenazine varies from 2 to 6 h, and the duration of action from 6 to 12 h. The onset of action of intramuscular and intravenous perphenazine is rapid, and the duration of action is the same as for the oral preparation.

---

* The phenothiazines also act as tranquilizers and are used as antipsychotic drugs. Their use in psychiatric treatment is discussed in Chapter 16.

Drug Interactions

Perphenazine interacts with numerous drugs. When perphenazine is taken with alcohol, antihypertensive agents, and nitrates, hypotension can result. There is an increase in central nervous system (CNS) depression when it is taken with alcohol, narcotics, sedative-hypnotics, and general anesthetics. Anticholinergic effects are increased when perphenazine is combined with antihistamines, anticholinergics such as atropine, and other phenothiazines. Laboratory test results may reveal increased levels of serum liver and cardiac enzymes, cholesterol, and blood glucose.

Side Effects and Adverse Reactions

Phenothiazines have antihistamine and anticholinergic properties. The side effects of phenothiazine antiemetics are moderate sedation, hypotension, extrapyramidal symptoms, which are those of parkinsonism, CNS effects (restlessness, weakness, dystonic reactions, agitation), and mild anticholinergic symptoms (dry mouth, urinary retention, constipation). Because the dose is lower for vomiting than for psychosis, the side effects are not as severe.

Table 36–2 lists the drug data for the phenothiazines along with other prescription antiemetics.

Benzodiazepines

Selected benzodiazepines indirectly control nausea and vomiting that may occur with cancer chemotherapy. Lorazepam is the choice drug. Previously, diazepam (Valium) was the desired benzodiazepine. Lorazepam may be given with an antiemetic such as metoclopramide.

Cannabinoids

Cannabinoids, the active ingredients in marijuana, had been approved for clinical use in 1985 to alleviate nausea and vomiting due to cancer treatment. These agents may be prescribed for clients receiving chemotherapy who do not respond to or are unable to take other antiemetics. They are contraindicated for clients with psychiatric disorders. Cannabinoids can be used as an appetite stimulant for clients with acquired immunodeficiency syndrome (AIDS). The two cannabinoids, dronabinol (Marinol) and nabilone (Cesamet), are described in Table 36–2.

FIGURE 36–2. Antiemetics: Phenothiazine

Phenothiazine Antiemetic	Dosage	**NURSING PROCESS**

Perphenazine
  (Trilafon)
Pregnancy Category: C
	A: PO: 8–16 mg/d in divided doses;
	  max: 24 mg
	IV: Max: 5 mg, diluted or slow IV
	  drip
	A&C > 12 y: IM: 5–10 mg PRN; max:
	  15 mg ambulatory care; max: 30 mg
	  acute care
		Assessment and Planning

Contraindications	Drug-Lab-Food Interactions	

Narrow-angle glaucoma, severe liver
  disease, intestinal obstruction, blood
  dyscrasias, bone marrow depression
Caution: Children < 12 y, seizures, car-
  diovascular disease
	Increase effects of alcohol, sedative-
	  hypnotics, beta-adrenergic blockers
	Decrease levodopa, lithium, other
	  phenothiazines
	Toxicity with epinephrine
	Lab: Increase liver and cardiac enzymes,
	  cholesterol, blood sugar
	Decrease hormones; false pregnancy test	

Pharmacokinetics	Pharmacodynamics	Interventions

Absorption: PO: Erratic absorption;
  liquid: absorption is increased
Distribution: PB: >90%
Metabolism: t½: 8 h
Excretion: In urine and feces
	PO: Onset: 2–6 h
	  Peak: 2–4 h
	  Duration: 6–12 h
	IM: Onset: 10 min
	  Peak: 1–2 h
	  Duration: 6–12 h
	IV: Onset: Rapid
	  Peak: UK
	  Duration:UK	

	Evaluation
Therapeutic Effects/Uses: To treat and prevent vomiting, especially from anticancer drug; to treat alcoholism. *Mode of Action:* Effects of dopamine changed in CNS; inhibits medullary chemoreceptor trigger zone as antiemetic; anticholinergic blocking agent.	

Side Effects	Adverse Reactions

Anorexia, dry mouth and eyes, consti-
pation, blurred vision, extrapyrami-
dal symptoms, rash, photosensitivity,
orthostatic hypotension, impotence,
weight gain, amenorrhea, gyneco-
mastia, transient leukopenia, pain at
IM injection site
	Extrapyramidal syndrome (tardive
	  dyskinesia, akathisia), tachycardia
	Life-threatening: Agranulocytosis, respi-
	  ratory depression, laryngospasm, al-
	  lergic reactions, cardiac arrest

KEY: A: adult; C: child; PO: by mouth; IM: intramuscular; PB: protein-binding; t½: half-life; IV: intravenous; >: greater than; UK: unknown.

Side Effects and Adverse Reactions

Side effects occurring as the result of cannabinoid use include mood changes, euphoria, drowsiness, dizziness, headaches, depersonalization, nightmares, confusion, incoordination, memory lapse, dry mouth, orthostatic hypotension or hypertension, and tachycardia. Less common symptoms are depression, anxiety, and manic psychosis.

Miscellaneous Antiemetics

Benzquinamide hydrochloride, metoclopramide hydrochloride (Reglan), diphenidol (Vontrol), and trimethobenzamide (Tigan) are several miscellaneous antiemetics because they do not act strictly as antihistamines, anticholinergics, or phenothiazides. These drugs suppress the impulses to the CTZ. Diphenidol also prevents vertigo by inhibiting impulses to the vestibular area.

Benzquinamide appears to have antiemetic, antihistaminic, and anticholinergic effects. It inhibits stimulation to the CTZ center and decreases activity in the vomiting center. This drug can also increase cardiac output and elevate blood pressure.

Side Effects and Adverse Reactions

The side effects and adverse reactions of the miscellaneous antiemetics are drowsiness and anticholinergic symptoms (dry mouth, increased heart rate, urine retention, constipation, blurred vision). Benzquinamide should be used cautiously in clients with cardiac problems such as dysrhythmias. Benzquinamide can cause CNS stimulation, including nervousness, excitement, and insomnia. Trimethobenzamide can cause hypotension, diarrhea, and extrapyramidal symptoms (abnormal involuntary movements, postural disturbances, and alteration in muscle tone). Metoclopramide can also cause extrapyramidal effects.

Table 36–2 lists the drug data for the miscellaneous antiemetics along with other prescription antiemetics.

TABLE 36–2 Prescription Antiemetics

Drug	Dosage	Uses & Considerations
Prescription Antihistamines Hydroxyzine (Vistaril, Atarax)	A: PO: IM: 25–100 mg, t.i.d. or q.i.d. PRN	For postoperative nausea and vomiting, vertigo (dizziness). Given preoperatively with narcotics to decrease nausea. Give hydroxyzine deep IM. Drowsiness and dry mouth usually occur. *Pregnancy category:* C; PB: UK; t½: 3 h
Promethazine (Phenergan)	A: PO: 12.5–25 mg, q4–6h, PRN C: PO: 0.25–0.5 mg/kg PRN Also suppository	Drug is a phenothiazine but has antihistamine effects. For postoperative nausea and vomiting, vertigo, motion sickness. *Pregnancy category:* C; PB: 60–90%; t½: UK
Anticholinergic Scopolamine (Transderm Scop)	A: transdermal patch Deliver: 0.5 mg in 3 d	For motion sickness. Has numerous anticholinergic side effects. One patch behind ear at least 4 h before antiemetic effect is required. Patch is effective for 3 d. Alternate ears if using for longer than 3 d. Wash hands after applying patch disc. Wear no more than one disc/patch at a time. *Pregnancy category:* C; PB: <25%; t½: 8 h
Phenothiazines Chlorpromazine (Thorazine)	A: PO: IM: 10–25 mg, q4–6h, PRN	Primarily used for psychosis but may be used to treat nausea and vomiting. Drowsiness, dizziness, EPS, and blurred vision may occur. *Pregnancy category:* C; PB: >90%; t½: biphasic: 2–30 h
Perphenazine (Trilafon)	See Prototype Drug Chart (Fig. 36–2)	For nausea and vomiting, especially due to chemotherapy (anticancer drug). Give before and after each cancer treatment. Side effects may include EPS, dry mouth and eyes, drowsiness, hypotension, dizziness, and syncope. *Pregnancy category:* C; PB: >90%; t½: 8 h
Prochlorperazine maleate (Compazine)	A: PO: IM: 5–10 mg, t.i.d./q.i.d., PRN (give deep IM) SR: 10 mg q12h Rect: 5–25 mg PRN C: PO: Rect: 2.5 mg b.i.d., t.i.d.	Primary use is for severe nausea and vomiting. Secondary use is to reduce anxiety and tension and for psychosis. Drowsiness, dizziness, EPS, dry mouth may occur. *Pregnancy category:* C; PB: >90%; t½: 23 h

TABLE 36–2 Prescription Antiemetics (*Continued*)

Drug	Dosage	Uses & Considerations
Thiethylperazine (Torecan, Norzine)	A: PO/IM/PR: 10 mg q.d./t.i.d.	To control nausea and vomiting by acting on CTZ and vomiting center. Same side effects as prochlorperazine. *Pregnancy category:* UK (X); PB: UK; t½: UK
Triflupromazine (Vesprin)	A: PO: 20–30 mg/d A: IM: 5–15 mg q4–6 h C: PO/IM: 0.2 mg/kg/d; *max:* 10 mg/d	For severe nausea and vomiting. Secondary use is for psychosis without depression. Similar to prochlorperazine. *Pregnancy category:* C; PB: >90%; t½: UK
Benzodiazepine Lorazepam (Ativan)	A: PO: 2–6 mg/d in 2–3 divided doses; *max:* 10 mg/d	For prevention of nausea and vomiting due to cancer chemotherapy. It is usually administered with an antiemetic such as metoclopramide. *Pregnancy category:* D; PB: 85%; t½: 10–20 h
Cannabinoids Dronabinol (Marinol) CSS II	Chemotherapy-induced nausea: A: PO: 5 mg/m² 1–3 h before chemotherapy; then q2–4h after; *max:* 15 mg/m²/dose	For nausea and vomiting due to cancer chemotherapy. Taken before and for 24 h after chemotherapy. It can be an appetite stimulant for clients with AIDS. Common side effects include drowsiness, dizziness, dry mouth, impaired thinking, and euphoria. *Pregnancy category:* B; PB: 98%; t½: 20–24 h
Nabilone (Cesamet) CSS II	Chemotherapy-induced nausea: A: PO: 1–2 mg b.i.d. 1–3 h before chemotherapy, continue for 48 h after	For chemotherapy-induced nausea and vomiting, especially for cisplatin chemotherapy. May be used when other antiemetics are ineffective. It is a synthetic derivative of marijuana. Alcohol and CNS depressants should be avoided. *Pregnancy category:* B; PB: UK; t½: 2 h
Miscellaneous Benzoquinamide HCl (Emete-con)	A&C > 12 y: IM: 50 mg q3–4h PRN IV: 25 mg or 0.2–0.4 mg/kg diluted in D₅W as one dose; give remainder of dose as IM	Treatment of nausea and vomiting due to anesthesia and postoperative surgery. It depresses the CTZ. It has anticholinergic, antihistamine, and sedative properties. Can cause drowsiness. *Pregnancy category:* C; PB: 60%; t½: 30–45 min
Diphenidol HCl (Vontrol)	Nausea, vomiting, vertigo: A: PO: 25–50 mg q4h C > 6 y: PO: 0.9 mg/kg; *max:* 5.5 mg/kg/d	For nausea, vomiting, and vertigo due to Ménière's disease and surgery of the middle ear. *Pregnancy category:* C; PB: UK; t½: 4 h
Droperidol (Inapsine)	A: IM/IV: 2.5–10 mg, 0.5–1h prior to surgery C 2–12 y: IM/IV: 0.088–0.165 mg/kg, 0.5–1h prior to surgery C < 2 y: Not recommended	Prevention of nausea and vomiting during surgical and diagnostic procedures. May cause hypotension, tachycardia, and EPS. *Pregnancy Category:* C; PB: UK: t½: 2.5 h
Granisectron (Kytril)	A: PO: 1 mg, b.i.d. (1 h before and 12 h after chemotherapy) A: IV: 10 μg/kg/30 min before chemotherapy	Prevention of nausea and vomiting due to cancer chemotherapy. Acts on the CTZ and vomiting centers. Headache may occur. *Pregnancy Category:* B; PB: 65%; t½: 4–10 h
Metoclopramide monohydrochloride monohydrate (Reglan)	A: PO: 10 mg a.c. and h.s. IV: 1–2 mg/kg 30 min before chemotherapy; then repeat q2h for 2 doses; then q3h for 3 doses; infuse diluted solution over not less than 15 min	For nausea and vomiting related to cancer chemtherapy treatment. It increases gastric and intestinal emptying. Avoid alcohol and CNS depressants. EPS may occur. *Pregnancy Category:* B; PB: 30%; t½: 4–7 h
Ondansetron HCl (Zofran)	A:PO: 8 mg, b.i.d. (1st dose 30 min before and 8 h after chemotherapy) or A: IV: 0.15 mg/kg 30 min before chemotherapy; then 4 and 8 h after (total, 3 doses)	For nausea and vomiting related to cancer chemotherapy, especially cisplatin. *Pregnancy Category:* B; PB: 70%–75%; t½: 4 h
Trimethobenzamide HCl (Tigan, Arrestin, Ticon)	A: PO: 250 mg t.i.d./q.i.d. IM/PR: 200 mg t.i.d./q.i.d. C 15–40 kg: PO/PR: 15–20 mg/kg/d divided in 3–4 doses or 100–200 mg, t.i.d., q.i.d.	For postoperative nausea and vomiting, motion sickness, and vertigo. Avoid if sensitive to benzocaine or similar local anesthetics, and with CNS depressants. *Pregnancy category:* C; PB: UK; t½: UK

KEY: A: adult; C: child; PO: by mouth; IM: intramuscular; IV: intravenous; PRN: whenever necessary; Rect: rectally; a.c.: before meals; h.s.: hour of sleep; EPS: extrapyramidal symptoms; CTZ: chemoreceptor trigger zone; UK: unknown; PB: protein-binding; t½: half-life; >: greater than; <: less than; CNS: central nervous system; CSS: Controlled Substance Schedule.

NURSING PROCESS: ANTIEMETICS

ASSESSMENT

- Obtain a history of the onset, frequency, and amount of vomiting and contents of the vomitus. If appropriate, elicit from the client possible causative factors such as food (seafood, mayonnaise).
- Obtain a history of present health problems. Clients with glaucoma should avoid many of the antiemetics.
- Assess vital signs (VS) for abnormalities and for future comparison.
- Assess urinalysis before and during therapy.

POTENTIAL NURSING DIAGNOSES

- Altered nutrition: less than body requirements
- High risk for fluid volume deficit related to vomiting

PLANNING

- Client will adhere to nonpharmacologic methods and/or drug regimen for alleviating vomiting.
- The underlying cause of vomiting is determined and corrected.

NURSING INTERVENTIONS

- Monitor VS. If vomiting is severe, dehydration may occur, and shock-like symptoms may be present.
- Monitor bowel sounds for hypoactivity or hyperactivity.
- Provide mouth care after vomiting. Encourage the client to maintain oral hygiene.

CLIENT TEACHING

General

- Instruct the client to store drug in tight, light-resistant container if required.
- Instruct the client to avoid over-the-counter (OTC) preparations.
- Instruct the client not to consume alcohol while taking antiemetics. Alcohol can intensify the sedative effect.
- Advise pregnant women to avoid antiemetics during the first trimester due to possible teratogenic effect on the fetus. Encourage them to seek medical advice about OTC or prescription antiemetics.

Side Effects

- Advise the client to report sore throat, fever, and mouth sores; notify health care provider and have blood drawn for a CBC.
- Instruct the client to avoid driving a motor vehicle or engaging in dangerous activities because drowsiness is common with antiemetics. If drowsiness becomes a problem, a decrease in dosage may be indicated.
- Advise the client with a hepatic disorder to seek medical advice before taking phenothiazines. Instruct the client to report dizziness.
- Suggest to the client nonpharmacologic methods of alleviating nausea and vomiting such as flattened carbonated beverages, weak tea, crackers, and dry toast.

EVALUATION

- Evaluate the effectiveness of the nonpharmacologic methods or antiemetic by noting the absence of vomiting. Identify any side effects that may result from drug.

EMETICS

When an individual has consumed certain toxic substances, induced vomiting (emesis) may be indicated to expel the substance before absorption occurs. There are many ways to induce vomiting without using drugs, such as putting the finger in the back part of the throat.

Vomiting should not be induced if caustic substances have been ingested, such as ammonia, chlorine bleach, lye, toilet cleaners, or battery acid. Regurgitating these substances can cause additional injury to the esophagus. To prevent aspiration, vomiting should also be avoided if petroleum distillates are ingested; these include gasoline, kerosene, paint thinners, and lighter fluid. Activated charcoal is given when emesis is contraindicated.

IPECAC

Ipecac is an OTC drug. Most health care providers instruct parents to keep ipecac in the household; however, it should be kept out of reach of children. When the client is purchasing ipecac, instruct the client to get ipecac syrup and *not* ipecac fluid extract, which is more potent. Ipecac syrup induces vomiting by stimulating the CTZ in the medulla and acting directly on the gastric mucosa. Ipecac should be taken with a glass of water or other fluid (do not give milk or carbonated beverages.) If vomiting does not occur in 20 to 30 minutes, the dose could be repeated. Ipecac can be toxic if it does not induce vomiting and is absorbed; treat with activated charcoal and/or gastric lavage and give cardiovascular support if necessary. Figure 36–3 gives the drug data for ipecac.

Pharmacokinetics

Following a dose of ipecac, eight or more ounces of tepid water or juice should be given. The absorption of ipecac is minimal. The protein-binding is unknown, and the half-life is short.

Pharmacodynamics

Ipecac acts on the chemotherapeutic trigger zone (CTZ) in the medulla and on the gastric mucosa to induce vomiting. The onset of action for ipecac is

FIGURE 36–3. Emetics

Emetic	Dosage	**NURSING PROCESS** Assessment and Planning
Ipecac Syrup *Pregnancy Category:* C	A: PO: 15–30 mL, followed by 200–300 mL tepid water C: >1–12 y: PO: 15 mL, followed by 200–300 mL tepid water C: <1 y: PO: 5–10 mL, followed by 100–200 mL tepid water Repeat initial dose if vomiting does not occur within 30 min only if the child is older than 1 yr	
Contraindications	**Drug-Lab-Food Interactions**	
Hypersensitivity, depressed gag reflex, unconsciousness or semiconsciousness, poisoning with caustic or petroleum products, convulsions	*Decrease* effect with activated charcoal, carbonated beverages, or milk	
Pharmacokinetics	**Pharmacodynamics**	Interventions
Absorption: Minimal *Distribution:* PB: UK *Metabolism:* t½: 2 h *Excretion:* GI	PO: Onset: 15–30 min Peak: UK Duration: 20–25 min	

	Evaluation
Therapeutic Effects/Uses: To induce vomiting after poisoning *Mode of Action:* Acts on chemoreceptor trigger zone (induces vomiting) and irritates gastric mucosa.	

Side Effects	Adverse Reactions
Diarrhea, sedation, lethargy, protracted vomiting	*Life-threatening:* Cardiotoxicity if ipecac is not vomited (hypotension, tachycardia, chest pain)

KEY: A: adult; C: child; >: greater than; <: less than; PO: by mouth; UK: unknown; PB: protein-binding; t½: half-life.

TABLE 36–3 Emetics and Adsorbent

Generic (Brand)	Route and Dosage	Uses & Considerations
Emetics Apomorphine CSS II	A: SC: 4–10 mg C: SC: 0.07–0.1 mg / kg; 100–200 mL of water or evaporated milk before injection; do not repeat	To induce vomiting. Dose should *not* be repeated if vomiting does not occur. Schedule II drug. Fluids should be given before injection. Large doses could cause CNS depression (bradycardia and decreased respirations). *Pregnancy category:* C; PB: UK; t½: UK
Ipecac syrup (OTC preparation)	See Prototype Drug Chart (Fig. 36–3)	To induce vomiting; contraindicated when caustic or petroleum substances have been ingested. Give with water (at least 200 mL). If vomiting does not occur, give activated charcoal to absorb ipecac and substance or gastric lavage. *Pregnancy category:* C; PB: UK; t½: UK
Adsorbent Charcoal (Charcoaid, CharcoCaps)	*For Poisoning:* *Charcoaid:* A: PO: 30–100 g dose in 6–8 oz of water *For Flatus:* *CharcoCaps:* A: PO: 520 mg, after meals; repeat PRN; *max:* 4 g/d	Promotes absorption of poison / toxic substances. Promotes absorption of intestinal gas. Both drugs are not systemically absorbed. *Pregnancy category:* C; PB: NA; t½: NA

KEY: *A: adult; C: child; PO: by mouth; SC: subcutaneous; >: greater than; UK: unknown; NA: not applicable; PB: protein-binding; t½: half-life; max: maximum; PRN: as necessary; OTC: over-the-counter; CNS: central nervous system; CSS: Controlled Substance Schedule.*

15 to 30 minutes and the duration of action is 20 to 25 minutes.

APOMORPHINE

Apomorphine is a morphine-derived emetic that can be administered subcutaneously or intramuscularly. Fluids are given prior to the injection, and vomiting should occur within 15 min. The drug is classified as a narcotic and can depress the respiratory center and decrease blood pressure; therefore, it is not used for narcosis due to CNS depressants, such as opiates, barbiturates, and alcohol. Side effects of apomorphine include restlessness, tremors, euphoria, tachycardia, hypotension, nausea, increased salivation, perspiration, and lacrimation. Table 36–3 presents the drug data for ipecac syrup and apomorphine.

NURSING PROCESS: EMETIC: Ipecac Syrup

ASSESSMENT

- Determine the toxic substance ingested. Do *not* induce vomiting if caustics or petroleum products have been ingested.
- Determine the time elapsed since the ingestion; lavage may be indicated.
- Check the client's vital signs (VS). Report abnormal findings.

POTENTIAL NURSING DIAGNOSES

- Potential risk for absorption of toxic substance
- Potential risk for infection

PLANNING

- Toxic substance will be expelled before absorption. There will be no bodily harm due to the toxic substance.

- Client will be closely monitored for adverse effects of the toxic substance for 24 to 48 h depending on the substance.

NURSING INTERVENTIONS

- Call the poison control center to report the toxic ingestion and for instructions.
- Monitor VS. Report changes.
- Offer sufficient fluids with ipecac syrup; warm clear liquids are best: *no* milk or milk products. Have client in high Fowler's position. Fluids dilute the toxic substance and are vehicles for expelling the substance; avoid carbonated beverages as they cause abdominal distention. If emetic is unsuccessful, gastric lavage may be performed or activated charcoal given to adsorb the toxic substances.
- Do not offer ipecac syrup or fluids to a semiconscious or unconscious person because of the

danger of aspiration. Gastric lavage is usually performed in such cases.

- Do not induce vomiting if the toxic substance is a caustic or a petroleum distillate.
- Prepare for forceful vomiting; have large basin ready, and move clothing to protected area.

General

- Instruct the parent or other family member to have ipecac syrup on hand. Explain that ipecac syrup is an OTC drug.
- Explain to the parent that ipecac should be given with sufficient fluids. Advise that ipecac syrup is *not* given if the toxic substance is a caustic or petroleum product.

- Advise the client or parents to *never* remove toxic substances from original labeled containers. Instruct parents on the use of child safety caps for future prevention.
- Advise the parent to keep readily available the telephone numbers of the poison control center and all emergency services.

EVALUATION

- Evaluate the effectiveness of ipecac syrup for inducing vomiting.
- Continue monitoring VS.
- Continue monitoring for signs and symptoms related to effect of ingested substance.

ANTIDIARRHEAL DRUGS

Diarrhea (frequent liquid stool) is a symptom of an intestinal disorder. Causes include (1) foods (spicy, spoiled), (2) fecal impaction, (3) bacterial or viral toxins, (4) drug reaction, (5) laxative abuse, (6) malabsorption syndrome due to lack of digestive enzymes, (7) stress and anxiety, (8) bowel tumor, and (9) inflammatory bowel disease, such as ulcerative colitis or Crohn's disease. Diarrhea can be mild to severe.

Because intestinal fluids are rich in water, sodium, potassium, and bicarbonate, diarrhea can cause minor or severe dehydration and electrolyte imbalances. The loss of bicarbonate places the client at risk for developing metabolic acidosis. Clients with diarrhea should avoid foods rich in fat and milk products. Diarrhea can develop very quickly and can be life-threatening to the young and elderly, who may not be able to compensate for the fluid and electrolyte losses.

NONPHARMACOLOGIC MEASURES

The cause of diarrhea should be identified. Nonpharmacologic treatment for diarrhea is recommended until the underlying cause can be determined. This includes use of clear liquids and oral solutions (Gatorade, Pedialyte or Ricolyte [children]) and intravenous electrolyte solutions. Antidiarrheal drugs are frequently used in combination with nonpharmacologic treatment.

ANTIDIARRHEALS

There are various antidiarrheals for treating diarrhea and decreasing hypermotility (increased peristalsis). Usually there is an underlying cause of the diarrhea that needs to be corrected as well. The antidiarrheals are classified as (1) **opiates,** (2) opiate-related agents, (3) **adsorbents,** and (4) antidiarrheal combinations.

Opiates

Opiates decrease intestinal motility, thus decreasing peristalsis. Constipation is a common side effect of opium preparations. Examples are tincture of opium, paregoric (camphorated opium tincture), and codeine. Opiates are frequently combined with other antidiarrheal agents. Opium antidiarrheals can cause CNS depression when taken with alcohol, sedatives, or tranquilizers. Duration of action of opiates is approximately 2 h.

Opiate-Related Agents

Diphenoxylate (Lomotil) and loperamide (Imodium) are synthetic drugs that are chemically related to the narcotic meperidine (Demerol). They decrease intestinal motility (peristalsis) and are taken for "traveler's diarrhea." Loperamide causes less CNS depression than diphenoxylate and can be purchased as an OTC drug. These drugs can cause nausea, vomiting, drowsiness, and abdominal distention. Tachycardia, paralytic ileus, urinary retention, decreased secretions, and physical dependence can occur with prolonged use.

Anticholinergic drugs decrease cramping, intestinal motility, and hypersecretion. They can be used in combination with opiates. Diphenoxylate product is approximately 50% atropine. (Atropine is added to discourage abuse; the amount of atropine is subtherapeutic.) The action and effects of diphenoxylate with atropine are shown in Figure 36–4.

FIGURE 36–4. Antidiarrheals

Diphenoxylate with Atropine	Dosage	**NURSING PROCESS** Assessment and Planning

Diphenoxylate with atropine
(Lomotil)
Pregnancy Category: C
CSS V
	A: PO: 2.5–5 mg b.i.d./q.i.d.
	C: >2 y: PO: 0.3–0.4 mg/kg daily in 4
	   divided doses or 2 mg 3–5 ×/d
	   (use liquid form only)	

Contraindications	**Drug-Lab-Food Interactions**	
Severe hepatic or renal disease, glaucoma, severe electrolyte imbalance, child <2 y	*Increase* CNS depression with alcohol, antihistamines, narcotics, sedative-hypnotics. MAOIs may *enhance* hypertensive crisis *Lab: Increase* serum liver enzymes, amylase	
Pharmacokinetics	**Pharmacodynamics**	Interventions

Absorption: PO: Well absorbed
Distribution: PB: UK
Metabolism: t½: 2.5 h
Excretion: In feces and urine
	PO: Onset: 45–60 min
	   Peak: 2 h
	   Duration: 3–4 h	

	Evaluation
Therapeutic Effects/Uses: To treat diarrhea by slowing intestinal motility. *Mode of Action:* Inhibition of gastric motility.	

Side Effects	Adverse Reactions
Drowsiness, dizziness, constipation, dry mouth, weakness, flushing, rash, blurred vision, mydriasis, urine retention	Angioneurotic edema *Life-threatening:* Paralytic ileus, toxic megacolon, severe allergic reaction

KEY: A: adult; C: child; PO: by mouth; >: greater than; <: less than; UK: unknown; PB: protein-binding; t½: half-life; MAOIs: monoamine oxidase inhibitors.

Pharmacokinetics

Diphenoxylate with atropine is well-absorbed from the GI tract. The diphenoxylate is metabolized by the liver mainly as metabolites. There are two half-lives: 2½ h for diphenoxylate and 3 to 20 h for the diphenoxylate metabolites. The drug is excreted in the feces and urine.

Pharmacodynamics

Diphenoxylate with atropine is an opium agonist with anticholinergic properties (atropine) that decreases GI motility (peristalsis). It has a moderate onset of action time of 45 to 60 min, and the duration of action is 3 to 4 h. Many side effects are due to the anticholinergic atropine. Clients with severe glaucoma should take another antidiarrheal that does not have an anticholinergic effect. If this drug is taken with alcohol, narcotics, or sedative-hypnotics, CNS depression can occur.

Adsorbents

Adsorbent antidiarrheals include kaolin and pectin. These agents are combined in Kaopectate, a mild or moderate antidiarrheal that can be purchased OTC and used in combination with other antidiarrheals. An example is Parepectolin which contains paregoric (an opiate) and Kaopectate (an adsorbent). Bismuth salts (Pepto-Bismol) is considered an adsorbent because it absorbs bacterial toxins. Bismuth salts can also be used for gastric discomfort. It is an

TABLE 36–4 Antidiarrheals: Opiates, Opiate Related, Adsorbents, and Miscellaneous

Generic (Brand)	Route and Dosage	Uses & Considerations
Opiates		
Deodorized opium tincture CSS II	A: PO: 0.6 mL or 10 gtt q.i.d. mixed with water; max: 6 mL/d C: PO: 0.005–0.01 mL/kg/dose q3–4 h; max: 6 doses/d	For acute, nonspecific diarrhea. To treat withdrawal symptoms in neonates of mothers who are addicted to opiates. Not to be used for diarrhea caused by poison. Avoid taking alcohol and CNS depressants. *Pregnancy category:* B (D at term); PB: UK; t½: 2–3 h
Camphorated opium tincture (paregoric) CSS III	Camphorated: 5–10 mL b.i.d./q.i.d. C: PO: 0.25–0.5 mL/kg daily–q.i.d.	To decrease incidence of diarrhea. Decreases GI peristalsis. *Pregnancy category:* B (D at term); PB: UK; t½: 2–3 h
Opiate Related		
Diphenoxylate with atropine (Lomotil) CSS V	A: PO: 2.5–5 mg b.i.d.–q.i.d. C > 2 y: 0.3–0.4 mg/kg daily in 4 divided doses or 2 mg 3–5 × d	For acute, nonspecific diarrhea. Inhibits GI motility. Diphenoxylate is a synthetic narcotic; atropine prevents possible narcotic abuse and decreases GI motility. Contraindicated in glaucoma, ulcerative colitis. *Pregnancy category:* C; PB: UK; t½: 2.5 h
Loperamide HCl (Imodium)	A: PO: Initially: 4 mg; then 2 mg after each loose stool; *max:* 16 mg/d C 2–5 y: PO: 1 mg, t.i.d.; 6–8 y: 2 mg, b.i.d.; 9–12 y: 2 mg, t.i.d.	For diarrhea. Newest OTC drug. Does not affect the CNS. Less than 1% reaches systemic circulation. *Pregnancy category:* B; PB: 98%; t½: 7–12 h
Adsorbents		
Bismuth salts (Pepto-Bismol)	*Prevention of travelers' diarrhea:* A: PO: 2 tab q.i.d. a.c. and h.s. *Treatment:* A: PO: 2 tab or 30 mL q30–60 min PRN	For diarrhea, gastric distress, OTC liquid and tablet form. *Pregnancy category:* UK; PB: UK; t½: UK
Kaolin-pectin (Kapectolin, Kaopectate)	A: 60–120 mL after each loose stool C 6–12 y: 30–60 mL after each loose stool	For diarrhea. Administered after each loose stool. OTC drug. *Pregnancy category:* B; PB: 97%; t½: 7–14 h
Miscellaneous		
Colistin sulfate (Coly-Mycin S)	Infants & children: PO: 5–15 mg/kg/d in 3 divided doses q8h	For diarrhea in infants and children. Has a bactericidal effect. *Pregnancy category:* C; PB: UK; t½: 3–5 h
Furazolidone (Furoxone)	A: PO: 100 mg q.i.d.; *max:* 400 mg/d C > 1 mo: PO: 5–8 mg/kg/d in 4 divided doses	Management of diarrhea and enteritis due to bacteria or protozoa. Common side effects include nausea and vomiting. *Pregnancy category:* C; PB: UK; t½: UK
Lactobacillus acidophilus and Lactobacillus bulgaricus (one or both) (Bacid [plus carboxymethylcellulose sodium], Lactinix, More-Dophilus)	A&C > 3 y: PO: 2 cap 2–9×/d Granules: 1 pkg with cereal, food, water t.i.d./q.i.d. Powder: 1 tsp daily with fluid C < 3 y: Not recommended	Management of diarrhea due to bacteria. *Pregnancy category:* UK; PB: UK; t½: UK
Octreotide acetate (Sandostatin)	*Diarrhea related to carcinoid tumors:* A: SC: Initially: 0.05 mg/d in divided doses for 2 wk; then increase according to response; *max:* 0.75 mg/d	For severe diarrhea due to metastatic carcinoid tumors. It suppresses secretion of serotonin, gastrin, and pancreatic peptides. *Pregnancy category:* B; PB: 65%; t½: 1.5 h
Combinations		
Difenoxin and atropine (Motofen) CSS IV	A: PO: Initially: 2 mg; then 1 mg after each loose stool; *max:* 8 mg/d for 2 d C < 2 y: Not recommended	For acute nonspecific and chronic diarrhea. Combination of a synthetic narcotic and atropine. Avoid use in narrow-angle glaucoma. Dry mouth, flushing, and tachycardia may occur. *Pregnancy category:* C; PB: UK; t½: 12–24 h
Diphenoxylate with atropine (Lomotil)	See Prototype Drug Chart (Fig. 36–4)	Similar to difenoxin and atropine
Parepectolin CSS V	A&C > 12 y: 15–30 mL after each loose stool; *max:* 120 mL/d C 6–12 y: 5–10 mL after each loose stool; *max:* 40 mL/d	Contains paregoric (an opiate) and kaopectate. OTC drug; however, must be signed at pharmacy for drug because it contains opium. *Pregnancy category:* D; PB: UK; t½: UK

KEY: A: adult; C: child; PO: by mouth; OTC: over-the-counter; <: less than; >: greater than; PB: protein-binding; t½: half-life; CNS: central nervous system; UK: unknown; CSS: Controlled Substance Schedule.

OTC drug that is used for "traveler's diarrhea." Table 36–4 lists the drug data for the commonly used antidiarrheals.

Miscellaneous Antidiarrheals

There are various miscellaneous antidiarrheals that are prescribed to control diarrhea. These drugs are colistin sulfate, furazolidone, loperamide (Imodium), lactobacillus, and octreotide acetate. Combination drugs with brand names are used to alleviate diarrhea and these include Lomotil (diphenoxylate HCl with atropine sulfate) and Parepectolin (paregoric, kaolin, pectin, alcohol). Most of these combination drugs contain a synthetic narcotic ingredient. Table 36–4 includes these drugs.

NURSING PROCESS: ANTIDIARRHEALS

ASSESSMENT

- Obtain a history of any viral or bacterial infection, drugs taken, and foods ingested that could be contributing factors to diarrhea. Many of the antidiarrheals are contraindicated if the client has liver disease, narcotic dependence, ulcerative colitis, or glaucoma.
- Check vital signs (VS) to provide baseline for future comparison and to determine body fluid and electrolyte losses.
- Assess frequency and consistency of bowel movements.
- Assess bowel sounds. Hyperactive sounds can indicate increased intestinal motility.
- Report if the client has a narcotic drug history. If opiate or opiate-related antidiarrheals are given, drug misuse or abuse may occur.

POTENTIAL NURSING DIAGNOSES

- Diarrhea
- Altered nutrition
- Alteration in fluid volume

PLANNING

- Client's bowel movements will no longer be diarrhea.
- Client's body fluids will be restored.

NURSING INTERVENTIONS

- Monitor VS. Report tachycardia or a systolic blood pressure decrease of 10 to 15 mmHg. Monitor respirations. Opiates and opiate-related drugs can cause CNS depression.
- Monitor the frequency of bowel movements and bowel sounds. Notify the health care provider if intestinal hypoactivity occurs when taking drug.
- Check for signs and symptoms of dehydration due to persistent diarrhea. Fluid replacement may be necessary. With prolonged diarrhea, check serum electrolytes.
- Administer antidiarrheals cautiously to clients with glaucoma, liver disorders, or ulcerative colitis or who are pregnant.
- Recognize that drug may need to be withheld if diarrhea continues for more than 48 h or acute abdominal pain develops.

CLIENT TEACHING

General
- Instruct the client not to take sedatives, tranquilizers, or other narcotics with drug. CNS depression may occur.
- Advise the client to avoid over-the-counter (OTC) preparations; they may contain alcohol.
- Instruct the client to take the drug only as prescribed. Drug may be habit forming; do not exceed recommended dose.
- Encourage the client to drink clear liquids. Advise the client not to ingest fried foods or milk products until after the diarrhea has stopped.
- Advise the client that constipation can result from the overuse of this drug.

EVALUATION

- Evaluate the effectiveness of the drug; diarrhea has stopped.
- Monitor long-term use of opiates and opiate-related drugs for possible abuse and physical dependence.
- Continue to monitor VS. Report abnormal changes.

CONSTIPATION

Constipation (accumulation of hard fecal material in the large intestine) is a relatively common complaint and a major problem of the elderly. Insufficient water intake and poor dietary habits are contributing factors. Other causes include (1) fecal impaction, (2) bowel obstruction, (3) chronic laxative use, (4) neurologic disorders (paraplegia), (5) ignoring the urge to have a bowel movement, (6) lack of exercise, and (7) selected drugs, such as anticholinergics, narcotics, and certain antacids.

NONPHARMACOLOGIC MEASURES

Nonpharmacologic management includes a diet that contains bulk (fiber) and water, exercise, and routine bowel habits. A "normal" number of bowel movements is one to three a day to three a week. What is normal varies from person to person; the nurse should determine what "normal" bowel habits are for the individual. At times, a laxative may be needed, but the client should also use nonpharmacologic measures to prevent constipation.

LAXATIVES

Laxatives and **cathartics** are used to eliminate fecal matter. Laxatives promote a soft stool and cathartics result in a soft to watery stool with some cramping. Frequently, the dosage determines whether the drug acts as a laxative or cathartic.* A **purgative** is a "harsh" cathartic, causing a watery stool with abdominal cramping. There are four types of laxatives: (1) osmotics (saline), (2) contact (previously called stimulants or irritants), (3) bulk-forming, and (4) emollients.

Laxatives should be avoided if there is any question that the client has an intestinal obstruction. Most laxatives stimulate peristalsis. Laxative abuse due to chronic use of laxatives is a common problem, especially with the elderly. Laxative dependence can be a problem, so client teaching is an important nursing responsibility.

Osmotic Laxatives

Osmotics (hyperosmolar laxatives) include salts or saline products, lactulose, and glycerin. The saline products are composed of sodium or magnesium, and a small amount is systemically absorbed. Serum electrolytes should be monitored to avoid electrolyte imbalance. The hyperosmolar salts pull water into the colon and increase water in the feces to increase bulk, which stimulates peristalsis. Saline cathartics cause a semiformed to watery stool. Good renal function is needed to excrete any excess salts. Saline cathartics are contraindicated for clients with congestive heart failure.

Lactulose, another saline laxative that is not absorbed, draws water into the intestines and promotes water and electrolyte retention. It decreases the serum ammonia level and is useful in liver diseases, such as cirrhosis. Glycerin acts like lactulose, increasing water in the feces in the large intestine. The bulk that results from the increased water in the feces stimulates peristalsis and defecation.

Side Effects and Adverse Reactions

Adequate renal function is needed to excrete excess magnesium. Clients who have renal insufficiency should avoid magnesium salts. Hypermagnesemia can result from continuous use of magnesium salts, causing symptoms such as drowsiness, weakness, paralysis, complete heart block, hypotension, flushing, and respiratory depression.

The side effects of lactulose from excess use include flatulence, diarrhea, abdominal cramps, nausea, and vomiting. Clients who have diabetes mellitus should avoid lactulose because it contains glucose and fructose.

Contact Laxatives

Contact (stimulant, or irritant) laxatives increase peristalsis by irritating sensory nerve endings in the intestinal mucosa. Types include those containing phenolphthalein (Ex-Lax, Feen-A-Mint, Correctol), bisacodyl (Dulcolax), cascara sagrada, senna (Senokot), and castor oil (purgative). Bisacodyl and several other of these drugs are used to empty the bowel prior to diagnostic tests (barium enema) and surgery. Figure 36–5 gives the pharmacologic data for the contact/stimulant laxative bisacodyl.

Pharmacokinetics

The contact laxative bisacodyl is minimally absorbed from the GI tract. It is excreted in the feces, but due to the small amount of bisacodyl absorption, a portion is excreted in the urine.

Pharmacodynamics

Bisacodyl promotes defecation. Bisacodyl irritates the colon, causing defecation, and psyllium com-

---

* These terms are often used interchangeably: laxative is used and refers to both terms in this chapter.

FIGURE 36–5. Laxatives: Contact

Contact Laxative	Dosage	NURSING PROCESS
Bisacodyl (Dulcolax); 🍁 Apo-Bisacodyl, Bisco-Lax *Pregnancy Category:* C	A: PO: 10–15 mg in a.m./p.m.; max: 30 mg C: >3 y: PO: 5–10 mg; 0.3 mg/kg/d A&C: >2 y: Rectal supp: 5–10 mg/d C <2 y & infants: 5 mg	Assessment and Planning
Contraindications	**Drug-Lab-Food Interactions**	
Hypersensitivity, fecal impaction, intestinal/biliary obstruction, appendicitis, abdominal pain, nausea, vomiting, rectal fissures	*Decrease* effect with antacids, histamine$_2$ blockers, milk	
Pharmacokinetics	**Pharmacodynamics**	Interventions

Absorption: Minimal absorption (5–15%)
Distribution: PB: UK
Metabolism: t½: UK
Excretion: In bile and urine
	PO: Onset: 10–15 min; act: 6–12 h
	    Peak: UK
	    Duration: UK
	Rect: Onset: 15–60 min
	    Peak: UK
	    Duration: UK	

Therapeutic Effects/Uses: Short-term treatment for constipation: bowel preparation for diagnostic tests.

Mode of Action: Increases peristalsis by direct effect on smooth muscle of intestine.

Evaluation

Side Effects	Adverse Reactions
Anorexia, nausea, vomiting, cramps, diarrhea	Dependence, hypokalemia *Life-threatening:* Tetany

KEY: A: adult; C: child; PO: by mouth; >: greater than; <: less than; UK: unknown; PB: protein-binding; t½: half-life; 🍁: Canadian drug names.

pounds increase fecal bulk and peristalsis. The onset of action of oral bisacodyl occurs within 6 to 12 h and within 15 to 60 min with the suppository (rectal administration).

Side Effects and Adverse Reactions

CONTACT LAXATIVES

Side effects include nausea, abdominal cramps, weakness, and reddish-brown urine due to excretion of phenolphthalein, senna, or cascara.

With excessive and chronic use of bisacodyl, fluid and electrolyte (especially potassium and calcium) imbalances are likely to occur. Systemic effects occur infrequently because of minimal absorption of bisacodyl. Mild cramping and diarrhea are side effects of bisacodyl.

Castor oil should not be used in early pregnancy because it stimulates uterine contraction. Spontaneous abortion may result. Prolonged use of senna can damage nerves, which may result in loss of intestinal muscular tone. Table 36–5 lists the osmotic and contact laxatives.

TABLE 36–5 Laxatives: Osmotic and Contact

Generic (Brand)	Route and Dosage	Uses & Considerations
Osmotics: Saline		
Glycerin	A: Supp: 3 g C < 6 y: Supp: 1–1.5 g	To relieve constipation. Use with caution for clients with cardiac, renal, or liver disease and for the elderly or for those who are dehydrated. *Pregnancy category:* C; PB: UK; t½: 30–45 min
Lactulose (Cephulac, Cholac, Constilec, Enulose)	*Chronic Constipation:* A: PO: 30–60 mL/d PRN C: PO: 7.5 mL/d after breakfast	For constipation. Also used in liver disease for ammonia elimination. May be used for constipation after barium studies. Poorly absorbed. *Pregnancy category:* C; PB: UK; t½: UK
Magnesium citrate (Citroma, Evac-Q-Mag)	A: PO: 120–240 mL C: PO: 4 mL/kg/dose or ½ adult dose	For constipation or to complete bowel elimination prior to diagnostic procedures and surgery. *Pregnancy category:* UK; PB: UK; t½: UK
Magnesium hydroxide (milk of magnesia)	A: PO: 20–60 mL/d C: PO: 0.5 mL/kg/dose	For constipation. Take with a glass of water in morning or evening. With frequent use, good renal function is necessary. *Pregnancy category:* B; PB: UK; t½: UK
Magnesium oxide (Maox, Mag-Ox)	A: PO: 2–4 g h.s. with 8 oz water Do not use in client with renal failure	Similar to magnesium hydroxide. *Pregnancy category:* B; PB: UK; t½: UK
Magnesium SO₄ (Epsom salts)	A: PO: 10–15 g in 8 oz water C: PO: 5–10 mg in water	For complete bowel elimination before surgery. Hypermagnesemia can occur if used frequently. Also used in pregnancy to control seizures with severe toxemia of pregnancy (given IV). Caution for use in renal dysfunction. *Pregnancy category:* B; PB: UK; t½: UK
Sodium biphosphate (Fleet Phospho-Soda)	A: PO: 15–30 mL mixed in water	For constipation or bowel preparation. Contraindicated with CHF. *Pregnancy category:* UK; PB: UK; t½: UK
Sodium phosphate with sodium biphosphate (Fleet Enema)	*Enema:* A: 60–120 mL C: 30–60 mL	For constipation or bowel preparation for diagnostic procedures. Frequent Fleet Enema may cause fluid imbalance in the elderly. *Pregnancy category:* UK; PB: UK; t½: UK
Contact		
Bisacodyl (Dulcolax)	See Prototype Drug Chart (Fig. 36–5)	For constipation or bowel preparation for diagnostic procedures. Onset: 6–8 h for oral and 15–30 min for suppository. Used for clients with decreased colon (motor) response due to spinal cord damage. *Pregnancy category:* C; PB: UK; t½: UK
Cascara sagrada	A: PO: Tab: 325 mg/d Fluid extract: 1 mL/d Aromatic fluid extract: 5 mL/d	For acute constipation or bowel preparation. Can be mixed with milk of magnesia. Onset: 6–12 h. *Pregnancy category:* C; PB: UK; t½: UK
Castor oil (Emulsoil, Neoloid, Purge)	A: PO: 15–60 mL C 6–12 y: 5–15 mL	For bowel preparation for diagnostic tests. Harsh cathartic or purgative. Not commonly used for constipation. *Pregnancy category:* X; PB: UK; t½: UK
Phenolphthalein (Ex-Lax, Feen-A-Mint, Correctal)	A&C > 12 y: 60–240 mg/d C 6–12 y: 30–60 mg	For acute constipation. Onset: 6–10 h. Urine is reddish color. *Pregnancy category:* C; PB: UK; t½: UK
Senna (Senokot)	A: PO: 2 tab or 1–4 tsp (granules) diluted in water; *max:* 8 tab/d	For constipation. Available in granules, syrup, and suppository. Prolonged use may cause fluid and electrolyte imbalances. Flatus and abdominal cramps may occur. *Pregnancy category:* C; PB: UK; t½: UK

KEY: *A: adult; C: child; PO: by mouth; >: greater than; <: less than; UK: unknown; PB: protein-binding; t½: half-life; CHF: congestive heart failure.*

NURSING PROCESS: LAXATIVES: Contact

ASSESSMENT

- Obtain a history of constipation and possible causes such as insufficient water/fluid intake, diet deficient in bulk or fiber, or inactivity; a history of the frequency and consistency of stools; and the general health status.
- Obtain baseline vital signs (VS) for identification of abnormalities and for future comparisons.
- Assess renal function.
- Assess electrolyte balance of clients with frequent laxative use.

POTENTIAL NURSING DIAGNOSES

- Constipation
- Altered nutrition
- High risk for fluid deficit
- Knowledge deficit related to overuse of laxatives
- Altered health maintenance

PLANNING

- Client will be free of constipation.
- Client will exercise, eat foods high in fiber, and have adequate fluid intake to avoid constipation.

NURSING INTERVENTIONS

- Monitor fluid intake and output. Note signs and symptoms of fluid and electrolyte imbalances that may result from watery stools. Habitual use of laxatives can cause fluid volume deficit and electrolyte losses. Also, it can cause a loss of urge for defecation.

CLIENT TEACHING

General

- Instruct the client to increase water intake, if not contraindicated, which will decrease hard, dry stools.
- Advise the client to avoid overuse of laxatives, which can lead to fluid and electrolyte imbalances and drug dependence. Suggest exercise to help increase peristalsis.
- Instruct the client not to chew the tablets; swallow them whole.
- Advise the client to store suppositories at <86°F.
- Advise the client to take the drug only with water to increase absorption.
- Instruct the client not to take drug within 1 h of any other drug.
- Remind the client that drug is not for long-term use; tone of bowel may be lost.
- Instruct the client to time administration of drug so as to not interfere with activities or sleep.

Diet

- Advise the client to increase foods rich in fiber such as bran, grains, and fruits.

Side Effects

- Instruct the client to discontinue use if rectal bleeding, nausea, vomiting, or cramping occurs.

EVALUATION

- Evaluate the effectiveness of nonpharmacologic methods for alleviating constipation.
- Evaluate the client's use of laxatives in managing constipation; constipation will be alleviated. Identify laxative abuse.

Bulk-Forming Laxatives

Bulk-forming laxatives are natural fibrous substances that promote large, soft stools by absorbing water into the intestine, increasing fecal bulk and peristalsis. Defecation usually occurs within 8 to 24 h; however, it may take up to 3 d after drug therapy is started for the stool to be soft and well formed. Bulk-forming laxatives, which come in flavored and sugar-free forms, should be mixed in a glass of water or juice, stirred, and drunk immediately, followed by a half to a full glass of water. Insufficient fluid intake can cause the drug to solidify in the GI tract, which can result in intestinal obstruction. This group of laxatives does not cause laxative dependence.

Calcium polycarbophil (FiberCon), methylcellulose (Citrucel), and psyllium hydrophilic muciloid (Metamucil) are examples of bulk-forming laxatives. Clients with hypercalcemia should avoid calcium polycarbophil due to the calcium in the drug. Figure 36–6 presents the bulk-forming laxative psyllium (Metamucil).

Pharmacokinetics

The bulk-forming laxative Metamucil is a nondigestible and nonabsorbent substance that, when mixed with water, becomes a viscous solution. Because it is not absorbed, there is no protein-binding or half-life for the drug. Metamucil is excreted in the feces.

Pharmacodynamics

The onset of action for Metamucil is 10 to 24 h. Peak action is 1 to 3 d. The duration of action is unknown.

Emollients

Emollients are stool softeners (surface-acting drugs) and lubricants used to prevent constipation.

These drugs decrease straining during defecation. Stool softeners work by promoting water accumulation in the intestine. They are frequently prescribed for clients following myocardial infarction or surgery. They are also given prior to administration of other laxatives in treating fecal impaction. Docusate calcium (Surfak), docusate potassium (Dialose), docusate sodium (Colace), and docusate sodium with casanthranol (Peri-Colace) are examples of stool softeners.

Lubricants such as mineral oil increase water retention in the stool. Mineral oil absorbs essential fat-soluble vitamins A, D, E, and K. Some of the minerals can be absorbed into the lymphatic system.

FIGURE 36–6. Laxatives: Bulk Forming

Bulk-Forming Laxative	Dosage	NURSING PROCESS Assessment and Planning
Psyllium hydrophilic muciloid (Metamucil, Naturacil); 🍁 Karasil *Pregnancy Category:* C	A: PO: 1–2 tsp in 8 oz water/d followed by 8 oz water C: >6 y: PO: 0.5–1 tsp in 4 oz water, followed by ≥4 oz water	
Contraindications	**Drug-Lab-Food Interactions**	
Hypersensitivity, fecal impaction, intestinal obstruction, abdominal pain	*Decrease* absorption of oral anticoagulants, aspirin, digoxin, nitrofurantoin	
Pharmacokinetics	**Pharmacodynamics**	Interventions
Absorption: Not absorbed *Distribution:* PB: UK *Metabolism:* t½: UK *Excretion:* In feces	PO: Onset: 10–24 h Peak: 1–3 d Duration: UK	

Therapeutic Effects/Uses: To control chronic constipation. *Mode of Action:* Bulk-forming laxative by drawing water into the intestine.	Evaluation

Side Effects	Adverse Reactions
Anorexia, nausea, vomiting, cramps, diarrhea	Esophageal/and or intestinal obstruction if not taken with adequate water *Life-threatening:* Bronchospasm, anaphylaxis

KEY: A: adult; C: child; PO: by mouth; >: greater than; UK: unknown; PB: protein-binding; t½: half-life; 🍁: Canadian drug name.

Side Effects and Adverse Reactions

Bulk-Forming

Bulk-forming laxatives are not systemically absorbed; therefore, there is no systemic effect. If bulk-forming laxatives are excessively used, nausea, vomiting, flatus, or diarrhea may occur. Abdominal cramps may occur if the drug is used in dry form.

Emollients

Side effects include nausea, vomiting, diarrhea, and abdominal cramping. This drug is not indicated for children, the elderly, or clients with debilitating diseases because they might aspirate the mineral oil, resulting in lipid pneumonia.

The docusate group of drugs may cause mild cramping.

TABLE 36–6 Laxatives: Bulk Forming, Emollients, and Evacuants

Generic (Brand)	Route and Dosage	Uses & Considerations
Bulk Forming		
Calcium polycarbophil (FiberCon, Fiberall, Mitrolan)	A: PO: 1 g, qid *max:* 6 g/d C 6–12 y: PO: 500 mg/d t.i.d.; *max:* 3 g C 2–5 y: PO: 500 mg/d b.i.d.; *max:* 1.5 g/d	Prevention of constipation. Also used to treat acute nonspecific diarrhea or diarrhea associated with irritable bowel syndrome. For diarrhea, it absorbs water and produces a formed stool. For constipation, chew tablet and follow with a full glass of water. *Pregnancy category:* C; PB: NA; t½: NA
Methylcellulose (Cologel, Citrucel)	A: PO: 5–20 mL t.i.d. in 8–10 oz water C: 5–10 mL b.i.d. with 8 oz water	For constipation. Effects are similar to Metamucil. Mix in at least 8 oz of water and take immediately. *Pregnancy category:* UK; PB: NA; t½: NA
Psyllium hydrophilic muciloid (Metamucil)	See Prototype Drug Chart (Fig. 36–6)	For preventing constipation. Dry fiber should be diluted in full glass of water and taken immediately to prevent solidification; follow with extra water. Insufficient water may cause bowel obstruction. Available as OTC with sugar or sugar-free. *Pregnancy category:* C; PB: UK; t½: UK
Emollient: Stool Softeners		
Docusate calcium (Surfak)	A: PO: 240 mg/d C: PO: 60–120 mg/d	Prevention of constipation. Softens the stool. Acts on the small and large intestines and has little absorption. When first used it may take 1–5 d for effectiveness. Available with calcium, potassium, or sodium. Drug should not be taken if CHF is present because of the sodium content. *Pregnancy category:* C; PB: NA; t½: NA
Docusate potassium (Dialose)	A: PO: 100–300 mg/d	
Docusate sodium (Colace)	A: PO: 50–300 mg/d C > 6 y: 40–120 mg/d	
Docusate sodium with casanthranol (Peri-Colace)	A: PO: 1–2 cap/d C: PO: 1 cap/d	For preventing constipation. Combination drug: docusate sodium 100 mg with casanthranol 30 mg. *Pregnancy category:* C; PB: NA; t½: NA
Emollient: Lubricant Mineral oil	A: PO: 15–45 mL/h.s. C 6–12 y: PO: 5–20 mL	Relief of constipation and fecal impaction. May be useful for those with cardiac disorder and following anorectal surgery. Avoid prolonged use because vitamins A, D, E, and K may be lost. *Pregnancy category:* UK; PB: NA; t½: NA
Evacuant/Bowel Prep Polyethylene glycol-electrolyte solution (CoLyte, GoLYTELY)	Prep for GI exam requires 4 h; fasting for 3–4 h A: PO: 240 mL q10–15 min for total of 4 L C: PO: 25–40 mL/kg/h for 4–10 h Administer via NGT to those unable or unwilling to drink solution (prepared with tap water and refrigerated)	For bowel preparation before GI examination. *Pregnancy category:* C; PB: NA; t½: NA

KEY: A: adult; C: child; PO: by mouth; UK: unknown; NA: not applicable; >: greater than; <: less than; NGT: nasogastric tube; t½: half-life; OTC: over-the-counter; CHF: congestive heart failure; PB: protein-binding.

Contraindications

Contraindications to the use of laxatives include inflammatory disorders of the GI tract, such as appendicitis, ulcerative colitis, undiagnosed severe pain that could be due to an inflammation of the intestine (diverticulitis, appendicitis), pregnancy, spastic colon, or bowel obstruction. Laxatives are contraindicated when any of these conditions is suspected.

Table 36–6 presents the drug data for the laxatives.

NURSING PROCESS: LAXATIVE: Bulk Forming

ASSESSMENT

- Obtain a history of constipation and possible causes such as insufficient water/fluid intake, diet deficient in bulk or fiber, or inactivity; a history of the frequency and consistency of stools; and the general health status.
- Obtain baseline vital signs (VS) for identification of abnormalities and for future comparisons.
- Assess renal function, urine output, BUN, and serum creatinine.

POTENTIAL NURSING DIAGNOSES

- Constipation
- High risk for fluid deficit

PLANNING

- Client will be free of constipation.
- Client will exercise, eat foods high in fiber, and have adequate fluid intake to avoid constipation.

NURSING INTERVENTIONS

- Monitor fluid intake and output. Note signs and symptoms of fluid and electrolyte imbalances that may result from watery stools. Habitual use of laxatives can cause fluid volume deficit and electrolyte losses.
- Monitor bowel sounds.
- Identify the cause of constipation.
- Avoid inhalation of psyllium dust.

 CLIENT TEACHING

General
- Instruct the client to mix drug with water immediately before use.
- Instruct the client to *not* swallow the drug in dry form.
- Advise the client to avoid overuse of laxatives, which can lead to fluid and electrolyte imbalances and drug dependence. Suggest exercise to help increase peristalsis.
- Advise the client to avoid inhaling psyllium dust; it may cause watery eyes, runny nose and wheezing.

Diet
- Instruct the client to increase water intake, which will decrease hard, dry stools. Drink at least eight 8-oz glasses of fluids per day.
- Instruct the client to mix the drug in 8 to 10 oz of water, stir, and drink immediately. A least one glass of extra water should follow. Insufficient water can cause the drug to solidify and cause fecal impaction.
- Advise the client to increase foods rich in fiber such as bran, grains, and fruits.

Side Effects
- Instruct client to discontinue use if nausea, vomiting, cramping, or rectal bleeding occurs.

EVALUATION

- Evaluate the effectiveness of nonpharmacologic methods for alleviating constipation.
- Evaluate the client's use of laxatives in managing constipation. Identify laxative abuse.

■ CASE STUDY

C.S., 34 years old, has been vomiting for 48 hours. In the last 12 hours, C.S. has had diarrhea. Prochlorperazine (Compazine) 10 mg was administered intramuscularly.

1. What nonpharmacologic measures should the nurse suggest when vomiting occurs?
2. What type of antiemetic is prochlorperazine?
3. Why was C.S. given prochlorperazine intramuscularly and not orally or rectally? Prochlorperazine should be given deep intramuscularly. Why?

4. What electrolyte imbalances may occur due to vomiting and diarrhea? Explain.
5. What are the side effects of prochlorperazine?

C.S. was prescribed diphenoxylate with atropine (Lomotil), 2.5 mg, t.i.d.

6. Is the Lomotil dosage for C.S. within the normal prescribed range? What is the normal range?
7. What clinical conditions are contraindicated for the use of Lomotil?
8. What are some of the combination drugs that may be prescribed to control diarrhea?
9. Name at lease two over-the-counter (OTC) antidiarrheals.
10. Give an example of an adsorbent. Do you think C.S. should receive an adsorbent? Explain.

STUDY QUESTIONS

1. The client complains of motion sickness. What types of drugs might be suggested? What are the side effects?

2. Certain phenothiazines are prescribed for vomiting. What are the pharmacodynamics (actions)? Give examples of phenothiazine antiemetics.
3. What is ipecac syrup? How is it administered? For what conditions is ipecac contraindicated?
4. The client is taking paregoric for diarrhea. How does this drug differ from opium tincture? What type of antidiarrheal is paregoric?
5. Diphenoxylate (Lomotil) is what type of drug? What are the side effects?
6. What is the difference between laxatives and cathartics? What is the action of contact (irritant) laxatives? What are the side effects?
7. The client is taking a bulk-forming laxative. What instructions should you give?

Chapter 37

Antiulcer Drugs

OUTLINE

Objectives
Terms
Introduction
Predisposing Factors in Peptic
  Ulcer Disease
    Gastroesophageal Reflux
      Disease (GERD)
Nonpharmacologic Measures:

Peptic Ulcer and GERD
Antiulcer Drugs
  Tranquilizers
  Anticholinergics
  Antacids
    Nursing Process
  Histamine$_2$ Blockers
    Nursing Process

Gastric Acid Secretion In-
  hibitor
Pepsin Inhibitor
  Nursing Process
Prostaglandin Analog
Case Study
Study Questions

OBJECTIVES

Identify the predisposing factors for peptic ulcers.

Define peptic ulcer, gastric ulcer, and duodenal ulcer.

Describe the actions of five groups of antiulcer drugs used in the treatment of peptic ulcer: tranquilizers, anticholinergics, antacids, histamine$_2$ blockers, and pepsin inhibitor.

Identify at least two drugs from each of the following drug groups: anticholinergics, antacids, and H$_2$ blockers.

Describe the side effects of anticholinergics and systemic and nonsystemic antacids.

Describe the nursing process, with client teaching, related to antiulcer drugs.

TERMS

antacids
duodenal ulcer
esophageal ulcer
gastric mucosal barrier
  (GMB)

gastric ulcer
histamine$_2$ receptor antagonists
hydrochloric acid
pepsin

peptic ulcer
stress ulcer

INTRODUCTION

Peptic ulcer is a broad term for an ulcer occurring in the esophagus, stomach, or duodenum within the upper gastrointestinal (GI) tract. The ulcers are more specifically named according to the site of involvement: esophageal, gastric, and duodenal ulcers. Duodenal ulcers occur ten times more frequently than gastric and esophageal ulcers. The release of **hydrochloric acid** (HCl) from the parietal cells of the stomach is influenced by histamine, gastrin, and acetylcholine. Peptic ulcers are caused by hypersecretion of hydrochloric acid and pepsin, which erode the GI mucosal lining.

The gastric secretions in the stomach strive to maintain a pH of 2 to 5. **Pepsin**, a digestive enzyme, is activated at a pH of 2, and the acid-pepsin complex of gastric secretions can cause mucosal damage. If the pH of gastric secretion rises to pH 5, the activity of pepsin declines. The **gastric mucosal barrier** (GMB) is a thick, viscous, mucous material that provides a barrier between the mucosal lining and the acidic gastric secretions. The GMB maintains the integrity of the gastric mucosal lining and is a defense against corrosive substances. The two sphincter muscles—the cardiac, located at the upper portion of the stomach, and the pyloric, located at the lower portion of the stomach—act as barriers to prevent reflux of acid into the esophagus and the duodenum. Figure 37–1 illustrates the stomach, sphincter muscles, and common sites of peptic ulcers.

Esophageal ulcers result from reflux of acidic gastric secretion into the esophagus due to a defective or incompetent cardiac sphincter. **Duodenal ulcers** are caused by hypersecretion of acid from the stomach that passes to the duodenum due to (1) insufficient buffers to neutralize the gastric acid in the stomach, (2) a defective or incompetent pyloric sphincter, or (3) hypermotility of the stomach. **Gastric ulcers** frequently occur because of a breakdown of the GMB.

PREDISPOSING FACTORS IN PEPTIC ULCER DISEASE

The nurse needs to assist the client in identifying possible causes of the ulcer and to teach ways to alleviate them. Predisposing factors include mechanical disturbances, genetic influences, environmental factors, and certain drugs. Healing of an ulcer takes 4 to 8 weeks. Complications can occur as the result of scar tissue. Table 37–1 lists the predisposing factors for peptic ulcers and their effects.

The classic symptom of peptic ulcers is gnawing, aching pain. With a gastric ulcer, pain occurs 30 min to 1½ h after eating, and with a duodenal ulcer, 2 to 3 h after eating. Small, frequent meals of nonirritating foods decrease the pain. With treatment, pain usually subsides in 10 days; however, the healing process takes 1 to 2 months.

A **stress ulcer** usually follows a critical situation such as extensive trauma or major surgery (e.g., burns, cardiac surgery). Prophylactic use of antiulcer drugs decreases the incidence of stress ulcers.

A common bacterium, *Helicobacter pylori* (*H. pylori*), is linked with the development of peptic ulcers. Treatment to eradicate this bacterial infection includes using either a dual, triple, or quadruple drug therapy program in a variety of combinations of the drugs—colloidal bismuth subcitrate, omeprazole, metronidazole, amoxicillin, ampicillin, and tetracycline—for 7 to 14 days. After completion of the treatment regimen, 6 weeks of standard acid suppression (e.g., histamine$_2$ blocker) therapy has been recommended.

GASTROESOPHAGEAL REFLUX DISEASE

Gastroesophageal reflux disease (GERD), also called reflux esophagitis, is inflammation of the esophageal mucosa due to a reflux of gastric acid content into the esophagus. Its main cause is an incompetent lower esophageal sphincter. Smoking and obesity tend to accelerate the disease process. The medical treatment for GERD is similar to the treatment for peptic ulcers, which includes the use of antiulcer drugs to neutralize gastric contents and to reduce gastric acid secretion.

NONPHARMACOLOGIC MEASURES: PEPTIC ULCER AND GERD

With a GI disorder, nonpharmacologic measures, along with drug therapy, are an important part of

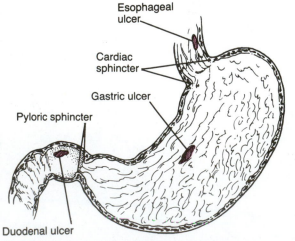

FIGURE 37–1 Common sites of stomach and peptic ulcers.

TABLE 37–1 Predisposing Factors in Peptic Ulcer Disease

Predisposing Factors	Effects
Mechanical disturbances	Hypersecretion of acid and pepsin. Inadequate GMB mucus secretion. Impaired GMB resistance. Hypermotility of the stomach. Incompetent (defective) cardiac or pyloric sphincter.
Genetic influences	Increased number of parietal cells in the stomach. Susceptibility of mucosal lining to acid penetration. Susceptibility to excess acetylcholine and histamine. Excess hydrochloric acid due to external stimuli.
Environmental influences	Foods and liquids containing caffeine; fatty, fried, and highly spiced foods; alcohol. Nicotine products, including cigarettes. Stressful situations. Pregnancy, massive trauma, major surgery.
Drugs	NSAIDs, including aspirin and aspirin compounds, ibuprofen (Motrin, Advil, Nuprin), and indomethacin (Indocin); corticosteroids (cortisone, prednisone); potassium salts; antineoplastic drugs.

KEY: GMB: gastric-mucosal barrier; NSAIDs: nonsteroidal antiinflammatory drugs.

the treatment. Once the GI problem is resolved, the client should continue to follow nonpharmacologic measures in order to avoid recurrence of the GI disorder.

Avoiding smoking and alcohol can decrease gastric secretions. With GERD, nicotine relaxes the lower esophageal sphincter, thus permitting gastric acid reflux. Obesity enhances the problem of GERD. Weight loss is helpful in decreasing symptoms. The client should avoid hot, spicy, and greasy foods, which could aggravate the gastric problem. Nonsteroidal antiinflammatory drugs (NSAIDs), which include aspirin, should be taken with food or in a decreased dosage. Glucocorticoids can cause gastric ulceration, and food should be taken with these drugs.

To relieve symptoms of GERD, the client should raise the head of his or her bed, not eat before bedtime, and wear loose-fitting clothing.

ANTIULCER DRUGS

There are eight groups of antiulcer agents: (1) tranquilizers, which decrease vagal activity; (2) anticholinergic drugs, which decrease acetylcholine by blocking the cholinergic receptors; (3) antacids, which neutralize gastric acid; (4) histamine$_2$ (H$_2$) blockers, which block the histamine$_2$ receptor; (5) the gastric acid secretion omeprazole, which inhibits gastric acid secretion regardless of acetylcholine or histamine release; (6) the pepsin inhibitor sucralfate; (7) the prostaglandin E$_1$ analog misoprostol, which inhibits gastric acid secretion and protects the mucosa; and (8) GI stimulants such as cisapride (Propulsid), which increase the lower esophagus sphincter pressure and lower esophagus peristalsis. Figure 37–2 illustrates the action of the eight antiulcer drug groups, each of which will be discussed separately.

TRANQUILIZERS

Tranquilizers have minimal effect in preventing and treating ulcers; they reduce vagal stimulation and decrease anxiety. Librax, a combination of the anxiolytic chlordiazepoxide (Librium) and the anticholinergic clidinium (Quarzan), is used in the treatment of ulcers.

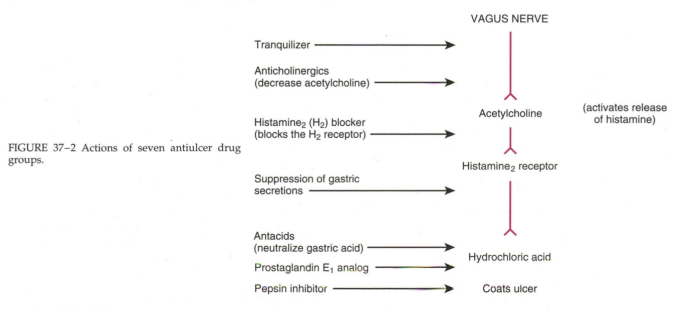

FIGURE 37–2 Actions of seven antiulcer drug groups.

TABLE 37–2 Antiulcer: Anticholinergics

Generic (Brand)	Route and Dosage	Uses and Considerations
Belladonna tincture	A: PO: 0.3–1 mL t.i.d./q.i.d.	For peptic ulcers; decreases gastric secretions. Contraindicated in narrow-angle glaucoma, myasthenia gravis, paralytic ileus, urinary retention. Dry mouth and constipation can occur. *Pregnancy category:* C; PB: UK; t½: 18–36 h
Clidinium bromide and chlordiazepoxide HCl (Librax)	A: PO 1–2 cap t.i.d./q.i.d. a.c., h.s.	Decreases anxiety and GI distress. Contains a benzodiazepine. *Pregnancy category:* C; PB: UK; t½: UK
Glycopyrrolate (Robinul)	A: PO: 1 mg b.i.d./t.i.d. IM/IV: 0.1–0.2 mg (100–200 µg) t.i.d./q.i.d.	For peptic ulcers and gastric disorder due to hyperacidity. Used as one of the preanesthetic drugs. Same contraindications as belladonna. *Pregnancy category:* B; PB: UK; t½: UK
Propantheline bromine (Pro-Banthine)	A: PO: 15 mg t.i.d. 30 min a.c. and 30 mg h.s.	For peptic ulcers; decreases gastric secretions, irritable bowel syndrome, pancreatitis, and urinary bladder spasm. Standard anticholinergic side effects. *Pregnancy category:* C; PB: UK; t½: 9 h
Tridihexethyl chloride (Pathilon)	A: PO: 25–50 mg t.i.d./q.i.d. a.c. and h.s.	For peptic ulcers; decreases gastric secretions. *Pregnancy category:* C; PB: UK; t½: UK

KEY: A: adult; PO: by mouth; a.c.: before meals; h.s.: hour of sleep; UK: unknown; PB: protein-binding; t½: half-life.

ANTICHOLINERGICS

Anticholinergics (antimuscarinics, parasympatholytics) and antacids were for many years the drugs of choice for peptic ulcers. However, with the introduction of histamine$_2$ blockers in 1975, anticholinergic use has declined. These drugs relieve pain by decreasing GI motility and secretion; they act by inhibiting acetylcholine and blocking histamine and hydrochloric acid. Anticholinergics delay gastric emptying time, so they are used more frequently for duodenal ulcers than for gastric ulcers. A new anticholinergic, pirenzepine (Gastrozepine), available in Canada, inhibits gastric secretions and does not cause tachycardia or decrease GI motility. Its action is selective for gastric acid secretory cells.

Anticholinergics should be taken before meals to decrease the acid secretion that occurs with eating. Antacids can slow the absorption of anticholinergics and should therefore be taken 2 h after anticholinergic administration.

Table 37–2 lists selected anticholinergic drugs that are used in the treatment of peptic ulcer. Anticholinergics should be used as adjunctive therapy and not as the only antiulcer drug. Anticholinergics are discussed in more detail in Chapter 19.

Side Effects and Adverse Reactions

Anticholinergics have many side effects, including dry mouth, decreased secretions, tachycardia, urinary retention, and constipation. Because anticholinergics decrease GI motility, the gastric emptying time is delayed, which can stimulate gastric secretions and aggravate the ulceration.

ANTACIDS

Antacids promote ulcer healing by neutralizing hydrochloric acid and reducing pepsin activity; they do not coat the ulcer. There are two types of antacids: those that have a systemic effect and those that have a nonsystemic effect.

Sodium bicarbonate, a systemically absorbed antacid, was one of the first antiulcer drugs. Because it has many side effects (sodium excess, causing hypernatremia and water retention; metabolic alkalosis due to the excess bicarbonate; and acid rebound [excess acid secretion]), sodium bicarbonate is seldom used for treating peptic ulcers. Examples of sodium bicarbonate compounds are Bromo Seltzer and Alka Seltzer.

Calcium carbonate is most effective in neutralizing acid; however, ⅓ to ½ of the drug can be systemically absorbed and cause acid rebound. Hypercalcemia and "milk-alkali syndrome" can result from excessive use of calcium carbonate. Milk-alkali syndrome is intensified if milk products are ingested with calcium carbonate. It is identified by the presence of alkalosis, hypercalcemia and, in severe cases, crystalluria and renal failure.

The nonsystemic antacids are composed of alkaline salts such as aluminum (aluminum hydroxide, aluminum carbonate) and magnesium (magnesium hydroxide, magnesium carbonate, magnesium trisilicate, and magnesium phosphate). There is a small degree of systemic absorption with these drugs, mainly of aluminum. Magnesium hydroxide has greater neutralizing power than aluminum hydroxide. Magnesium compounds can cause diarrhea, and aluminum and calcium compounds can cause constipation with long-term use. A combination of magnesium and aluminum salts neutralizes gastric acid without causing constipation or severe diarrhea. Simethicone (an antigas agent) is found in many antacids, including Mylanta II, Maalox Plus, and Gelusil II.

Figure 37–3 gives the drug data for the aluminum hydroxide antacid (Amphojel).

Pharmacokinetics

Aluminum hydroxide (Amphojel) was one of the first antacids used for neutralizing hydrochloric acid. Aluminum products are frequently used to lower high serum phosphate (hyperphosphatemia). Because aluminum hydroxide alone can cause constipation and magnesium products alone can cause diarrhea, combination drugs, such as aluminum hydroxide and magnesium hydroxide (Maalox), have become popular.

Only a very small amount of Amphojel is absorbed from the GI tract. It is primarily bound to phosphate and excreted in the feces. The small portion that is absorbed is excreted in the urine.

Pharmacodynamics

Amphojel neutralizes gastric acid, including hydrochloric acid, and increases the pH of gastric se-

FIGURE 37–3. Antiulcer: Antacids

Antacid	Dosage	**NURSING PROCESS** Assessment and Planning
Aluminum hydroxide (Amphojel, ALternaGEL, Alu-Tab) *Pregnancy Category:* C	*Antacid:* A: PO: 600 mg 1 h p.c. and h.s.; chewed with water or milk Susp: 5–10 mL 1 h p.c. and h.s. *Hyperphosphatemia:* A: PO: 2 cap or 12.5 mL t.i.d./q.i.d. with meals	
Contraindications	**Drug-Lab-Food Interactions**	
Hypersensitivity to aluminum products, hypophosphatemia *Caution:* In elderly	*Decrease effects* with tetracycline, phenothiazine, isoniazid, phenytoin, digitalis, quinidine, amphetamines; may *increase* effect of benzodiazepines *Lab:* Increase urine pH	
Pharmacokinetics	**Pharmacodynamics**	Interventions
Absorption: PO: Small amount absorbed *Distribution:* PB: UK *Metabolism:* t½: UK *Excretion:* In feces; small amount in urine	PO: Onset: 15–30 min Peak: 0.5 h Duration: 1–3 h	

Therapeutic Effects/Uses: To treat hyperacidity, peptic ulcer, and reflux esophagitis; to reduce hyperphosphatemia. *Mode of Action:* Neutralization of gastric acidity.	Evaluation

Side Effects	Adverse Reactions
Constipation	Hypophosphatemia; long term: GI obstruction

KEY: A: adult; PO: by mouth; UK: unknown; PB: protein-binding; *t½*: half-life; p.c.: after meals; h.s.: at bedtime.

cretions (an elevated pH inactivates pepsin). The onset of action is fairly rapid, but the duration of action varies depending on whether the antacid is taken with or without food. If the antacid is taken after a meal, the duration of action may be up to 3 h because food delays gastric emptying time. Frequent dosing may be necessary if the antacid is given during a fasting state or early in the course of treatment.

The ideal dosing interval for antacids is 1 and

TABLE 37-3 Antiulcers: Antacids

Generic (Brand)	Route and Dosage	Uses and Considerations
Aluminum carbonate (Basaljel)	A: PO: 10–30 mL or 2 tab/cap q2h Extra strength 5–15 mL	To alleviate gastric hyperacidity related to gastritis, gastric and duodenal ulcers, esophageal reflux, and hiatal hernia. Increases gastric pH and inhibits pepsin activity. Also is used to decrease hyperphosphatemia for clients with renal dysfunction. Duration of action is 2 to 3 h when taken 1 h after meals. *Pregnancy category:* C; PB: UK; t½: UK
Aluminum hydroxide (Amphojel, ALternaGEL)	A: PO: 30 mL, 1–3 h p.c. and h.s. *Peptic ulcer disease:* A: PO: 15–45 mL 1–3 h p.c. and h.s. C: PO: 5–15 mL 1–3 h p.c. and h.s. *Prophylaxis GI bleeding:* A: PO: 30–60 mL qh C: PO: 5–15 mL q1–2h; maintain gastric pH >5	Same as aluminum carbonate. Constipation can occur. *Pregnancy category:* C; PB: UK; t½: UK
Calcium carbonate (Tums, Dicarbosil)	A: PO: 2 tab or 10 mL q2h; *max:* 12 doses/d	To alleviate heartburn, acid indigestion, esophagitis, and hiatal hernia due to hyperacidity. Also to treat hyperphosphatemia for clients with renal disorders. OTC drug. One-third of the drug dose is absorbed from GI tract. Constipation can be a problem. *Pregnancy category:* C; PB: UK; t½: UK
Dihydroxyaluminum sodium carbonate (Rolaids Antacid)	A: PO: Chew 1–2 tab PRN	Similar to calcium carbonate except it contains sodium instead of calcium. *Pregnancy category:* C; PB: UK; t½: UK
Magaldrate (Riopan, Lowsium [plus simethicone])	A: PO: 5–15 mL PRN; *max:* 100 mL/d; or 1–2 tab PRN; *max:* 20 tab/d	To alleviate heartburn, gastritis, esophagitis, peptic ulcers due to hyperacidity. Contains aluminum and magnesium hydroxide. Low sodium content. Simethicone decreases flatus. Drug is minimally absorbed. *Pregnancy category:* C; PB: UK; t½: UK
Magnesium hydroxide and aluminum hydroxide (Maalox)	A: PO: 2–4 tab PRN; *max:* 16 tab/d or 10–30 mL, 1–3 h p.c. and h.s.	Same as magaldrate. Caution for clients with renal disorder due to the magnesium content. OTC drug. *Pregnancy category:* UK; PB: UK; t½: UK
Magnesium hydroxide, aluminum hydroxide, and calcium carbonate (Camalox)	A: PO: 10–20 mL PRN; *max:* 80 mL/d; or 2–4 tab PRN; *max:* 16 tab	Same as magaldrate except it also contains calcium. *Pregnancy category:* UK; PB: UK; t½: UK
Magnesium hydroxide and aluminum hydroxide with simethicone (Aludrox, Mylanta, Mylanta III, Maalox Plus, Gelusil-I, Gelusil-II, Gelusil-M, Di-Gel)	A: PO: 10–20 mL PRN; *max:* 120 mL/d; or 2–4 tab PRN; *max:* 24 tab	Same as magaldrate. It also contains simethicone, which decreases flatus. OTC drug. *Pregnancy category:* UK; PB: UK; t½: UK
Magnesium trisilicate (Gaviscon)	A: PO: 1–2 tab PRN; *max:* 8 tab/d	To relieve gastric disorders due to hyperacidity. OTC drug. Contains magnesium trisilicate and aluminum hydroxide. *Pregnancy category:* UK; PB: UK; t½: UK
Sodium bicarbonate	A: PO: 0.5 tsp of powder in 8 oz water	Previously used for gastric hyperacidity. It is a short-acting, potent antacid that is systemically absorbed. Acid-base imbalance could occur. *Pregnancy category:* C; PB: UK; t½: UK

KEY: *A: adult; C: child; PO: by mouth; PB: protein-binding; t½: half-life; PRN: as necessary; >: greater than; OTC: over-the-counter; UK: unknown.*

3 h after meals (maximum acid secretion occurs after eating) and at bedtime. Antacids taken on an empty stomach are effective for 30 to 60 min before passing into the duodenum. Chewable tablets should be followed by water. Liquid antacids should also be taken with water (2 to 4 oz) to ensure that the drug reaches the stomach; however, no more than 4 oz of water should be taken, because water quickens gastric emptying time.

The dosage for antacids is determined according to the health care provider's order or the directions on the drug label (1 to 2 tsp or 5 to 10 mL).

Overuse or overdosing can result in side effects and some systemic absorption. Table 37–3 lists the drug data for antacids.

Antacids containing magnesium salts are contraindicated in clients with impaired renal function because of the risk of hypermagnesemia. Prolonged use of aluminum hydroxides can cause hypophosphatemia (low serum phosphate). If hyperphosphatemia occurs because of poor renal function, aluminum hydroxide can be given to decrease the phosphate level. In clients with renal insufficiency, aluminum salt ingestion can cause encephalopathy from accumulation of aluminum in the brain.

NURSING PROCESS: ANTIULCER: Antacids

ASSESSMENT

- Assess the client's pain, including the type, duration, severity, and frequency.
- Assess the client's renal function.
- Assess for fluid and electrolyte imbalances, especially serum phosphate and calcium levels.
- Obtain drug history; report probable drug-drug interactions.

POTENTIAL NURSING DIAGNOSES

- Pain
- Knowledge deficit related to (mis)use of antacids

PLANNING

- Client will be free of abdominal pain after 1 to 2 wk of antiulcer drug management.

NURSING INTERVENTIONS

- Avoid administering antacids with other oral drugs, because antacids can delay their absorption. An antacid should definitely not be given with tetracycline, digoxin, or quinidine because it binds with and inactivates most of the drug. Antacids are given 1 to 2 h after other medications.
- Shake suspension well before administering: follow with water.
- Monitor urinary pH, calcium, and phosphate levels, and electrolytes.

CLIENT TEACHING

General
- Instruct the client to report pain, coughing, or vomiting of blood.
- Encourage client to drink 1 oz of water after antacid to ensure that the drug reaches the stomach.

- Advise the client to take the antacid 1 to 3 h after meals and at bedtime. Do not take antacids at mealtime; they slow gastric emptying time, causing increased GI activity and gastric secretions.
- Advise the client to notify the health care provider if constipation or diarrhea occurs; the antacid may have to be changed. Self-treatment should be avoided.
- Stress that antacids are not candy and that an unlimited amount is contraindicated.
- Advise the client to avoid taking acids with milk or foods high in vitamin D.
- Instruct the client to avoid taking antacids within 1 to 2 h of other oral medications because there may be interference with absorption.
- Advise the client to check antacid labels for sodium content if on a sodium-restricted diet.
- Alert the client to consult with the health care provider before taking self-prescribed antacids for longer than 2 wk.
- Instruct the client on the use of relaxation techniques.

Skill
- Instruct the client how to take antacids correctly. Chewable tablets should be thoroughly chewed and followed with water. With liquid antacid, 2 to 4 oz of water should follow the antacid.

Side Effects
- Advise the client to avoid foods and liquids that can cause gastric irritation, such as caffeine-containing beverages, alcohol, and spices.
- Advise that stools may become speckled or white.

EVALUATION

- Determine the effectiveness of the antiulcer treatment and the presence of side effects. The client should be free of pain, and healing should be progressing.

HISTAMINE₂ BLOCKERS

The **histamine₂ (H₂) blockers** (histamine₂ receptor antagonists) are the most popular drugs used in the treatment of gastric and duodenal ulcers. H₂ blockers prevent acid reflux in the esophagus (reflux esophagitis). These drugs block the H₂ receptors of the parietal cells in the stomach, thus reducing gastric acid secretion and concentration. Antihistamines, used to treat allergic conditions, act against histamine₁ (H₁); they are not the same as H₂ blockers.

The first H₂ blocker was cimetidine (Tagamet), introduced in 1975. Cimetidine, which has a short half-life and a short duration of action, blocks about 70% of acid secretion for 4 h. Good kidney function is necessary, because approximately 50% to 80% of the drug is excreted unchanged in the urine. If renal insufficiency is present, cimetidine dose and frequency may need to be reduced. Antacids can be given an hour before or after cimetidine as part of the antiulcer drug regimen; however, if they are given at the same time they decrease the effectiveness of the H₂ blocker.

Three H₂ blockers, ranitidine (Zantac, 1983), famotidine (Pepcid, 1986), and nizatidine (Axid, 1988), are more potent than cimetidine. In addition to blocking gastric acid secretions, they also pro-

FIGURE 37–4. Antiulcer: Histamine₂ Blockers

Histamine₂ blocker	Dosage	NURSING PROCESS
		Assessment and Planning
Ranitidine (Zantac) *Pregnancy Category:* B	A: PO: 150 mg q12h or 300 mg h.s.; maint: 300 mg h.s. IM: 50 mg q6–8 h IV: 50 mg q6–8 h diluted C: PO: 2–4 mg/kg/d divided q12h IV: 1–2 mg/kg/d divided q6–8 h	
Contraindications	**Drug-Lab-Food Interactions**	
Hypersensitivity, severe renal or liver disease *Caution:* Pregnancy, lactation	*Decrease* absorption with antacids; *decrease* absorption of ketoconazole; *toxicity* with metoprolol *Lab: Increase* serum alkaline phosphatase	
Pharmacokinetics	**Pharmacodynamics**	Interventions
Absorption: PO: Well absorbed, 50% *Distribution:* PB: 15% *Metabolism:* t½: 2–3 h *Excretion:* In urine and feces	PO: Onset: 15 min Peak: 1–3 h Duration: 8–12 h IM/IV: Onset: 10–15 min Peak: 15 min Duration: 8–12 h	

Therapeutic Effects/Uses: To prevent and treat peptic ulcers, gastroesophageal reflux, and stress ulcers.

Mode of Action: Inhibition of gastric acid secretion by inhibiting histamine at histamine₂ receptors in parietal cells.

Evaluation

Side Effects	Adverse Reactions
Headache, confusion, nausea, vertigo, diarrhea or constipation, depression, rash, blurred vision, malaise	*Life-threatening:* Hepatotoxicity, cardiac dysrhythmias, blood dyscrasias

KEY: A: adult; C: child; PO: by mouth; IM: intramuscular; IV: intravenous; PB: protein-binding; t½: half-life; h.s.: at bedtime.

mote healing of the ulcer by eliminating its cause. Their duration of action is longer, thus decreasing the frequency of dosing, and they have fewer side effects and fewer drug interactions than cimetidine. Figure 37–4 gives the pharmacologic data for ranitidine (Zantac), the most popular H$_2$ blocker.

Pharmacokinetics

Ranitidine is 5 to 12 times more potent than cimetidine; however, it is less potent than famotidine. It is rapidly absorbed and reaches its peak concentration after a single dose in 1 to 3 h. Ranitidine has a low protein-binding power and a short half-life. With liver disease, ranitidine's half-life is prolonged. About 50% of the absorbed drug is excreted unchanged in the urine.

Ulcer healing occurs in 4 weeks for 70% of clients and in 8 weeks for 90% of clients taking ranitidine. Large doses of ranitidine are effective for controlling Zollinger-Ellison syndrome, whereas cimetidine is not effective in controlling the symptoms of this disorder.

Pharmacodynamics

Ranitidine inhibits histamine at the H$_2$ receptor site. The drug is effective in treating gastric and duodenal ulcers and can be used prophylactically. It is also useful in relieving symptoms of reflux

esophagitis, preventing stress ulcers that can occur following major surgery, and preventing aspiration pneumonitis that can result from aspiration of gastric acid secretions.

Ranitidine has a longer onset of action and duration of action (up to 12 h) than cimetidine. Because cimetidine has a duration of action of only 4 to 5 h, it is frequently given three to four times a day.

Cimetidine increases the effects of theophylline, beta blockers, oral anticoagulants, anticonvulsants (phenytoin), diazepam (Valium), and the antidysrhythmics. Cimetidine can cause an increase in blood urea nitrogen (BUN), serum creatinine, and serum alkaline phosphatase. Neither cimetidine nor ranitidine should be taken with antacids because their H$_2$ blocking action could be decreased. Ranitidine can increase the effect of oral anticoagulants.

Famotidine is 50% to 80% more potent than cimetidine and is five to eight times more potent than ranitidine. It is indicated for short-term use (4 to 8 weeks) for duodenal ulcer and for Zollinger-Ellison syndrome.

Side Effects and Adverse Reactions

Side effects and adverse reactions of H$_2$ blockers include headaches, dizziness, constipation, pruritus, skin rash, gynecomastia, decreased libido, and impotence.

TABLE 37–4 Antiulcers: Histamine$_2$ Blockers

Generic (Brand)	Route and Dosage	Uses and Considerations
Cimetidine (Tagamet)	A: PO: 300 mg q.i.d. with meals and h.s. or 800 mg h.s.; maint: 300 mg h.s. IV: 300 mg q6–8h diluted in 50 mL (administered over 15–30 min) IV: continuous infusion: 37.5 mg/h over 24 h; *max:* 900 mg/d C: PO/IV: 10–40 mg/kg/d divided q6h	For peptic ulcers (gastric and duodenal). The first H$_2$ blocker marketed. Has many drug interaction and side effects. Duration of action is 4–6 h. *Pregnancy category:* B; PB: 20%; t½: 2 h
Famotidine (Pepcid)	A: PO: 20 mg q12h or 40 mg h.s.; maint: 20 mg h.s. IV: 20 mg q12h diluted C: PO: 1 mg/kg/d divided q8–12h C: IV: 0.6–0.8 mg/kg/d divided q8–12h	For treatment of active duodenal ulcer. Inhibits gastric secretion. More potent than cimetidine. *Pregnancy category:* B; PB: 15%–20%; t½: 2.5–4 h
Nizatidine (Axid)	A: PO: 150 mg q12h or 300 mg h.s.; maint: 150 mg h.s.	Same as famotidine. Also to treat gastroesophageal reflux. Give drug after meals or at bedtime. Do not give within 1 h of antacids. *Pregnancy category:* B; PB: 35%; t½: 1–2 h
Ranitidine (Zantac)	See Prototype Drug Chart (Fig. 37–4)	Commonly prescribed H$_2$ blocker. To treat peptic ulcers (gastric and duodenal) and gastroesophageal reflux disease (GERD). Administer after meals or at bedtime. Do not give within 1 h of antacids. If creatinine clearance is <50 mL/min, dose should be decreased. Drug is more potent than cimetidine. *Pregnancy category:* B; PB: 15%; t½: 2–3 h

KEY: A: adult; C: child; h.s.: hour of sleep; IV: intravenous; PB: protein-binding; PO: by mouth; t½: half-life.

Drug Interactions

Cimetidine interacts with many drugs. By inhibiting hepatic drug metabolism, it enhances the effects of oral anticoagulants, theophylline, caffeine, phenytoin (Dilantin), diazepam (Valium), propranolol (Inderal), phenobarbital, and calcium channel blockers. Ranitidine and famotidine have fewer side effects than cimetidine. Table 37–4 lists the drug data for the H_2 blockers.

NURSING PROCESS: ANTIULCER: Histamine$_2$ Blocker

ASSESSMENT

- Assess the client's pain, including the type, duration, severity, frequency, and location.
- Assess GI complaints.
- Assess mental status.
- Assess fluid and electrolyte imbalances, including intake and output.
- Assess gastric pH (>5 is desired), BUN, and creatinine.
- Assess drug history; report probable drug-drug interactions.

POTENTIAL NURSING DIAGNOSES

- Pain related to gastric dysfunction

PLANNING

- Client will no longer experience abdominal pain after 1 to 2 wk of drug therapy.

NURSING INTERVENTIONS

- Do not confuse drug with alprazolam (Xanax).
- Administer drug just before meals to decrease food-induced acid secretion or at bedtime.
- Be alert that reduced doses of drug are needed by the elderly, who have less gastric acid; need to prevent metabolic acidosis.
- Administer drug intravenously in 20 to 100 mL of IV solution.

CLIENT TEACHING

General
- Instruct the client to report pain, coughing, or vomiting of blood.
- Advise the client to avoid smoking because it can hamper the effectiveness of the drug.
- Remind the client that the drug must be taken exactly as prescribed to be effective.
- Instruct the client to separate ranitidine and antacid dosage by at least 1 h, if possible.
- Instruct the client not to drive a motor vehicle or engage in dangerous activities until stabilized on the drug.
- Tell the client that drug-induced impotence and gynecomastia are reversible.
- Instruct the client on the use of relaxation techniques to decrease anxiety.

Diet
- Advise the client to eat foods rich in vitamin B_{12} to avoid deficiency as a result of drug therapy.
- Advise the client to avoid foods and liquids that can cause gastric irritation, such as caffeine-containing beverages, alcohol, and spices.

EVALUATION

- Determine the effectiveness of the drug therapy and the presence of any side effects or adverse reactions. The client should be free of pain, and healing should be progressing.

GASTRIC ACID SECRETION INHIBITOR

Omeprazole (Prilosec) inhibits gastric acid secretion (up to 90%) to a greater extent than histamine antagonists. It is metabolized by the liver, reaches peak levels in 2 to 5 h, and is primarily eliminated by the kidneys. Omeprazole is highly protein bound; has a half-life of 0.5 to 1.5 h; however, action is of long duration (4 to 72 h), possibly because of distribution to tissues, especially to the parietal cells. The general dose is 20 mg daily; this dose may be increased. Possible side effects include diarrhea, dry mouth, numbness, dizziness, and weakness.

PEPSIN INHIBITOR

Sucralfate (Carafate), a complex of sulfated sucrose and aluminum hydroxide, is classified as a pepsin inhibitor, or mucosal protective drug. It is nonabsorbable and combines with protein to form a viscous substance that covers the ulcer and protects it from acid and pepsin. This drug does not neutralize acid or decrease acid secretions.

The dosage of sucralfate is 1 g, usually 4 times a day before meals and at bedtime. If antacids are added to decrease pain, they should be given either 30 min before or after the administration of sucralfate. Because sucralfate is not systemically absorbed, side effects are few; however, it can cause constipation. If the drug is stored at room temperature in a tight container, it will remain stable for up to 2 years.

The action and effects of sucralfate are shown in Figure 37–5.

Pharmacokinetics

Less than 5% of sucralfate is absorbed by the GI tract. It has a half-life of 6 to 20 h. Ninety percent of the drug is excreted in the feces.

Pharmacodynamics

Sucralfate promotes healing by adhering to the ulcer surface. The onset of action occurs within 30 min, and the duration of action is short. Sucralfate decreases the absorption of tetracycline, phenytoin, fat-soluble vitamins, and the antibacterial agents ciprofloxacin and norfloxacin. Antacids decrease the effects of sucralfate.

FIGURE 37–5. Antiulcer: Pepsin Inhibitor

Pepsin Inhibitor	Dosage	**NURSING PROCESS** Assessment and Planning
Sucralfate (Carafate), 🍁: Sulcrate *Pregnancy Category:* B	*Active Disease:* A: PO: 1 g q.i.d. 1 h a.c. and h.s. *Maintenance:* A: PO: 1 g b.i.d.	
Contraindications	**Drug-Lab-Food Interactions**	
Hypersensitivity *Caution:* Renal failure	*Decrease* effects with tetracycline, phenytoin, fat-soluble vitamins, digoxin; *altered absorption* with ciprofloxacin, norfloxacin, antacids	
Pharmacokinetics	**Pharmacodynamics**	Interventions
Absorption: PO: Minimal absorption (<5%) *Distribution:* PB: UK *Metabolism:* $t\frac{1}{2}$: 6–20 h *Excretion:* In urine	PO: Onset: 30 min Peak: UK Duration: 5 h	

Therapeutic Effects/Uses: To prevent gastric mucosal injury from drug-induced ulcers (aspirin, NSAIDs); to manage ulcers.

Mode of Action: In combination with gastric acid forms a protective covering on the ulcer surface.

Evaluation

Side Effects	Adverse Reactions
Dizziness, nausea, constipation, dry mouth, rash, pruritus, back pain, sleepiness	None significant

KEY: A: adult; PO: by mouth; UK: unknown; PB: protein-binding; $t\frac{1}{2}$: half-life; a.c.: before meal; h.s.: at bedtime; 🍁 : Canadian drug names.

TABLE 37–5 Antiulcers: Pepsin Inhibitor, Gastric Acid Secretion Inhibitor, Prostaglandin Analog, and GI Stimulant

Generic (Brand)	Route and Dosage	Uses and Considerations
Pepsin Inhibitor Sucralfate (Carafate)	See Prototype Drug Chart (Fig. 37–5)	Management of duodenal ulcer. May be used for aspirin-induced gastric ulcer. Produces a pasty substance to protect the damaged mucosa. May cause nausea and constipation. *Pregnancy category:* B; PB: UK; t½: 6–20 h
Gastric Acid Secretion Inhibitor Lansoprazole (Prevacid)	*Duodenal Ulcer:* A: PO: 15 mg/d a.c. for 4 wk *Erosive Esophagitis:* A: PO: 30 mg/d a.c. for 8 wk	Short-term treatment for duodenal ulcer and erosive esophagitis. Also effective for treating Zollinger-Ellison syndrome. Swallow capsule whole (do not chew or crush). *Pregnancy category:* B; PB: UK; t½: UK
Omeprazole (Prilosec)	*Gastroesophageal reflux disease (GERD):* A: PO: 20 mg/d for 4–8 wk *Hypersecretory:* A: PO: Initially: 60 mg daily; may increase to 120 mg t.i.d. in divided doses	Treatment of gastroesophageal reflux disease, including esophagitis and Zollinger-Ellison syndrome. Poorly absorbed with only 35%–40% in circulation. Antacids can be taken with drug. *Pregnancy category:* C; PB: 95%; t½: 0.5–1.5 h
Prostaglandin Analog Misoprostol (Cytotec)	A: PO: 100–200 µg q.i.d. with food C < 18 y: PO: Safety and efficacy not established	Prevention of NSAID-induced gastric ulcer. May be taken during NSAID therapy, including with aspirin. Side effects include diarrhea, abdominal pain, flatulence, nausea and vomiting, constipation, menstrual spotting. Has a short duration of action. *Pregnancy category:* X; PB: 85%; t½: 1.5 h
GI Stimulants Cisapride (Propulsid)	*Heartburn and GERD:* A: PO: 10 mg, 15 min a.c. and h.s.	For nocturnal heartburn and gastroesophageal reflux disease (GERD). Avoid alcohol intake with drug. *Pregnancy category:* C; PB: 98%; t½: 8–10 h

KEY: A: adult; C: child; h.s.: hour of sleep; PB: protein-binding; PO: by mouth; t½: half-life; <: less than.

PROSTAGLANDIN ANALOG ANTIULCER DRUG

Misoprostol, a synthetic prostaglandin analog, is a new drug for prevention and treatment of peptic ulcer. It appears to suppress gastric acid secretion and increases cytoprotective mucus in the GI tract. It causes a moderate decrease in pepsin secretion. Misoprostol is considered to be as effective as cimetidine. Clients having complaints of gastric distress from taking NSAIDs, such as aspirin or indomethacin prescribed for long-term therapy, can benefit from use of misoprostol. When the client is taking high doses of NSAIDs, misoprostol is frequently recommended for the duration of the NSAID therapy. Misoprostol is contraindicated during pregnancy and for women of child-bearing age. Table 37–5 lists drug data for sucralfate, omeprazole, and misoprostol.

■ CASE STUDY
Client with a Peptic Ulcer

J.H., 48 years old, complained of a gnawing, aching pain in the abdominal area that usually occurs sev-

eral hours after eating. He said that Tums helped some, but the pain has recently intensified. Diagnostic tests indicated that the client has a duodenal ulcer.

1. What is a duodenal ulcer? How is it related to a peptic ulcer? Is it the same as a gastric ulcer?
2. A nursing history is taken. What are some predisposing factors related to peptic ulcers?
3. What nonpharmacologic measures can you suggest for alleviating symptoms related to peptic ulcer?

The health care provider prescribed Mylanta 2 tsp to be taken 2 h after meals, and ranitidine (Zantac) 150 mg, b.i.d. Mylanta is to be taken either 1 h before or 1 h after the ranitidine.

4. What type of drug is Mylanta? What are its ingredients?
5. The health care provider may suggest that the client take ranitidine with meals. Why? Why should Mylanta and ranitidine not be taken at the same time?
6. In what ways are ranitidine and cimetidine the same and how do they differ? Explain.

NURSING PROCESS: ANTIULCERS: Pepsin Inhibitor

ASSESSMENT

- Assess the client's pain, including the type, duration, severity, and frequency. Ulcer pain usually occurs after meals and during the night.
- Assess the client's renal function. Report urine output of <600 mL/d or < 25 mL/h.
- Assess for fluid and electrolyte imbalances.
- Assess gastric pH (>5 is desired).

POTENTIAL NURSING DIAGNOSES

- Pain related to GI dysfunction

PLANNING

- Client will be free of abdominal pain after 1 to 2 wk of antiulcer drug management.

NURSING INTERVENTIONS

- Administer drug on empty stomach.
- Administer an antacid 30 min before or after sucralfate. Allow 1 to 2 h to elapse between sucralfate and other prescribed drugs; sucralfate binds with certain drugs such as tetracycline, phenytoin, thus reducing the effect of the other drugs.

CLIENT TEACHING

General
- Advise client to take drug exactly as ordered. Therapy usually requires 4 to 8 wk for optimal ulcer healing. Advise the client to continue to take drug even if feeling better.
- Increase fluids, dietary bulk, and exercise to relieve constipation.
- Instruct the client on the use of relaxation techniques.
- Monitor for severe, persistent constipation.
- Stress need for follow-up medical care.
- Emphasize cessation of smoking, as indicated.

Diet
- Advise the client to avoid foods and liquids that can cause gastric irritation, such as caffeine-containing beverages, alcohol, and spices.

Side Effects
- Instruct the client to report pain, coughing, or vomiting of blood.

EVALUATION

- Determine the effectiveness of the antiulcer treatment and the presence of any side effects. The client should be free of pain, and healing should be progressing.

---

7. What side effects are associated with ranitidine?

The client states he drinks beer at lunch and has two gin and tonics in the midafternoon. He states that these drinks help him to relax.

8. What nursing intervention should be taken in regard to his alcoholic intake?
9. What foods should he avoid?

A week later the client states that he discontinued the prescribed medications because he "felt better." However, the pain recurred and he asked if he should resume taking the medications.

10. What would your response be? What client teaching should be included?

STUDY QUESTIONS

1. What is the action of antacids used in the treatment and control of peptic ulcers?
2. Your client is taking Maalox 15 mL four times a day. At what times should the drug be taken? What would the duration of action be if the drug were taken with food and without food? How should it be taken?
3. What is a major side effect of antacids containing aluminum salts and magnesium salts?
4. Your client is taking ranitidine (Zantac). What type of drug is ranitidine?
5. What is sucralfate (Carafate)? What is its action in treating peptic ulcer?
6. What are the actions of omeprazole and misoprostol?

Unit X

Eye, Ear, and Skin Agents

Many of the drugs used in the treatment of eye and ear disorders are discussed in other chapters of this text, for example, antibiotics in Chapters 22, 23, and 24. Of particular interest and importance in Chapter 38 are drugs used in the treatment of glaucoma and ocular infections.

OVERVIEW OF THE EYE

The eyeballs, protected within the orbits of the skull, are controlled by the third, fourth, and sixth cranial nerves, connected to six extraocular muscles. The eye has three layers: (1) the cornea and sclera, (2) the choroid, iris, and ciliary body, and (3) the retina. Figure X–1 illustrates the basic structures of the eye.

The cornea, the anterior covering of the eye, is transparent, enabling the light to enter the eye. The cornea, which has no blood vessels, receives nutrition from the aqueous humor. An abraded cornea is susceptible to infection. Loss of corneal transparency is generally caused by increased intraocular pressure.

The sclera is the opaque, white fibrous envelope of the eye. Within the sclera are the posterior chamber and the anterior chamber. The posterior chamber has a blind spot (not sensitive to light) around the optic nerve. The lens, held in place by ligaments, separates these two chambers. The normally transparent lens focuses light on the retina by changing its shape through a process called accommodation.

The anterior chamber, filled with aqueous humor secreted by the ciliary body, lies in front of the lens. The fluid flows into the anterior chamber through a space between the lens and iris. The excess fluid drains into the canal of Schlemm. A rise in intraocular pressure, resulting in glaucoma, occurs with increased production or decreased drainage of aqueous humor.

The choroid, iris, and ciliary body (thickened part of vascular covering of the eye; provides attachment to ligaments and support to lens) constitute the second layer. The choroid absorbs light. The iris, which surrounds the pupil and gives the eye its color, controls the quantity of light reaching the lens through dilation and constriction.

The retina, the third layer, is composed of nerves, rods, and cones that serve as visual sensory receptors. The retina is connected to the brain via the optic nerve.

The eyebrows, eyelashes, eyelids, tears, and corneal and conjunctival reflexes all serve to protect the eye. Bilateral blinking occurs every few seconds during waking hours to keep the eye moist and free of foreign material.

OVERVIEW OF THE EAR

The ear is divided into the external, middle, and inner ear. Figure X–2 illustrates the basic structures of the ear.

The **external ear** consists of the pinna and the external auditory canal. The external audi-

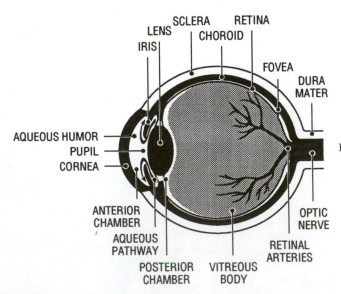

FIGURE X–1 Basic structures of the eye.

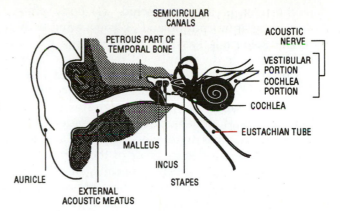

FIGURE X–2 Basic structures of the ear.

tory canal transmits sound to the tympanic membrane (eardrum), a transparent partition between the external and middle ear. The eardrum in turn transmits sound to the bones of the middle ear and also serves a protective function.

The three auditory ossicles (malleus, incus, and stapes) transmit sound waves to the inner ear and are located in the **middle ear,** an air-filled cavity. The tip of the malleus is attached to the eardrum; its head is attached to the incus, which is attached to the stapes. The eustachian tube provides a direct connection to the nasopharynx and equalizes air pressure on both sides of the eardrum to prevent it from rupturing. Swallowing, yawning, and chewing gum help the eustachian tube to relieve pressure changes on airplane flights.

The **inner ear,** a series of labyrinths (canals), consists of a bony section and a membranous section. The vestibule, cochlea, and semicircular canals make up the bony labyrinth. The vestibular area is responsible for maintaining equilibrium and balance. The cochlea is the principal hearing organ.

Professional evaluation of ear problems is essential because hearing loss can result from untreated disorders. Middle ear problems require prescription medications and are not treated with over-the-counter preparations.

SKIN

Skin, the largest organ of the body, is composed of two major layers: the epidermis, which is the outer layer of the skin; and the dermis, which is the layer of skin beneath the epidermis.

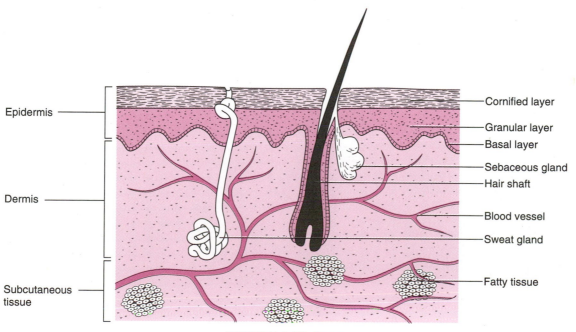

FIGURE X–3 Skin layers.

579

The functions of the skin include (1) body protection from the environment, (2) aiding in body temperature control, and (3) preventing body fluid loss.

The epidermis has four layers (1) the basal layer (stratum germinativum), the deepest layer lying over the dermis, (2) the spinous layer (stratum spinosum), (3) the granular layer (stratum granulosum), and (4) the cornified layer (stratum corneum), the outer layer of the epidermis. As the epidermal cells migrate to the surface, they die and their cytoplasm is converted to keratin (hard and rough texture), forming keratinocytes. Eventually the keratinocytes slough off as new layers of epidermal cells migrate upward.

The dermis has two layers: the papillary layer, next to the epidermis; and the reticular layer, which is the deeper layer of the dermis. The dermal layers consist of fibroblasts, collagen fibers, and elastic fibers. The collagen and elastic fibers give the skin its strength and elasticity. Within the dermal layer, there are sweat glands, hair follicles, sebaceous glands, blood vessels, and sensory nerve terminals. Figure X–3 shows the layers of the skin.

The subcutaneous tissue, primarily fatty tissue, lies under the dermis. Besides fatty cells, subcutaneous tissue contains blood and lymphatic vessels, nerve fibers, and elastic fibers. It supports and protects the dermis.

Chapter 38

Drugs for Disorders of the Eye and the Ear

OUTLINE

Objectives
Terms
Introduction
Drugs for Disorders of the Eye
    Diagnostic Aids
    Topical Anesthetics
    Antiinfectives
    Lubricants
    Miotics
      Nursing Process
    Carbonic Anhydrase In-
      hibitors
      Nursing Process

Osmotics
    Nursing Process
Anticholinergic Mydriatics
   and Cycloplegics
Administration of Eye
   Drops and Ointments
Clients with Eye Disorders:
   General Suggestions for
   Client Teaching
Drugs for Disorders of the Ear
   Antiinfectives
     Nursing Process

Antihistamine-Deconges-
   tants
Combination Products
Ceruminolytics
Administration of Ear Med-
   ications
Clients with Ear Disorders:
   General Suggestions for
   Client Teaching
Case Study
Study Questions

OBJECTIVES

Identify medication groups commonly used for disorders of the eye and the ear.

List mechanisms of action, route, side effects and adverse reactions, and contraindications for selected drugs in each group.

Describe content of teaching plans for groups of drugs presented.

Describe the nursing process, including client teaching, related to disorders of the eye and ear.

TERMS

carbonic anhydrase in-
  hibitors
cerumen
ceruminolytic
conjunctivitis

cycloplegics
lacrimal duct
miosis
miotics
mydriatics

ophthalmic
optic
osmotics
otic

INTRODUCTION

This chapter describes the most commonly used drugs for eye and ear disorders. Many of these drugs have other uses and are discussed in greater detail in other chapters.

DRUGS FOR DISORDERS OF THE EYE

DIAGNOSTIC AIDS

Diagnostic aids are used frequently to locate lesions or foreign objects and to provide local anesthesia to the area. Drugs commonly used as diagnostic aids are presented in Table 38–1.

TOPICAL ANESTHETICS

Topical anesthetics are used in selected aspects of a comprehensive eye examination and in the removal of foreign bodies from the eye. The two most common topical anesthetics are proparacaine hydrochloride (Ophthaine, Ophthetic) and tetracaine hydrochloride (Pontocaine).

Corneal anesthesia is achieved within 1 min and generally lasts about 15 min. The blink reflex is temporarily lost; therefore, the corneal epithelium is not kept moist. To protect the eye, a patch is usually worn over the eye until the effects of the drug are gone. These drugs are not to be self-administered by the client. Repeated doses are given only under strict medical supervision.

TABLE 38–1 Diagnostic Aids for Eye Disorders

Diagnostic Aids	Purpose
Fluorescein sodium	A dye used to demonstrate defects in corneal epithelium. Corneal scratches turn bright green; foreign bodies are surrounded by green ring. Loss of conjunctiva shows orange yellow. Dye appears in nasal secretions if lacrimal duct patent.
Fluress (fluorescein and benoxinate)	Used for short corneal and conjunctival procedures, including removal of foreign bodies. Dye and local anesthetic.

ANTIINFECTIVES

Antiinfectives are frequently used for eye infections. **Conjunctivitis** (inflammation of the delicate membrane covering the eyeball and lining the eyelid) and local skin and eye irritation are possible side effects of topical **ophthalmic** antiinfective drugs. Screen for previous allergic reactions. Conjunctivitis is also one type of eye infection that can be bacterial or viral in origin. For more comprehensive information on antiinfectives, see Chapters 22, 23, and 24. The drug data for optic antiinfectives are presented in Table 38–2; antiinflammatory drug data are presented in Table 38–3.

LUBRICANTS

Both healthy and ill persons may need to use eye lubricants. Healthy clients who complain of "dry-

---

TABLE 38–2 Ophthalmic: Antiinfectives

Generic (Brand)	Route and Dosage*	Uses and Considerations
Antibacterials		
Chloramphenicol (AK-Chlor, Chloromycetin Ophthalmic)	A&C: Ophthalmic: Instill 1–2 gtt or ½ inch oint q3–4 h for 48 h; increase interval to b.i.d./t.i.d.	Effective against both gram-negative and gram-positive bacteria. For treatment of severe infections or when other antibacterials not effective. Continue treatment for at least 48 h after eye appears normal. *Pregnancy category:* C; PB: NA; t½: NA
Ciprofloxacin HCl (Cipro)	Day 1: 2 gtt q15min for 6 h then 2 gtt q30min for the rest of the day Day 2: 2 gtt qh Days 3–14: 2 gtt q4h	Effective against bacterial conjunctivitis. To treat corneal ulceration. Minimal absorption through cornea or conjunctiva. *Pregnancy category:* C; PB: NA; t½: NA
Erythromycin (Ilotycin)	Oint 0.5%: 0.5–1 cm q.d./q.i.d.	Most commonly used antibacterial; for superficial ocular infections and prevention of ophthalmia neonatorum. *Pregnancy category:* B; PB: NA; t½: NA
Gentamicin sulfate (Garamycin Ophthalmic)	A&C: Sol 0.3%: 1–2 gtt q4h; may increase to 2 gtt q1h for severe infections Oint 0.3%: ½ inch ribbon b.i.d./t.i.d.	For infections of the external eye. *Pregnancy category:* C; PB: NA; t½: NA
Norfloxacin (Chibroxin)	A&C > 1 y: Sol 3%: instill 1–2 gtt in affected eye(s) q.i.d. for ≤ 7 d	For treatment of conjunctivitis. *Pregnancy category:* C; PB: NA; t½: NA

TABLE 38–2 Ophthalmic: Antiinfectives *(Continued)*

Generic (Brand)	Route and Dosage*	Uses and Considerations
Tobramycin (Nebcin, Tobrex)	0.3% oint: ½ inch b.i.d./t.i.d. 0.3% Sol: 1–2 gtt q4h *For severe infections:* Oint: ½ inch q 3–4 hours Sol: 2 gtt q 30–60 min until improvement, then decrease frequency	*Pregnancy category:* D; PB: NA; t½: NA
Silver-nitrate 1% (Dey-Drop)	Neonate: Instill 2 gtt in each eye within 1 h of birth	For prevention and treatment of ophthalmia neonatorum. *Pregnancy category:* C; PB: NA; t½: NA
Tetracycline HCl (Achromycin Ophthalmic)	A: Instill 1–2 gtt b.i.d./q.i.d. A: Oint: Instill ½ inch q2–12h	Bacteriostatic action; alternative to silver nitrate for prevention of ophthalmia neonatorum. *Pregnancy category:* D; PB: NA; t½: NA
Antifungal Natamycin (Natacyn Ophthalmic)	A&C: Sol 5%: 1 gt q2h for 3–4 d; then 1 gt q3h for 14–21 d	May cause transient stinging or temporary blurring of vision. *Pregnancy category:* C; PB: NA; t½: NA
Antiviral Idoxuridine (IDU, Herplex Liquifilm)	A&C: Sol (1%): Initially: 1 gt q1h during the day and q2h at night; when definite improvement occurs, use 1 gt q2h during the day and q4h at night; continue 3–7 d after healing occurs 0.5% oint: place ½ inch q4h while awake	To treat cytomegalovirus or herpes simplex keratitis. Store in refrigerator; do not mix with boric acid. If no response in 1 week, discontinue. *Pregnancy category:* C; PB: NA; t½: NA
Trifluridine (Viroptic)	A: 1% sol: Instill 1 gt into infected eye q2h while awake; max: 9 gtt/d until corneal ulcer reepithelialized; then 1 gt q4h for 7 d; max: 21 d of treatment	For treatment of keratoconjunctivitis caused by herpes simplex virus types 1 and 2; herpetic ophthalmic infections. *Pregnancy category:* C; PB: NA; t½: NA
Vidarabine Vira-A ophthalmic	A&C: Oint 3%: ½ inch 5 × d at 3-h intervals	For treatment of keratoconjunctivitis and herpes simplex keratitis. *Pregnancy category:* C; PB: NA; t½: NA

* To minimize systemic absorption, apply gentle pressure on inner canthus.
KEY: A: adult; C: child; gt: drop; gtt: drops; oint: ointment; PB: protein-binding; sol: solution; t½: half-life; UK: unknown.

TABLE 38–3 Ophthalmic: Antiinflammatories

Generic (Brand)	Route and Dosage*	Uses and Considerations
Dexamethasone (AK-Dex Ophthalmic, Maridex Ophthalmic)	A&C: Oint: Apply into conjunctival sac t.i.d./q.i.d.; gradually decrease to discontinue Susp: Instill 2 gtt qh while awake and q2h during night; taper to q3–4h; then t.i.d./q.i.d.	For uveitis, allergic conditions, and inflammation of conjunctiva, cornea, and lids. Should not be used for minor abrasions and wounds. *Pregnancy category:* C; PB: NA; t½: NA
Diclofenac Na (Voltaren)	A: 1 gt to affected eye q.i.d. for 2 wk; start 24 h after cataract surgery	*Pregnancy category:* B; PB: NA; t½: NA
Flurbiprofen Na (Ocufen)	A: Instill 1 gt q30 min 2 h before surgery, total dose is 4 gtt	To decrease corneal edema; miosis. *Pregnancy category:* C; PB: NA; t½: NA
Suprofen (Profenal)	*Preoperative:* A: Instill 2 gtt in sac q4h while awake on day preceding surgery; instill 2 gtt in conjunctival sac at 3, 2, and 1 h before surgery	Used to prevent intraoperative miosis. *Pregnancy category:* C; PB: NA; t½: NA
Ketorolac tromethamine (Acular)	A: 0.5% sol: Instill 1 gt q.i.d.	Nonsteroidal. Efficacy has not been established beyond 1 wk of therapy. Used for the relief of itching associated with seasonal allergic conjunctivitis. *Pregnancy category:* C; PB: NA; t½: NA

Table continued on following page

TABLE 38–3 Ophthalmic: Antiinflammatories *(Continued)*

Generic (Brand)	Route and Dosage*	Uses and Considerations
Medrysone (HMS Liquifilm)	A&C: Susp: Initially: Instill 1 gt in conjunctival sac q1–2h (1–2 d); then 1 gt b.i.d./q.i.d.	To treat allergic conditions, burns, inflammation of conjunctiva, cornea, and lids. *Pregnancy category:* C; PB: NA; t½: NA
Prednisolone acetate (Econopred, Predforte)	A: Initially: Instill 1–2 gtt in conjunctival sac qh while awake, q2h during night until desired effect; maint: 1 gt q4h Susp: 0.125% and 1%	Steroidal. To treat uveitis, allergic conditions, burns, inflammation of conjunctiva, cornea, and lids. *Pregnancy category:* C; PB: NA; t½: NA
Prednisolone Na phosphate (AK-Pred, Inflamase)	Sol: 0.125% and 1%	

* To minimize systemic absorption, apply gentle pressure to inner canthus.
KEY: A: adult; C: child; gt: drop; gtt: drops; oint: ointment; PB: protein-binding: sol: solution; susp: suspension; t½: half-life; NA: not applicable.

ness of the eyes" use lubricants as artificial tears; lubricants are also used to moisten contact lenses or artificial eyes. Lubricants are used to alleviate discomfort associated with dryness and to maintain integrity of the epithelial surface. Lubricants are also used during anesthesia and in acute or chronic central nervous system (CNS) disorders that result in unconsciousness or decreased blinking.

Most lubricants are available over-the-counter (OTC) in both liquid and ointment form. Popular lubricants are Isopto Tears, Tearisol, Ultra Tears, Tears Naturale, Tears Plus, Lens Mate, and Lacri-Lube. Be alert to allergic response to preservatives in lubricants.

MIOTICS

In open-angle glaucoma, miotics are used to lower the intraocular pressure, thereby increasing blood flow to the retina and decreasing retinal damage and loss of vision. Direct-acting cholinergics and cholinesterase inhibitors, the two types of miotics, differ in their mechanism of action. Miotics cause a contraction of the ciliary muscle and widening of trabecular meshwork. Figure 38–1 illustrates increased intraocular pressure resulting in glaucoma.

Table 38–4 presents the drug data for miotics.

Pharmacokinetics

Systemic absorption is possible but not common with the use of miotics. Pilocarpine binds to the ocular tissues; its half-life is unknown. The metabolism and elimination of this drug are also currently unknown.

Pharmacodynamics

Pilocarpine produces **miosis** and decreases intraocular pressure. The onset of action, peak, and duration of action vary with the dose, desired effect, and form. The onset of action of pilocarpine given to produce miosis is 10 to 30 min, the time of peak action is unknown, and the duration of action is 4 to 8 h. When used to reduce intraocular pressure, ophthalmic pilocarpine has an unknown onset of action, peak time of 75 min, and duration of action of 4 to 14 h. With the ocular therapeutic system Ocusert, the onset of action is unknown, the peak is 1.5 to 2 h, and the duration of action is 7 d.

Ocusert is a wafer-thin disk impregnated with time-release pilocarpine. The disk is replaced every 7 d. Clients should check for presence of the Ocusert disk in the conjunctival sac daily at bedtime and on arising.

The drug data for pilocarpine are shown in Figure 38–2.

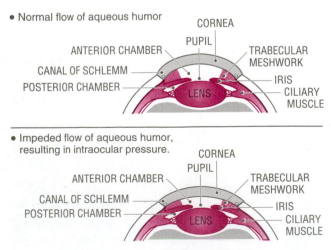

FIGURE 38–1 Increased intraocular pressure.

TABLE 38–4 Miotics: Cholinergics and Beta-Adrenergic Blockers

Generic (Brand)	Route and Dosage	Uses and Considerations
Direct-Acting Cholinergics Acetylcholine Cl (Miochol)	A: Intraocular: 0.5–2 ml of 1% sol injected in anterior chamber before or after suturing	To achieve miosis in cataract and other anterior segment surgery. *Pregnancy category:* C; PB: NA; t½: NA
Carbachol intraocular (Miostat)	A: Ophthalmic: 1–2 gtt 1–4 × d A: IO: 0.5 mL into anterior chamber before or after suturing	For miosis during eye surgery. To reduce intraocular pressure, especially when pilocarpine is ineffective. *Pregnancy category:* C; PB: NA; t½: NA
Pilocarpine HCl (Isopto Carpine)	See Prototype Drug Chart (Fig. 38–2)	
Pilocarpine nitrate (Ocusert Pilo-20, Pilo-40)	See Prototype Drug Chart (Fig. 38–2)	
Echothiophate iodide (Phospholine Iodide)	A: 0.03%–0.25% sol: 1 gt daily/b.i.d.	Used to treat chronic open-angle glaucoma and glaucoma following cataract surgery. *Pregnancy category:* C, PB: NA; t½: NA
Indirect-Acting Cholinesterase Inhibitors: Short Acting Physostigmine salicylate (Isopto Eserine)	A&C: Oint 0.25%: ¼ inch up to 3 × d Sol 0.25–0.5%: 1–2 gtt daily/q.i.d.	For wide-angle glaucoma. *Pregnancy category:* C; PB: NA; t½: NA
Long-Acting Demecarium bromide (Humorsol)	A: Sol 0.125–0.25%: 1–2 gtt 2 × wk or 1–2 gtt b.i.d.	Used for open-angle glaucoma when shorter-acting agents have been unsuccessful, conditions affecting aqueous outflow, accommodative strabismus. *Pregnancy category:* C; PB: NA; t½: NA
Isoflurophate (Floropryl)	A&C: Oint 0.025%: 0.5 cm daily for 2 wk, then eventually decrease to q2–7d.	For primary open-angle glaucoma and conditions with obstructed aqueous outflow. Also for convergent strabismus. To maintain potency, keep tip of tube dry. *Pregnancy category:* C; PB: NA; t½: NA
Beta-Adrenergic Blockers Betaxolol HCl (Betoptic)	0.25% susp or 0.5% sol: Usual dose: 1 gt b.i.d.	Beta blockers. Used to decrease elevated intraocular pressure in chronic open-angle glaucoma and ocular hypertension. Contraindicated in clients with asthma due to increased airway resistance from systemic absorption. Use caution in clients receiving oral beta blockers. *Pregnancy category:* C; PB: NA; t½: NA
Levobunolol HCl (Betagan Liquifilm)	0.25%–0.5% sol: 1–2 gtt daily/b.i.d.	Lowers intraocular pressure. *Pregnancy category:* C; PB: NA; t½: NA
Timolol maleate (Timoptic)	A: Sol 0.25%–0.5% initially: 1 gt b.i.d.; maint: 1 drop daily once response occurs with initial dosage	Reduces production of aqueous humor. Monitor vital signs during initial therapy. Concurrent use of similar drugs must be individualized. Blurred vision decreases with use. *Pregnancy category:* C; PB: NA; t½: NA

KEY: A: adult; C: child; NA: not applicable; oint: ointment; PB: protein-binding; sol: solution; susp: suspension; t½: half-life; gt: drop; gtt: drops.

Contraindications

Contraindications to pilocarpine include retinal detachment, adhesions between the iris and lens, and acute ocular infections. Caution is advised for clients with the following conditions: asthma, hypertension, corneal abrasion, hyperthyroidism, coronary vascular disease, urinary tract obstruction, gastrointestinal (GI) obstruction, ulcer disease, parkinsonism, and bradycardia.

FIGURE 38–2. Direct-acting Miotic

Miotic	Dosage	NURSING PROCESS
Pilocarpine (Isopto Carpine, Pilopine HS, Ocusert Pilo-20 and -40) *Pregnancy Category:* C	A&C: sol: 1–2%, 1–2 gtt, t.i.d./q.i.d. Gel: Apply 0.5-in ribbon in lower eyelid at bedtime Ocusert: Replaced q7d	Assessment and Planning

Contraindications	Drug-Lab-Food Interactions
Retinal detachment, adhesions between iris and lens, acute ocular inflammation; must avoid systemic absorption of drug with coronary artery disease, obstruction of GI/GU tract, epilepsy, asthma	Avoid use with carbachol and echothiophate *Decrease* antiglaucoma effects with belladonna alkaloids, *decrease* dilation with phenylephrine

Pharmacokinetics	Pharmacodynamics	Interventions
Absorption: PO: Some systemic absorption *Distribution:* PB: UK *Metabolism:* $t\frac{1}{2}$: UK; binds to ocular tissue *Excretion:* UK	*Miosis:* Ophthalmic: Onset: 10–30 min Peak: 20 min Duration: 4–8 h *Reduce IOP:* Ophthalmic: Onset: 45–60 min Peak: 75 min Duration: 4–14 h Ocusert: Onset: 1 h Peak: 1.5–2 h Duration: 7 d Gel: Onset: 1 h Peak: 3–12 h Duration: 18–24 h	

	Evaluation
Therapeutic Effects/Uses: To induce miosis; to decrease IOP in glaucoma. *Mode of Action:* Stimulation of pupillary and ciliary sphincter muscles.	

Side Effects	Adverse Reactions
Blurred vision, eye pain, headache, eye irritation, brow ache, stinging and burning, nausea, vomiting, diarrhea, increased salivation and sweating, muscle tremors, contact allergy Conjunctival irritation with Ocusert	Dyspnea, hypertension, tachycardia, retinal detachment; long term: bronchospasm Corneal abrasion and visual impairment potential with Ocusert

KEY: A: adult; C: child; IOP: intraocular pressure; PB: protein-binding; sol: solution; $t\frac{1}{2}$: half-life; UK: unknown.

Drug Interactions

Ophthalmic epinephrine, timolol, levobunolol, betaxolol, and systemic carbonic anhydrase inhibitors have the added effect of lowering intraocular pressure. Cyclopentolate, ophthalmic belladonna alkaloids, and antidepressants antagonize the therapeutic effects.

Use of beta-adrenergic blockers, such as betaxolol hydrochloride, levobunolol hydrochloride, and timolol maleate, represents the most recent approach to the treatment of open-angle glaucoma. Refer to

Chapter 18 for a comprehensive discussion of adrenergic blockers. The commonly prescribed miotics are listed in Table 38–4. Figure 38–2 presents the actions and effects of pilocarpine.

Side Effects and Adverse Reactions

Miotic side effects include headache, eye pain, decreased vision, brow pain, and, less frequently, hyperemia of the conjunctiva. Systemic absorption can cause nausea, vomiting, diarrhea, frequent urination, precipitation of attacks in asthma clients, increased salivation, diaphoresis, muscle weakness, and respiratory difficulty. Manifestations of toxicity include vertigo, bradycardia, tremors, hypotension, syncope, cardiac dysrhythmias, and seizures. Atropine sulfate must be available in case of systemic toxicity.

NURSING PROCESS: MIOTICS

ASSESSMENT

- Obtain medical and drug history. Miotics are contraindicated in clients with narrow-angle glaucoma, acute inflammation of the eye, heart block, coronary artery disease, obstruction of the GI and/or urinary tracts, and asthma.
- Check vital signs (VS). Baseline VS can be compared with future findings.
- Assess the client's level of anxiety. The possibility of diminished vision or blindness increases anxiety.
- Assess client's eye pigment; clients with dark, heavily pigmented eyes may benefit from a pilocarpine concentration greater than 4%.

POTENTIAL NURSING DIAGNOSES

- Altered visual perception
- High risk for injury

PLANNING

- Client will take miotics as prescribed.
- Client's intraocular pressure will decrease and be within the accepted range.

NURSING INTERVENTIONS

- When administering eye drops, apply gentle pressure to the inner canthus to prevent or minimize systemic absorption.
- Monitor VS. Heart rate and blood pressure may decrease with large doses of cholinergics.
- Monitor for side effects such as headache, eye pain, and decreased vision.
- Monitor for postural hypotension. Instruct client to rise slowly from a recumbent position.
- Check breath sounds for rales and rhonchi; cholinergic drugs can cause bronchospasms and increase bronchial secretions.
- Maintain oral hygiene with excessive salivation.
- Have atropine available as antidote for pilocarpine.

- Instruct the client or family on correct administration of eye drops and ointment; include return demonstration. See Figures 3–6 and 3–7.
- Instruct client on need for regular and ongoing medical supervision.
- Instruct the client not to stop medication suddenly without prior approval of the health care provider.
- Advise client to avoid driving or operating machinery while vision is impaired.
- Instruct the client on the use of relaxation techniques for decreasing anxiety, if appropriate.
- Instruct the client with glaucoma to avoid atropine-like drugs, which increase intraocular pressure. Clients should check labels on OTC drugs or check with a pharmacist.

Ocular Therapeutic Systems (Ocusert)
- Instruct clients to follow instructions related to insertion and removal.
- Store drug in refrigerator.
- Instruct clients to check for presence of disk in conjunctival sac at bedtime and when arising.
- Discard damaged or contaminated discs.
- Explain that the myopia is minimized by bedtime insertion in the upper conjunctival sac.
- Explain that temporary stinging is expected; notify health care provider if blurred vision or brow pain occurs.

Cholinesterase Inhibitors
- First dose should be administered by health care provider and followed by tonometry reading.
- Instruct client to tightly cap tube because ointment is inactivated by water.

EVALUATION

- Evaluate the effectiveness of drug therapy and the presence of side effects. Intraocular pressure will be within desired range or reduced.

TABLE 38–5 Carbonic Anhydrase Inhibitors

Drug	Dosage	Uses and Considerations
Acetazolamide (Diamox)	A: PO: 250–1000 mg daily given in divided doses for amounts >250 mg; doses >1000 mg show no increased benefit	To reduce aqueous humor formation, thus lowering intraocular pressure. Monitor for dehydration and postural hypotension. Monitor electrolytes. Avoid hazardous activities due to drowsiness. Most frequently prescribed. *Pregnancy category:* C; PB: UK; t½: 2–6 h
Dichlorphenamide (Daranide)	A: PO: Initially: 100–200 mg followed by 100 mg q12h until desired response is obtained	As above. Can cause confusion, especially in elderly. *Pregnancy category:* C; PB: UK; t½: UK
Dorzolamide (Trusopt)	A: 2% sol: 1 gt t.i.d.	Do not use with oral carbonic anhydrase inhibitors. Side effects include burning, stinging, bitter taste. *Pregnancy category:* UK; PB: UK; t½: UK
Methazolamide (Neptazane)	A: 50–100 mg, b.i.d. or t.i.d.	Similar to Diamox and Darenide. Increases action of amphetamines. Increases effects of salicylates, lithium, and barbiturates. *Pregnancy category:* C; PB: UK; t½: 14 h

KEY: *A: adult; C: child; gt: drop; PB: protein-binding; PO: by mouth; t½: half-life; UK: unknown.*

CARBONIC ANHYDRASE INHIBITORS

Carbonic anhydrase inhibitors interfere with production of carbonic acid, which leads to decreased aqueous humor formation and decreased intraocular pressure. These drugs, which were developed as diuretics, are now used for the long-term treatment of open-angle glaucoma. It is recommended that they be used only when pilocarpine, beta blockers, epinephrine, and cholinesterase inhibitors have not been effective. Table 38–5 presents the drug data for carbonic anhydrase inhibitors.

Side Effects and Adverse Reactions

Side effects include lethargy, anorexia, drowsiness, paresthesia, depression, polyuria, nausea, vomiting, hypokalemia, and renal calculi. Clients frequently discontinue medications because of the side effects. These drugs are contraindicated during the first trimester of pregnancy. Do not use in persons allergic to sulfonamides; carbonic anhydrase inhibitors can also cause photosensitivity.

NURSING PROCESS: CARBONIC ANHYDRASE INHIBITORS

ASSESSMENT

- Obtain medical and drug history. Use is contraindicated during first trimester of pregnancy.
- Check vital signs (VS). Baseline VS can be compared with future readings.
- Assess level of anxiety. Eye disorders carrying the possibility of blindness promote high anxiety state in clients.

POTENTIAL NURSING DIAGNOSES

- Altered visual perception
- High risk for injury

PLANNING

- Client will take carbonic anhydrase inhibitors as prescribed.
- Client's intraocular pressure will decrease to within the desired range.

NURSING INTERVENTIONS

- Monitor for side effects such as lethargy, anorexia, drowsiness, polyuria, nausea, and vomiting.
- Monitor electrolytes because drug can cause hypokalemia.
- Increase fluid intake, unless contraindicated. Record intake and output; weigh daily.
- Maintain oral hygiene.

- Instruct client or family on the correct administration of eye drops and ointment. Include return demonstration. See Figures 3–6 and 3–7.
- Encourage use of artificial tears for "dry eyes."
- Encourage client to maintain oral hygiene if mouth is dry; ice chips and sugarless gum are recommended.
- Instruct client not to abruptly discontinue medication. Clients frequently discontinue drug because of side effects.

- Instruct client on need for regular and ongoing medical supervision.
- Advise client to avoid driving or operating hazardous machinery while vision is impaired.
- Advise client to avoid prolonged exposure to sunlight because of the potential for photosensitivity.

EVALUATION

- Determine effectiveness of drug therapy and presence of side effects. Intraocular pressure will be within desired range.

OSMOTICS

Osmotics are generally used preoperatively and postoperatively to decrease vitreous humor volume, thereby reducing intraocular pressure. These drugs are used primarily in the emergency treatment of acute closed-angle glaucoma because of their ability to rapidly reduce intraocular pressure. Commonly prescribed osmotic drugs are presented in Table 38–6.

Side Effects and Adverse Reactions
Osmotic medications can cause headache, nausea,

vomiting, and diarrhea. Disorientation, especially in the elderly due to electrolyte imbalances, can result from use of mannitol and urea.

ANTICHOLINERGIC MYDRIATICS AND CYCLOPLEGICS

Mydriatics dilate the pupils; **cycloplegics** paralyze the muscles of accommodation. Both are used in diagnostic procedures and ophthalmic surgery. (Refer to Chapters 17 and 19 for a review of the autonomic nervous system and comprehensive discus-

NURSING PROCESS: OSMOTICS

ASSESSMENT

- Obtain medical and drug history.
- Check vital signs (VS). Obtain baseline data to compare with future findings.
- Assess level of anxiety. Possibility of blindness increases anxiety.

POTENTIAL NURSING DIAGNOSES

- Altered visual perception
- High risk for injury

PLANNING

- Client's intraocular pressure will be lowered.

NURSING INTERVENTIONS

- Monitor for side effects.
- Monitor for potassium depletion and electrolyte imbalances.

- Increase fluid intake, unless contraindicated. Record input and output and weigh daily.
- Monitor changes in level of orientation, especially in the elderly.

- Instruct client regarding side effects of drugs.
- Osmotics are usually administered intravenously in a health care setting.

EVALUATION

- Determine the effectiveness of drug therapy and presence of side effects. Intraocular pressure will be within desired range.

TABLE 38–6 Osmotics

Drug	Dosage	Uses and Considerations
Glycerin	A: PO: 1–1.5 g/kg given 1–1.5 h prior to surgery	Decreases volume of intraocular fluid, thus lowering ocular tension. Carbohydrate; use with caution in diabetics. *Pregnancy category:* C; PB: UK; t½: 30–45 min
Isosorbide (Ismotic)	A: 45% sol, 1.5–3 g/kg, b.i.d.–q.i.d.	Monitor I&O and electrolytes. *Pregnancy category:* C; PB: UK; t½: 5–9.5 h
Mannitol (Osmitrol)	A: IV: 15–20% sol, 1.5–2 g/kg over 0.5–1h	Monitor I&O; weigh daily. Contraindicated in severe pulmonary congestion, anuria, and dehydration. Use with caution in clients with CHF. *Pregnancy category:* C; PB: UK; t½: 15–100 min
Urea (Ureaphil)	A: IV: 30% sol, 1–1.5 g/kg over 1–3 h; max: 4 mL/min C > 2y: IV: 0.5–1.5 g/kg up to 4 mL/min C < 2y: IV: 0.1 g/kg up to 4 mL/min	Monitor I&O; weigh daily. Do *not* mix with any other medication or blood. Contraindicated with intracranial bleeding and dehydration. *Pregnancy category:* C; PB: UK; t½: < 60 min

KEY: A: adult; C: child; sol: solution; IV: intravenous; I&O: intake and output; <: less than; PB: protein-binding; t½: half-life; UK: unknown; PO: by mouth; CHF: congestive heart failure.

sion of anticholinergics.) Anticholinergics cause both dilation of the pupils and paralysis of the muscles of accommodation by relaxing the ciliary and dilator muscles of the iris by blocking acetylcholine. Commonly prescribed anticholinergic mydriatics and cycloplegics are presented in Table 38–7.

Side Effects and Adverse Reactions

Cycloplegics

Cycloplegics can cause tachycardia, photophobia, dryness of the mouth, edema, conjunctivitis, and dermatitis. Symptoms of atropine toxicity include dry mouth, blurred vision, photophobia, constipation, fever, tachycardia, confusion, hallucinations, delirium, and coma. Toxicity is treated with physostigmine. Cycloplegics are contraindicated in clients with glaucoma because of increased intraocular pressure.

Adrenergic Mydriatics

Side effects include headache, brow pain, allergic reaction, and worsening of narrow-angle glaucoma. Adrenergic mydriatics are contraindicated in cardiac dysrhythmias and cerebral atherosclerosis and should be used with caution in the elderly and clients with prostatic hypertrophy, diabetes mellitus, or parkinsonism. Notify the health careprovider of blurring of vision or loss of sight, difficulty in breathing, sweating, or flushing.

ADMINISTRATION OF EYE DROPS AND OINTMENTS

The techniques for administering eye drops and ointments are described in Tables 3–5 and 3–6 and illustrated in Figures 3–6 and 3–7.

CLIENTS WITH EYE DISORDERS: GENERAL SUGGESTIONS FOR CLIENT TEACHING

- Eye disorders carrying the possibility of blindness promote a high anxiety state in clients. Provide time, instructions, and return demonstration in all teaching plans.
- Use caution with confused or forgetful clients in order to prevent overdose.
- Instruct client or family in proper administration of eye drops or ointment. Maintain sterile technique and prevent dropper contamination. Expect some blurriness from ointments. Apply at bedtime, if possible, to avoid safety problems from diminished vision.
- Instruct client to report changes in vision, blurring, loss of vision, difficulty in breathing, or flushing.
- Instruct client to store drug in light-resistant container away from heat.
- Instruct client not to suddenly stop medication without *prior* approval from the prescribing health care provider.
- Instruct client to record medications administered. Prepare a chart so the client can record when eye medications were given.
- Instruct client with glaucoma to avoid atropine-like drugs, which increase intraocular pressure. Some drugs for glaucoma are long acting and re-

TABLE 38–7 Mydriatics and Cycloplegics

Generic (Brand)	Route and Dosage*	Uses and Considerations
Atropine sulfate (BufOpto-atropine, Isopto-atropine)	A: Sol 1%: 1–2 gtt up to q.i.d. C: Sol 0.5% 1–2 gtt up to t.i.d. 1% oint: Apply in lower eyelid sac up to t.i.d.	Most potent cycloplegic. For refraction, especially in children; for iritis and uveitis. *Not* for use with glaucoma or tachycardia. Wait 5 min before using other drugs. *Pregnancy category:* C; PB: NA; t½: NA
Cyclopentolate HCl (Cyclogyl)	A: Sol 0.5%–2%: 1–2 gtt; then 1 gt in 5 min C: 1–2 gtt × 1; may repeat × 1 in 5–10 min with 0.5% or 1% sol	Mydriasis and cycloplegia for eye examination. *Pregnancy category:* C; PB: NA; t½: NA
Dipivefrin HCl (Propine)	A: Sol 0.1%; 1 gt q12h	Control of intraocular pressure in chronic open-angle glaucoma. *Pregnancy category:* B; PB: NA; t½: NA
Epinephrine HCl (Epifrin, Glaucon)	A&C: Sol 0.1%–2%: 1–2 gtt daily/b.i.d.	For open-angle glaucoma and during eye surgery. Discard brown or precipitate solution. *Pregnancy category:* C; PB: NA; t½: NA
Epinephrine borate (Epinal, Eppy/N)	*Surgery:* A: 0.5–1% sol: Instill 1–2 gtt ≤ 3 × *Open-angle glaucoma:* A: 0.5% or 1.0% sol: Instill 1 gt in eye b.i.d.	For treatment of open-angle glaucoma and during ocular surgery. Contraindicated in narrow-angle glaucoma. Monitor tonometer readings with long-term use. Increased pressor effects. *Pregnancy category:* C; PB: UK; t½: UK
Homatropine hydrobromide (Isopto Homatropine)	A&C: Sol 2% and 5%: 1–2 gtt q3–4h Cy: Use only 2%	Similar to atropine, but faster onset and shorter duration. Mydriasis and cycloplegia for eye examination. *Pregnancy category:* C; PB: NA; t½: NA
Phenylephrine HCl (AK-Dilate)	*Mydriasis:* A&C: 2.5% or 10% sol: Instill 1 gt in eye before examination *Mydriasis with vasoconstriction:* A&C >12 y: Instill 1 gt in eye; repeat × 1 in 1h PRN Cy: 2.5% sol: Instill 1 gt in eye; repeat × 1 in 1h PRN	For eye examination or surgery; treatment of wide-angle glaucoma and uveitis. *Pregnancy category:* C; PB: UK; t½: UK
Scopolamine hydrobromide (Isopto Hyoscine)	A: Sol: 0.25% 1–2 gtt 1 h before exam; 1–2 gtt for treatment up to q.i.d.	Used for clients sensitive to atropine sulfate. More rapid onset and shorter duration than atropine. *Pregnancy category:* C; PB: NA; t½: NA
Tropicamide (Mydriacyl Ophthalmic)	*Refraction:* 1%: 1–2 gtt; repeat in 5 min *Fundus exam:* 0.5%: 1–2 gtt 15–20 min before exam	Mydriasis and cycloplegia for eye exam. *Pregnancy category:* C; PB: NA; t½: NA

* To minimize systemic absorption, apply gentle pressure to lacrimal duct.
KEY: Cy: cycloplegic; A: adult; C: child; gt: drop; gtt: drops; oint: ointment; sol: solution; PB: protein-binding; t½: half-life; NA: not applicable; UK: unknown; PRN: as necessary.

quire only daily dosing if client is forgetful or needs family member or other to administer. Clients should be alerted to check labels on OTC drugs with pharmacist.

- Instruct client to carry a medical alert identification card or bracelet at all times if allergic to any medications.
- Encourage client to keep health care appointments.

DRUGS FOR DISORDERS OF THE EAR
The medications most often used to treat **otic** disorders are the same preparations used to treat similar problems in other areas of the body; e.g., antiinfectives. Refer to the appropriate chapter(s) in the text

for a comprehensive discussion of the specific drug group.

ANTIBACTERIALS
Several antibacterials are commonly prescribed for external use for otic disorders. Refer to Chapters 22, 23, and 24 on antibiotics. Table 38–8 presents the drug data for selected antibacterial medications.

Side Effects and Adverse Reactions
Side effects include overgrowth of nonsusceptible organisms. Prior hypersensitivity is a contraindication.

TABLE 38–8 Otic: Antiinfectives

Generic (Brand)	Route and Dosage	Uses and Considerations
External		
Acetic acid and aluminum acetate (Otic Domeboro)	A&C: Sol 2%: Insert saturated wick, keep moist × 24h; instill 4–6 gtt q2–3h	Provides an acid medium; has antibacterial activity. Low cost. *Pregnancy category:* UK; PB: NA; t½: NA
Boric acid (Ear-Dry) Carbamide peroxide (Debrox)	A&C > 12 y: Instill 5–10 gtt b.i.d.; tilt head to unaffected side to keep gtt in ear or put cotton plug in outer ear	OTC preparations to dry the ear canal and to loosen and remove impacted wax (cerumen) from the ear canal. Debrox—instill for up to 4 d. If no improvement, call health care provider. *Pregnancy category:* C; PB: NA; t½: NA
Chloramphenicol (Chloromycetin Otic)	A&C: 0.5% otic sol: Instill 2–3 gtt into ear t.i.d.	Topically for infections of ear canal. *Pregnancy category:* C; PB: NA; t½: NA
Polymyxin B	A&C: 3–4 gtt t.i.d./q.i.d. for 7–10 d	Usually given in combination with neomycin and hydrocortisone. For disorders of external ear. Discontinue after 10 d to prevent fungal overgrowth. *Pregnancy category:* B; PB: NA; t½: NA
Tetracycline (Achromycin)	A&C: 1–2 gtt b.i.d./q.i.d.	Similar to polymyxin B. *Pregnancy category:* D; PB: NA; t½: NA
Trolamine polypeptide oleate-condensate (Cerumenex)	A&C: Fill ear canal and insert cotton plug for 15–30 min; flush ear with lukewarm water; repeat × 1 if needed.	To loosen and remove impacted wax (cerumen) from the ear canal. *Pregnancy category:* C; PB: NA; t½: NA
Internal		
Amoxicillin (Amoxil, Augmentin)	A: PO: 250–500 mg q8h C: PO: 20–40 mg/kg/d in 3 divided doses	For treatment of otitis media. Eighty percent absorbed by mouth; food does not prevent absorption. Long duration of action. *Pregnancy category:* B; PB: 20%; t½: 1–1.5 h
Ampicillin trihydrate (Polycillin)	A: PO: 250–500 mg q6h IM/IV: 2–8 g/d in divided doses C: PO: 50–200 mg/kg/d in divided doses IM/IV: 50–200 mg/kg/d in divided doses	First broad-spectrum penicillin. Fifty percent of drug absorbed by GI tract. Effective against gram-negative and gram-positive bacteria. Individuals allergic to penicillin may also be allergic to ampicillin. *Pregnancy category:* B; PB: 15%–28%; t½: 1–2 h
Cefaclor (Ceclor)	A: PO: 250–500 mg q8h; *max,* 4 g/d C: PO: 20–40 mg/kg/d in 3 divided doses; *max:* 1 g/d	Second-generation cephalosporin. To treat ampicillin-resistant and gram-negative strains. Third-line drug for otitis media. Not for infants < 1 mo. Monitor electrolytes in long-term therapy. *Pregnancy category:* B; PB: 25%; t½: 0.5–1 h
Erythromycin (E-Mycin)	A: PO: 250–500 mg q6h IV: 1–4 g/d in 4 divided doses C: PO: 30–50 mg/kg/d in 4 divided doses IV: 20–50 mg/kg/d in 4 divided doses	To treat gram-positive and gram-negative bacterial infections in clients allergic to penicillin. Enteric-coated tablet to prevent gastric acid from destroying drug. *Pregnancy category:* B; PB: 65%; t½: PO, 1–2 h; IV, 3–5 h
Penicillin (Pentids, Pen-V)	*Penicillin G:* A: PO: 200,000–500,000 U q6h IM: 500,000–5 million U/d in divided doses IV: 4–20 million U/d in divided doses diluted in IV solution C: PO: 25,000–90,000 U/d in divided doses IV: 50,000–100,000 U/kg/d in divided doses *Penicillin V:* A: PO: 125–500 mg q6h C: PO: 15–50 mg/kg/d in 3–4 divided doses	For otitis media and mastoiditis. Take before or after meals. Penicillin G: electrolytes should be monitored; injectable solution is clear. Penicillin V: not recommended in renal failure. *Pregnancy category:* B; PB: (G) 60%, (V) 80%; t½: (G) 0.5–1 h, (V) 0.5 h

TABLE 38–8 Otic: Antiinfectives *(Continued)*

Generic (Brand)	Route and Dosage	Uses and Considerations
Sulfonamides (Azulfidine [sulfasalazine], Gantrisin [sulfisoxazole], Bactrim [trimethoprim and sulfamethoxazole])	Dose and route vary See Chapter 24	Most are highly protein-bound. Increase fluid intake to decrease crystalluria. Side effects include allergic response. Blood disorders may result from long-term use and high doses. Avoid in third trimester of pregnancy. *Pregnancy category:* B, D; PB: 50–95%; t½: 4.5–12 h
Clarithromycin (Biaxin)	A: PO: 250–500 mg q12h C: PO: 7.5 mg/kg q12h	For otitis media. Cautious use in renal impairment. Efficacy not established in children < 12 y. *Pregnancy category:* C; PB: UK; t½: 3–5 h
Amoxicillin and potassium clavulanate (Augmentin)	A: PO: 250 mg q8h C: PO: 40 mg/kg/day divided q8h	For otitis media. Clavulanate inhibits beta lactamase degradation of amoxicillin. *Pregnancy category:* B; PB: UK; t½: 1–3 h
Loracarbef (Lorabid)	A: PO: 200 mg q12h C: PO: 30 mg/kg/day q12h	For otitis media. Second-generation cephalosporin. Cautious use in renal impairment and seizures. *Pregnancy category:* B; PB: UK; t½: 45–60 min

KEY: A: adult; C: child; PO: by mouth; IM: intramuscular; IV: intravenous; gtt: drops; sol: solution; <: less than; PB: protein-binding; t½: half-life; NA: not applicable; UK: unknown; OTC: over-the-counter.

NURSING PROCESS: ANTIINFECTIVES FOR EAR DISORDERS

ASSESSMENT

- Obtain a medical and drug history including any allergies.
- Check vital signs (VS). Obtain baseline data that can be compared with future findings.

POTENTIAL NURSING DIAGNOSES

- Altered auditory perception
- Pain

PLANNING

- Client will be free of ear infection after completion of drug regimen.

NURSING INTERVENTIONS

- Complete culture and sensitivity before starting drug.
- Monitor input and output.
- Report hematuria or oliguria. High doses of antibacterials are nephrotoxic.
- Relief of associated pain, if present.
- Monitor renal function, liver studies, and blood studies (white cell count, red cell count, hemoglobin and hematocrit, bleeding time).
- Store medication in airtight container.
- Report dizziness to health care provider.
- Report fatigue, fever, or sore throat, any of which could indicate superimposed infection.

CLIENT TEACHING

- Instruct client to complete entire course of medication (10 to 14 d) and *not* to stop medication when he or she "feels better."
- Encourage client to eat yogurt or buttermilk to maintain intestinal flora.
- If client is prone to otitis secondary to swimming or in warm weather, instruct him or her to keep ear canals dry; instillation of drops of alcohol into the ear canal may be helpful. Check with the health care provider.
- Instruct client to have medical alert identification with him or her at all times if allergic to medications.

EVALUATION

- Determine the effectiveness of drug therapy and the presence of side effects.

ANTIHISTAMINE-DECONGESTANTS

Antihistamine-decongestants are thought to reduce nasal and middle ear congestion in acute otitis media. (Refer to Chapter 30 for a comprehensive discussion of upper respiratory agents.) Reduction of the edema around the orifice of the eustachian tube promotes drainage from the middle ear. There are numerous antihistamine-decongestant medications on the market, including Actifed, Allerest, Dimetapp, Drixoral, Novafed, Ornade, Phenergan, and Triaminic. Common side effects are drowsiness, blurred vision, and dry mucous membranes.

COMBINATION PRODUCTS

Combination products such as Cortisporin Otic are not held in high regard by most health care providers. This is based on the maxim that only what is needed should be used. These drugs combine local anesthetics or antiinflammatory drugs with antiinfectives.

CERUMINOLYTICS

Cerumen (earwax), produced by glands in the outer half of the ear canal, usually moves to the external os by itself and is washed away. However, **ceruminolytics** are sometimes needed to loosen and remove impacted cerumen from the ear canal. Irrigation with hydrogen peroxide solution (3% diluted to half strength with water) can be done to flush cerumen deposits out of the ear canal. For chronic impaction, 1 to 2 gtt of olive oil or mineral oil will soften the wax. Cerumenex (prescription) and Debrox (OTC) cost more and are no more effective than hydrogen peroxide solution.

ADMINISTRATION OF EAR MEDICATIONS

Ear medications are generally contained in a liquid vehicle for ease of administration. Guidelines for the administration of ear drops are given in Table 3–7 and Figure 3–8A and B.

Irrigation

Irrigations of the ear may also be ordered. Irrigation is best accomplished when there is direct visualization of the tympanic membrane (eardrum). It must be done *gently* to avoid damage to the eardrum. Frequently used irrigating solutions include Burow's solution, hydrogen peroxide 3% (with water), hypertonic sodium chloride solution 3%, and acetic acid (vinegar) solution. Contraindications include perforation of the eardrum and prior hypersensitivity.

CLIENTS WITH EAR DISORDERS: GENERAL SUGGESTIONS FOR CLIENT TEACHING

- Instruct client not to insert any foreign objects into the ear canal.
- Instruct client to take drug as prescribed.
- Instruct client to keep drug in light-resistant container.
- Instruct client about expected effect of drug, dosage, and side effects, and when to notify health care provider.
- Encourage client to keep follow-up appointments.

■ CASE STUDY
Pediatric Client with an Ear Infection

Mrs. Z. brings 7-year-old Chris to the HMO practice because he has been complaining of "pain in my ear" for 2 days. Following an assessment, the health care provider determines that Chris has an infection in the external right ear canal. Polymyxin B is prescribed to be administered 3 to 4 gtt, t.i.d. for 14 days.

1. Is the drug regimen appropriate for Chris? What is the nurse's responsibility?
2. What is a consequence of long-term use of this drug?
3. What drug may be used in combination to decrease edema, itching, and redness?

Client teaching is an integral part of the therapeutic drug regimen. Explain the role of the nurse in relation to the following:

4. What position should Chris be in to receive the drugs?
5. What instructions would you give Mrs. Z. regarding the administration of ear drops, including the actual positioning of the ear prior to administering the drops? In what way would you modify these instructions if the child were 2 years old?
6. What advice do you give Chris about putting things in his ear?

STUDY QUESTIONS

1. Miotics are used in the treatment of what disorders? What is the mechanism of action of miotics?
2. What information would be required in a teaching plan for a client receiving pilocarpine?
3. What drug is the most potent cycloplegic? What are the nursing implications of the use of this medication?
4. The client E.H., aged 85 years, was just started on acetazolamide. What category of drug is this? What is the brand name? What are the nursing interventions associated with clients receiving this drug?
5. Mrs. H. has been on pilocarpine for several days. She tells you that she must need new glasses because newsprint and TV picture are a bit "fuzzy." Is any action indicated? If so, what?
6. Mannitol is a commonly used osmotic. What are the contraindications for use of this drug?
7. Your client is being prepared for an eye examination. In taking the health history, you discover she is sensitive to atropine sulfate. What drug might be used instead for the examination?
8. Describe appropriate general teaching strategies for clients with eye disorders.
9. What is included in the nursing assessment of the client prior to the start of an antibacterial drug for the treatment of an ear infection?

Chapter 39

Drugs for Dermatologic Disorders

OUTLINE

Objectives
Terms
Introduction
Acne Vulgaris
Psoriasis
    Side Effects and Adverse
      Reactions
    Nursing Process

Drug-Induced Dermatitis
Contact Dermatitis
Hair Loss and Baldness
Burns and Burn Preparations
    Mafenide Acetate
    Silver Sulfadiazine
    Nursing Process

Study Questions

OBJECTIVES

Define acne vulgaris, psoriasis, drug-induced dermatitis, and contact dermatitis.

Describe nonpharmacologic measures for treating mild acne vulgaris.

List three drugs that can cause drug-induced dermatitis and their characteristic symptoms.

Identify the topical antibacterial agents used in prevention and treatment of burn tissue infection.

Describe nursing process, including client teaching, related to commonly used drugs for acne vulgaris, psoriasis, and burns.

TERMS

acne vulgaris
contact dermatitis
macule

papule
plaques
psoriasis

tinea capitis
tinea pedis
vesicle

INTRODUCTION

There are numerous skin lesions and eruptions requiring mild to aggressive drug therapy. Some of the skin disorders include acne vulgaris, psoriasis, eczema dermatitis, contact dermatitis, drug-induced dermatitis, and burn infection. Skin eruptions may result from viral infections (e.g., herpes simplex, herpes zoster) and from fungal infections (e.g., **tinea pedis** [athlete's foot], **tinea capitis** [ringworm]), as well as from bacterial infections. These skin eruptions may be treated with over-the-counter (OTC) drugs and will not be discussed in this chapter. Antiviral drugs are presented in Chapter 26.

Most of the treatments for skin eruptions include topical creams, ointments, pastes, lotions, and solutions. Skin lesions may appear as **macules** (flat with varying colors), **papules** (raised, palpable, and less than 1 cm in diameter), **vesicles** (raised, filled with fluid, and less than 1 cm in diameter), or **plaques** (hard, rough raised, and flat on top). Selected skin disorders and their drug therapy regimens are discussed separately.

ACNE VULGARIS

Acne vulgaris is the formation of papules, nodules, and cysts on the face, neck, shoulders, and back resulting from keratin plugs at the base of the pilosebaceous oil glands near the hair follicles. Ninety percent of persons with acne are adolescents. The increase in androgen production that occurs during adolescence increases the production of sebum, an oily skin lubricant. The sebum combines with keratin to form a plug.

Nonpharmacologic measures should be tried before drug therapy is initiated. A prescribed or suggested cleansing agent is necessary with all types of acne. Skin should be gently cleansed several times a day. Vigorous scrubbing should be avoided. Well-balanced diet is indicated. Megadoses of vitamin A were once used for treating acne. Vitamin A is fat-soluble and is retained in tissues, especially the liver, for long periods; excessive doses of vitamin A, therefore, can be highly toxic, so megadosing with vitamin A is no longer a valid therapy for treating acne. High doses of vitamin A may also cause teratogenic effects to a fetus. Decreasing emotional stress and increasing emotional support are suggested. If drug therapy is necessary, the nonpharmacologic measures should be maintained.

Mild acne may require gentle cleansing and the use of keratolytics (keratin dissolvers, such as ben-zoyl peroxide, resorcinol, salicylic acid). Benzoyl peroxide is applied as a cream, lotion, or gel once or twice a day. This agent loosens the outer, horny layer of the epidermis. Moderate acne requires a stronger concentration of benzoyl peroxide (10%), and topical antibiotics, such as tetracycline, erythromycin, clindamycin, or meclocycline, may be used. Erythromycin and clindomycin are most frequently prescribed with fewest side effects. Oral tetracycline may be part of the drug regimen. For severe acne, oral antibiotics (tetracycline [drug of choice] or erythromycin), and topical glucocorticoids may be prescribed. Tetracycline inhibits bacterial protein synthesis. It is used in the treatment of acne with a lower maintenance dose over a period of months. Tetracycline should not be taken with antacids or milk products, because these bind the tetracycline into an insoluble compound, thus decreasing its absorption. A major side effect of tetracycline is photosensitivity. Exposure to the sun can result in a severe sunburn. Tetracycline should not be taken when pregnant because of possible teratogenic effects on the fetus.

PSORIASIS

Psoriasis is a chronic skin disorder that affects 1% to 2% of the U.S. population. It is more common in whites than blacks. Onset of psoriasis may be as early as at age 10 years but usually appears before the age of 30 years. Psoriasis is characterized by erythematous papules and plaques covered with silvery scales. It appears on the scalp, elbows, palms of the hands, knees, and soles of the feet. With psoriasis, epidermal cell growth and epidermal turnover is accelerated to approximately five times the normal expected epidermal growth. Antipsoriatic drug therapy uses preparations such as coal tar products and anthralin to keep the psoriasis in check; however, there are usually periods of remission and exacerbation.

The psoriatic scales may be loosened with keratolytics (salicylic acid, sulfur). Topical glucocorticoids are used at times for mild psoriasis. The anticancer drug methotrexate, which slows high growth fraction, is prescribed to decrease the acceleration of epidermal cell growth in severe psoriasis. Ultraviolet light may be used to suppress mitotic (cell division) activity. Photochemotherapy, a combination of ultraviolet radiation with methoxsalen (photosensitive drug), is used to decrease proliferation of epidermal cells. Table 39–1 lists the drugs used for controlling psoriasis and acne vulgaris.

TABLE 39–1 Drugs for Acne Vulgaris and Psoriasis

Drug	Dosage	Uses and Considerations
Acne Vulgaris		
Systemic Preparations		
Tetracycline (Sumycin)	A: PO: 250–500 mg, b.i.d.	For moderate to severe acne. Inexpensive. Should not be taken during pregnancy. Should not be taken with milk products or antacids. *Pregnancy category:* D; PB: 65%; t½: 6–12 h
Erythromycin (E-Mycin)	A: PO: 250–500 mg, b.i.d.	For moderate to severe acne. A substitute for tetracycline. *Pregnancy category:* B; PB: 75%–90%; t½: 1.5–2 h
Isotretinoin (Accutane)	A: PO: 0.5–2 mg/kg/d, in 2 divided doses, for 15 wk	For severe acne. Decreases sebum secretion. Used when oral antibiotics have failed. Avoid use with tetracycline and vitamin A to reduce toxic effects. *Pregnancy category:* X; PB: 99%; t½: 10–20 h
Topical Preparations		
Keratolytic Agents		
Benzoyl peroxide (Benzac, Persa-Gel)	2.5%–10%, once to four times/d (cream, gel, or lotion)	For mild to moderate acne. Promotes keratolysis (removal of horny layer of the epidermis). May cause skin irritation (burning, blistering, or swelling)
Salicylic acid (Sebulex)	*Antiacne/antiseborrheic:* 2%–10%, cream, gel, shampoo Use as directed	For mild to moderate acne. Promotes desquamation
Resorcinol (Bicozene)	1%–10% cream, ointment, lotion, and shampoo	For mild to moderate acne
Resorcinol and sulfur	2% resorcinol + 5% sulfur 2% resorcin + 8% sulfur Use as directed	For mild to moderate acne
Antibiotics		
Tetracycline	Ointment: 3%; sol: 2.2 mg/mL	For moderate acne. *Pregnancy category:* B
Erythromycin	Ointment: 2%; gel: 1.5%–2%	
Clindamycin (Cleocin)	Gel: ⅕; lotion: 1%; sol: 1%	
Meclocycline (Meclan)	Ointment, b.i.d.	
Tretinoin (Retin-A)	Cream: 0.05%–0.1% Gel: 0.025%–0.1% Liquid: 0.05% daily, h.s.	For mild to moderate acne. Vitamin A derivative. May be used with benzoyl peroxide or topical antibiotic. Should not be applied to open wounds. Area should be cleansed first. *Pregnancy category:* B
Psoriasis		
Methoxsalen (Oxsoralen)	A: PO: 10–20 mg, 2 h before exposure to therapeutic ultraviolet rays. Topical application before exposure to ultraviolet rays	For severe psoriasis. Systemic antimetabolite drug. Avoid during pregnancy. Avoid sunlight during drug therapy; sunlight could cause burning and blistering. *Pregnancy category:* C; PB: 80%–90%; t½: >2 h
Etretinate (Tegison)	A: PO: 0.5–0.75 mg/kg/d, in divided doses, not to exceed 1.5 mg/kg/d	For recalcitrant psoriasis. Related to vitamin A. It may take up to 1–6 mo for a response to treatment. *Pregnancy category:* X; PB: 99%; t½: 4–8 d
Topical Preparations		
Coal Tar (Estar, Psorigel)	Shampoos, creams, gel, paste, soap, ointment, lotion, solution	For mild to moderate psoriasis. Suppresses DNA synthesis, decreasing mitotic activity. May stain clothing, skin, and hair
Anthralin (Anthra-Derm)	0.1%–1.0% ointment and creams	For moderate-type psoriasis. It inhibits DNA synthesis, thus suppressing proliferation of the epidermal cells. It can stain clothing, skin, and hair
Keratolytic Drugs		
Salicylic acid, sulfur, resorcinol		See acne vulgaris

KEY: *A: adult; PO: by mouth; PB: protein-binding; sol: solution; t½: half-life; >: greater than.*

SIDE EFFECTS AND ADVERSE REACTIONS

Acne Vulgaris

Tetracycline

Nausea, vomiting, diarrhea, rash, urticaria, photosensitivity. **Adverse Reactions:** Oral candidiasis, superinfection, blood dyscrasias, hepatotoxicity, and nephrotoxicity.

Isotretinoin

Nosebleeds; dryness of the nose, mouth, especially in corners of mouth, and skin; inflamed eyes; pruritus; photosensitivity; anorexia, nausea, vomiting; elevated liver enzymes. **Adverse Reactions:** Thrombocytopenia, hematuria.

Benzoyl Peroxide

Dry and irritated skin with burning, scaling, and swelling.

Tretinoin

Skin irritation, such as burning, swelling, blistering, and peeling.

Psoriasis

Coal Tar

Skin irritation, such as burning; photosensitivity; and staining effect.

Anthralin

Erythema (redness) to normal skin, inflamed eyes, and staining effect.

Methoxsalen

Nausea, headache, vertigo, rash, pruritus, burning and peeling of skin. **Adverse Reactions:** Anemia, leukopenia, thrombocytopenia, ulcerative stomatitis, bleeding; alopecia, cystitis.

Etretinate

Anorexia, vomiting, dry skin and nasal mucosa, rash, pruritus, fatigue, bone or joint pain, peeling of skin, photosensitivity. **Adverse Reactions:** Alopecia, cardiac dysrhythmias, hepatitis, hematuria.

NURSING PROCESS: ACNE VULGARIS AND PSORIASIS

ASSESSMENT

- Obtain a history from the client of the onset of skin lesions. Note if there is a familial history of the skin disorder.
- Assess the client's skin eruptions. Describe the lesions, location, and drainage, if present.
- Assess the psychologic effect from skin lesions and changes in body image.
- Obtain a culture of a purulent draining skin lesion.
- Obtain baseline vital signs (VS). Report any elevation in temperature.

POTENTIAL NURSING DIAGNOSES

- High risk for impaired skin integrity
- High risk for infection
- Body image disturbance related to skin lesions.

PLANNING

- The client's skin lesions will be decreased in size or will be absent after drug therapy and skin care.

NURSING INTERVENTIONS

- Apply topical medications to the skin lesions using aseptic technique.
- Monitor VS and report abnormal findings.
- Check the lesion sites during drug therapy for improvement or adverse reactions to the drug therapy, such as blistering, swelling, or scaling.

CLIENT TEACHING

- Instruct the client not to use harsh cleansers on the skin. Tell the client to clean the skin several times a day.
- Teach the client how to apply topical ointments and creams using a clean technique.
- Teach the client about the side effects and adverse reactions associated with the drugs being taken.
- Tell the client to report abnormal findings immediately. Inform the client not to take milk or antacids with tetracycline.
- Inform the client to alert the health care provider if pregnant or there is a possibility of pregnancy.

Many agents for treating acne can cause terato-genic effects on the fetus.

• Instruct the client to keep health care appointments and have laboratory tests performed as prescribed.

EVALUATION

• Evaluate the effectiveness of the drug therapy on the skin lesions. If improvement is not apparent, drug therapy and skin care regimen may need to be changed.

DRUG-INDUCED DERMATITIS

An adverse reaction to drug therapy may result in skin lesions, which may vary from a rash, urticaria, papules, and vesicles, to life-threatening skin eruptions, such as erythema multiforme (red blisters over a large portion of the body) or Stevens-Johnson syndrome (large blisters in the oral and anogenital mucosa, pharynx, eyes, and viscera). The hypersensitive reaction to a drug is caused by the formation of sensitizing lymphocytes. If multiple drug therapy is used, the last drug given may be the cause of the hypersensitivity and skin eruptions. The usual skin reactions are a rash that may take several hours or a day to appear, and urticarias (hives), which usually take a few minutes to appear. Certain drugs, such as penicillin, are known to cause hypersensitivity.

Other drug-induced dermatitides include discoid lupus erythematosus (DLE) and exfoliative dermatitis. Hydralazine hydrochloride (Apresoline); isoniazid (INH); phenothiazines; anticonvulsants; and antidysrhythmics, such as procainamide (Pronestyl), may cause lupus-like symptoms. If lupus symptoms occur, the drug should be discontinued. Certain antibacterials and anticonvulsants may cause exfoliative dermatitis resulting in erythema of the skin, itching, scaling, and loss of body hair.

CONTACT DERMATITIS

Contact dermatitis, also called exogenous dermatitis, is caused by chemical or plant irritation. It is characterized by a skin rash with itching, swelling, blistering, oozing, or scaling at the affected skin sites. The chemical contact may include cosmetics, cleansing products (such as soaps and detergents), perfume, clothing, dyes, and topical drugs. Plant contacts include poison ivy, oak, or sumac.

Nonpharmacologic measures include avoiding direct contact with the causative irritant. Protective gloves or clothing may be necessary if the chemical is associated with work. Cleanse the skin area that has been in contact with the irritant immediately. Patch testing may be needed to determine the causal factor.

Treatment may consist of wet dressings containing Burow's solution (aluminum acetate); lotions, such as calamine, that contain zinc oxide; calcium hydroxide solution; and glycerin. Calamine lotion may contain the antihistamine diphenhydramine, and is used primarily for plant irritations. If itching persists, antipruritics (topical or systemic diphenhydramine [Benadryl]) may be used. Topical antipruritics should not be applied to open wounds or near the eyes or genital area. Other agents used as antipruritics are

1. Systemic drugs, such as cyproheptadine hydrochloride (Periactin), and trimeprazine tartrate (Temaril)
2. Antipruritic baths of oatmeal or Alpha-Keri
3. Solutions of potassium permanganate, aluminum subacetate, or normal saline
4. Glucocorticoid ointments, creams, or gels

Dexamethasone (Decadron) cream, hydrocortisone ointment or cream, methylprednisolone acetate (Medrol) ointment, triamcinolone acetonide (Aristocort), and flurandrenolide (Cordran) are examples of topical glucocorticoids that aid in alleviating dermatitis. Table 39–2 lists selected topical glucocorticoids according to their potency for relieving the itching and inflammation associated with dermatitis.

A portion of topical glucocorticoids can be systemically absorbed into the circulation, the amount and rate of absorption depending on the vehicle (cream, lotion), drug concentration, drug composition, and skin area to which the glucocorticoid is applied. Absorption is greater where the skin is more permeable: at the face, scalp, eyelids, neck, axilla, and genital area. Side effects and adverse reactions may occur with prolonged use of the topical drug and if the drug is continuously covered with a dressing. Prolonged use of topical glucocorticoids can cause thinning of the skin with atrophy of the epidermis and dermis, and purpura from small-vessel eruptions.

HAIR LOSS AND BALDNESS

When the hair shaft is lost and the hair follicle cannot regenerate, male pattern baldness, or alopecia, occurs. Permanent hair loss is associated with a familial history and occurs during the aging process, earlier in some individuals than others. Drugs and

TABLE 39–2 Topical Glucocorticoids

Potency	Drug Name	Drug Form
High	Amcinonide 0.1% (Cyclocort)	Cream, ointment
	Betamethasone dipropionate 0.05% (Diprosone)	Cream, ointment, lotion
	Desoximetasone 0.25% (Topicort)	Cream, ointment
	Desoximetasone 0.05%	Gel
	Diflorasone diacetate 0.05% (Florone)	Cream, ointment
	Halcinonide 0.1% (Halog)	Cream, ointment
	Triamcinolone acetonide 0.5% (Aristocort A, Kenalog)	Cream, ointment
Moderate	Betamethasone benzoate 0.025% (Benisone)	Cream, ointment
	Betamethasone valerate 0.1% (Valisone)	Cream, ointment, lotion
	Desoximetasone 0.05% (Topicort LP)	Cream, gel
	Fluocinolone acetonide 0.025% (Fluonid)	Cream, ointment
	Flurandrenolide 0.025% (Cordran, Cordran SP)	Cream, ointment, lotion
	Halcinonide 0.025% (Halog)	Cream, ointment
	Hydrocortisone valerate 0.2% (Westcort)	Cream, ointment
	Mometasone furoate 0.1% (Elocon)	Cream, ointment, lotion
	Triamcinolone acetonide 0.025%–0.1% (Aristocort A, Kenalog)	Cream, ointment, lotion
Low	Dexamethasone 0.1% (Decadron)	Cream
	Desonide 0.05% (Tridesilon)	Cream
	Fluocinolone acetonide 0.01% (Fluonid)	Solution
	Hydrocortisone 0.25%, 0.5%, 1.0%, 2.5% (Cortef, Hytone)	Cream, ointment
	Methylprednisolone acetate 0.25%, 1.0% (Medrol)	Ointment

health conditions that are also known to cause alopecia include the anticancer (antineoplastic) agents, gold salts, sulfonamides, anticonvulsants, aminoglycosides, and some of the nonsteroidal antiflammatory drugs (NSAIDs), such as indomethacin. Severe febrile illnesses, pregnancy, myxedema (condition resulting from hypothyroidism), and cancer therapies are some of the conditions contributing to temporary hair loss.

A 2% minoxidil (Rogaine) solution has been approved by the Food and Drug Administration (FDA) for treating male pattern baldness. Minoxidil causes vasodilation, thus increasing cutaneous blood flow. The increased blood flow tends to stimulate hair follicle growth. When the drug is discontinued, however, hair loss occurs within 3 to 4 months. Systemic absorption of minoxidil is minimal, so adverse reactions seldom occur. Occasionally, there may be headaches and a slight drop in systolic blood pressure.

BURNS AND BURN PREPARATIONS

Burns from heat (thermal burns), electricity (electrical burns), and chemical agents (chemical burns) can cause skin lesions. Burns are classified according to degree and tissue depth of burns and are described in Table 39–3.

A moderately severe sunburn is an example of a first-degree burn. A severe sunburn can result in a second-degree burn. A burn needs immediate attention regardless of the degree and tissue depth of the burn.

For first-degree and minor burns, cold wet compress should be applied to the burned area to constrict blood vessels and decrease swelling. This treatment also decreases the amount of pain. The quicker the burn area is cooled, the less tissue damage occurs. A nonprescription antibiotic, such as bacitracin with polymyxin B (Polysporin), may be used for minor burns. Polymyxin B and neomycin, used separately, are not drugs of choice because they do not have a broad-spectrum effect. With chemical burns, the clothing should be removed immediately and the skin thoroughly flushed with water.

Persons with second- and third-degree burns that involve dermis and subcutaneous tissue should be treated in a burn center or other hospital setting. Intravenous therapy is started immediately and a non-narcotic or narcotic analgesic is given for pain. Burn areas are cleansed with sterile saline solution

TABLE 39–3 Degree and Tissue Depth of Burns

Type	Degree	Depth	Characteristics
Superficial epidermal	First	Epidermis	Erythema (redness), painful
Partial thickness superficial	First–second	Epidermis, upper dermis	Blistering, very painful
Deep thickness	Second	Epidermis, lower dermis	Mottled, blistering, intense pain
Full thickness	Third	Epidermis, dermis, nerve ending involvement, subcutaneous tissue	Pearly white skin, charred, no pain

and an antiseptic, such as povidone-iodine (Betadine). If a povidone-iodine solution is used, it should be determined that the client is not allergic to iodine or seafood. Broad-spectrum topical antibacterials, usually effective against many gram-positive and gram-negative as well as yeast infections, are applied to burn areas to prevent infection. Examples of these antibacterials include mafenide acetate (Sulfamylon), silver sulfadiazine (Silvadene), silver nitrate 0.5% solution, and nitrofurazone (Furacin). Figure 39–1 lists the drug data for the antibacterial agent mafenide acetate (Sulfamylon).

MAFENIDE ACETATE

Pharmacokinetics

Mafenide acetate is absorbed through the skin and is metabolized by the liver to a metabolite. The drug is excreted in the urine. The drug and its metabolite are strong carbonic anhydrase inhibitors, which may lead to acid-base imbalances, such as metabolic acidosis and respiratory alkalosis, and fluid loss due to the mild diuretic effect. If respiration becomes rapid, labored, or shallow, the cream should be discontinued for a few days until the acid-base balance is restored.

Pharmacodynamics

Mafenide, a sulfonamide derivative, interferes with bacterial cell wall synthesis and metabolism and is bacteriostatic. It is used as a topical water-soluble antibacterial agent to prevent or combat a burn infection. After the burn is cleansed and debrided, 1/16 in. of mafenide cream is applied to the affected area daily or twice a day, and covered lightly with a dressing. The client may complain of a burning sensation when the drug is applied.

FIGURE 39–1. Antiinfectives: Burns

Antiinfective: Sulfonamide	Dosage	NURSING PROCESS Assessment and Planning
Mafenide acetate (Sulfamylon) *Pregnancy Category:* C	A & C: Topical: Apply ¹⁄₁₆-inch layer evenly to affected area daily/b.i.d; reapply as necessary	
Contraindications	**Drug-Lab-Food Interactions**	
Hypersensitivity, inhalation injury	None known	
Pharmacokinetics	**Pharmacodynamics**	Interventions
Absorption: Some absorbed *Distribution:* PB: UK *Metabolism:* t½: UK *Excretion:* In urine	PO: Onset: On contact Peak: 2–4 h Duration: As long as applied	

Therapeutic Effects/Uses: To treat second- and third-degree burns; to prevent organism invasion of burned tissue areas; to treat burn infections.

Mode of Action: Inhibits bacterial cell wall synthesis.

Evaluation

Side Effects	Adverse Reactions
Rash, burning sensation, urticaria, pruritus, swelling	Metabolic acidosis, respiratory alkalosis, blistering, superinfection *Life-threatening:* Bone marrow suppression, fatal hemolytic anemia

KEY: A: adult; C: child; UK: unknown; PB: protein-binding; t½: half-life.

TABLE 39–4 Topical Antiinfectives: Burns

Generic (Brand)	Route and Dosage	Uses and Considerations
Burns Nitrofurazone (Furacin)	0.2% cream, ointment, sol *Adjunctive therapy:* Apply directly or to dressing daily for 2°–3° burns; q4–5d for 2° burns with scant exudate	For second- and third-degree burns. Can cause photosensitivity, so avoid sunlight. May cause contact dermatitis. *Pregnancy category:* C; PB: NA; t½: NA
Mafenide acetate (Sulfamy-lon)	See Prototype Drug Chart (Fig. 39–1)	For prevention and treatment of sepsis due to second- or third-degree burns. Pain and burning on application are common side effects. Allergic reaction (itching, rash, edema) may occur 10–14 d after use of mafenide. *Pregnancy category:* C; PB: UK; t½: UK
Silver nitrate	0.5 sol; 10%, 25% sticks; apply only to affected area 2–3 ×/wk for 2–3 wk	For second- and third-degree burns. Dressings are soaked in 0.5% silver nitrate solution and the dressings are removed before they dry. Effective against some gram-negative organisms. May cause electrolyte imbalance (hypokalemia) if used extensively. *Pregnancy category:* C; PB: NA; t½: NA
Silver sulfadiazine (Sil-vadene, SSD)	1% cream, apply daily—b.i.d. in ¹⁄₁₆-inch layer	Prevent and treat infection of second- and third-degree burns. Ten percent of the drug is absorbed. Excessive use or extensive application area may cause sulfa crystals (crystalluria). *Pregnancy category:* C; PB: NA; t½: NA

KEY: NA: nonapplicable; UK: unknown; <: less than; PB: protein-binding; t½: half-life; sol: solution.

Aseptic technique should be used when caring for the burn site and applying the topical antibacterial agent. Table 39–4 lists the topical medications for burns, their strengths, uses, and considerations.

SILVER SULFADIAZINE

Silver sulfadiazine (Silvadene, SSD) is becoming more popular for the prevention and treatment of sepsis in second- and third-degree burns than other antibacterial agents. It acts on the cell membrane and cell wall to produce bactericidal effects. Unlike mafenide, it is *not* a carbonic anydrase inhibitor. It is contraindicated at or near term pregnancy.

One percent or less of the silver is absorbed and up to 10% of sulfadiazine is absorbed. Side and adverse effects may include skin discoloration, burning sensation, rashes, erythema multiforme, skin necrosis, and possible leukopenia.

NURSING PROCESS: TOPICAL ANTIINFECTIVES: Burns

ASSESSMENT

- Assess burned tissue for infection. Culture an oozing wound.
- Check client's vital signs (VS). Report abnormal findings such as an elevated temperature.
- Assess fluid status. Report signs and symptoms of hypovolemia or hypervolemia.

POTENTIAL NURSING DIAGNOSES

- High risk for infection related to loss of skin integrity
- Pain related to thermal injury
- Body image disturbance

PLANNING

- Aseptic technique will be enforced when caring for burned tissue, and tissue will be free from infection.

NURSING INTERVENTIONS

- Administer prescribed analgesia before application, if needed.
- Cleanse burned tissue sites using aseptic technique.
- Apply topical antibacterial drug and dressing with sterile technique.
- Monitor client's fluid balance and renal function.
- Monitor client for side effects of and adverse reactions to topical drug.

- Monitor client's VS and be alert for signs of infection. Use with caution in client with acute renal failure.
- Closely monitor client's acid-base balance, especially in the presence of pulmonary or renal dysfunction.
- Store drug in dry place at room temperature.

CLIENT TEACHING

General

- Instruct client and family about changes in respiratory status.

Skill

- Explain to client and family the care given to the burned tissue areas, using aseptic technique.
- Instruct client and family to apply topical agent and dressings to the burned areas.

EVALUATION

- Evaluate effectiveness of treatment interventions to burned tissue areas by determining if healing is proceeding and sites are free from infection.

STUDY QUESTIONS

1. M. G., who is 15 years old, complains of numerous "blackheads" and large raised "pimples" on her face. What nonpharmacologic measures would you teach her in caring for her facial skin problem?
2. M. G.'s skin disorder does not improve. Her health care provider said she has acne and has prescribed benzoyl peroxide and oral tetracycline.
   a. What is benzoyl peroxide and how is it used?
   b. What should be included in a teaching program about the use of oral tetracycline?
3. T. H. has psoriasis. A coal tar preparation has been suggested and anthralin has been prescribed by the health care provider. T. H. wants to know how these agents will help him. How would you respond?
4. R. Q. has poison ivy. Poison ivy is classified as what type of skin disorder? What nondrug and drug regimen may be used to alleviate the poison ivy?
5. What drug is used to treat male pattern baldness? How is it administered and how does it achieve hair follicle growth?
6. B. R. has second- and third-degree burns over 25% of his body. Mafenide acetate has been ordered. How is it administered? What care is taken prior to its administration? What acid-base imbalance can result from its use?

Unit XI

Endocrine Agents

INTRODUCTION

The endocrine system is composed of ductless glands that secrete hormones into the bloodstream. **Hormones** are chemical substances synthesized from amino acids and cholesterol that act on body tissues and organs and affect cellular activity. Hormones can be divided into two categories: (1) proteins or small peptides, and (2) steroids. Hormones from the adrenal glands and the gonads are steroid hormones; the others are protein hormones. The **endocrine glands** include the pituitary (hypophysis), thyroid, parathyroid, adrenal, gonads, and pancreas. Figure XI–1 illustrates the location and functions of these glands. This unit discusses the hormonal activity of the endocrine glands.

PITUITARY GLAND

The pituitary gland, or hypophysis, located at the base of the brain, has two lobes, the anterior pituitary (adenohypophysis) and the posterior pituitary (neurohypophysis). The anterior pituitary gland is called the *master gland*, because it secretes hormones that stimulate the release of other hormones from target glands, including the thyroid, parathyroids, adrenals, and gonads. The posterior pituitary gland secretes two neurohormones, antidiuretic hormone

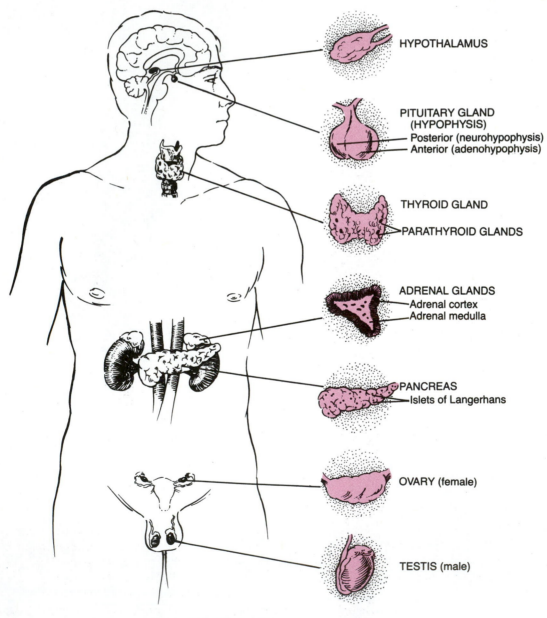

FIGURE XI–1 The endocrine glands.

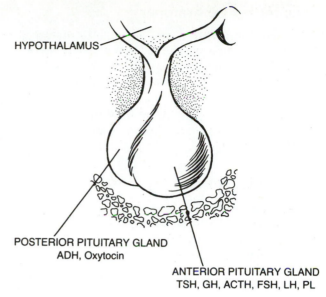

FIGURE XI–2 The anterior and posterior pituitary glands. (Key: ADH: antidiuretic hormone; TSH: thyroid-stimulating hormone; GH: growth hormone; ACTH: adrenocorticotropic hormone; FSH: follicle-stimulating hormone; LH: luteinizing hormone; PL: prolactin.)

HYPOTHALAMUS

POSTERIOR PITUITARY GLAND
ADH, Oxytocin

ANTERIOR PITUITARY GLAND
TSH, GH, ACTH, FSH, LH, PL

(ADH), or vasopressin, and oxytocin. Figure XI–2 shows the anterior and posterior pituitary gland and the types of hormones that are secreted.

ANTERIOR PITUITARY GLAND

The anterior pituitary hormones are (1) thyroid-stimulating hormone (TSH), (2) adrenocorticotropic hormone (ACTH), and (3) the gonadotropins (follicle-stimulating hormone [FSH] and luteinizing hormone [LH]). They control the synthesis and release of hormones from the thyroid, adrenals, and ovaries. Other hormones secreted from the anterior pituitary (adenohypophysis) include growth hormone (GH), prolactin, and melanocyte-stimulating hormone (MSH). The amount of each hormone secreted from the anterior pituitary is regulated by a negative feedback system. If excess hormone is secreted from the target gland, hormonal release from the anterior pituitary will be suppressed. If there is a lack of hormone secretion from the target gland, there will be an increase in that particular anterior pituitary hormone.

Thyroid-Stimulating Hormone

The anterior pituitary gland secretes thyroid-stimulating hormone (TSH) in response to thyroid-releasing hormone (TRH) from the hypothalamus. TSH, or thyrotropic hormone, stimulates the release of levothyroxine (T_4) and triiodothyronine (T_3) from the thyroid gland. Hypersecretion of TSH can cause hyperthyroidism and thyroid enlargement, and hyposecretion can cause hypothyroidism. Serum TSH levels should be checked to determine whether there is a TSH deficit or excess. TSH and T_4 levels are frequently measured to differentiate pituitary from thyroid dysfunction. A decreased T_4 level and a normal or elevated TSH level can indicate a thyroid disorder.

Adrenocorticotropic Hormone

Secretion of adrenocorticotropic hormone (ACTH) occurs in response to corticotropin-releasing factor (CRF) from the hypothalamus. ACTH from the anterior pituitary stimulates the release of glucocorticoids (cortisol), mineralocorticoids (aldosterone), and androgen from the adrenal cortex (adrenal glands). Elevated serum cortisol from the adrenal cortex inhibits ACTH and CRH release. When the cortisol level is low, ACTH secretion is stimulated, which in turn stimulates the adrenal cortex to release more cortisol. More ACTH is secreted in the morning than in the evening.

Gonadotropic Hormones

The gonadotropic hormones regulate hormone secretion from the ovaries and testes (the gonads). Follicle-stimulating hormone (FSH), luteinizing hormone (LH), and prolactin are the gonadotropic hormones secreted from the anterior pituitary gland. FSH promotes the maturation of follicles in the ovaries and initiates sperm production in the testes. LH combines with FSH in follicle maturation and estrogen production and promotes secretion of androgens from the testes. Prolactin stimulates milk formation in the glandular breast tissue after delivery. Estrogen, progesterone, and testosterone are discussed in Chapters 42, 43, and 44, respectively.

Growth Hormone

Growth hormone (GH), or somatotropic hormone (STH), acts on all body tissues, but particularly the bones and skeletal muscles. The amount of growth hormone secreted is regulated by growth hormone-releasing hormone (GHRH) and growth hormone-inhibiting hormone (GHIH, or somatostatin) from the hypothalamus. Sympathomimetics, serotonin, and glucocorticoids can inhibit the secretion of growth hormone.

POSTERIOR PITUITARY GLAND

The posterior pituitary gland (neurohypophysis) secretes antidiuretic hormone (ADH, vasopressin) and oxytocin. Interconnecting nerve fibers between the hypothalamus and the posterior pituitary gland allow ADH and oxytocin to be synthesized in the hypothalamus and stored in the posterior pituitary gland. ADH increases the reabsorption of water from the renal tubules, thus returning it to the systemic circulation. Secretion of ADH is regulated by the serum osmolality (concentration of the vascular fluid). An increase in serum osmolality increases the release of ADH from the posterior pituitary; more water is then absorbed from the renal tubules to dilute the vascular fluid. Excess ADH can overload the vascular system. A decrease in serum osmolality decreases the release of ADH, promoting more water excretion from the renal tubules. Oxytocin stimulates contraction of the smooth muscles of the uterus; it is discussed in Chapters 42 and 43.

THYROID GLAND

Located anterior to the trachea, the thyroid gland has two lobes that are connected by a bridge of thyroid tissue. The thyroid gland secretes two hormones, thyroxine (T_4) and triiodothyronine (T_3 liothyronine). These hormones affect nearly every tissue and organ by controlling their metabolic rate and activity. Stimulation by the thyroid hormones results in an increase in cardiac output, oxygen consumption, carbohydrate utilization, protein synthesis, and breakdown of fat (lipolysis). Body heat regulation and the menstrual cycle are also affected by thyroid hormones. Thyroid hormone levels in the blood are regulated by negative feedback. The anterior pituitary gland secretes thyroid-stimulating hormone (TSH), which stimulates the thyroid gland to produce T_4 and T_3. An increased amount of circulating thyroid hormones suppresses the release of TSH, and a decreased amount increases the release of TSH by the adenohypophysis.

PARATHYROID GLANDS

There are four parathyroid glands (two pairs) that lie on the dorsal surface of the thyroid gland. The parathyroid gland secretes parathormone, or parathyroid hormone (PTH), which regulates calcium levels in the blood. A decrease in serum calcium stimulates the release of PTH. PTH increases calcium levels by (1) mobilizing calcium from the bone, (2) promoting calcium absorption from the intestine, and (3) promoting calcium reabsorption from the renal tubules. Calcitonin, a hormone produced primarily by the thyroid gland and to a lesser extent by the parathyroid and thymus glands, inhibits calcium reabsorption by bone and increases renal excretion of calcium. Calcitonin counteracts the action of PTH.

ADRENAL GLANDS

The adrenal glands, located at the top of each kidney, are composed of two separate sections: the adrenal medulla (the inner section) and the adrenal cortex (the section surrounding the adrenal medulla). The adrenal medulla releases the catecholamines epinephrine and norepinephrine and is linked with the sympathetic nervous system. The adrenal cortex produces two major types of hormones (corticosteroids), glucocorticoids and mineralocorticoids. The principal glucocorticoid is cortisol and the principal mineralocorticoid is aldosterone. In addition, the adrenal cortex produces small amounts of androgen, estrogen, and progestin. Glucocorticoids have a profound influence on electrolytes, and carbohydrate, protein, and fat metabolism, and deficiencies can result in serious illness and even death.

PANCREAS

The pancreas, located to the left of and behind the stomach, is both an exocrine and an endocrine gland. The exocrine section of the pancreas secretes digestive enzymes into the duodenum; these enzymes are discussed in Unit IX. The endocrine section has cell clusters called islets of Langerhans. The alpha islet cells produce glucagon, which breaks down glycogen to glucose in the liver, and the beta cells secrete insulin, which regulates glucose metabolism. Insulin, an antidiabetic agent, is used to control diabetes mellitus. Antidiabetic agents are discussed in Chapter 41.

DRUGS FOR ENDOCRINE DISORDERS

Chapters 40 and 41 discuss the drugs used in diagnosing and treating endocrine disorders. In Chapter 40, the agents for disorders involving the pituitary gland, thyroid gland, parathyroid gland, adrenal gland, and antidiuretic hormone (ADH) are discussed. The parenteral and oral antidiabetic drugs (hypoglycemic drugs) are described in Chapter 41.

Drugs discussed in Chapter 40 are used for pituitary disorders and include (1) drugs for growth hormone replacement and a drug that suppresses the release of GH and prolactin; (2) a thyroid-stimulating hormone agent for diagnosing the cause of hypothyroidism; (3) ACTH agents, used for diagnosing and treating adrenal insufficiency, and (4) drugs used to control diabetes insipidus resulting from ADH insufficiency. Hypothyroidism and hyperthyroidism are discussed in relation to their drug therapy. The use of glucocorticoids as antiinflammatory agents and in diagnosing and treating adrenocortical insufficiency is presented.

In Chapter 41, insulin and oral antidiabetic (hypoglycemic) drugs are presented. Recognition of hypoglycemia, insulin injection sites, and client teaching are emphasized. The nursing process format is applied throughout both chapters.

Chapter 40

Endocrine Pharmacology: Pituitary, Thyroid, Parathyroids, and Adrenals

OUTLINE

Objectives
Terms
Introduction
Pituitary Gland
    Anterior
    Growth Hormone
    Thyroid-Stimulating Hormone
    Adrenocorticotropic Hormone

Posterior
    Nursing Process
Thyroid Gland
    Hypothyroidism
    Hyperthyroidism
    Nursing Process
Parathyroids
    Calcitriol
    Nursing Process
Adrenals

Glucocorticoids
Mineralocorticoids
    Nursing Process
Case Study
Study Questions

OBJECTIVES

Define hormone, hypophysis, thyroxine, and glucocorticoids.

Name the hormones secreted from the adenohypophysis and the neurohypophysis.

Identify the actions, uses, and side effects of the pituitary hormones, T_4, T_3, PTH, and glucocorticoids.

Describe the nursing process, including client teaching, of drug therapy related to hormonal replacement or hormonal inhibition for the pituitary, thyroid, parathyroid, and adrenal glands.

TERMS

acromegaly
Addison's disease
adenohypophysis
adrenal glands
adrenocorticotropic hormone
antidiuretic hormone (ADH)
corticosteroids
cretinism
Cushing's syndrome

diabetes insipidus
endocrine
exocrine
gigantism
glucocorticoids
Graves' disease
hyperthyroidism
hypophysis
hypothyroidism

mineralocorticoids
myxedema
neurohypophysis
parathyroid hormone
thyroid-stimulating hormone
thyrotoxicosis
thyroxine (T_4)
triiodothyronine (T_3)

INTRODUCTION

This chapter describes drugs used for hormonal replacement and for inhibition of hormonal secretion from the pituitary, thyroid, parathyroid, and adrenal glands. The gonadal, or sex, hormones are discussed in Chapters 42 through 46. Before reading Chapters 40 and 41, the student or nurse should review the introduction to Unit XI, which describes the locations of the endocrine glands and the hormones that they secrete. Knowledge of the various endocrine hormones and their functions facilitates an understanding of the drugs that act on the endocrine glands.

PITUITARY GLAND

ANTERIOR

The pituitary gland (hypophysis) has an anterior and a posterior lobe. The anterior pituitary gland, called the adenohypophysis, secretes various hormones that target glands and tissues: (1) growth hormone (GH), which stimulates growth in tissue and bone; (2) thyroid-stimulating hormone (TSH), which acts on the thyroid gland; (3) adrenocorticotropic hormone (ACTH), which stimulates the adrenal gland; and (4) gonadotropins (follicle-stimulating hormone [FSH] and luteinizing hormone [LH]), which affect the ovaries. FSH and LH are discussed in Chapter 42. The drugs with adenohypophyseal properties used to stimulate or inhibit glandular activity are discussed according to their drug use. The negative feedback system that controls the amount of hormonal secretion from the pituitary gland and the target gland is discussed in the introduction to Unit XI.

GROWTH HORMONE

Two hypothalamic hormones regulate growth hormone (GH): (1) growth hormone releasing hormone (GHRH), and (2) growth hormone release-inhibiting hormone (somatostatin or SIH). GH does not have a specific target gland; it affects body tissues and bone. GH replacement stimulates linear growth when there is a growth hormone deficiency. Enzymes in the gastrointestinal (GI) tract inactivate GH, thus requiring subcutaneous or intramuscular administration of GH.

If a child's height is well below the standard for a specified age, GH deficiency may be diagnosed and dwarfism can result. Because GH replacement is very expensive, various tests are performed to determine if this therapy is essential. Because GH acts on newly forming bone, it must be adminis-

tered before the epiphyses are fused. Administration of GH over a period of several years can increase height by a foot. Prolonged GH therapy can antagonize insulin secretion and eventually cause diabetes mellitus. Because of its effects on blood sugar and other side effects, athletes should be advised not to take GH to build muscle and physique.

Gigantism (during childhood) and **acromegaly** (after puberty) can occur with GH hypersecretion, and are frequently caused by a pituitary tumor. If the tumor cannot be destroyed by radiation, bromocriptine, a prolactin-release inhibitor, can inhibit the release of GH from the pituitary. Table 40–1 lists the drugs that are used to replace or inhibit the growth hormone.

THYROID-STIMULATING HORMONE

The adenohypophysis secretes **thyroid-stimulating hormone** (TSH) in response to thyroid-releasing hormone (TRH) from the hypothalamus. TSH stimulates the thyroid gland to release levothyroxine (T_4) and triiodothyronine (liothyronine) (T_3). Excess TSH secretion can cause hyperthyroidism, and a TSH deficit can cause hypothyroidism. Hypothyroidism may be due to a thyroid gland disorder (primary cause) or a decrease in TSH secretion (secondary cause). Thyrotropin (Thytropar), a purified extract of TSH, is used as a diagnostic agent to differentiate between primary and secondary hypothyroidism (see Table 40–1).

ADRENOCORTICOTROPIC HORMONE

The hypothalamus releases corticotropin-releasing factor (CRF), which stimulates the pituitary corticotrophs to secrete **adrenocorticotropic hormone** (ACTH). ACTH secretion stimulates the release of glucocorticoids (cortisol), mineralocorticoids (aldosterone), and androgen from the adrenal cortex. Usually ACTH, and cortisol secretions follow a diurnal rhythm in which cortisol secretion is higher in the early morning and then decreases through the day. Stresses such as surgery, sepsis, and trauma override the diurnal rhythm, causing an increase in secretions of ACTH and cortisol.

The ACTH drug corticotropin (ACTHAR) is used in the diagnosis of adrenal gland disorders, for treating adrenal gland insufficiency, and as an anti-inflammatory drug in the treatment of an allergic response. ACTH decreases the symptoms of multiple sclerosis during its exacerbation phase. Figure 40–1 lists the actions and effects of corticotropin (ACTHAR).

TABLE 40–1 Anterior and Posterior Pituitary Hormones

Generic (Brand)	Route and Dosage	Uses and Considerations
Anterior: Growth Hormone (GH)		
Sermorelin acetate (Geref)	*Diagnostic:* A&C: IV: 0.3–1 µg/kg	Diagnostic test to determine if the pituitary gland secretes growth hormone.
Somatrem (Protropin)	*Growth hormone deficiency:* C: SC/IM: 100 µg/kg (0.1 mg/kg) 3 × wk or 0.2 U/kg 3 × wk; 48-h interval is recommended between doses	For growth hormone replacement for treating dwarfism. It affects growth of most body tissues, and promotes bone growth at epiphyseal plates of long bones. *Pregnancy category:* C; PB: UK; t½: 20–30 min
Somatropin (Humatrope)	C: SC/IM: 60 µg/kg (0.06 mg/kg) 3 × wk or 0.16 IU/kg 3 × wk; 48-h interval is recommended between doses	For treating growth hormone deficiency. Promotes bone growth at epiphyseal plates of long bones. *Pregnancy category:* D; PB: UK; t½: 15–60 min
Thyroid-Stimulating Hormone (TSH)		
Thyrotropin (Thytropar)	*Hypothyroidism and treatment of thyroid cancer:* A: SC/IM: 10 IU/d for 1–3 d; cancer treatment: 3–8d	For diagnosing cause of hypothyroidism (pituitary or thyroid). Radioiodine study follows last injection. *Pregnancy category:* C; PB: UK; t½: 35 min with normal thyroid
Adrenocorticotropic Hormone (ACTH)		
Corticotropin (Acthar)	See Prototype Drug Chart (Fig. 40–1)	For diagnostic test to evaluate adrenocortical function and ACTH replacement. For acute exacerbations of multiple sclerosis. Long-term therapy can cause side effects similar to glucocorticoids. Repository injections have long duration of action (12 to 24 h), IM. *Pregnancy category:* C; PB: UK; t½: UK
Corticotropin repository (Acthar gel)	A: SC/IM: 40–80 U/q24–72h	
Cosyntropin (Cortrosyn)	A: C > 2 y: IM: 0.25–0.75 mg IV: 0.25 mg C < 2 y: IM: 0.125 mg IV: 0.125 mg (0.04 mg/h)	For diagnostic testing to differentiate between pituitary and adrenal cause of adrenal insufficiency. Obtain a plasma cortisol level before and 30 min after cosyntropin administration. *Pregnancy category:* C; PB: UK; t½: 15 min
Posterior: Antidiuretic Hormone (ADH)		
Desmopressin acetate (DDAVP)	*Diabetes Insipidus:* A: Intranasal: 0.1–0.4 mL/d in divided doses C < 12 y: Intranasal: 0.05–0.3 mL/d in divided doses	For treating diabetes insipidus, hemophilia A, von Willebrand's disease. Can have a long duration of action (5 to 21 h). *Pregnancy category:* B; PB: UK; t½: 1.25 h
Desmopressin (Stimate)	A: SC/IV: 2–4 µg, in 2 divided doses C < 12 y: Inf: 0.3 µg/kg diluted in 10 mL of NSS over 15–30 min	Same as above
Lypressin (Diapid)	*Diabetes insipidus:* A&C: Intranasal: 1–2 sprays per nostril q.i.d.	Prevention or control of diabetes insipidus caused by insufficient ADH. To decrease polydipsia, polyuria, and dehydration. Duration of action is 3–8 h. *Pregnancy category:* B; PB: UK; t½: 15 min
Vasopressin (aqueous) (Pitressin)	*Diabetes insipidus:* A: SC/IM: 5–10 U b.i.d./q.i.d. C: SC/IM: 2.5–10 U b.i.d./q.i.d.	For treating diabetes insipidus. For relief of intestinal distention. Decreases GI bleeding from esophageal varices. Can also be given intranasally. Promotes reabsorption of water from the renal tubules. Duration of action is 2–8 h. *Pregnancy category:* X; PB: UK; t½: 15 min
Vasopressin tanate/oil (Pitressin Tannate)	A: IM: 1.5–5.0 U q2–3d C: IM: 1.25–2.5 U q2–3d	Same as for vasopressin. Action is longer due to the oil.

KEY: A: adult; C: child; inf: infusion; IM: intramuscular; IV: intravenous; SC: subcutaneous; PB: protein-binding; t½: half-life; UK: unknown.

FIGURE 40–1. Pituitary: Adrenocorticotropic Hormone (ACTH)

Adrenocorticotropic Hormone (ACTH)	Dosage	NURSING PROCESS Assessment and Planning
Corticotropin (Acthar, ACTH) *Corticotropin repository* (Acthar Gel, cortigel) *Corticotropin zinc hydroxide* (Cortrophin Zinc) *Pregnancy Category:* C	*Diagnostic testing:* A: IV: 10–25 U in 500 mL D$_5$W q8h SC/IM: 20 U, q.i.d. *Repository injection:* A: SC/IM; 40–80 U, q24–72 h *Acute Multiple Sclerosis* A: SC/IM: 80–120 U/d for 2–3 wk	
Contraindications	**Drug-Lab-Food Interactions**	
Severe fungal infection, CHF, peptic ulcer *Caution:* Hepatic disease, psychiatric disorders, myasthenia gravis	*Increase* ulcer formation with aspirin; may *increase* effect of potassium-wasting diuretics *Decrease* effects of oral antidiabetics (hypoglycemics) or insulin	
Pharmacokinetics	**Pharmacodynamics**	Interventions

Absorption: IM: Well absorbed
Distribution: PB: UK
Metabolism: t½: 15–20 min
Excretion: In urine
	IM: Onset: <6 h
	  Peak: 6–18 h
	  Duration: 12–24 h
	IV: Onset: UK
	  Peak: 1 h
	  Duration: UK	

Therapeutic Effects/Uses: To diagnose adrenocortical disorders; acts as an antiinflammatory agent; to treat acute multiple sclerosis (MS). *Mode of Action:* Stimulation of the adrenal cortex to secrete cortisol.	Evaluation

Side Effects	Adverse Reactions
Nausea, vomiting, increased appetite, mood swing (euphoria to depression), petechiae, water and sodium retention, hypokalemia, hypocalcemia	Edema, ecchymosis, osteoporosis, muscle atrophy, growth retardation, decreased wound healing, cataracts, glaucoma, menstrual irregularities *Life-threatening:* Ulcer perforation, pancreatitis

KEY: A: adult; SC: subcutaneous; IM: intramuscular; IV: intravenous; UK: unknown; PB: protein-binding; t½: half-life.

Pharmacokinetics

Corticotropin stimulates the adrenal gland to secrete corticosteroids. The aqueous and gel preparations are well-absorbed into the circulation. Zinc is added to some formulations to slow the absorption rate. A portion of the drug is bound to protein; however, the percent is unknown. The half-life of the drug is 15 to 20 min. It is excreted in the urine.

Pharmacodynamics

Corticotropin suppresses the inflammatory and immune responses. The drug is administered intramuscularly and intravenously (IV). By intramuscular injection, its onset of action, peak concentration time, and duration of action are prolonged. The IV preparation is in an aqueous form; therefore, its actions are faster than those of the gel and zinc-additive preparations.

Drug Interactions

Corticotropin has numerous drug interactions. Diuretics and anti-*Pseudomonas* penicillins such as piperacillin can decrease the serum potassium level (hypokalemia). If the client is taking a digitalis preparation and hypokalemia is present, digitalis toxicity can result. Phenytoin, rifampin, and barbiturates increase the metabolic rate, which can decrease the effect of the ACTH drug. Diabetics may need increased insulin and oral antidiabetic (hypoglycemic) drugs, because ACTH stimulates cortisol secretion, which increases the blood sugar level.

POSTERIOR

The posterior pituitary gland, known as the **neurohypophysis**, secretes **antidiuretic hormone** (ADH, vasopressin) and oxytocin. (Oxytocin is discussed in Chapter 42).

ADH promotes water reabsorption from the renal tubules to maintain water balance in the body fluids. When there is a deficiency of ADH, large amounts of water are excreted by the kidneys. This condition, **diabetes insipidus** (DI), can lead to severe fluid volume deficit and electrolyte imbalances. Head injury and brain tumors resulting in trauma to the hypothalamus and pituitary gland can also cause diabetes insipidus. Fluid and electrolyte balance must be closely monitored in these clients, and ADH replacement may be needed. The ADH preparations vasopressin (Pitressin) and desmopressin acetate (DDAVP) can be administered intranasally or by injection.

Table 40–1 lists the drugs used for pituitary disorders, their dosages, and uses and considerations.

NURSING PROCESS: PITUITARY HORMONES

ASSESSMENT

- Obtain baseline vital signs (VS) for future comparison. Report abnormal results.
- Assess the client's urinary output and weight.
- Assess the client for an infectious process. Corticotropin can suppress signs and symptoms of infection.
- Assess the client's physical growth. Compare child's growth with reported standards. Report findings.

POTENTIAL NURSING DIAGNOSES

- Altered health maintenance
- Altered growth and development

PLANNING

- Client will be free of pituitary disorder with appropriate drug regimen.

NURSING INTERVENTIONS

Antidiuretic Hormone (ADH)
- Monitor VS. Increased heart rate and decreased systolic pressure can indicate fluid volume loss due to decreased ADH production. With less ADH secretion, more water is excreted, decreasing vascular fluid (hypovolemia).
- Monitor urinary output. Increased output can indicate fluid loss due to a decrease in ADH.

Adrenocorticotropic Hormone (ACTH), Corticotropin
- **Avoid** administering corticotropin to clients with adrenocortical hyperfunction. Corticotropin stimulates the release of cortisol from the adrenal glands.
- Monitor the growth and development of a child receiving corticotropin.
- Monitor the client's weight. If a weight gain occurs, check for edema. A side effect of corticotropin (ACTH) is sodium and water retention.
- Monitor for adverse effects when corticotropin is discontinued. Dose should be tapered and not stopped abruptly because adrenal hypofunction may result.
- Check laboratory findings, especially electrolyte levels. Electrolyte replacement may be necessary.

Growth Hormone (GH)
- Monitor blood sugar and electrolyte levels in clients receiving GH. Hyperglycemia can occur with high doses.

CLIENT TEACHING

ACTH
- Advise the client to adhere to the drug regimen. Discontinuation of certain drugs, such as corticotropin, can cause hypofunction of the gland being stimulated.
- Advise the client to decrease salt intake to decrease or avoid edema. Potassium supplement may be needed.

- Instruct the client to report side effects, such as muscle weakness, edema, petechiae, ecchymosis, decrease in growth, decreased wound healing, and menstrual irregularities.

Growth Hormone

- Advise athletes not to take GH due to its side effects. GH can be effective for children whose height is markedly below the expected norm for their age. Because GH acts on the newly forming bone, it should be administered before the epiphyses are fused.
- Inform the diabetic client to closely monitor blood sugar levels. Insulin regulation may be necessary.
- Suggest that the client or family monitors the client's growth rate.

EVALUATION

- Evaluate the effectiveness of the drug therapy.

THYROID GLAND

Thyroxine (T_4) and **triiodothyronine** (T_3) are secreted by the thyroid gland. The functions of T_4 and T_3 are to regulate protein synthesis and enzyme activity and to stimulate mitochondrial oxidation. Approximately 20% of circulating T_3 is secreted from the thyroid gland and 80% of T_3 comes from the degradation of about 40% of T_4, which occurs in the periphery. T_4 and T_3 are carried in the blood by thyroxine-binding globulin (TBG) and albumin, which protects the hormones from being degraded. T_3 is more potent than T_4, and only unbound free T_3 and T_4 are active and produce a hormonal response.

T_4 and T_3 secretion from the thyroid gland is regulated by the feedback mechanisms. The hypothalamus releases thyrotropin-releasing hormone (TRH), which stimulates the release of thyroid-stimulating hormone (TSH) from the pituitary gland. TSH stimulates the synthesis and release of T_4 and T_3 from the thyroid gland. Excess free T_4 and T_3 inhibit the hypothalamus-pituitary-thyroid (HPT) axis, which results in decreased TRH and TSH secretion. Likewise, too low T_4 and T_3 increases the function of the HPT axis.

When there is a thyroid deficiency (hypothyroidism), synthetic T_4 and T_3 may be prescribed, either alone or in combination. When the thyroid gland is secreting an overabundance of thyroid hormones (hyperthyroidism), antithyroid drugs are usually indicated.

HYPOTHYROIDISM

Hypothyroidism, a decrease in thyroid hormone secretion, can have a primary (thyroid gland disorder) or a secondary cause (lack of TSH secretion). Primary hypothyroidism occurs more frequently. Decreased T_4 and elevated TSH levels indicate primary hypothyroidism, the causes of which are acute or chronic inflammation of the thyroid gland, radioiodine therapy, excess intake of antithyroid drugs, and surgery. **Myxedema** is severe hypothyroidism; symptoms include lethargy, apathy, memory impairment, emotional changes, slow speech, deep coarse voice, edema of the eyelids and face, thick dry skin, cold intolerance, slow pulse, constipation, weight gain, and abnormal menses. In children, hypothyroidism can have a congenital (cretinism) or prepubertal (juvenile hypothyroidism) onset. Drugs containing T_4 and T_3 alone or in combination, are used to treat hypothyroidism. Figure 40–2 presents the drug data for the synthetic thyroid drug levothyroxine.

Pharmacokinetics

Levothyroxine (T_4) is a synthetic thyroid hormone preparation. Fifty to 75 percent of levothyroxine is absorbed by the gastrointestinal (GI) mucosa. T_4 is highly protein-bound, and when administered with other highly protein-bound drugs like oral anticoagulants, side effects can result. The half-life of levothyroxine is longer than that of liothyronine. Levothyroxine is excreted in the bile and feces.

Pharmacodynamics

Levothyroxine increases metabolic rate, cardiac output, protein synthesis, and glycogen utilization. The peak concentration time and duration of action are much longer with levothyroxine than with liothyronine. Liotrix is a combination of T_4 and T_3 with a greater concentration of T_4.

Drug Interactions

There are many drug interactions associated with T_4 and T_3 drugs. They increase the effect of oral anticoagulants because of drug displacement from the

FIGURE 40–2. Thyroid Hormone: Replacement

Thyroid Synthetic Hormone

Levothyroxine sodium, T_4, (Canadian) Eltroxin (Synthroid, Levothroid)
Pregnancy Category: A

Dosage

A: PO: Initially: 50 μg/d (0.05 mg/d); maint: 50–200 μg/d (0.05–0.2 mg/d)
IV: 0.2–0.5 mg initial dose
C: >3 y: PO: 50–100 μg/d (0.05–0.1 mg/d)

NURSING PROCESS
Assessment and Planning

Contraindications

Thyrotoxicosis, MI, severe renal disease
Caution: Cardiovascular disease, hypertension, angina pectoris

Drug-Lab-Food Interactions

Increase cardiac insufficiency with epinephrine; *increase* effects of anticoagulants, tricyclic antidepressants, vasopressors, decongestants
Decrease effects of antidiabetics (oral and insulin), digitalis products; *decrease* absorption with cholestyramine, colestipol

Pharmacokinetics

Absorption: PO: 50–75%
Distribution: PB: 99%
Metabolism: t½: 6–7 d
Excretion: In bile and feces

Pharmacodynamics

PO: Onset: UK
Peak: 24 h–1 wk
Duration: 1–3 wk
IV: Onset: 6–8 h
Peak: 24–48 h
Duration: UK

Interventions

Therapeutic Effects/Uses: To treat hypothyroidism, myxedema, and cretinism.

Mode of Action: Increase metabolic rate, oxygen consumption, and body growth.

Evaluation

Side Effects

Nausea, vomiting, diarrhea, cramps, tremors, nervousness, insomnia, headache, weight loss

Adverse Reactions

Tachycardia, hypertension, palpitations
Life-threatening: Thyroid crisis, angina pectoris, cardiac dysrhythmias, cardiovascular collapse

KEY: A: adult; C: child; PO: by mouth; IV: intravenous; UK: unknown; PB: protein-binding; t½: half-life; (Canadian): Canadian drug name.

protein-binding sites. When either of these drugs is taken with an adrenergic agent, such as a decongestant or vasopressor, the cardiac and central nervous system (CNS) actions are increased. Levothyroxine and liothyronine can decrease the effectiveness of digitalis preparations. Estrogen can increase the effect of liothyronine. Insulin and oral antidiabetic drug dosages may need to be increased.

Table 40–2 lists the drug data for natural and synthetic thyroid preparations.

HYPERTHYROIDISM

Hyperthyroidism is an increase in circulating T_4 and T_3 levels, which results from an overactive thyroid gland or excessive output of thyroid hormones from one or more thyroid nodules. Hyperthyroidism may be mild with few symptoms or severe, as in thyroid storm in which death may occur from vascular collapse. **Graves' disease,** or **thyrotoxicosis,** is the most common type of hyperthyroidism due to hyperfunction of the thyroid gland. It is

TABLE 40–2 Thyroid Hormone: Replacements and Antithyroid Drugs

Generic (Brand)	Route and Dosage	Uses and Considerations
Thyroid Replacements: Hypothyroidism		
Levothyroxine Na (Synthroid)	See Prototype Drug Chart (Fig. 40–2)	For primary hypothyroidism. Synthetic T_4 drug. Onset of action is very slow. Effects occur in 1–3 wk. IV use for myxedema coma. Common side effects include nervousness, tachycardia, and weight loss. *Pregnancy category:* A; PB: 99%; t½: 6–7 d
Liothyronine Na (Cytomel)	A: PO: Initially: 5–25 μg/d; maint: 25–100 μg/d C: PO: Initially: 5 μg/d, > 3 y: 50–100 μg/d	For hypothyroidism. Synthetic T_3 drug. Onset: faster acting than other thyroid drugs; Effects in 24–72 h. Cardiac side effects. *Pregnancy category:* A; PB: 99%; t½: 1–1.5 h
Liotrix (Euthroid, Thyrolar)	A: PO: Initially: 15–30 μg/d, *increase* q2–3wk; maint: 60–120 μg/d C: PO: Initially: same as adult C 6–12 y: 75–150 μg/d	For hypothyroidism. Synthetic T_4 and T_3 drug: 4:1 ratio. Onset of action is immediate. Duration of action is 72 h. Common side effects include irritability, nervousness, insomnia, tachycardia, weight loss. *Pregnancy category:* A; PB: 99%; t½: <7 d
Thyroglobulin (Proloid)	A: PO: Initially: 32 mg/d; maint: 32–200 mg/d Elderly: Initially: 16 mg/d	For hypothyroidism. From extract of hog thyroid. T_4 and T_3: 2.5:1 ratio. Seldom used. *Pregnancy category:* A; PB: 99%; t½: 6–7 d
Thyroid (Armour Thyroid, Thyrar)	A: PO: Initially: 15–60 mg/d, *increase* monthly as needed; maint: 60–180 mg/d C: PO: 15 mg/d, *increase* q2wk as needed	For hypothyroidism, to reduce goiter size. Natural form obtained from animals. T_4 and T_3: 4:1 ratio. Onset of action is slow; long duration of action (wks). Common side effects include irritability, nervousness, insomnia, tachycardia and weight loss. *Pregnancy category:* A; PB: 99%; t½: <7d (T_3: 1–2 h, T_4: 6–7 h)
Antithyroid Drugs: Hyperthyroidism		
Methimazole (Tapazole)	A: PO: Initially: 15–60 mg/d in 3 divided doses; maint: 5–15 mg/d C: PO: Initially: 0.4 mg/kg/d in divided doses; maint: 0.2 mg/kg/d in divided doses	For treating hyperthyroidism. Inhibits thyroid hormone synthesis. Onset of action: 1 wk for effect. Rash, urticaria, headache, GI upset may occur. *Pregnancy category:* D; PB: 0%; t½: 5–13 h
Thioamide: Propylthiouracil (PTU)	A: PO: Initially: 300–400 mg/d in divided doses; maint: 100–300 mg/d C: 6–10 y: PO: 50–150 mg/d > 10 y: PO: Same as adult or 150 mg/m²/d	For hyperthyroidism, Graves' disease. Inhibits conversion of T_4 and T_3. May be used prior to surgery or radioactive iodine treatment and palliative control of toxic goiter. *Pregnancy category:* D; PB: 75%–80%; t½: 1–2 h
Iodine: strong iodine solution (Lugol solution, potassium iodide solution)	A&C: PO: 0.1–0.3 mL (3–5 drops) t.i.d. *Thyroid crisis:* A&C: PO: 1 mL in water p.c. t.i.d.	For hyperthyroidism. To reduce size and vascularity of thyroid gland. Dilute drug and administer after meals; sip through straw to avoid discoloration of teeth. Maximum effect after 10–15 d. *Pregnancy category:* D; PB: UK; t½: UK

KEY: *A: adult; C: child; PO: by mouth; PB: protein-binding; t½: half-life; UK; unknown.*

characterized by a rapid pulse (tachycardia), palpitations, excessive perspiration, heat intolerance, nervousness, irritability, exophthalmos (bulging eyes), and weight loss.

Hyperthyroidism can be treated by surgical removal of a portion of the thyroid gland (subtotal thyroidectomy), radioactive iodine therapy, or antithyroid drugs, which inhibit either the synthesis or the release of thyroid hormone. Any of these treatments can cause hypothyroidism. Propranolol (Inderal) can control the cardiac symptoms, such as palpitations and tachycardia, that result from hyperthyroidism. Table 40–2 gives the drug data for the antithyroid drugs used to treat hyperthyroidism.

Drug Interactions

Thyroid drugs interact with many other drugs. When used with oral anticoagulants (warfarin [Coumadin]), they can cause an increase in the anticoagulating effect. In addition, thyroid drugs decrease the effect of insulin and oral antidiabetics; digoxin and lithium increase the action of thyroid drugs; and phenytoin (Dilantin) increases serum T_3 level.

NURSING PROCESS: THYROID HORMONE: Replacement and Antithyroid Drugs

ASSESSMENT

- Obtain baseline vital signs (VS) to compare with future data. Report abnormal results.
- Check serum T_3, T_4, and TSH levels. Report abnormal results.

Thyroid Replacement

- Obtain a history of drugs the client is currently taking. Be aware that thyroid drugs enhance the action of oral anticoagulants, sympathomimetics, and antidepressants and decrease the action of insulin, oral hypoglycemics, and digitalis preparation. Phenytoin and aspirin can enhance the action of thyroid hormone.

Antithyroid Drugs

- Assess for signs and symptoms of a thyroid crisis (thyroid storm), which includes tachycardia, dysrhythmias, fever, heart failure, flushed skin, apathy, confusion, behavioral changes, and later hypotension and vascular collapse. Thyroid crisis can result from a thyroidectomy (excess thyroid hormones released), abrupt withdrawal of antithyroid drug, excess ingestion of thyroid hormone, or failure to give antithyroid medication before thyroid surgery.

POTENTIAL NURSING DIAGNOSES

- Altered health maintenance
- Altered tissue perfusion

PLANNING

- Client's signs and symptoms of hypothyroidism will be alleviated within 2 to 4 wk with prescribed thyroid drug replacement, and the client will not experience side effects.
- Client's signs and symptoms of hyperthyroidism will be alleviated in 1 to 3 wk with the prescribed antithyroid drug.

NURSING INTERVENTIONS

- Monitor VS. With hypothyroidism, the temperature, heart rate, and blood pressure are usually decreased. With hyperthyroidism, tachycardia and palpitations usually occur.
- Monitor the client's weight. Weight gain commonly occurs in clients with hypothyroidism.

CLIENT TEACHING

Thyroid Drug Replacement for Hypothyroidism

- Instruct the client to take the drug at the same time each day, preferably before breakfast. Food will hamper absorption rate.
- Advise the client to check cautions on labels of OTC drugs. Avoid OTC drugs that caution against use by persons with heart or thyroid disease.
- Advise the client to report symptoms of hyperthyroidism (tachycardia, chest pain, palpitations, excess sweating) due to drug accumulation or overdosing.
- Suggest that the client carry a medical alert card, tag, or bracelet with health condition and thyroid drug listed.

Diet

- Instruct the client to avoid foods that can inhibit thyroid secretion, such as strawberries, peaches, pears, cabbage, turnips, spinach, kale, Brussels sprouts, cauliflower, radishes, and peas.

Antithyroid Drugs for Hyperthyroidism

- Instruct the client to take the drug with meals to decrease GI symptoms.
- Advise the client about the effects of iodine and its presence in iodized salt, shellfish, and OTC cough medicines.
- Emphasize the importance of drug compliance; abruptly stopping the antithyroid drug could bring on a thyroid crisis.
- Teach the client the signs and symptoms of hypothyroidism: lethargy, puffy eyelids and face, thick tongue, slow speech with hoarseness, lack of perspiration, and slow pulse. Hypothyroidism can result from treatment of hyperthyroidism.
- Advise the client to avoid antithyroid drugs if pregnant or breast feeding. Antithyroid drugs taken during pregnancy can cause hypothyroidism in the fetus or infant.

Skill

- Demonstrate to the client how to take a pulse rate. Instruct the client to monitor the pulse rate and report increases or marked decreases in pulse rate.

Side Effects

- Teach the client the side effects of antithyroid drugs, such as skin rash, hives, nausea, alopecia, loss of hair pigment, petechiae or ecchymoses, and weakness.

- Advise the client to contact the health care provider if a sore throat and fever occur while taking antithyroid drugs. A serious adverse reaction of antithyroid drugs is agranulocytosis (loss of WBCs). CBC should be monitored for leukopenia.

EVALUATION

Thyroid Replacement

- Evaluate the effectiveness of the thyroid drug and drug compliance

- Continue monitoring for side effects from drug accumulation or overdosing.

Antithyroid Drugs

- Evaluate the effectiveness of the antithyroid drug in decreasing signs and symptoms of hyperthyroidism. If signs and symptoms persist after 2 to 3 wk of therapy, other methods for correcting hyperthyroidism may be necessary.

PARATHYROIDS

The parathyroid glands secrete **parathyroid hormone** (PTH), which regulates calcium levels in the blood. A decrease in serum calcium stimulates the release of PTH. Calcitonin decreases serum calcium levels by promoting renal excretion of calcium. The functions of PTH and calcitonin are discussed in the introduction to Unit XI.

PTH agents treat hypoparathyroidism and synthetic calcitonin treats hyperparathyroidism. Hypocalcemia (serum calcium deficit) can be caused by PTH deficiency, vitamin D deficiency, renal impairment, or diuretic therapy. PTH replacement will help to correct the calcium deficit. PTH promotes calcium absorption from the GI tract, promotes reabsorption of calcium from the renal tubules and activates vitamin D.

CALCITRIOL

Calcitriol is a vitamin D analog that promotes calcium absorption from the GI tract and secretion of

calcium from bone to the blood stream. Figure 40–3 describes the drug data related to calcitriol.

Pharmacokinetics

Calcitriol is readily absorbed from the GI tract. Half-life is moderate (3 to 8 h). Most of the drug is excreted in the feces.

Pharmacodynamics

Calcitriol is given for the management of hypocalcemia. It increases serum calcium levels by promoting calcium absorption from the intestines and from the renal tubules. Calcitriol has a long onset of action, peak action, and duration of action.

Hyperparathyroidism can be caused by malignancies of the parathyroid glands or ectopic PTH hormone secretion from lung cancer, hyperthyroidism, or prolonged immobility during which calcium is lost from bone. Table 40–3 lists the drugs used for treating hypoparathyroidism and hyperparathyroidism.

TABLE 40–3 Parathyroid Hormones: Replacements and Supplements

Generic (Brand)	Route and Dosage	Uses and Considerations
Hypoparathyroidism and Hypocalcemia: Vitamin D Analogs		
Calcifediol (Calderol)	A: PO: Initially: 300–350 µg/wk PO: 50–100 µg/d or 100–200 µg q.o.d.	For bone disease and hypocalcemia associated with chronic renal disease and dialysis. *Pregnancy category:* C; PB: UK; t½: 12–22 d
Calcitriol (Rocaltrol)	A: PO: 0.25 µg/d; may increase 0.25 µg q4wk; *max:* 1.0 µg/d IV: 0.5 µg 3 × wk at end of dialysis C: PO: 0.014–0.041 µg/kg/d	For pseudohypoparathyroidism, hypoparathyroidism, and hypocalcemia in chronic renal disease. It is a synthetic form of vitamin D₃. It promotes calcium absorption from the GI tract and regulates calcium homeostasis. *Pregnancy category:* C; PB: UK; t½: 3–8 h
Ergocalciferol (Drisdol Drops)	A&C: PO: 50,000–200,000 IU/d or 1.25–5.0 µg/d	For hypoparathyroidism and rickets. A larger dose may be required in vitamin D-resistant rickets. It enhances calcium and phosphorus absorption. It has a long duration of action. *Pregnancy category:* C; PB: UK; t½: 12–24 h

Table continued on following page

TABLE 40–3 Parathyroid Hormones: Replacements and Supplements (*Continued*)

Generic (Brand)	Route and Dosage	Uses and Considerations
Hyperparathyroidism and Hypercalcemia		
Calcitonin (human) (Cibacalcin)	A: SC: Initially: 0.5 mg/d; maint: 0.25 mg daily–0.5 mg b.i.d.	For treating Paget's disease of the bone (osteitis deformans), hyperparathyroidism, and hypercalcemia. Calcitonin salmon is more potent than calcitonin human. Calcitonin decreases serum calcium by binding at receptor sites on osteoclast. *Pregnancy category:* C; PB: UK; t½: 1–1.5 h
Calcitonin (salmon) (Calcimar)	A: SC/IM: Initially: 4 IU/kg/d; maint: 4–8 IU/kg q12h.	
Etidronate (Didronel)	A: PO: 5–10 mg/kg/d *Max:* 20 mg/kg/d	For Paget's disease; for hypercalcemia due to antineoplastic therapy. *Pregnancy category:* B; PB: UK; t½: 6 h

KEY: A: adult; C: child; IM: intramuscular; PO: by mouth; SC: subcutaneous; PB: protein-binding; t½: half-life; UK: unknown.

FIGURE 40–3. Parathyroid Hormone

Vitamin D Analog	**Dosage**	**NURSING PROCESS** Assessment and Planning
Calcitriol (Rocaltrol) *Pregnancy Category:* C	A: PO: 0.25 µg/d	

Contraindications	**Drug-Lab-Food Interactions**	
Hypersensitivity, hypercalcemia, hyperphosphatemia, hypervitaminosis D, malabsorption syndrome *Caution:* Cardiovascular disease, renal calculi	*Increase* cardiac dysrhythmias with digoxin, verapamil *Decrease* calcitriol absorption with cholestyramine *Lab: Increase* serum calcium with thiazide diuretics, calcium supplements	

Pharmacokinetics	**Pharmacodynamics**	Interventions
Absorption: PO: Well absorbed *Distribution:* PB: UK; crosses the placenta *Metabolism:* t½: 3–8 h *Excretion:* Mostly in feces	PO: Onset: 2–6 h Peak: 10–12 h Duration: 3–5 d	

Therapeutic Effects/Uses: To treat hypocalcemia in chronic renal failure.

Mode of Action: Enhancement of calcium deposits in bones.

Evaluation

Side Effects	**Adverse Reactions**
Anorexia, nausea, vomiting, diarrhea, cramps, drowsiness, headache, dizziness, lethargy, photophobia	Hypercalciuria, hyperphosphatemia, hematuria

KEY: *A: adult; PO: by mouth; UK: unknown; PB: protein-binding; t½: half-life.*

NURSING PROCESS: PARATHYROID HORMONE

ASSESSMENT

- Assess serum calcium level. Report abnormal results.
- Assess for symptoms of tetany in hypocalcemia: twitching of the mouth, tingling and numbness of the fingers, carpopedal spasm, spasmodic contractions, and laryngeal spasm.

POTENTIAL NURSING DIAGNOSES

- High risk for impaired tissue integrity
- Altered health maintenance

PLANNING

- The client's serum calcium level will be within the normal range.

NURSING INTERVENTIONS

- Monitor the serum calcium level. Normal reference value is 8.5 to 10.5 mg/dL, or 4.5 to 5.5 mEq/L. A serum calcium level <8.5 mg/dL, or <4.5 mEq/L, indicates hypocalcemia, and a serum calcium level >10.5 mg/dL, or >5.5 mEq/L, indicates hypercalcemia. Serum ionized calcium levels are usually used because much of the calcium is protein-bound and is nonionized and nonactive.

Hypoparathyroidism
- Advise the client to report symptoms of tetany (see Assessment).

Hyperparathyroidism
- Advise the client to report signs and symptoms of hypercalcemia: bone pain, anorexia, nausea, vomiting, thirst, constipation, lethargy, bradycardia, and polyuria.
- Instruct women to inform their health care provider about pregnancy status before taking calcitonin preparation.
- Advise the client to check OTC drugs for possible calcium content, especially if the client has an elevated serum calcium level. Some vitamins and antacids contain calcium. Tell the client to contact the health care provider before taking drugs with calcium.

EVALUATION

- Monitor the effectiveness of drug therapy.
- Continue monitoring for signs and symptoms of hypocalcemia (tetany) when commercially prepared calcitonin has been given.

ADRENALS

The paired **adrenal glands** are composed of the adrenal medulla and the adrenal cortex. The adrenal cortex produces two types of hormones, or corticosteroids: **glucocorticoids** (cortisol) and **mineralocorticoids** (aldosterone). Cortisol secreted by the adrenal glands is in response to the hypothalamus-pituitary-adrenal (HPA) axis as a result of the feedback mechanism. A decrease in the serum cortisol levels increases CRF and ACTH secretions, which stimulate the adrenal glands to secrete and release cortisol. An increased serum cortisol level exerts the negative feedback mechanism, which inhibits the HPA axis and less cortisol is released. Additional physiologic functions related to the hormones secreted from the adrenal medulla and adrenal cortex are described in the introduction to Unit XI.

The **corticosteroids** promote sodium retention and potassium excretion. A sodium ion is reabsorbed from the renal tubules in exchange for a potassium ion; the potassium ion is then excreted. Due to their influence on electrolytes and carbohydrate, protein, and fat metabolism, a deficiency of corticosteroids can result in serious illness or death. A decrease in corticosteroid secretion is known as adrenal hyposecretion (adrenal insufficiency, or **Addison's disease**) and an increase in corticosteroid secretion is called adrenal hypersecretion (**Cushing's syndrome**).

GLUCOCORTICOIDS

Glucocorticoids are influenced by ACTH, released from the anterior pituitary gland. They affect carbohydrate, protein, and fat metabolism, as well as muscle and blood cell activity. Due to their many mineralocorticoid effects, glucocorticoids can cause sodium absorption from the kidney, resulting in water retention, potassium loss, and increased blood pressure. Cortisol, the main glucocorticoid, has antiinflammatory, antiallergic, and antistress effects. Indications for glucocorticoid therapy include trauma, surgery, infections, emotional upsets, and anxiety. Table 40–4 lists the physiologic aspects of adrenal hyposecretion (Addison's disease) and hypersecretion (Cushing's syndrome).

Most of the wide variety of glucocorticoid drugs, frequently called *cortisone* drugs, are synthetically produced. These drugs have several routes of administration: oral, parenteral (intramuscular or intravenous), topical (creams, ointments, lotions) and aerosol (inhaler). The intramuscular form, although seldom used, should be administered deep in the muscle. The subcutaneous route is not recommended.

Glucocorticoids are used to treat many diseases and health problems including inflammatory, allergic, and debilitating conditions. Among the inflammatory conditions that may require glucocorticoids are autoimmune disorders such as multiple sclerosis, rheumatoid arthritis, and myasthenia gravis; ulcerative colitis; glomerulonephritis; shock; ocular and vascular inflammations; head trauma with cerebral edema; polyarteritis nodosa; and hepatitis. Allergic conditions include asthma, drug reactions, contact dermatitis, and anaphylaxis. Debilitating conditions are mainly due to malignancies. Organ transplant recipients may require glucocorticoids to prevent organ rejection.

There are many glucocorticoids, some more potent than others. Dexamethasone (Decadron) has been used for severe inflammatory response due to head trauma or allergic reactions. An inexpensive glucocorticoid that is frequently prescribed is prednisone. Figure 40–4 describes the pharmacologic data for prednisone.

Pharmacokinetics

Prednisone is readily absorbed from the GI tract. It has a short half-life of 3 to 4 h, and it has a moderately high protein-binding power. Prednisone is excreted primarily in the urine.

Pharmacodynamics

The major actions of prednisone are to suppress an acute inflammatory process and for immunosuppression. It prevents cell-mediated immune reactions. Prednisone should not be confused with prednisolone. Peak action occurs in 1 to 2 h, and its duration of action is long (1 to 1.5 d).

Commonly used glucocorticoid drugs are listed in Table 40–5. Most of the glucocorticoids are pregnancy category C drugs. Agents used for adrenocortical insufficiency contain both glucocorticoids and mineralocorticoids, whereas drugs for antiinflammatory or immunosuppressive use contain mostly glucocorticoids.

Side Effects and Adverse Reactions

The side effects and adverse reactions of glucocorticoids due to high doses or prolonged use include increased blood sugar, abnormal fat deposits in the

TABLE 40–4 Adrenal Hyposecretion and Hypersecretion

| Body System | Systemic Effects | |
	Hyposecretion	*Hypersecretion*

Metabolism
  Glucose
  Protein
  Fat
	Hypoglycemia
	Muscle weakness
		Hyperglycemia
		Muscle wasting; thinning of the skin; poor wound healing; osteoporosis; fat accumulation in face, neck, and trunk (protruding abdomen, buffalo hump); hyperlipidemia; high cholesterol

Central nervous system	Apathy, depression, fatigue	Increased neural activity; mood elevation; irritability; seizures
Gastrointestinal	Nausea, vomiting, abdominal pain	Peptic ulcers
Cardiovascular	Tachycardia, hypotension, cardiovascular collapse	Hypertension; edema; heart failure
Eyes	None	Cataract formation
Fluids and electrolytes	Hypovolemia; hyponatremia; hyperkalemia	Hypervolemia; hypernatremia; hypokalemia
Blood cells	Anemia	Increased RBCs and neutrophils; impaired clotting.

FIGURE 40–4. Adrenal Hormone

Glucocorticoid	Dosage	NURSING PROCESS
		Assessment and Planning
Prednisone (Deltasone, Meticorten, Orasone, Panasol-S), ✹ Apo-Prednisone, Winpred *Pregnancy Category:* C	A: PO: 5–60 mg/d in divided doses C: PO: 0.1–0.15 mg/kg/d in 2–4 divided doses or 4–5 mg/m²/d in 2 doses	
Contraindications	**Drug-Lab-Food Interactions**	
Hypersensitivity, psychosis, fungal infection *Caution:* Diabetes mellitus	*Increase* effect with barbiturates, phenytoin, rifampin, ephedrine, theophylline *Decrease* effects of aspirin, anticonvulsants, isoniazid (INH), antidiabetics, vaccines	
Pharmacokinetics	**Pharmacodynamics**	Interventions
Absorption: PO: Well absorbed *Distribution:* PB: 65–91%; crosses the placenta *Metabolism:* t½: 3–4 h *Excretion:* In urine	PO: Onset: UK Peak: 1–2 h Duration: 24–36 d	

Therapeutic Effects/Uses: To decrease inflammatory occurrence; as an immunosuppressant; to treat dermatologic disorders.

Mode of Action: Suppression of inflammation and adrenal function.

Evaluation

Side Effects	Adverse Reactions
Nausea, diarrhea, abdominal distention, increased appetite, sweating, headache, depression, flushing, mood changes	Petechiae, ecchymosis, hypertension, tachycardia, osteoporosis, muscle wasting *Life-threatening:* GI hemorrhage, pancreatitis, circulatory collapse, thrombophlebitis, embolism

KEY: A: adult; C: child; PO: by mouth; PB: protein-binding; UK: unknown; t½: half-life; GI: gastrointestinal; ✹: Canadian drug names.

face and trunk (moon face and buffalo hump) and decreased extremity size, muscle wasting, edema, sodium and water retention, hypertension, euphoria or psychosis, thinned skin with purpura, increased intraocular pressure (glaucoma), peptic ulcers, and growth retardation. Long-term use of glucocorticoid drugs can cause adrenal atrophy (loss of adrenal gland function). When drug therapy is discontinued, the dose should be tapered to allow the adrenal cortex to produce cortisol and other corticosteroids. An abrupt withdrawal of the drug can result in severe adrenocortical insufficiency.

Drug Interactions

Glucocorticoids increase the potency of drugs taken concurrently, including aspirin and nonsteroidal antiinflammatory drugs (NSAIDs), thus increasing the risk of GI bleeding and ulceration. Use of potassium-wasting diuretics (HydroDIURIL, Lasix) with

TABLE 40–5 Adrenal Hormones: Glucocorticoids

Generic (Brand)	Route and Dosage	Uses and Considerations
Beclomethasone Dipropionate (Vanceril)	A: Inhal: 2 puffs b.i.d./q.i.d.	Inhalation for treating bronchial asthma and bronchial inflammation. Also to treat seasonal rhinitis. *Like all glucocorticoid inhalants, it is for prophylactic use and not for acute asthmatic attack.* Pregnancy category: C; PB: 87%; t½: 5–15 h
Betamethasone (Celestone, Celestone Phosphate)	A: PO: 0.6–7.2 mg/d in single or divided doses IM/IV: 1–9 mg/d; *max:* IM: 12 mg/d	Potent antiinflammatory steroid drug. It may be injected in joints. Effective for treating bronchial asthma, arthritis, severe allergic reactions, and cerebral edema. Should be taken with food. *Pregnancy category:* C; PB: 64%–90%; t½: 3–5 h
Cortisone acetate (Cortone Acetate, Cortistan)	A: PO/IM: 25–300 mg/d; decrease dose periodically	For adrenocortical insufficiency. Contains glucocorticoid and mineralocorticoid. Decreases inflammatory process. Oral dose is rapidly absorbed from the GI tract. Administer deep intramuscularly. With oral dose, give with food. *Pregnancy category:* C; PB: UK; t½: 0.5–12 h
Dexamethasone (Decadron)	*Inflammation:* A: PO: 0.25–4 mg b.i.d./q.i.d. IM: 4–16 mg q1–3wk C: PO: 0.2 mg/kg/d in divided doses *Shock:* A: IV: 1–6 mg/kg as a single dose (IV push in IV fluids)	Potent antiinflammatory drug. For acute allergic disorders; asthmatic attack; cerebral edema; unresponsive shock. For diagnosis of Cushing's syndrome and depression. Can be administered by IV push or in IV fluids. With oral dose, give with food. *Pregnancy category:* C; PB: 80%–90%; t½: 3–4 h
Fludrocortisone acetate (Florinef Acetate)	A&C: PO: 0.1–0.2 mg/d	For treating adrenocortical insufficiency as in Addison's disease. Also for salt-losing adrenogenital syndrome. Used only for its mineralocorticoid effects. *Pregnancy category:* C; PB: 92%; t½: 3.5 h
Hydrocortisone (Cortef, Hydrocortone)	A: PO: 20–240 mg/d in 2–4 divided doses IV: 15–240 mg (phosphate) q12h Rectal supp: 10–25 mg	For adrenocortical insufficiency and inflammation. Hydrocortisone sodium phosphate is parenteral form. Acetate form of drug may be injected into joints. Available in cream, ointment, lotion, and spray. *Pregnancy category:* C; PB: 79%; t½: 2–12 h
Methylprednisolone (Medrol, Solu-Medrol [sodium succinate] Depo-Medrol [acetate])	A: PO: 4–48 mg/d in one or more divided doses IM/IV: Succinate: 10–250 mg q6h IM: Acetate: 40–80 mg/wk	For treating inflammatory conditions such as arthritis, bronchial asthma, allergic reactions, cerebral edema. *Pregnancy category:* C; PB: UK; t½: 3.5 h
Paramethasone acetate (Haldrone)	A: PO: 0.5–6 mg t.i.d./q.i.d. C: PO: 58–200 μg/kg/d in 3–4 divided doses	For treating inflammatory conditions and allergic reactions. Similar to prednisone. Give with food. Do not abruptly stop dosing with long-term therapy. *Pregnancy category:* C; PB: 95%; t½: 3–45 h
Prednisolone (Delta-Cortef, Hydeltrasol [phosphate])	A: PO: 2.5–15 mg b.i.d./q.i.d. IV: Phosphate: 2–30 mg q12h C: PO: 0.14–2 mg/kg/d in a single or divided doses	For antiinflammatory or immunosuppressive effect. For parenteral use. It can be injected into joints and soft tissue. Potent steroid. *Pregnancy category:* C; PB: 80%–90%; t½: 3.5 h (tissue: 18–36 h)
Prednisone	See Prototype Drug Chart (Fig. 40–4)	For antiinflammatory or immunosuppressive effect. Inexpensive drug. This oral glucocorticoid is drug of choice. Take with food. Drug should not be abruptly stopped. *Pregnancy category:* C; PB: UK; t½: 3–4 h
Triamcinolone (Aristocort, Kenacort, Azmacort, Kenalog)	A: PO: 4–48 mg/d in 2–4 divided doses Inhal: 2 puffs, t.i.d., q.i.d. Topical preparations: cream, ointment	For antiinflammatory or immunosuppressive effect. *Pregnancy category:* C; PB: UK; t½: 2–5 h

KEY: *A: adult; C: child; PO: by mouth; Inhal: inhalation; IV: intravenous; PB: protein-binding; t½: half-life; UK: unknown.*

glucocorticoids increases potassium loss resulting in hypokalemia. Glucocorticoids can decrease the effect of oral anticoagulants (warfarin [Coumadin]). Barbiturates, phenytoin, and rifampin decrease the effect of prednisone. Prolonged use of prednisone can cause severe muscle weakness.

Dexamethasone, a potent glucocorticoid, interacts with many drugs. Phenytoin, theophylline, rifampin, barbiturates, and antacids decrease the action of dexamethasone, whereas NSAIDs, including aspirin, and estrogen increase it. Dexamethasone decreases the effects of oral anticoagulants and oral antidiabetics. When the drug is given with diuretics and/or anti-*Pseudomonas* penicillin preparations, the serum potassium level may decrease markedly. Glucocorticoids can increase the blood sugar levels; thus, insulin or oral antidiabetic drug dosage may need to be increased.

MINERALOCORTICOIDS

Mineralocorticoids, the second type of corticosteroid, secrete aldosterone. These hormones maintain fluid balance by promoting the reabsorption of sodium from the renal tubules. Sodium attracts water, resulting in water retention. When hypovolemia (decrease in circulating fluid) occurs, more aldosterone is secreted to increase sodium and water retention and to restore fluid balance. With sodium reabsorption, potassium is lost and hypokalemia (potassium deficit) can occur. Some glucocorticoid drugs also contain mineralocorticoids; these include cortisone and hydrocortisone. A severe decrease in the mineralocorticoid aldosterone leads to hypotension and vascular collapse, as seen in Addison's disease. Mineralocorticoid deficiency usually occurs with glucocorticoid deficiency, frequently called *corticosteroid deficiency.*

Fludrocortisone (Florinef) is an oral mineralocorticoid that can be given with a glucocorticoid. It can cause a negative nitrogen balance, so a high-protein diet is usually indicated. Because potassium excretion occurs with the use of mineralocorticoids and glucocorticoids, the serum potassium level should be monitored.

NURSING PROCESS: ADRENAL HORMONE: Glucocorticoids

ASSESSMENT

- Obtain baseline vital signs (VS) for future comparison.
- Assess laboratory test results, especially serum electrolytes and blood sugar. Serum potassium level usually decreases and blood sugar level increases when a glucocorticoid such as prednisone is taken over an extensive period of time.
- Obtain the client's weight and urine output to use for future comparison.
- Assess the client's medical history. Report if the client has glaucoma, cataracts, peptic ulcer, psychiatric problems, or diabetes mellitus. Glucocorticoids can intensify these health problems.

POTENTIAL NURSING DIAGNOSES

- Fluid volume excess
- High risk for impaired tissue integrity

PLANNING

- The client's inflammatory process will abate. Side effects of glucocorticoid will be minimal.

NURSING INTERVENTIONS

- Monitor VS. Glucocorticoids such as prednisone can increase blood pressure and sodium and water retention.
- Administer glucocorticoids only as ordered. Routes of administration include PO, IM (not in the deltoid muscle), IV, aerosol, and topical. Topical glucocorticoid drugs should be applied in thin layers. Rashes, infection, and purpura should be noted and reported.
- Monitor weight. Report weight gain of 5 lb in several days; this would most likely be due to water retention.
- Monitor laboratory values, especially serum electrolytes and blood sugar. Serum potassium level could decrease to <3.5 mEq/L, and blood sugar level would probably increase.
- Observe for signs and symptoms of hypokalemia, such as nausea, vomiting, muscular weakness, abdominal distention, paralytic ileus, and irregular heart rate.
- Observe for side effects from glucocorticoid drugs when therapy has lasted >10 d and the drug is taken in high dosages. The cortisone preparation should not be abruptly stopped because adrenal crisis can result.
- Monitor older adults for signs and symptoms of increased osteoporosis. Glucocorticoids promote calcium loss from the bone.
- Report changes in muscle strength. High doses of glucocorticoids promote loss of muscle tone.

CLIENT TEACHING

General

- Advise the client to take the drug as prescribed. Instruct the client *not* to abruptly stop the drug. When the drug is discontinued, the dose is tapered over 1 to 2 wk.

- For short-term use (<10 d) of glucocorticoids such as prednisone or other cortisone preparations, the drug dose still needs to be tapered. Prepare a schedule for the client to decrease the dose over a period of 4 to 5 d. For example, take 1 tab q.i.d.; the next day take 1 tab t.i.d.; the next day, take 1 tab b.i.d.; and then take 1 tab daily.
- Advise the client not to take cortisone preparations (PO or topical) during pregnancy unless necessary and prescribed by the health care provider. These drugs may be harmful to the fetus.
- Instruct the client to avoid persons with respiratory infections since these drugs suppress the immune system. This is especially important if the client is receiving a high dose of glucocorticoids.
- Advise the client receiving glucocorticoids to inform other health care providers of all drugs taken, especially before surgery.
- Advise the client to have a medical alert card, tag, or bracelet stating the glucocorticoid drug being taken.

Skill

- Teach the client how to use an aerosol nebulizer. Warn the client against overuse of the aerosol to avoid possible rebound effect.

Diet

- Instruct the client to take cortisone preparations at mealtime or with food. Glucocorticoid drugs can irritate the gastric mucosa and cause a peptic ulcer.
- Advise the client to eat foods rich in potassium, such as fresh and dried fruits, vegetables, meats, and nuts. Prednisone promotes potassium loss and, thus, hypokalemia.

Side Effects

- Teach the client to report signs and symptoms of drug overdose or Cushing's syndrome, including a moon face, puffy eyelids, edema in the feet, increased bruising, dizziness, bleeding, and menstrual irregularity.

EVALUATION

- Evaluate the effectiveness of glucocorticoid drug therapy. If the inflammation has not improved, a change in drug therapy may be necessary.
- Continue monitoring for side effects, especially when the client is receiving high doses of glucocorticoids.

■ CASE STUDY

M. P., age 68 years, had a severe allergic reaction to shellfish. She is taken to the emergency room. A single dose of dexamethasone 100 mg IV (direct IV over 30 seconds) was ordered. M. P. weighs 65 kg.

1. What type of drug is dexamethasone?
2. Is the dosage within safe therapeutic range? Explain.
3. Is the route for administering dexamethasone correct? Describe the various intravenous means of administration.

Twenty-one tablets of prednisone, 5 mg each, were prescribed to be taken over 5 days, with tapering daily doses. First day would be 10 mg, 4 times a day; second day 10 mg, 3 times a day; third day 10 mg, 2 times a day; fourth day 10 mg once a day; and the fifth day 5 mg once a day.

4. Why was prednisone ordered and not oral dexamethasone? Explain.
5. What is the purpose for tapering prednisone doses? Explain.

6. Is the drug dose within safe therapeutic range? Explain.
7. Should M. P. have side effects such as peripheral edema due to water and sodium retention with tapering prednisone doses? Explain.
8. What is the difference between prednisone and prednisolone?
9. What are the adverse reactions from prolonged use of prednisone?
10. What are the nursing interventions and client teaching for M. P. and clients taking prednisone?

STUDY QUESTIONS

1. What hormones are secreted by the anterior pituitary gland (adenohypophysis) and what are their functions?
2. What is the action of ACTH? What are the nursing interventions and client teaching for clients receiving ACTH?
3. The client has diabetes insipidus. Is this the

same as diabetes mellitus? Explain. What are the symptoms of diabetes insipidus? What drug is used to control this health problem?

4. What are the two hormones secreted by the thyroid gland? Differentiate between levothyroxine (Synthroid) and liothyronine (Cytomel). What are their actions?

5. For what disorders are the antithyroid drugs used? What severe side effects can result from their use?

6. What electrolyte is directly influenced by parathyroid hormone?

7. What are the physiologic effects of hypersecretion and hyposecretion of parathyroid hormone?

8. What are the subgroups of corticosteroids? What are four signs and symptoms of prolonged use of corticosteroids (cortisone)? What are the nursing implications of discontinuing a cortisone preparation? What instructions should the client receive?

9. A deficiency of the hormone cortisol leads to what health problem? What are the symptoms of this disease? What type of drug is used to control this disease?

Chapter 41

Antidiabetic Drugs

OUTLINE

Objectives
Terms
Introduction
Diabetes Mellitus
   Insulin
     Nursing Process

Oral Antidiabetic Drugs
   (Oral Hypoglycemic
   Drugs): Sulfonylureas
Second-Generation
   Sulfonylureas

Nonsulfonylureas: Newer
   Drugs
Hyperglycemic Drugs
Nursing Process
Case Study
Study Questions

OBJECTIVES

Define diabetes mellitus, IDDM (type I), NIDDM (type II), insulin, oral hypoglycemic agents, and glucagon.

Identify the symptoms of diabetes mellitus.

Explain a hypoglycemic reaction and describe the symptoms.

Differentiate among rapid-acting, intermediate-acting, and long-acting insulin.

Identify the peak concentration time for the three types of insulin action and when a hypoglycemic action is most likely to occur.

Identify the action of oral hypoglycemic drugs and their side effects.

Describe the nursing process including client teaching, for insulin and oral hypoglycemic agents.

TERMS

diabetes mellitus
hypoglycemic reaction
IDDM
insulin

insulin shock
ketoacidosis
lipodystrophy
NIDDM

oral hypoglycemic drugs
polydipsia
polyphagia
polyuria

INTRODUCTION

Antidiabetic drugs are used primarily to control diabetes mellitus, a chronic disease that affects carbohydrate metabolism. There are two groups of antidiabetic agents: (1) insulin, and (2) oral hypoglycemic drugs. Oral hypoglycemic drugs are synthetic preparations that stimulate insulin release or otherwise alter the metabolic response to hyperglycemia. **Insulin,** a protein secreted from the beta cells of the pancreas, is necessary for carbohydrate metabolism and also plays an important role in protein and fat metabolism. The beta cells make up 75% of the pancreas, and the alpha cells that secrete glucagon, a hyperglycemic substance, occupy approximately 20% of the pancreas.

DIABETES MELLITUS

Diabetes mellitus, a chronic disease resulting from deficient glucose metabolism, is caused by insufficient insulin secretion from the beta cells.* This results in high blood sugar (hyperglycemia). Diabetes mellitus is characterized by the three Ps: **polyuria** (increased urine output), **polydipsia** (increased thirst), and **polyphagia** (increased hunger). The two forms of diabetes are (1) insulin-dependent diabetes mellitus (IDDM), or type I diabetes mellitus (also referred to as juvenile-onset diabetes with no insulin secretion), and (2) non–insulin-dependent diabetes mellitus (NIDDM), or type II diabetes mellitus (also known as maturity-onset or adult-onset diabetes with some insulin secretion).

How the lack of insulin causes diabetes mellitus is not fully understood. Some authorities suggest that viral infections may contribute to the onset of IDDM, and heredity is a major factor in NIDDM. In NIDDM, there is some beta cell function with varying amounts of insulin secretion, and hyperglycemia can be controlled with oral antidiabetic drugs and a diet prescribed by the American Diabetic Association. However, insulin may be required during times of stress (surgery, trauma, infection, pregnancy). A person with NIDDM whose diabetes is controlled by an oral hypoglycemic drug can become insulin-dependent years later.

Certain drugs increase blood sugar and can cause hyperglycemia in prediabetic persons. These include glucocorticoids (cortisone, prednisone), thiazide diuretics (hydrochlorothiazide [Hydro-DIURIL]), and epinephrine. Usually the blood sugar level returns to normal after the drug is discontinued.

---

* Diabetes mellitus is a disorder of the pancreas; diabetes insipidus is a disorder of the posterior pituitary gland.

INSULIN

Insulin is released from the beta cells of the islets of Langerhans in response to an increase in blood glucose. Oral glucose load is more effective in raising the serum insulin level than an intravenous glucose load. This is partly due to an increase in GI hormones. Insulin promotes the uptake of glucose, amino acids, and fatty acids and converts them to substances that are stored in body cells. Glucose is converted to glycogen for future glucose needs in the liver and muscle, thereby lowering the blood glucose level. The normal range for blood glucose is 60 to 100 mg/dL and, for serum glucose, 70 to 110 mg/dL. When the blood glucose level is greater than 180 mg/dL, glycosuria (sugar in the urine) can occur. Increased blood sugar acts as an osmotic diuretic, causing polyuria. When blood sugar remains elevated (>200 mg/dL), diabetes mellitus occurs.

The beta cells in the pancreas secrete approximately 0.2 to 0.5 U/kg/d. A client weighing 70 kg (154 pounds) would secrete 14 to 35 U of insulin a day. More insulin secretion may occur if the person consumes a greater caloric intake. A client with diabetes mellitus may require 0.2 to 1.0 U/kg/d. The higher range may be due to obesity, stress, or tissue insulin resistance.

Parenteral (injectable) insulin is obtained from pork and beef pancreas when the animals are slaughtered. Pork insulin is closely related to human insulin, having only one different amino acid; beef insulin has four different amino acids. Human insulin (Humulin) was introduced in 1983 and is produced by two separate methods: (1) changing the different amino acid of pork insulin or (2) using DNA technology. Pork insulin is a weaker allergen than beef insulin, and the use of human insulin has a very low incidence of allergic effects and insulin resistance. Insulin is now purer than previously, especially the Humulin produced by DNA technology, resulting in fewer side effects. Today, newly diagnosed clients with insulin-dependent diabetes are usually prescribed human insulin. If a client has been taking animal (pork or beef) insulin without having any untoward effects, then it is not necessary to change to human insulin.

Insulin should be kept in a cool place or refrigerated once opened. The concentration of insulin is 40 or 100 U/mL (U40/mL, U100/mL) and the insulin is packaged in a 10 mL vial (see figures on insulin in Chapter 4D). Insulin syringes are marked in units to a maximum of 100 U per 1 mL. Insulin syringes must be used for accurate dosing. To prevent dosage errors, the nurse must be certain that there is a match of the insulin concentration with the calibration of units on the insulin syringe. Before use, the client or nurse must roll, not shake, the bottle to ensure that the insulin and its ingredients are well mixed. Shaking a bottle of insulin can cause bubbles and an inaccurate dose. Insulin requirements vary; usually less insulin is needed with increased exercise and more insulin with infections and high fever.

There are three types of insulin: rapid-acting, intermediate-acting, and long-acting. Rapid-acting insulin is called regular (crystalline) insulin and is a clear solution without any added substance to prolong the insulin action. The onset of action is 1/2 to 1 h, peak action occurs in 2 to 4 h, and the duration of action is 6 to 8 h. The onset of intermediate-acting insulin is 1 to 2 h, peak is 6 to 12 h, and the duration of action is 18 to 24 h. Long-acting insulin acts in 4 to 8 h, peaks in 14 to 20 h, and lasts for 24 to 36 h.

Insulin is a protein and *cannot* be administered orally because gastrointestinal (GI) secretions destroy the insulin structure. It is administered subcutaneously, at a 45- to 90-angle. The 90-angle is made by raising the skin and fatty tissue; the insulin is injected into the pocket between the fat and the muscle. In a thin person with little fatty tissue, the 45- to 60-angle is used. Regular insulin is the *only* type that can be administered intravenously.

The site and depth of insulin injection affect absorption. Insulin absorption is greater when given in the deltoid and abdominal areas than when given in the thighs and buttock areas. Insulin administered subcutaneously has a slower absorption rate than if administered intramuscularly. Heat and massage could increase subcutaneous absorption. Cooling the subcutaneous area can decrease absorption.

Insulin is usually given in the morning before breakfast. It can be given several times a day. Insulin injection sites should be rotated to prevent **lipodystrophy** (tissue atrophy or hypertrophy), which can interfere with insulin absorption. Lipoatrophy (tissue atrophy) is a depression under the skin surface. A frequent cause of an atrophied area is due to the use of animal insulins (beef and pork). Lipohypertrophy (tissue hypertrophy) is a raised lump or knot on the skin surface. It frequently is caused by repeated injections into the same subcutaneous site. The client needs to develop a "site rotation pattern" in order to avoid lipodystrophy and to promote insulin absorption. There are various insulin rotation programs, such as an 8-day rotation schedule (insulin is given at a different site each day). The American Diabetic Association suggests that insulin should be injected daily at a chosen site for 1 week. Injections should be 1½ inches apart (a knuckle length) at a site area each day. If a client has to take two insulin injections a day (morning and evening), one site should be chosen on the right side (morning) and one site on the left side (evening). Figure 41–1 illustrates sites for insulin injections. A record of injection area sites and dates administered should be kept.

Obesity can be a causative factor of insulin resistance. Persons taking animal insulin will develop antibodies over time. This can slow the onset of insulin action and extend its duration of action. Antibody development can cause insulin resistance and insulin allergy. Skin tests with different insulin preparations may be performed to determine if there is an allergic effect. Human and regular insulins produce fewer allergens.

Illness and stress increase the need for insulin. Insulin doses should *not* be withheld during illness, including infections and stress. Hyperglycemia and ketoacidosis may result from withholding insulin.

To prolong the action, intermediate-acting and long-acting insulins are used, which contain protamine or zinc or both in addition to regular or crystalline insulin. The lente insulins contain zinc, neutral-protamine-Hagedorn (NPH) insulin contains protamine, and protamine-zinc insulin (PZI) contains both protamine and zinc. Regular insulin can be mixed in the same syringe with protamine or zinc insulin. Mixing insulin can alter absorption rate. When regular insulin is mixed with lente insulin, a portion of the regular insulin effect is lost.

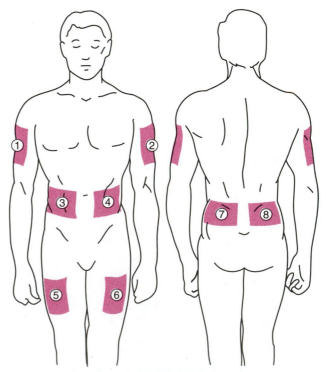

FIGURE 41–1 Sites for insulin injection.

FIGURE 41–2. Antidiabetic: Insulins

Regular and NPH Insulin	Dosage	NURSING PROCESS
Regular Insulin *NPH Insulin* Injectable insulins *Pregnancy Category:* B	Varies according to client's blood sugar	**Assessment and Planning**

Contraindications	**Drug-Lab-Food Interactions**	
Hypersensitivity to beef, zinc, prota- mine insulins	*Increase* hypoglycemic effect with as- pirin, oral anticoagulant, alcohol, oral hypoglycemics, beta blockers, tricyclic antidepressants, MAOIs, tetracycline *Decrease* hypoglycemic effect with thi- azides, glucocorticoids, oral contra- ceptives, thyroid drugs, smoking	

Pharmacokinetics	**Pharmacodynamics**	Interventions

Absorption: SC, IV (regular)
Distribution: PB: UK
Metabolism: t½: Regular IV insulin: 5–9
  min; varies with type of insulin
Excretion: Mostly in urine
	Regular Insulin:
	SC: Onset: 0.5–1 h
	    Peak: 2–4 h
	    Duration: 4–8 h
	IV: Onset: 10–20 min
	    Peak: 15–30 min
	    Duration: 1–2 h
	NPH Insulin:
	SC: Onset: 1–2 h
	    Peak: 6–12 h (8–9 h average)
	    Duration: 18–24 h	

Therapeutic Effects/Uses: To control diabetes mellitus; to lower blood sugar. *Mode of Action:* Insulin promotes utilization of glucose by body cells.	Evaluation

Side Effects	**Adverse Reactions**
Hunger, tremors, weakness, headache, lethargy, fatigue, redness, irritation or swelling at insulin injection site, flushing, confusion, agitation	Urticaria, tachycardia, palpitations, hy- poglycemic reaction, rebound hyper- glycemia (Somogyi effect), lipodys- trophy *Life-threatening:* Shock; anaphylaxis

KEY: SC: subcutaneous; IV: intravenous; UK: unknown; PB: protein-binding; t½: half-life;
MAOIs: monoamine oxidase inhibitors.

Less regular insulin is lost when mixed with NPH insulin than if mixed with lente. Figure 41–2 compares regular insulin to NPH insulin.

Pharmacokinetics

Regular and NPH insulins are well absorbed with all routes of administration. Both insulins can be administered subcutaneously, but only regular insulin can be given intravenously. The half-life varies. Insulin is metabolized by the liver and muscle and excreted in the urine.

Pharmacodynamics

Insulin lowers blood sugar by promoting utilization of glucose by the body cells. It also stores glucose as glycogen in muscles. The onset of action of regular insulin given subcutaneously is ½ to 1 h and given intravenously, 10 to 30 min. The onset of action of NPH is 1 to 2 h. The peak action time of insulins is very important because of the possibility of hypoglycemic reaction (insulin shock) occurring during that time. The peak time for regular insulin is 2 to 4 h and 6 to 12 h for NPH insulin. The nurse needs to assess for signs and symptoms of hypoglycemic reaction, such as nervousness, tremors, confusion, sweating, and increased pulse rate. Orange juice, sugar-sweetened beverages, or hard candy should be kept available and given if a reaction occurs.

Regular insulin can be given several times a day, especially during the regulation of insulin dosage. NPH insulin is usually administered once a day. Regular insulin (3 to 15 U) can be mixed with an intermediate-acting insulin (NPH or lente), especially if rapid onset of action is needed. Long-acting insulins are seldom ordered because their peak action time occurs during the night or early morning. When switching from pork to human insulin, the client may require an adjustment of insulin dose, because human insulin has a shorter duration of action.

Drug Interactions

Drugs such as thiazide diuretics, glucocorticoids (cortisone preparations), thyroid agents, and estrogen increase the blood sugar, and insulin dosage may need adjustment. Drugs that decrease insulin needs are tricyclic antidepressants, monoamine oxidase (MAO) inhibitors, aspirin products, and oral anticoagulants.

Table 41–1 lists the drug data for the rapid-acting, intermediate-acting, and long-acting insulins.

TABLE 41–1 Antidiabetics: Insulins

Generic (Brand)	Route and Dosage	Pregnancy Category	Half-life	Protein-Binding	Action		
					Onset	*Peak*	*Duration*
Rapid-Acting							
Humulin R Regular	Same as regular insulin A & C: SC/IV: 100 U/mL; dose is individualized according to blood sugar	B	10 min–1 h	UK	0.5–1 h	2–4 h	6–8 h
Semilente	A & C: SC: 100 U/mL; dose is individualized according to blood sugar	B	<13 h	UK	30–45 min	4–6 h	12–16 h
Intermediate-Acting							
Humulin L insulin	Same as lente	B	13 h	UK	1–2 h	8–12 h	18–28 h
Humulin N insulin	Same as NPH insulin	B	13 h	UK	1–2 h	8–12 h	18–24 h
Lente insulin	A & C: SC: 100 U/mL; dose is individualized according to blood sugar	B	13 h	UK	1–2 h	8–12 h	18–28 h
NPH insulin	See Prototype Drug Chart (Fig. 41–2)	B	13 h	UK	1–2 h	6–12 h	18–24 h
Long-Acting							
PZI insulin*	Same as lente	B	13 h	UK	4–8 h	14–20 h	24–36 h
Ultralente insulin	Same as lente	B	13 h	UK	5–8 h	14–20 h	30–36 h

KEY: *IV: intravenous; NPH: neutral-protamine-Hagedorn; PZI: protamine-zinc insulin; SC: subcutaneous; UK: unknown.*
* *Protamine and zinc suspensions are added to regular insulin.*

Side Effects and Adverse Reactions: Hypoglycemic Reactions and Ketoacidosis

When more insulin is administered than is needed for glucose metabolism, **a hypoglycemic reaction,** or **insulin shock,** occurs. The person may become nervous, trembling, and uncoordinated, with cold and clammy skin, and may complain of a headache. Giving sugar orally or intravenously increases the utilization of insulin, and the symptoms disappear immediately.

With an inadequate amount of insulin, the sugar cannot be metabolized and fat catabolism occurs. The use of fatty acids (ketones) for energy causes **ketoacidosis** (diabetic acidosis or diabetic coma). Table 41–2 gives the signs and symptoms of hypoglycemic reaction and ketoacidosis.

TABLE 41–2 Hypoglycemic Reaction and Diabetic Ketoacidosis

Reaction	Signs and Symptoms
Hypoglycemic reaction (insulin shock)	Headache, lightheadedness Nervousness, apprehension Tremor Excess perspiration; cold, clammy skin Tachycardia Slurred speech Memory lapse, confusion, seizures Blood sugar level < 60 mg/dL
Diabetic ketoacidosis (hyperglycemic reaction)	Extreme thirst Polyuria Fruity breath odor Kussmaul breathing (deep, rapid, labored, distressing, dyspnea) Rapid, thready pulse Dry mucous membranes, poor skin turgor Blood sugar level > 250 mg/dL

NURSING PROCESS: ANTIDIABETICS: Insulin

ASSESSMENT

- Assess the drugs the client is currently taking. Certain drugs, such as alcohol, aspirin, oral anticoagulants, oral hypoglycemics, beta blockers, tricyclic antidepressants, MAOIs, and tetracycline, increase the hypoglycemic effect when taken with insulin. Note that thiazides, glucocorticoids, oral contraceptives, thyroid drugs, and smoking can increase blood sugar.
- Assess the type of insulin and dosage. Note if it is given once or twice a day.
- Check vital signs (VS) and blood sugar levels. Report abnormal findings.
- Assess the client's knowledge of diabetes mellitus and the use of insulins.
- Assess for signs and symptoms of a hypoglycemic reaction (insulin shock) and hyperglycemia or ketoacidosis.

POTENTIAL NURSING DIAGNOSES

- High risk for impaired tissue integrity
- Altered nutrition: more or less than body requirements
- High risk for injury

PLANNING

- Client's blood sugar will be within the normal values (70 to 110 mg/dL).

NURSING INTERVENTIONS

- Monitor VS. Tachycardia can occur during an insulin reaction.
- Monitor blood glucose levels and report changes. The reference value is 60 to 100 mg/dL for blood glucose and 70 to 110 mg/dL for serum glucose.
- Prepare a teaching plan based on the client's knowledge of the health problem, diet, and drug therapy.

CLIENT TEACHING

General

- Instruct the client to report immediately symptoms of a hypoglycemic (insulin) reaction, such as headache, nervousness, sweating, tremors, and rapid pulse, and symptoms of a hyperglycemic reaction (diabetic acidosis), such as thirst, increased urine output, and sweet fruity breath odor.
- Advise the client that hypoglycemic reactions are more likely to occur during the peak action time. Most diabetics know if they are having a hypoglycemic reaction; however, some have a higher tolerance to low blood sugar and can have a severe hypoglycemic reaction without realizing it.
- Explain that orange juice, sugar-containing drinks, and hard candy may be used when a hypoglycemic reaction begins.
- Instruct family members in administering

glucagon by injection if the client has a hypoglycemic reaction and cannot drink sugar-containing fluid.
- Instruct the client about the necessity for compliance to prescribed insulin and diet.
- Advise the client to obtain a medical alert card, tag, and/or bracelet indicating the health problem and insulin dosage.

Skill
- Instruct the client how to check the blood sugar using Chemstrip bG test.
- Instruct the client in the care of the insulin bottle and syringes. Inform the client taking NPH or lente insulin with regular insulin that the regular

insulin should be drawn up before the NPH or lente insulin.

Diet
- Advise the client taking insulin to eat the prescribed diet on schedule. The diet may be from the American Diabetic Association (ADA).

EVALUATION

- Evaluate the effectiveness of the insulin therapy by noting whether blood sugar level is within the accepted range.
- Evaluate the client's knowledge of the signs and symptoms of hypoglycemic or hyperglycemic reaction.

ORAL ANTIDIABETIC DRUGS (ORAL HYPOGLYCEMIC DRUGS): SULFONYLUREAS

Oral antidiabetic drugs, also called **oral hypoglycemics,** were discovered in the 1950s. These drugs are used by persons with NIDDM. They should **not** be used by persons with IDDM. Persons with NIDDM have some degree of insulin secretion by the pancreas. The sulfonylureas, a group of antidiabetics that are chemically related to sulfonamides but lack antibacterial activity, stimulate the beta cells to secrete more insulin. This increases the insulin cell receptors, thus increasing the cells' ability to bind insulin for glucose metabolism.

The sulfonylureas are classified as first- and second-generations. The first-generation sulfonylureas are divided into short-acting, intermediate-acting, and long-acting antidiabetics. Figure 41–3 lists the actions and effects of the first-generation, intermediate-acting sulfonylurea, acetohexamide (Dymelor).

Pharmacokinetics

Acetohexamide is well absorbed from the GI tract and is highly protein-bound. Acetohexamide is metabolized by the liver with 50% converted to a metabolite. There are two half-lives: the half-life of the drug metabolite is three times as long as that of the pure drug. The kidneys excrete the drug unchanged in the urine.

Pharmacodynamics

Acetohexamide is prescribed to control NIDDM. It lowers the blood sugar by stimulating the beta cells in the pancreas to secrete insulin. Acetohexamide's onset of action usually occurs within 1 h, and the

peak action time is between 2 and 6 h. The drug is usually given once a day in the morning due to its long duration of action.

SECOND-GENERATION SULFONYLUREAS

The second-generation sulfonylureas were first used in Europe, and in 1984 were approved by the Food and Drug Administration for use in the United States. The newer sulfonylureas increase the tissue response to insulin and decrease glucose production by the liver. They have a greater hypoglycemic potency than the first-generation sulfonylureas. Effective doses for the second-generation drugs are less than the dosages of the first generation. The second-generation drugs have less displacement potential from protein-binding sites by other highly protein-bound drugs, such as salicylates and warfarin (Coumadin), than those of the first-generation drugs. The second-generation sulfonylureas should not be used when liver or kidney dysfunction is present. A hypoglycemic reaction is more likely to occur in the elderly.

Table 41–3 lists the drug data for the sulfonylureas.

Side Effects, Adverse Reactions, and Contraindications

The side effects are similar to those of insulin. Taking antidiabetic drugs without adequate food can lead to an insulin reaction with signs and symptoms such as nervousness, tremors, and confusion. Adverse reactions are those of hematologic disorders: aplastic anemia, leukopenia, and thrombocytopenia. Sulfonylureas are contraindicated in IDDM

FIGURE 41–3. Antidiabetics: Sulfonylurea

Sulfonylurea	Dosage	NURSING PROCESS Assessment and Planning
Acetohexamide (Dymelor) ✳ Dimelor Oral hypoglycemic drug *Pregnancy Category:* C	A: PO: 250–1000 mg/d in 1 or 2 di- vided doses; max: 1.5 g/d; Maint: 1000 mg/d	
Contraindications	**Drug-Lab-Food Interactions**	

Diabetes mellitus (DM) type IDDM; se-
vere renal, hepatic, cardiac, or thy-
roid disease; unstable DM
	Increase hypoglycemic effect with
	  aspirin, alcohol, anticoagulants, some
	  NSAIDs, anticonvulsants,
	  sulfonamides, oral contraceptives,
	  MAOIs
	Decrease hypoglycemic effect with
	  glucocorticoids (cortisone), thiazide
	  diuretics, estrogen, calcium channel
	  blockers, phenytoin, thyroid drugs	

Pharmacokinetics	**Pharmacodynamics**	Interventions

Absorption: PO: Well absorbed
Distribution: PB: 90%
Metabolism: t½: Drug: 1–1.5 h metabo-
  lite; 5–7 h
Excretion: Unchanged in urine
	PO: Onset: 1 h
	  Peak: 2–6 h
	  Duration: 12–24 h	

	Evaluation
Therapeutic Effects/Uses: To control DM type II (maturity-onset diabetes); to lower blood sugar. *Mode of Action:* Stimulation of beta cells to secrete insulin.	

Side Effects	Adverse Reactions
Nausea, vomiting, diarrhea, rash, pru- ritus, headache, photosensitivity	Hypoglycemic reaction *Life-threatening:* Aplastic anemia, leukopenia, thrombocytopenia

KEY: A: adult; PO: by mouth; PB: protein-binding; t½: half-life; NSAIDs: nonsteroidal anti-inflammatory drugs; MAOIs: monoamine oxidase inhibitors; ✳ : Canadian drug name.

(no functioning beta cells), pregnancy, breast-feeding, and during stress, surgery, or severe infection.

Drug Interactions

Aspirin, anticoagulants, anticonvulsants, sulfonamides, and some NSAIDs can increase the action of sulfonylureas by binding to the plasma protein and displacing sulfonylureas. Because this causes increased free sulfonylurea, an insulin reaction can result. Sulfonylureas also enhance the action of thiazide diuretics, phenothiazines, and barbiturates. Sulfonylureas decrease the action of thyroid replacement drugs. Clients should be alerted not to drink alcohol while taking sulfonylureas because alcohol increases the half-life and a hypoglycemic reaction can result.

There are many drug interactions associated with acetohexamide. Glucocorticoids (cortisone), thiazide diuretics, calcium channel blockers, thyroid drugs, estrogen, and phenytoin (Dilantin) can decrease the effectiveness of acetohexamide. When acetohexa-

TABLE 41–3 Antidiabetics: Sulfonylureas

Generic (Brand)	Route and Dosage	Uses and Considerations
First-Generation: Short-Acting Tolbutamide (Orinase)	A: PO: 500–3000 mg/d in 2–3 divided doses	For managing non–insulin-dependent diabetes mellitus (NIDDM) or type II diabetes. Drug is chemically related to sulfonamides with no antiinfective effect. Hypoglycemic reaction may occur if overdosed. *Pregnancy category:* C; PB: >90%; t½: 4–7 h
First-Generation: Intermediate-Acting Acetohexamide (Dymelor)	See Prototype Drug Chart (Fig. 41–3)	For managing NIDDM or type II diabetes. May be given with selected type I diabetes clients. Doses >1000 mg are given twice a day. Has a diuretic effect. Duration of action is 12–24 h. *Pregnancy category:* C; PB: 90%; t½: 5–7 h
Tolazamide (Tolinase)	A: PO: 100–250 mg/d in 1–2 divided doses; *max:* 1 g/d	Same as acetohexamide. Diet and exercise should be a part of diabetic therapy. Duration of action is 10–20 h. *Pregnancy category:* C; PB: 90%; t½: 7 h
First-Generation: Long-Acting Chlorpropamide (Diabinese)	A: PO: Initially: 100–250 mg/d; maint: 100–500 mg/d in 1–2 divided doses; *max:* 750 mg/d	For managing NIDDM or type II diabetes. May be given to selected type I diabetics for reducing insulin doses. Diet and exercise should be a part of diabetic therapy. Duration of action is 24 h. May cause water and sodium retention. *Pregnancy category:* C; PB: 95%; t½: 36 h
Second-Generation: Glipizide (Glucotrol)	A: PO: Initially: 2.5–5.0 mg a.c. daily/b.i.d.; maint: 10–15 mg/d (dose should be divided if >15 mg), *max:* 40 mg/d	Same as acetohexamide and chlorpropamide. Duration of action is 10–24 h. Potent drug. *Pregnancy category:* C; PB: 90%–95%; t½: 2.5–5 h
Glyburide nonmicronized (DiaBeta, Micronase)	A: PO: Initially: 1.25–5 mg/d; maint: 1.25–20 mg q.d./b.i.d.; *max:* 20 mg/d	Same as chlorpropamide. Potent drug. Duration of action is 10–24 h. *Pregnancy category:* B; PB: 90%–95%; t½: 10 h
Glyburide micronized (Glynase)	A: PO: 1.5–3 mg/d in AM; maint: 3–4.5 mg/d; *max:* 12 mg/d in 1 or 2 divided doses	For NIDDM. Same as glyburide nonmicronized.
Nonsulfonylurease Metformin (Glucophage)	A: PO: Initial: 500 mg, daily/b.i.d.; increase dose gradually; *max:* 2500 mg/d	For NIDDM when no response to sulfonylureas. Take with meals. May be combined with sulfonylurea (dose reduction of metformin would be needed). *Pregnancy category:* B; PB: 0%; t½: 6.2 h
Acarbose (Precose)	A: PO: 25 mg, t.i.d.; *max:* 300 mg/d	For NIDDM. Client may experience diarrhea, abdominal distention, and/or flatulence. *Pregnancy category:* C; PB: UK; t½: UK

KEY: A: adult; PB: protein-binding; PO: by mouth; t½: half-life; UK; unknown; >: greater than.

mide is taken with sulfonamides, aspirin, NSAIDs, MAO inhibitors, cimetidine (Tagamet), alcohol, or insulin, a hypoglycemic reaction can occur.

NONSULFONYLUREAS: NEWER DRUGS

Expanding knowledge of glucose metabolism has revealed new mechanisms for the management of NIDDM or type II diabetes. These new drugs, metformin and acarbose, use different methods to control serum glucose levels following a meal. Unlike the sulfonylureas, which enhance insulin release and receptor interaction, these drugs affect the hepatic and gastrointestinal production of glucose.

Metformin (Glucophage)

Metformin is a biguanide compound that acts by decreasing hepatic production of glucose from stored glycogen. This diminishes the rise in serum glucose following a meal and blunts the degree of postprandial hyperglycemia. Metformin also decreases the absorption of glucose from the small intestine. There is also evidence that it increases insulin receptor sensitivity as well as peripheral glucose uptake at the cellular level. Unlike sulfonylureas, metformin does not produce hypoglycemia or hyperglycemia.

Metformin is 50% to 60% bioavailable and is absorbed primarily from the small intestine. It does not undergo hepatic metabolism and is eliminated unchanged in the urine. It is not recommended for clients with renal impairment. Monotherapy with metformin is effective; however, when combined with a sulfonylurea, the drug is useful in cases resistant to oral antidiabetics (oral hypoglycemics).

Acarbose (Precose)

Acarbose acts by inhibiting the digestive enzyme in the small intestine responsible for the release of glucose from the complex carbohydrates (CHO) in the diet. By inhibiting alpha glucosidase, the CHO cannot be absorbed and they pass into the large intestine. Acarbose has no demonstrated systemic effects and is not absorbed into the body in significant amounts.

Acarbose is intended for use in clients who do not achieve results on diet alone. Because the dietary carbohydrates pass into the large intestine, the normal flora ferments them, producing considerable gas. The diet selected should be a standard diabetic diet with reduced complex carbohydrates.

Guidelines for Oral Hypoglycemic (Antidiabetic) Use in NIDDM

The following are criteria for the use of oral hypoglycemics:

1. Onset of diabetes mellitus at age 40 years or older
2. Diagnosis of diabetes for less than 5 years
3. Normal or overweight
4. Fasting blood glucose equal to or less than 200 mg/dL
5. Less than 40 units of insulin required per day
6. Normal renal and hepatic function

HYPERGLYCEMIC DRUGS

Glucagon

Glucagon is a hyperglycemic hormone secreted by the alpha cells of the islets of Langerhans in the pancreas. Glucagon increases blood sugar by stimulating glycogenolysis (glycogen breakdown) in the liver. It protects the body cells, especially those in the brain and retina, by providing the nutrients and energy needed to maintain body function.

Glucagon is available for parenteral use (subcutaneous, intramuscular, and intravenous). It is used to treat insulin-induced hypoglycemia when other methods of providing glucose are not available. For example, the client may be semiconscious or unconscious and unable to ingest sugar-containing products. Diabetics who are prone to severe hypoglycemic reactions (insulin shock) should keep glucagon in the home, and family members should be taught how to administer subcutaneous or intramuscular injections during an emergency hypoglycemic reaction. The blood glucose level begins to increase within 5 to 20 min after administration. Recently, IV glucagon has been used in the acute treatment of beta blocker overdose and profound shock.

Diazoxide

Oral diazoxide (Proglycem), which is chemically related to thiazide diuretics, increases blood sugar by inhibiting insulin release from the beta cells and stimulating release of epinephrine (Adrenalin) from the adrenal medulla. This drug is not indicated for hypoglycemic reactions; rather, it is used to treat chronic hypoglycemia caused by hyperinsulinism due to islet cell cancer or hyperplasia. The parenteral form of diazoxide (Hyperstat) is prescribed for malignant hypertension. Hypotension usually does not occur with oral diazoxide.

Diazoxide has a long half-life and is highly protein-bound. Its onset of action is 1 h and the duration of action is 8 h. Most of the drug is excreted unchanged in the urine.

NURSING PROCESS: ANTIDIABETICS: Sulfonylureas

ASSESSMENT

- Assess the drugs the client is currently taking. Aspirin, alcohol, sulfonamides, oral contraceptives, and MAOIs increase the hypoglycemic effect; decrease in oral hypoglycemic drug may be needed. Glucocorticoids (cortisone), thiazide diuretics, and estrogen increase blood sugar.
- Assess vital signs (VS) and blood sugar levels. Report abnormal findings.

- Assess the client's knowledge of diabetes mellitus and the use of oral antidiabetics (sulfonylurea).

POTENTIAL NURSING DIAGNOSES

- High risk for impaired tissue integrity
- Altered nutrition: more or less than body requirements

PLANNING

- Client's blood sugar will be within normal serum levels (70 to 100 mg/dL).
- Client will adhere to prescribed diet, blood testing, and drug.

NURSING INTERVENTIONS

- Monitor VS. Sulfonylureas increase cardiac function and oxygen consumption, which can lead to cardiac dysrhythmias.
- Administer oral antidiabetics with food to minimize gastric upset.
- Monitor blood glucose levels and report changes. The reference value is 60 to 100 mg/dL for blood glucose and 70 to 110 mg/dL for serum glucose.
- Prepare a teaching plan based on the client's knowledge of health problems, diet, and drug therapy.

CLIENT TEACHING

General

- Advise the client that hypoglycemic (insulin) reaction can occur when taking an oral hypoglycemic drug. This drug stimulates the release of insulin from the beta cells of the pancreas. Oral antidiabetics are *not* insulin. Normally, clients with diabetes mellitus type I do not have functioning beta cells and should *not* take oral antidiabetics, only insulin. Sulfonylureas are prescribed for clients with diabetes mellitus type II.
- Instruct the client to recognize symptoms of hypoglycemic reaction (headache, nervousness, sweating, tremors, rapid pulse), and symptoms of hyperglycemic reaction (thirst, increased urine output, sweet fruity breath odor).

- Explain that insulin might be needed instead of an oral antidiabetic drug during stress, surgery, or serious infection. Blood sugar levels are usually elevated during stressful times.
- Instruct the client about the necessity for compliance to diet and drug.
- Advise the client to obtain a medical alert card, tag, and/or bracelet indicating the health problem and insulin dosage.

Skill

- Instruct the client how to check the blood sugar level using a Chemstrip bG test. Client should record and report abnormal results.

Diet

- To avoid a hypoglycemic reaction, instruct the client not to ingest alcohol with sulfonylurea drugs. Food taken with oral antidiabetics will decrease gastric irritation.
- Advise the client taking sulfonylurea to eat the prescribed diet on schedule. Delaying or missing a meal can cause hypoglycemia.
- Explain the use of orange juice, sugar-containing drinks, and hard candy when a hypoglycemic reaction begins.

Side Effects

- Instruct the client to report side effects, such as vomiting, diarrhea, rash.

EVALUATION

- Evaluate the effectiveness of drug therapy by noting whether blood sugar levels are within the accepted range.

■ CASE STUDY:
Client with Diabetes Mellitus

T. C., 32 years old, was diagnosed as having diabetes mellitus after the birth of her first child; her blood sugar level was 180 mg/dL. Her serum glucose level has been maintained within the normal range with acetohexamide (Dymelor) 250 mg/d.

1. What type of drug is acetohexamide? What is its action? Why is it taken only once a day?
2. Acetohexamide is indicated for what type of diabetes mellitus? When should acetohexamide not be taken?
3. Should acetohexamide be taken with sulfon-

amides, aspirin, NSAIDs, cimetidine, alcohol or insulin? Why or why not?
4. Why should T. C. monitor her blood sugar using Chemstrip bG?

Two years ago, T. C. became pregnant again. Acetohexamide was discontinued and Humulin N insulin 25 U prescribed. Since the birth of her second child, she has remained on Humulin N 25 U daily.

5. Give a possible reason why the health care provider changed the antidiabetic drug to insulin when T. C. became pregnant.
6. Humulin N is similar to what other type of insulin? How do these two types differ?
7. Give the onset, peak, and duration of action for

Humulin N insulin. When is an insulin reaction most likely to occur with Humulin N?

8. What are the signs and symptoms of a hypoglycemic reaction?

9. What should be included in client teaching?

T. C. asks the nurse if she can take acetohexamide again instead of insulin because she is eating the "right foods."

10. What should your response be?

STUDY QUESTIONS

1. Virginia, 13 years old, has been recently diagnosed with diabetes mellitus. She is receiving 35 units of NPH insulin daily. She asks why she has to take insulin when other diabetics she knows do not. What should your response be?

2. Prepare a teaching plan for Virginia, regarding the type of insulin, sites for injections, checking the blood sugar, and recognizing the signs and symptoms of a hypoglycemic reaction.

3. Shirley is taking the sulfonylurea tolbutamide (Orinase). What generation and what type of sulfonylurea is tolbutamide?

4. Develop a nursing plan for Shirley focusing on tolbutamide. What are the side effects of this drug? How often is it usually taken? What drug interactions should she be aware of?

Unit XII

Reproductive and Gender-Related Agents

This unit is comprised of five chapters that focus on reproductive and gender-related drugs. Chapters 42, 43, and 44 address agents specifically associated with female health and disorders. Drugs used throughout the female reproductive cycle, including pregnancy, preterm neonate, and labor and delivery are comprehensively discussed in Chapter 42. Chapter 43 focuses on the pharmacology of the postpartum and neonatal period. Chapter 44 details the variety of oral contraceptive products and the drugs used to treat uterine dysfunction, including premenstrual syndrome, endometriosis, and menopausal discomforts. Chapter 45 describes androgens and anabolic steroids, antiandrogens, and other drugs related to male reproductive health and disorders. Chapter 46 concludes this unit with a discussion of drugs used for sexually transmitted diseases and infertility.

Each chapter uses the nursing process to illustrate the nurses' role in pharmacologic therapy. Thought-provoking study questions and case studies provide the opportunity for application of the material presented.

Chapter 42

Drugs Associated with the Female Reproductive Cycle: Pregnancy, Preterm Neonate, Labor, and Delivery

Jane Purnell Taylor

OUTLINE

Objectives
Terms
Introduction
Pregnancy Physiology
Therapeutic Drug Use in
  Pregnancy
    Iron
    Folic Acid
    Multiple Vitamins
    Drugs for Minor Discomforts of Pregnancy
    Nursing Process
Drugs That Decrease Uterine
  Motility

Preterm Labor
  Tocolytic Therapy
  Nursing Process
Corticosteroid Therapy in
  Preterm Labor
    Betamethasone
    Nursing Process
Surfactant Therapy in
  Preterm Birth
    Synthetic Surfactant
    Nursing Process
Drugs for Pregnancy-Induced
  Hypertension
    Nursing Process

Drugs for Pain Control During
  Labor
    Analgesia
    Nursing Process
    Anesthesia
    Nursing Process
Drugs That Enhance Uterine
  Motility
    Oxytocin
    Ergot Alkaloids
    Nursing Processes
Case Study
Study Questions

OBJECTIVES

Explain potential health-promoting and detrimental effects of substances taken by the mother during the prenatal period.

Describe the drugs that alter uterine motility.

Describe drug therapy to decrease the incidence or degree of postnatal respiratory dysfunction during preterm labor.

Describe systemic and regional medications for pain control during labor.

Describe the drugs used in pregnancy-induced hypertension.

Describe the nursing process, including client teaching, associated with the drugs used during pregnancy, labor, and delivery.

TERMS

ataractic drug
eclampsia
ergot alkaloids
ergotism
HELLP syndrome
labor augmentation
labor induction
L/S (lecithin/sphingomyelin) ratio

multiparous
neural tube defect
oxytocic drugs
preeclampsia
pregnancy-induced hypertension
preterm labor
primiparous
progesterone

respiratory distress syndrome
ripening
surfactant
teratogen
tocolytic therapy
uterine atony
uterine inertia
uterine motility

INTRODUCTION

This chapter focuses on the pharmacologic aspects of pregnancy, labor, and delivery. Topics include prenatal health promotion, fetal effects of drugs, and drugs for uterine dysfunction during labor and delivery, for respiratory distress in prematurity, for pain control during labor, and for pregnancy-induced hypertension.

PREGNANCY PHYSIOLOGY

The use of prescription and nonprescription medications raises concern throughout pregnancy and into the postpartum period. The many maternal physiologic changes that occur during pregnancy affect drug action and utilization; these include the influence of circulating steroid hormones on liver metabolism of drugs, more rapid renal excretion of drugs due to the increased glomerular filtration rate and increased renal perfusion, dilution of drugs within the expanded maternal circulatory system, and changes in the actual clearance of drugs in later pregnancy, resulting in decreases in the levels of serum and tissue concentrations of drugs. The result is that therapeutically prescribed drugs may not be ordered in lower doses with longer intervals between doses.

Medication effects are influenced by additional factors. Some drugs have shorter half-lives (e.g., antibiotics, barbiturates) during late pregnancy; events such as labor can actually increase the half-life of some drugs (e.g., analgesics, hypnotics, antibiotics), because drug clearance is believed to decrease due to reduced blood flow associated with transient uterine contractions and maternal positioning (decreased with supine or recumbent position). Increased drug accumulation is a concern in disorders with decreased renal perfusion, such as diabetes and hypertension in pregnancy.

The placenta plays an important role in drug utilization and metabolism. It allows substances to transfer quickly or slowly between mother and fetus, depending on variables such as quality of uteroplacental blood flow, the molecular weight of the substance (low-weight substances cross more easily), the level of ionization of the drug molecules (more highly ionized substances cross less readily), and the degree to which the drug is bound to maternal plasma protein (highly bound drugs do not readily cross) versus fetal plasma protein. In addition, the placenta performs its own enzymatic activity in the biotransformation of a drug into metabolites that can affect the fetus. Thus, the belief that the placenta acts as a protective barrier to keep substances from entering the fetal circulation has proved erroneous.

Guidelines for medication administration during pregnancy must include determination that the benefits of prescribing a drug outweigh potential short- or long-term risks to the maternal–fetal system. Careful selection and monitoring for the minimum effective dose for the shortest interval in the therapeutic range with consideration given to alterations related to pregnancy physiology are required.

Drug effects may be more evident and last longer in the fetus than in the mother, because drug excretion is slower in the fetus due to the immaturity of the fetal liver. The degree of fetal exposure to a drug and its breakdown products is more important to fetal outcome than the rate at which the drug is transported to the fetus.

The mechanisms by which drugs cross the placenta are analogous to the way in which drugs infiltrate breast tissue. Lactation results in increased blood flow to the breasts, and drugs accumulate in adipose breast tissue through simple diffusion. Long-term effects on infants from drugs in breast milk are unknown.

Despite public service announcements and information conveyed through the popular press, use of licit and illicit drugs by pregnant women continues. In addition, health care providers may prescribe drugs for maternal disorders that indirectly affect the fetus. About one-half of the medications taken are over-the-counter (OTC) drugs. The most commonly ingested drugs during pregnancy (other than illicit drugs) are iron and vitamins, antiemetics, antacids, nasal decongestants, mild analgesics, and antibiotics.

Drugs determined conclusively to be safe for the embryo are limited in number. Many more are possible or known **teratogens** (substances that cause developmental abnormalities). Timing, dose, and duration of exposure are of crucial importance in determining the teratogenicity of a given drug. In the human, the teratogenic period lasts from a few days past the first missed menstrual period through 10 weeks from the last period, the period of organogenesis (development of major structures and organs). Examples of adverse effects of selected substances commonly abused during pregnancy are presented in Table 42–1.

THERAPEUTIC DRUG USE IN PREGNANCY

The most common indications for therapeutic use of drugs during pregnancy are nutritional supplementation with iron, vitamins, and minerals and treatment of nausea and vomiting, gastric acidity, and mild pain.

TABLE 42–1 General Adverse Effects of Selected Substances Commonly Abused During Pregnancy

Substance	Maternal Effects	Fetal Effects*
Alcohol (high risk: 6 oz or more/d)	1 oz (2 drinks) absolute alcohol 2×wk: increased risk of spontaneous abortion (2–4 times)	1 oz (2 drinks) absolute alcohol 2×wk: fetal alcohol syndrome (FAS): mild to moderate mental retardation, altered facial features, growth retardation, low birth weight, small head circumference, hypotonia, poor motor coordination. Full FAS seen only in some children; others display only fetal alcohol effect (FAE)
Caffeine	2 cups increases epinephrine concentrations after 30 min and decreases intervillous blood flow with potential for spontaneous abortion (dosage and gestational period related)	Excess consumption (>6–8 cups/d) likely toxic to embryo. No evidence of teratogenicity
Cocaine	48-h clearance via urine. Increased incidence of spontaneous abortion in first trimester. Continued use or sporadic use related to premature delivery and abruptio placentae secondary to placental vasoconstriction and hyperextension	4–5 d clearance time via urine of newborn due to liver immaturity and lack of cholinesterase. Intrauterine growth retardation, decreased head circumference, intrauterine cerebral infarction. No true withdrawal syndrome but increased irritability, hyperreflexia, tremulousness. Deficient organization and interactive abilities. By 4 mo, still exhibits hypertonicity, tremulousness, and impaired motor development. By 6 mo, effects may appear to be self-limited, but long-term research needed
Heroin	First trimester spontaneous abortion, premature delivery, inadequate maternal calorie and protein intake	Neonatal meconium aspiration syndrome; decreased weight and length through 9th postnatal month (weight and length catch up by 12 mo); smaller head circumference (with no catch up); impaired interactive abilities (hard to console and engage); inconsistent behavioral responses; increased tremulousness and irritability
Marijuana	Heavy use (5 or more joints per week). Shortened gestation (<37 wk). May hasten delivery through uterine stimulation	No higher incidence of serious birth defects due solely to marijuana. Higher incidence of meconium passage during labor
Tobacco/Nicotine	Degenerative placental lesions with areas of poor O_2 exchange; higher incidence of abruptio placentae, placenta previa, vaginal bleeding during pregnancy; possible PROM; possible amnionitis; less likely to choose to breast feed	Short stature, smaller head-arm circumferences, no increase in mortality rate or congenital anomalies (some evidence of increased oral clefts); increased respiratory infections beyond the perinatal period; possibly shorter attention span beyond perinatal period
Methadone	If taken prior to pregnancy will need to slow detoxification during pregnancy and decrease dose 5 mg every 2 wk. Do not detoxify prior to 14 wk gestation due to increased risk of spontaneous abortion	Smaller weight through 9 mo postnatally; smaller length through 9 mo postnatally (catch up on weight and length by 12 mo); smaller head circumference (no catch up)*; withdrawal-induced fetal distress if mother detoxifies after 32 wk gestation
Barbiturates	CNS depression; lethargy; sleepiness; subtle mood alterations and impaired judgment/fine motor skills for 24 h. No known inhibitory effect on uterine tone or contractility. Selective anticonvulsant activity without anesthesia effects may warrant use in pregnancy for seizure disorders. Active labor with imminent delivery is a contraindication since no antagonist drug is available	Rapidly cross placenta and cause CNS depression with excessive use/high doses leading to respiratory depression, hyperactivity, decreased sucking reflex
Tranquilizers	Dose-dependent; toxic reactions include ataxia, syncope, vertigo, drowsiness; control of acute eclamptic seizures during labor	Benzodiazepine (diazepam [Valium]) use in 1st trimester not associated with oral clefts or other anomalies. Chronic 3rd trimester or labor exposure in high doses associated with hypotonia, hypothermia, hyperbilirubinemia, poor sucking reflex. Effects may be enhanced if systemic analgesics also given to mother

KEY: PROM: premature rupture of fetal membranes; <: less than.
   * Narcotic-exposed infants show downward trend in development score by age 2, suggesting that lack of environmental stimulation may be the major variable based on the Bayley Scales of Development.

IRON

During pregnancy, approximately twice the normal amount of iron is needed to meet fetal and maternal daily requirements. Most of the required iron is needed during the last 20 weeks of pregnancy. Supplementation is not generally necessary until the second trimester, when the fetus begins to store iron; the goal is to prevent maternal deficiency, not to supply the fetus. The fetus is adequately supplied through the placenta even though the mother is deficient; the time of greatest demand is during the third trimester.

Although normal diet generally will provide the 18 mg recommended daily allowance (RDA) for nonpregnant clients, nonanemic pregnant women usually are instructed to supplement using a dosage that provides 60 mg of elemental iron; anemic clients receive 120 mg of elemental iron. Clients are advised to continue supplements during the 6 weeks postpartum.

Pregnant women generally have hematocrit increased early in the third trimester; those under 30% have iron increased and complete blood counts with platelet and ferritin measured. In those found with true iron deficiency anemia, response to iron supplementation is usually noted within 2 weeks. No teratogenic effects have been reported with physiologic doses. Numerous OTC and prescription iron products are available in varying dosages, which differ in the amount of elemental iron contained in the form of iron salt. Examples are shown in Table 42–2.

Side Effects and Adverse Reactions

Common side effects include nausea, constipation, black or red tarry stools, epigastric pain, vomiting, and diarrhea. In addition, if liquid forms are not diluted and are not administered through a plastic straw, there may be temporary discoloration of the teeth.

FOLIC ACID

During pregnancy, folic acid (vitamin B_6, folacin) is needed in increased amounts. Folic acid deficiency early in pregnancy can result in spontaneous abortion or birth defects (e.g., **neural tube defects**), premature birth, low birth weight, and premature separation of the placenta (abruptio placentae).

The RDA for folic acid in the nonpregnant client is 180 μg. The RDA for folic acid during pregnancy is 400 to 800 μg. Pregnancy risk factor is classified as A (note: factor is C if dosage exceeds RDA recommendation).

Side Effects and Adverse Reactions

Side effects include allergic bronchospasm, rash, pruritus, erythema, and general malaise.

MULTIPLE VITAMINS

Prenatal vitamin preparations are routinely recommended for pregnant women. These preparations generally supply vitamins A, D, E, C, B complex

TABLE 42–2 Iron Products

Drug	Dosage	Uses and Considerations
Ferrous sulfate (Fer-In-Sol, Feosol, Fero-Gradumet, Mol-Iron, Fer-Iron)	A: PO: 300–600 mg/day in divided doses 325 mg daily sufficient to meet needs of non–iron-deficient pregnant client; with iron deficiency, should receive 325 mg 2–3×d	Hematinic; for iron deficiency anemia; prophylaxis for iron deficiency in pregnancy; replaces iron stores needed for RBC development; half-life: UK; PB: UK; onset: 4 d; peak reticulocytosis: 5–10 d; hemoglobin values increase: 2–4 wk. Duration: 3–4 mo. Absorption PO is 5%–30% in intestines; therefore GI side effects; toxic reactions include pallor, hematemesis, shock, cardiovascular collapse, metabolic acidosis; contraindicated in hypersensitivity and peptic ulcer; decreased absorption of tetracycline, penicillamine, antacids; increased absorption with ascorbic acid; decreased absorption with eggs, milk, coffee, tea; can reduce availability of zinc from the diet Nursing implications: use straw (elixir); swallow tablet/capsule whole; take with water on empty stomach, sit upright 30 min after dose to decrease reflux; increase fluids, activity, and dietary bulk; keep away from children; *Pregnancy category:* A
Ferrous gluconate (Fergon, Ferralet, Simron, Fetinic)	A: PO: 200–600 mg, t.i.d.	Same as above
Ferrous fumarate (Fumasorb, Eldofe, Fecot, Femiron, Feostat, Fumerin)	A: PO: 200 mg, t.i.d. or q.i.d.	Same as above

KEY: *A: adult; GI: gastrointestinal; PO: by mouth; UK: unknown.*

(B_1, B_2, B_3, B_5, B_6), B_{12}, iron, calcium, and other minerals. Recommended daily allowances for vitamins and minerals during pregnancy are presented in Appendix D. Studies indicate that folic acid-containing multivitamins in recommended doses prior to and during the early gestational period may reduce the risk of neural tube defects. The role of prenatal vitamins in prevention of other congenital defects (e.g., cleft lip/palate, limb defects) remains unanswered.

It must be stressed that poor food habits cannot be rectified through supplements alone; vitamins are used most effectively by the body when taken with meals. Calories and protein are not supplied by supplements.

Vitamin and mineral megadoses during pregnancy will not improve health and may cause harm.

Practitioners should consider *cultural* food practices and beliefs in regard to the use of prenatal vitamins. For example, in Mexico, some view vitamins as a *hot* food that should not be ingested while pregnant.

DRUGS FOR MINOR DISCOMFORTS OF PREGNANCY

The average prenatal client takes three drugs during pregnancy, two of which are vitamin and mineral supplements. Drug ingestion is most likely during the first and the third trimesters, the time when the minor discomforts of pregnancy tend to be most bothersome.

Nausea and Vomiting

Nausea and vomiting during early pregnancy is a major complaint for most (about 88%) pregnant women, possibly because of increased levels of human chorionic gonadotropin, changes in the metabolism of carbohydrates, and emotional changes. Nonpharmacologic measures to decrease nausea and vomiting to be suggested before drugs are used include (1) eating crackers, dry toast or bread, dry cereal, or other carbohydrate before rising; (2) avoiding fatty or highly seasoned foods; (3) eating small, frequent meals; (4) drinking fluids between meals rather than with meals; (5) drinking apple juice or flat carbonated beverages between meals; (6) eating a high-protein bedtime snack; and (7) stopping or cutting down on smoking. These measures work well for most women, but if vomiting is severe, fluid replacement and pharmacologic measures may be necessary. The incidence of hyperemesis is approximately 3.5 in every 1000 pregnancies, and about 1% exhibit persistent vomiting across a variety of countries and cultures. Table 42–3 presents examples of the most commonly used drugs for management of nausea and vomiting during pregnancy. It must be noted that the

TABLE 42–3 Examples of Drugs That Have Been Used for Management of Nausea and Vomiting During Pregnancy (Recommendation Not Implied)

Drug	Dosage	Uses and Considerations
Anticholinergics/ Antihistamines		
Meclizine (Antivert, Bonamine, Vertol)	PO: 20–50 mg daily	No evidence of teratogenesis; in use since 1956; considered mild; available as OTC drug; site of action is labyrinth, CNS; blocks chemoreceptor trigger zone (CTZ), which acts on vomiting center; onset of action: 1–2 h; duration of 8–24 h; metabolized in liver and excreted unchanged in feces and as metabolites in urine; t½: 6 h; increased effect of alcohol, tranquilizers, narcotics; *Pregnancy category:* B *Side Effects:* Dizziness, drowsiness, dry mouth and nose, blurred vision, diplopia, urinary retention, urticaria, rash, and headache. Cardiovascular effects can include hypotension, palpitations, and tachycardia *Contraindications:* Hypersensitivity to drug or any component *Warning Precautions:* Use with angle-closure glaucoma
Other		
Trimethobenzamide (Tigan, T-Gen)	200 mg rectally, q6–8h	Obscure action; may be mediated through CTZ; does not inhibit direct impulse to vomiting center; chemically classified as an ethanolamine derivative; precautions include use in client with cardiac dysrhythmias, narrow-angle glaucoma, asthma, and pyloroduodenal obstruction. Rectal doses of the drug are more unpredictable *Side Effects:* Drowsiness, headache, blurred vision, diarrhea, depression, hypotension, muscle cramps, allergic reactions, and extrapyramidal symptoms; blood dyscrasias *Contraindications:* Benzocaine, hypersensitivity to drug; children: suppository form in neonates or preterm infants *Warning:* Avoid use in acute emesis to avoid masking of symptoms *Interactions with* phenothiazines/barbiturates, belladonna. *Pregnancy category:* C; t½: UK; onset: PO/PR: 10–40 min; IM: 15–35 min; duration: 3–4 h

KEY: PO: by mouth; PR: by rectum; t½: half-life; IM: intramuscular; UK: unknown.

Food and Drug Administration (FDA) has *not* given approval for any drug for use in morning sickness, nor is there consensus among those few health care providers who do prescribe drug therapy as to the best agent(s); the literature reminds the reader that antiemetic drug studies often find that affected individuals rate even placebo agents as "helpful."

Women who experience nausea and vomiting may experience gastric distress if they are also taking supplemental iron; temporary suspension of iron therapy may help. It is suggested that prenatal vitamins be taken at the time of day the client is least likely to vomit. Salting food to taste may help replace vomited chloride; foods rich in potassium and magnesium may also help replace lost nutrients.

Those clients whose symptoms persist and who experience severe weight loss and dehydration may require IV rehydration, including replacement of electrolytes and vitamins. Antiemetic therapy (probably with phenothiazines) may be used.

Heartburn

Heartburn (pyrosis) is a burning sensation perceived in the epigastric and sternal region that occurs with reflux of acid stomach contents. Pregnant clients experience decreased motility in the gastrointestinal (GI) tract as a result of the normal increase in the hormone **progesterone.** Progesterone also relaxes the cardiac sphincter (sphincter leading into the stomach from the esophagus), making reflux activity (reverse peristalsis) more likely. Digestion and gastric emptying are slower than in the nonpregnant state. Heartburn is common when a pregnant client sits or lies down soon after eating a normal meal, only to have her enlarged abdomen exert upward force on her stomach, causing increased reflux activity and the perception of hyperacidity. Heartburn is a disorder of the second and third trimesters of pregnancy.

Nonpharmacologic measures are preferred in the management of heartburn. These include (1) limiting the volume of food at each feeding; (2) avoiding highly seasoned, fried, or greasy foods; (3) avoiding gas-forming foods; (4) eating slowly and chewing thoroughly; (5) avoiding citrus juices; (6) drinking adequate fluids but not with meals; and (7) avoiding reclining immediately after eating. Antacids should be considered part of the therapeutic regimen only if conservative therapy is unsuccessful.

Most clients do not realize that remedies commonly used by nonpregnant individuals (e.g., baking soda [sodium bicarbonate], antacids such as Alka-Seltzer, Bromo-Seltzer, Rolaids) can be harmful during pregnancy. Clients are usually unaware that selection of the wrong antacid can result in diarrhea, constipation, or electrolyte imbalance. The combination of nonpharmacologic measures plus minimal use of safe antacids should effectively meet the pregnant client's need.

The antacids of choice for the pregnant client include nonsystemic low-sodium products (those considered dietetically sodium free) containing aluminum and magnesium (in the form of hydroxide) in combination. These two ingredients can also be found in combination in the form of malgaldrate (also known as hydroxymagnesium aluminate). Some products also include simethicone (an antiflatulent to decrease the surface tension of GI gas bubbles, burst them, and promote rapid gas expulsion). Calcium carbonate antacid preparations are avoided in pregnancy because of the rebound effect following acid neutralization by the antacid, in which hypersecretion of more acid occurs.

Liquid antacids are the preparations most commonly used in pregnancy owing to their even and uniform dissolution, their rapid action, and their greater activity. Tablets are also acceptable, particularly for convenience, provided these are thoroughly chewed and the client maintains an adequate fluid intake. Table 42–4 presents antacids commonly used during pregnancy.

Pain

Headaches (up through week 26 due to emotional factors, hormonally induced bodily changes, sinus congestion, or eye strain), backaches, joint pains, round ligament pain resulting in mild abdominal aches and pains, and minor injuries are common in pregnancy. Nonpharmacologic pain relief measures should be tried first. These include rest, nonstimulatory environment, relaxation exercises, alteration in routine, mental imagery, ice packs, warm-moist heat, postural changes, better body mechanics for tasks at hand, and changes in the height and style of footwear.

Acetaminophen

Acetaminophen (Tylenol, Datril), a para-aminophenol analgesic, is a pregnancy category B drug. It is the most commonly ingested nonprescription drug during pregnancy. Chapter 14 (Fig. 14–1) presents a drug chart for in-depth review of pharmacokinetics.

Acetaminophen is routinely used during all trimesters of pregnancy in therapeutic doses on a

TABLE 42–4 OTC Antacids Commonly Used in Pregnancy

Drug	Dosage	Uses and Considerations
Aluminum hydroxide (Amphojel)	A: PO: as directed*	Contains aluminum hydroxide gel (320 mg) per 300 mg tablet or per 5 mL; ANC 8; contains saccharin and sorbitol. OTC preparation Use: heartburn secondary to reflux; action: neutralization of gastric acidity; side effects: constipation; adverse reactions: dehydration, hypophosphatemia (long-term use), GI obstruction; *Decrease* effects with: tetracycline, phenothiazine, benzodiazepines, isoniazid, digoxin; follow dose with water; *Pregnancy category:* C; t½: UK; PB: UK; Onset: 15–30 min; peak: 0.5 h; duration: 1–3 h
Magnesium hydroxide and aluminum hydroxide with Simethicone (Maalox Plus, Extra Strength Maalox Plus Suspension, Mylanta Liquid, Mylanta II)	As directed*	*Maalox Plus Tablets:* Each tablet contains magnesium hydroxide (200 mg), aluminum hydroxide (200 mg), and Simethicone (25 mg); ANC 11, 4; chewable; contains saccharin and sorbitol; OTC *Extra Strength Maalox Plus Suspension:* Each 5 mL contains magnesium hydroxide (450 mg), aluminum hydroxide (500 mg), and Simethicone (40 mg); ANC 28; contains saccharin and sorbitol; OTC *Mylanta Liquid:* Each 5 mL contains magnesium hydroxide (200 mg), aluminum hydroxide (200 mg) and Simethicone (25 mg); ANC 12.7; contains sorbitol; OTC *Mylanta II:* Each 5 mL contains magnesium hydroxide (400 mg), aluminum hydroxide (400 mg), and Simethicone (40 mg); ANC 23; OTC; use: same as above with addition of antiflatulence action; interactions: same with addition of allopurinol, quinolones, ketoconazole; *Pregnancy category:* C; PB: UK; t½: UK
Magaldrate with Simethicone (Riopan Plus Tablets, Riopan Plus Suspension)	As directed*	*Riopan Plus Tablets:* Each contains Magaldrate (480 mg) and Simethicone (20 mg); ANC 13.5; chewable; contains sorbitol *Riopan Plus Suspension:* Each 5 mL contains Magaldrate (540 mg) and Simethicone (20 mg); ANC 15.0; contains saccharin; use: same as above; action: same as above; side effects: same as above; adverse reactions: same as above; interaction: decreased absorption of phenothiazines, isoniazid, fluroquinolones, tetracyclines. *Pregnancy category:* C; t½: UK; PB: UK; onset: immediate; peak: UK; duration: prolonged

* Dosage recommendations for antacid preparations should be clarified by the health care provider; however, as a general rule, not more than 12 tablets or 12 tsp should be taken in a 24-h period depending on the strength of the product. Major side effects are a change in bowel habits (diarrhea or constipation), nausea, vomiting, alkalosis, and hypermagnesemia.

Antacids figure in numerous drug interactions owing to their action on gastric pH (increased) and their propensity to bind with other drugs to form poorly absorbed complexes. Antacids should not be given within 2 h of iron, digitalis products, or tetracycline. Likewise, when a client is taking a phenothiazine as an antiemetic, 2 h should elapse between administration of these drugs.

KEY: ANC: acid-neutralizing capacity (per tablet or 5 mL); GI: gastrointestinal; OTC: over-the-counter; PB: protein-binding; PO: by mouth; t½: half-life; UK: unknown.

short-term basis, generally for its analgesic and antipyretic effects. The drug has no significant antiinflammatory effect. Acetaminophen is 20% to 50% protein-bound and crosses the placenta during pregnancy; it also is found in low concentrations in breast milk. To date, there is no concrete evidence of fetal anomalies associated with use of the drug, and no adverse effects have been noted in infants who nurse from mothers who use or did use the drug.

Use of acetaminophen during pregnancy should not exceed 12 tablets per 24 h of a 325-mg formulation (regular strength) or 8 tablets per 24 h of a 500-mg (extra strength) formulation. The drug should be taken at 4- to 6-h intervals. Onset of effects following oral ingestion occurs within 10 to 30 min; peak action occurs at 1 to 2 h; duration of drug effects is from 3 to 5 h.

Side Effects and Adverse Reactions

Most clients *without* preexisting renal or hepatic disease tolerate acetaminophen quite well. Obvi-

ously, clients with hypersensitivity to the compound should not use it. Use cautiously in clients at risk for infection due to possibility of masked signs and symptoms. The most frequently seen side effects are skin eruptions, urticaria, unusual bruising, erythema, hypoglycemia, jaundice, hemolytic anemia, neutropenia, leukopenia, pancytopenia, and thrombocytopenia.

Aspirin

Aspirin (A.S.A., Bayer, Astrin, Ecotrin), a salicylate, is classified as a mild analgesic. Aspirin is a pregnancy category C drug (which changes to category D if full-dose aspirin is used in the third trimester). Aspirin is presented in drug chart form in Chapter 14 for review.

Aspirin is a prostaglandin synthetase inhibitor that has antipyretic, analgesic, and antiinflammatory properties. Teratogenic effects have not been shown conclusively, and the risk of anomalies is perceived to be small.

Aspirin can inhibit the initiation of labor and actually prolong labor through effects on uterine contractility; therefore, its use is not recommended during pregnancy. In addition, aspirin use late in pregnancy is associated with greater maternal blood loss at delivery. There may be increased risk of anemia in pregnancy and of antepartum hemorrhage as well. Hemostasis is affected in the newborn whose mother ingested aspirin during the last 2 months of pregnancy (even without use during the actual week of delivery). The platelets are unable to aggregate to form clots, and it appears that this is not a reversible effect after delivery; the baby has to wait for the bone marrow to produce new platelets. Most recently, aspirin continues to be investigated as a drug that may prevent or treat preeclampsia when given in a low-dose form.

NURSING PROCESS: ANTEPARTUM DRUGS

ASSESSMENT

- Gather comprehensive medical and drug histories.
- Obtain baseline vital signs for comparison with future findings during the prenatal period.
- Identify clients at high risk for substance abuse and plan strategies to minimize risks in collaboration with other professionals.
- Assess drug history to determine if there will be any interference with absorption because of antacids.
- Review history on admission of client in labor in relation to aspirin use during pregnancy. If aspirin has been used, alert the staff and prepare to handle possible increased bleeding.
- Obtain a medical history of alcoholism, liver disease, viral infection, and renal deficiencies. Acetaminophen should be used cautiously in these clients.

POTENTIAL NURSING DIAGNOSIS

- Knowledge deficit related to health maintenance needs during pregnancy
- Knowledge deficit related to potential outcome(s) from exposure to teratogens during pregnancy

PLANNING

- Client will take drugs during pregnancy as advised.

NURSING INTERVENTIONS

General
- Be cognizant that drug use may be part of multiple substance abuse and may also involve maternal-neonatal infections.
- Stress prenatal care and discuss fears the client may have about health care professionals and concerns about legal action in the event of substance abuse.

Specific
- Instruct on strategies to relieve common pregnancy discomforts.
- Refer to smoking or drug treatment program if appropriate.
- Instruct on nutrition/therapeutic supplements needed during pregnancy.
- Monitor hemoglobin during prenatal visits.

Iron
- Question client about nausea, constipation, and bowel habit changes if taking iron preparations.
- Give diluted liquid iron preparation through a plastic straw to prevent discoloration of teeth.
- Store iron in a light-resistant container.
- Be cognizant that client may have false-positive occult blood in stool if taking iron.

CLIENT TEACHING

General
- Advise pregnant woman that smoking, drinking alcohol, and heavy caffeine use may have adverse effects on the fetus.
- Stress that OTC drugs should be used sparingly: the smallest dose for the shortest time.
- Advise client not to plan to breast feed if she is using illicit drugs.

Aspirin/Acetaminophen
- Advise the client not to take aspirin during pregnancy, particularly not during the third trimester.
- Instruct the client not to take nonsteroidal antiinflammatory drugs (NSAIDs) with acetaminophen.

Diet
Caffeine/Alcohol/Nicotine
- Teach client to limit coffee to 1 to 2 cups per day and to consider other sources of caffeine (tea, cola, soft drinks, chocolate, certain drugs).
- Teach client to space limited caffeine intake evenly through the day because caffeine passes readily to the fetus, who cannot metabolize it.

Caffeine can decrease intervillous placental blood flow.

- Suggest that client use decaffeinated products or make drinks weaker.
- Suggest that client use herbal teas carefully because of occasionally harmful ingredients.
- If the client plans to breast feed, tell her that 1% of the caffeine she consumes will appear in her breast milk within 15 min. Therefore, while a cup of coffee is not a problem, it is not wise to drink several cups of coffee in succession; excess caffeine will accumulate in the baby's tissues. The baby lacks enzymes to adequately clear the caffeine for 7 to 9 months after birth.
- Instruct client not to drink alcohol if she is pregnant, because no safe level of alcohol has been determined and even moderate exposure has resulted in fetal alcohol effect.
- Advise client that nicotine is to be avoided.
- Advise client that smoking can cause the loss of nutrients such as vitamins A and C, folic acid, cobalamin, and calcium.

Iron

- Instruct the client about dietary sources of iron, which include organ meats (liver), nuts and seeds, wheat germ, spinach, broccoli, prunes, and cereals.
- Explain to the client that if iron is taken between meals, increased absorption (and also increased side effects) may result. Taking iron 1 h before meals is suggested. Give with juice or water, but not with milk, antacids, or eggs.

Skill
Iron

- Advise the client to swallow the iron tablets whole and not to crush them. Liquid iron preparations should be drunk with a plastic straw.

- Caution the client not to take antacids with iron because antacids impair absorption and are generally discouraged during pregnancy. Iron and antacids should be taken 2 h apart if both are prescribed.

Antacids

- Stress that antacids should not be taken within 1 h of taking an enteric-coated tablet because the acid-resistant coating may dissolve in the increased alkaline condition of the stomach, and the medication will not be released in the intestine as intended. Stomach upset may result.
- Advise the client to store antacid liquid suspension at room temperature, not to let it freeze, and to shake the bottle well before pouring.

Side Effects
Iron

- Advise the client to keep iron tablets away from children. Iron tablets look like candy and death has been reported in small children who have ingested 2 g or less of ferrous sulfate.
- Advise the client that there may be a change in bowel habits when taking antacids. Aluminum products can cause constipation, while magnesium products can cause diarrhea. Many antacids contain both ingredients.

EVALUATION

- Evaluate the effectiveness of the prescribed drug therapy. Report side effects.
- Evaluate the client's understanding of possible effects on the fetus of illegal drugs, alcohol, and smoking.

DRUGS THAT DECREASE UTERINE MOTILITY

The uterus is a pear-shaped, hollow, but very muscular organ located in the pelvic cavity between the rectum and the bladder; it is connected to the vagina by the cervix (Fig. 42–1). Three distinct layers compose the uterine wall: the outer layer, the perimetrium; the muscular middle layer, the myometrium; and the inner mucosal layer, the endometrium.

The myometrium is a network of involuntary (smooth) muscles divided into three layers, with the muscles of each layer configured in different patterns. For example, the outer muscles are arranged longitudinally to assist with cervical effacement (thinning and shortening) and to expel the fetus at the time of delivery. Muscles in the middle layer are arranged in a figure-8 design. These muscles are extremely important in the control of bleeding (hemostasis). Blood vessels are threaded throughout these muscles, and when a contraction occurs the vessels are compressed, which creates a hemostatic effect. Circular muscle fibers are found in the area of the internal os and help control its sphincter. This keeps the fetus contained in the uterus for the normal gestational period. It is these muscles that stretch (dilate) the cervix to a diameter of 10 cm during labor. When all three muscle layers work together during labor,

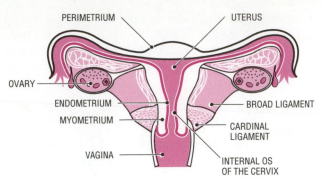

FIGURE 42–1 Anatomy of the female reproductive system.

contractions cause cervical dilatation and the delivery of the products of conception.

PRETERM LABOR (PTL)

Preterm labor is labor that occurs between 20 and 37 weeks of pregnancy involving a fetus with an estimated weight between 500 and 2499 g. Regular contractions occur at less than 10-min intervals over a 30- to 60-min period that are strong enough to result in 2-cm cervical dilatation and 80% effacement. PTL occurs in approximately 5% to 10% of all births. Preterm infants who survive early delivery have significant physiologic impediments to overcome. Preterm labor that progresses to preterm delivery accounts for the majority of perinatal morbidity and mortality (excluding fetuses with anomalies) in the United States.

Although preterm labor has no single known cause, certain risk factors have been identified: maternal age of under 16 or over 35 years, low socioeconomic status, previous history (17% to 50% chance of recurrence), intrauterine infections, polyhydramnios, maternal sepsis due to release of endotoxin with uterine irritation, multiple gestation, uterine anomalies, antepartum hemorrhage, smoking, drug use, urinary tract infections, and incompetent cervix. Attempts to arrest preterm labor are *absolutely contraindicated* in (1) pregnancy less than 20 weeks' gestation (confirmed by ultrasound); (2) bulging or premature rupture of membranes (PROM); (3) confirmed fetal death or anomalies incompatible with life; (4) maternal hemorrhage and evidence of severe fetal compromise; and (6) chorioamnionitis.

TOCOLYTIC THERAPY

When clients in preterm labor have no contraindications, they become candidates for **tocolytic therapy** (drug therapy to decrease uterine motility) using beta-adrenergic agents (e.g., Ritodrine HCl [Yutopar]; terbutaline [Brethine], or the calcium an-

tagonist magnesium sulfate [MgSO$_4$]). The goal in tocolytic therapy is to decrease the level of **uterine motility** (spontaneous movement) in order to interrupt or inhibit labor to create additional time for fetal maturation within the uterine environment.

Table 42–5 lists the drugs most commonly used to decrease uterine motility.

Ritodrine

The beta-sympathomimetic drugs act by stimulating the beta$_2$ receptors in smooth muscle. The frequency and intensity of uterine contractions decrease as the muscle relaxes. The two beta-adrenergic agents ritodrine (Yutopar) and terbutaline (Brethine) are widely used; of these, ritodrine is the only FDA approved (1980) tocolytic drug; terbutaline is approved for medicinal use but not specifically as a tocolytic. These beta-adrenergic drugs effectively decrease uterine contractions 60% to 80%. However, the literature indicates that knowledge about the long-term cumulative effects of these drugs is still lacking.

The action and effects of ritodrine are presented in Figure 42–2 and the nursing process related to the drug.

Pharmacokinetics

Ritodrine (Yutopar) has an absorption rate of 30% following oral administration. It is 32% protein-bound and has a multiphasic variable half-life. With oral administration, the half-life has two phases, 1.3 h and 12 to 20 h, and with IV administration it has three phases, 7 to 9 min, 1.5 to 2.8 h, and 15 to 17 h. Ritodrine is metabolized by the liver and excreted by the kidneys.

Clients who present with mild contractions may be given a subcutaneous course of terbutaline initially, followed by administration of ritodrine or terbutaline IV if contraction strength is enhanced. Clients are monitored to determine if and when contractions diminish or cease; oral therapy with ritodrine or terbutaline and/or subcutaneous pump therapy with terbutaline may be employed for long-term maintenance.

Pharmacodynamics

Oral ritodrine has an onset of action of 30 min, a peak plasma/serum concentration of 30 to 60 min, and a duration of action of 4 to 6 h. Oral administration of ritodrine is initiated 30 min prior to discontinuing the IV administration. The 10 to 20 mg

TABLE 42–5 Drugs Used to Decrease Uterine Motility

Drug	Dosage	Uses and Considerations
Beta-Adrenergic Agents		
Ritodrine (Yutopar)	See Prototype Drug Chart (Fig. 42–2)	Sympathomimetic beta$_2$-adrenergic agonist. If long-acting corticosteroids are taken simultaneously, pulmonary edema is risk (discontinue both drugs); sufficient time must elapse before another sympathomimetic amine drug is given due to additive effect; cardiovascular effects potentiated by magnesium sulfate, meperidine, and diazoxide; beta-adrenergic blockers inhibit action of ritodrine (avoid concurrent use); IV use elevates plasma insulin and glucose and decreases plasma potassium concentrations; expect increase in maternal pulse of 20–40 bpm; expect increase in FHR of 10 bpm; more expensive than terbutaline; FDA approved; *Pregnancy category:* B; rapidly crosses placenta; absorption rate 30% (PO); PB: 32%; t½: 15 h (is multiphasic and varies with route); metabolized by liver; excreted by kidneys; breast feeding not contraindicated due to short half-life
Terbutaline (Brethine)	Follow agency protocols for specific directives plus individual health care provider's order; only drug that may be given SC; usual therapy is 0.25 mg SC initially (repeat as necessary); then 0.1 mg SC q 4h for maintenance; then 2.5–5 mg PO q 4–6 h starting with last SC dose. Some agencies begin therapy IV using 10 μg/min, increasing to 5 μg/min q 10 min until contractions stop	Sympathomimetic beta$_2$-adrenergic agonist; action onset is within 15 min IV/SC and 30–45 min PO; peak serum levels reached in 0.5–1 h IV/SC and 1–2 h PO; *Pregnancy category* B; partially metabolized in the liver; excreted by the kidneys; not FDA approved for labor inhibition and requires written consent; less expensive than ritodrine; 40%–50% rate of tocolytic breakthrough and recurrence of preterm labor 3 wk after start of PO therapy may require repeat therapy (may be due to desensitization of beta receptors over time); current research focused on use of low-dose continuous SC pumps that are portable and can deliver intermittent bolus doses based on data reflecting peak need periods; pumps are cost effective with high client satisfaction; drug interactions same as for ritodrine; expected increases in maternal pulse and FHR same as for ritodrine; rapidly crosses placenta; breast feeding not contraindicated due to short half-life; duration of drug effects 4–8 h PO and 1.5–4 h SC
Calcium Antagonist		
Magnesium sulfate	Follow agency protocols for specific directives plus individual physician orders for concentration and mL/h IV: usual LD: 4–6 g in 50–100 mL over 20–30 min Maintenance: 40 g in 1 L of IVF at 2–4 g/h. Dose based on serum magnesium levels and deep tendon reflex assessment	Calcium antagonist and CNS depressant; relaxes uterine smooth muscle through calcium displacement. Must be given by infusion pump for accurate dosage; *Pregnancy category:* B; onset: IV: immediate; duration: 30 min; freely crosses placenta; few contraindications allow for use in clients who exhibit life-threatening complications; maternal magnesium levels readily monitored through serum analyses, reflexes, respiratory rate, and urinary output (extreme care needed with decreased output!); antidote: calcium gluconate; elevated levels may be evident in newborn for 7 d; observe newborn for 24–48 h for signs of toxicity if mother treated close to delivery; breast feeding not contraindicated

KEY: bpm: beats per minute; LD: loading dose; IVF: intravenous fluid; IV: intravenous; PB: protein-binding; PO: by mouth; SC: subcutaneous; t½: half-life; >: greater than.

oral dose is administered every 1 to 6 h until tocolysis is no longer needed.

Intravenously administered ritodrine has an onset of action of 5 min, a peak plasma/serum concentration of 50 to 60 min, and a duration of action of 30 min.

See physician's orders and agency protocols for administration. Common therapy is to mix 150 mg ritodrine in 500 mL IV fluid (it is thought that dextrose decreases the incidence of pulmonary edema) to infuse at 10 to 20 mL/h. Increase by 10 mL/h every 15 min until contractions are more than 15 min apart. The maximum dose is 70 mL/h. Decrease therapy as contractions taper off. Initiate oral therapy 30 min before discontinuing IV administration to ensure adequate serum levels.

Side Effects and Adverse Reactions

Side effects include tremors, malaise, weakness, dyspnea, tachycardia (maternal and fetal), increased systolic pressure and decreased diastolic pressure, chest pain, nausea, vomiting, diarrhea, constipation, erythema, sweating, hyperglycemia, and hypokalemia. More serious adverse reactions include pulmonary edema, dysrhythmias, ketoacidosis, and anaphylactic shock.

Ritodrine must be used cautiously in clients with premature rupture of the membranes, diabetes mellitus, or mild to moderate preeclampsia.

Ritodrine can cause tachycardia in the fetus and hypoglycemia in the neonate. Because the half-life is short, breast feeding is not contraindicated.

FIGURE 42–2. Sympathomimetic Beta-Adrenergic Agonists: Ritodrine

Ritodrine HCl	**Dosage**	**NURSING PROCESS** Assessment and Planning
Ritodrine HCl (Yutopar) Adrenergic *Pregnancy Category:* B	IV: Mix 150 mg in 500 mL D_5W and infuse at 10–20 mL/h; increase by 10 mL/h q15 min until contractions >15 min apart; max: 70 mL/h; decrease therapy as contractions taper off Initiate PO therapy 10–20 mg 30 min before stopping IV drug; PO dose q1–6h until tocolysis not needed Refer to specific protocol.	
Contraindications	**Drug-Lab-Food Interactions**	
Before 20th week of gestation, condition in which maintenance of pregnancy is hazardous, eg., antepartal hemorrhage and intrauterine fetal death; selected preexisting maternal conditions, e.g., uncontrolled hypertension or diabetes	*Increase* effects of ritodrine with diazoxide, meperidine, potent general anesthetics, magnesium sulfate; *increase* effects of sympathomimetic amines *Decrease* effects of ritodrine with beta blockers	
Pharmacokinetics	**Pharmacodynamics**	Interventions
Absorption: PO: 30% *Distribution:* PB: 32%, crosses placenta; probably crosses blood–brain barrier *Metabolism:* $t\frac{1}{2}$: 15 h *Excretion:* In urine	PO: Onset: 30 min Peak: 30–60 min Duration: 4–6 h IV: Onset: Within 5 min Peak: 50–60 min Duration: 30 min	

	Evaluation
Therapeutic Effects/Uses: To inhibit uterine contractions. *Mode of Action:* Stimulation of receptors in smooth muscles of uterus, thereby decreasing intensity and frequency of contractions.	

Side Effects	**Adverse Reactions**
Malaise, weakness, dyspnea, tachycardia (maternal and fetal), palpitations, increased chest pain, nausea, vomiting, diarrhea, hyperglycemia, hypokalemia	Ketoacidosis *Life-threatening:* Long term: pulmonary edema, anaphylactic shock

KEY: IV: intraveneous; PO: by mouth; PB: protein binding; $t\frac{1}{2}$: half-life.

Drug Interactions

The increased effects of general anesthetics can produce additive hypotension. Pulmonary edema can occur with concurrent use of corticosteroids. Cardiovascular effects may be additive with other sympathomimetic drugs, such as epinephrine, al-buterol, and isoproterenol. Ritodrine is antagonized by beta-adrenergic blocking agents.

Magnesium Sulfate

Magnesium sulfate, a calcium antagonist and central nervous system depressant, relaxes the smooth muscle of the uterus through calcium displacement. Administered intravenously, the drug has a direct depressant effect on contractility. The drug also decreases blood pressure and increases perfusion through the uterus, which has a therapeutic effect on the fetus. This drug, which is also less expensive, may be safer to use than the beta-sympathomimetics because it has fewer adverse effects; it can also be used when beta-sympathomimetics are contraindicated (e.g., in diabetes and cardiovascular disease). The drug is excreted by the kidneys and does cross the placenta. A loading dose of from 4 to 6 gm IV over 20 to 30 minutes is given initially, followed by gradual increase (approximately 0.5 gm/h q 30 min until contractions decrease to less than six per hour or cease) to a dosage level of 3.0 gm/h; the maintenance dose must be titrated to deep tendon reflexes (checked q 1 to 2 h) and magnesium levels are drawn based on the clinical response of the client. The effective maternal serum level range for tocolysis is 5 to 8 mg/dL. Generally, once the client is stable for 12 hours, the client may be switched to PO medication (magnesium chloride, magnesium oxide, or magnesium gluconate). Magnesium sulfate therapy is contraindicated in clients who have myasthenia gravis; impaired kidney function and recent myocardial infarction are relative contraindications; clients with renal impairment require adjusted dosages.

Side Effects and Adverse Reactions

Dosage-related side effects in the maternal client include flushing, feelings of increased warmth, sweating, dizziness, nausea, headache, lethargy, slurred speech, sluggishness, nasal congestion, heavy eyelids, blurred vision, decreased GI action, increased pulse rate, and hypotension; increased severity is evidenced by depressed reflexes, confusion, and magnesium toxicity (respiratory depression and arrest, circulatory collapse, cardiac arrest). Side effects in the fetus and neonate include slight hypotonia with diminished reflexes and lethargy for 24 to 48 hours; in general, the drug is considered safe.

In the event maternal neurologic, respiratory, or cardiac depression is evidenced, the antidote is calcium gluconate (10 mg IV push over 3 min) or calcium chloride (10 mL of 10% solution IV push over 10 min at a rate of 1 mL/min).

NURSING PROCESS: BETA-ADRENERGIC AGONISTS: Ritodrine

ASSESSMENT

- Identify clients at risk for preterm labor early in pregnancy.
- Obtain a history, complete physical assessment, vital signs (VS), fetal heart rate (FHR), and urine specimen for infection screening.

POTENTIAL NURSING DIAGNOSES

- High risk for activity intolerance
- Altered health maintenance
- Knowledge deficit related to information gap about etiology and interventions for preterm labor
- Fear related to potential for early labor and birth

PLANNING

- Client's preterm contractions will be eliminated by resting in left side lying position, increasing fluid intake, and tocolytic therapy as needed.
- No cervical change from initial examination.

NURSING INTERVENTIONS

- Monitor and assess uterine activity and FHR before, during, and for 1 h after discontinuing IV infusion.
- Maintain client in left lateral position as much as possible.
- Monitor maternal and fetal VS every 15 min when the client is receiving IV dose. Report if systolic blood pressure drops to <90 mmHg or is >140 mmHg, if diastolic blood pressure is <50 mmHg, or if pulse increases to >120 beats per minute. If any of these occur, place client in Trendelenburg position and increase the infusion rate of primary IV (*not* of the piggyback IV containing the drug).
- Report auscultated cardiac dysrhythmias. An ECG may be ordered.
- Auscultate breath sounds every 4 h. Notify health care provider if respirations are >30/min or there is a change in quality (wheezes, rales, coughing).
- Monitor daily weight to assess fluid overload; monitor strict input and output every 8 h.
- Provide passive range of motion of legs every 1 to 2 h.

- Report fetal baseline heart rate >180 beats per min.
- Report persistence of frequent contractions despite tocolytic therapy.
- Report rupture of membranes, vaginal bleeding, or sudden complaints of rectal pressure, suggesting impending delivery.
- Be alert to presence of hypoglycemia and hypoglycemia in the newborn delivered within 5 h of discontinued beta-sympathomimetic drugs.
- Administer only clear solutions of drugs if using IV route.
- Assist clients on home tocolytic therapy plan for assistance with self-care and family responsibilities.

CLIENT TEACHING

General
- Teach client the signs and symptoms of impending preterm labor (menstrual type cramps, sensation of pelvic pressure, low backache, and increased vaginal discharge).
- Instruct client that if she experiences preterm labor contractions at home, she should void, recline on her left side to increase uterine blood flow, drink extra fluids to decrease the release of antidiuretic hormone (ADH) and oxytocin from the posterior pituitary, rest for 30 min, and then attempt to resume her activities if asymptomatic. Stress that she should notify her health care provider if the contractions do not end or if they return.
- Tell client that she may return to her normal activities after 36 to 48 h without contractions; check with health care provider.
- Explain the effects of beta-sympathomimetic drugs; the contractions should be arrested. Report heart palpitations or dizziness.
- Instruct client to take the drug as directed.
- Advise the client to contact the health care provider before taking any other drugs while on tocolysis.
- Instruct the client that if she misses a dose and <1 h has elapsed, she should take the missed dose. However, if >1 h has elapsed, she should wait until the next regularly scheduled dose.

EVALUATION

- Evaluate the effectiveness of the tocolytic drug by noting the absence of six or more contractions in 1 h.
- Evaluate the client's understanding of nonpharmacologic measures for decreasing preterm contractions, such as increasing fluid intake and resting on the left side.
- Continue monitoring the client's and fetal VS. Report any change immediately.

ADDITIONAL NURSING CONSIDERATIONS

Tocolytic Therapy: Magnesium Sulfate
- Monitor VS every ½ h and FHR every 15 min. Client's respirations should be above 12/min or she may be toxic.
- Monitor I & O every hour. Report if the urinary output is less than 30 mL/h.
- Check breath and bowel sounds every 4 h.
- Assess reflexes prior to initiation of therapy and then every hour. Notify health care provider of change.
- Weigh daily.
- Monitor serum magnesium levels (therapeutic level is 4 to 7 mg/dL).
- Have available calcium gluconate or calcium chloride as an antidote for overdosing of magnesium sulfate.
- Observe newborn for 24 to 49 hours for magnesium toxicity if drug was given to mother shortly before birth.

CORTICOSTEROID THERAPY IN PRETERM LABOR

The best client outcome from tocolytic therapy is prevention or cessation of preterm labor. Maternity clients 24 to 34 weeks' gestation at risk for, or who experience, preterm labor are recommended to receive antenatal corticosteroid therapy with betamethasone or dexamethasone to accelerate lung maturation with resultant surfactant development in the fetus in utero, thereby decreasing the inci- dence and severity of respiratory distress syndrome (RDS) with increased survival of preterm infants. **Surfactant** is made up of two major phospholipids, sphingomyelin and lecithin. Sphingomyelin develops in greater quantity initially (from about the 24th week) than lecithin. However, by the 33rd to 35th weeks of gestation, lecithin production peaks, making the ratio of the two substances about 2:1 in favor of lecithin. This is referred to as the **L/S (lecithin/sphingomyelin) ratio,** measured in the amniotic fluid, and it is an

TABLE 42–6 Prenatal Therapy for Surfactant Development

Drug	Dosage	Uses and Considerations
Betamethasone (Celestone, Soluspan)	IM: 12 mg q 12h×2	Corticosteroid; given to prevent RDS in preterm infants by injecting mother prior to delivery to stimulate surfactant production in the fetal lung. Not effective in treating preterm infant after delivery. Most effective if given at least 24 h (preferably 48–72 h) but less than 7 d prior to delivery in 33rd wk or before. May be repeated if baby not delivered within 7 d. Contraindicated in severe PIH and in systemic fungal infection. Simultaneous use with terbutaline may enhance risk of pulmonary edema. Drug can mask signs of chorioamnionitis; therefore, drug not given with ruptured membranes. Metabolized in the liver and excreted by the kidneys; crosses the placenta; enters breast milk; onset of action is 1–3 h. Therapy less effective with multifetal birth and with male infants. No data available related to breast feeding. *Pregnancy category:* C; PB: 64%; t½: 6.5 h; Peak: IV: 10–36 min

KEY: *IM: intramuscular; PB: protein binding; PIH: pregnancy-induced hypertension; RDS: respiratory distress syndrome; t¹/₂: half-life.*

important predictor of fetal lung maturity, because it implies that the alveoli will not collapse after birth.

Clients with pregnancy-induced hypertension (PIH), premature rupture of the membranes, placental insufficiency, some types of diabetes, or narcotic abuse may have amniotic fluid with higher than expected L/S ratios for gestational date because of a stress-induced increase in corticosteroid production. It would appear that nature tries to prepare stressed fetuses for early extrauterine life.

Betamethasone

When preterm labor occurs prior to the 33rd week of gestation, corticosteroid therapy with betamethasone suspension may be prescribed. Table 42–6 provides the data for this drug.

SIDE EFFECTS AND ADVERSE REACTIONS. Side effects of betamethasone suspension include seizures, headache, vertigo, edema, hypertension, increased sweating, petechiae, ecchymoses, and facial erythema.

NURSING PROCESS: BETAMETHASONE

ASSESSMENT

- Assess for history of hypersensitivity.
- Assess vital signs, and report abnormal findings.
- Assess fetal heart rate (FHR).
- Assess visual status.

POTENTIAL NURSING DIAGNOSES

- Fear related to potential for early labor and birth with uncertain fetal outcome secondary to fetal immaturity
- Infection, risk for

PLANNING

- Client will not deliver within 24 h of receiving betamethasone.

NURSING INTERVENTIONS

- Observe for respiratory difficulties.
- Maintain accurate I & O records.

- Shake the suspension well. Avoid exposing it to excess heat or light.
- Inject in large muscle mass, not the deltoid, to avoid high incidence of local atrophy.
- Check blood glucose if used for diabetic.
- Assess lab data for electrolytes.

CLIENT TEACHING

General
- Instruct the client to avoid exposure to infections.
- Remind diabetic client to carefully screen her glucose.

Diet
- Advise the client to avoid alcohol and to severely restrict caffeine.

Side Effects
- Instruct the client to report immediately any breathing difficulty, weakness, or dizziness.

- Instruct client to report changes in stool, easy bruising, bleeding, blurred vision, unusual weight gain, emotional changes.

- Continue monitoring FHR. Report changes.
- Monitor fetus/neonate for hypoglycemia and presence of neonatal sepsis.

EVALUATION

- Continue monitoring the client's vital signs. Report changes.

SURFACTANT THERAPY IN PRETERM BIRTH

SYNTHETIC SURFACTANT

A second approach to addressing respiratory difficulties in the preterm infant is surfactant replacement therapy. This is done to prevent the development of **respiratory distress syndrome** (RDS), also known as hyaline membrane disease (HMD). Clinical findings in RDS include stiff, inflexible lungs due to lack of surfactant, dyspnea with cyanosis, inspiratory dilatation of the nares, expiratory grunt, atelectasis with each expiration, harsh breath sounds or fine rales, significant inspiratory retractions (suprasternal, substernal, intercostal, subcostal), respiratory acidosis, and metabolic acidosis. Surfactant therapy is also used to decrease the severity of RDS following diagnosis.

The deficit in the amount of endogenous surfactant available to maintain distention of the alveolar sacs is the focus of this therapy.

Five major types of surfactant therapy have been under investigation during the past decade. Currently, the FDA has approved the use of Exosurf Pediatric, a protein-free synthetic pulmonary surfactant which, following reconstitution, contains in 1 mL, 13.5 mg colfosceril palmitate (DPPC) (the major lipid component of natural surfactant). Berastant (Survanta) intratracheal suspension, a natural bovine lung extract, contains phospholipids, neutral lipids, fatty acids, and surfactant-associated proteins to which colfosceril palmitate (DPPC) palmitic acid and tripalmitin are added; thus, each mL of Survanta contains 25 mg of phospholipids. Survanta does not require reconstitution.

Each of these two products defines *prophylactic* and *rescue* use slightly differently (Table 42–7) and has different dosing and administration requirements.

Both products require a patent endotracheal (ET) tube for administration and special positioning of the infant with specified alterations throughout the procedure. These very precise position changes during the procedure allow gravity to assist in the distribution of product in the lungs, particularly at the alveolar surface.

Rales and moist breath sounds may be a transient finding following administration of these products. Unless very obvious signs of airway obstruction are noted, suctioning should not be performed for 2 h following administration.

Surfactant replacement therapy has been found effective in reducing the severity of RDS; rapid improvements in lung compliance and oxygenation that may require immediate decreases in ventilator settings (to prevent lung overdistention and pulmonary air leak) may occur, requiring close monitoring; overall, mortality has been reduced and some studies indicate that a decrease in the incidence of bronchopulmonary dysplasia is occurring since the introduction of these products.

Side Effects and Adverse Reactions

Side effects during administration have included some incidents of reflux of product up the ET tube with decreases in oxygenation. Dosing is slowed or halted if the infant becomes dusky in color or agitated or experiences transient bradycardia, or oxygen saturation decreases more than 15%. Rapid improvement in underlying pathology may occur as well, requiring astute monitoring of ventilated lung function. Pulmonary hemorrhage has been seen in 2% to 4% of treated infants with Exosurf. Suctioning prior to dosing lessens the chance for endotracheal tube blockage during dosing. No long-term complications or sequelae of Exosurf Pediatric or Survanta therapy have been found.

Future Directions

Current research using *perfluorocarbon liquids ventilation* (PFC liquids) with respiratory-compromised infants is also being conducted as a proposed alternative to adjunctive approach. It is hoped that PFC liquids might distribute throughout the alveolar surface in a very uniform manner and offer assistance to the area where atelectasis has occurred.

TABLE 42–7 Postnatal Surfactant Therapy for Prevention and Treatment of Respiratory Distress Syndrome

Drug	Dosage	Uses and Considerations
Exosurf Pediatric	5 ml/kg per dose ET in one of two modes: *Prophylaxis:* 1 dose immediately following birth; 2 additional doses (if indicated) at 12 h and 24 h to mechanically ventilated infants *Rescue:* 1 dose as soon as RDS diagnosis is made, followed by 2nd dose 12 h later to infants who remain on mechanical ventilation After endotracheal (ET) suctioning, administered in two 2.5 mL/kg doses via special ET tube adapter supplied with product without interrupting mechanical ventilation	FDA-approved synthetic, protein-free surfactant (artificial) given by a ventilator-experienced neonatologist as *prevention* or *rescue* in treatment of RDS; for intratracheal use only; treated infants must be on intermittent mechanical ventilation *Prophylaxis* defined as infants under 1350 g at high risk for RDS or larger infants with pulmonary immaturity. *Rescue* defined as treatment of infants with moderate to severe RDS defined in clinical trials as an arterial:alveolar oxygen tension ratio (a/A) of less than 0.22. Absorbed from alveolus into lung tissue, where extensively catabolized and reutilized for further phospholipid synthesis and secretion. Due to RDS based interruption of alveolar surface integrity, some surfactant may escape to systemic circulation; more even distribution of surfactants observed following immediate prophylaxis at birth due to initial availability of lung fluids. t½: UK (however, t½ of natural human surfactant ranges from 20–36 h; not known if generalizable to drug form). Well-tolerated in clinical trials; lesser need for ventilatory support; adverse reactions: possible reflux up ET tube during dosing (slow dosing or halt if dusky, agitated, transient bradycardia or decrease of 15% in O_2 saturation); astute monitoring of lung functioning in relation to ventilator settings required; supplied as white powder; must be reconstituted with 8 mL of supplied sterile H_2O; suspension pH 5–7; store at 15°–30°C (59°–86°F) in dry place. Stable after reconstituted for 12 h (if stored about 2°–30°C); contains no antibacterial preservatives. No known contraindications to drug use
Survanta (beractant) Intratracheal Suspension	4 mL/kg per dose ET (divided into 4 aliquots) in one of two modes: *Prophylaxis:* 1 dose within 15 min of birth if possible; 3 additional doses in 1st 48 h (6 h apart) *Rescue:* Up to 4 doses in 1st 48 h of life no more frequently than q 6h; 1st dose immediately following diagnosis; preferably give by 8 h of age; DO NOT SHAKE	FDA-approved natural bovine lung extract containing phospholipids, neutral lipids, fatty acids and surfactant-associated proteins to which colfosceril palmitate (DPPC), palmitic acid, and tripalmitin are added; each mL contains 2.5 mg phospholipids; does not require reconstitution; must be given by a ventilator-experienced neonatologist as *prevention* or *rescue* in treatment of RDS; administered through a 5F end-hole catheter as a dosing catheter inserted into ET tube. Following administration of each quarter dose, catheter removed from ET tube and infant ventilated for 30 sec until stable. *Prophylaxis* defined as infants under 1250 g at high risk for RDS or larger infants with evidence of pulmonary immaturity. *Rescue* defined as treatment of infants with moderate to severe RDS (defined in clinical trials as need for mechanical ventilation and fractional inspired oxygen concentration [FiO_2] above 0.40). Biophysical effects occur at the alveolar surface; lowers surface tension on alveolar surfaces during respiration and stabilizes alveoli against collapse at resting pressures. Infants receiving it should be frequently monitored with arterial or transcutaneous measurement of systemic O_2 or CO_2. No known contraindications. Adverse reactions associated with dosing procedure (transient bradycardia, O_2 desaturation): less than 1% experience ET tube reflux, blockage, pallor, vasoconstriction, hypotension, hypocarbia, hypercarbia, and apnea. All reactions resolve with symptomatic treatment; drug should appear off-white to light brown; swirl vial gently; DO NOT SHAKE; foaming at surface normal; store at 2°–8°C; warm 20 min at room temperature or in hand for at least 8 min (DO NOT ARTIFICIALLY WARM); for prevention dose, begin preparation prior to infant's birth; do not warm and return drug to refrigerator more than once; protect from light

NURSING PROCESS: EXOSURF PEDIATRIC/SURVANTA

ASSESSMENT

- Check for signed consent; need separate consents if multifetal birth.
- Check infant's vital signs (VS).

POTENTIAL NURSING DIAGNOSES

- Impaired gas exchange related to inadequate lung surfactant

PLANNING

- Infant's oxygen requirement and respiratory effort will decrease.
- Infant's need for alteration in mechanical ventilation settings will be quickly noted and accomplished.

NURSING INTERVENTIONS

Exosurf Pediatric

- Prepare drug within 20 min of use.
- *Reconstitute* with 8 mL supplied sterile H₂O; draw dose from beneath the foamy layer.
- Assist with the positioning of the baby after each half-dose as detailed in the protocol.
- Store drug at 15° to 30°C in dry place; document time of reconstitution and use within 12 h.

Survanta

- Prepare drug in adequate time for drug to warm at room temperature for 20 min or in hand or at least 8 min.
- Do not artificially warm drug.
- Do not shake drug.
- Provide only off-white–light brown product for use in procedure.
- Have 5F end-hole catheter available.
- Assist with the positioning of the baby after each quarter dose as detailed in protocol.

Both Exosurf Pediatric and Survanta

- Expect the baby's lungs to sound wet after administration; do not suction through the endotracheal tube for 2 h.
- Monitor infant carefully for chest expansion, color, arterial blood gases, oxygen saturation, heart rate, facial expression, ET tube patency, blood pressure, ECG.
- Monitor ventilator pressure readings and breath sounds.

General

- Explain to client what RDS is and why it is risky for the baby.
- Explain to client how surfactant helps the baby.
- Explain to client the purpose of monitoring the baby with a quantity of monitoring devices to reduce fear of devices and translation that baby may be more ill than he or she is in reality.

Side Effects

- Encourage client to verbalize her understanding about the risks associated with the use of the drug (harsh breath sounds on transient basis; occasional mucous plugs in some babies).

EVALUATION

- Evaluate preadministration breath sounds and ventilator pressure readings in comparison with postadministration findings.

DRUGS FOR PREGNANCY-INDUCED HYPERTENSION

Pregnancy-induced hypertension (PIH), the most common serious complication of pregnancy, can have devastating maternal and fetal effects. However, with proper management, the prognosis for both mother and baby is good. Hypertensive disorders occur in about 6% to 30% of all pregnant clients, with about 5% to 7% of all pregnancies reflecting incidence of PIH. The condition is most often observed during the last 10 gestational weeks, throughout labor, and during the first 72 hours postpartum. The cause of PIH remains unknown, although numerous theories exist. The major predisposing risk factors for the development of PIH are listed in Table 42–8.

PIH is divided into two categories based on clinical manifestations: **Preeclampsia** is defined as the presence of hypertension, proteinuria, and edema in a previously normotensive prepregnant client after the 20th week of gestation. Preeclampsia is subdivided into *mild* preeclampsia and *severe* preeclampsia (see Table 42–9 for comparison).

About 5% of preeclamptic clients, notably those without adequate prenatal care, progress to the second major PIH category, **eclampsia,** in which seizure activity occurs and perinatal mortality is about 20%. Fortunately, early diagnosis of PIH with appropriate treatment keeps most preeclamptic clients from progressing to this stage. About 25% of eclampsia occurs postpartum.

TABLE 42–8 Predisposing Factors for Pregnancy-Induced Hypertension

Black

Primigravida

<20 or >35 years of age (especially as primigravida)

Multifetal gestation

Family history of PIH

Lower socioeconomic class

Gestational trophoblastic disease

Diabetes mellitus

Preexisting hypertensive, vascular, renal disease

Underweight or overweight

TABLE 42–9 Comparison of Mild and Severe Preeclampsia and Eclampsia

Mild Preeclampsia	Severe Preeclampsia	Eclampsia
Blood pressure increase of more than 30 but less than 60 mmHg (systolic) and more than 15 but less than 30 mmHg (diastolic) or >140/90 but <160/110	Blood pressure increase of more than 60 mmHg (systolic) and more than 30 mmHg (diastolic) over baseline or >160/110 on two occasions at least 6 h apart (client on bedrest)	All signs and symptoms to left plus progression to seizure activity
Proteinuria >500 mg in 24 h or +1 or +2; edema not generalized; noted in hands, feet	Proteinuria >5 g in 24 h or +3 or +4; edema generalized; found in face (puffy eyes, coarse features), hands, lower abdomen	
Weight gain >1 lb/wk before 32 wk or >2.5 lb/wk after 34 wk	Weight gain up to 10 lb in 1 wk	
Deep tendon reflexes in arms and legs only slightly increased (0: no response; 1+: sluggish/low; 2+: normal active; 3+: brisk)	Deep tendon reflexes (DTRs) in arms and legs hyperactive (4+: hyperactive/transient clonus; 5+: brisk; clonus sustained)	
Adequate urinary output	Oliguria present (<400 mL per 24 h)	
No major cerebral or visual symptoms	Cerebral or visual symptoms, particularly blurred vision, spots, flashing lights, and/or persistent, severe headache in frontal area	
No epigastric pain	Epigastric pain may be present in very severe preeclampsia; pulmonary edema, cyanosis	

A severe sequela of PIH is known as **HELLP syndrome** (defined by *H*emolysis, *E*levated *L*iver enzymes and *L*ow *P*latelet count being present), which occurs in about 2% to 12% of clients with PIH. Clients who manifest severe preeclampsia are the most likely to also present with HELLP syndrome. At the present time, there is no effective cure for PIH. Current research using calcium supplementation and low-dose aspirin may hold some promise as a prevention strategy in the future, but is still experimental.

Two primary treatment goals in PIH, in addition to delivery of an uncompromised fetus and psychological support for the client and her family, are prevention of seizures and reduction of vasospasm.

Thus, medically prescribed, supervised home care with nursing management, fetal well-being testing, and laboratory screening commonly is instituted until term is reached or the client's condition deteriorates, necessitating additional intervention.

Delivery of the infant is the only known treatment. Vaginal delivery is preferred in order not to add anesthesia or surgical risks. Those clients with HELLP syndrome may have their labor induced for a vaginal delivery at 32 or more weeks' gestation if the fetus exhibits lung maturity and well-being (based on biophysical profile score) and the client has a ripe (inducible) cervix based on a Bishop's score. For those clients with HELLP syndrome and less than 32 weeks' gestation, a cesarean birth will be considered.

Should a client's disease progress to the point of maternal seizure, delivery is generally postponed for 1 to 3 hours. The induction or cesarean section is an additional stressor for the client who exhibits acidosis and hypoxia due to the seizure. Anesthesia and surgery are not well tolerated; once vital signs are stable with improved urinary output and decreased acidosis/hypoxia, delivery is pursued.

Table 42–10 presents the drug data for the two most commonly used drugs for treating severe preeclampsia: magnesium sulfate and hydralazine.

SIDE EFFECTS AND ADVERSE REACTIONS

Magnesium Sulfate

Early signs of increased magnesium levels in the client include flushing, feelings of increased warmth, sweating, thirst, sedation, heavy eyelids, slurred speech, hypotension, depressed reflexes, and decreased muscle tone. Adverse reactions generally occur with serum levels greater than 10 mEq/L. Magnesium toxicity is manifested by a rapid drop in blood pressure and respiratory paralysis. Reflexes may be absent. Heart block has been reported occasionally with levels lower than 10 mEq/L.

Decreased beat-to-beat variability may be seen on the FHR tracing. If the client received magnesium sulfate close to the time of delivery, the neonate may exhibit low Apgar scores, hypotonia, lethargy,

TABLE 42–10 Drugs Used in Severe Preeclampsia

Drug	Dosage	Uses and Considerations
Magnesium sulfate	Loading dose: 4 g in 20–30 min IV; piggyback using infusion pump/controller Maintenance dose: 1–2 g/h IV using constant infusion pump in piggyback mode	Prevention and treatment of seizures related to PIH; acts as CNS depressant; decreases acetylcholine from motor nerves, which blocks neuromuscular transmission and decreased incidence of seizures Secondarily affects peripheral vascular system with increased uterine blood flow due to vasodilation and some transient BP decrease during first hour; also inhibits uterine contractions. Depresses deep tendon reflexes and respiration; maintenance dose depends on reflexes, respiratory rate, urinary output, and magnesium level. Production of abnormally high magnesium level is main risk; therapeutic levels range from 2.5 to 6.7 mEq/L; levels of 4–7.5 mEq/L are effective in preventing seizures. Client is at risk if respiratory rate < 12, output < 30 ml/h, deep tendon reflex (knee jerk) is absent. Antidote: calcium gluconate 10 ml of 10% solution (1 g) slow IV push by physician over 3 min. Can be given IV or IM. Should not be given parenterally to clients with heart block, myocardial damage, or renal impairment. Contraindicated in myasthenia gravis. IV: Immediate onset; duration: 30 min; IM: onset 1 h; duration: 3–4 h. Absorbed magnesium is excreted by kidney; excreted in breast milk but not contraindication to breast feeding. *Pregnancy category: B; t½: UK; infusion usually stopped 24 h postpartum*
Hydralazine hydrochloride (Apresoline)	IV: 100 mg in 1000 mL normal saline by infusion pump titrated at 6–12 mg/h to maintain elected BP IV Push: 5–10 mg slow IV; additional 5–10 mg doses q 20 min PRN; single dose should not be more than 20 mg IM: 5–10 mg PO: 100 mg/d in 4 divided doses	Antihypertensive agent. Acts by causing arteriolar vasodilation. Usually lowers diastolic BP more than systolic BP. Objective of treatment is to maintain diastolic BP between 90 and 110 mmHg. Usually not given to pregnant PIH client with diastolic BP < 105 mmHg due to risk of reduced intervillous blood flow. Clients with impaired renal function may require lower doses. Parenteral: onset of action 5–20 min; peak action 10–80 min; duration of action 2–6 h; well-tolerated; maternal tachycardia and increased cardiac output and oxygen consumption may occur. Oral: onset: 20–30 min; peak: 1–2 h; duration: 2–4 h

KEY: BP: blood pressure; IM: intramuscular; IV: intravenous; PO: by mouth; PIH: pregnancy-induced hypertension; PRN: as needed; t½: half-life; UK; unknown; <: less than.

weakness, and potential respiratory distress. The fetal level of magnesium generally reaches more than 90% of maternal levels within 3 h of administration. There is no evidence linking congenital defects and maternal hypocalcemia or hypermagnesemia. The greater risk to the fetus is from maternal PIH: decreased placental blood flow and intrauterine growth retardation.

HYDRALAZINE

Observe the client for headache, nausea, vomiting, nasal congestion, dizziness, tachycardia, palpitations, and angina pectoris. In the fetus and neonate, observe for a sudden fall in maternal blood pressure, which may cause fetal hypoxia. Hydralazine has no known adverse effects on the fetus.

NURSING PROCESS: PREGNANCY-INDUCED HYPERTENSION

ASSESSMENT

- Obtain baseline vital signs during early pregnancy to compare with future findings.
- Identify client factors that may predispose to PIH.

POTENTIAL NURSING DIAGNOSES

- Fluid volume deficit related to shift of intravascular fluid to extravascular space as outcome of vasospasm with subsequent elevated arterial hypertension

- Knowledge deficit related to information gap about PIH, diagnosis, treatment modalities, common outcomes for mother and baby
- Potential for inadequate placental perfusion secondary to vasospasm with risk to fetal well-being
- Potential for maternal injury related to seizure activity
- Potential for maternal injury related to magnesium toxicity

PLANNING

- Client's blood pressure will be within acceptable ranges.

- Client will verbalize content in her own words that demonstrates accurate grasp of PIH-related information.
- Client will comply with planned PIH treatment regimen.
- Fetus will tolerate disease-altered intrauterine environment and subsequent delivery without injury.
- Mother will maintain therapeutic magnesium levels.
- Plan for magnesium sulfate infusion for at least 24 h postpartum and continue to check respirations and urinary output from Foley catheter hourly; also assess DTRs.

HYDRALAZINE

- Take pulse and BP every 5 min when drug is administered or constantly by use of an electronic monitor until stabilized and then every 15 min.
- Maintain diastolic BP between 90 and 110 mmHg; check with health care provider.
- Observe for change in level of consciousness if BP decreases too rapidly.
- Monitor I & O to avoid hypotensive episodes or overload.
- Monitor fetus.
- Do not mix with any other medications in same bag.

CLIENT TEACHING

General

- Teach client information about PIH and implications for mother, fetus, and newborn.
- Provide client information about potential treatment modalities for PIH.

Safety

- Teach client how and why to rest in the left lateral recumbent position.
- Teach the client signs and symptoms of further deterioration due to progressive PIH and when and why to seek medical assistance.
- Explain to client that fetal well-being will be assessed through biophysical profile studies, a nonstress test, or contraction stress test at determined frequencies.
- Educate family regarding possibility of convulsions and appropriate actions to take if convulsions should occur when with client.

Diet

- Provide nutritional counseling in regard to need for additional protein intake due to protein losses, normal sodium diet, and importance of adequate fluid intake.

- Explain to client why her weight must be obtained each day.

Magnesium Sulfate
General

- Explain to the client why she will have a Foley catheter, infusion pump, and continuous fetal monitoring.
- Tell the client that therapy will extend into the postpartum period, including the Foley catheter.

Safety

- Explain to the client that she will be in a low-stimulation room but will not be left alone.

Side Effects

- Tell the client that she will likely experience hot flashes and possibly nausea and vomiting with the loading dose.
- Tell client that evidence of magnesium levels that are within therapeutic range include decreased appetite, awkwardness when moving about, and some speech slurring to reduce her potential anxiety.
- Tell client to report any swallowing difficulties or drooling (occur at lower end of toxic range).

Hydralazine
Safety

- Explain to client that nurses will be monitoring pulse and BP almost constantly until she becomes stable after administration, and then every 15 min. Explain that an electronic monitor may be used to obtain constant readings.
- Explain to client need for monitoring I & O.

NURSING INTERVENTIONS

Magnesium Sulfate

- Continuous electronic fetal monitoring is required; document evaluations of tracings every 15 min.
- Have available airway suction and resuscitation equipment and emergency drugs.
- Antidote must be at bedside. Calcium gluconate (1 g) is usual antidote, but calcium chloride may also be used. Usual therapy is 10 mL of 10% calcium gluconate or 5 mL of 10% calcium chloride by IV push over 3 min by personnel as specified in agency protocol.
- Maintain client in left lateral recumbent position in low-stimulation environment. Do not leave client alone.
- For IM administration, must use Z-track technique and rotate sites (drug is painful and irritating).

- Monitor BP, pulse, respiratory rate (every 15 to 30 min), deep tendon reflexes (every 1 to 2 h), and hourly I & O (PO and IV; Foley catheter output).
- Monitor temperature, breath sounds, and bowel sounds every 4 h.
- Check urine for albumin every hour.
- Check for epigastric pain, headache, visual symptoms, sensory changes, edema, level of consciousness, and seizure activity on ongoing basis.
- Monitor serum magnesium levels every 4 h or according to agency protocol for range between 4 and 7 mEq/L.
- Notify physician if following observed:
    Respirations less than 12/min
    Absence of patellar reflexes
    Urinary output less than 30 mL/h
    Systolic BP less than or equal to 160 mmHg, unless ordered
    Magnesium level greater than 7 mEq/L
    Absent bowel sounds or altered breath sounds
    Epigastric pain, headache, visual symptoms, sensory changes, change in affect or level of consciousness, seizure activity

- Monitor laboratory reports for evidence of low platelet count, and if present, observe for excessive bleeding. This is important because some women with preeclampsia develop HELLP syndrome (hemolysis, elevated liver enzymes, low platelet count), which involves many organs and is life threatening.
- Monitor fetal status.
- Postpartum fundal status must be monitored due to increased risk of hemorrhage.

EVALUATION

- Evaluate the effectiveness of drug therapy to reduce BP.
- Continue monitoring vital signs. Report changes.
- Document effect of teaching/learning opportunity upon client's knowledge deficit about PIH treatment modalities, and outcomes.
- Note status of fetal well-being secondary to treatment with drugs as evidenced by fetal monitoring strips.
- Monitor changes that occur in magnesium level per laboratory results as compared with behavioral cues.

DRUGS FOR PAIN CONTROL DURING LABOR

Labor and delivery, a stressful event for most clients, is divided into three major stages. During the *first stage* cervical effacement and dilatation occur; the cervix becomes fully dilated at 10 cm. The *second stage* is the period of pushing, during which expulsion of the fetus occurs. During the *third stage* the placenta separates from the uterine wall, is expelled, and initial recovery begins. It is beyond the scope of this chapter to discuss the many physical and behavioral changes observable during each of these stages. However, it is important to recognize that, as the first stage of labor progresses, uterine contractions become stronger in quality and longer in duration and the interval between them becomes shorter.

Physical causes of labor pain include uterine muscle hypoxia, cervical effacement and dilatation, referred pain, and distention of the bladder, vagina, and perineum. Possible psychological causes include past experience with pain, anticipation of pain, high anxiety, knowledge deficit about what to expect, and lack of a support person.

If pharmacologic intervention is needed for pain relief, drugs should be used sparingly and as an adjunct to ongoing nonpharmacologic measures. Examples of nonpharmacologic comfort and pain relief measures useful throughout labor and delivery are (1) mobility within the environment, (2) positioning supportive of the gravid uterus and promoting uterine perfusion, (3) hygiene and comfort measures, (4) presence of support person, and (5) use of relaxation techniques.

Drugs should be selected to decrease the client's pain but, at the same time, to eliminate or minimize side effects of these drugs for the fetus/newborn and the mother throughout the rest of her labor and delivery. Remember, the placenta is not an effective barrier for fetal protection.

Pain relief in labor and delivery can be obtained through the use of systemic analgesics and regional inhalation, or general anesthesia. Inhalation and general anesthesia are not discussed in this chapter. Analgesics alter the client's perception and sensation of pain without producing unconsciousness.

ANALGESIA

Systemic medications (drugs that enter the circulatory system and are distributed throughout the body and brain) employed for pain control during labor include sedative-hypnotics, narcotic agonists, and mixed narcotic agonist-antagonists.

The sedative-hypnotic drugs are generally given when an apprehensive client is in false labor or very early labor, or has ruptured membranes but no true labor. These drugs allow the mother to rest and relax and reduce her fears and anxiety. The sedative drugs most commonly used are barbiturates, generally secobarbital sodium (Seconal) and pentobarbital sodium (Nembutal). Other drugs in this category include several that can be given alone during early labor or combined with narcotic agonists and given later when the client is in active labor. Used this way, these drugs have an **ataractic** effect (potentiating the analgesic action of a low-dose narcotic) in addition to decreasing anxiety and apprehension. These drugs include promethazine (Phenergan), a sedative-antihistamine; hydroxyzine hydrochloride (Vistaril, Atarax), a sedative-hypnotic; and promazine (Sparine), an antipsychotic-neuroleptic.

The most commonly used narcotic agonist for pain relief during labor is meperidine hydrochloride (Demerol), a synthetic narcotic. Morphine sulfate is seldom used in labor. These drugs interfere with pain impulses at the subcortical level of the brain. Secondary effects include sedation and de-creased anxiety. Meperidine is generally not given before a **primiparous** (first pregnancy) client is 5 to 6 cm dilated, or before a **multiparous** (more than one pregnancy) client is 3 to 4 cm dilated. In practice, the narcotic agonists are not given after a primiparous client is fully dilated or a multiparous client is 7 to 8 cm dilated. These restrictions arise because of the fact that narcotics received by the mother 1 to 3 h before delivery may result in neonatal respiratory depression, as noted in 10-min Apgar scores.

The third group of systemic medications used for pain relief in labor are the mixed narcotic agonist-antagonists. These drugs must be used cautiously with other CNS depressant drugs because they potentiate their respiratory depressant effects. If a client is addicted to narcotics, this group of drugs may cause her to exhibit extreme withdrawal symptoms. An example of a common drug from this group is butorphanol tartrate (Stadol).

Table 42–11 presents additional information about these three groups of systemic medications used during labor.

TABLE 42–11 Common Systemic Medications Used for Pain Relief in Labor

Drug	Dosage	Uses and Considerations
Sedative-Hypnotics		
Secobarbital (Seconal)	IM: 50–100 mg PO: 100–200 mg	Used to decrease anxiety during early latent phase of labor; onset: 10–30 min; peak: 20–30 min; duration: 4–8 h; no effects on uterine tone or contractility; rapidly crosses placenta; can cause decreased variability in FHR (pseudo-sinusoidal pattern) due to decreased CNS control over heart rate. Since no antagonist for barbiturates, contraindicated if delivery is imminent
		Generally administered only if delivery not expected for 24–48 h. May have prolonged depressant effects on neonate. Excreted into breast milk. Compatible with breast feeding. May increase CNS depression with alcohol, narcotics, antihistamines, tranquilizers, and MAOIs. *Pregnancy category:* D; t½: 15–30 h; PB: UK
Pentobarbital (Nembutal)	PO: 20–30 mg	Short-acting barbiturate. *Pregnancy category:* D; see Prototype Drug Chart (Fig. 13–2)
Ataractics		
Promethazine HCL (Phenergan)	IM/IV: 12.5–25 mg q 4–6 h or IM: 25–50 mg with 25–75 mg meperidine or IV: 15–25 mg with 25–75 mg meperidine; repeat if needed Maximum dose: no more than 100 mg in 24 h	A phenothiazine antihistamine; used as adjunct to narcotic analgesics during first stage of labor; antiemetic properties; onset: PO: 20 min; IM: 3–5 min; IV: 1–2 min; used alone to promote rest and sleep; potentiates action of narcotic agonists reducing narcotic doses; may cause decreased variability in FHR; contraindicated during lactation; at term, rapidly crosses placenta; fetal and maternal blood concentrations in equilibrium in 15 min, with infant levels persisting for 4 h; transient hypotension, lethargy and electroencephalographic changes for 3 d in newborn; may cause maternal tachycardia; may impair newborn platelet aggregation. If given with meperidine, give slowly at beginning of contraction over several minutes to decrease amount of drug perfused immediately to the fetus via placenta. Other adverse reactions: dizziness, dry mouth, excessive sedation, weakness, blurred vision, restlessness. Do not give subcutaneous or intraarterially. *Pregnancy category:* C; PB: UK; t½: UK
Hydroxyzine pamoate (Vistaril, Atarax)	IM: 25–50 mg, q 4–6 h; repeat if needed	Antianxiety agent; antihistamine; antiemetic; sedative-hypnotic; used alone early in labor or later to potentiate action of narcotic agonists; can cause decreased variability in FHR; use Z-track injection for IM to reduce pain; no data available about breast feeding; onset: 15–30 min; peak: <2 h; duration: 4–6 h. Intraarterial, SC, or IV administration *not* recommended (thrombus and digital gangrene can occur); extravasation can result in sterile abscesses and marked tissue induration; use with caution in clients with chronic obstructive pulmonary

Table continued on following page

TABLE 42–11 Common Systemic Medications Used for Pain Relief in Labor (*Continued*)

Drug	Dosage	Uses and Considerations
		disease and asthma. Adverse reactions: hypotension, drowsiness, dizziness, headache, dry mouth, pain at injection site, weakness, ataxia; may cause CNS depression with alcohol, analgesics, barbiturates, narcotics; may decrease effects of epinephrine. No effect on labor or neonatal Apgar scores. *Pregnancy category:* C; PB: UK; t½: 3 h
Promazine (Sparine)	IM: 25–50 mg	A propylamino phenothiazine related to chlorpromazine; antipsychotic-neuroleptic antiemetic; IV route not recommended but can use in concentrations <25 mg/mL; potentiates narcotic agonists; can cause decreased variability in FHR; onset 15 min, peaks in 1 h, duration 4–6 h. Readily crosses placenta; increases effect with CNS depressants, epinephrine, anticholinergics; side effects observed include drowsiness, headache, rash, dry mouth, nausea, vomiting, anorexia, constipation, and orthostatic hypotension. Excreted into breast milk but little data available on effects (with related drug, chlorpromazine, drowsiness and lethargy in infant if high milk-drug concentration). *Pregnancy category:* C; PB: >90%; t½: >24 h
Narcotic Agonists Meperidine hydrochloride (Demerol)	IM: 50–100 mg, q 3–4 h IV (slow push): 25–50 mg	Synthetic morphine-like narcotic agonist alters pain perception and depresses pain impulses by binding to opiate receptor in CNS; onset IM is 10 min with peak in 40–60 min and duration of 2–4 h; onset IV is 30 sec with peak in 5–7 min and duration of 1–2 h; crosses placenta and appears in fetus in 1–2 min after IV dose; can cause decreased variability in FHR; caution needed for use with cardiac clients due to tachycardia; well absorbed; excreted in urine as metabolites. Adverse reactions: bradycardia, severe hypotension, convulsion, respiratory depression, cardiovascular collapse, increased intracranial pressure. Respiratory depression in the newborn following use during labor is time and dose dependent; naloxone should be available; newborn may exhibit moderate CNS and mild behavioral depression. Mother may have nausea, vomiting, drowsiness, sedation, confusion. May increase or decrease uterine activity. Give drug at beginning of contraction to prevent fetal bolus of drug. *Pregnancy category:* B; PB: 60%–70%; t½: 3–8 h
Mixed Narcotic Agonists/ Antagonists Butorphanol tartrate (Stadol)	IM: 2 mg, q 3–4 h IV: 1 mg, q 3–4 h	Potent nonnarcotic analgesic (2 mg dose approximately equivalent to 10–15 mg morphine); has mixed narcotic agonist-antagonist mechanism of action with central analgesic actions; binds to CNS opiate receptors and inhibits ascending pain pathways. Used for relief of moderate to severe pain, for preoperative medication, supplement to anesthesia. *Pregnancy category:* B (D, if prolonged use or high at-term dose); PB: >90%; t½: 2.5–4 h; onset: IM: 10–30 min; IV: 1–2 min; peak: IM: 0.5–1 h; IV: 4–5 min; duration: IM: 3–4 h; IV: 2–4 h. Additive effects with CNS depressants; may see withdrawal symptoms in narcotic-dependent clients; may cause drowsiness and respiratory depression, sedation, euphoria, hallucinations, headache, palpitations. Do not give SC; have naloxone available as antidote. Do not give if respirations <12/min. Use with caution in client having preterm baby because fetus may exhibit decreased beat-to-beat variability on FHR monitor; newborn may have moderate CNS depression, hypotonia at birth, and mild behavioral depression

KEY: FHR: fetal heart rate; IM: intramuscular; IV: intravenous; PB: protein-binding; PO: by mouth; SC: subcutaneous(ly); t½: half-life; UK: unknown; <: less than.

Side Effects and Adverse Reactions

Side effects of sedative-hypnotic drugs (secobarbital, pentobarbital) for the client include paradoxically increased pain and excitability, lethargy, subdued mood, decreased sensory perception, and hypotension. Side effects include decreased beat-to-beat variability in the heart rate in the fetus and respiratory depression, sleepiness, hypotonia, delayed breast feeding with poor sucking response (number of sucks/amount of sucking pressure) for up to 4 days in the neonate.

Side effects of ataractic drugs (promethazine, hydroxyzine, promazine) for the client include confusion, disorientation, excess sedation, dizziness, hypotension, tachycardia, blurred vision, headache, restlessness, weakness, and urinary retention with *promethazine;* drowsiness, dry mouth, dizziness, headache, blurred vision, dysuria, urinary retention, and constipation with *hydroxyzine;* and drowsiness, headache, rash, dry mouth, nausea, vomiting, anorexia, constipation, and orthostatic hypotension with *promazine.* Decreased beat-to-beat variability can be seen in the fetus, and the neonate can experience moderate CNS depression, hypotonia, lethargy, poor feeding, and hypothermia.

Side effects of narcotic agonist drugs (meperidine) for the client include orthostatic hypotension, nausea, vomiting, headache, sedation, hypotension, and confusion. Neonatal CNS depression and decreased beat-to-beat variability on the FHR monitor can occur with meperidine.

In the client, mixed narcotic agonist-antagonists can cause nausea, clamminess, sweating, sedation, respiratory depression, vertigo, lethargy, headache, and flushing. Side effects in the fetus and neonate include decreased beat-to-beat variability on the FHR monitor, moderate CNS depression, hypotonia at birth, and mild behavioral depression.

NURSING PROCESS: PAIN CONTROL DRUGS

ASSESSMENT

- Assess the client's laboring behavior for degree of relaxation and pattern of labor in relation to expected norms.
- Assess the client's verbal and nonverbal behavior for data supportive or nonsupportive of positive coping with labor.
- Obtain baseline data for vital signs, blood pressure (BP), breath sounds, quality of contractions, degree of effacement and dilatation, and fetal heart rate prior to administering the analgesic for later comparison to determine effectiveness (pain scale).
- Screen for drug history to ascertain potential for drug-drug interactions.
- Assess for cultural expectations related to pain experiences.

POTENTIAL NURSING DIAGNOSIS

- Pain related to progressive labor
- Fear of pain related to progressive labor
- Anxiety related to uncertainty about labor experience and personal coping ability

PLANNING

- The client's pain during labor will be controlled without severe side effects.

NURSING INTERVENTIONS

- Offer appropriate analgesia for stage and phase of labor and the anticipated method of delivery. Encourage the client and her support person to participate in the discussion and decision-making about accepting analgesia. Make certain that the client knows that the choice is hers.
- Record administration of the drug on the fetal monitoring strip.
- Provide appropriate safety measures after administration of drugs that may alter sensorium (side rails, call bell).
- Check compatibility chart for any mixing of drugs.

- Verify that correct antidote drugs for selected drugs are available.
- Within agency protocols and safe obstetric practice, administer drugs prior to maximum intensity pain/anxiety.

Sedative-Hypnotics: Barbiturates
- Consider the amount of time likely until delivery; do not give if delivery is imminent because narcotic antagonists will not counteract respiratory depression and no other antidote is available. Observe FHR tracing for decreased beat-to-beat variability.

Ataractics: Promethazine, Hydroxyzine, Promazine
- *Promethazine:* If IV, give at beginning of contraction over several minutes; do not give SC or intraarterially; screen for allergy to sulfites; administer at 25 mg/min or lower rate.
- Monitor amount of promethazine the client receives in 24 h; monitor for maternal heart rate following administration; observe FHR strip for beat-to-beat variability.
- *Hydroxyzine:* Do not give SC, intraarterially, or IV; use IM Z-track technique; observe FHR strip for beat-to-beat variability.
- *Promazine:* Usually do not give IV (if is to be given, use in concentration <25 mg/mL); observe FHR strip for beat-to-beat variability.
- Recall that all three drugs have limited data concerning breast feeding, although they are not specifically contraindicated.

Narcotic Agonists and Mixed Narcotic Agonist-Antagonists
- Consider parity (number of fetuses gestated to viability) of client, and relationship to likely amount of time remaining until delivery. Consider general rule that these drugs are not given *after* a primiparous client is fully dilated or a multiparous client is 7 to 8 cm dilated.
- Do not give when delivery is likely within 1 to 3 h, because of greater chance of depressed fetus or neonate (i.e., birth should occur within 1 h or after 3 to 4 h following administration).
- Monitor voiding status carefully.

- Observe FHR strip for decreased beat-to-beat variability.

Meperidine

- Generally not given before a primiparous client is 5 to 6 cm dilated or a multiparous client is 3 to 4 cm dilated. Be certain a narcotic antagonist (naloxone) is available as antidote if needed.
- If drug is administered intravenously, give very slowly at beginning of a contraction over several minutes to decrease the amount of drug perfused immediately to the fetus via the placenta.
- Check for respirations >12 prior to administration.
- IM: inject deep into muscle.
- Provide calm, nonstimulating environment as adjunctive therapy.
- Keep bedrails up when client is nonambulatory and have client solicit assistance if she does ambulate.
- Observe FHR strip.
- Have naloxone readily available in neonatal form.

Butorphanol Tartrate

- Observe for signs of narcotic withdrawal in narcotic-dependent clients.
- Do not administer SC.
- Observe for respiratory depression.
- Ascertain respirations >12 prior to administration.
- IM: inject deep into muscle.
- Provide low-stimulation environment.
- Observe FHR strip.
- Have naloxone readily available in neonatal form.
- If given IV, give slowly at beginning of contraction.

General
- Instruct client concerning
  - Drugs ordered
  - Route to be administered and reason
  - Expected effects of drug on labor
  - Potential drug effects on fetus/newborn
- Tell the client that most drugs used for pain relief in labor and delivery are not given PO because the GI tract functions more slowly during labor and thus drug absorption is decreased. Tell her that feelings of nausea might be heightened if oral medications are used.

Safety
- Instruct client about restrictions that will be placed on her while receiving the drug, including
  - Positioning in bed
  - Side rails up
  - Bed rest

EVALUATION

- Evaluate the effectiveness of the particular drug in lessening or alleviating the pain using pain scale within expectations for a normally progressing labor.
- Evaluate fear and anxiety levels in regard to pain and ability to cope with the labor experience.
- Monitor respirations, heart rate, blood pressure, and FHR strip for alterations from baseline and stability. Report deviations beyond those expected with a normally progressing labor.
- Document findings using agency protocols and obstetric standard of care.

ANESTHESIA

Anesthesia in labor and delivery represents the loss of painful sensations with or without the loss of consciousness, depending on the approach used. There are two types of pain experienced in childbirth: The pain of labor arises from nociceptors in the uterine and perineal structures. *Somatic* pain due to stretching of the perineum and vagina travels to sacral 2, 3, and 4 by way of the pudendal nerve. Visceral pain from the cervix and uterus is carried by nerves together with sympathetic fibers and enters the neuraxis at the thoracic 10, 11, 12, and lumbar 1 spinal level.

Regional Anesthesia

Regional anesthesia achieves pain relief during labor and delivery (depending on the form of anesthesia selected) without loss of consciousness through temporarily blocking the conduction of painful impulses along sensory nerve pathways to the brain through the use of injected local anesthetics. The use of regional anesthesia allows an awake and aware client to experience labor and the birth of her baby more fully with lack of discomfort in the blocked area. Regional anesthesia may also inhibit the urge to push, which can help prevent some babies from too rapid delivery.

Local anesthetics most commonly used for regional anesthesia are chemically related to cocaine, considered to be the first natural anesthetic substance found. The chemically related drugs that have evolved since that time are much less toxic and more potent and have longer lasting therapeutic effects. Names of frequently used local anesthetics of the amide type (metabolized in the liver) include mepivacaine (Carbocaine), lidocaine (Xylocaine), and bupivacaine (Marcaine). These potent agents have a long duration of action. They cross the placenta and, depending on the degree to which they are protein-bound, can enter the fetal circulation. The fetal effects last for 24 to 48 h after delivery. The ester type agents are rapidly metabolized by plasma pseudocholinesterase, rather than the liver. Thus, the mother's drug level is lower, and less anesthetic is placentally transferred to the fetus. Chloroprocaine (Nesacaine) is an example of an ester type agent.

Side effects from local anesthetic agents depend on their chemical properties. These include palpitations, dizziness, confusion, headache, off-taste in the mouth, nausea, vomiting, hypotension, seizures, and coma. Where there is concern, a small test dose can be tried. IV fluids are generally infused or are kept available, particularly to help with hypotension should this complication occur.

The following is an overview of the forms in which local anesthetic agents are administered to obstetric clients to assist with pain management.

Subarachnoid Block

SPINAL BLOCK

Indication: Need for high degree of pain relief for delivery. Preferred for surgery, seldom used for labor today.

When given: Immediately prior to delivery; late in second stage when fetal head is on the perineum.

Area blocked: Umbilicus to toes.

Injection site: With client side lying, injected into subarachnoid space at L4–L5.

Considerations: Client needs to be well hydrated. Anesthetic has to be given immediately after a contraction to avoid impairing respiratory efforts. Client generally in curled side-lying position for administration. Contraindicated if skin over lumbar region is infected or client has severe coagulopathy, severe hypovolemia, or severe BP abnormalities.

Side effects: For client: hypotension; occasional spinal headache. For fetus or neonate: none, unless secondary to maternal hypotension. *Note:* Headache is now less common due to small size (25 gauge) of needle used; may have nausea, backache, urinary retention. Contraindicated in the preeclamptic client.

SADDLE BLOCK

Indication: Pain relief for delivery with perineal anesthesia, forceps delivery, and episiotomy repair.

When given: Same as for spinal block.

Area blocked: Perineal area, buttocks, inner area of thighs (for true saddle block); uterus and perineum (for modified saddle block).

Injection site: With client sitting, injected in S1–S5 (true saddle) or T1–S5 (modified saddle).

Advantage: Can be used for cesarean birth if injected to T4.

Considerations: Same as for spinal block.

Side effects: For client none. For fetus and neonate: none.

Lumbar Epidural

LUMBAR EPIDURAL BLOCK (ONE DOSE)

Indication: Pain relief in first and second stages of labor.

When given: Active phase of labor.

Area blocked: T12–S5 (entire pelvis) in area of dorsal root ganglion with motor and sensory loss.

Injection site: Epidural space (potential space between the dura mater and vertebral canal from cranium to sacrum) between L2–L3 or L3–L5 or L4–L5; *not* into the dura. Never put in above L1. Note that L1–L2 is where the spinal cord ends. Nerves run off and down into the spinal canal. Nerve free floats and can move out of the way of the epidural needle. The goal is to bathe the nerves with the dispersed local anesthetic.

Considerations: Loss of bearing-down reflex means forceps or vacuum extractor will be needed. May slow labor. Contraindicated in clients with skin infection in lumbar region or with severe coagulopathy.

Side effects: For client: dural puncture with leak of spinal fluid creates a true spinal block (level drug reaches determines the degree of side effects); hypotension (severe); convulsions; local anesthetic, coma, respiratory arrest. For fetus or neonate: few effects unless severe maternal hypotension occurs (late decelerations in FHR); may depend on the anesthetic agent used.

Note: Test dose (not in quantity to cause seizure) used to determine placement; if local anesthetic is injected into vein, client may experience dizziness, ringing in ears, numb mouth, toxic response.

CONTINUOUS LUMBAR EPIDURAL BLOCK (REPEAT DOSES USING INDWELLING CATHETER IN EPIDURAL SPACE)

Indication: Pain relief during first and second stages. Most useful for prolonged labors.

When given: 3 to 4 cm dilation in multigravida; 4 to 6 cm in primigravida.

Note: Prior to 4 cm dilation, there is risk of arresting the first stage of labor.

This is the most widely used and acceptable method for labor pain management today.

Area blocked: Same as for lumbar epidural block.

Injection site: Same as for lumbar epidural block.

Advantages: Provides continuous anesthesia from stage 1 through delivery and perineal repair. Client can feel movement and pressure but no pain. Can be used for vaginal delivery or cesarean birth. Sensory level can be altered and the density of the block can be manipulated. Can be used to deliver epidural morphine PF (Duramorph) or fentanyl (Sublimaze) into epidural space for regional analgesia (highly effective); used less often now because of the large number of clients who experience itching that is not effectively relieved using diphenhydramine (Benadryl) (naloxone [Narcan] infusions also do not relieve this itch) and therefore, clients are returning to PCA pumps and traditional forms of postpartum pain relief. Preserves motor and sensory function but blocks pain perception; requires smaller doses than systemic drugs because it begins to work without the liver being involved. Has slow onset of action (15 to 60 min).

Considerations: Forceps will be needed. Requires a large amount of local agent. Bupivacaine must be used in low concentration (0.25% to 0.5%).

Complications: Same as for lumbar epidural block.

Side effects: For client and fetus or neonate: pruritus (in 2 to 3 h when drug reaches upper thoracic segments), respiratory depression (before 1 h and after 6 h), urinary retention, and nausea and vomiting.

Caudal (A Type of Epidural Anesthesia)

Indication: Pain in first and second stages of labor.

When given: Active phase of labor.

Area blocked: Perineum; masks uterine contractions.

Injection site: Epidural space through sacral hiatus (S4).

Advantages: Useful for women with metabolic, lung, and heart disease. Very rapid perineal anesthesia and muscle relaxation. No puncture of the dura occurs routinely. Can be used continuously. Client can move about in bed after catheter is inserted.

Considerations: Hard to administer. Painful until needle is correctly placed. Increased need to use forceps. Loss of urge to push. Risk of systemic toxic reactions; level of anesthesia difficult to obtain.

Side effects: None. Used infrequently today.

Paracervical Block

Indication: Pain during first stage.

Time given: Active phase of first stage; repeated periodically until 8 cm dilated.

Area blocked: Uterus, cervix, and vagina; masks contractions.

Injection site: Transvaginally, adjacent to rim of cervix.

Advantages: Rapid onset. Lasts 60 to 90 min. Relieves pain of cervical dilatation and contractions. Does not block lower vagina or perineum. Many clients can sleep through contractions.

Considerations: Rapid absorption (because injected into vascular area). Skilled health professional required for administration. Does not last long enough to help with delivery or episiotomy. Has variable effects on labor progress.

Side effects: For client: hematomas in tissue around injection site. For fetus and neonate: mild to severe bradycardia common with decreased beat-to-beat variability (nonreassuring sign) for approximately 15 min.

Pudendal

Indication: For outlet forceps episiotomy and repair.

When given: Immediately before birth.

Area blocked: Perineum; pudendal nerves numbed.

Injection site: Inside birth canal deep into lower sides of vagina to bathe the pudendal nerves.

Considerations: None.

Side effects: None.

Local Infiltration

Indication: For episiotomy repair to be done when pudendal anesthesia not possible because of timing and position of fetal head.

When given: Just prior to delivery.

Area blocked: Perineum.

Injection site: Perineal subcutaneous tissue.

Advantage: No effect on FHR or client's vital signs.

Considerations: May not get complete relief of pain, and may need additional drug; requires large amount of agent.

Side effects: For client: drug may sting. For fetus or neonate: none.

Contraindications

There are some contraindications to regional anesthesia:

- Morbid obesity
- Tocolysis with terbutaline

- Severe pregnancy-induced hypertension (PIH) (due to increased risk of profound hypotension and risk of disseminated intravascular coagulation, secondary to poor hydration [hypovolemia] associated with underlying disease state)

- Coagulation disorders (client should have a normal PTZ and platelet counts)
- Generalized sepsis or local infection at needle insertion site.

NURSING PROCESS: REGIONAL ANESTHETICS

ASSESSMENT

- Check history for drug sensitivity to local agents. May need to use a test dose before large-scale administration.
- Assess for presence of a "labor plan" with expectations for performance in labor and beliefs about use of analgesia/anesthesia.
- Assess knowledge level about regional anesthesia.
- Determine extent of cervical dilatation and extent of labor progress.
- Review fetal status in utero.
- Review history for presence of any contraindications to regional anesthesia.

POTENTIAL NURSING DIAGNOSES

- Pain related to progressive progress in labor with diminished coping ability
- Knowledge deficit related to inexperience with regional anesthesia/analgesia
- Potential for impaired gas exchange to fetus should maternal hypotension occur secondary to use of local anesthetic
- Impaired physical mobility secondary to bed rest restriction during epidural anesthesia
- Potential for altered urinary retention (less than) secondary to epidural anesthesia

PLANNING

- Client will have relief of discomfort during labor.
- Client will remain normotensive and maintain a normal pulse rate; FHR will remain within normal limits.
- Client will not experience bladder distention.
- Client will be able to discuss specifics of regional anesthesia correctly.

NURSING INTERVENTIONS

General
- Review hydration status of client before regional anesthesia is started because of the possible need to counteract hypotensive effects.

- Position the client on her left side. Keep her off her back in order to avoid pressure on the inferior vena cava, which would cause maternal hypotension and decreased placental perfusion.
- Monitor the progress of labor for a decrease in frequency and intensity of contractions and decrease in BP. Monitor vital signs and for fetal bradycardia.
- Be certain that atropine, antihistamines, O_2, and resuscitation equipment are readily available
- Be aware of the size of needle used for subarachnoid block and any leakage of cerebrospinal fluid (CSF) that might indicate risk of postspinal headache.
- Be aware of how to operate the client's bed and how to place the client in Trendelenburg position if necessary.

Spinal
- Be certain to accurately determine when the client is having contractions, because the anesthetic agent must be given immediately after a contraction, not before or during.
- Check BP every 1 to 2 min × 10 min, then every 5 to 10 min for an hour for hypotensive effects after injection. Keep O_2 with bag and mask ventilation with positive pressure readily available.
- Apply tight abdominal binder when the client is upright after delivery if it is known that she had a leakage of CSF at the time of the injection or if she reports headache symptoms. The binder will increase the intraabdominal pressure, which will be transmitted to the epidural space with engorgement of veins and an increase in pressure of CSF and decreased headache. Also encourage PO fluids. Assess for validity of headache through sitting client up (headache present) and lying her down (headache goes away).

Epidural
- Ascertain that the client is in the active phase of labor prior to administration. Check client's fluid status. Recommend that client have 500 to 1000 mL of an isotonic solution IV prior to the procedure in order to increase circulatory volume.
- Have client on a fetal heart monitor and observe closely. Monitor progress of labor and recall that too much anesthetic can inhibit fetal descent.

- If hypotension occurs, turn client on left side and increase rate of IV fluids. Notify health care provider.
- Check bladder status carefully. Prior to allowing client to ambulate after delivery, be sure that adequate sensation has returned.
- Conduct ongoing pain assessment. When nature of pain changes, contact the anesthesia department to re-inject anesthetic.
- Perform stat and 1 min blood pressure when epidural anesthesia is used for cesarean delivery.
- Position client in slightly elevated manner, tipped to left side postepidural.
- Document procedure on FHR strip.

Caudal

- Place client in lateral Sims' position for administration. Client can move about in bed after injection.

Paracervical Block

- Maintain close FHR monitoring for fetal bradycardia for 5 min after administration and carefully monitor maternal BP.

CLIENT TEACHING

- Discuss technique, potential benefits, and side effects of client's particular method of anesthesia.

Side Effects

- Tell the client that regional anesthetics may slow labor and that some clients may need a drug to enhance uterine motility.

Spinal
Side Effects

- Explain to the client who develops a headache that epidural blood patches are used to seal the injection site hole and reduce headache.

Epidural
Skill

- Teach client how to curl into position for administration. Tell her that forceps or vacuum extractor will be needed for delivery (due to loss of "urge to push" sensation).

Safety

- Tell the client she will have an IV line for her safety should hypotension occur. Also tell her that she will have an FHR monitor to allow observation of the quality of her contractions and the effect of the anesthetic agent on the fetus.

Caudal
Skill

- Show the client how to assume the left lateral Sims' position.

EVALUATION

- Evaluate blood pressure compared with preprocedure baseline; also FHR strips for alterations in beat-to-beat variability and for any decelerations.
- Evaluate the effectiveness of the anesthetic in relief of discomfort; also for uniformity of coverage (if difference in sides of body, have anesthesia service reposition catheter).
- Evaluate urinary output and palpate for bladder distention.
- Evaluate the fundus for atony.
- Evaluate blocked areas for return of sensation.

DRUGS THAT ENHANCE UTERINE MOTILITY

Oxytocic drugs enhance uterine motility by stimulating the smooth muscle of the uterus to contract. Oxytocin, the ergot alkaloids, and some prostaglandins make up this group of drugs.

Oxytocin is synthesized in the hypothalamus and transported to nerve endings in the posterior pituitary. The hormone is released by the nerve endings under appropriate stimulation; capillaries absorb the substance and carry it into the general circulation where it facilitates smooth muscle contraction. When the effects of natural oxytocin are inadequate or medical indications warrant an induced (planned) labor, synthetic oxytocin products, prostaglandin formulations, and an inflated Foley bulb can be used.

In the presence of adequate estrogen levels (those normally achieved by the third trimester), intravenous oxytocin acts on the uterus to initiate labor contractions. This is useful for clients and their fetuses who have medical indications for such a procedure owing to risks associated with continuing the pregnancy. Table 42–12 presents common medical reasons for induction.

Before a labor is induced, the status of both the client and her fetus must be assessed. The gestational age and level of maturity of the fetus must be accurately determined, together with a determination of the position of the fetus inside the uterus (head down and engaged) and the size of the head

TABLE 42–12 Indications for Labor Induction

Pregnancy-induced hypertension

Chronic maternal hypertension

Fetal membrane rupture >24 h previously

Chorioamnionitis

Postmaturity (>42 wk gestation)

Intrauterine growth retardation

Positive oxytocin challenge test (CST)

Maternal diabetes mellitus (classes B–F)

Maternal renal disease

Rh isoimmunization

Intrauterine fetal death

KEY: CST: contraction stress test.

TABLE 42–13 Contraindications to Labor Induction

Disproportion between fetal head and pelvis (cephalopelvic disproportion)

Nonfavorable fetal presentation (transverse or breech)

Unfavorable fetal position in utero

Documented fetal distress

Prematurity

Placenta previa and/or suspected abruptio placentae

Severe pregnancy-induced hypertension

Grand multiparity

Multifetal gestation

History of uterine trauma

Previous major surgery in the area of the cervix or uterus

Excessive amniotic fluid causing overdistended uterus

in relation to the client's pelvis. The client's cervix must also appear ripe (softening with progress in effacement and partial dilatation). An objective scoring system called the Bishop score is used to objectively assess readiness for induction. The higher the client's score, the more likely is a positive response to induction.

Some clients are not suitable candidates for labor induction because the risks of the procedure outweigh the potential benefits. Table 42–13 presents some of the major contraindications to labor induction.

Two approaches are frequently employed to ripen, efface, and begin cervical dilatation in pregnant women at term (or near term) with a medical or obstetric need for labor induction. One method involves insertion by the physician of a Foley bulb into the cervix, which is then inflated 30 cc to dilate the cervix 3 to 4 cm in size; when the Foley "falls out," the client is started on intravenous oxytocin. The second approach employs prefilled syringes of dinoprostone cervical gel 0.5 mg (Prepidil Gel). Dinoprostone is the naturally occurring form of prostaglandin E_2 (PGE_2). It is thought that endocervically administered PGE_2 gel acts to create effacement and softening by a combination of contraction-inducing and cervical-ripening properties, possibly secondary to collagen degradation resulting from collagenase secretion in response to PGE_2. Table 42–14 presents the dosage and uses and considerations for dinoprostone.

Intravenous oxytocin can be used to augment rather than initiate labor. It facilitates smooth muscle contraction in the uterus of a client already in

TABLE 42–14 Dinoprostone for Cervical Ripening

Drug	Dosage	Uses and Considerations
Dinoprostone Cervical Gel, 0.5 mg (Prepidil Gel)	Endocervical: supplied in 3 g prefilled syringe applicators; 3 doses (1 dose q6h) 6 h after last dose IV oxytocin administered Maximum: 1.5 mg of drug/24 h (7.5 mL or 3 syringes)	A naturally occurring form of prostaglandin E_2 (PGE_2). Must be administered in a hospital with intensive care and acute surgical facilities by a physician. *Pregnancy category:* C. Used to ripen unfavorable cervix at or near term in pregnant women needing labor induction. Metabolized in lung, liver, and kidney; eliminated by kidney. Must be used with caution in clients with renal or hepatic dysfunction. Safety in clients with ruptured membranes has not been determined. Use with caution in asthma, glaucoma or increased intraocular pressure. Not recommended for clients in whom oxytocic drugs are contraindicated or with prolonged uterine contractions; not recommended in clients with placenta previa or active genital herpes (vaginal delivery not indicated). Drug must *not* be placed above level of cervix os. Drug may augment other oxytocic agents; therefore, no concomitant use; sequential use 6–12 h following gel is recommended. Adverse reactions include uterine hyperstimulation, nausea, vomiting, diarrhea, back pain, fetal distress. Clients should have a reactive nonstress test prior to first dose. Client is to remain recumbent 1 h following each dose. Monitor uterine activity and fetal heart rate (FHR); suggest a 20 min FHR strip prior to doses. Must be used at room temperature prior to administration.

labor but experiencing poor uterine contractility with nonprogressive dilation of the cervix and inadequate descent of the presenting part of the fetus. The client with **uterine inertia** may be more responsive to oxytocin than the client who has not begun labor, and a lower starting dose may be needed.

In both labor induction and labor augmentation, oxytocin is infused at a prescribed individualized dosage rate, and this rate is increased, decreased, or maintained at fixed intervals based on client vital signs, uterine response, and FHR. The objective is to establish an adequate contraction pattern that promotes labor progress, generally represented by contractions every 2 to 3 min that last for 50 to 60 sec with moderate intensification. It is an important goal that the client receiving oxytocin not experience uterine hyperstimulation and tetanic contractions, which cause markedly increased pain. The fetus will likely respond with nonreassuring heart rate patterns as hypoxia and acidosis occur owing to interference with placental perfusion should tetanic contractions occur. Continuous observation for impending complications during induction/augmentation is critical. The need for accurate control of infusion flow requires the use of an infusion pump. Once cervical dilatation has reached 5 to 6 cm and an adequate contraction pattern is evident, the rate of oxytocin infusion can be gradually slowed and stopped. The client is then allowed to continue to labor spontaneously.

Following delivery, oxytocin can be added to an existing intravenous electrolyte or dextrose solution to help the uterus contract to close the uterine sinuses. The drug can also be given as a single IM injection following the delivery of the placenta.

Oxytocin is prepared in synthetic form and marketed as Pitocin and Syntocinon. Oxytocin is an FDA-approved drug for labor induction and labor augmentation.

Figure 42–3 shows the actions and effects of oxytocin.

OXYTOCIN

Pharmacokinetics

Oxytocin (Pitocin, Syntocinon) is well absorbed from the nasal mucosa when administered intranasally for milk letdown. The protein-binding percent is low, and the half-life is 1 to 9 min. It is rapidly metabolized and excreted by the liver.

Pharmacodynamics

The onset of action of intramuscularly administered oxytocin occurs in 3 to 5 min, the peak concentration time is unknown, and the duration of action is 2 to 3 h. The onset of action of intravenously administered oxytocin is immediate, the peak concentration time is unknown, and the duration of action is 1 h. The onset of action of intranasally administered oxytocin is a few minutes, the peak concentration time is unknown, and the duration of action is 20 min.

The medication is administered intravenously for induction or enhancement of labor. Pitocin is diluted in 1000 mL lactated Ringer's solution to 10 mU/mL. This is added as a secondary IV line to a control IV. The initial dose is 0.5 mU/min titrated at a rate of 0.2 to 2.5 mU every 15 to 30 min until contractions are approximately 3 min apart and of acceptable quality.

For the prevention and control of hemorrhage due to uterine atony, 10 U of oxytocin is added to a 1 L electrolyte or dextrose solution (10 mU/mL) to infuse at a rate to control atony. Oxytocin is administered intramuscularly (10 U) after the delivery of the placenta.

Side Effects and Adverse Reactions

Maternal effects are seen with IV use only and include hypotension, hypertension, nausea, vomiting, decreased uterine blood flow, rash, and anorexia. Adverse reactions include uterine tetany, anaphylaxis, asphyxia, seizures, coma, intracranial hemorrhage, water intoxication, and dysrhythmias. In the fetus, owing to the induced uterine motility, oxytocin can cause bradycardia, premature ventricular contractions, and other arrhythmias, and rarely fetal death. Low Apgar scores at 5 min, jaundice, and retinal hemorrhage have been reported in the neonate.

Drug Interactions

Concurrent use of vasopressors can result in severe hypertension. Hypotension can occur with concurrent use of cyclopropane anesthesia.

ERGOT ALKALOIDS

The **ergot alkaloids** act by direct smooth-muscle cell receptor stimulation. These drugs are extremely powerful and are used when the uterus does not contract effectively after delivery (**uterine atony**). These drugs are not used during labor because of their propensity to cause sustained uterine contractions (tetanic contractions), which can result in fetal

FIGURE 42–3. Oxytocic Drug: Oxytocin

Oxytocin	Dosage	NURSING PROCESS
		Assessment and Planning

Oxytocin

Oxytocin
  (Pitocin, Syntocinon)
Oxytocic
Pregnancy Category: X

Dosage

A: IV: 10 Units (1 amp) diluted in 1000 mL lactated Ringer's to 10 mU/mL; connect to control IV line at the needle site of main IV line, as a secondary line; start at 0.5 mU/min (3 mL/h) and titate at rate of 0.5–2.5 mU every 15–30 min until contractions are approximately 3 min apart and adequate
IV: 10 Units added to 1 L electrolyte or dextrose solution; infuse at rate to control atony
  (IM: 10 Units after delivery of the placenta if no IV)
Nasal spray: 1 spray into 1 or both nostrils 2–3 min before nursing or pumping

Contraindications

Toxemia, cephalopelvic disproportionment, fetal distress, hypersensitivity, anticipated nonvaginal delivery, pregnancy (intranasal spray)

Drug-Lab-Food Interactions

Hypertension with vasopressors, cyclopropane anesthetics

Pharmacokinetics

Absorption: PO: Well absorbed
Distribution: PB: Low; widely distributed in extracellular fluid; minute amounts in fetal circulation
Metabolism: t½: 1–9 min; rapidly metabolized by liver
Excretion: In urine

Pharmacodynamics

IM: Onset: 3–5 min
  Peak: UK
  Duration: 2–3 h
IV: Onset: Immediate
  Peak: UK
  Duration: 1h
Intranasal: Onset: Few minutes
  Peak: UK
  Duration: 20 min

Interventions

Therapeutic Effects/Uses: To induce/augment labor contractions; to treat uterine atony; milk letdown (intranasal spray)

Mode of Action: Action of myofibrils to stimulate letdown of milk and promote uterine contractions.

Evaluation

Side Effects

Maternal effects with IV use only:
  Hypotension, hypertension, nausea, vomiting, constipation, decreased uterine blood flow, rash, anorexia

Adverse Reactions

Seizures, water intoxication
Life-threatening: Intracranial hemorrhage, cardiac dysrhythmias asphyxia; fetus: jaundice, hypoxia

KEY: A: adult; IV: intraveneous; IM: intramuscular; PO: by mouth; PB: protein binding; t½: half-life; UK: unknown.

TABLE 42–15 Oxytocic Drugs Commonly Used to Enhance Uterine Motility

Drug	Dosage	Uses and Considerations
Oxytocin (Pitocin, Syntocinon)	See Prototype Drug Chart (Fig. 42–3)	
Ergonovine maleate (Ergotrate)	PO: 0.2–0.4 mg (1–2 tablets) q 6–12 h over 48 h IM: 0.2 mg q 2–4 h; maximum 5 doses IV: 0.2 mg (only for severe bleeding) over 1 min while BP and uterine contractions are monitored	Oxytocic; ergot alkaloid; directly stimulates vascular smooth muscle to vasoconstrict peripheral and cerebral vessels Prevention and treatment of postpartum or postabortion hemorrhage caused by uterine atony or subinvolution IV only for true emergencies. Limit use in clients with coronary artery disease, hypertension, PIH; contraindicated before delivery of placenta. *Pregnancy risk factor: X* IV: Immediate onset, 45 min duration IM: 2–5 min onset, 3 h duration PO: 6–15 min onset, 3 h duration $t^{1/2}$: 2 h Use with caution in sepsis, hepatic or renal impairment Adverse reactions: diaphoresis, palpitations, transient chest pain, thrombophlebitis, seizures, cerebrovascular accidents, dizziness, headache, nausea, vomiting, tinnitus, dyspnea Metabolized in liver; excreted in urine Oxytocic
Methylergonovine maleate (Methergine)	PO: 0.2–0.4 mg, q 6–12 h; maximum of 1 wk IM: 0.2 mg after delivery of anterior shoulder (if full obstetric supervision), after delivery of placenta, or post partum; repeat q 2–4 h; oral doses may follow parenteral IV: Same as for IM; but slowly over 1 min with careful monitoring of BP	Prevention and treatment of postpartum hemorrhage; subinvolution and postabortion hemorrhage *Pregnancy risk factor: C* IV: Immediate onset, 45 min duration IM: 2–5 min onset; 3 h duration PO: 5–25 min onset; 3 h duration $t^{1/2}$: (biphasic): Initial: 1–5 min; terminal: 30 min–2 h Metabolized in liver; eliminated in urine Adverse reactions: transient hypertension, diaphoresis, palpitations, dizziness, headache, nausea, vomiting, tinnitus, transient chest pain, dyspnea. Exhibits similar smooth muscle action to ergotamine but affects primarily smooth muscle, producing *sustained* contractions, and thus shortens the 3rd stage of labor. Not administered IV routinely due to possibility of sudden hypertensive and cerebrovascular accidents; limit use with clients with hypertension (especially IV); contraindicated with maternal sepsis, labor induction, threatened spontaneous abortion; do not use with vasopressors, other ergot alkaloids, or vasoconstrictors; appears in breast milk but interference with breast feeding is less than with ergonovine

KEY: *BP: blood pressure; IM: intramuscular; IV: intravenous; PIH: pregnancy-induced hypertension; PO: by mouth; $t^{1/2}$: half-life.*

hypoxia and rupture of the uterus. Following delivery, however, long-sustained contractions are extremely useful for prevention or control of postpartum hemorrhage and promotion of uterine involution. If given too soon after delivery, these drugs can cause the placenta to become trapped inside the uterus.

The two most commonly used ergot derivatives in obstetrics are ergonovine maleate (Ergotrate) and methylergonovine maleate (Methergine). These preparations can be given intramuscularly, PO, or intravenously (IV administration is recommended only for true hemorrhagic emergencies). Transient elevations in BP can occur, particularly after IV infusion of either drug, and clients with pregnancy-related hypertension or peripheral vascular dis-

eases should not receive these products. Table 42–15 presents the most commonly used oxytocic drugs to enhance uterine motility.

Side Effects and Adverse Reactions

Side effects include uterine cramping, nausea and vomiting (mostly after IV dose), dizziness, hypertension (particularly with IV administration), sweating, tinnitus, chest pain, dyspnea, itching, and sudden severe headache. Signs of ergot toxicity (**ergotism**) include pain in arms, legs, and lower back, numbness, cold hands and feet, muscular weakness, diarrhea, hallucinations, seizures, and blood hypercoagulability.

NURSING PROCESS: ENHANCEMENT OF UTERINE MOTILITY: Oxytocins

ASSESSMENT

For induction or augmentation of labor:

- Collect accurate baseline data before beginning infusion, including maternal pulse and blood pressure, uterine activity, and fetal heart rate (FHR).
- Record assessment results on FHR monitor graph paper in addition to other agency records.

POTENTIAL NURSING DIAGNOSIS

- Knowledge deficit

PLANNING

- Oxytocin will enhance uterine contractions without adverse effects.
- Client's vital signs (VS) will be within acceptable ranges during the therapy.

NURSING INTERVENTIONS

- Have magnesium sulfate and/or other tocolytic agents and oxygen readily available in case hypertonicity occurs.

- Monitor I & O every 2 h. Fluids should not exceed 1000 mL/8 h.
- Monitor maternal pulse and blood pressure, uterine activity, and FHR before increasing oxytocin infusion.
- Maintain the client in the lateral recumbent position or sitting to promote placental infusion.
- Be alert for signs of uterine rupture (very infrequent), which include sudden increased pain, loss of contractions and decreased or absent FHR, hemorrhage, and rapidly developing hypovolemic shock.

CLIENT TEACHING

- Explain to the client that the drug is given intravenously to adjust dosage in response to contraction pattern.
- For milk letdown: Teach client timing and method of nasal administration.

EVALUATION

- Evaluate the effectiveness of the drug. Labor progresses.
- Continue monitoring VS. Report changes in VS or vaginal bleeding.

NURSING PROCESS: OTHER OXYTOCICS

ASSESSMENT

Ergonovine and Methylergonovine
- Assess lochia and status of uterus before giving ergonovine or methylergonovine.
- Recognize that these two drugs have a vasoconstrictive effect on blood vessels, which may cause hypertension. Ergonovine is more vasoconstrictive than methylergonovine.
- Recognize that the client may have increased risk of thrombosis if on bedrest during the postpartum period.

NURSING INTERVENTIONS

Ergonovine and Methylergonovine
- Monitor the client's BP before and during drug administration consistent with agency protocol, but every 15 min if the client has a known vascular disorder (hypotension, hypertension).

- Monitor status of the uterus (height, tone) before giving.
- Assess client's lochial discharge for color, odor, and amount before giving.
- Protect drugs from light exposure.
- Observe for side effects or symptoms of ergot toxicity (ergotism). Notify physician if systolic BP increases by 25 mmHg or diastolic BP by 20 mmHg over baseline.

CLIENT TEACHING

Ergonovine and Methylergonovine
- Explain to the client that she may feel uterine cramps after receiving the drug but may receive analgesics for pain.

Safety
- Advise the client to avoid smoking. Nicotine increases the vasoconstrictive properties of these drugs.

Side Effects

- If the client is breast feeding, explain that the drug lowers serum prolactin levels with potential to inhibit postpartum lactation; note that ergonovine is more likely to do so than methylergonovine.

EVALUATION

- Evaluate the effectiveness of the drug.
- Continue monitoring vital signs. Report changes in vital signs or vaginal bleeding.

■ CASE STUDY
Induction/Augmentation of Labor

Tanya, a pregnant client (para 0, gravida 3), discovers her health care provider plans to induce her labor since she is at 42 weeks' gestation at this prenatal visit and experiencing pregnancy-induced hypertension. Tanya tells the nurse, "He said, if necessary, he may first use some kind of gel in my cervix followed by medicine in an IV in my arm." She further states, "Can you help me understand all this?"

1. What objective tool (scoring system) will be used to predict the extent to which Tanya's cervix is "ripe" and therefore favorable for successful induction?

If Tanya's health care provider orders Prepadil Gel be used in her cervix, the nurse will need to be prepared to address the following aspects of the therapy for Tanya:

2. Why is the gel being used (what is to be accomplished)?
3. Who will administer the gel?
4. How often will the gel be administered?
5. How long after the last dose of gel before the intravenous oxytocic medication can be started to induce labor?
6. Why is there a period of waiting prior to starting the oxytocic?

It is now 16 hours since Tanya first had the gel inserted. Answering Tanya's call light, the nurse finds her in the bathroom upset that she seems to be feeling nauseous, occasionally vomiting a little bit of stomach fluid, and complaining that her stool seems "really watery." "Is something wrong?" Tanya wails.

7. Analysis of the data about Tanya's symptoms would support what conclusion about what is occurring?
8. Explain what nursing actions might be taken to support her and address the issue?
9. When Tanya returns to her bed and is reattached to the external fetal monitor, what electronic and physical data should the nurse collect and record?

In one-half hour it will be time for the third dose of gel for Tanya.

10. According to the protocol, what specific activities will need to take place in preparation for Tanya, for the fetus, in preparation of the dose, and for the health care provider?

Twenty-four hours have elapsed since Tanya had her first gel instillation; it has been 6 hours since her last insertion. A vaginal examination is completed. Tanya's cervix is soft and 50% effaced and dilated 3 cm, and the baby is at −3 station. Contractions are 5 minutes apart and of slight intensity. The health care provider elects to begin an oxytocin infusion.

11. Tanya asks how a medicine "running into my arm is able to make my uterus contract?" How would you explain the mode of action of oxytocin to Tanya?
12. What are the purpose and value of running the oxytocin infusion through a secondary line attached as a "piggyback" to the primary line? At which port along the primary line is the piggyback inserted? Why at this location rather than higher up?
13. Why is it necessary to administer oxytocin via an infusion pump?
14. What actions in regard to the IV equipment setup should be taken as safety measures prior to starting the oxytocin drip?
15. What drug(s) would you want nearby in the event of an emergency with the oxytocin?
16. What information would you record on the fetal monitoring strip? Why is the strip an important source of documented data?
17. A young nurse being oriented stops to chat with you while you are setting up the oxytocin infusion. She asks you what criteria you will use to know when success has occurred and allow you to slow the rate of infusion and stop it. These criteria are:

    Contractions _____ min apart; _____ intense
    Cervix _____ cm dilated

18. Considering that you know that Tanya has a history of active pregnancy-induced hypertension, explain why vigilance for uterine hyperstimulation during the oxytocin infusion is es-

sential for the fetus. How are the stressors for the fetus in utero similar in both instances?

19. Should uterine hyperstimulation occur, explain how you would handle the situation to protect mother and baby. Address the following:

Position Tanya _____

      Rationale _____

IV Fluids _____

      Rationale _____

Oxygen _____

      Rationale _____

20. Tanya asks when she might be eligible to receive a continuous epidural. She is now 3 cm dilated. As the nurse, you could correctly state that: Prior to _____ cm, there is risk of arresting the first stage of labor.

STUDY QUESTIONS

1. What is the main reason drug use is discouraged during pregnancy and breast feeding?

2. What are the nursing responsibilities associated with the administration of the drugs used during tocolysis?

3. What are two drugs used to protect and promote respiratory function for the neonate experiencing premature labor? What is the expected effect of each?

4. A client who initially planned to have "natural childbirth with nothing for pain" has changed her mind. What information will she need about analgesics used in labor?

5. What are potential complications of an oxytocin infusion to induce labor?

6. What are the two most commonly used drugs in the treatment of pregnancy-induced hypertension?

7. What are five nursing interventions associated with oxytocin induction or augmentation?

Chapter 43

Drugs Associated with the Postpartum and the Newborn

Jane Purnell Taylor

OUTLINE

Objectives
Terms
Introduction
Drugs Used During the Postpartum Period
    Pain Relief for Uterine Contractions
    Pain Relief for Perineal Wounds and Hemorrhoids
        Nursing Process

Lactation Suppression
Promotion of Bowel Function
    Nursing Process
Immunizations
    Rh_0 (D) Immune Globulin
        Nursing Process
    Rubella Vaccine
        Nursing Process
Drugs Administered to the Newborn Immediately After Delivery

Side Effects and Adverse Reactions
Nursing Process
Immunization During the Newborn Period Prior to Discharge
    Nursing Process
Case Study
Study Questions

OBJECTIVES

Identify drugs commonly administered during the postpartum period and explain their uses.

Identify the purpose of the drugs administered to the newborn immediately after delivery.

Describe the nursing process, including client teaching, related to drugs used during the postpartum period and for the newborn immediately after delivery.

TERMS

absorption
amide-type anesthetics
anoderm
anorectal
antiflatulent
contact dermatitis
congenital rubella syndrome
denuded
dependence
engorgement

episiotomy
folliculitis
hydrolyzed
lactation
lyophilized
necrosis
occlusive
percutaneous
perineal
permeability

prolactin
protrusion
puerperium
recombinant
Rh_0 (D) immune globulin
Rh sensitization
sensitization
seroconvert
titer
urticaria

INTRODUCTION

This chapter focuses on the pharmacologic considerations for both mother and infant after delivery. Nonpharmacologic measures and pharmacologic agents related to the relief of common discomforts during the postpartum period are described. In addition, drugs commonly administered to newborns immediately after delivery are included.

DRUGS USED DURING THE POSTPARTUM PERIOD

During the **puerperium** (the period from delivery of the baby and the placenta until 6 weeks postpartum), the maternal body physically recovers from antepartal and intrapartal stressors and returns to its prepregnant state.

Pharmacologic and nonpharmacologic measures commonly employed during the postpartum period can have five main purposes: (1) prevention of uterine atony and postpartum hemorrhage (discussed in Chapter 42; (2) pain relief (from uterine contractions, perineal wounds, and hemorrhoids); (3) enhancement or suppression of lactation; (4) promotion of bowel function; and (5) enhancement of immunity.

Table 43–1 lists the nonpharmacologic measures commonly used during the postpartum period. As during pregnancy, whenever possible nonpharmacologic measures are preferred to the use of drugs or are used in conjunction with drugs.

Postpartum nursing care ideally occurs as a client-caregiver partnership. In an effort to enhance health and wellness, the nurse collaborates with the client to strengthen the new mother's self-confidence and ability to handle her own health challenges. One major challenge is management of postdelivery discomfort(s). An emerging trend is for postpartum mothers to be provided self-medication administration packets that contain appropriate medications (for either vaginal- or cesarean-delivered clients) with printed instructions for self-directed use in the hospital and later at home. Thus, the "well client" admitted to the hospital to deliver her baby and recover during a limited time period is not placed in a dependent "sick-role" position; instead, the mother uses her supplied medications (within instructional guidelines) when she determines the need for pain management. The nurse's role in this system is fourfold: (1) to provide astute physical and pain assessment with the client to determine healing progress within a standard and effectiveness of self-administered medications; (2) to directly administer medications for

TABLE 43–1 Nonpharmacologic Measures for Common Postpartum Needs

Indication	Measure
	Pain relief
Uterine contractions	Position client on abdomen with pillow under abdomen periodically for 3–4 d
	Distraction, breathing techniques, therapeutic touch, relaxation, guided imagery, ambulation
	Do not apply heat to abdomen due to risk of uterine relaxation and increased bleeding
Perineal wound due to episiotomy or laceration	Apply ice for 6–8 h after delivery covered in thin, absorbent material (to protect tissue, collect lochial flow, and keep area cold) backed by peripad
	Position on side as much as possible with pillow between legs
	Early and frequent ambulation
	Perineal exercises
	Warm sitz bath 12–24 h after delivery 3–4 × d for approximately 20 min
	Cleanse area front to back using perispray squeeze bottle, cleansing shower, or Surgi-Gator
	Instruct client to squeeze buttocks together before sitting and to sit tall and flat, not rolled back onto coccyx
	Perineal heat lamp with 40-watt or less bulb approximately 18 inches from perineal area
	Do not use tampons, douche, or feminine hygiene sprays
	No intercourse until after bleeding has stopped and preferably when client has been seen first by health care provider
Hemorrhoids	As above, plus most particularly: Ice
	Sims' position in bed to help increase venous return
	Warm, moist heat; sitz bath

those clients unable to take their own due to nursing assessment of cognitive, psychomotor, or physiological deficits; (3) to directly administer narcotic analgesics (as prescribed) when pain control by nonnarcotic products is determined ineffective due to breakthrough pain episodes; and (4) to distribute the correct self-administration packet to each client based on allergy/sensitivity history to contained products and to obtain signed consent forms for client participation.

Analysis of data collected from facilities employing self-medication administration programs indicates that clients use fewer narcotics overall and report satisfaction with products included in the packets for promoting comfort. Table 43–2 presents contents of a typical self-medication packet.

TABLE 43–2 Prototype Self-Medication Administration Packet Contents

Vaginal Delivery
Witch hazel pads (Tucks)
Perineal spray (Dermoplast; Americaine)
Acetaminophen 500 mg or ibuprofen 200 mg
Docusate with casanthranol tablets

Cesarean Delivery
Acetaminophen 500 mg or ibuprofen 200 mg
Docusate with casanthranol tablets
Simethicone chewable tablets

TABLE 43–3 Commonly Used Postpartum Systemic Analgesics

Acetaminophen (Tylenol)
Propoxyphene (Darvon)
Ibuprofen (Motrin)
Acetaminophen with codeine (Tylenol with codeine)
Codeine sulfate
Meperidine (Demerol)
Morphine sulfate (Pectoral)
Oxycodone hydrochloride (Percocet)

PAIN RELIEF FOR UTERINE CONTRACTIONS

"Afterbirth pains" occur during the first few days postpartum when uterine tissue experiences ischemia during contractions. Table 43–3 presents a list of systemic analgesics commonly used during the postpartum period. Narcotic agents are generally reserved for more severe pain such as that experienced by the client after cesarean birth or tubal ligation. The specific drugs are described in Chapter 14.

TABLE 43–4 Drugs Used for Pain Relief from Perineal Wounds and Hemorrhoids

Agent	Dosage	Uses and Considerations
Perineal Wounds (episiotomy or laceration) Benzocaine (Americaine, Dermoplast OTC)	Spray liberally t.i.d. or q.i.d. 6–12 inches from perineum following perineal cleansing Supplied as aerosol; benzocaine 20%	Local anesthetic inhibits impulses from sensory nerves as a result of alteration of cell membrane permeability to ions. Contraindicated in secondary bacterial infection of tissue and known hypersensitivity. 1-min peak effect, 30–60 min duration. Hydrolyzed in the plasma and (to lesser extent) in the liver by cholinesterase; eliminated as metabolites in urine. Well absorbed from mucous membranes and traumatized skin; apply 6–12 inches from affected area (side-lying with upper leg lifted helpful)
Witch hazel pads (Tucks [50% witch hazel with glycerine, water, and methylparaben])	Apply premoistened pads t.i.d. or q.i.d. to wound site	Precipitates protein, causing tissue to contract. May be chilled on ice in original container for additional comfort. If liquid, pour over ice and dip absorbent pads into solution; change when diluted. Supplied 40 pads per container. Medical intervention should be sought if rectal bleeding is present. Side effect: local irritation (discontinue use)
Hemorrhoids Hydrocortisone acetate 10 mg (Anusol HC, Anusol Ointment [Promoxine HCl 1%, mineral oil 46.7%, zinc oxide 12.5%])	One suppository b.i.d. for 3–6 d	Relieves pain and itching from irritated anorectal tissue. Contains hydrocortisone acetate. Acts as an antiinflammatory agent. Available without hydrocortisone. Contraindicated with hypersensitivity. If secondary infection in tissue, discontinue. Not known if excreted in breast milk; use cautiously. *Pregnancy category:* C. If anorectal symptoms do not improve in 7 d or if bleeding, protrusion, or seepage occurs, inform health care provider. Wear gloves. Onset: UK; peak: UK; duration: UK
Hydrocortisone acetate 1% and promazine HCl 1% topical aerosol (Proctofoam-HC)	1 applicator transferred to a 2 × 2 pad and placed against rectum inside peripad b.i.d. or t.i.d. and after bowel movements	Topical corticosteroid aerosol foam with same action and considerations as above. Also available in nonsteroidal preparation. Shake foam aerosol before use. Extent of percutaneous absorption of topical corticosteroids is determined by vehicle integrity of epidermal barrier and use of occlusive dressings (not known if any quantity detectable in breast milk). Side effects: burning, itching, irritation, dryness, infrequent folliculitis reactions. Onset: UK; peak: UK; duration: UK
Dibucaine ointment, USP 1% (Nupercaine)	Apply as above t.i.d. or q.i.d., using no more than 1 tube in 24 h	Local anesthetic ointment containing dibucaine 1%. Action same as benzocaine. Do not use if rectal bleeding is present. *Pregnancy category:* C. Onset: within 15 min; peak: UK; duration: 2–4 h. Do not use near the eyes or over denuded surfaces or blistered areas. Side effects: burning, tenderness, irritation, inflammation, contact dermatitis, urticaria, cutaneous lesions, edema. Do not use if known hypersensitivity to amide-type anesthetics

KEY: UK: unknown.

Because some systemic analgesics (codeine, meperidine, and oxycodone) can cause decreased alertness, it is important that the nurse observe the client when she is caring for her newborn, to ensure safety. Clients who receive codeine sulfate or ibuprofen need to be assessed for bowel function and GI irritation, respectively. Clients who receive codeine or morphine need evaluation for respiratory status.

PAIN RELIEF FOR PERINEAL WOUNDS AND HEMORRHOIDS

The process of birth is a stressor on the perineal soft tissue. The tissue may become bruised and/or edematous. The tissue may be further stressed, with the potential for bruising, edema, and pain if episiotomy or laceration occurred as an outcome of the delivery. Clients may also have developed hem-

orrhoids during pregnancy, which may be exacerbated as a result of pushing during the labor process. Comfort measures and selected topical agents may be helpful.

Drugs used for relief of pain from perineal wounds and hemorrhoids are presented in Table 43–4.

Side Effects and Adverse Reactions

The most commonly reported side effects of local or topical agents ("caine" family drugs and witch hazel) include burning, stinging, tenderness, swelling, rash, tissue irritation, sloughing, and tissue necrosis. The most commonly reported side effects of hydrocortisone local or topical drugs include burning, itching, irritation, dryness, folliculitis, allergic contact dermatitis, and secondary infection. These side effects are more likely to be observed if occlusive dressings are used.

NURSING PROCESS: PAIN RELIEF FROM PERINEAL WOUNDS AND HEMORRHOIDS

ASSESSMENT

- Assess the perineal area for wounds and hemorrhoids (size, color, location, pain scale).
- Check the expiration dates on topical spray cans, bottles, and ointment tubes.
- Assess for presence of infection in perineal site in order to prevent use of benzocaine on perineal tissue postpartum.

POTENTIAL NURSING DIAGNOSES

- Alteration in comfort: pain related to episiotomy or hemorrhoids
- Knowledge deficit related to cause of discomfort and how long client may expect pain to last when products are used as directed

PLANNING

- Client's perineal discomfort will be alleviated by use of topical sprays, compresses, and ointment.
- Client will not experience side effects.

NURSING INTERVENTIONS

- Do not use benzocaine spray when infections are present.
- Shake benzocaine spray can. Administer 6 to 12 inches from perineum with client lying on her side with top leg up and forward to provide maximum exposure.

- Use witch hazel compresses (Tucks and/or witch hazel solution) with an ice pack and a peripad to provide cold in addition to the active agent.
- Store Anusol HC suppositories below 86°F, but protect from freezing. Use gloves for administration. Progress client to nonhydrocortisone preparation as quickly as possible based on assessment if breast feeding.
- Check for lot numbers and expiration date.
- Use of Proctoloam HC needs to be explained carefully to the client because directions refer to placing agent inside the anus and this is not generally done with OB clients who may have extensive perineal wounds extending into the anus.

CLIENT TEACHING

Perineal Wounds: Topical Spray Containing Benzocaine
General
- Explain expected effects.
- Tell the client that the drug is not for prolonged use (no more than 7 days) or application to a large area.
- Advise the client with bleeding hemorrhoids to use the drug carefully and to keep her health care provider informed.

Skill
- Apply three to four times daily or as directed.
- Apply without touching sensitive area.

- Hold can 6 to 12 inches from affected area; side-lying in bed with upper leg lifted and spraying from behind is helpful for many clients.

Safety
- Advise the client to avoid contact with eyes.
- Instruct the client not to apply anesthetic and then use a perineal heat lamp, because this could cause tissue burns.
- If condition worsens or symptoms occur again within a few days, notify the health care provider and discontinue use until directed.
- Keep out of reach of visiting children in postpartum unit and later at home. Contact poison control immediately if ingested.
- Do not store above 120°F.
- Do not puncture or incinerate can when disposing of empty can.

Witch Hazel Compresses
General
- Explain expected effects of product (relief of itching, burning, irritation in episiotomy site or hemorrhoid with cooling, soothing sensation).
- Notify health care provider if condition worsens or does not improve within 7 days.

Skill
- If using liquid witch hazel, client may pour over chipped ice and place soft, clean absorbent squares in solution; fold and place moist square (squeezing square very slightly to eliminate excess [not all] moisture) against episiotomy/hemorrhoids.
- If using commercial medicated pads, entire container may be placed on ice.
- Instruct the client not to touch the surface of the pad that will be placed next to the perineal wound.
- Tell the client when to change the compress and show how to place an ice bag and peripad over the compress.

Safety
- Do not insert medicated pads into the rectum.
- Keep product away from children.
- Do not use if rectal bleeding is present (requires medical intervention).

Side Effects
- Discontinue use if local irritation occurs.

Hemorrhoids: Anusol Ointment and Anusol Suppositories (HC and Plain)
General
- Explain expected effects of product use (relief of

burning, itching, discomfort from irritated anorectal tissues with soothing, lubricating, coating action of mucous membranes).
- Explain that surface analgesia lasts for several hours after use.
- Tell the client to store below 86°F so suppositories do not melt. Do not freeze.

Skill
- Apply externally in postpartum period (ointment); lower portion of anal canal (suppositories) (products usually not inserted rectally with a 3- or 4-degree type episiotomy).
- Express small quantity *ointment* into 2 × 2 gauze square and place against swollen anorectal tissue (approximately five times per day) inside peripad.
- If *suppository* form is ordered, tell client to keep refrigerated but not to freeze; remove wrapper before inserting in rectum (hold suppository upright and peel evenly down sides); do not hold suppository for prolonged period (it will melt); if the suppository softens before use, hold in foil wrapper under cold water for 2 to 3 min.

Safety
- Tell the client to avoid contact with eyes.
- Ascertain any client hypersensitivity to any of the components of the ointment (i.e., promazine HCl 1%, mineral oil 46.7%, zinc oxide 12.5%, etc.).

Side Effects
- Ointment may cause burning sensation occasionally in some clients—especially if anoderm is *not* intact.
- Although rare, some persons may develop sensitivity/allergic reactions to ingredients. Discontinue use if this occurs.
- If redness, irritation, swelling, or pain develops or increases, discontinue use and consult health care provider; also notify health care provider if bleeding occurs.

Promazine and Hydrocortisone (Proctofoam HC) and Promazine Hydrochloride (Proctofoam—OTC)
General
- Explain expected effects of product use.
- Explain that promazine HCl is not chemically related to "caine" type local anesthetics and there is a decreased chance of cross-sensitivity reactions in clients allergic to other local anesthetics.

Skill
- Tell client that product is for anal or perianal use only. In postpartum clients, product is not inserted into rectum.

- Shake foam aerosol vigorously before use.
- Do not insert any part of aerosol container into anus.
- Tell client to hold the aerosol can upright to fill applicator and to have the plunger fully extended prior to filling.
- Express contents of applicator onto a 2 × 2 gauze pad and place against rectum inside peripad b.i.d. or t.i.d. and after bowel movement.
- Tell the client to take the applicator apart after each use and wash with warm water.

Safety
- Keep aerosol container away from visiting children in postpartum unit and later at home.
- Store below 120°F.
- Do not puncture or burn aerosol container.

Side Effects
- Tell client it is not known whether topical administration of corticosteroids could result in sufficient systemic absorption to produce detectable quantities in breast milk.
- Burning, itching, irritation, dryness, folliculitis reactions, especially if occlusive dressings are used, may occur as local adverse reactions *infrequently.*

Dibucaine Ointment 1% (Nupercainal Ointment)
General
- Explain that the ointment is poorly absorbed through intact skin but that it is well absorbed through mucous membrane and excoriated skin.
- Explain that effects should begin to be perceived within 15 min and last for 2 to 4 h.

Skill
- Instruct the client not to place the applicator in the rectum. Instead place medication from the applicator on a tissue or 2 × 2 pad and place against the anus.

Safety
- Stress not using product near the eyes, over denuded surface or blistered areas, or if there is rectal bleeding.
- Tell the client not to use more than 1 tube (30 g size) in 24 h.
- Keep product out of the reach of children.

Side Effects
- Ask if client has any known hypersensitivity to amide-type anesthetics; if so, product is contraindicated.
- Tell client local effects may include burning, tenderness, irritation, inflammation, and contact dermatitis; client should inform her health care provider if these should occur.
- Other adverse effects may include edema, cutaneous lesions, and/or urticaria.

EVALUATION

- Evaluate pain for tolerable level using pain scale following use of product(s).
- Evaluate content of client communications for need for additional pain relief.
- Reevaluate characteristics of perineal/anal tissues for integrity and healing progress within accepted standard; also evaluate for lack of side effects.

LACTATION SUPPRESSION

In Table 43–1, nonpharmacologic measures for **lactation** (milk formation and secretion) suppression were presented. Until very recently, lactation was commonly controlled through drug therapy by use of one of three agents: chlorotrianisene (TACE), Deladumone OB (combination of estrogen plus androgen in the form of estradiol valerate and testosterone enanthate), or bromocriptine mesylate (Parlodel). The first two agents are estrogenic substances that suppress lactation through localized inhibitory effects on the alveolar breast cells responsible for milk secretion. The third agent, a dopamine receptor agonist, is nonhormonal and acts at a systemic level on the anterior pituitary gland to inhibit the secretion of **prolactin,** which causes the milk glands to produce milk. High levels are necessary to initiate lactation. Estrogenic substances are much less popular today than in the past because of the increased incidence of thrombophlebitis associated with the dosage needed to suppress lactation, as well as concerns about potential carcinogenic effects. In August 1994, the Food and Drug Administration (FDA) officially withdrew its support for the use of bromocriptine as a lactation suppressant because of severe hypertension secondary to vasospasm in some clients, ineffectiveness of the drug in some, and a rebound effect (lactation occurrence) in some. The drug is still approved for other medical conditions.

PROMOTION OF BOWEL FUNCTION

Constipation is common during the postpartum period because of the residual effects of progesterone on smooth muscle coupled with decreased peristalsis and relaxation of the abdominal muscles. Nonpharmacologic measures (high-fiber foods, early ambulation, at least 64 oz of fluids a day, prompt response to the defecation urge) are generally instituted after delivery.

Pharmacologic measures include the use of stool softeners, laxative stimulants, and, for the postcesarean client, antiflatulents. Table 43–5 presents examples of agents used to promote bowel function during the postpartum period. (See Chapter 36 for additional information about these drug groups.)

Side Effects and Adverse Reactions

The following side effects have been reported: *docusate sodium*: bitter taste, throat irritation, rash; *casanthranol and docusate sodium*: nausea, abdominal cramping, diarrhea, and rash; *bisacodyl suppositories*: proctitis and inflammation; *magnesium hydroxide*: abdominal cramps and nausea; *senna*: nausea, vomiting, diarrhea, abdominal cramps, can also result in diarrhea in breast-fed infants; *mineral oil*: nausea, vomiting, diarrhea, abdominal cramps, also lipid pneumonitis (if aspirated).

TABLE 43–5 Drugs Used to Promote Postpartum Bowel Function

Drug	Dosage	Uses and Considerations
Docusate sodium (Colace) 50 mg or 100 mg capsule Docusate calcium (Surfak) 240 mg capsule	50–200 mg PO daily usually h.s.; 50–400 mg PO daily in 1–4 divided doses	Reduces surface tension of the oil-water interface of the stool, resulting in enhanced incorporation of water and fat, allowing for stool softening. PB: NA; onset: 12–72 h; t½: NA. Docusate salts are interchangeable (amount of Na, Ca, or K per dosage is clinically insignificant). *Pregnancy category*: C. Do not use concomitantly with mineral oil. Contraindicated if intestinal obstruction, acute abdominal pain, nausea, or vomiting present. Do not use >1 wk. Prolonged, frequent, or excessive use may cause bowel dependence or electrolyte imbalance. Side effects: rash. Compatible with breast feeding
Casanthranol with docusate sodium (Peri-Colace); docusate sodium, 100 mg; casanthranol, 30 mg	1–2 capsules PO, usually h.s.	Mild stimulant laxative. Do not use if abdominal pain, nausea, or vomiting present. Effect on stool in 8–12 h, but may require up to 24 h. *Pregnancy category*: C. Should be taken with full glass of water. Adverse reactions: rash, abdominal cramping, diarrhea, nausea. Compatible with breast feeding. PB: NA; t½: NA
Docusate potassium (Dialose)	1 capsule PO, daily/b.i.d.	Stool softener. Sodium free. *Pregnancy category*: C. Onset 12–72 h. See docusate sodium for additional information.
Casanthranol with docusate potassium (Dialose Plus)	1 capsule PO, b.i.d.	Mild stimulant laxation. Sodium. *Pregnancy category*: C. Onset 8–12 h, but may require up to 24 h. See casanthranol with docusate sodium for additional information
Bisacodyl USP (Dulcolax) (suppository 10 mg or tablet 5 mg)	2–3 tablets PO or 1 suppository	Stimulant laxative. Irritates smooth muscle of the intestine, possibly the colon and intramural plexus; alters water and electrolyte secretion, increasing intestinal fluid and producing laxative effect. Onset: 6–10 h PO; 15 min–1 h rectally. Absorption: <5% absorbed systemically following oral or rectal form. Metabolized in the liver to conjugated metabolites; eliminated in breast milk, bile, and urine. Do not crush tablets (enteric coated). Do not administer within 1 h of milk or antacid because enteric coating may dissolve, resulting in abdominal cramping and vomiting. Side effects: abdominal cramps, nausea, vomiting, rectal burning, electrolyte and fluid acidosis or alkalosis, hypocalcemia. *Pregnancy category*: C
Magnesium hydroxide (Milk of Magnesia)	15–60 mL PO h.s.	Laxative. Acts by increasing and retaining water in intestinal lumen, causing distention that stimulates peristalsis and bowel elimination. Poses risk to client with renal failure because 15%–30% of magnesium is systemically absorbed. Use with caution in patients with impaired renal function because hypermagnesemia and toxicity may occur due to decreased renal clearance of absorbed magnesium. *Pregnancy category*: B. Contraindicated in clients with colostomy, ileostomy, abdominal pain, nausea, vomiting, fecal impaction, renal failure. Drug interactions may occur with tetracyclines, digoxin, indomethacin, or iron salts, isoniazid. Milk of Magnesia concentrate is 3 × as potent as regular-strength product. Side effects: abdominal cramps, nausea. Other adverse reactions include hypotension, hypermagnesemia, muscle weakness, and respiratory depression. Onset: 4–8 h. Excreted by kidneys (absorbed portion); unabsorbed portion excreted in feces
Magnesium hydroxide with mineral oil (Haley's M-O)	15–30 mL PO h.s.	Mild saline laxative. Acts by drawing H_2O into gut, increasing intraluminal pressure and intestinal motility. Onset: 0.5–6 h. *Pregnancy category*: B. Equivalent to magnesium hydroxide

TABLE 43–5 Drugs Used to Promote Postpartum Bowel Function (*Continued*)

Drug	Dosage	Uses and Considerations
Mineral oil (Agoral)	15–45 mL PO once daily or in divided doses	Lubricant laxative eases passages of stool by decreasing water absorption and lubricating the intestine. *Pregnancy category:* C. Onset: 6–8 h; t½: NA; PB: NA; peak: UK; duration: UK. May impair absorption of fat-soluble vitamins (A, D, E, K), oral contraceptives, coumarin, sulfonamides. Generally recommend avoidance of bedtime doses due to risk of aspiration (lipid pneumonitis). Contraindicated in clients with ileostomy, colostomy, appendicitis, ulcerative colitis, diverticulitis. Best administered on an empty stomach. Do not give with food or meals because of risk of aspiration and decreased fat-soluble vitamin absorption. Side effects: nausea, vomiting, diarrhea, abdominal cramps
Senna (Senokot)	10–15 mL syrup h.s.; 2–4 tablets PO b.i.d.	Stimulant laxative. Acts by local irritant effect on colon to promote peristalsis and bowel evacuation. Also increases moisture content of stool by accumulating fluids in intestine. Contraindicated in clients with fluid and electrolyte disturbances, abdominal pain, nausea and vomiting. Excreted in breast milk. *Pregnancy category:* C. Onset: 6–24 h; metabolized in the liver; eliminated in the feces (viable) and in urine. t½: NA. Drug interactions may occur with monoamine oxidase (MAO) inhibitors, disulfiram, metronidazole, procarbazine. May discolor urine or feces; liquid syrups contain 7% alcohol. May create laxative dependence and loss of bowel function with prolonged use
Simethicone (Mylicon) (chewable tablets 40 mg, 80 mg)	1 tablet q.i.d. p.c. and h.s. up to 6 × d as needed	Antiflatulent. Acts by dispersing and preventing formation of mucus-surrounded gas pockets in GI tract; changes surface tension of gas bubbles and allows them to coalesce, making them easier to eliminate as belching and rectal flatus. *Pregnancy category:* C. Onset: UK; t½: UK. Excreted unchanged in the feces. May interfere with results of guaiac tests of gastric aspirates; must be chewed thoroughly before swallowing; suggest client drink a full glass of water after tablets are chewed. Double doses should not be taken to make up for missed doses. No known side effects; store below 40°C (104°F) in well-closed container

KEY: *NA: not applicable; PB: protein-binding; t½: half-life; UK: unknown.*

NURSING PROCESS: LAXATIVES

ASSESSMENT

- Note time of delivery, predelivery food intake, predelivery bowel emptying measures used (if any).
- Obtain history of bowel problems.
- Assess the client for bowel sounds in all four quadrants (particularly postcesarean section delivery) and abdominal distention.

POTENTIAL NURSING DIAGNOSES

- Potential for altered bowel elimination: high risk for constipation related to perineal discomfort and decreased peristalsis
- Fear of discomfort at time of first postdelivery bowel movement (especially if extensive episiotomy or hemorrhoids present)

PLANNING

- Client will have a bowel movement by 2 to 4 days postpartum.
- Client will resume normal prepregnancy bowel elimination pattern within 6 weeks.

NURSING INTERVENTIONS

Docusate Sodium and Casanthranol with Docusate Sodium; Docusate Potassium and Casanthranol with Docusate Potassium

- Store at room temperature.
- If a liquid preparation is ordered, give with milk or fruit juice to mask bitter taste.
- Assess client for any history of laxative dependence.
- Drug interaction may occur with mineral oil, phenolphthalein, aspirin.

Bisacodyl USP

- Store tablets and suppositories below 77°F and avoid excess humidity.
- Do not crush tablets.
- Do not administer within 1 h of milk or antacid because enteric coating may dissolve, resulting in abdominal cramping and vomiting.

Mineral Oil

- Do not give with or immediately after meals.
- Give with fruit juice or carbonated drinks to disguise taste.

Magnesium Hydroxide
- Shake container well.
- Do not give 1 to 2 h before or after PO drugs because of effects on absorption.
- Note that milk of magnesia concentrate is three times as potent as regular-strength product.

Senna
- Protect from light and heat.

Simethicone
- Administer after meals and at bedtime.

CLIENT TEACHING

General
- Explain that oral stool softeners are not given to cause bowel evacuation, but to provide for a bowel movement without straining.
- Caution all clients against becoming laxative dependent.
- Instruct clients regarding temperature and storage requirements for particular drugs.

Docusate Sodium and Casanthranol with Docusate Sodium and Docusate Potassium and Casanthranol with Docusate Potassium
Diet
- Drink at least six 8-oz glasses of liquid daily to make stool softer. Drink one glass with each dose.
- If dosage form ordered is liquid, take with milk or fruit juice to mask bitter taste.
- Explain that many laxatives contain sodium. Tell client to check with health care provider or pharmacist before using laxative if on a low-sodium diet.

Safety
- Tell client not to take drug if she is already taking mineral oil or having acute abdominal pain, nausea, vomiting, or signs of intestinal obstruction.

Side Effects
- Tell client she should not use products for longer than 1 week and that prolonged, frequent, or excessive use may result in dependence on drug or electrolyte imbalance.
- Tell client to report to health care provider if skin rash occurs. If stomach or intestinal cramping occurs and does not diminish, inform health care provider.

Senna
Side Effects
- Tell client that drug may discolor urine or feces.
- Tell client to discontinue the drug if abdominal pain occurs.
- Tell client syrup form is 7% alcohol.

Mineral Oil
General
- Tell client not to take other laxatives (for example, docusate products) if she is already taking mineral oil.

Diet
- Tell client to take mineral oil on an empty stomach; do not take with food or meals because of risk of aspiration and decreased fat-soluble vitamin absorption.

Safety
- Avoid bedtime doses because of risk of aspiration.

Side Effects
- Tell client to report any occurrence of nausea, vomiting, diarrhea, or abdominal cramp.

Magnesium Hydroxide
General
- Tell client that laxative action generally occurs in 4 to 8 h.

Safety
- Tell client to be aware of whether she is using regular strength or concentrated form of drug, because concentrate is three times as potent as regular strength.
- Tell client that drug may interact with tetracyclines, digoxin, indomethacin, iron salts, isoniazid; be certain any health care provider seen is aware of the use of this or any drug.

Side Effects
- Tell client to report any muscular weakness, diarrhea, or abdominal cramps.

Simethicone
General
- Tell client that drug will help relieve gas pains in the stomach and intestines.

Skill
- Explain the need to chew tablets thoroughly and to take after meals. Drink a full glass of water after chewing the tablets.
- Tell client that if a dose is missed, to take it as soon as possible; however, if the time is close to next scheduled dose, skip the missed dose and take the scheduled dose. Do not double doses.

EVALUATION

- Evaluate the effectiveness of the drug. Return of prepregnant regular bowel function occurs.

TABLE 43–6 RH$_0$ (D) Immune Globulin (RhoGAM)

Dose and Route	Uses and Considerations
Given IM in deltoid	A sterile concentrated solution of gamma globulin prepared from human serum containing antibodies to the Rh factor (D antigen), also expressed as anti-Rh$_0$ (D). Administered to nonsensitized Rh-negative clients. Action is to suppress active antibody response and formation of anti-Rh$_0$ (D) in Rh-negative clients exposed to RH-positive blood. Promotes destruction of Rh-positive fetal cells in maternal serum before mother can make antibodies that would cause hemolysis of RBCs in Rh-positive fetuses and newborns in subsequent pregnancies. Never give IV. *Pregnancy category:* C. Use with caution in thrombocytopenia or bleeding disorders and in IGA deficiency. Contraindicated in clients with known hypersensitivity to immune globulins or thimerosal, transfusion of Rh$_0$ (D)-positive blood in previous 3 mon or prior sensitization to Rh$_0$ (D). Adverse reactions: lethargy, splenomegaly, elevated bilirubin, myalgia, temperature elevation; most commonly (rare) fever and pain at injection site. Appears in breast milk (not absorbed by infant). t½: 23–26 d. 1 vial (300 μg) prevents maternal sensitization if fetal red cell volume that entered maternal circulation is < 15 mL. Additional vials given if more.
300 μg (1 vial) (standard dose)	Standard dose given at 28 wk gestation as prophylaxis and again after normal delivery (within 72 h) based on titer. Also given after amniocentesis. Larger than standard dose may be given if tests show large fetal-maternal blood transfusion has occurred.
50 μg (1 vial) (microdose)	Microdose given after abortion (less than 12 wk gestation). Because it is a blood product, some clients may refuse due to religious beliefs.

KEY: *IM: intramuscular; IV: intravenous; t½: half-life.*

IMMUNIZATIONS

RH$_0$ (D) IMMUNE GLOBULIN

During pregnancy, an Rh-negative client who lacks the Rh factor in her own blood may carry a fetus who is either Rh-negative or Rh-positive. The circulatory systems of client and baby do not mix during pregnancy unless an event occurs that allows some fetal blood cells to enter the maternal blood stream. Such a situation can happen with early spontaneous or induced abortions, ectopic pregnancy, amniocentesis, chorionic villus sampling, prenatal bleeding due to abruptio placentae, and separation of the placenta from the uterine wall at delivery. If the client and fetus are both Rh-negative, there is no difficulty. However, if the fetus is Rh-positive, the Rh-negative client is at risk for **Rh sensitization** (i.e., the development of protective antibodies against Rh-positive blood) unless preventive measures are employed. The reason why it is important to prevent formation of these antibodies is that, once created, they remain throughout life and will create hemolytic difficulties for fetuses in subsequent pregnancies. Although the circulatory systems of the client and fetus do not normally mix, the protective antibodies that have been formed against Rh-positive blood are small enough to cross the placenta and cause rapid hemolysis in any Rh-positive fetus.

The Rh sensitization process can be prevented through the administration of **Rh$_0$ (D) immune globulin** (RhoGAM) to nonsensitized Rh-negative clients following each actual or potential exposure to Rh-positive blood. Table 43–6 presents the drug data for Rh$_0$ (D) immune globulin.

Side Effects and Adverse Reactions

Side effects are rare, but include fever and pain at the injection site.

NURSING PROCESS: RH$_0$ (D) IMMUNE GLOBULIN

ASSESSMENT

- Determine blood type and Rh status of all prenatal clients.
- Assess the client for the meaning of her Rh status and her partner's Rh status to her.
- Ask the client if she has had previous pregnancies and their outcome; ask if she has ever received Rh$_0$ (D) immune globulin.
- Follow agency protocols for Rh blood work-up for client and baby at time of delivery.

- Postpartum, assess data about newborn's Rh type (if baby is Rh negative, no need for drug; if baby is Rh positive [mother negative], and mother is *not* sensitized [indirect Coomb's test negative] and the baby is direct Coomb's test negative, the mother is a candidate to receive the injection [to *prevent* antibody production, i.e., "sensitization"]).
- Obtain client's permission to receive the drug. A refusal form is required in some institutions if the drug is declined.

- Assess for history of allergy to immune globulin products.

POTENTIAL NURSING DIAGNOSES

- Knowledge deficit related to Rh incompatibility and sensitization
- Knowledge deficit related to Rh_0 (D) immune globulin and when and why drug is needed

PLANNING

- Client will receive Rh_0 (D) immune globulin as indicated within 72 h after delivery or miscarriage.
- Client will be able to explain the Rh process and actions client will need to take in subsequent pregnancies.

NURSING INTERVENTIONS

- Document Rh work-up data and eligibility of client to receive drug in written client record using agency protocol and convey in verbal report.

- Carefully check any lot numbers on vial and lab slip for agreement prior to administration; also check expiration date. Check ID band and lab slip for matching numbers. Return required slips to lab or blood bank.
- Give drug as soon as possible postpartum (within 3 h if possible but definitely within 72 h).
- Give drug IM in deltoid.
- Drug needs to be stored at 36° to 46°F.

General
- Explain to the client the purposes of the drug and review the literature with her.
- Provide the client with written documentation of date of administration for client's personal health record.

EVALUATION

- Evaluate client's understanding of the need for Rh_0 (D) immune globulin.

RUBELLA VACCINE

Rubella is a potentially devastating infection for the fetus, depending on gestational age. If a nonimmunized client contracts the virus during the first trimester, a high rate of abortion and neurologic and developmental sequelae associated with **congenital rubella syndrome** may result. Cataracts, glaucoma, deafness, heart defects, and mental retardation are seen. When infection occurs later in pregnancy, there is less risk of fetal damage because of the developmental stage of the fetus. There is no treatment for maternal or congenital rubella infection, so the goal is prevention of rubella in the childbearing population. Table 43–7 presents the drug data for rubella vaccine.

Side Effects and Adverse Reactions

Side effects are generally mild and temporary. Burning or stinging at the injection site is due to the acidic pH of the vaccine. Regional lymphadenopathy, urticaria, rash, malaise, sore throat, fever, headache, polyneuritis, arthralgia, and moderate fever are also seen.

TABLE 43–7 Rubella Virus Vaccine, Live, MSD (Meruvax II) (Ra27/3 Strain)

Dose and Route	Uses and Considerations
Given subcutaneously: 0.5 mL into outer aspect of upper arm	Live virus vaccine for immunization against German measles. Dose is the same for all persons, using either single dose or multidose vials. Do not give immune serum globulin (ISG) concurrent with vaccine. Contraindicated in pregnant females and clients with anaphylactoid reactions to neomycin, febrile respiratory illness or other febrile infection, active untreated TB, or immune deficiency conditions. Vaccinated persons can shed but not transmit the virus. Defer vaccination for 3 mon after blood or plasma transfusions; also after human ISG. Postpartum clients who received blood products may be vaccinated if repeat titer is drawn 6–8 wk later to ensure that seroconversion occurred. Excreted in breast milk; use caution. *Pregnancy category:* X. Side effects: burning, stinging at injection site; malaise; fever; headache; slight rash 2–4 wk after injection; joint pain 1–3 d within 1–10 wk of injection.

NURSING PROCESS: RUBELLA VACCINE

ASSESSMENT

- Obtain a history and laboratory results indicating a need for rubella vaccine. Pregnant clients should not receive the rubella vaccine.
- Women with a rubella titer of less than 1:10 (or who are ELISA antibody negative) are considered to be suitable postpartum recipients for the vaccine.
- Interview client and/or conduct chart review to determine if client has
  - Received blood transfusions within past 3 mon, plasma transfusion, or human immune serum globulin.
  - Anaphylactic or anaphylactoid reactions to neomycin (dose contains 25 μg of neomycin).
  - Received other virus vaccines within 1 mon. (Do not give <1 mon before or after other virus vaccines.)
  - Active, untreated tuberculosis (TB).
  - Exhibited a primary or acquired immunodeficiency state (AIDS or other clinical manifestations of human immunodeficiency virus [HIV] infection).
  - Any febrile or respiratory illness or other active febrile infection.
- Rubella vaccine is contraindicated if any of the above exist.
- Determine if client is also a candidate to receive Rh$_0$ (D) immune globulin (RhoGAM).
- Outcome may be suppression of rubella antibodies with need to recheck titer in approximately 3 mon.

POTENTIAL NURSING DIAGNOSES

- Knowledge deficit related to rubella infection and its prevention
- High risk for injury related to rubella infection in subsequent pregnancy secondary to lack of immunity

PLANNING

- Client will receive the rubella vaccine to protect against rubella (also known as German measles).
- Client will state in her own words the specific plan she has to prevent pregnancy for 3 mon following injection and accurately describe how to use pregnancy prevention method(s).

NURSING INTERVENTIONS

- Protect vaccine from light and store it at 35.6 to 46.4°F before reconstitution.

- Use only the supplied diluent to reconstitute and use within 8 h.
- Give SC only; never inject IV.
- If tuberculin test is to be done, administer it before or simultaneously with rubella vaccine (may have temporary depression in tuberculin skin sensitivity).

Skill: Reconstitution
- Single-dose vial: withdraw entire amount of diluent into syringe.
- Inject total volume into vial of lyophilized vaccine and agitate to mix thoroughly.
- Withdraw entire contents into syringe and inject total volume of restored vaccine.
- Have epinephrine readily available in case of anaphylactic shock.
- Clearly convey in writing and verbal report that vaccination has occurred.
- Record date of administration, lot number, manufacturer, name, and title to comply with federal law.

CLIENT TEACHING

General
- Discuss the importance of immunity to rubella with client and help her understand the need to obtain titers to determine immune status.
- Teach client measures to ensure adequate birth control for 3 mon postvaccine injection.
- Tell client that there is no risk to her from being near small children who received the injection even if she is pregnant and not immune.

Side Effects
- Tell client that the most common side effect is burning or stinging at site of injection; some also experience malaise, fever, headache, slight rash about 2 to 4 wk after injection; some also experience joint pain 1 to 10 wk after injection that lasts 1 to 3 days in some clients.

Safety
- Recommend that client have titer rechecked if she also received RhoGAM.

EVALUATION

- Evaluate the need for rubella vaccine.

TABLE 43–8 Drugs Administered to the Newborn Immediately After Delivery

Drug	Dosage	Uses and Considerations
Erythromycin ophthalmic ointment	½ inch ribbon of ointment placed in lower conjunctival sac of each eye within 1 h of delivery	Prevention of gonococcal conjunctivitis (ophthalmia neonatorum), which can cause blindness. Also prevents chlamydial conjunctivitis. Origin of infection from vagina. Contains antibiotic (erythromycin) in sterile base of mineral oil and white petrolatum. Has bactericidal or bacteriostatic action based on concentration per gram and the target organisms present. Side effects: chemical conjunctivitis (swelling, inflammation 24–48 h)
Phytonadione (Vitamin K$_1$, Mephyton, Aquamephyton, Konakion)	0.5–1.0 mg IM into anterior or lateral thigh within 1 h after birth	Oral anticoagulant antagonist. An aqueous colloidal solution of vitamin K$_1$. Newborn does not receive adequate vitamin K transplacentally and is unable to initially synthesize vitamin due to limited intestinal flora; therefore production of clotting factors in liver is hindered and low prothrombin levels are evidenced. Phytonadione facilitates production of clotting factors equal to natural vitamin K. Newborns of mothers who received oral anticoagulants or anticonvulsants during pregnancy may need higher dosage. Dose may be repeated in 6–8 h. Side effects: pain and edema at injection site; possible allergic reactions include urticaria and rash; those who receive larger doses may exhibit hyperbilirubinemia and jaundice

KEY: IM: intramuscular.

DRUGS ADMINISTERED TO THE NEWBORN IMMEDIATELY AFTER DELIVERY

The typical neonate receives few drugs after birth. Drugs routinely administered to the newborn are erythromycin ophthalmic ointment to provide prophylaxis against eye infections (legally required in the U.S.), and vitamin K, to prevent hemorrhagic disease. In addition, a disinfectant is usually applied to the umbilical area during the first few hours after birth. Table 43–8 presents the drug data for drugs administered to the newborn immediately after delivery.

SIDE EFFECTS AND ADVERSE REACTIONS

Erythromycin Ophthalmic Ointment

Side effects include chemical conjunctivitis in about 20% of newborns, which manifests as swelling and inflammation lasting about 24 to 48 h. This may interfere slightly with eye-to-eye contact between parents and newborn.

Phytonadione (Vitamin K$_1$)

Side effects include pain and edema at the site of the injection. Some allergic reactions, manifested by urticaria and rash, have been reported. Babies who receive larger doses may exhibit hyperbilirubinemia and jaundice due to competition for binding sites.

NURSING PROCESS: DRUGS ADMINISTERED TO THE NEWBORN AFTER DELIVERY

ASSESSMENT

Erythromycin Ophthalmic Ointment
• Assess baby for signs of hypersensitivity.

Phytonadione (Vitamin K$_1$)
• Assess newborn for bleeding from umbilical cord, circumcision site, nose, and GI tract, and for generalized ecchymoses.

POTENTIAL NURSING DIAGNOSIS

• Potential risk of injury related to infectious process (congenital) and/or transient low prothrombin levels in the newborn

PLANNING

• Newborn will receive the drugs as prescribed after delivery.

NURSING INTERVENTIONS

Erythromycin Ophthalmic Ointment
• See procedure for administration of eye ointments (see Chapter 3).
• Delay instillation no more than 1 h; promote eye contact between parents and the baby during this period.
• Wear gloves for handling the newborn during instillations.

- Do not place tube of ointment under radiant warmer with baby prior to administration.
- Do not irrigate eyes following instillation.

Phytonadione (Vitamin K₁)
- Protect from light due to photosensitivity of the preparation.
- Wear gloves for handling the newborn during injection.
- Observe injection site for swelling and inflammation.

CLIENT TEACHING

General
Erythromycin Ophthalmic Ointment
- Tell parents that any swelling around eyes will usually disappear within 24 to 48 h.

- Explain that administration of eye prophylaxis is a legal requirement and that there is no harm to vision from the ointment.

Phytonadione (Vitamin K₁)
- Explain the need for the drug to parents so they do not think there is something wrong with their baby when they see an injection being given.

EVALUATION

- Evaluate documentation of required drugs.

IMMUNIZATION DURING THE NEWBORN PERIOD PRIOR TO DISCHARGE

Since 1991, the American Academy of Pediatrics and the Centers for Disease Control and Prevention (CDC) have recommended that immunization against hepatitis B virus (HBV) begin in the newborn period. The goal is prevention of HBV infection that may result in serious long-term liver disease, cancer, and death in adulthood (caused by transmission of HBV in blood and body fluids) for the entire population over time through the reduction of chronic carriers of the virus.

In pregnancy, HBV transmission occurs vertically, primarily at the time of delivery. For those infants born to HBsAg-positive mothers, it is believed that infection can be prevented in 90% through postdelivery screening and injection of both hepatitis B immune globulin (HBIG) and hepatitis B vaccine.

The current recommendation is that newborn infants be given three injections intramuscularly in the anterolateral thigh following a protocol based on their mother's HBsAg-positive or -negative status. Table 43–9 presents hepatitis B vaccine data for the newborn.

TABLE 43–9 Hepatitis B Immunization in the Newborn Period

Drug	Dosage	Uses and Considerations
Hepatitis B vaccine (Engerix B)	For newborns of HBsAg-*positive* mothers: 0.5 mL (10 μg) IM *within* 12 h after birth (first dose); repeated at 1 mon and 6 mon. (In addition, hepatitis B immune globulin [HBIG] is given with the first dose of hepatitis B vaccine for infants of infected mothers.) For newborns of HBsAG-*negative* mothers: 0.5 mL (10 μg) IM before discharge but no later than 2 mon of age; followed by repeat doses at 1–2 mon and 6–18 mon. (If unlikely to return for routine immunizations, may give repeat doses at 4 mon and 6–18 mon).	Product is a recombinant hepatitis B vaccine used for immunization against infection caused by hepatitis B virus (HBV). Given to all infants regardless of HBsAg status of mother. Unvaccinated infants *less than* 12 mon old with a mother or primary care giver with acute hepatitis B should be given HBIG because of risk of becoming an HBV carrier following infection (also start HBV vaccine series). Must be injected IM into anterolateral thigh; never inject IV. Following three doses >90% of infants and children will seroconvert. Protection in those who seroconvert will last 3–7 y with a single booster. Contraindicated if hypersensitivity to any component of vaccine (e.g., yeast)—no reports of problems published. Neonatal side effects: soreness at injection site with swelling, warmth, redness, and induration. *Pregnancy category:* C

NURSING PROCESS: HEPATITIS B VACCINE

ASSESSMENT

- Review laboratory data for HBsAg-negative or -positive status of mother.
- Validate whether infant is to receive hepatitis B vaccine singly or in consort with HBIG.

POTENTIAL NURSING DIAGNOSES

- Injury, risk for hepatitis B infection
- Knowledge deficit related to hepatitis B and prophylaxis (maternal)

PLANNING

- The newborn will receive correct dosage of hepatitis B vaccine prior to discharge, including HBIG, if indicated.
- The primary health care provider will be informed when the client is to return for repeat doses.

NURSING INTERVENTIONS

Skill
- Do not dilute.
- Shake well before withdrawal.
- Discard if other than slightly opaque white suspension.

- Have epinephrine available if allergic reaction.
- Use full recommended dose of the vaccine.
- Monitor baby's temperature postinjection.

Safety
- Give IM in anterolateral thigh.
- Document site used in chart.
- Record lot number, expiration date, name, title in chart.
- Store product at 2° to 8°C.
- Do not freeze (destroys potency).

CLIENT TEACHING

General
- Inform mother of implications of her HBsAg-positive or -negative status for her newborn and recommended interventions.
- Have mother read literature and sign permission for administration of vaccine (place copy in newborn's chart).
- Inform mother when repeat doses need to be given.

EVALUATION

- Evaluate mother's understanding of the need for hepatitis B vaccine for her baby.

■ CASE STUDY
Postpartum Client and Newborn

Tanya, age 17 years, is the client you planned care for during labor induction in Chapter 42. Tanya was sent to the hospital for labor induction/augmentation at 42 weeks' gestation by her doctor, who was concerned that she was moving into the "post-dates" period and also exhibiting pregnancy-induced hypertension. Tanya's mother arrived at the hospital when Tanya was dilated 8 cm, in time for the latter stages of Tanya's labor. Her mother remained as Tanya's support person throughout the delivery, which occurred at 0600 by vacuum extraction. Tanya had a continuous epidural for her labor and delivery. A fourth-degree episiotomy was necessary at the time the baby, an 8-pound 7-ounce girl, arrived. A cluster of hemorrhoids is evident. Although Tanya has had three pregnancies, this baby, Jessica, is the first pregnancy that has resulted in a live birth. Tanya is not married. She lives with her mother and has been going to high school and working part-time in a retail auto parts store.

Tanya plans to keep this baby. She would like to breast feed "for at least 3 months." She plans on finishing school and returning to work in 6 weeks. Baby Jessica had an Apgar score of 7 and 9. The baby is alert and active.

Immediately after the delivery, you conduct an assessment of Tanya, analyze the data, and determine and prioritize her nursing care needs. You do the same for the baby.

1. Based on the data supplied about the episiotomy, define a priority nursing diagnosis for Tanya.
2. Define an outcome-based goal for the diagnosis you stated.
3. Describe how you would intervene in regard to the episiotomy during the early postpartum period, integrating both pharmacologic and nonpharmacologic measures. Orders include benzocaine spray, witch hazel pads, Proctofoam HC, ibuprofen tablets (200 mg) at the bedside.

Baby Jessica must have eye prophylaxis and a vitamin K injection completed while still in the labor/delivery/recovery area. You are also trying to get the baby to bond with Tanya and her mother.

4. Within the standard, how could you promote bonding, including eye contact between mother and baby, and also handle eye prophylaxis?
5. State the steps you will follow to instill the ointment into the baby's eyes, including safety aspects for yourself.
6. What would you teach Tanya about the side effects of eye prophylaxis?
7. Describe the reason for the vitamin K_1 injection for the baby in terms Tanya can understand.
8. State the steps you will follow to prepare and give the vitamin K_1 injection, including safety aspects for yourself.

Tanya is Rh negative. The baby's father's blood type is unknown. A cord blood was drawn on the baby at the time of delivery. Based on Tanya's historical data:

9. What would you be concerned about in terms of defining her as a likely or unlikely RhoGAM candidate? What data about mother and baby will be needed to aid in the decision?

Assuming Tanya is a RhoGAM candidate:

10. Define a nursing diagnosis for Tanya.
11. Define an outcome-based goal for the diagnosis you stated.
12. State the timeframe in which you would want to administer the globulin and the rationale for this timeframe.
13. Explain what verbal and written documentation must be addressed in regard to RhoGAM administration, both prior to administration and following administration.
14. Tanya's chart reveals that her rubella titer is 1:6. What is the implication of this titer for Tanya?
15. While reviewing Tanya's medication administration record, you notice that in the section that addresses known allergies, neomycin is listed. Considering Tanya's titer, the standing health care provider's order, and your knowledge about this vaccine, describe how you would handle the situation.
16. In a situation in which a mother is both a rubella and RhoGAM candidate, with both products being administered, what is one major piece of information the nurse should share with the client in regard to the rubella titer?

Tanya is concerned about having a first bowel movement because of her episiotomy. You tell her that the docusate with casanthranol product she will be supplied will help.

17. Tanya says that she does not want to take the docusate because she plans to breast feed. What nursing diagnosis could you state based on Tanya's communication?
18. Describe how you might address Tanya's concerns based on your knowledge of the product and breast feeding.

Tanya asks what can be done about the hemorrhoids. You tell her about the mode of action of the ordered pharmacologic products. She states, "So I just have to insert this syringe-type applicator up my rectum once I fill it from the big can?"

19. Analyze Tanya's communication. What is correct and incorrect in regard to the content?
20. What nursing diagnosis is appropriate for Tanya on the basis of the data supplied?
21. Describe what client teaching you need to do as an outcome.

Baby Jessica is ordered to receive hepatitis B vaccine prior to discharge. Tanya is listed as being HbsAg negative.

22. Which babies are eligible to receive hepatitis B vaccine?
23. How many doses constitute the total series, and what is the time period for these?
24. What is the purpose of giving newborns this vaccine? Why is this important in today's society in particular?
25. Tanya asks how long the baby's immunity should last provided that seroconversion occurs. How would you answer Tanya?
26. Where would you expect to find the vaccine stored at the hospital?
27. Describe the written documentation required with administration of this vaccine as a part of the permanent record.

STUDY QUESTIONS

1. A client was supposed to chew her simethicone tablets at 0800 but she forgot. It is now 1115. She asks if she should chew them now or wait and take extra at the scheduled 1200 dose. What would you tell her? What is your rationale?
2. Describe what you would tell a newly admitted postpartum (vaginal delivery) client about the process of self-administered drugs and the specific products included. Why would you select this content to include?
3. What client data are required prior to postpartum administration of ergot derivatives (e.g., methergine)? (See Chapter 42.)

4. What should the nurse assess a client for prior to the client initiating laxative products?

5. Sarah is a 24-year-old woman who delivered her baby 24 h ago. She has a history of drug and alcohol abuse. Her health care provider ordered senna syrup for her as a stimulant laxative. What action would you take? Why?

6. Why are bedtime doses of mineral oil not generally recommended?

7. Your client complains during the postpartum period of "pain in my bottom where the doctor cut me." Her chart states that she has a fourth-degree episiotomy. What pharmacologic products are available to help this client, in addition to nonpharmacologic comfort measures? How will these help the client?

8. Mary, a postpartum client, has an order for promazine and hydrocortisone. You discover she has the product at her bedside but has not used it. When questioned, Mary said, "Oh, I forgot to tell you, I'm allergic to things like lidocaine, benzocaine." What response could you correctly make to Mary?

9. What are three aspects to evaluate concerning drugs/products for relief of pain from perineal wounds and hemorrhoids?

10. A client tells you she doesn't see any reason to use her dibucaine ointment because it "feels like nothing on my hand—not cooling or soothing—so it probably won't help my bottom." How could you correctly respond with factual information?

11. Why is a newborn given an injection of vitamin K_1 following delivery?

12. What prophylactic agent is used after delivery for newborn eye care? In what time period should it be given? How is it administered?

13. In what site would you administer hepatitis B vaccine to a newborn?

Chapter 44

Drugs Related to Women's Health and Disorders

Jane Purnell Taylor

OUTLINE

Objectives
Terms
Introduction
Oral Contraceptive Products
    Estrogen-Progestin Combination Products
    Progestin-Only Products

Nursing Process
Drugs Used to Treat Uterine Dysfunction
    The Menstrual Cycle
    Premenstrual Syndrome
        Nursing Process
    Endometriosis

Nursing Process
Menopause
    Nursing Process
Case Study
Study Questions

OBJECTIVES

Describe the types, expected actions, and side effects of oral contraceptive products.

Recognize new hormonal/pharmacologic products related to conception control.

Explain the expected effects of medications used to treat uterine dysfunction, including premenstrual syndrome, endometriosis, and menopause.

Describe nursing process, including client teaching, associated with the drugs used for women's health and disorders.

TERMS

dyspareunia
endometriosis
estrogen replacement
  therapy
follicular phase

hormone replacement
  therapy
luteal phase
menopause
oral contraceptives

ovulatory phase
premenstrual syndrome
progestin

INTRODUCTION

Oral contraceptive products and medications for uterine dysfunction and menopause are described in this chapter. Nursing interventions and client teaching are emphasized.

ORAL CONTRACEPTIVE PRODUCTS

Among the various methods of contraception available today, the **oral contraceptives** that employ hormone therapy enjoy wide popularity because of their ease of use and high degree of effectiveness with relative safety for most women. When these steroidal agents were first approved for use by the Food and Drug Administration (FDA) in 1960, little was known about the best combinations of drugs to use or optimum doses, and adverse side effects, particularly circulatory disorders, were frequent. Subsequent research has resulted in lower-dose drugs. Research continues to focus upon actual and potential short-and long-term benefits and risks associated with use of low-dose oral contraceptives and new administration forms (e.g., long-acting progestin-releasing subcutaneous implants), particularly in the areas of circulatory risks and carcinogenesis. Immunologic methods of contraception are another area of current research.

There are two main types of oral contraceptives: the estrogen-progestin combination products, often referred to as "the pill," and the progestin-only products, sometimes called "the mini-pill." The combination products have the lowest pregnancy rate.

ESTROGEN-PROGESTIN COMBINATION PRODUCTS

Combined estrogen-progestin oral contraceptive products prevent pregnancy by suppressing pituitary release of follicle-stimulating hormone (FSH) and luteinizing hormone (LH), which are needed to mature a graafian follicle in the ovary, thereby inhibiting ovulation. These agents also create changes in the endometrium that make it less favorable for implantation of a fertilized ovum. In addition, the quantity and viscosity of the cervical mucus is changed by progestins, making it hostile to sperm. Alterations in motility within the fallopian tube may also impede the movement of the ova.

The most commonly prescribed oral contraceptive products are the estrogen-progestin combinations. These formulations are differentiated based on the strength of the individual components and whether estrogen or progesterone effects predominate. The amount of estrogen varies among the available products. Low-dose combination products have 35 μg or less of ethinyl estradiol, or 50 μg or less of mestranol. The higher-dose combination products (no longer available as of 1988) contained 50 to 100 μg of one of these estrogens and had more severe estrogen-linked side effects. The synthetic progesterone **progestin** incorporated in the combination products is employed to reduce the effects of estrogen. The goal of therapy is to identify the product that offers the best contraceptive protection throughout the menstrual cycle with the fewest unwanted side effects due to either the estrogen or the progestin component.

There are three types of combination products: monophasic, biphasic, and triphasic. The monophasics, the most common, consist of products that provide a fixed ratio of estrogen to progestin throughout the menstrual cycle. In biphasics, the amount of estrogen is fixed throughout the cycle, but the amount of progesterone varies (reduced in the first half and increased in the second half) to provide for proliferation of the endometrium and secretory development similar to the physiologic process. Ortho-Novum 10/11-21 is an example of a biphasic. The triphasics, the newest combination products, deliver low doses of both hormones with minimal side effects, including breakthrough bleeding. With triphasics, the amount of both estrogen and progestin varies throughout the cycle in different ratios during three phases. Examples include Ortho-Novum 7/7/7, Tri-Norinyl, and Triphasil.

PROGESTIN-ONLY PRODUCTS

The progestin-only oral contraceptive, referred to as "the mini-pill," acts mainly by altering the cervical mucus, and secondarily by altering the endometrium to inhibit implantation. Ovulation is also inhibited in some clients through blockage of LH release. These products were designed to further decrease circulatory side effects. There is, however, a lower pregnancy prevention rate, further increased if clients miss a pill, because these drugs do not suppress activity of the hypothalamus and pituitary to the same degree as the combination products. An increase in the amount of breakthrough bleeding is also noted. Examples of progestin-only products include Ovrette, Micronor, and Nor-QD. Table 44–1 presents selected examples of the various oral contraceptive formulations.

Pharmacokinetics

Ethinyl estradiol is rapidly absorbed orally. It undergoes significant first-pass metabolism and elimination via the liver. Mestranol is converted in the liver to ethinyl estradiol, which is 97% to 98% bound to plasma proteins. The half-life varies from 6 to 20 h. Excretion is via bile and urine in a conjugated form. There is some enterohepatic recirculation.

TABLE 44–1 Oral Contraceptives

Product	Amount of Estrogen (μg)	Amount of Progestin (mg)	Product	Amount of Estrogen (μg)	Amount of Progestin (mg)
Combination Products: Listed by Decreasing Estrogen Content			N.E.E. 10/11	*Phase II:* 11 d	
Monophasic Products				35 ethinyl estradiol	1.0 norethindrone
Norinyl 1 + 50 (21 d)	50 mestranol	1 norethindrone			
Genora 1/50	50 mestranol	1 norethindrone	Nelova 10/11	*Phase I:* 10 d	
Ovcon 50	50 ethinyl estradiol	1 norethindrone		35 ethinyl estradiol	0.5 norethindrone
Norlestrin 1/50	50 ethinyl estradiol	1 norethindrone acetate		*Phase II:* 11 d	
				35 ethinyl estradiol	1 norethindrone
Demulen 1/50	50 ethinyl estradiol	1 ethynodiol diacetate	Ortho-Novum 10/11	Same formulation as above but different colors for tablets	
Norlestrin 21 2.5/50	50 ethinyl estradiol	2.5 norethindrone acetate	**Triphasic Products**		
			Tri-Norinyl	*Phase I:* 7 d	
Ovral	50 ethinyl estradiol	0.5 norgestrel		35 ethinyl estradiol	0.5 norethindrone
Genora 1/35	35 ethinyl estradiol	1 norethindrone		*Phase II:* 9 d	
Norcept-E 1/35	35 ethinyl estradiol	1 norethindrone		35 ethinyl estradiol	1 norethindrone
Ortho Novum 1/35	35 ethinyl estradiol	1 norethindrone		*Phase III:* 5 d	
				35 ethinyl estradiol	0.5 norethindrone
N.E.E. 1/35	35 ethinyl estradiol	1 norethindrone	Ortho Tri-Cyclen	*Phase I:* 7 d	
Norethin 1/35 E	35 ethinyl estradiol	1 norethindrone		35 ethinyl estradiol	0.18 norgestimate
Norinyl 1 + 35	35 ethinyl estradiol	1 norethindrone		*Phase II:* 7 d	
Modicon	35 ethinyl estradiol	0.5 norethindrone		35 ethinyl estradiol	0.215 norgestimate
Brevicon	35 ethinyl estradiol	0.5 norethindrone		*Phase III:* 7 d	
				35 ethinyl estradiol	0.25 norgestimate
Nelova	35 ethinyl estradiol	0.5 norethindrone	Ortho-Novum 7/7/7	*Phase I:* 7 d	
Ovcon 35	35 ethinyl estradiol	0.4 norethindrone		35 ethinyl estradiol	0.5 norethindrone
Demulen 1/35	35 ethinyl estradiol	1 ethynodiol diacetate		*Phase II:* 7 d	
				35 ethinyl estradiol	0.75 norethindrone
Desogen	30 ethinyl estradiol	0.15 desogestrel		*Phase III:* 7 d	
Loestrin 21 1.5/30	30 ethinyl estradiol	1.5 norethindrone acetate		35 ethinyl estradiol	1 norethindrone
Lo/Ovral	30 ethinyl estradiol	0.3 norgestrel	Tri-Levlen	*Phase I:* 6 d	
Levlen	30 ethinyl estradiol	0.15 levonorgestrel		30 ethinyl estradiol	0.05 levonorgestrel
Nordette	30 ethinyl estradiol	0.15 levonorgestrel		*Phase II:* 5 d	
Loestrin 21 1/20	20 ethinyl estradiol	1 norethindrone acetate		40 ethinyl estradiol	0.075 levonorgestrel
				Phase III: 10 d	
				30 ethinyl estradiol	0.125 levonorgestrel
Biphasic Products			Triphasil	Same as above	
Jenest 28	*Phase I:* 7 d				
	35 ethinyl estradiol	0.5 norethindrone	**Progestin-Only Products: Listed by Decreasing Progestin Content**		
	Phase II: 14 d				
	35 ethinyl estradiol	1.0 norethindrone	Micronor		0.35 norethindrone
N.E.E. 10/11	*Phase I:* 10 d		Nor-QD		0.35 norethindrone
	35 ethinyl estradiol	0.5 norethindrone	Ovrette		0.075 norgestrel

Progestins are also well absorbed orally. Peak plasma levels occur from 0.5 to 4 h after ingestion, depending on the particular compound. Norethynodrel and ethynodiol diacetate are converted to norethindrone. Levonorgestrel is bioavailable and does not undergo first-pass liver metabolism; norethindrone undergoes first-pass metabolism and is 65% available. The progestins are bound to plasma proteins and to sex hormone-binding globulin. The half-life of norethindrone varies from 5 to 14 h; that of levonorgestrel from 11 to 45 h.

Dosage Schedule
Combination Products

Most monophasic products are available in 21- and 28-tablet packages. The 28-tablet packages include seven non–hormone-containing tablets (some contain iron) so that the client continues to take one tablet each day, rather than having to remember starting and stopping times. Clients are given instructions to take one tablet every day at approximately the same time each day. Many products require the client to start the tablets on the Sunday following the first day of menstruation. If menstruation actually starts on Sunday, the client starts her tablets that day. Other products instruct the client to start her tablets on day 5 of the menstrual cycle (day 1 is the day she begins her period). If the client is on a 21-day regimen, she restarts her next cycle following a 7-day break whether her bleeding has stopped or not.

The biphasic and triphasic products are taken in phases and are color-coded to assist the client. They, too, are available in 21- and 28-day regimens and are started within the guidelines previously presented. For example, the biphasic Ortho-Novum 10/11 requires 10 white tablets for 10 days, followed by 11 peach tablets for 11 days. With a 21-day regimen, the client stops for 7 days; with a 28-day regimen, the client takes seven green inert tablets during this period before beginning the next cycle. The triphasic Ortho-Novum 7/7/7 works similarly. White tablets are taken for 7 days, light peach for 7 days, darker peach for 7 days, followed by 7 days off or 7 green inert tablets. Exceptions to these guidelines include the triphasics Triphasil 21 and Tri-Levulen 21, which are started on the first day of the menstrual cycle with the designated color code followed for 6 days, 5 days, and 10 days, respectively. These, too, are available in 21- and 28-day packaging.

Progestin-Only Products

The progestin-only products are taken one tablet at the same time daily all year without interruption. The tablets are started on the first day of menstruation.

Missed Doses

Clients occasionally miss a tablet. If only one tablet is missed, it is fairly unlikely that ovulation will occur. However, the risk increases with each additional missed dose. Table 44–2 presents guidelines for missed doses of oral contraceptives.

TABLE 44–2 Guidelines for Missed Doses of Oral Contraceptives

Missed Dose	Recommendations
Combination Products	

One tablet	Take tablet as soon as realized
	  or
	take two tablets the next day
	  or
	take one tablet and discard missed tablet and continue schedule but use secondary form of contraception until menses begin

Two tablets	Take two tablets as soon as realized with next tablet at the usual time or take two tablets daily for the next 2 d and resume regular schedule plus use a secondary form of contraception for the rest of the cycle.
Three tablets	Start a new package of tablets 7 d after the last tablet was taken. Use another form of contraception until tablets have been taken for 7 consecutive d.
Progestin-Only Products	
One tablet	Take tablet as soon as realized; follow with next tablet at regular time plus consider secondary form of contraception
Two tablets	Take one of the missed tablets; discard the second missed tablet; follow with next scheduled tablet at regular time plus use secondary form of contraception until menstruation occurs or a pregnancy is tested for.
Three tablets	Discontinue use of tablets and employ another form of birth control. Observe for return of menstruation and test for pregnancy

TABLE 44–3 Contraindications for Oral Contraceptives

Absolute Contraindications
Thromboembolic disease—history or actual
Breast cancer
Cerebrovascular disease
Myocardial infarction
Coronary artery disease
Estrogen-dependent tumors
Hepatic tumors (benign or malignant) originating during use of any estrogen product
Markedly impaired liver function
History of obstructive jaundice during pregnancy
Genital bleeding of unknown origin
Pregnancy—confirmed or suspected
Hyperlipidemia

Cautious Use
Women over age 35 who smoke
Women over age 40 who do not smoke
Women (any age) who smoke >15 cigarettes per day
Varicose veins
Diabetes or history suggesting possibility
Preexisting fibroid tumors of the uterus
Hypertension
Obesity
Anemia
Migraine headaches
Epilepsy
Elective surgery
Porphyria

Contraindications

Not every client should take oral contraceptives. Table 44–3 lists contraindications to their use.

Drug Interactions

The effectiveness of some drugs is impaired by oral contraceptives; other drugs impair the effectiveness of oral contraceptives. Table 44–4 lists examples of drugs for which the nurse should maintain a high index of suspicion for interactive effects with oral contraceptives. Clients receiving low-dose formulations of oral contraceptives need to be particularly cautious about potential interactions.

Side Effects and Adverse Reactions

The risk of death from the use of oral contraceptives is less than the risk from pregnancy, especially if the client does not exhibit contraindications listed in Table 44–3. Most side effects are related to differences in the estrogen-progestin ratio of the products and the client's response.

Side effects due primarily to an excess of estrogen include nausea, vomiting, dizziness, fluid retention, edema, bloating, breast enlargement, breast tenderness, chloasma (slightly more in dark-skinned clients exposed to sunlight on higher dose tablets), leg cramps, decreased tearing, corneal curvature alteration, visual changes, vascular head-

ache, and hypertension (in about 1% to 5% of previously normotensive clients within the first few months).

Side effects due primarily to estrogen deficiency include vaginal bleeding (breakthrough bleeding) while taking the tablets (especially in the first few cycles after starting therapy) lasting several days (usually during days 1 to 14), oligomenorrhea (especially after long-term use), nervousness, and dyspareunia secondary to atrophic vaginitis.

Side effects due primarily to an excess of progestin include increased appetite, weight gain, oily skin and scalp, acne, depression, vaginitis due to yeast (Candida), excess hair growth, and amenorrhea after cessation of use (1% to 2%), decreased breast size.

Side effects due primarily to progestin deficiency include dysmenorrhea, bleeding late in the cycle (days 15 to 21), and heavy menstrual flow with clots, or amenorrhea.

There may also be changes in laboratory values, including thyroid and liver function, blood glucose, and triglycerides.

TABLE 44–4 Drug Interactions with Oral Contraceptives*

Analgesics: acetaminophen, meperidine, salicylates

Antibiotics and antibacterials: ampicillin, chloramphenicol, griseofulvin, penicillins, rifampicin, sulfonamides, tetracycline

Anticoagulants (oral)

Anticonvulsants: phenytoin, phenobarbital, primidone, carbamazepine, valproic acid

Antifibrinolytic agents: aminocaproic acid

Antihistamines and decongestants

Antihypertensive agents: metoprolol

Antitubercular drugs

Benzodiazepines: lorazepam, oxazepam, temazepam

Caffeine

Cholesterol-lowering drugs: clofibrate

Corticosteroids

Mineral oil

Nonsteroidal antiinflammatory drugs (phenylbutazone, naproxon)

Theophyllines

Tricyclic antidepressants

* Contraceptive effectiveness may be affected by some interactions involving one or more of these drugs. Secondary forms of contraception may be temporarily needed.

Adverse reactions of a more severe nature include increased risk of superficial and deep venous thrombosis, pulmonary embolism, cerebrovascular accident (thrombotic stroke), myocardial infarction, and acceleration of preexisting but nondiagnosed breast tumors.

NURSING PROCESS: ORAL CONTRACEPTIVES

ASSESSMENT

- Obtain baseline blood pressure (BP), weight, and liver enzyme tests. Report abnormal findings. Interview about pregnancy status.
- Recognize the need for periodic reassessment of baseline data and side effects. Most clients should be seen in 1 to 3 months after beginning regimen.

POTENTIAL NURSING DIAGNOSES

- Knowledge deficit related to fertility pattern
- Knowledge deficit related to oral contraceptive method(s)
- Potential for noncompliance with oral contraceptive method selected

PLANNING

- Client will take oral contraceptives as prescribed and will report side effects if they occur.

NURSING INTERVENTIONS

General

- Separate personal views from those of the client regarding contraception and use of specific products.
- Recognize that about 50% to 70% of clients on oral contraceptives abandon the method within a year; therefore, plan to provide the client with alternatives.

CLIENT TEACHING

- Remind client that these drugs should be used only under a health care provider's direction.
- Review with client the following aspects of oral contraceptives.

Advantages

- Easy to use and have low failure rate.
- Minimal risks for teens and those in twenties.
- Contraception is not linked to the sexual act.
- Suppressed pain at ovulation.
- Decreased dysmenorrhea.

- Lighter, shorter menstrual flow.
- Regular, predictable menses.
- Decreased pregnancy fears may increase sexual responsiveness.
- Decreased iron-deficiency anemia due to decreased menstrual flow.
- 80% to 90% reduced risk of functional ovarian cysts.
- May provide protection against benign breast lesions and uterine and ovarian cancers.
- Reduced risk of pelvic inflammatory disease.
- Lower risk of ectopic pregnancy.
- Decreased menstrual migraine type headache.
- No concrete supportive evidence that breast cancer is caused or increased by use of oral contraceptives.
- Decreased chance of endometrial cancer (possibly due to progestin) in younger women not past menopause; protection may last up to 10 years after pills have been stopped if a client has used them long-term.
- Benign functional ovarian cysts are less common.
- Thromboembolism risk does not appear related to duration of oral contraceptive use, rather to the dose of estrogen (lower dose products less risky).

Disadvantages

- If nonmonogamous, there is increased risk of acquiring sexually transmitted diseases, because no barrier is involved.
- Extremely risky for fetus if pregnancy should occur.
- Some clients may perceive specific side effects as particularly bothersome.
- Requires medical follow-up every 6 months, which may, in addition to cost of tablets, be perceived as expensive in terms of both time and money by some clients.

Side Effects

- Acquaint client with the rare but possible side effects that are considered serious, including thrombophlebitis, pulmonary embolus, myocardial infarction, cerebral vascular accident, and retinal vein thrombosis.
- As an outcome of discussion about serious side

effects, teach client the acronym ACHES for dangerous side effects that must be reported to a health care provider:

A = *A*bdominal pain (severe)

C = *C*hest pain or shortness of breath

H = *H*eadaches that are severe; dizziness, weakness, numbness, speech difficulties

E = *E*ye disorders including blurring or loss of vision.

S = *S*evere leg pain or swelling in the calf or thigh

More Common Side Effects

- Inform the client that her menstrual flow may be less in amount and duration due to thinning of the endometrial lining.
- Check to see if the client wears contact lenses and discuss how to handle dry eyes due to decreased tearing and alterations in the shape of the cornea.
- Tell the client who experiences postpill amenorrhea that 95% of women have regular periods within 12 to 18 months. Also tell her that those who participate in endurance fitness activities may have increased postpill amenorrhea.

Safety

- Counsel the client not to smoke tobacco due to increased cardiovascular risks.
- Advise the client to use barrier method of contraception during the first month of oral contraceptive use and for 3 months after discontinuing prior to trying to conceive.
- Provide instructions about handling missed pills (see Table 44–2).
- Tell the client to report any effects from the pill to a health professional so that the therapy can be adjusted to suit her own particular needs. Encourage her not to give up and discontinue use of the pills.
- Tell the client to report breakthrough bleeding or spotting, because she may need a change in dose of oral contraceptive.
- Tell the client to always report that she takes oral contraceptives when seeing a health care provider due to possible synergistic or antagonistic responses to other therapies.
- Nursing mothers should delay use of oral contraceptives until after breast feeding is completed; another method should be selected.

Skill

- Ask the client to weigh herself at home and observe for any edema.
- Teach the client to do a monthly breast self-examination.

Diet

- Counsel the client to moderate caffeine intake because elimination may be decreased due to the oral contraceptives.
- Tell the client to take her pill with a snack at night or after meals to help eliminate nausea and to take the pill at the same time each 24 h.

General

- Nonnursing mothers can begin combination oral contraceptives 3 to 4 weeks postpartum, regardless of whether menstruation has spontaneously occurred.
- Tell the client about new forms of hormone therapy that have long-lasting but reversible contraceptive effects such as Norplant (approved in December, 1990), which employs low-dose levonorgestrel in six matchstick-shaped silastic implants placed under the skin of the upper arm. Norplant is considered effective for 5 years and has the advantage of not requiring conscious daily awareness of contraception. However, the method is being requested less frequently because of side effects that include reports of rods being visible and some rods travelling up the arm, scars on the arm, breakthrough and uncontrolled bleeding, hirsutism, weight gain, increased ovarian cysts, and removal difficulties in some clients that requires a minor surgical procedure.
- Inform the client about long-acting injectable progestin known as medroxyprogesterone acetate (Depo-Provera), which is gaining favor today because it only requires injections every 3 months (based on a wheel-type calculator that determines injection dates, taking lengths of months into account). The method is considered safe for postpartum clients to receive prior to discharge following delivery; clients may also breast feed. The most common side effects reported include initially irregular periods and spotting (periods may cease in about 1 year). Women who smoke may complain of headaches on Depo-Provera (usually relieved by acetaminophen). In addition, other side effects include weight gain, bloating, decreased libido, hair loss, and depression. Like oral contraceptives, there is no protection against sexually transmitted diseases. The injection, given deep IM in the gluteus, is relatively inexpensive. The site of the injection is documented in order to rotate every other injection. The client is provided with a personalized calendar for subsequent doses. The injection acts by suppressing ovulation and changing the pH of the vaginal mucosa to an environment less hospitable to sperm. In

some clients, resumption of fertility may be delayed (when the injections are discontinued) for a year or more. In a rare instance, some serious side effects may occur, including chest pain, hemoptysis, abdominal pain, shortness of breath, and numbness in the extremities. The drug is contraindicated in cases of undiagnosed vaginal bleeding or known or suspected pregnancy.

- Inform the client about hormone-releasing intrauterine devices.
- Clarify information in lay literature concerning contraception as clients ask about, or exhibit misinformation in regard to substances such as RU486 (Mefepristone), a progesterone antagonist used in France (not available in the U.S. at this time) both as a contraceptive agent and an abortifacient (when taken within 1 month following a missed menstrual period). Note that as debate continues about introducing RU486 in the United States, combinations of other drugs already on the market are being studied with an eye toward seeking FDA approval. Two drugs in combination currently being studied for medically induced abortion purposes are methotrexate (a chemotherapeutic agent) and misoprostol (an ulcer drug). The first agent destabilizes the uterine lining; the second agent, given a week later, triggers contractions that shed the lining within about 24 h.

EVALUATION

- Evaluate the client's compliance with the oral contraceptive regimen.

DRUGS USED TO TREAT UTERINE DYSFUNCTION

Uterine dysfunction is common in premenstrual syndrome, endometriosis, and menopause. This section briefly addresses these entities and presents current pharmacologic approaches to management.

THE MENSTRUAL CYCLE

The reproductive cycle is hormonally controlled by interactions between the endocrine and reproductive systems, particularly the hypothalamus secretes gonadotropin-releasing hormone (GnRH), which stimulates the anterior pituitary to synthesize and release follicle-stimulating hormone (FSH) and luteinizing hormone (LH). These gonadotropins stimulate the ovaries to produce estrogen and progesterone.

In most women, the menstrual cycle lasts 28 days (range, 22 to 34 days). The ovarian hormones estrogen and progesterone regulate changes in the cycle, which has three ovarian phases, follicular, ovulatory, and luteal. Endometrial phases occur simultaneously with these ovarian phases. The **follicular phase** occurs during days 1 to 14 of the cycle. Days 1 to 6 of this period constitute the menstrual phase and days 6 to 14, the proliferative phase. During the total 14-day period, FSH increases and follicles begin to mature within the ovary. One graafian follicle from the group matures and swells by days 12 to 13, ruptures on day 14, and releases the ovum to the fallopian tube. The **ovulatory phase** occurs on day 14 when the ovum is released. The **luteal phase** occurs from days 15 to 28 and includes the secretory phase of the endometrial cycle. During this period, estrogen and progesterone are produced by the ovarian corpus luteum (the ruptured graafian follicle), reaching peak levels 8 days into the phase. Changes in the endometrium for optimal implantation of the ovum (if ovum is fertilized) occur. FSH and LH levels decrease, mediated somewhat by dopamine, norepinephrine, and serotonin. Estrogen and progesterone are withdrawn immediately prior to menstruation and the endometrial prostaglandin level increases. The cycle begins anew with the follicular phase. In cycles that are nonovulatory, hormonal secretion of estrogen, FSH, and LH is erratic; there is also an alteration in the usual amount of progesterone. These physiologic changes become the basis for the pharmacologic interventions employed.

PREMENSTRUAL SYNDROME

Premenstrual syndrome (PMS), first formally described and named in 1931, comprises a collection of varied physical, emotional, and behavioral symptoms. Table 44–5 lists a few of the commonly reported physical and psychobehavioral symptoms in PMS. Over 150 symptoms have been reported in the literature.

Premenstrual syndrome is often disruptive to normal life, resulting in decreased work effectiveness and impaired interpersonal relationships. PMS affects 40% of all adult women (4 to 5 million in the U.S.) to some degree, with about 5% exhibiting debilitating symptoms. There is a family history associated with the syndrome, but it is not hereditary. The syndrome is seen most commonly in women in their thirties and early forties, but it also affects

TABLE 44–5 Physical and Psychobehavioral Symptoms of Premenstrual Syndrome

Bloating in lower abdomen
Weight gain
Headache (migraine)
Increased appetite
Cravings for foods high in sugar or salt
Breast soreness
Fatigue
Sleep disorders
Backaches
Acne
Joint pain
Constipation
Feelings of being out of control
Emotional liability
Tension
Anxiety
Difficulty with concentration
Irritability
Agitation
Depression
Suicidal thoughts
Rage

adolescents. Premenstrual syndrome occurs in a repetitive regular pattern during the luteal phase (days 15 to 28) of the menstrual cycle; it decreases during the follicular phase.

There is no universal agreement about the definition, etiology, symptoms, or treatment of PMS. The most widely held theory is that PMS is linked to estrogen and progesterone levels (and the relationship of these hormones to other brain chemicals) because the symptoms are observed during the luteal phase (when levels are high) and decrease when drugs that inhibit gonadotropin-releasing hormone (GnRH) and ovulation are used. Other hypotheses center on the release of endogenous opiates (beta-endorphins), disruptions in CNS neurotransmitters, resulting in mood swings, and the role of prolactin secretion.

Diagnosis of PMS is made when the client's symptoms can be documented as consistently occurring at about the same time and in the same way over a defined number of menstrual periods. It also helps when other endocrine abnormalities can be ruled out. One difficulty encountered is that PMS is not consistent, because every cycle is not the same. Thus, measurement is problematic, particularly because every symptom that occurs associated with a menstrual period is not PMS.

Treatment of PMS includes both nonpharmacologic and pharmacologic measures. There is not one curative therapy nor any way to know what therapy may be best for a particular client other than trial and error.

Nonpharmacologic treatment includes expression of empathy for what the client is experiencing, support from family and others, correction of knowledge deficits about PMS and the menstrual cycle, exercise, dietary changes (limited salty foods, alcohol, caffeine, chocolate, concentrated sweets; four to six small high-carbohydrate, low-fat meals; rice cakes, vegetables, bagels and fresh fruit; also pancakes and syrup [without butter], pasta, soups, cereals). These foods help stabilize blood sugar levels and, as a side benefit, enhance mood. Stress reduction is also helpful, as is heightened aerobic exercise, which is believed to have a regulatory effect on estrogen and progesterone secondary to hypothalamic stimulation. These measures may help the client to feel more proactive in regard to her situation, give her a sense of overall well-being, and improve her general health. Also, endorphin levels are naturally heightened, which is found helpful.

Pharmacologic treatment remains largely empirical because research has not consistently used double-blind, placebo-controlled conditions. Some clients experience improvement with selected symptoms through use of vitamin B_6 (popular with self-help groups but not found superior to placebo) or vaginal or rectal progesterone suppositories (200 to 400 mg b.i.d.), which are commonly used but not documented as being effective and have uncommon long-term effects; in addition, individuals who exhibit depressive symptoms tend to get worse on progesterone due to its depressant effects. Also tried have been diuretics (not recommended) and prostaglandin inhibitors; bromocriptine (Parlodel) (2.5 mg b.i.d. started on day 10 of cycle and taken until menstruation begins) for breast soreness; and alprazolam (Xanax) (0.25 mg t.i.d. from day 20 of cycle to day 2 of menses, followed by one tablet per day) for treatment of anxiety, irritability, and depression. Oral contraceptives have been experimentally employed to interrupt the menstrual cycle as a form of anovulatory therapy but are not approved for this purpose. Breast tenderness is helped by caffeine reduction in the diet more than by pharmacologic intervention. Lastly, it is theorized and being studied that stronger antiprostaglandins (NSAIDs) taken when symptoms begin through the beginning of the menstrual period will prove useful in conjunction with vitamin therapy with a product that contains magnesium, calcium, pyridoxine, vitamin E, and zinc.

Recently a Canadian study demonstrated symptom reduction using fluoxetine (Prozac) (thought to work through regulating serotonin use by the brain). More study is needed, and the use of Prozac may be reserved for the most severely affected clients with protracted symptoms.

NURSING PROCESS: PREMENSTRUAL SYNDROME

ASSESSMENT

- Obtain history of PMS symptoms such as bloating, weight gain, headache, and increased appetite.

POTENTIAL NURSING DIAGNOSES

- Knowledge deficit related to the menstrual cycle and etiology of chronic alterations in mood and comfort
- Individual coping ineffective
- Family processes altered

PLANNING

- Client will receive relief from PMS from nonpharmacologic and pharmacologic measures.

NURSING INTERVENTIONS

- Provide quality client and family education in a supportive manner that encourages family communication.

CLIENT TEACHING

General
- Express that symptoms experienced are reality based and that "crazy feelings" do not mean the client is crazy.
- Explain menstrual cycle and current knowledge about PMS verbally, in writing, and graphically.
- Share current research findings regarding PMS and treatment modalities as these become better known and understood, with the client, her family, and community groups.
- Encourage client to plan to include regular aerobic exercise in her activity pattern three to five times each week.
- Review and discuss stress-reduction activities.
- Encourage family communication regarding PMS symptoms experienced by the client so that the family can understand and not personalize the client's behavior.
- Suggest sources for, and potential value of, support groups.

Diet
- Encourage client to take vitamin and mineral supplements with meals in nontoxic quantities.
- Encourage planning low-fat, low-salt, high-carbohydrate (four to six small meals) diet. Suggest suitable portable snacks for low periods (bagels, rice cakes).
- Decrease use of caffeine and increase water consumption.
- Limit intake of alcoholic beverages that may precipitate headaches.

Skill
- Have the client keep a record of what she experiences and when during her menstrual cycle to better link events with symptoms.
- If alprazolam (Xanax) is ordered, discuss issues of dependency and withdrawal.
- If danazol (Danocrine) is ordered, see the guidelines included below for use of the drug in endometriosis.

TABLE 44–6 Drug Therapy for Endometriosis

Drug	Dosage	Uses and Considerations
Danazol (Danocrine)	PO: 400 mg, b.i.d. for 4–6 mon. Can extend to 9 mon. Can restart if symptoms return.	Pituitary gonadotropin inhibitory agent. No estrogenic or progestational action. Suppresses and atrophies intra- and extrauterine tissue; menses cease during therapy and no ovulation occurs; pain is relieved. Ovulation/menses usually recur within 90 d after treatment. Commonly used for women with infertility associated with endometriosis. Used for PMS on investigational basis. Contraindicated in pregnancy, breast feeding, abnormal genital bleeding, impaired heart, liver, or kidney function, severe hypertension. Can alter some laboratory values (e.g., decreased HDL, increased LDL). Can increase insulin requirements and, if given with warfarin, cause a prolonged PT. Therapy started during menstruation or after pregnancy ruled out. If therapy is for fibrocystic breast disease, breast carcinoma must also be ruled out before treatment. Pharmacokinetics: Absorbed well orally; 2–4 h peak action; 4.5 h half-life; biotransformed by liver. Therapeutic effects occur within 3 wk of daily therapy. Excreted in the urine. *Pregnancy category:* X.

TABLE 44–6 Drug Therapy for Endometriosis (*Continued*)

Drug	Dosage	Uses and Considerations
		Adverse effects: thrombocytopenia, hypertension, depression, headache, *hot flashes, weight gain,* androgenic effects, hemorrhagic cystitis, hematuria, hepatotoxicity, cholestatic hepatitis, acne, rashes, oily skin, hirsutism, bloating, *muscle cramps,* voice deepening (irreversible), hearing loss, mood swings, anxiety, fatigue, nausea, vomiting, diarrhea, constipation. Also produces atherogenic lipid profile. Many clients cannot tolerate side effects and discontinue drug. Alternate doses may be used for clients with hereditary angioedema and fibrocystic breast disease.
Gonadotropin-Releasing Hormone (GnRH) Agonists Leuprolide acetate for depot suspension (Lupron Depot 3.75)	IM: 3.75 mg q mon for up to 6 mon	As an agonist, initially stimulates FSH and LH, but over time, creates prolonged suppression, which causes decreased ovarian secretion of estrogen/progesterone, resulting in a hypoestrogenic state. Lack of hormonal stimulation causes regression of displaced endometrial tissue. Contains no androgen. Found as effective as danazol in reducing extent of endometriosis. Normal function returns in 4 to 12 wk after treatment discontinued. Contraindicated in actual or potential pregnancy, undiagnosed vaginal bleeding and breast feeding since is not known if excreted in breast milk. FDA classification 3B.* *Pregnancy category:* X. Pharmacokinetics: Therapeutic levels detected for at least 4 wk after injection; 85%–100% released within 4 wk with no accumulation. $t\frac{1}{2}$: 3–4.2 s h; PB: 46%. Side effects: hot flashes, headaches, decreased libido, dry vagina, night sweats, mood changes, mild bone loss (usually regained within 6 mon of finishing treatment). Initial dose best given during day 1–3 of menstrual cycle to avoid affecting a pregnancy. Barrier contraceptives should be used during treatment because pregnancy is possible. Minimal changes produced in lipid profile. Retreatment not recommended because safety data beyond 6 mon are not available.
Nafarelin acetate (Synarel Nasal Solution)	400 μg daily, administered as one spray (200 μg) into one nostril in morning and one spray (200 μg) into other nostril for up to 6 mon	Contains no androgen. Controlled studies comparing Synarel (400 μg) and danazol (600 or 800 μg/d) found higher hypoestrogenic (therapeutic state) but less androgenic side effects. Found comparable in reducing extent of endometriosis and in effect on associated client symptoms. Maintains LDL/HDL ratio. Return of normal function in 4–12 wk after treatment discontinued. Contraindicated in those sensitive to GnRH, GnRH analogs, or inert substances included in product; other contraindications include actual or potential pregnancy, undiagnosed vaginal bleeding, and breast feeding. Clients with rhinitis should have a topical decongestant prescribed by health care provider and use at least 30 min after Synarel. FDA classification 1B.† Pharmacokinetics: Maximum serum concentrations achieved in 10–40 min; serum half-life approximately 3 h (range, 0.8–10 h); 80% bound to plasma proteins; drug elimination after intranasal administration has not been studied. Side effects are those seen in a natural menopause due to a hypoestrogenic state, notably hot flashes, vaginal dryness, decreased libido, headaches, and emotional lability.

KEY: *FSH: follicle-stimulating hormone; GnRH: gonadotropin-releasing hormone; HDL: high-density lipoproteins; IM: intramuscular; LDL: low-density lipoproteins; LH: luteinizing hormone; PB: protein-binding; PO: by mouth; PT: prothrombin time; t½: half-life.*
* *A new formulation of a compound already on the market which offers a modest therapeutic gain over currently available agents.*
† *A new chemical entity that offers a modest therapeutic gain over currently available agents.*

Two other forms of experimental (not FDA approved) hormonal anovulatory treatment are danazol (Danocrine) and GnRH agonists. These formulations are presented in Table 44–6 following the discussion of endometriosis, for which these agents are approved therapy.

ENDOMETRIOSIS

Endometriosis is the abnormal location of endometrical tissue outside of the uterus in the pelvic cavity; it has no single, clearly identifiable cause.

Possible etiologies are retrograde menstruation (backward movement of endometrial cells through the fallopian tubes out into the abdomen) or spread through the lymphatic or vascular systems. Regardless of cause, the displaced endometrial tissue is generally found affixed to the ovaries, on the posterior surface of the uterus, the uterosacral ligaments, the broad ligaments, or the bowel. The displaced tissue responds to hormonal control, particularly estrogen, from the ovaries in the same way as the tissue inside the uterus. Thus, when menstruation occurs, this extrauterine tissue also bleeds. As the number of menstrual cycles experienced by the client increases, the result is inflammation, scar tissue formation, and adhesions.

Clients with endometriosis may be symptomatic (about 75%) or asymptomatic (those diagnosed during infertility work-ups). The diagnosis is made based on symptoms presented and laparoscopic evidence of endometrial tissue. Symptoms include severe low-back and pelvic pain that increases with menstruation. Painful, sometimes bloody bowel movements during menstruation have been reported, as has painful sexual intercourse (**dyspareunia**). Irregular bleeding (spotting) pre- and postmenses is common. Long term, there is an association with primary or secondary infertility; about 25% to 40% of infertile women exhibit the condition. Endometriosis may obstruct or affect the motility of the fallopian tubes. There is also a risk that nearby organs (e.g., urinary and gastrointestinal tracts) may become obstructed due to invasion by endometrial tissue.

Endometriosis is found most often in women who have delayed childbearing until their thirties, although it may occur during adolescence. There is an increased prevalence rate of 7% for siblings and daughters of affected women. Approximately 5 million women are affected in the United States. Affected women may exhibit increased ectopic pregnancy rates and difficult pregnancies and labors.

Some success is being achieved in treating endometriosis using a laser during operative lap-aroscopy to remove or destroy endometrial growths.

Three drugs are approved for use in endometriosis: danazol (Danocrine) and two gonadotropin-releasing hormone (GnRH) agonists, leuprolide acetate (Lupron Depot) and nafarelin acetate (Synarel). Danazol has been the drug of choice, but use of the GnRH agonists is increasing. These three drugs are presented in Table 44–6.

In long-term and highly painful endometriosis that has not been controlled with drug therapy or laparoscopy, hysterectomy (including ovary removal) may be elected.

NURSING PROCESS: ENDOMETRIOSIS

ASSESSMENT

- Obtain a complete client history, including menstrual history.
- Identify the client's fertility plans.
- Review chart to see if baseline liver function studies have been obtained.

Side Effects and Adverse Reactions

Danazol

Side effects due to mild androgenic properties include weight gain, acne, mild hirsutism, oily skin and hair, decrease in breast size, deepening of the voice, and increased appetite. Side effects due to hypoestrogenic properties include hot flashes or flushing, sweating, vaginitis (itching, dryness, burning), and mood swing. A few clients may also exhibit emotional depression, anxiety, fatigue, nausea, vomiting, diarrhea, and constipation. The incidence of side effects is reduced with lower doses (<800 mg/d). The drug may also result in decreased high-density lipoprotein (HDL) and increased low-density lipoprotein (LDL) levels. There is a 4% chance of conceiving during a given cycle.

In general, the side effects of the GnRH agonists that follow are better tolerated by women than are the side effects of Danazol. However, estrogen levels are more suppressed with the GnRH agonists; thus, hypoestrogenic effects are more pronounced.

Leuprolide Acetate (Lupron Depot 3.75)

Side effects include vasodilation (hot flashes), vaginal dryness, decreased libido, headache, nervousness, dizziness, and depression. Transient minor localized irritation at the injection site may occur. The major risk is potential loss of bone density; the degree of reversibility after the treatment is under study.

Nafarelin Acetate (Synarel Nasal Solution)

Side effects are related to the drug's hypoestrogenic effects and include vasodilation (hot flashes), vaginal dryness, decreased libido, headaches, and emotional lability.

Because the GnRH agonists as a group are generally well tolerated, there is less discontinuation of therapy related to side effects. In some cases an oral progestin or clonidine may be added to address the vasomotor symptoms experienced.

- Check to see if a pregnancy test has been done before starting the drug.

Leuprolide Acetate
- Review the client's history for risk factors associated with major bone loss for which the drug may pose an additional risk.

POTENTIAL NURSING DIAGNOSES

- Discomfort (acute and chronic) related to hormonally controlled displaced endometrial tissue
- Activity limitation secondary to painful menstrual cycles
- Knowledge deficit related to menstrual cycle, displaced endometrial tissue, etiology of pain, and treatment options

PLANNING

- Client will be free of pain/discomfort due to endometriosis with the use of danazol, leuprolide acetate, or nafarelin acetate.

NURSING INTERVENTIONS

Danazol
- Observe the client for signs of anxiety about potential loss of fertility and amount of time involved in treatment.
- Recall that the drug must be started during the client's menstrual period.

Leuprolide Acetate
- Store product and diluent at room temperature.
- Must be reconstituted and used immediately (no preservatives). Reconstituted product must be shaken to create a milky suspension. Use supplied syringe.

CLIENT TEACHING

Danazol
- Discuss the purpose, action, and side effects of the drug with the client. Explain that the medication is expensive. Explain length of treatment.
- Plan with the client for the use of a back-up nonhormonal form of birth control.
- Tell the client that menses will usually return in 2 to 3 months after treatment.
- Tell the client to have one menstrual cycle after treatment is completed before trying to become pregnant.

Diet
- Ask the client to keep a food history. Suggest increased exercise to help offset weight gain that is experienced by 75% (average, 4 kg); suggest caloric control plan based on history.
- Increase water consumption.

Skill
- Teach the client breast self-examination.

Side Effects
- Suggest that the client carry minipads for spotting

during the first month of therapy. Tell the client to report any bleeding to her health care provider.
- Discuss removal of unwanted hair and skin care for acne prevention.
- Suggest client wash her face and hair more often due to oily scalp and skin and use oil-free makeup and shampoo.
- If acne occurs, consult a dermatologist.
- If muscle cramps occur, try warm-up exercises prior to active workout and gradually increase exertion.

Leuprolide Acetate
- Explain to the client that drug causes a temporary state of menopause.
- Explain that the treatment process requires one injection each month.
- Explain that the drug is palliative and temporarily effective in reducing symptoms. It does not create a change in basic physiology, metabolism, or hormone production. When treatment is complete, whatever is normal for the client will return over time.
- Advise the client that initially there may be an increase in clinical signs and symptoms of endometriosis. These will disappear.
- Explain that 6 months is the accepted duration of therapy for GnRH agonists. Safety data are available only for 6-month use. Retreatment is not recommended.

Skill
- Remind client that she must use a nonhormonal contraceptive method during treatment.

Side Effects
- If the client is concerned about potential bone loss, state that one 6-month course of treatment has been found to cause only a small loss. However, clients who are at higher risk for bone loss due to chronic alcoholism, tobacco use, strong family history of osteoporosis, or chronic use of anticonvulsants or corticosteroids should carefully discuss the decision for or against therapy with this drug.
- Stress that the client must be consistent in receiving her doses of the drug, or breakthrough bleeding or ovulation can occur.
- Tell the client to inform the health care provider if menstruation persists while being treated.
- Suggest client add weight-bearing exercise and walking or low-impact aerobics to offset bone loss.
- Discuss mood changes secondary to hormonal changes with drug and possible emotional lability; suggest support network and resource groups.

- If vaginal dryness occurs, suggest client use water-based lubricants and try alternate sexual positions for intercourse.
- If night sweats occur, suggest cotton bedclothes, change of clothes, resist chilling by gradually exposing body to room air from under bed covers; also, contact health care provider if sleep disturbances persist.

Diet
- Suggest increased calcium-based food products.

Nafarelin Acetate
- Explain that precise guidelines must be followed by the client if the treatment is to be effective.
- Ask the client if she is allergic to any component of the drug including nafarelin base, benzalkonium chloride, acetic acid, sodium hydroxide, hydrochloride, or sorbitol.
- Tell the client that the action of the drug, guidelines for birth control use, hypoestrogenic effects, and return of normal function are the same as for leuprolide.
- Advise the client that the medication is expensive and is provided as a 30-day supply. She will need to be sure she can absorb the expense of 6 months of therapy so that treatment is not interrupted.

Skill
- Stress that the client must use the drug twice a day (every 12 h) for the full duration of treatment.
- Tell the client to start the drug between days 2 and 4 of the menstrual period.
- The client must be told of the need to prime the spray pump only before the first use. The sprayer is designed to deliver the exact correct dose each time. A fine spray will occur after 7 to 10 pushes on the pump. If a thin stream occurs, she should call her pharmacist immediately. Directions and diagrams are included.
- Tell the client to store the bottle upright below 86°F out of light. Because she must use it every 12 h, it is suggested she put it in a place that will remind her, such as near her toothbrush or a commonly used product (morning and night) that is kept out of direct light.
- Tell the client she should record each dose on a supplied chart and to refill prescription so as not to miss any doses.
- Tell the client it is permissible to use a nasal decongestant spray (with health care provider's knowledge) while on Synarel. Use the Synarel spray first and allow 30 minutes to elapse before using the decongestant spray.
- The client should blow her nose to clear both nostrils before using the drug. She should bend forward and place the spray tip in one nostril aimed at the back and outer side of her nose. She should close the other nostril with her finger and then spray one time while sniffing gently, then tilt her head back to spread the drug over the back of the nose. She must be told *not* to spray in the second nostril unless told to do so by her doctor. The other side is used for the next dose.

Side Effects
- Advise the client that she may note irregular vaginal spotting or bleeding, which should decrease and stop on its own unless doses are missed.
- See Leuprolide—similar effects and potential remedial actions.

Diet
- See Leuprolide—same recommendations.

EVALUATION
- Evaluate the effectiveness of the drug regimen. If pain or discomfort is still present, notify the health care provider. Drug dose adjustment may be necessary.

MENOPAUSE

The transitional process experienced by women as they move from the reproductive into the nonreproductive stage of life is called the female climacteric, a natural event. The "change of life" experience is perceived by women in an individualized way on a continuum from no difficulty to severe difficulty. This phase of life occurs for most women somewhere between the late thirties to the late fifties. The climacteric can be divided into premenopause, menopause, and postmenopause, during which certain physiologic events occur.

Menopause is defined as the actual or permanent end of menstruation due to decreased ovarian function. The average age at menopause is about 50 years (range 45 to 55). Women who experience menopause before age 40 years are referred to as having premature menopause. This natural event is documented as having occurred once a woman has had no menstrual periods for 1 year. The triggering event for the onset of natural menopause is not known. Menopause can also occur abruptly as a secondary effect of surgical removal of the ovaries (oophorectomy), radiologic procedures in which ovarian function is destroyed, severe infection, ovarian tumors, or as a temporarily induced state for treatment of entities such as endometriosis.

The premenopausal period may last for over 5 years before true menopause occurs. During this period, menstrual variations begin to be evident. For example, menstrual periods may occur as usual; be lighter in flow; or last shorter time. They may begin, stop, and then start again, or be of longer duration, with a heavier flow that may contain blood clots. Sudden episodes of vasodilation (hot flashes) can also begin to occur periodically in some women. Others experience vaginal dryness. These unpredictable changes may last for several years and are probably due to alterations in the hypothalamic-pituitary-ovarian feedback system.

Postmenopause is the period when the body tries to adapt to a new hormonal environment. Although the production of estrogen and progesterone from the ovaries decreases during the late premenopausal and early postmenopausal periods, the ovary is able to secrete androgens (testosterone) in varying amounts due to the influence of increased LH levels. During this period, androstenedione (the main androgen secreted by the ovaries and adrenal cortex, which is present in reduced amounts postmenopause) is converted into estrone (a naturally occurring estrogen formed in extraglandular tissue of the brain, liver, kidney, and adipose tissue), which represents the main source of available estrogen once the ovaries lose the ability to produce estradiol. Table 44–7 presents common physical effects associated with the climacteric.

Hormone Replacement Therapy

Hormone replacement therapy (HRT) is the most prevalent treatment for relief of vasodilation and vaginal dryness and for prevention of cardiovascular disease and osteoporosis. Oral estrogen, most commonly in the form of conjugated estrogens, is taken by the client together with the synthetic hor-

TABLE 44–7 Common Physical Effects Associated with the Female Climacteric

Hypoestrogenic State	Effects
Irregular menstruation	Variable frequency, duration, intensity
Vasodilation	Hot flashes or transient sensations of intense heat in upper chest, neck and head; visible flushing; sweating; chills; tachycardia; sleep disruption
Vaginal alterations	Dryness; decreased lubrication during sexual stimulation; thinning. Decreased acidity and increased irritation response to stressors such as intercourse can cause increased vaginitis (itching, burning, discharge). Increased incidence of prolapse/cystocele
Decreased bone mass (osteoporosis)	Backache, reduced height, sudden fracture, particularly in thin, fair, small-boned women and those with a family history, no pregnancies, sedentary lifestyle, inadequate diet, smoking, alcohol use, or use of drugs that increase calcium loss (anticonvulsants, corticosteroids). Most rapid decrease in mass (particularly in hips, spine and torso) occurs in first 3–5 y postmenopause and slows after age 65
Additional Effects Due to Menopause Combined with Natural Aging	
Urethral disorders	Loss of urethral tone, painful urination, urgency, frequency, and stress incontinence
Decreased breast size	
Decreased skin elasticity	Facial, neck, and hand wrinkling; variations in quantity and distribution of body hair
Lower HDL levels	Increased risk (3×) for cardiovascular disease postmenopause as LDLs rise
Abdominal fat development	Greater degree of central android abdominal fat accumulates due to altered peripheral resistance to insulin and increase in type II diabetes as aging progresses (lower incidence in estrogen users)
Hyperinsulinemia	
Short-term memory loss	In some women (estrogen may have some stabilizing effect on maintenance of short-term memory)

KEY: HDL: high-density lipoproteins; LDL: low-density lipoproteins.

mone progestin in one of several possible, but still controversial, treatment regimens. The progestin is added to minimize the risk of endometrial hyperplasia, endometrial cancer, and breast cancer from the use of estrogen alone. The progestin, however, has potential negative effects, including potential PMS-type symptoms, breast pathology, and alterations in lipid metabolism. Thus, progestin partially blunts the beneficial effects of estrogen and the client has much to consider when deciding the course of action she wants to elect.

In the United States, the typical approach in HRT is to use an oral estrogen in the lowest dose to control symptoms (most commonly 0.625 mg/d), for days 1 to 25 of the month, with the addition of progesterone (Provera) 10 mg from days 16 to 25. In Europe, it is common for the estrogen and progesterone to be taken together every day without any days off.

Currently, there is no one absolutely correct HRT management regimen. Healthy care providers continue to experiment with either cyclic or continuous estrogen with progestin (for 12 days per month) or a combined continuous approach in which both the estrogen and progestin are taken daily without interruption.

Regardless of approach, the goal is to use the lowest effective dose of the least metabolically active progestin to oppose the stimulation of the endometrium.

When **estrogen replacement therapy** (ERT) is selected, in conjunction with nonpharmacologic measures (see Client Teaching) to prevent bone loss, it is important to start the regimen early in menopause and continue for at least 10 years following menopause. Clients who select HRT often taper off after 2 or 3 years and the menopausal symptoms, such as vaginal changes and hot flashes, return at some point.

Compliance with treatment regimens shifts with the health reports in the lay press that bring the latest piece of worrisome or hopeful news. For example, the two major reasons women choose not to use estrogen therapy or to decrease their compliance are fear of breast cancer and resumption of withdrawal bleeding. Women may often deemphasize the tremendous preventive health care benefits.

Dosage forms in estrogen replacement therapy include oral, transdermal, vaginal cream, injections, and pellets, along with a variety of types of estrogen. The natural or biologic estrogens (comprised of estrones [including conjugated equine estrogens, esterified estrogens and piperazine estrone sulfate] and estradiols [including micronized estradiol and estradiol valerate or 17β-estradiol]) are preferred for use in postmenopausal clients over the synthetic estrogens (ethinyl estradiol, mestranol) used for oral contraception. Synthetic estrogens are believed to be more taxing to the renal and hepatic systems than biologic estrogens. Conjugated estrogens, mixtures of natural estrogens isolated from the urine of pregnant mares, are the most commonly used preparations for estrogen replacement therapy. Premarin is the most frequently used conjugated estrogen product and is presented in Figure 44–1.

The goal of replacement therapy has bearing on the dosage form. For example, bone protection requires extended systemic therapy, while treatment of hot flashes may involve shorter-term therapy. Vaginal changes may be treated with local or systemic therapy, or both.

Contraindications

Contraindications to estrogen replacement therapy include pregnancy, history of endometrial or breast cancer within the last 5 years, history of thromboembolic disorders, acute liver disease or chronic impaired liver function, gallbladder or pancreatic disease, poorly controlled hypertension, undiagnosed genital bleeding, and endometriosis. Lifestyle factors, such as smoking, known to enhance risk of thromboembolism should be considered in the treatment decision. The client with a history of fibroid tumors is not started on estrogen replacement for a full year after the last period, because estrogen would likely result in further growth. The hypoestrogenic state associated with natural menopause usually causes existing fibroids to shrink. The presence of fibrocystic breast disease, diabetes, or obesity may require extra caution. Estrogen is not thought to cause breast cancer, but the promotion of growth in an incipient breast cancer is a possibility. Doses used in estrogen replacement therapy are generally low.

Contraindications to progestin replacement in conjunction with estrogen replacement therapy are the same as those for estrogen. It is extremely important to rule out the presence of known or suspected breast cancer before progestins are used.

Dosage Forms

The oral route is the most commonly employed; it is well tolerated by most clients and relatively easy to use but does require daily dosing. Some clients will experience GI upsets, particularly nausea and vomiting. Clients with GI disorders such as colitis, irritable bowel syndrome, peptic ulcer, or malabsorption may receive inconsistent doses with oral

FIGURE 44–1. Estrogen Replacements

Conjugated Estrogens	Dosage	NURSING PROCESS
		Assessment and Planning
Conjugated estrogens (Premarin, PMB, Milprem-400) Hormone replacement therapy (HRT) *Pregnancy Category X*	A: PO: 0.3–1.25 mg/d cyclically (with or without progestins); most often, 0.625 mg/d)	
Contraindications	**Drug-Lab-Food Interactions**	
Breast or reproductive cancer, undiagnosed genital bleeding, pregnancy, lactation, thromboembolitic disorders, smoking *Caution:* Cardiovascular disease, severe renal or hepatic disease, smoking, diabetes mellitus	*Increase* effects with corticosteroids *Decrease* effects of anticoagulants, oral hypoglycemics; *decrease* effects with rifampin, anticonvulsants, barbiturates Toxicity with tricyclic antidepressants	
Pharmacokinetics	**Pharmacodynamics**	Interventions

Absorption: PO: Well absorbed
Distribution: PB: Widely distributed; crosses placenta and enters breast milk
Metabolism: t½: UK
Excretion: In urine and bile
	PO/IV: Onset: Rapid
	          Peak: UK
	          Duration: UK
	IM: Onset: Delayed
	          Peak: UK
	          Duration: UK	

	Evaluation
Therapeutic Effects/Uses: To relieve vasodilation, hot flashes, and vaginal dryness, to prevent cardiovascular disease and osteoporosis. *Mode of Action:* Development and maintenance of female genital system, breast, and secondary sex characteristics; increased synthesis of protein.	

Side Effects	Adverse Reactions
Nausea, vomiting, fluid retention, breast tenderness, leg cramps and breakthrough bleeding, chloasma	Jaundice, thromboembolic disorders, depression, hypercalcemia, gall bladder disease *Life-threatening:* Thromboembolism, cerebrovascular accident, pulmonary embolism, MI, endometrial cancer

KEY: A: adult; PO: by mouth; tab: tablet; inj: injection; PB: protein-binding; UK: unknown; t½: half-life; MI: myocardial infarction.

administration, necessitating the use of another dosage form. Oral estrogens have a particularly beneficial effect on lipids by increasing high-density lipoproteins. Although the oral route does result in complete absorption from the GI tract, there is greater impact upon liver proteins.

The transdermal skin patch (the Estraderm Transdermal System) is a convenient method because it does not require daily dosing. The patch is applied to intact skin in the prescribed dosage.

Generally the lower abdomen is used, but other sites (except for the breasts) may be employed. The patch is applied twice a week for 3 weeks, with rotation of sites, followed by 1 week without use of the patch to allow for normal withdrawal bleeding. The transdermal patch allows for absorption of the estrogen (17β estradiol) directly into the blood stream through a membrane that limits the absorption rate. The advantage is that the GI tract and liver are bypassed initially, which results in less

TABLE 44–8 Estrogens and Progestins

Generic (Brand)	Route and Dosage	Pregnancy Category
Conjugated Estrogens		
Premarin	See Prototype Drug Chart (Fig. 44–1)	
Steroidal Estrogens		
Estradiol (Estrace, Estraderm)	*Menopausal/hypogonadism:*	X
	PO: 1–2 mg/d for 21 d; then, 7–10 d off cycle; may repeat cycle	
	Patch: 10–20 cm² system 2×/wk, in above cycle	
	Breast cancer:	
	10 mg t.i.d.	
	Prostate cancer:	
	1–2 mg t.i.d.	
	Atrophic vaginitis:	
	Cream: 2–4 g/d for 1–2 wk; maint: 1 g 2×/wk	
Estradiol cypionate (Depo-Estradiol Cypionate)	*Menopausal symptoms:*	X
	IM: 1–4 mg q3–4 wk	
	Hypogonadism:	
	IM: 1.5–2 mg q mon	
Esterified estrogens (Estratab, Menest)	*Menopausal symptoms:*	X
	PO: 0.3–1.25 mg/d for 3 wk; then 7–10 d off cycle	
	Breast cancer:	
	PO: 10 mg t.i.d.	
	Prostate cancer:	
	1.25–2.5 mg t.i.d.	
Estrone (Theelin, Kestrone 5)	*Hypogonadism:*	X
	0.1–2 mg/wk	
	Prostate cancer:	
	2–4 mg 3×/wk	
Estropipate SO₄ (Ogen, Ortho-Est)	*Hypogonadism:*	X
	1.25–7.5 mg/d for 3 wk; then 7–10 d off cycle	
Nonsteroidal Estrogens		
Chlorotrianisene (Tace)	*Menopausal/hypogonadism:*	X
	12–25 mg/d for 21 d; then, 10 d off cycle; repeat cycle	
	Prostate cancer:	
	12–25 mg/d	
Dienestrol (DV)	*Atrophic vaginitis:*	X
	Cream: Apply q.d./b.i.d. for 1–2 wk; maint: 1–3×/wk	
Diethylstilbestrol	*Breast cancer:*	X
	15 mg/d	
	Prostate cancer:	
	1–3 mg t.i.d.	
Quinestrol (Estrovis)	*Menopausal/hypogonadism:*	X
	100 μg daily for 7 d; then 7 d off cycle; maint: q wk	
Progestins		
Progesterone	*DUB:*	X
	IM: 5–10 mg/d for 7 d	
	Amenorrhea:	
	IM: 5–10 mg/d for 6–8 d	
Medroxyprogesterone acetate (Amen, Curretab, Provera, Cycrin, Depo-Provera)	*DUB/amenorrhea:*	X
	5–10 mg/d for 5–10 d	
	Endometriosis:	
	IM: 150 mg q3mon	
Megestrol acetate (Megace)	*Breast cancer:*	X
	PO: 40 mg q.i.d.	
	Endometrial cancer:	
	40–320 mg/d in divided doses	
Norethindrone (Norlutin)	*DUB/amenorrhea:*	X
	5–20 mg/d on days 5–25 of menstrual cycle	

nausea and vomiting and less impact upon liver proteins.

Vaginal cream preparations are used in the treatment of vaginal atrophy, which causes painful intercourse and urinary difficulties. Vaginal cream preparations containing conjugated estrogens are rapidly absorbed into the blood stream via the mucous membrane that lines the vagina. There is some question as to the amount of estrogen that is systemically absorbed through this route; thus, it is not usually used to provide protection against bone loss. It can be used in conjunction with another method, such as tablets or the transdermal patch.

Medroxyprogesterone acetate (Provera), the progestin most often administered in combination with the estrogen, is taken orally. Examples of products employed in estrogen replacement therapy are given in Table 44–8.

Pharmacokinetics

The natural estrogens are completely and rapidly absorbed from the GI tract and rapidly metabolized by the liver, necessitating daily doses when oral products that are nonesterified (a process that delays metabolism and lengthens action) are used. About 80% of estradiol is bound to sex hormone binding globulin, with 2% unbound and the rest bound to albumin. Estradiol is converted to estrone in the enterohepatic circulation, and is conjugated and excreted via the urine. Progestin (Provera) is rapidly absorbed and metabolized primarily in the liver with excretion via the kidney; distribution of the agent is not well described.

Side Effects and Adverse Reactions

ESTROGEN

After being screened for contraindications, most individuals using low-dose biologic estrogen have few, if any, side effects. Occasional clients experience nausea and vomiting, fluid retention, breast tenderness, leg cramps, and breakthrough bleeding.

Serious adverse reactions to estrogen include thromboembolic disorders (higher incidence in women over age 40, even after discontinuing the therapy), stroke, pulmonary embolism, myocardial infarction, endometrial carcinoma (dose- and duration-related, especially if estrogen is not given cyclically with progestin), acceleration of preexisting but nondiagnosed breast tumors, and gallbladder disease.

PROGESTIN

Side effects are infrequent but include leg cramps, fluid retention, bloating, GI distress, mood swings, and depression. All are dose related. Serious adverse reactions include thrombophlebitis, pulmonary embolism, hypersensitivity, visual disturbances, migraine headache, severe depression, cholestatic jaundice, and hyperglycemia.

NURSING PROCESS: ESTROGEN REPLACEMENTS

ASSESSMENT

- Assess the client for baseline data, including height, weight, usual physical activity, diet, family history, and personal risk factors regarding osteoporosis, family and personal risk of cardiovascular disease, and the nature of the family members' climacteric experience, the client's menstrual history, and current experience with the climacteric and the drugs the client is using.
- Assess the client's perception of menopause.
- Assess the client's attitude toward resumption of menstrual periods.

POTENTIAL NURSING DIAGNOSES

- Sexual dysfunction
- Body image disturbance
- Health-seeking behaviors

PLANNING

- Client will know menopausal symptoms and the nonpharmacologic and pharmacologic measures that may aid in alleviating symptoms.

NURSING INTERVENTIONS

- Educate women about the nature of the climacteric, its potential effects, and nonpharmacologic as well as pharmacologic treatment. Place current educational materials in health and community sites.
- Indicate on the laboratory slip or specimen that the client is taking hormone replacement therapy (HRT).
- Administer IM route at bedtime to decrease adverse effects.
- Administer IV route slowly to avoid flushing reaction.

CLIENT TEACHING

General
- Review the risk-to-benefit ratio for deciding to use or not to use estrogen replacement therapy.
- Review the contraindications to this HRT.
- Advise the client to have a thorough breast examination, pelvic examination, Pap test, and endometrial biopsy before starting HRT.
- Tell the client that warm weather and stress exacerbate vasodilation/hot flashes.
- Advise the client to use a fan, drink cool liquids,

wear layered cotton clothes, decrease intake of caffeine and spicy foods, and talk with her health care provider about the use of vitamin E to cope more comfortably with vasodilation. Individuals with diabetes, hypertension, or rheumatic heart disease should use vitamin E in low doses with the health care provider's approval.

- Encourage the client on HRT to have medical follow-up every 6 to 12 mo, including blood pressure check and breast and pelvic examinations.
- Suggest that the client carry sanitary pads or tampons for breakthrough bleeding or irregular periods.
- Stress the need to use nonhormonal birth control because irregular periods may create anxiety about pregnancy. Tell the client to plan to use birth control for 2 y. If she has progesterone-induced bleeding, the only way to determine whether she is truly menopausal is by hormone assay.
- Suggest to the client that she use a water-soluble vaginal lubricant to reduce painful intercourse (dyspareunia) and prevent trauma.
- Advise the client to decrease use of antihistamines and decongestants if she is experiencing vaginal dryness.
- Advise the client to wear cotton underwear and pantyhose with a cotton liner and to avoid douche and feminine hygiene products.
- Suggest that client take Premarin after meals together with progestin to avoid nausea and vomiting.
- Tell the client to report any heavy bleeding (flooding) and to have her hematocrit and hemoglobin evaluated for anemia.
- Tell the client to report bleeding that occurs between periods or return of bleeding after cessation of menstruation. A cancer work-up may be indicated.
- Advise the client starting on HRT that the withdrawal bleeding that occurs from days 25 to 30 is normal and not the same as the cyclic menstrual periods she had secondary to ovulation. Tell her that this bleeding will usually last only 2 to 3 d and that she will not experience the same degree of premenstrual symptoms she may have had with regular periods.
- Advise the client to report if bleeding occurs other than on days 25 to 30 once she has started on HRT.
- Tell her that the withdrawal bleeding does not

signify that she can become pregnant (since she is not fertile).
- Advise the client that after HRT is discontinued, there may be a recurrence of menopausal signs and symptoms such as hot flashes.

Diet

- Discuss the use of yogurt containing *Acidophilus* or *Lactobacillus* as a way of maintaining normal bacterial flora in the vagina.
- Tell the client that she may experience an occasional hot flash on days 25 to 30 when she is going through withdrawal bleeding. Instruct the client to stop treatment and contact health care provider if she has headache, visual disturbances, signs of thrombophlebitis, heaviness in legs, chest pain, or breast lumps.
- Tell the client that if she wants to stop HRT, she should do so with guidance of her health care provider.
- Suggest that the client at risk for osteoporosis have consistent exercise such as walking or bicycling, eat a well-balanced diet (low in red meat and sugar) with 1200 mg calcium/d if premenopausal or 1200 to 1500 mg/d if menopausal, and avoid smoking and alcohol.

Skill

- Teach the client to perform breast self-examination consistently.
- If the client is using vaginal cream, review the application procedure and suggest that she wear minipads.
- If the client is using the transdermal patch, tell her to open the package and apply it immediately, holding it in place for about 10 s; to check the edges to ensure adequate contact; to use the abdomen (except waistline) for the patch; to rotate the sites with at least 1 wk before reuse of a site; to not use the breast as a site; to not put the patch on an irritated or oily area; to reapply the patch if it loosens or put on a new one; and to follow the same cycle schedule.

EVALUATION

- Evaluate the effectiveness of the nonpharmacologic or pharmacologic measures for premenopausal symptoms.
- Determine whether side effects are occurring. Plan with the client alternative measures to control menopausal symptoms.

■ CASE STUDY

Tanya, following delivery of baby Jessica (presented in Chapter 43), is ready to leave the hospital. She has had three pregnancies, one birth. She developed pregnancy-induced hypertension during the pregnancy but has no prior history of hypertension. She plans to breast feed for 3 months. She does not want to become pregnant again soon. She asks you questions about hormonally controlled birth control methods.

1. Tanya asks if she can take combination birth control pills and also breast feed. Describe a nursing diagnosis for Tanya based on her communication to you.

2. You tell her that she may breast feed and start using combination pills in about 6 weeks once the milk flow is established although she might wish to consider another method. This information is:
   Correct:_____ Why? _____
   Incorrect:_____ Why? _____

3. Tanya asks you if there are any advantages to the use of the oral contraceptives instead of using a diaphragm. List four arguments for and four against the products that a nurse could include in her discussions with clients about birth control.

4. Tanya tells you that she smokes about ¾ of a pack of cigarettes per day. Describe how this piece of information might impact the decision for or against oral contraceptive use.

5. Tanya starts to use combination birth control pills and calls the clinic upset that she has forgotten to take one pill. What would you expect the clinic nurse to tell Tanya to do? How might the nurse in the postpartum unit prepare Tanya for this eventuality ahead of time?

6. Because milk flow needs to become established prior to starting on the combination birth control pills for at least 6 weeks (should she elect this method), what would you recommend to Tanya about contraception upon leaving the hospital? Consider that Tanya had a fourth-degree episiotomy and hemorrhoids.

7. Tanya states that when she has "bad allergies" she sometimes takes over-the-counter antihistamines. You know that she plans to use oral contraceptives. Do you raise any concerns about this with Tanya? Why?

8. When would you suggest Tanya take her birth control pills and what advantage might this offer her?

9. Considering Tanya's age, you decide to raise the issue of injectable progestin (Depo-Provera) with her as an alternative method.

10. What advantage might this product have for Tanya instead of using oral products?

11. Can Tanya breast feed while using this product?

12. You recall that Tanya smokes. What implication does this have in regard to known side effects with Depo-Provera?

13. Should Tanya elect to use this method, why should you document the site in which the injection is given?

14. How would you explain the way Depo-Provera works to Tanya?

15. She asks how long it will take to regain her fertility once she quits using the method. You can correctly respond with what information?

STUDY QUESTIONS

1. What key factors should the nurse cover in a teaching plan for oral contraceptive use? What is the degree of effectiveness of oral contraceptives? What are the advantages and disadvantages of this method?

2. What are some common symptoms associated with PMS? What are effective treatment modalities for the symptoms?

3. Explain the expected effects of drug therapy for endometriosis using danazol or gonadotropin-releasing hormone agonists.

4. A client asks you about hormonal replacement therapy. What information would you share with her in regard to (a) indications for hormone therapy, (b) routes of administration, (c) types of therapy, (d) expected duration of therapy, (e) contraindications, (f) side effects?

Chapter 45

Drugs Related to Reproductive Health: Male Reproductive Disorders

Nancy C. Sharts-Hopko

OUTLINE

Objectives
Terms
Introduction
Drugs Related to Male Reproductive Disorders

Male Reproductive Processes
Androgens and Anabolic Steroids
   Nursing Process

Antiandrogens
Drugs Used in Other Male Reproductive Disorders
Case Study
Study Questions

OBJECTIVES

Describe the feedback loop comprising hypothalamic, anterior pituitary, and gonadal hormones.

Describe the role of testosterone in development of primary and secondary male sex characteristics and in spermatogenesis.

Identify common conditions for which androgen therapy and antiandrogen therapy are indicated.

Identify clients for whom androgen therapy is particularly risky.

Assess clients for therapeutic and adverse effects of androgen therapy.

Identify commonly prescribed medications that can impair male sexual function.

Explain the nursing process, including client teaching, related to drugs for male reproductive disorders.

TERMS

Addison's disease
anabolic steroids
androgens
antiandrogens
buccal tablet
cryptorchidism
Cushing's syndrome

delayed puberty
ejaculatory dysfunction
erectile dysfunction
gynecomastia
hirsutism
hyperthyroidism
hypogonadism

hypothyroidism
inhibited sexual desire
orchitis
priapism
spermatogenesis
testosterone
virilization

INTRODUCTION

This chapter discusses drug regimens for various alterations in male reproductive health other than the sexually transmitted diseases, which, because of their association with infertility, particularly among women, will be addressed in Chapter 46.

Reproductive health requires the production of adequate quantities of various hypothalamic, pituitary, and gonadal hormones, as well as the appropriate hormone receptors. It requires normal development and patency of the reproductive tract. In addition, reproductive health implies that men and women of developmentally appropriate lifestages are fertile; that is, able to produce gametes (sperm or eggs). Finally, reproductive health entails the ability to engage in sexual intercourse with ejaculation by the male.

Alterations in reproductive health reflect a wide range of developmental, endocrine, infectious, inflammatory, hypertrophic, malignant, and psychoemotional processes. To gain a better understanding of ways in which reproductive health can be affected, reproductive processes are reviewed.

The drug family most clearly associated with male reproductive processes is the androgens. In addition, anabolic steroids and the antiandrogens are discussed.

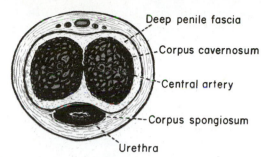

FIGURE 45–2 Erectile tissue of the penis. (*Source:* Guyton AC: *Human Physiology and Mechanisms of Disease,* 4th ed. Philadelphia: WB Saunders, 1987, p. 623.)

Male Reproductive Anatomy and Physiology

The anatomy of the male sexual organs is depicted in Figure 45–1. The external reproductive organs include the penis, the scrotum, and the testes. The penis is composed of three cylindrical bodies of erectile tissue: two corpora cavernosa and the corpus spongiosum. With sexual excitement, the vascular spaces fill with blood to produce an erection (Fig. 45–2).

The scrotum has two compartments, each of which holds a testis, epididymis, and spermatic

DRUGS RELATED TO MALE REPRODUCTIVE DISORDERS
MALE REPRODUCTIVE PROCESSES

There are three male reproductive processes: **spermatogenesis,** or sperm production; regulation of male sexual functioning; and sexual intercourse.

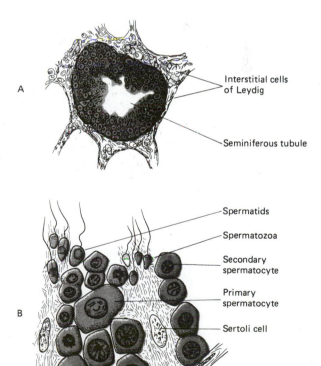

FIGURE 45–3 (*A*) Cross section of a seminiferous tubule. (*B*) Spermatogenesis. (*Source:* Guyton AC: *Human Physiology and Mechanisms of Disease,* 4th ed. Philadelphia: WB Saunders, 1987, p. 620.)

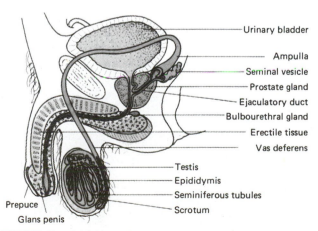

FIGURE 45–1 Male reproductive anatomy. (*Source:* Guyton AC: *Human Physiology and Mechanisms of Disease,* 4th ed. Philadelphia: WB Saunders, 1987, p. 620.)

cord. The spermatic cord supports the testis and includes the vas deferens, blood vessels, nerves, and muscle fibers.

Each testis contains seminiferous tubules in which spermatogenesis occurs (Fig. 45–3). The sperm then move into the epididymis. This leads into the vas deferens, the source of about 20% of ejaculate, or semen. On either side of the prostate gland, a seminal vesicle empties seminal fluid, which contains fructose to provide energy for the sperm, prostaglandins, fibrinogen, and a sperm-activating factor, into the ampulla.

The contents of the ampulla and the seminal vesicles empty into an ejaculatory duct that leads through the body of the prostate to empty into the urethra. Prostatic fluid, which constitutes about 20% of semen, empties from the prostate gland into the ejaculatory duct. The urethra carries semen to its distal end. The urethral glands along the length of the urethra and the bulbourethral glands near the prostatic end of the urethra supply the urethra with mucus. The bulbourethral glands secrete alkaline preejaculatory fluid to protect sperm from the acidity of the urethra.

Hormonal Regulation of Male Reproductive Functioning and Spermatogenesis

Gonadotropin-releasing hormone (GnRH) from the hypothalamus stimulates the anterior pituitary gland to secrete two major gonadotropins, follicle-stimulating hormone (FSH) and luteinizing hormone (LH), in both males and females. LH stimulates the interstitial Leydig cells of the testes to mature and produce testosterone. There is a direct relationship between the amount of circulating LH and the amount of testosterone produced. Testosterone is also produced to a lesser extent in the adrenal cortex, and in the ovaries of females.

In males, FSH stimulates the Sertoli cells to begin conversion of spermatids into mature sperm. In addition, the Sertoli cells are stimulated to secrete estrogens, which may promote spermatogenesis. For spermatogenesis to be complete, testosterone must be secreted simultaneously by the Leydig cells (Fig. 45–4) and diffuse into the seminiferous tubules.

Testosterone is the precursor of two classes of sex steroids: 5-alpha-reduced androgens and estrogens. The net effect of endogenous androgens is the sum of the effects of the 5-alpha-reduced metabolite *dihydrotestosterone* and its estrogen derivative, *estradiol* (Fig. 45–5). Most testosterone is loosely bound by plasma protein and circulates for 15 to 30 minutes before it is fixed to target tissues or metabolized.

FIGURE 45–4 Interstitial cells of Leydig located between the seminiferous tubules. (*Source:* Guyton AC: *Human Physiology and Mechanisms of Disease,* 4th ed. Philadelphia: WB Saunders, 1987, p. 624.)

Most testosterone fixed to target cells is converted to its active form, dihydrotestosterone.

The rate of testosterone production is controlled by a negative feedback loop. With increased testosterone, the hypothalamus decreases production of GnRH (Fig. 45–6). Also, with sperm production the Sertoli cells release a hormone called inhibin, which suppresses FSH production by the anterior pituitary, thus maintaining a constant rate of spermatogenesis. It is not known how, before puberty, the brain stimulates the hypothalamus to begin GnRH secretion, but if the brain is not intact, this may not occur.

Sexual Function

The human sexual response cycle consists of five phases: desire, excitement, plateau, orgasm, and resolution. Sexual desire is the stimulus that causes an individual to initiate or be receptive to sexual activity. During the excitement phase, the male ex-

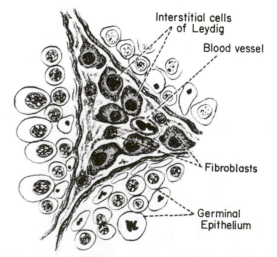

FIGURE 45–5 Testosterone and its metabolite dihydrotestosterone. (*Source:* Guyton AC: *Human Physiology and Mechanisms of Disease,* 4th ed. Philadelphia: WB Saunders, 1987, p. 624.)

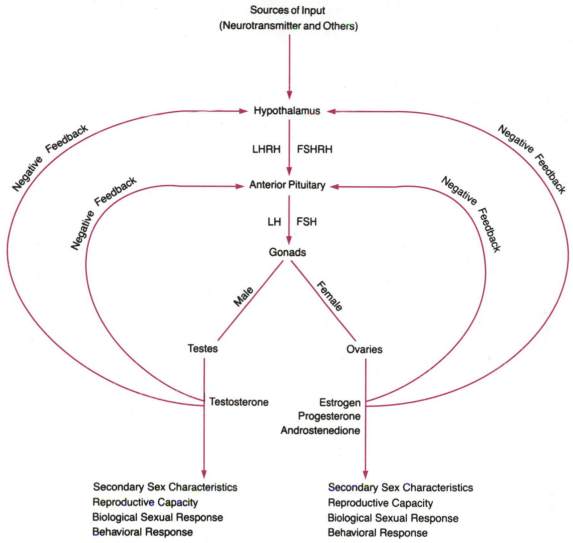

FIGURE 45–6 Hypothalamic-pituitary-gonadal feedback loops. (*Source:* Fogel CI, Lauver D: *Sexual Health Promotion.* Philadelphia: WB Saunders, 1990, p. 339.)

periences penile erection. Males are incapable of engaging in sexual intercourse without this arousal. The plateau phase is characterized by genital enlargement, mucus secretion, generalized muscle tension, hyperventilation, tachycardia, and increased blood pressure. During the orgasmic phase, the vas deferens, seminal vesicles, ejaculatory duct, and penile urethra contract three or four times over a few seconds and the male ejaculates. During resolution, there is a refractory period in which pelvic vasocongestion declines and generalized muscle relaxation takes place.

ANDROGENS AND ANABOLIC STEROIDS

Androgens, or male sex hormones, affect sexual processes, accessory sexual organs, cellular metabolism, and bone and muscle growth. The actions and

effects of natural androgens are listed in Figure 45–7. Testosterone, the main androgen, is synthesized primarily in the testes and, to a lesser extent, in the adrenal cortex. In women, the ovaries synthesize small amounts of testosterone. In men, normal plasma concentrations of testosterone are 250 to 1000 mg/dL, with circadian fluctuations.

Pharmacokinetics

In men, about 98% of circulating testosterone is bound to protein. It is the unbound fraction that is biologically active. Estrogen elevates the production of sex hormone-binding globulin; therefore, more circulating testosterone is bound in women.

The half-life of endogenous free testosterone in the blood is 10 to 20 minutes. Exogenous testosterone is absorbed orally, but because as much as 50% is metabolized on its first pass through the he-

FIGURE 45–7. Androgens

		NURSING PROCESS Assessment and Planning

Testosterone

Testosterone
(Andro-Cyp 100, depAndro 100,
Depotest 100, Duratest 100,
DEPO-Testosterone,
Testred Cypionate 200, Virilon,
depAndrogyn, Everone)
Pregnancy Category: X
CSS III

Dosage

Androgen Replacement
PO: 10–40 mg daily
Buccal: 5–20 mg daily
SC: 150–450 mg q3–6mo
IM: 10–30 mg 2–3×/wk

Metastatic Carcinoma of the Breast:
PO: 200 mg daily
Buccal: 200 mg daily
IM: 100 3×/wk

Contraindications

Pregnancy, nephrosis, hypercalcemia,
pituitary insufficiency, hepatic
dysfuction, benign prostatic
hypertrophy, prostatic cancer, history
of myocardial infarction, prepubertal
status, non–estrogen-dependent
breast cancer

Caution: Hypertension, hypercholesterolemia, coronary artery disease,
gynecomastia, renal disease, seizure
disorders, before puberty, older
adults

Drug-Lab-Food Interactions

Increases effects of anticogulants
Decreases effect with barbiturates,
phenytoin, phenylbutazone
Antagonizes calcitonin, parathyroid
Corticosteroids exacerbate edema
Lab: Decreases blood glucose in
diabetics: *increases* serum cholesterol,
thyroid, liver function, hematocrit

Pharmacokinetics

Absorption: IM: Well absorbed
Distribution: PB: 98%
Metabolism: t½: 10–100 min
Excretion: In urine and bile

Pharmacodynamics

IM: Onset: UK
Peak: UK
Duration: cypionate enanthate:
2–4 wk
Base, propionate: 1–3 d

Interventions

Therapeutic Effects/Uses: To achieve normal androgen levels; to slow progress of estrogen-
dependent breast cancers.

Mode of Action: Development and maintenance of male sex organs and secondary sex
characteristics.

Evaluation

Side Effects

Abdominal pain, nausea, diarrhea, constipation, hives, irritation at injection
site, increased salivation, mouth
soreness, increased or decreased
libido, insomnia, aggressive behavior, weakness, dizziness, pruritus

Adverse Reactions

Acne, masculinization, irregular
menses, urinary urgency,
gynecomastia, priapism, red skin,
jaundice, sodium and water
retention, allergic reaction,
depression
Life-threatening: Hepatic necrosis,
hepatitis, hepatic tumors, respiratory
distress

KEY: SC: subcutaneous; IM: intramuscular; PO: by mouth; PB: protein-binding; t½: half-life; UK:
unknown.

patic circulation, high doses are needed to achieve effective plasma levels. Synthetic androgens have longer half-lives. Testosterone can be combined with esters to form esterified testosterone, in an oil base, to achieve a duration of action of up to 4 weeks.

Testosterone is excreted mainly in the urine as the metabolites androsterone and etiocholanolone. About 6% of the hormone is excreted unaltered in the feces. Synthetic androgens may be excreted as unaltered hormone or as metabolites. In some tissues, the action of testosterone depends on its reduction to 5-alpha-dihydrotestosterone, whereas in other tissues testosterone itself is the active hormone. In the central nervous system, it is the metabolite estradiol that effects hormonal action.

Pharmacodynamics

Testosterone is responsible for the development of male characteristics. These include the fetal development and the maturation of the male reproductive system and the development of secondary sex characteristics such as pubic hair growth, beard and body hair growth, baldness, deepening of the male voice, thickening of the skin, sebaceous gland activity, increased musculature, bone development, and red blood cell formation.

The mechanism for these effects may be increased protein formation in the target cells. Dehydrotestosterone with its receptor acts at binding sites on the chromosomes. Increased RNA polymerase activity and increased synthesis of specific RNA and proteins result, accounting for testosterone's anabolic effects.

The testes produce testosterone in utero. After birth until just before puberty, production is negligible. During puberty production increases rapidly and continues until later adulthood. As men age, the number of Leydig cells decreases, sperm production declines, and LH and FSH levels rise. Levels of unbound testosterone are reduced in elderly men to one-third to one-fifth the peak value. Although a "male menopause" does not occur, some men do experience temporary vasomotor flushing that may be alleviated by testosterone replacement therapy.

Indications for Androgen Therapy

Various androgens and their uses are identified in Table 45–1.

Hypogonadism

The clearest indication for androgen therapy is insufficient testosterone production by the testes, or

hypogonadism. Hypogonadism can be primary, reflecting testicular abnormality, or secondary, reflecting hypothalamic or pituitary failure. Most severely affected males do not experience puberty. Mild hypogonadism may result in lack of libido or the onset of vasomotor flushing. The timing and extent of treatment depend on the clinical manifestations.

Induction of puberty will be undertaken after boys reach 15 to 17 years of age. Hypothalamic and pituitary function is assessed. A 4- to 6-month trial of androgen therapy is indicated, followed by a like period of rest for reevaluation. If prolonged therapy is required, testosterone cypionate or testosterone enanthate is given, starting with 100 mg IM every 2 weeks for 6 to 12 months, with a gradual increase to 200 mg every 2 weeks. It takes 3 or 4 years for sexual development to occur. Plasma testosterone levels should be monitored and dosages adjusted as needed in order to maintain normal levels.

A transdermal testosterone skin patch for daily application to the scrotum, which eliminates the need for injections, is under investigation. This delivery system provides circadian fluctuations in dosage.

Micropenis

Neonates occasionally demonstrate inadequate penile development. Intramuscular or topical administration of low concentrations of testosterone for no longer than 3 months may promote penile growth. Treatment may be repeated later in childhood.

Constitutional Growth Delay

A height of two or more standard deviations below the mean for age and sex occurs in 2.5% of normal children. It tends to be of greater concern for boys. Delay in bone growth seems to be of little consequence by the time boys reach the age of 20 years, but in some families delayed growth causes significant emotional distress despite reassurance from health professionals. Treatment is not initiated before the age of 14 years. Therapy for 3 to 6 months or less before epiphyseal closure may result in linear growth without adverse permanent effects on hypothalamic, pituitary, or gonadal maturation. It is not known whether treatment has an effect on final adult height.

The selection of an androgen or anabolic steroid depends on the balance of growth and sexual maturation that is desired, as well as the preferred route of administration. The effectiveness of oxandrolone for this purpose has been demonstrated.

TABLE 45–1 Androgens

Drug	Dosage	Uses and Considerations
Natural Androgens		
Testosterone (Histerone, Tesamone, Testopel pellets, testosterone aqueous, testosterone powder)	IM: 10–25 mg 2–3 × w SC: 150–450 mg q3–6m IM: 100 mg 3 × w	Androgen replacement, delayed puberty, senile or postmenopausal osteoporosis. Carcinoma of the breast *Pregnancy category:* X; PB: 98%; t½: 10–100 min
Testosterone cypionate (Andro-Cyp, Andronate, depAndro, Depotest, DEPO-Testosterone, Duratest, Testred cypionate, Virilon IM)	IM: 50–400 mg q2–6w	Androgen replacement, delayed puberty. *Pregnancy category:* X; PB: 98%; t½: 10–100 min
Testosterone enanthate (Andro I.A., Andropository, Delatest, Delatestryl, Durathate, Everone, Testrin)	IM: 50–400 mg q2–6w	Androgen replacement, delayed puberty. *Pregnancy category:* X; PB: 98%; t½: 10–100 min
Testosterone propionate (Testex, testosterone propionate powder)	IM: 50 mg 3 × w	Androgen replacement. *Pregnancy category:* X; PB: 98%; t½: 10–100 min
Synthetic Androgens		
Danazol (Danocrine)	PO: 100–800 mg daily divided in two doses initially	Endometriosis, fibrocystic breast disease, angioedema. Initial doses are gradually reduced on an individual basis. Endometriosis therapy lasts 6–9 mon; fibrocystic breast disease therapy lasts 4–6 mon. *Pregnancy category:* X; PB: UK; t½: 4.5 h
Fluoxymesterone (Halotestin)	PO: 10–30 mg daily divided in 1–4 doses	Androgen deficiency, carcinoma of the breast. *Pregnancy category:* X; PB: 98%; t½: 20–100 min
Methyltestosterone (Android, Oreton Methyl, Testred, Virilon)	PO: 10–50 mg daily in divided doses initially, reduced for maintenance Buccal: 5–25 mg daily in divided doses PO: 50–200 mg daily Buccal: 2–25 mg daily in divided doses	Androgen deficiency Carcinoma of the breast *Pregnancy category:* X; PB: UK; t½: UK
Anabolic Steroids		
Nandrolone decanoate (Androlone-D, Deca-Durabolin, Hybolin Decanoate, Neo-Durabolic)	IM: 50–200 mg q1–4w C: IM: 25–50 mg q3–4w	Anemia of renal disease. *Pregnancy category:* X; PB: UK; t½: UK
Nandrolone phenpropionate (Durabolin, Hybolin improved, Nandrobolic)	IM: 50–100 mg/w	Carcinoma of the breast. *Pregnancy category:* X; PB: UK; t½: 1–9 h
Oxandrolone (Oxandrin)	PO: 5–20 mg daily, divided C: PO: 0.1 mg/kg/d	Delayed growth/puberty, osteoporotic pain, short stature, Turner's syndrome, alcoholic hepatitis. *Pregnancy category:* X; PB: UK; t½: 1–9 h
Oxymetholone (Anadrol-50)	PO: 1–5 mg/kg/d	Anemias of deficient RBC production. *Pregnancy category:* X; PB: UK; t½: 9 h
Stanozolol (Winstrol)	PO: 2–6 mg/d	t½: UK

KEY: IM: intramuscular; PO: by mouth; SC: subcutaneous; C: child; PB: protein-binding; UK: unknown; t½: half-life.

Testosterone enanthate, 50 mg/month IM, has been effective, and a sublingual testosterone preparation (Andro Test-SL) is currently undergoing clinical trials.

Other Uses

Other uses of androgens include treatment of refractory anemias in men and women; the autosomal clotting disorder, hereditary angioneurotic edema; tissue wasting associated with severe or chronic illness; advanced carcinoma of the breast in women; and endometriosis. The effectiveness of androgens for treatment of cryptorchidism and impotence has not been established. Androgens may be used in combination with estrogens for management of severe menopausal symptoms (see Chapter 44).

Side Effects

Side effects of androgen therapy include abdominal pain, nausea, insomnia, diarrhea or constipation, hives or redness at the injection site, increased salivation, mouth soreness, and increased or decreased sexual desire. If side effects persist, worsen, or disturb the individual, the health care provider should be notified.

Adverse Effects

Virilizing effects (the development of secondary male sex characteristics) are inappropriate when the client is not a hypogonadal adult male. Women risk such manifestations as acne and skin oiliness, the growth of facial hair, and vocal huskiness. Menstrual irregularities or amenorrhea, suppressed ovulation or lactation, baldness or increased hair growth, and hypertrophy of the clitoris may develop in women undergoing androgen therapy. Although most adverse effects slowly reverse themselves after short-term therapy is completed, vocal changes may be permanent. With long-term therapy, as in the treatment of breast cancer, adverse effects may be irreversible.

Children may experience profound virilization or feminization, as well as impaired bone growth. During pregnancy, androgens can cross the placenta and cause masculinization of the fetus.

Hypogonadal males may experience frequent or continuous erection, called **priapism; gynecomastia,** or breast swelling or soreness; and urinary urgency. Continued use of androgens by normal men can halt spermatogenesis. The sperm count may be low for 3 or more months after therapy.

Less frequent adverse effects include dizziness, weakness, changes in skin color, frequent headaches, confusion, respiratory distress, depression, pruritus, allergic skin rash, edema of the lower extremities, jaundice, bleeding, paresthesias, chills, polycythemia, muscle cramps, and sodium and water retention. Hepatic carcinoma can occur in clients who have received 17-alpha-alkyl substituted androgens over prolonged periods (i.e., 1 to 7 years).

Serum cholesterol may become elevated during androgen therapy. Other alterations in laboratory tests include altered thyroid and liver function tests, elevated urine 17-ketosteroids, and increased hematocrit.

Rare complications of long-term therapy include hepatic necrosis, hepatic peliosis, hepatic tumors, and leukopenia.

Contraindications

Androgen therapy is contraindicated during pregnancy and in individuals with nephrosis or the nephrotic phase of nephritis, hypercalcemia, pituitary insufficiency, hepatic dysfunction, benign prostatic hypertrophy, or prostate cancer. Men with breast cancer are not treated with androgens, nor are women whose breast cancer is not estrogen-dependent. A history of myocardial infarction is a contraindication.

Caution must be exercised in using androgen therapy in individuals with hypertension, hypercholesterolemia, coronary artery disease, gynecomastia, renal disease, or seizure disorder. It is used with caution in infants and prepubertal children because of the potential for growth disturbances and in geriatric males because of their increased risk for benign prostatic hypertrophy and prostate cancer.

Anabolic Steroids

Anabolic steroids are testosterone derivatives developed to maximize the androgens' anabolic effects and minimize their androgenic effects. Abuse of these drugs by athletes is a growing problem. Some athletes and trainers believe these drugs enhance aerobic performance, strength, lean body mass, and muscular development. Other perceived benefits include euphoria and enhanced sexual performance. However, the dosages used may be up to 30 times the therapeutic amount, and numerous serious and sometimes irreversible adverse effects have been reported. Moreover, the adverse effects may not be recognized until several decades have passed. Because most of these drugs are obtained illegally, young people socialized to this pattern of use may be at risk for abuse of other illegal drugs. All major athletic organizations prohibit the use of anabolic steroids.

Drug Interactions

Androgens potentiate the effects of oral anticoagulants, necessitating a decrease in anticoagulant dosage. Androgens antagonize calcitonin and parathyroid hormones. Because androgens can decrease blood glucose in diabetics, dosages of insulin or other antidiabetic agents may need to be reduced. Concurrent use of corticosteroids exacerbates the edema that can occur with androgen therapy. Barbiturates, phenytoin, and phenylbutazone decrease the effects of androgens.

NURSING PROCESS

ASSESSMENT

- Assess the reason for androgen therapy and the client's perception of it. If delayed puberty is the indication, the nurse will assess the client's and family's attitudes about the condition.
- Monitor the client's weight, blood pressure, liver and thyroid function, hemoglobin and hematocrit, creatinine, clotting factors, glucose tolerance, serum lipids and electrolytes, and blood count before and throughout treatment. The presence of liver or endocrine dysfunction is noted.
- Determine the pregnancy status of fertile women. Concomitant anticoagulant therapy should be noted. When a prepubertal child is treated, x-rays are taken before, every 6 months during, and after treatment to monitor growth.
- Appraise the client's affect during therapy, particularly aggressiveness in clients taking large doses. Self-concept is an important consideration in the client on androgen therapy, particularly in children with delayed puberty and in women.

NURSING DIAGNOSES

- Body image disturbance
- Altered growth and development
- Self-esteem disturbance
- Sexual dysfunction
- Altered sexuality patterns
- Knowledge deficit regarding the treatment protocol

PLANNING

- Nursing goals for clients include adherence to the prescribed regimen for taking the medication and for monitoring.
- Long-term goals include appropriate use of the medication, avoidance of preventable adverse effects, and maintenance of a positive self-concept.

NURSING INTERVENTIONS

General

- The client and family need instruction on proper administration of the medications, their reasons for use, and potential undesired effects. They are apprised of those effects that warrant prompt medical attention (e.g., urinary problems, priapism, and respiratory distress).
- If an intermittent approach to treatment is used, the client needs to understand that this allows for monitoring of endocrine status between courses of androgen therapy. The need to return to the health care facility for monitoring is explained, and the client's ability to do so is determined. Social service referrals are made if necessary.

Specific

- The nutritional intake of individuals with anemia, osteoporosis, or tissue wasting is assessed and revised as needed to ensure adequate intake of calories, protein, vitamins, iron, and other minerals.
- Sodium may need to be restricted if edema develops. The client will be instructed to record body weight several times per week.
- Individuals with elevated serum calcium need 3 to 4 L of fluid per day to prevent kidney stones. Individuals on bedrest need range-of-motion exercises, whereas ambulatory clients need to engage in active weight bearing. Indicators of hypercalcemia are shown in Table 45–2.

TABLE 45–2 Signs of Hypercalcemia

Nausea and vomiting

Lethargy

Decreased muscle tone

Polyuria

Increased urine and serum calcium

Hypercalcemia needs prompt medical attention because it can lead to cardiac arrest.

- Individuals being treated for tissue wasting are urged to reduce environmental stressors and promote rest and relaxation, because stress hormones are catabolic. Muscle strength will be monitored during treatment.

- Oral androgens should be taken with food to decrease gastric distress.
- Families pursuing treatment for a client with delayed puberty are instructed about the range of normal development.
- Women and prepubertal clients need instruction on good skin hygiene to decrease the severity of acne.
- Men undergoing androgen therapy are instructed to report priapism (painful, continuous erection) promptly. The drug dosage will be reduced to avoid subsequent erectile dysfunction. In addition, they are taught to report decreased

urinary stream promptly because androgens can stimulate prostatic hypertrophy.

EVALUATION

- The client's ability to adhere to the treatment regimen and response to prescribed drugs will be monitored.
- The client will be asked about therapeutic and adverse drug effects on follow-up visits. Monitoring of weight, blood pressure, and laboratory tests will continue throughout therapy, with alterations in the plan of care as needed.
- Youngsters and women who experience virilizing effects or acne will be periodically assessed for the ability to cope with these changes and maintain a positive self-concept.
- Sexual function is assessed when appropriate.
- The client's ability to adhere to the treatment plan and to discuss the treatment and its effects knowledgeably suggests that teaching has been effective and that the client accepts the treatment.

ANTIANDROGENS

Antiandrogens, or androgen antagonists, block the synthesis or action of androgens (Table 45–3). These drugs may be useful in the management of benign prostatic hypertrophy and carcinoma of the prostate. They have been used to treat male-pattern baldness, acne, hirsutism, virilization syndrome in women, and precocious puberty in boys, although their effectiveness is not well established. The effectiveness of these drugs on the inhibition of sex drive in men who are sex offenders is controversial and not well documented.

GnRH, or an analog such as leuprolide, is the most effective inhibitor of testosterone synthesis. When such agents are given over time, LH and testosterone levels fall. Ketoconazole is under investigation for treatment of prostatic carcinoma because of its inhibition of adrenal and gonadal steroid synthesis.

Two types of drugs have been developed to block testosterone action: androgen-receptor antagonists and agents that block conversion of testosterone to its active form, dihydrotestosterone. Cyproterone acetate, an orally active progesterone, is a potent androgen antagonist. It also suppresses LH and FSH secretion and has progestational qualities. Cyproterone acetate competes with dihydrotestosterone for binding to the androgen receptor. Cyproterone acetate can stunt growth in youngsters. Acne and baldness have been reported.

Flutamide (Eulexin) is a nonsteroidal drug that competes with androgens at androgen receptors. Men receiving flutamide show elevations in plasma LH and testosterone levels. Flutamide is used along with GnRH blockade or estrogen in the treatment of prostate cancer. Spironolactone also competes with dihydrotestosterone at the receptor site. It is used in doses of 50 to 100 mg/d for treatment of hirsutism in women.

Finasteride, a steroid, inhibits conversion of testosterone to dihydrotestosterone. This orally ac-

TABLE 45–3 Antiandrogens

Mechanism	Drugs
Elevation of GnRH level	Goserelin (Zoladex) Nafarelin (Synarel) Leuprolide acetate (Lupron, Lupron Depot)
Inhibition of testosterone synthesis	Ketoconazole (Nizoral)
Blocks conversion of testosterone to dihydrotestosterone	Finasteride (Proscar)
Receptor inhibitors	Cyproterone, cyproterone acetate (orphan drug status in U.S.A.) Flutamide (Eulexin) Spironolactone (generic, Aldactone)

tive agent decreases the concentration of dihydrotestosterone in plasma and in the prostate without elevated plasma concentrations of LH or testosterone. Finasteride is used for the treatment of benign prostatic hypertrophy. Other uses are under investigation.

DRUGS USED IN OTHER MALE REPRODUCTIVE DISORDERS

Developmental Disorders

The hormones testosterone and human chorionic gonadotropin (hCG) are often used to treat boys with **cryptorchidism** (failure of the testes to descend into the scrotum by birth). Undescended testes are associated with subsequent infertility and testicular cancer. Treatment is usually initiated before the age of 6 years. The dosage of hCG in boys is 500 to 4000 IU intramuscularly two to three times per week for several weeks. Adverse reactions include headache, irritability, precocious puberty, gynecomastia, and edema. The nurse will need to inspect the boy's genitalia for evidence of early puberty. If drug therapy is ineffective, surgery will be planned.

Delayed Puberty

In up to 5% of cases of delayed puberty, there is insufficient secretion of GnRH, LH, or FSH. Once the cause is determined, GnRH, LH, or FSH replacement therapy is instituted.

Pituitary, Thyroid, and Adrenal Disorders

Inadequate pituitary function can result in hypogonadism. In a prepubertal male, it results in lack of secondary sex characteristics and infertility; adult men may experience testicular atrophy and decreased libido, decreased potency, decreased beard growth, and decreased muscle tone. Menotropins (Pergonal), one ampule of which contains 75 IU each of LH and FSH, injected IM three times weekly over a period of years, can stimulate testosterone production. Menotropins is indicated when both LH and FSH levels are low. It is given concomitantly with hCG 2000 IU intramuscularly twice per week. Adverse effects include nausea, vomiting, diarrhea, gynecomastia, and fever. Reconstituted with 1 to 2 mL sterile saline, the drug must be used immediately.

Hypothyroidism, a deficiency in thyroid hormone, can be the result of insufficient thyroid hormone production or resistance to its effects at the target organs. The problem could be congenital. It can cause inhibited sexual desire and erectile dysfunction. In **Addison's disease,** there is a deficit of both cortisol and the mineralocorticoid aldosterone. Men with Addison's disease may experience inhibited sexual desire, erectile dysfunction, or diminished fertility. Both of these conditions are highly responsive to replacement therapy with the appropriate hormones (see Chapter 40).

Sexual Dysfunction

Sexual dysfunction is the inability to experience sexual desire, erection, ejaculation, and detumescence—the phases of the sexual response cycle. **Inhibited sexual desire** can result from androgen deficiency, an affective disorder, or discord in the sexual relationship. **Erectile dysfunction** may be due to psychoemotional problems, vascular insufficiency, neurologic disorders, androgen deficiency or resistance, or diseases of the penis. **Ejaculatory dysfunction** can be psychogenic or a result of drug therapy, androgen deficiency, or sympathetic degeneration. **Failure of detumescence** is most commonly caused by penile disease or systemic disease. Male sexual dysfunction may result from the use of various drugs, as shown in Table 45–4.

L-dopa, used in the treatment of Parkinson's syndrome, has shown effectiveness in stimulating libido and treating erectile dysfunctions in non-Parkinson's clients. Individuals who experience premature ejaculation related to excessive anxiety about sexual intercourse may be helped by treatment with one of the monoamine oxidase (MAO) inhibitors in conjunction with psychotherapy (see Chapter 16). Erectile dysfunction due to vascular insufficiency is occasionally treated on a short-term basis by local vasoactive drugs, including papaverine, phentolamine, prostaglandin E, nitroglycerin, or yohimbine, a systemic vasoactive drug.

Certain drugs are often abused by individuals seeking a heightened sexual experience. Amyl nitrate is commonly believed to be an aphrodisiac. Sudden death, myocardial infarction, and methemoglobinemia have been reported with its use. Cantharides (Spanish fly) causes bladder and urethral irritation, accounting for its use as a sexual stimulant. Permanent penile damage has been reported with its use.

Nonsexually Transmitted Infections

Urinary tract infections are addressed in Chapter 27. If left untreated, acute or chronic prostatitis, orchitis, or epididymitis can develop.

TABLE 45–4 Drugs Causing Sexual Dysfunction in Males

Drug Category	Drugs or Drug Families
Anticholinergics	Atropine Scopolamine Benztropine Trihexyphenidyl
Antidepressants	Tricyclic antidepressants Monoamine oxidase inhibitors
Antihistamines	Cimetidine Diphenhydramine Hydroxyzine
Antihypertensives	Central sympathetic ganglion blockers Postganglionic blockers Alpha- and beta-receptor blockers Diuretics
Antipsychotics	Phenothiazines Thioxanthenes Butyrophenone Lithium
Sedatives and social drugs	Alcohol Barbiturates Diazepam Chlordiazepoxide Cannabis Cocaine Opiates Methadone
Others	Aminocaproic acid Baclofen Steroids Ethionamide Perhexiline Digoxin Chemotherapeutic agents

Malignant and Benign Tumors

Prostatic cancer accounts for about 10% of all cancer deaths among American men. Most prostatic cancers are adenocarcinomas. Metastasis to lymph nodes, bone, lungs, liver, and adrenal glands is common. Prostatic cancer is often asymptomatic, but urinary obstruction is commonly the first sign. Treatment may include a combination of surgical resection, cryotherapy, estrogen administration, radiation therapy, chemotherapy, and pain relief.

Testicular tumors peak in early adulthood. They include malignant germinal cell tumors and benign Leydig or Sertoli cell tumors. Treatment depends on the type and stage of tumor. Surgical excision, radiation therapy, and chemotherapy are used singly or in combination.

Males account for 1% of breast cancer cases.

Breast cancer in men occurs most commonly after the age of 60 years. Treatment, which is similar for men and women, entails surgery, radiation therapy, chemotherapy, and endocrine therapy. Carcinoma of the penis represents less than 1% of all malignancies among males. In situ, treatment entails local excision, radiation therapy, and local application of 5-fluorouracil cream or solution. Invasive carcinoma is treated by surgical resection of the penis and involved nodes. Radiation and chemotherapy follow as needed. Antineoplastic therapies are discussed in Unit 6.

■ CASE STUDY
Client with Male Reproductive Disorder

Matt is a 16-year-old high school junior who is 5'3" and weighs 126 lbs. He has increased feelings of discomfort about not fitting in with other students in his school because he has not yet begun sexual maturation. He is a good student and an accomplished violinist in the school orchestra. His only brother is younger than he is. His father states that he also was a "late bloomer," but he and his wife are concerned about their son's increasing social withdrawal and seem determined to seek medical intervention for him. The nurse in the clinic assesses the needs and status of Matt and his family.

1. What is the client's primary complaint? What concerns his family?
2. What information must be included in the history and physical examination?
3. What teaching should the nurse do prior to the parents making the decision to allow their son to start on androgen therapy?

The decision is made to prescribe methyltestosterone 5 mg/d by **buccal tablet** (held inside the cheek until it dissolves). Matt will be on this regimen for 4 months, during which time he is to come to the clinic at monthly intervals.

4. Matt asks why he will be treated for 4 months. What will the nurse reply?
5. About what adverse effects do Matt and his parents need to be taught?
6. What physical and psychosocial parameters will be monitored at his monthly visits?
7. What special hygiene needs does Matt have while on this regimen?
8. When should he have x-rays? Why?
9. During a clinic visit, Matt mentions that he has heard that the use of anabolic steroids might improve his chances of making the wrestling team.

What should he be told about the safety and efficacy of anabolic steroid use?

STUDY QUESTIONS

1. Explain the relationships among gonadotropin-releasing hormone, follicle-stimulating hormone, luteinizing hormone, and the gonadal hormones.
2. What are some desired effects of androgen therapy?
3. Why would healthy adolescents abuse androgens?
4. What is the role of androgen therapy in treatment of breast cancer?
5. What physical parameters are measured during androgen therapy?
6. In what groups must extra care be taken when androgen therapy is used?
7. What is an indication for antiandrogen therapy?
8. What are two reasons for treatment of cryptorchidism early in life?
9. What are long-term implications of infection of the male reproductive tract?
10. Identify the stages of the sexual response cycle, and identify which are most important for fertility in males and in females.
11. Identify 10 commonly used medications that can impair male sexual function.

Chapter 46

Drugs Related to Reproductive Health: Infertility and Sexually Transmitted Diseases

Nancy C. Sharts-Hopko

OUTLINE

Objectives
Terms
Introduction
Drugs Related to Infertility
  Treatment
    Process of Fertilization
    Infertility Management
      Nursing Process

Drugs Used in the Treatment of
  Sexually Transmitted
  Diseases
    Transmission and Risk
    HIV Disease
    Occupational Exposure of
      Health Workers
    Nursing Process

Summary
Case Study
Study Questions

OBJECTIVES

Describe male, female, and couple causes of infertility.

Instruct couples on the relationships among ovulatory stimulation therapy, fertility awareness, and timing of coitus.

Describe the way in which ovulatory stimulants promote fertility.

Identify clients at risk for STDs.

Describe the relationship among STDs and infertility.

Instruct clients in regimens for common STDs.

Plan management for STDs for which cures do not exist.

Counsel health care workers about management of worksite exposure to blood-borne STDs.

Describe the nursing process, including client teaching, related to drugs for infertility and sexually transmitted diseases.

TERMS

autoimmune
blastocyst
fertilization
gumma
implantation

infertility, primary,
  secondary
ovulation
perinatal infection
placenta

sexually transmitted disease
trophoblast
vertical transmission
zygote

INTRODUCTION

This chapter discusses drug regimens for two broad categories of reproductive health alterations that are often interrelated: infertility and sexually transmitted diseases. Alterations in fertility reflect a wide range of developmental, endocrine, infectious, inflammatory, hypertrophic, and psychoemotional processes. As a basis for understanding infertility, the process of fertilization is reviewed. Drug therapies used in the management of female and, more briefly, male infertility are addressed, with emphasis on ovulation stimulants.

The broad category of diseases that are sexually transmitted in general constitutes a threat to reproductive tract integrity and functioning, as well as to neonatal health. Some, such as human immunodeficiency virus (HIV) disease, are life-threatening in and of themselves. Drug therapies for these conditions are reviewed briefly.

DRUGS RELATED TO INFERTILITY TREATMENT

Infertility is defined as the inability to conceive a child after 12 months of unprotected sexual intercourse. Women over 35 years of age may be treated after a shorter trial. Infertility is considered **primary** if a couple have never borne a live infant, and **secondary** if they have.

PROCESS OF FERTILIZATION

Fertilization, or **conception,** occurs when a sperm penetrates an ovum, usually in the distal third of the fallopian tube (Fig. 46–1).

In a single ejaculation, between 200 and 400 million spermatozoa are deposited in the vagina. Sperm move up the female reproductive tract by the flagellar motion of their tails. It takes an average of 4 to 6 hours for the sperm to reach the distal fallopian tube. Semen contains prostaglandins that may enhance uterine motility to facilitate sperm migration. The ciliary action of the fallopian tubes enhances migration of the ovum to the uterus and of sperm toward the ovary.

Uterine enzymes capacitate the sperm by altering their glycoprotein coat. In an acrosomal reaction, the sperm release an enzyme, hyaluronidase, that breaks through the outer layer of the ovum. The moment one sperm penetrates the ovum a chemical reaction occurs that blocks other sperm from entering. Cellular division begins immediately in what is now called the **zygote,** or fertilized egg.

After 3 days the zygote enters the uterus. It has now differentiated into an inner solid mass of cells, the **blastocyst,** and an outer layer, the **trophoblast.**

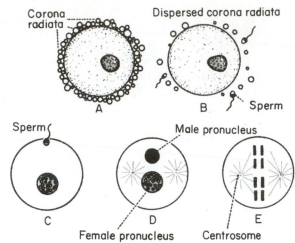

FIGURE 46–1 Fertilization of an ovum by a sperm. (*A*) Corona radiata is the outermost layer of the ovum. (*B*) Acrosomal reaction of the sperm breaks through the corona radiata. (*C*) One sperm penetrates the ovum. (*D* and *E*) Genetic reorganization begins immediately, allowing for cellular replication. (*Source:* Guyton AC: *Textbook of Medical Physiology,* 6th ed. Philadelphia: WB Saunders, 1981, p. 1022.)

Progesterone secreted by the corpus luteum of the ovary maintains a favorable uterine environment to nourish the blastocyst until **implantation** in the uterine lining occurs (Fig. 46–2). The blastocyst develops into the embryo and the amniotic membrane, whereas the trophoblast develops into the chorionic membrane and the fetal side of the placenta. The maternal portion of the placenta develops under the site of the blastocyst's implantation. The **placenta** is the structure through which oxygen, nutrients, and metabolic wastes pass between the maternal and fetal circulations for the duration of pregnancy. The placenta begins to function by the fourth week of pregnancy. Within the first 8 weeks of pregnancy, organ systems are differentiated, and it is during this period that the fetus is

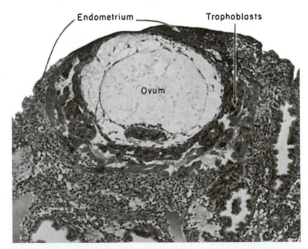

FIGURE 46–2 Implantation of the blastocyst and trophoblast development. (*Source:* Guyton AC: *Textbook of Medical Physiology,* 6th ed. Philadelphia, WB Saunders, 1981, p. 1023.)

most threatened by teratogens. Growth of the fetus throughout pregnancy depends on adequate oxygenation and nutrition, the metabolic environment, freedom from infection, and integrity of the mother's reproductive tract.

INFERTILITY MANAGEMENT
Assessing Infertility

Causes of infertility, listed in Table 46–1, are numerous. In about 15% of cases, no specific cause can be found. Up to 40% of cases are the result of sexually transmitted diseases, which may result in neonatal death or altered reproductive tract integrity. Treatment of infertility depends on assessment of the cause.

General health is assessed; nutritional, reproductive, and sexual histories are taken; and physical examinations with routine laboratory tests are conducted on both partners. Common tests to determine specific causes of infertility are shown in Table 46–2.

TABLE 46–1 Causes of Infertility

Female Factors	
Genetic	Chromosomal abnormalities, enzyme defects
Tubal or peritoneal	Infection, occlusion, fimbrial damage, pelvic adhesions, endometriosis
Ovarian	Anovulation/oligoovulation, inadequate luteal phase, polycystic ovaries
Cervical	Cervicitis, poor quality cervical mucus, diethylstilbestrol exposure
Uterine	Uterine fibromas, congenital malformations, adhesions, endometrial abnormalities
Endocrine	Panhypopituitarism, hypothyroidism, adrenal insufficiency, congenital adrenal hyperplasia, Cushing's disease, cirrhosis, hormone receptor defects
Other	Age, drugs, malnutrition, excess alcohol intake, smoking
Male Factors	
Genetic	Klinefelter's syndrome, Reifenstein's syndrome, chromosomal abnormalities
Seminal	Failure of semen to liquefy, inadequate volume, low sperm count, decreased or erratic sperm motility, sperm dysmorphology, varicocele
Transport	Hypospadias, micropenis, retrograde ejaculation, epididymitis, impotence, ductal occlusion, ductal adhesions
Testicular	Oligospermia/azoospermia, cryptorchidism, testicular agenesis, history of high fever, postpubertal orchitis
Endocrine	Panhypopituitarism, hypothyroidism, adrenal insufficiency, congenital adrenal hyperplasia, Cushing's disease, cirrhosis, hormone receptor abnormalities
Other	Age, drugs, excess alcohol intake, smoking, pollution, malnutrition, scrotal heat exposure, autoimmunity to sperm, infectious processes
Couple Factors	Sexual technique, inappropriate timing of intercourse, immune response to sperm

TABLE 46–2 Common Tests for Infertility

Test	Purpose
Physical examination	Assess reproductive tract function and patency by gross examination
Hematology, liver and renal function	Rule out disease processes
Hysterosalpingogram, tubal insufflation	Evaluate fallopian tube patency
Postcoital examination of cervical mucus	Assess mucus viscosity, its effect on sperm motility
Plasma progesterone	Assess function of corpus luteum
Endometrial biopsy	Assess ovulatory status or adequacy of corpus luteum
Semen analysis	Check number, structure, movement of sperm
Basal body temperature	Determine if ovulation occurs; chart
Sperm penetration assay	Determine sperm's ability to penetrate and fertilize ovum
Laparoscopy	Visualize female pelvic organs
Hysteroscopy	Visualize uterus
Echohysteroscopy	Assess structure of woman's internal reproductive organs
Hormone assays	GnRH, FSH, LH, progesterone, estrogen, prolactin, testosterone, thyroid hormone levels
Immunologic testing	Assess cervical immunity against sperm, seminal fluid immunity against sperm, serum antisperm antibodies in either partner
Imaging	Pituitary integrity

KEY: FSH: follicle-stimulating hormone; GnRH: gonadotropin-releasing hormone; LH: luteinizing hormone.

Induction of Ovulation

Clomiphene citrate (Serophene, Clomid), an estrogen antagonist, blocks the negative hypothalamic-pituitary-gonadal feedback loop. The precise mechanism of action is not understood, but increased gonadotropin-releasing hormone (GnRH) release increases luteinizing hormone (LH) and follicle-stimulating hormone (FSH) output. It is the most commonly used ovulation stimulant (Fig. 46–3). Some women on clomiphene citrate therapy require the addition of glucocorticoid therapy such as dexamethasone or prednisone.

Human menopausal gonadotropin (hMG) and human chorionic gonadotropin (hCG) replace or supplement FSH and LH (Table 46–3). These drugs normalize LH and FSH levels in order to stimulate follicle maturation, ovulation, and development of the corpus luteum. In a small percentage of amenorrheic women, an elevated level of prolactin is the causative factor. A portion of these women can be treated with the ergot derivative bromocriptine 2.5 mg two or three times a day. Bromocriptine binds to dopamine receptors in the pituitary and inhibits prolactin secretion, and treatment should lead to the onset of menses in 3 to 5 weeks. Chemically, drugs in the category of ovulation stimulants are not similar.

FIGURE 46–3. Ovulation Stimulant: Clomiphene Citrate

Clomiphene Citrate	Dosage	NURSING PROCESS Assessment and Planning
Clomiphene Citrate (Clomid, Milophene, Serophene) Ovulation stimulant *Pregnancy Category:* X	A: PO: 50–250 mg/d for days 5–9 of cycle If ovulation does not occur with 50 mg/d, increase next course to 100 mg/d	
Contraindications	**Drug-Lab-Food Interactions**	
Pregnancy, undiagnosed vaginal bleeding, depression, fibroids, hepatic dysfunction, thrombophlebitis, primary pituitary or ovarian failure	None are significant; Danazol may inhibit response; *decrease* effects of ethinyl estradiol *Lab: Increase* in serum thyroxine	
Pharmacokinetics	**Pharmacodynamics**	Interventions
Absorption: Readily absorbed from GI tract *Distribution:* PB: UK *Metabolism:* t½: 5–8 d *Excretion:* In feces	PO: Onset: 5–14 d Peak: UK Duration: UK	

	Evaluation
Therapeutic Effects/Uses: To stimulate ovarian follicle growth. *Mode of Action:* Stimulates release of follicle-stimulating hormone (FSH) and luteinizing hormone (LH).	

Side Effects	Adverse Reactions
Breast discomfort, fatigue, dizziness, depression, anxiety, nausea, vomiting, constipation, increased appetite, headache, flatulence, multiple gestation, hot flashes, fluid retention	Visual disturbances, abdominal pain, weight gain, hair loss, major congenital anomalies, ovarian hyperstimulation, anxiety, ovarian cysts

KEY: PO: by mouth; PB: protein-binding; UK: unknown; t½: half-life.

TABLE 46–3 Ovulatory Stimulants

Drug	Dosage	Use and Considerations
Bromocriptine mesylate (Parlodel)	Up to 7.5 mg/d in divided doses	Normalizes prolactin levels. Possibly teratogenic. *Pregnancy category:* C; PB: 92%; t½: 50 h
Clomiphene citrate (Clomid, Serophene)	50–250 mg/d PO days 5–9 of cycle	Stimulates follicle growth. May be teratogenic. May impede fertilization. *Pregnancy category:* X; PB: UK; t½: 5–8 d
GnRH	1–10 μg/60–120 min via pump	Induces ovulation in women with hypothalamic amenorrhea. Ovarian hyperstimulation is a risk. Pregnancy loss is common. *Pregnancy category:* X; PB: UK; t½: 11–23 h
Human menopausal gonadotropin, menotropins and FSH, urofollitropin (Pergonal, Metrodin)	IM: 1–2 ampules/d × 5–12 d until follicle maturation; next day, hCG (5000–10,000 IU IM) administered	These contain various ratios of FSH and LH. Ovarian hyperstimulation is a risk. Ectopic pregnancy and spontaneous abortion may occur. *Pregnancy category:* X; PB: UK; t½: 4–70 h

KEY: *PO: by mouth; IM: intramuscular; FSH: follicle-stimulating hormone; LH: luteinizing hormone; hCG: human chorionic gonadotropin; PB: protein-binding; UK: unknown; t½: half-life.*

Pharmacokinetics

Data on the pharmacokinetics of clomiphene citrate are limited, but clomiphene is readily absorbed from the gastrointestinal (GI) tract. It is partially metabolized in the liver and excreted in the feces via biliary elimination. Clomiphene has a half-life of about 5 days.

Pharmacodynamics

The mechanism of action of clomiphene is unknown, but it is hypothesized that it competes with estrogen at receptor sites. The perception of decreased circulating estrogen by the hypothalamus and pituitary triggers the negative feedback response of increasing the secretion of FSH and LH. The result is ovarian stimulation, maturation of the ovarian follicle, and development of the corpus luteum.

Side Effects

Side effects of clomiphene citrate include breast discomfort, fatigue, dizziness, depression, nausea, vomiting, increased appetite, weight gain, dermatitis, urticaria, anxiety, restlessness, weakness, heavier menses, vasomotor flushing, abdominal bloating or pain, and gas (Table 46–4). Antiestrogenic effects include interference with endometrial maturation and cervical mucus production. Paradoxically, this may interfere with fertilization or implantation.

Adverse Effects

Adverse effects include photophobia, mastalgia, diplopia, and decreased visual acuity. Ovarian hy-

perstimulation may result in ovarian enlargement, midcycle ovarian pain, and cysts. Reversible hair loss has been noted. Multiple gestation occurs in up to 12% of women who become pregnant. The effect of clomiphene citrate on fetal development is unclear. Neural tube defects have been reported, but have not been confirmed by controlled studies. Adverse effects of other ovulatory stimulants are shown in Table 46–4.

Contraindications

Contraindications for treatment with clomiphene citrate include undiagnosed vaginal bleeding, pregnancy, uterine fibroids, mental depression, history of hepatic dysfunction or thromboembolic disease, and primary pituitary or ovarian failure. If the woman has ovarian cysts, clomiphene citrate may cause them to enlarge. Contraindications to the use of other ovulatory stimulants are shown in Table 46–3.

Interactions

There are no known significant drug interactions with clomiphene citrate. Danazol may inhibit client response to clomiphene citrate, and clomiphene citrate may suppress response to ethinyl estradiol. There are no known drug interactions with hMG or hCG.

Other Drug Treatments

Other pharmacologic approaches for treatment of women with infertility include the use of pulsatile

TABLE 46–4 Side Effects, Adverse Effects and Contraindications for Selected Infertility Drugs

Side Effects	Adverse Effects	Contraindications
Human menopausal gonadotropin Breast pain, abdominal bloating or pain	Ovarian enlargement, ovarian hyperstimulation syndrome, fever, nausea, vomiting, diarrhea, hemoperitoneum, arterial thromboembolism, ovarian cysts, multiple births	Primary ovarian failure, pregnancy, ovarian cysts, enlargement not due to polycystic ovaries, thyroid or adrenal dysfunction, intracranial lesion, abnormal bleeding of unknown origin, infertility not due to anovulation
Urofollitropin Bloating, nausea, vomiting, diarrhea, cramping, headache, breast pain, aches, fatigue, malaise, dry skin	Ovarian enlargement, ovarian hyperstimulation syndrome, hair loss, ectopic pregnancy, thromboembolism, ascites, pleural effusion, multiple births	High levels FSH, LH, thyroid or adrenal dysfunction, intracranial lesions, abnormal bleeding of unknown origin, ovarian cysts not due to polycystic ovary syndrome, pregnancy. Used with caution in persons with thromboembolism and nursing mothers
Human chorionic gonadotropin Headache, irritability, restlessness, fatigue, depression, fluid retention, pain at injection site	Ovarian hyperstimulation syndrome, rupture of ovarian cysts, multiple births, arterial thromboembolism	Androgen-dependent neoplasms. Caution in asthma, cardiac or renal disease, epilepsy, migraine
Bromocriptine mesylate Nausea, vomiting, headache, dizziness, drowsiness, fatigue, lightheadedness, nasal congestion, diarrhea, insomnia, depression	Confusion, visual disturbances, vertigo, shortness of breath, abdominal discomfort, involuntary movements, hypotension, anxiety, dysphagia, paresthesia, blepharospasm, mottling, urinary frequency, epileptiform seizures, ergotism, transient elevations in BUN, SGOT, SGPT, creatine phosphokinase, alkaline phosphatase, serum uric acid	Ischemic heart disease, peripheral vascular disease, pregnancy, lactation, ergot nervousness, sensitivity. Caution in hypotension, epilepsy, psychoses, cardiac arrhythmia, impaired hepatic or renal function

exogenous GnRH. In addition, hypo- or hyperthyroidism and adrenal dysfunction must be treated. Endometriosis can be treated with a course of danazol to suppress gonadotropin output. Women with inadequate luteal-phase progesterone output are treated with progesterone 25 mg twice daily intravaginally or 12.5 mg IM.

Drug Therapy for Male Infertility

For the majority of men with infertility, no specific causal factor can be identified. They are identified as having idiopathic oligospermia and asthenospermia. There is no documented cost-effective treatment for this large group of people. Most drug regimens that have been used have never been evaluated in controlled studies. Drugs that have been tried include testosterone; hCG; GnRH; mesterolone, a synthetic androgen; antiestrogenic agents, including clomiphene citrate and tamoxifen; and testolactone, which inhibits the conversion of testosterone to estradiol. Assisted reproductive techniques currently appear to hold more promise than drug therapy.

NURSING PROCESS: Infertility

Infertility management is a highly specialized field. Nurses are most likely to encounter clients when they are in the process of trying to identify the possible causes of their infertility. Nurses need to be sensitive to the guilt, decreased self-esteem, and embarrassment that infertility may cause. Treatment of infertility requires that a couple's sexual life be directed by the health care team. Evaluation and intervention are often uncomfortable and expensive, and there is no guarantee that a viable pregnancy will result. The process is emotionally and economically draining for the couple.

ASSESSMENT

- A general health history and physical examination are required. The clients' reproductive and sexual histories are assessed, with attention to the timing and technique of coitus.
- The couple undergo an exhaustive battery of di-

agnostic tests to evaluate the cause of infertility. Once this is determined, conditions that contraindicate the treatment of choice are ruled out.

- It is particularly important that the couple's interpretation of their infertility be explored, along with its impact on their relationship. Placing blame on one another or their families can be devastating.

POTENTIAL NURSING DIAGNOSES

- Altered sexuality patterns
- Altered sexual functioning
- Body image disturbance
- Low self-esteem
- Knowledge deficit related to treatment regimen

PLANNING

- Short-term goals include the clients' adherence to the medical regimen with minimal adverse effects.
- The long-term goal is the achievement of pregnancy or the consideration of alternatives to pregnancy with the partners' self-esteem and relationship intact.

NURSING INTERVENTIONS

General

- Interventions are aimed at helping clients understand the interrelationships among and timing of menses, ovulation, and coitus as they relate to conception. In addition, they need to know sexual techniques that enhance fertilization, such as

---

1. Purchase a special thermometer calibrated in tenths of degrees between 96 and 100° F.
2. Place the thermometer under the tongue for at least a full 3 minutes (preferably 5 minutes) after waking in the morning and before *any* activity (e.g., lifting your head off the pillow, shaking thermometer down, intercourse, or urinating).
3. If you forget to take your temperature and have already gotten up, *do not take it*. Write *missed* on that day.
4. Take your temperature in the same manner about the same time each day.
5. Carefully record the reading on the graph by placing a dot at the proper location. Start this chart on the first day of your period.
6. Insert the month and day in the space provided.
7. The first day of menstrual flow is considered to be the start of a cycle (day 1). Each day of flow should be indicated with an M on the graph, starting at extreme left under number 1 day of cycle.
8. Record any obvious reason for temperature variation such as a cold, flu, or infection on the graph above the reading for that day.
9. If you are placed on medication, please indicate it in the space labeled medications on the days you take it.
10. If you feel you have menstrually related symptoms, such as breast tenderness or cramping, note these also.
11. If intercourse has taken place during the previous 24 hours, mark it with an (X).

Calendar for Thermal Method of Fertility Awareness

Day of Cycle: 1 2 3 4 5 6 7 8 9 10 11 12 13 14 15 16 17 18 19 20 21 22 23 24 25 26 27 28 29 30 31

Temperature
99.0
98.8
98.6
98.4
98.2
98.0
97.8
97.6
97.4
97.2
97.0

Menses (M):
Intercourse (X):

Mucus
    Color
    Consistency
    Amount

Other factors
    Medications
    Breast tenderness
    Cramps

FIGURE 46–4 Record-keeping for basal body temperature, timing of coitus, and ovulatory effect of clomiphene citrate. (Source: Fogel CI, Lauver D: *Sexual Health Promotion.* Philadelphia: WB Saunders, 1990, p. 100.)

the placement of a pillow under the woman's hips during coitus and her remaining supine with hips elevated for about 30 min after her partner ejaculates. In addition, clients and their partners need to understand the treatment regimen.

Specific

- The female client is taught to report adverse effects such as abdominal pain or visual disturbances to her infertility specialist at once, and to be cautious with tasks that require alertness. If she misses a dose of her medication, she should call her infertility specialist.
- Clients need to understand that treatment increases the chance of multiple births.

CLIENT TEACHING

- Couples need to be taught how to evaluate and record basal body temperature and cervical mucus changes on a chart. The first day of menses is day 1 of the cycle. Ovulation is predicted by a 0.5°F drop in basal body temperature followed by a 1°F rise. In addition, over-the-counter diagnostic kits for assessing ovulatory status can be used to time coitus. The couple is advised to engage in coitus no more frequently than every

other day from 4 days before to 3 days after ovulation, to maximize the man's sperm count (Fig. 46–4).

- The man is advised to wear boxer shorts during infertility treatment, because briefs hold the scrotum close to the body and the heat reduces the sperm count. For the same reason, if he is seated all day in his work, he is counseled to take breaks every hour or so to walk about. Some women have been helped to conceive by taking guaifenesin (Robitussin) for its effect of thinning cervical mucus.
- The woman is advised to take her medication at the same time each day to maintain steady blood levels.

EVALUATION

- Successful outcomes of fertility treatment include avoidance of ovarian hyperstimulation, as well as other untoward effects. The achievement of pregnancy that results in the birth of a live infant fulfills the objectives of treatment. If pregnancy is not achieved, then intervention is aimed at helping the couple to consider alternatives to childbearing without adverse impact on their self-esteem or harm to their relationship.

DRUGS USED IN THE TREATMENT OF SEXUALLY TRANSMITTED DISEASES

Sexually transmitted diseases (STDs) are infections that are transmitted during sexual contact. Some pathogens are spread primarily through sexual contact. Others, such as *Shigella*, hepatitis A, or *Candida*, are transmitted primarily by other ways but can be spread sexually. Pathogens implicated in sexually transmitted diseases are shown in Table 46–5. If not treated, STDs can result in damage to the male and female reproductive tracts that impairs fertility, in life-threatening illness and death, and in neonatal illness and death. The last 30 years have seen a dramatic increase in this problem. The emergence of STDs that are incurable or lethal in adults, such as genital herpes and HIV infection, has led to growing awareness of the seriousness of STDs, even in affluent, industrialized countries. Several infections, including those caused by HIV, human papillomavirus, human T-lymphotrophic virus, and Epstein-Barr virus, are associated with malignancies.

TRANSMISSION AND RISK

Sexual transmission of pathogens can occur through breaks in the vaginal or cervical mucosa or the skin covering the shaft or glans of the penis.

Recent research to better understand mechanisms of HIV transmission demonstrates that each act of coitus results in tiny, friction-induced fissures on these surfaces. This problem is exacerbated by inadequate vaginal lubrication, which may occur postmenopausally, postpartally, just following menses, or when the woman is not sufficiently aroused before penetration.

Semen, sperm cells themselves, vaginal secretions, blood, and other body fluids can carry pathogens. Skin and mucosal lesions not only can be penetrated by microorganisms but can also shed them. Sexual contact can involve skin to skin, mouth to mouth, oral-genital, oral-anal, or hand-anal transmission of pathogens through breaks in the skin or mucosal surfaces or from inoculation by infectious body fluids. Anal penetration is particularly risky because of the likelihood of tissue trauma that results in the partner's exposure to enteric microorganisms.

One practice that places individuals at high risk for the transmission of STDs, particularly HIV, is engaging in sexual activity with multiple partners. Investigators at the National Institutes of Health suggest that risk of STDs is markedly increased among individuals who have more than one sexual partner per year versus those who have fewer partners. Other high-risk practices are anal or vaginal

TABLE 46–5 Pathogens Causing Sexually Transmitted Diseases

| Pathogen | Mode of Transmission | | |
	Predominantly Sexual	*Can be Sexual*	*Sexual Contact with Oral-Fecal Exposure*
Bacteria	*Calymmatobacterium granulomatis* *Chlamydia trachomatis* *Haemophilus ducreyi* *Neisseria gonorrhoeae* *Treponema pallidum* *Ureaplasma urealyticum*	*Escherichia coli* *Gardnerella vaginalis* Other vaginal bacteria Group B streptococcus *Mycoplasma hominis*	*Shigella* *Campylobacter*
Viruses	Cytomegalovirus HIV-1, HIV-2 Hepatitis B Herpes simplex virus type 2 Human papillomavirus Molluscum contagiosum virus	HTLV-1 Hepatitis C, D Herpes simplex virus type 1 Epstein-Barr virus	Hepatitis A
Protozoa, fungi, ectoparasites	*Trichomonas vaginalis* *Phthirus pubis* *Sarcoptes scabei*	*Candida albicans*	*Giardia lamblia* *Entamoeba histolytica*

intercourse without a condom, hand-anal contact, blood contact during sexual activity during menses, the use of an enema before anal intercourse, and urination on broken skin or inside the body. Risk-reducing behaviors are shown in Table 46–6.

STDs are often manifested as multiple infections. Individuals undergoing treatment for one STD should be assessed for others, including HIV. This is especially true if genital or perianal ulcerations are present.

Vertical transmission, or **perinatal infection,** occurs when a fetus or neonate is infected by the mother. Microbes can travel up the reproductive tract from the vagina or cervix and enter the intrauterine environment. Transmission can occur through contact with the mother's blood at birth or through breast milk, as in the cases of HIV and hepatitis B virus. Organisms that are of little consequence to healthy adults can be devastating to a fetus. Many STDs, such as syphilis, are transmitted transplacentally. Others, such as infection with herpes simplex virus type 2, require actual contact by the infant with microorganisms in the birth canal.

Common STD syndromes and their causative pathogens are listed in Table 46–7. Current guidelines from the Centers for Disease Control and Prevention (CDC) for the primary treatment of various STDs are listed in Table 46–8. All sexual contacts of an infected individual should be informed of their exposure and treated. Partners should refrain from sexual activity until each is clear of infection on follow-up evaluation or, at the very least, condoms should be used.

HIV DISEASE

HIV infection, which leads to acquired immunodeficiency syndrome (AIDS), is one of several diseases known to be caused by a retrovirus. Retroviruses known to cause illness in humans include HTLV-1, HTLV-2, HIV-1, and HIV-2. The retrovirus most clearly associated with AIDS is HIV-1.

Because retroviruses are able to penetrate the nucleus of the host cell, become integrated into its DNA, and replicate as the cell divides, retroviral infections last the lifetime of the infected person. The host cells that these retroviruses prefer are human T lymphocytes.

HTLV-1 is associated with adult T-cell leukemia and lymphoma. No drug regimen has yet been es-

TABLE 46–6 Risk-Reducing Behaviors for Avoidance of STDs

Sexual abstinence or sexual contact with one faithful partner

Washing and urinating before and after intercourse

Consistent use of a condom treated with nonoxynol-9

Avoiding sex with someone with genital or anal lesions

Reduction of use of alcohol or drugs, both of which impair judgment about sexual risk and immune response

Avoidance of sexual contact with HIV-infected persons, users of intravenous drugs, immigrants from high-prevalence regions, or sexual partners of all such individuals

Never sharing hypodermic needles or razors

TABLE 46–7 Common STD Syndromes and Their Causative Pathogens

Syndrome	Pathogens
Acute arthritis	*Neisseria gonorrhoeae, Chlamydia trachomatis*, hepatitis B virus (HBV), human immunodeficiency virus (HIV)
AIDS	HIV-1, HIV-2, and opportunistic pathogens
Cervicitis	*C. trachomatis, N. gonorrhoeae*, Herpes simplex virus (HSV), *Candida albicans*
Cystitis, urethritis (female)	Gram-negative bacilli, Gram-positive cocci, *C. trachomatis, N. gonorrhoeae*
Epididymitis	*C. trachomatis, N. gonorrhoeae*
Genital, anal warts	Human papillomavirus (HPV)
Lymphadenopathy	Cytomegalovirus (CMV), HIV, Epstein-Barr virus (EBV)
Neoplasias Squamous cell cancers of cervix, anus, vulva, penis	HPV
Kaposi's sarcoma	HIV, EBV
Lymphoid neoplasia, hepatocellular carcinoma	HIV, human T-lymphotrophic virus (HTLV-1)
Pelvic inflammatory disease	*Trichomonas vaginalis, N. gonorrhoeae, C. trachomatis, Bacteroides* spp, peptostreptococci, *Escherichia coli*, streptococci groups B and D, bacterial vaginitis-associated pathogens
Proctitis, proctocolitis or enterocolitis, enteritis	*N. gonorrhoeae*, HSV, *C. trachomatis, Treponema pallidum, Giardia lamblia, Campylobacter* spp, *Shigella* spp, *Entamoeba histolytica, Mycobacterium avium-intracellulare, Salmonella* spp, *Cryptosporidium, Isospora* (ingestion of intestinal flora)
Pubic lice	*Phthirus pubis*
Scabies	*Sarcoptes scabei*
Ulcerative lesions of the genitalia	HSV-1, HSV-2, *T. pallidum, C. trachomatis, Calymmatobacterium granulomatis*, HPV, *Haemophilus ducreyi*, molluscum contagiosum virus
Urethritis, male	*N. gonorrhoeae, C. trachomatis, T. vaginalis*, HSV, *Ureaplasma urealyticum, Mycoplasma hominis, Bacteroides urealyticum*
Vulvovaginitis	Bacterial vaginosis: *Gardnerella vaginitis (Haemophilus vaginalis), M. hominis, U. urealyticum, Mobiluncus curtisii, Mobiluncus mulieris, Bacteroides* spp, peptostreptococci, *T. vaginalis, C. albicans, Torulopsis oflabrata*

tablished to treat HTLV-1 infection. HTLV-2 infection is endemic among drug-addicted populations. Its role in disease is unclear. It may have a synergistic effect on HIV that hastens the development of AIDS.

HIV-2 is the most recently discovered human retrovirus. It is a less common, less efficient cause of AIDS. Its spread is less rapid than HIV-1.

The retrovirus of gravest concern among health care professionals is HIV-1. Over 300,000 Americans have been diagnosed with AIDS since 1981, and millions more have been infected with HIV.

The primary syndrome is a self-limiting episode characterized by rash, fever, and arthralgia, with or without meningitis and encephalitis. However, the primary infection may be asymptomatic. Most infected individuals develop detectable antibodies within 3 months, but this can take 12 months or longer. Many asymptomatic infected persons do not suspect that they are infected; thus, they do not seek testing or take precautions against spread of the disease.

HIV is spread by sexual contact, by contact with contaminated blood, transplacentally, and via breast milk. By destroying T lymphocytes, particularly the T_4 type, HIV depresses immunity to infectious diseases. HIV also directly affects the central nervous system (CNS) to produce polyneuropathy, transverse myelopathy, and, most commonly, an encephalopathy resulting in dementia.

Death due to one or more of the complicating conditions shown in Table 46–9 typically occurs within 10 years of HIV infection. The disease may enjoy a long period of latency, even more than a decade, and hence its spread is insidious and there is concern for educating the public about its prevention.

Current CDC criteria for the diagnosis of AIDS

TABLE 46–8 Current Guidelines for Primary Therapies for Common STDs

Disease	Primary Therapy	Notes
Acute urethral syndrome	Doxycycline 100 mg, PO, b.i.d. *or* sulfamethoxazole 1.6 g plus trimethoprim 320 mg, PO, single dose	
Bacterial vaginosis	Metronidazole 500 mg PO b.i.d. ×7d, *or* 2 g PO, single dose	Avoid alcohol during therapy; contraindicated in pregnancy
Candidiasis	Miconazole nitrate 200 mg vaginal suppository, qhs, × 3 d *or* miconazole nitrate 2% vaginal cream, 5 g, qhs × 3 d *or* clotrimazole 200 mg, vaginal suppository, daily × 3 d	Recurrent candidiasis may be indicative of other disease, such as diabetes or HIV infection
Chancroid	Azithromycin 1 g PO × 1 *or* ceftriaxone 250 mg IM × 1 *or* erythromycin base 500 mg PO q.i.d. × 7 d	Use compresses to remove necrotic material; clean ulcerative lesions t.i.d.
Chlamydia	Doxycycline 100 mg PO b.i.d. × 7–10 d *or* azithromycin 1 g PO × 1 *Children <45 kg:* Erythromycin 50 mg/kg/d PO divided in 4 doses, × 10–14 d *Children >45 kg:* Erythromycin base 500 mg PO q.i.d. × 7 d *or* erythromycin succinate 800 mg PO q.i.d. × 7 d *Infants:* Erythromycin 50 mg/kg/d PO divided into 4 doses × 10–14 d	A second course of therapy may be required
Epididymitis	Ceftriaxone 250 mg IM × 1 *and* doxycycline 100 mg PO b.i.d. × 10 d	
Genital warts	Cryotherapy *or* cryoprobe *or* podofilox 0.5% solution b.i.d. × 3 d, then 4 days off; repeat cycle × 4, *or* podophyllin 10–25% in compound tincture of benzoin × 1/w × 6 w	Nothing eradicates HPV; podophyllin contraindicated during pregnancy
Gonorrhea	Ceftriaxone 125 mg IM × 1 *or* ciprofloxacin 500 mg PO × 1 *or* cefixime 400 mg PO × 1 *or* ofloxacin 400 mg PO × 1 *Children < 45 kg:* Ceftriaxone 125 mg IM × 1 *or* ceftriaxone 50 mg/kg IM/IV (*max*, 1 g) daily × 7 d *Ophthalmia neonatorum:* Ceftriaxone 25–50 mg/kg IM/IV × 1 (*max*, 125 mg) *Ophthalmia neonatorum prophylaxis:* Silver nitrate (1%) aqueous × 1 *or* Erythromycin (0.5%) ophthalmic ointment × 1	Treat for *Chlamydia* as well Neonate may also have scalp abscess at site of fetal monitors, rhinitis, anorectal infection
Granuloma inguinale	Tetracycline hydrochloride 0.5 g PO b.i.d. × 21 d *or* streptomycin 0.5 g IM q.i.d. × 21 d *or* chloramphenicol 0.5 g PO t.i.d. × 21 d *or* gentamicin 40 mg IM b.i.d. × 21 d	
Hepatitis B	No specific therapy exists	HBV is the only STD for which a vaccine exists. The CDC recommends vaccination of all infants and adolescents. ACIP recommends vaccination of all persons with recent STD and those with more than 1 partner in the last 6 months
Herpes genitalis	*First episode, genital:* Acyclovir 200 mg PO × 5/d, × 7–10 d *Herpes proctitis, first episode:* Acyclovir 400 mg PO × 5/d, × 10 d *Recurrent:* Acyclovir 200 mg PO × 5/d	Types 1 and 2 cannot be distinguished clinically. No cure is known. Systemic disease is life-threatening to neonates, and neurologic damage may result. Viral shedding is most prevalent when symptomatic; sexual relations should be avoided

Table continued on following page

TABLE 46–8 Current Guidelines for Primary Therapies for Common STDs *(Continued)*

Disease	Primary Therapy	Notes
	Suppressive: Acyclovir 400 mg PO b.i.d. *Severe:* Acyclovir 5–10 mg / kg IV q8h × 5–7 d *HIV-infected:* Acyclovir 400 mg PO × 3–5/d until resolution *Neonatal:* Acyclovir 30 mg / kg / d	
Lymphogranuloma venereum	Doxycycline 100 mg PO b.i.d. × 21 d *or* tetracycline 500 mg PO q.i.d. × 21 d	
Molluscum contagiosum	Cryoanesthesia and curettage *or* caustic chemicals (podophyllin, trichloroacetic acid, silver nitrate) and cryotherapy	If all lesions not eradicated, may recur
Mucopurulent cervicitis Nongonococcal urethritis	Doxycycline 100 mg PO b.i.d. × 7–10 d Doxycycline 100 mg PO b.i.d. × 7 d *or* erythromycin 500 mg PO q.i.d. × 7 d	
Pelvic inflammatory disease (PID)	*Inpatient:* Doxycycline 100 mg IV b.i.d. *and* cefoxitin 2 g IV q.i.d. *or* defotetan 2 g IV q.i.d. *48 h after clinical improvement:* Doxycy- cline 100 mg PO b.i.d. for total of at least 14 d therapy *Ambulatory care:* Ofloxacin 400 mg b.i.d. *plus* either clindamycin 450 mg q.i.d. *or* metronidazole 500 mg b.i.d. × 14 d	Often polymicrobial. This regimen may not treat anaerobes, pelvic mass, or IUD-associated PID
Proctitis	Ceftriaxone 125 mg IM × 1 *and* doxycy- cline 100 mg PO b.i.d. × 7 d	
Pubic lice	Lindane 1% shampoo, apply for 4 min *or* Permethrin 1% creme rinse, apply for 10 min	Lindane not recommended for pregnant women or children < 2 years; decontaminate clothes, bedding
Scabies	Permethrin cream 5% applied to all affected areas from neck down, for 8–14 min *or* Lindane 1% applied to all affected areas from neck down for 8 h	
Sexual assault	Ceftriaxone 125 mg IM × 1 and metro- nidazole 2 g PO × 1 and doxycycline 100 mg PO b.i.d. × 7 d	Tetanus booster and gamma globulin, as well as base-line HIV testing and follow-up are recommended
Syphilis	*Primary, secondary, or <1 y duration:* Ben- zathine penicillin G, 2.4 million units IM *Unknown duration or >1 y:* Benzathine penicillin G, 7.2 million units divided in 2.4 million IM weekly ×3 *Allergic to penicillin:* Doxycycline 100 mg PO b.i.d. × 14–28 d *Penicillin-allergic pregnant women or doxy- cycline-intolerant:* Erythromycin (stearate, ethyl succinate or base) 500 mg PO q.i.d. × 2 w *Children:* Benzathine penicillin G 50,000 units / kg IM × 1, up to 2.4 million units; repeat × 3 if unknown or >1 y duration *Infants:* Aqueous crystalline penicillin G 200,000–300,000 units / kg / d IM / IV, × 10–14 d *Congenital:* Aqueous crystalline penicillin G 100,000–150,000 units / kg / d IV, × 10–14 d *or* procaine penicillin G 50,000 units / kg / d IM × 10–14 d	Some studies indicate that pregnant women should be treated with penicillin, on an incremental basis, with an emergency set-up at the bedside, if they are allergic to penicillin. In recent years CDC has recommended this approach
Trichomoniasis	Metronidazole 2 g PO × 1 *or* metronida- zole 500 mg PO b.i.d. × 7 d	Pregnant women can be treated after the first trimester

TABLE 46–9 Common Complications of Advanced HIV Infection

Reproductive tract cancers, accelerated

Human papillomavirus, exacerbated

Pneumonia, *Pneumocystis carinii,* and others

Mycobacterial infection

Tuberculosis

Meningitis

Encephalitis

Intracranial lymphoma

Kaposi's sarcoma

Herpes infection

Cytomegalovirus infection

Diarrhea, infectious or malabsorptive

Dysphagia

Sexually transmitted diseases, accelerated and/or fulminant

Gastrointestinal infections, opportunistic

Hepatic disease

Bowel obstruction

Biliary disease

Neuropathy

Shingles

Psoriasis

Arthritis

Seborrheic dermatitis

Autoimmune diseases, exacerbated

Encephalopathy

TABLE 46–10 Current CDC Criteria for Staging of HIV Infection and Diagnosis of AIDS

Category A: One of the following conditions:
Asymptomatic HIV
Persistent generalized lymphadenopathy
Acute (primary) HIV with accompanying illness or history of acute HIV infection
CD_4 cell categories: (1) 500/mm³ or more
               (2) 200–499/mm³
               (3) <200/mm³

Category B: Symptomatic conditions that meet one of the following criteria: (a) the conditions are attributed to HIV or indicate defect in cell-mediated immunity; (b) conditions considered to have clinical course complicated by HIV infection. Examples include:
Bacterial endocarditis, meningitis, pneumonia, sepsis
Candidiasis, vulvovaginitis, >1 mo or poorly responsive to therapy
Candidiasis, oropharyngeal
Cervical dysplasia, severe, or carcinoma
Constitutional syndromes, e.g. fever 38.5°C or more or diarrhea >1 mo
Hairy leukoplakia, oral
Herpes zoster, two distinct episodes or more than one dermatome
Idiopathic thrombocytopenic purpura
Listeriosis
M. tuberculosis, pulmonary
Nocardiosis
Pelvic inflammatory disease
Peripheral neuropathy
CD_4 categories: (1) 500/mm³ or more
           (2) 200–499/mm³
           (3) <200/mm³

Category C: Any condition in the 1987 AIDS case definition:
Candidiasis of bronchi, trachea, lungs
Candidiasis of esophagus
Coccidioidomycosis, disseminated or extrapulmonary
Cryptococcosis, extrapulmonary
Cryptosporidiosis, intestinal >1 mo
Cytomegalovirus (CMV) infection other than liver, spleen, or nodes
CMV retinitis with vision loss
HIV encephalopathy
Herpes simplex, ulcers >1 mo; bronchitis, pneumonitis, esophagitis
Histoplasmosis, disseminated or extrapulmonary
Isosporiasis, intestinal, >1 mo
Kaposi's sarcoma
Lymphoma, Burkitt's
Lymphoma, immunoblastic
Lymphoma, brain
Mycobacterium avium complex or *M. kansasii,* disseminated or extrapulmonary
M. tuberculosis, disseminated or extrapulmonary
Other spp, disseminated or extrapulmonary
Pneumocystis carinii pneumonia
Progressive multifocal leukoencephalopathy
Salmonella septicemia, recurrent
Toxoplasmosis of brain
Wasting syndrome due to HIV
CD_4 categories: (1) 500/mm³ or more
           (2) 200–499/mm³
           (3) <200/mm³

AIDS: Subcategories A3, B3, C1, C2, and C3

Source: *Centers for Disease Control and Prevention, U.S. Department of Health and Human Services: 1992 Revised Classification System for HIV Infection and Expanded AIDS Surveillance Case Definition for Adolescents and Adults, Nov. 15, 1991.*

are shown in Table 46–10. Because the disease has been studied mainly through the observation of males, common complications experienced by HIV-infected women are listed in Table 46–11.

Antiviral drugs currently in use to treat HIV and guidelines for their use are listed in Table 46–12 (see Chapter 26). Treatment is continued indefinitely. One major problem with HIV infection is that the virus mutates quickly within the same individual, rendering drug therapy less effective over time.

Clients are followed every 1 to 6 months, at which time a complete blood count, differential,

TABLE 46–11 Diseases Complicating HIV Infection in Women

Chronic vaginitis

Recurrent yeast infections

Pelvic inflammatory disease

Human papillomavirus, accelerated course

Cervical intraepithelial neoplasia, aggressive

Severe, persistent genital herpes

Syphilis, accelerated course

Cytomegalovirus infection of genital tract

Genital tuberculosis

Molluscum contagiosum

Postpartal infections

TABLE 46–12 Guidelines for Antiretroviral Treatment in HIV Infection

CD4 T lymphocytes>500/mm^3:
  No drug therapy
  Follow CD4 counts every 4–6 mon

CD4 T lymphocytes 200–500/mm^3:
  Begin antiretroviral therapy if symptomatic; if history of opportunistic infection; if cell count deteriorates

Initial therapy;
  Zidovudine (Retrovir) alone or in combination with didanosine (Videx) or zalcitabine (Hivid)

If patient tolerates ZDV for 4 or more months and has CD4 T lymphocyte count <300/mm^3, change to DDI.

If clinical or immmunologic deterioration on ZDV monotherapy:
  Begin combination therapy with DDC *or*
  Switch to DDI or DDC *or*
  Begin combination therapy with DDI

In pregnancy:
  A two-thirds reduction in perinatal transmission can be achieved if ZDV is begun at the 13th week; administered IV during labor and delivery; and administered to the neonate for 6–8 weeks after birth.

Sources: Rakel (Ed.), 1995 Conn's Current Therapy, Philadelphia: WB Saunders, p. 45; and CDC (1994), Recommendations of the US Public Health Service Task Force on the Use of Zidovudine to Reduce Perinatal Transmission of Human Immunodeficiency Virus, Morbid-

TABLE 46–13 Prevention and Management of Common Opportunistic Infections Associated with HIV Infection

Infection	Drugs and Dosages
Pneumocystis carinii	
Infection, acute	Trimethoprim 15 mg/kg/d + sulfamethoxazole 75–100 mg/kg/d PO or IV × 14–21 d *or* pentamidine 4 mg/kg/d IV × 14–21 d
Prophylaxis	Aerosolized pentamidine 300 mg/mo *or* trimethoprim + sulfamethoxazole PO, 1 DS daily or ×3/w
Toxoplasma encephalitis	
Acute	Pyrimethamine 50–100 mg/d PO + folinic acid 5–15 mg/d PO + sulfadiazine or trisulfapyrimidines 4–8 g/d PO × 6 w + leucovorin 10 mg PO daily
Suppressive	Pyrimethamine 25 mg PO daily + folic acid 5–15 mg/d + leucovorin 10 mg/d *or* sulfadiazine or trisulfapyrimidines 2–4 g/d PO or ×3–5/w
Cryptosporidiosis	Nutritional supplements, antidiarrheals
Isosporiasis	
Acute	Trimethoprim + sulfamethoxazole PO DS q.i.d. × 10–14 d *or* pyrimethamine 50–75 mg/d PO + folinic acid 5–10 mg/d × 1 mo
Suppressive	Trimethoprim + sulfamethoxazole 1–2 DS/d PO *or* pyrimethamine 25 mg + sulfadoxine 500 mg PO week *or* pyrimethamine 25 mg + folinic acid 5 mg/d
Candidiasis, thrush	Ketoconazole 200–400 mg PO b.i.d. ×7–14 d *or* nystatin 500,000 units ×5/d × 7–14 d *or* clotrimazole 10 mg ×5/d × 7–14 d *or* fluconazole 100 mg PO daily × 7–14 d
Candidiasis esophagitis	Fluconazole 200–400 mg/d PO × 14–21 d *or* amphotericin B 0.3 mg/kg/d IV
Cryptococcal meningitis	
Initial	Amphotericin B 0.5–1.0 mg/kg/d IV × 14 d *then* fluconazole 400 mg/d IV or PO × 8 w
Maintenance	Fluconazole 200 mg PO daily
Histoplasmosis, disseminated	
Initial	Amphotericin B 2–2.5 g total dose
Maintenance	Amphotericin B 1 mg/kg/w *or* ketoconazole 200 mg PO b.i.d. *or* itraconazole 200 mg PO daily

Table continued on following page

TABLE 46–13 Prevention and Management of Common Opportunistic Infections Associated with HIV Infection *(Continued)*

Coccidioidomycosis	
Initial	Amphotericin B 2–2.5 g total dose *or* fluconazole 200 mg PO b.i.d.
Maintenance	Amphotericin B 1 mg/kg/w *or* fluconazole 200 mg PO daily
Tuberculosis	
Active	INH 300 mg/d + RIF 600 mg/d + PZA 20–30 mg/kg/d × 2 m, then INH + RIF continued at least 9 mo and until 6 mo culture negative
Prophylaxis	INH 300 mg/d × 12 mo
M. avium complex, prophylaxis	Rifabutin 300 mg/d
Herpes simplex, mucocutaneous	
Initial, mild	Acyclovir 200 mg PO × 5/d × 10 d
Severe	Acyclovir 15 mg/kg/d IV *or* vidarabine 15 mg/kg/d IV *or* foscarnet 90 mg/kg/d IV
Maintenance	Acyclovir 200 mg PO t.i.d.
Visceral	Acyclovir 30 mg/kg/d IV × 10 d *or* vidarabine 15 mg/kg/d IV × 10 d
Herpes zoster	
Dermatomal	Acyclovir 30 mg/kg/d IV or 800 mg PO × 6/d at least × 7 d
Disseminated or visceral	Acyclovir 30 mg/kg/d IV for at least 7 d
Cytomegalovirus retinitis	
Initial	Ganciclovir 5 mg/kg/IV b.i.d. × 14–21 d *or* foscarnet 60 mg/kg IV q8h × 14–21 d
Maintenance	Ganciclovir 5 mg/kg IV daily × 5/w *or* foscarnet 90–120 mg/kg IV daily
Enteritis, colitis, esophagitis	Ganciclovir 5 mg/kg IV b.i.d. × 14–21 d (experimental)
Streptococcal pneumonia	Penicillin *or* erythromycin *or* cephalosporins
Influenza	Cefuroxime/cefamandole, ampicillin/amoxicillin *or* trimethoprim sulfamethoxazole cephalosporins
Salmonellosis	
Acute	Ampicillin 8–12 g/d IV × 1–4 w, then amoxicillin 500 mg PO t.i.d. to complete course *or* ciprofloxacin 500–750 mg PO b.i.d × 2–4 w *or* trimethoprim 5–10 mg/kg/d + sulfamethoxazole IV or PO × 4 w *or* cephalosporins, 3rd generation
Maintenance	Amoxicillin 250 mg PO b.i.d. *or* ciprofloxacin 500 mg PO daily or b.i.d. *or* trimethoprim + sulfamethoxazole 1 DS PO b.i.d.

platelet count, creatinine, transaminase, lactic dehydrogenase, and creatinine phosphokinase are evaluated. Bone marrow suppression is the most common adverse effect of treatment. When clients experience severe anemia, treatment may be halted or the individual may be transfused.

Treatments of common opportunistic infections found in individuals whose HIV infection has pro-

TABLE 46–14 Drugs Used in Management of Selected Complications Associated with HIV Infection*

Complication	Drug/Drug Category
GI: Anorexia	Megace 80 mg PO q.i.d.
	Dronabinol 5–20 mg/d divided into 2 doses, before lunch and supper
Cardiac: Cardiomyopathy	Solumedrol × 3 d, then prednisone
Pulmonary: Lipoid interstitial pneumonia	Corticosteroids
Renal: Nephropathy	Hemodialysis
Neurologic: Peripheral neuropathy	Nortriptyline, capsicin-containing ointments
Myopathy	Discontinue zidovudine × 3 w, NSAIDs, prednisone
AIDS dementia complex	Zidovudine, DDI, nimopidine, nitroglycerin, memantine (experimental)
Hematologic	
Idiopathic thrombocytopenia purpura	Prednisone, zidovudine, gamma globulin, splenectomy

Table continued on following page

TABLE 46–14 Drugs Used in Management of Selected Complications Associated with HIV Infection* (Continued)

Complication	Drug/Drug Category
Anemia	Transfusions, erythropoietin
Neutropenia	Granulocyte-macrophage colony-stimulating factor (experimental)
Malignancies	
Kaposi's sarcoma	Total liquid nitrogen, intralesional vinblastine, alpha-interferon, radiation, chemotherapy (bleomycin and vincristine +/− doxorubicin)
B-cell lymphoma	Cyclophosphamide, doxorubicin, vincristine, corticosteroids +/− cranial radiation
CNS lymphoma	Cranial radiation +/− chemotherapy
Dermatologic	
Molluscum contagiosum	Surgical extirpation, freezing
Dermatophytic fungi	Topical miconazole or clotrimazole, griseofulvin or ketoconazole × 1–3 mo
	Nails: griseofulvin × 6–15 mo
Eczema, psoriasis	Topical steroids, antipruritics
Seborrhea	Hydrocortisone 1% cream + topical ketoconazole, zirconium sulfide, salicylic acid, or coal tar shampoos
Oral	
Oral ulcers	Rinses: Miles' solution (60 mg hydrocortisone + 20 mL mycostatin + 2 g tetracycline + 120 mL viscous lidocaine)
	Dyclonine, Benadryl or viscous lidocaine 2%
	Prednisone 40 mg/d PO × 1–2 w then taper
Oral hairy leukoplakia	Acyclovir 200 mg PO × 5/d × 2–3 w
Gingivitis/periodontitis	Metronidazole 250 mg PO t.i.d. or 500 mg PO b.i.d. × 7–14 d
	Chlorhexidine gluconate 0.12% rinse b.i.d.
Diarrhea	Lomotil, loperamide, paregoric, as effective
	Nutritional formulas: Ensure, Sustacal, Enrich, Magnecal, 10 cans/d
	Vivonex T.E.N.
CMV enteritis, colitis	Ganciclovir 5 mg/kg b.i.d. × 3 w
Psychiatric, sleep disorders	
Anxiety	Lorazepam 1 mg b.i.d.
	Alprazolam 0.25 mg b.i.d.
	Buspirone 5 mg t.i.d. increased to 15–30 mg/d
Depression	Fluoxetine 20 mg daily
	Nortriptyline 25 mg h.s. increased to 75–150 mg/d PRN
Insomnia	Benadryl 25 mg h.s.
	Nortriptyline 25 mg h.s.
	Chloral hydrate 500 mg h.s.
Apathy	Ritalin 5–10 mg t.i.d.

Note: Drug dosages may not be given because of the rapidly changing, highly experimental, individualized and empirical nature of AIDS symptom management.

gressed to AIDS are shown in Table 46–13. Drugs that have been used to relieve other common symptoms and complications are shown in Table 46–14.

OCCUPATIONAL EXPOSURE OF HEALTH WORKERS

The Occupational Safety and Health Administration (OSHA) generated standards on blood-borne pathogens that make universal precautions mandatory for all health care workers. The new rules also require employers to offer the HBV vaccine free of charge to every employee who can reasonably be expected to have direct contact with blood or other infectious materials. Table 46–15 shows a protocol for worksite exposure currently being implemented at some large medical centers.

TABLE 46–15 Blood-borne Infections Postexposure Protocol for Health Care Workers

Thoroughly scrub skin exposure site, generously rinse mucosal exposure site.

Report to employee health or infection control department.

Perform baseline HIV test, with appropriate pre- and post-test counseling.

Inform client of worker exposure and request that client be tested; if client refuses, preexisting blood samples can be tested.

Begin zidovudine prophylaxis within 2 h (duration varies among medical centers).

Administer immunoglobulin and hepatitis B vaccine series if worker is not vaccinated.

If client HIV status cannot be determined or client is known to be infected, HIV testing is repeated q 3 mo × 1 y, then annually × 2 y.

NURSING PROCESS: Sexually Transmitted Disease

Nurses need to be sensitive to clients' reasons for seeking or avoiding care for STDs. Psychosocial reactions to a diagnosis of STD may include feelings of anger, depression, shame, guilt, hurt, fear, and concern. Clients need privacy during the interview and examination, with attention to their comfort, such as warming the speculum before a pelvic examination. A second health professional should be present in the examination room during the physical examination of a female client.

ASSESSMENT

- Before physical data are gathered, a history is elicited. Less sensitive issues are addressed first so that trust can be established. The term "partners" is used in discussing sexual activity rather than value-laden terms such as "wife" or "boyfriend."
- The history includes the chief complaint, a description of the course of illness, a review of systems and general health history, a reproductive history, a sexual history, a review of lifestyle and social habits, and identification of allergies.
- Physical examination includes inspection and palpation of the genitalia and other points of inoculation.
- Laboratory tests include wet slides with microbe-specific setting agents, urinalysis, cultures, pap smear, a complete blood count, syphilis serology, and herpes simplex virus 1 and 2 antibodies.

POTENTIAL NURSING DIAGNOSES

- Actual as well as potential infection
- Knowledge deficit with regard to transmission and prevention as well as treatment
- Noncompliance with known prevention strategies
- Pain
- Low self-esteem
- Altered sexuality patterns.

A medical diagnosis of HIV disease would bring with it additional nursing diagnoses:
- Fatigue
- Anxiety
- Anticipatory grieving
- Social isolation
- Self-care deficits and health maintenance needs

PLANNING

- Short-term goals include the client's adherence to the treatment regimen and avoidance of adverse effects.
- Long-term goals include the client's return for follow-up evaluation and adoption of risk-reducing sexual behaviors.

NURSING INTERVENTIONS

- The client needs to understand procedures performed during evaluation and how to administer prescribed medications and treatments. Side effects and adverse effects that require immediate intervention are reviewed.
- Specific interventions include providing needed support as the client deals with the fact that the infection is sexually transmitted.
- The client needs to notify sexual partners so that they can be evaluated and treated.
- Ideally, sexual contact is avoided during treatment. At the least, condoms should be used until both partners are clear of infection.
- Individuals are scheduled for follow-up visits from 4 days to 4 weeks, depending on the type of infection and treatment.
- Individuals with any STD are counseled about being tested for HIV infection.

CLIENT TEACHING

- The mode of transmission of STDs, the relationship of all STDs with HIV infection, and how HIV risk is avoided should all be reviewed.
- Individuals are advised to plan periodic reproductive health check-ups.

EVALUATION

- Intervention has been successful if the individual's infection is cleared up on reevaluation or, in the case of viral infections, the individual experiences quiescence of the virus.
- One important outcome to evaluate is that the infection is not transmitted to other individuals. Another is that the individual is able to avoid sexual practices that carry risk of STDs, including promiscuity, intercourse without the use of a condom, and traumatic sexual practices.

SUMMARY

Reproductive health and fertility require integrity of hormonal mechanisms and reproductive anatomy. Infertility can be caused by male, female, or couple factors. Often, the use of drugs to stimulate ovulation is effective treatment. Clients need to understand the treatment regimen, and they need support in dealing with the psychological impact of this condition.

Finally, STDs can constitute a threat to reproductive health, neonatal health, fertility, and even life. Early diagnosis and treatment are crucial but less effective than prevention. HIV/AIDS is complicated by numerous opportunistic infections and autoimmune processes. For some, drug therapies may offer relief, although ultimately this disease is fatal.

■ CASE STUDY

Clients with Infertility

Todd Johnson, a teacher, married Diane, age 32 years, 3 years ago. Diane is the only sexual partner Todd has ever had. For the last year they have been trying to conceive, without success. Diane's nurse practitioner learns when taking Diane's history that Diane had multiple sexual partners during her college years and that she was once treated for gonorrhea. Diane's menstrual history reveals an erratic pattern of unpredictable periods, about every 2 or 3 months. The nurse practitioner reviews the relationship between timing of coitus and conception, instructs Diane on taking her temperature each morning before she gets out of bed and maintaining an ovulation record, and suggests that a home test kit may be helpful in identifying when ovulation has occurred. Diane and Todd are referred to an infertility specialist.

1. What is the relevance of Diane's past sexual history to the current complaint?
2. Why would the infertility specialist consider cultures for *C. trachomatis* and *N. gonorrhoeae* years after exposure?
3. What other tests would reveal damage resulting from STDs?
4. What is positive about Diane's menstrual history? What about her menstrual pattern makes conception difficult?
5. How can Diane predict when she will ovulate?
6. After a complete evaluation of Todd and Diane, a course of clomiphene citrate is prescribed. What side effects can Diane expect?
7. When should Diane take the medication?
8. When should Todd and Diane have sexual intercourse?

9. Diane experiences midcycle abdominal pain. What should she do when this occurs? How will her infertility specialist interpret this?
10. Diane becomes pregnant after four cycles on clomiphene citrate. What is one potential risk factor with this pregnancy?

Diane becomes pregnant and has a baby boy following an uneventful pregnancy. The baby has numerous upper respiratory infections during his first 4 months of life, twice requiring hospitalization, and gains weight slowly. When the family is referred to a tertiary pediatric medical center, the medical staff ask Diane if she would consider being tested for HIV.

11. What in her history puts her at risk for HIV infection?
12. Why is it possible that Diane could test positive for HIV when she has shown no sign of infection for nearly a decade after her high-risk behavior?

STUDY QUESTIONS

1. What is the relationship between STDs and infertility?
2. How should a couple determine the timing of coitus when they are trying to conceive?
3. What should be the timing of coitus in relation to ovarian stimulation therapy?
4. What are some adverse effects of clomiphene citrate therapy?
5. What are some psychosocial effects of infertility therapy?
6. Which STDs cannot be cured?
7. Which STDs are associated with life-threatening illness?
8. Any time an individual is successfully treated for an STD, what should the nurse emphasize in client teaching?
9. What reproductive tract infections may or may not be sexually transmitted? What should the client tell his or her partner when such an infection occurs?
10. Why do ulcerative STDs place an individual at risk for HIV infection?
11. Why is AIDS still considered a terminal illness even though three antiretroviral medications have been licensed for use in its management?
12. What is the most profound adverse effect of zidovudine?

Unit XIII

Emergency Agents

This final unit focuses on adult and pediatric emergency drugs. The chapter considers pharmacologic treatment for five categories of emergency situations: (1) cardiac, (2) neurosurgical, (3) poisoning, (4) shock, and (5) hypertensive crisis. Specific drug protocols and dosages for the pediatric client are included.

Chapter 47

Adult and Pediatric Emergency Drugs

Linda Laskowski-Jones

OUTLINE

Objectives
Terms
Introduction
Emergency Drugs for Cardiac
  Disorders
    Nitroglycerin
    Morphine Sulfate
    Atropine Sulfate
    Isoproterenol
    Verapamil
    Diltiazem
    Adenosine
    Lidocaine
    Procainamide

Bretylium Tosylate
Epinephrine
Sodium Bicarbonate
Emergency Drugs for Neurosur-
  gical Disorders
    Mannitol
    Methylprednisolone
Emergency Drugs for Poisoning
    Naloxone
    Ipecac Syrup
    Activated Charcoal
    Magnesium Sulfate/Mag-
      nesium Citrate

Emergency Drugs for Shock
    Dopamine
    Dobutamine
    Norepinephrine
    Epinephrine
    Diphenhydramine Hy-
      drochloride
    Dextrose 50%
    Glucagon
Emergency Drugs for Hypertensive Crises
    Sodium Nitroprusside

OBJECTIVES

Describe indications for the emergency drugs listed in this chapter.

Explain how to administer the drugs properly.

List pertinent nursing considerations and actions specific for each agent.

Define the basic mechanism of action for each emergency drug.

Describe significant adverse effects of each drug.

TERMS

anaphylactic shock
angina pectoris
asthma
bradycardia
cathartic

dysrhythmias
emetic
extravasation
glycogenolysis
heart block

hypertensive crisis
hypovolemic shock
myocardial infarction
tachycardia

INTRODUCTION

The drugs described in this chapter are first-line agents commonly used to treat various medical emergencies. Nurses must have a ready knowledge of the indications and actions of these agents, because medical and surgical emergencies can occur in virtually any area of nursing practice. Learning key nursing implications prior to a crisis situation will enable the nurse to function at the highest possible level when the client requires life-saving intervention.

At the end of each group of emergency drugs there is a summary table of the drugs, their dosages, and indications. Common adult doses are listed in the tables; pediatric dosages may vary widely depending on the age and the weight of the child. The tables list only the most common indications and dosages for the emergency drugs discussed; the tables *do not* describe all possible uses and dosing regimens for the agents.

EMERGENCY DRUGS FOR CARDIAC DISORDERS

Drugs described in this section are indicated for cardiac emergencies such as angina, myocardial infarction, disturbances of cardiac rate or rhythm, and cardiac arrest. These drugs often must be prepared and administered rapidly. A sound knowledge base as well as easy access to the drugs and necessary equipment is essential for the best client outcome in cardiac emergency situations. These drugs are cross referenced to the specialty chapter.

NITROGLYCERIN

Nitroglycerin dilates coronary arteries and improves blood flow to ischemic myocardium. It is therefore the treatment of choice for **angina pectoris** (chest pain) and **myocardial infarction** (heart attack). Nitroglycerin is available in sublingual, oral, topical, and intravenous forms. Only the sublingual and intravenous preparations will be discussed.

Sublingual nitroglycerin (Nitrostat) (0.3 to 0.4 mg) is indicated for clients experiencing an acute anginal attack. The client is taught to place one sublingual nitroglycerin tablet under the tongue and allow it to dissolve slowly. Not all sublingual nitroglycerin preparations available today cause a burning sensation under the tongue, and this should not be relied on to indicate potency. If the chest pain is not relieved, sublingual nitroglycerin may be repeated at 5-min intervals until a total of three tablets has been taken. If pain persists, further

interventions are necessary in an emergency or critical care setting. An ambulance should be called if the client is outside of the hospital. Blood pressure and heart rate must be monitored closely. Hypotension is a common adverse effect, especially the first time a client takes nitroglycerin. Tachycardia or, uncommonly, bradycardia also may occur.

Intravenous nitroglycerin (Tridil) is reserved for clients with unstable angina or acute myocardial infarction. A continuous infusion is usually initiated at a rate of 10 to 20 μg/min and increased by 5 to 10 μg/min every 5 to 10 min based on chest pain and blood pressure response. Continuous blood pressure and heart monitoring are required because hypotension is a common adverse effect. Hypotension usually is treated by reducing or discontinuing the nitroglycerin infusion as ordered (see Chapter 32).

MORPHINE SULFATE

Morphine sulfate, a narcotic analgesic, is used to treat the chest pain associated with acute myocardial infarction. It also is indicated for acute pulmonary edema. Morphine relieves pain, dilates venous vessels, and reduces the workload on the heart. The standard dosage of morphine sulfate is 1 to 3 mg intravenously (IV) over 1 to 5 min repeated until chest pain is relieved. The nurse must be aware that respiratory depression and hypotension are common adverse effects; close client monitoring is essential. The narcotic antagonist naloxone (Narcan) may be ordered to reverse the action of morphine if adverse effects pose a significant risk to the client. The dose is 0.4 to 0.8 mg every 2 to 3 min as indicated (see Chapter 14).

ATROPINE SULFATE

Atropine sulfate is indicated in the treatment of hemodynamically significant **bradycardia** (slow heart rate) and **heart block** (e.g., low cardiac output, hypotension), as well as asystole. Atropine acts to increase heart rate by inhibiting the action of the vagus nerve (parasympatholytic effect). Atropine sulfate is also used as an emergency drug to reverse the toxic effects of organophosphate pesticide exposure, which include bradycardia and excessive secretions. In symptomatic bradycardia, atropine is administered intravenously in 0.5-mg doses at 5-min intervals until the desired heart rate is achieved or until 0.04 mg/kg or a total of 3 mg is given. In **asystole** (cardiac arrest), atropine is given as a 1.0-mg bolus dose IV, which may be repeated up to the dosing limits every 3 to 5 minutes.

The adult intravenous atropine dose should not be less than 0.5 mg or exceed 3 mg: doses below 0.5 mg can produce a paradoxical bradycardia; at doses of 3 mg or greater, vagal activity is considered completely blocked and further atropine administration may have no benefit. Atropine sulfate can be administered through an endotracheal tube if no venous access exists; 2 to 2.5 times the IV dose should be diluted in 10 mL of sterile water or normal saline and instilled deep into the endotracheal tube via a feeding tube attached to a syringe. After endotracheal administration, the client should be ventilated vigorously with an Ambu bag to enhance absorption of the drug.

Continuous cardiac and blood pressure monitoring is essential for the client who receives intravenous atropine sulfate. Significant adverse effects include cardiac dysrhythmias, tachycardia, myocardial ischemia, restlessness, anxiety, mydriasis, thirst, and urinary retention.

Pediatric Implications

Because cardiac output is dependent on heart rate in infants under 6 months, bradycardia (heart rate <80 beats per minute [bpm]) must be treated. Prior to administration of drugs, efforts should be targeted toward restoring adequate ventilation and oxygenation. If these maneuvers do not produce the desired clinical response, then atropine is indicated.

The pediatric dose of atropine is 0.02 mg/kg IV or via endotracheal tube (ETT) or intraosseous route. It is important to be cognizant that the minimum dose is 0.1 mg. The maximum total pediatric dose is 1.0 mg in a child and 2.0 mg in an adolescent. For the neonate in cardiac arrest or with a spontaneous heart rate of <80 bpm, epinephrine 0.01 to 0.03 mg/kg IV or via ETT every 3 to 5 minutes as indicated may be preferred to elevate the heart rate, because stressed neonates quickly deplete their own stores of catecholamines (see Chapter 19).

ISOPROTERENOL

Isoproterenol (Isuprel) is a beta-adrenergic drug given to increase heart rate. Typically, isoproterenol is considered only after the maximum dose of atropine (3 mg), dopamine and epinephrine infusions, and a transcutaneous pacemaker have failed to produce the desired clinical response in clients with third-degree heart block. Thus, the client who exhibits symptomatic refractory bradycardia is a candidate for isoproterenol. Isoproterenol is administered as an IV infusion, generally 1 mg diluted in 250 mL of 5% dextrose in water, at 2 to 10 $\mu g/min$ titrated to heart rate (usually 60 bpm). An electronic infusion device must be used to provide precise infusion control.

The nurse must carefully monitor the client receiving isoproterenol. Significant adverse effects include myocardial ischemia, tachycardia, and life-threatening dysrhythmias such as ventricular tachycardia and ventricular fibrillation. The nurse should alert the physician promptly if any increase in premature ventricular contractions is noted on the cardiac monitor or if the heart rate exceeds 100 bpm; the dosage may need to be decreased or the infusion stopped.

Pediatric Implications

Epinephrine infusions may be preferable to isoproterenol infusions to increase heart rate above 80 bpm in pediatric clients. Isoproterenol can cause a large fall in diastolic blood pressure. The initial dose is 0.5 $\mu g/kg/min$ titrated to the desired response. As in the adult client, isoproterenol should never be used in the cardiac arrest situation (see Chapter 18).

VERAPAMIL

Verapamil (Isoptin), a calcium channel blocker, is indicated for the treatment of **tachycardia** (rapid heart rate) originating above the ventricles (supraventricular tachycardia). Such heart rates generally exceed 150 bpm. Verapamil slows conduction through the heart and has negative inotropic and vasodilating effects. In emergency situations, verapamil is administered as an intravenous bolus in variable age- and weight-dependent dosages, which should not exceed 2.5 to 5 mg given slowly over a 1- to 2-min period. Repeat doses of 5 to 10 mg may be ordered in 15 to 30 minutes. The nurse must carefully monitor heart rate and rhythm as well as blood pressure. Cardiac conduction disturbances and profound hypotension can occur. An intravenous injection of calcium may be ordered to prevent or treat calcium channel blocker–induced hypotension (see Chapters 32 and 34).

DILTIAZEM

Diltiazem is a calcium channel blocker like verapamil that is administered as an intravenous bolus to treat supraventricular tachycardia and to slow the ventricular response rate in atrial fibrillation or flutter. Diltiazem has less of a negative inotropic effect than verapamil, but it has strong negative chronotropic actions. Therefore, IV diltiazem is less likely to cause cardiac depression but is very effective in controlling heart rate.

The usual initial bolus dose of IV diltiazem is 0.25 mg/kg given over 2 min. If the supraventricular tachycardia does not convert to a normal sinus rhythm in 15 minutes, a second IV bolus of 0.35 mg/kg may be necessary. For ongoing control of the ventricular rate in clients with atrial fibrillation or flutter, a continuous infusion of diltiazem is indicated at a dose range of 5 to 15 mg/h, titrated according to the desired heart rate for not longer than 24 hours.

The nurse must carefully monitor blood pressure and heart rate after administering IV diltiazem. Although mild, transient hypotension is common, significant hypotension may be treated with injection of intravenous calcium to elevate blood pressure. In clients who are hypotensive prior to calcium channel blocker administration, intravenous calcium may be ordered as a pretreatment to prevent the hypotensive response to the drug.

Diltiazem can raise serum digoxin levels, predisposing the client to digitalis toxicity. Simultaneous use of calcium channel blockers and beta blockers is contraindicated because their negative inotropic and negative chronotropic effects will be synergistic, causing myocardial depression and bradycardia. Other contraindications include heart block or sick sinus syndrome in the client without a pacemaker and severe heart failure. The nurse should be especially careful when administering calcium channel blockers to pediatric patients, because they may have preexisting myocardial dysfunction.

ADENOSINE

Adenosine (Adenocard) was introduced recently to treat paroxysmal supraventricular tachycardia (PSVT), a sudden, uncontrolled, rapid rhythm. A natural substance found in all body cells, adenosine slows impulse conduction through the heart's atrioventricular (AV) node, interrupts dysrhythmia-producing reentry pathways, and can restore a normal rhythm in clients with PSVT. Because the half-life is less than 5 sec, adenosine is administered rapidly as a 6-mg IV bolus over 1 to 3 sec. A 12-mg bolus may be given 1 to 2 min after the initial dose if PSVT persists and can be repeated once if necessary. Dosages greater than 12 mg are not recommended.

Nursing considerations include continuous cardiac monitoring and frequent assessment of vital signs. Adenosine is inhibited by methylxanthines such as caffeine and theophylline. Although few adverse reactions have been reported, hypotension and dyspnea may occur. In addition, a short period of asystole may follow administration (up to 15 sec). Spontaneous cardiac activity resumes. Adenosine is contraindicated in clients with second- and third-degree heart block and in clients with sick sinus syndrome, except those with functioning pacemakers (see Chapter 32).

LIDOCAINE

Lidocaine is the primary drug used to treat ventricular **dysrhythmias** (irregular heart beats), such as premature ventricular contractions (PVCs), ventricular tachycardia, and ventricular fibrillation. Lidocaine exerts a local anesthetic effect on the heart, thus decreasing myocardial irritability. For this reason, lidocaine is commonly prescribed following myocardial infarction as prophylaxis against dangerous ventricular dysrhythmias. Typically, a client with ventricular dysrhythmias is given a 1 mg/kg bolus of lidocaine, followed by 0.5 mg/kg every 5 to 10 min until the dysrhythmia is controlled or a total dose of 3 mg/kg has been administered. A continuous lidocaine infusion is initiated at a rate of 2 to 4 mg/min to maintain a therapeutic serum level. Lidocaine may also be administered via the endotracheal route in an amount 2 to 2.5 times the IV dose.

Important nursing considerations for the client receiving lidocaine include continuous cardiac monitoring and assessment for signs and symptoms of lidocaine toxicity (confusion, drowsiness, hearing impairment, cardiac conduction defects, myocardial depression, muscle twitching, and seizures). Because lidocaine is metabolized by the liver, clients with hepatic impairment, congestive heart failure, shock, and advanced age are at higher risk for toxicity. In these clients, the lidocaine dose may need to be reduced by as much as 50%.

Pediatric Implications

Ventricular ectopy is uncommon in children. Metabolic causes should be suspected if ventricular dysrhythmias occur. The pediatric dose of lidocaine is 1 mg/kg IV, ETT, or via the intraosseous route. A maintenance infusion of 20 to 50 μg/kg/min is recommended following the bolus dose (see Chapter 32). Drug data for lidocaine are presented in Figure 47–1.

PROCAINAMIDE

Procainamide (Pronestyl) is an antidysrhythmic agent often prescribed when lidocaine has failed to achieve the desired clinical response. Indications in-

FIGURE 47–1. Emergency Treatment of Cardiac States: Antidysrhythmic

Lidocaine HCl	Dosage	**NURSING PROCESS** Assessment and Planning
Lidocaine HCl (Xylocaine) Antidysrhythmic, class IB *Pregnancy Category:* C	A: IV: ETT*: 1–1.5 mg/kg; may repeat 0.5 mg/kg q 5–10 min up to 3 mg/kg (max) Drip: 1–4 mg/min C: IV: ETT* or IO: Initially: 1 mg/kg; maint: 30–50 μg/kg/min is recommended after bolus *Note: For *endotracheal* drug administration, dose should be 2 to 2.5 times IV dose in adults and up to 10 times the IV dose for pediatric arrest. *Therapeutic Range:* 1.5–5 μg/mL	
Contraindications	**Drug-Lab-Food Interactions**	
Hypersensitivity, advanced atrioventricular block *Caution:* Liver disease, congestive heart failure, elderly	*Increase* effects with phenytoin, quinidine, procainamide, propranolol; *increase* risk of toxicity with cimetidine, beta-adrenergic blockers	
Pharmacokinetics	**Pharmacodynamics**	Interventions
Absorption: *Distribution:* PB: 60–80%; concentrates in adipose tissue *Metabolism:* t½: Initial: 7–30 min; terminal: 9–120 min *Excretion:* Through the liver	PO: Onset: 45–60 s Peak: 45–60 s Duration: 10–20 min	

Therapeutic Effects/Uses: Primary drug to treat ventricular dysrhythmias such as premature ventricular contractions (PVCs), ventricular tachycardia, and ventricular fibrillation. *Mode of Action:* Decreases automaticity; increases electrical threshold of ventricle.	Evaluation

Side Effects	**Adverse Reactions**
Drowsiness, confusion, dyspnea, lethargy, hypotension, nausea, vomiting	*Life-threatening:* Seizures, cardiac arrest

KEY: IV: intravenous; ETT: endotracheal tube; PB: protein-binding; t½: half-life; s: seconds.

clude ventricular tachycardia, PVCs, and rapid supraventricular dysrhythmias. The typical intravenous loading dose of procainamide is 20–30 mg/min until the dysrhythmia is successfully treated. Other end points to procainamide administration include giving a total of 17 mg/kg of the drug, the development of hypotension, and specific changes on the electrocardiogram (ECG) (e.g., widening of the QRS complex by 50% or more). A continuous maintenance infusion of 1 to 4 mg/min may be ordered following the loading dose.

Procainamide administration can cause severe hypotension. Heart block, rhythm disturbances, and cardiac arrest can occur. Procainamide is contraindicated in clients with torsades de pointes. The drug is eliminated via the kidneys; therefore, clients in renal failure are at higher risk of adverse effects and often require a lower dosage (see Chapter 32).

BRETYLIUM TOSYLATE

Bretylium (Bretylol) is an antidysrhythmic agent used to treat ventricular tachycardia and ventricular fibrillation when lidocaine, electric countershock, or procainamide has been ineffective. How bretylium works is not well established. For ventricular fibrillation, bretylium is administered undiluted as a rapid intravenous 5-mg/kg bolus dose. After 5 min, the dosage may be increased to 10 mg/kg if necessary. Bretylium 10 mg/kg may be repeated every 5 to 30 min until a maximum dose of 35 mg/kg is given. For ventricular tachycardia, bretylium is usually diluted in 50 mL of dextrose 5% in water or normal saline solution, and 5 to 10 mg/kg is administered slowly over 8 to 10 min; rapid infusion may cause nausea, vomiting, and low blood pressure in a conscious client. Do not exceed the maximum total dose of 35 mg/kg over a 24-hour period. A continuous infusion of bretylium can be initiated at a rate of 2 mg/min. Bretylium may not take effect for up to 20 min after injection.

After bretylium administration, the nurse must monitor the client in ventricular fibrillation for return of pulses. In the client experiencing ventricular tachycardia, bretylium may cause an initial rise in blood pressure and heart rate, followed by orthostatic hypotension. Generally, placing the client in a supine position and administering IV fluids as ordered are appropriate interventions to treat the orthostatic hypotension.

Pediatric Implications

The use of bretylium in children is not well established.

EPINEPHRINE

Epinephrine is a catecholamine with both alpha- and beta-adrenergic effects. Indications for administration of intravenous epinephrine include profound bradycardia, asystole, pulseless ventricular tachycardia, and ventricular fibrillation. Epinephrine is thought to improve perfusion of the heart and brain in cardiac arrest states through constriction of peripheral blood vessels. In addition, epinephrine increases the chances for successful electrical countershock (defibrillation) in ventricular fibrillation. For bradycardia, an epinephrine infusion may be ordered at 2 to 10 μg/min. For asystole, pulseless ventricular tachycardia, and ventricular fibrillation, epinephrine is administered in 1-mg doses IV every 3 to 5 min until the desired clinical response is achieved (usually, return of effective cardiac activity). High-dose epinephrine (5 mg or 0.1 mg/kg) may be considered after the initial 1.0-mg dose. Epinephrine also may be given via the ETT route, as described for atropine sulfate.

Nursing implications for clients receiving epinephrine include constant cardiac and hemodynamic monitoring. Epinephrine can cause myocardial ischemia and cardiac dysrhythmias. Epinephrine should never be administered in the same site as an alkaline solution such as sodium bicarbonate; alkaline solutions inactivate epinephrine. In addition, the presence of metabolic or respiratory acidosis will decrease the effectiveness of epinephrine. All efforts should be made to correct acid-base imbalances in the client.

Pediatric Implications

The pediatric dose of epinephrine is 0.01 mg/kg (1:10,000 solution) given IV, ETT, or via the intraosseous route for cardiac arrest (see Chapter 18).

SODIUM BICARBONATE

Sodium bicarbonate is prescribed to treat the metabolic acidosis that often accompanies cardiac arrest. The current standard is to give sodium bicarbonate only after adequate ventilation, chest compressions, and drug therapy fail to correct the acidotic state. Sodium bicarbonate is rarely a first-line drug in cardiac arrest situations; it is preferentially given based on results of arterial blood gas analysis when acidosis is severe. In the event that a client has been in arrest for a prolonged period and blood gas analysis is not available, sodium bicarbonate may be ordered as part of the ongoing resuscitation attempt. The standard initial intravenous dose of sodium bicarbonate is 1 mEq/kg. The drug may be repeated at 0.5 mEq/kg every 10 min as needed.

Important nursing considerations relevant to sodium bicarbonate include careful monitoring of arterial blood gas analysis results. Sodium bicarbonate administration can lead to metabolic alkalosis. In addition, catecholamines such as epinephrine, norepinephrine, and dopamine should not be infused in the same site as sodium bicarbonate; catecholamines are inactivated by solutions containing sodium bicarbonate. Table 47–1 lists emergency cardiac drugs, their dosages, and indications.

Pediatric Implications

If metabolic acidosis persists after attention has been directed at maintaining optimal ventilation and oxygenation, sodium bicarbonate may be given to the pediatric client in a 1 mEq/kg dose via the IV or intraosseous route. Subsequent doses of 0.5

TABLE 47–1 Cardiac Emergency Drugs

Generic (Brand)	Route and Dosage	Uses & Considerations
Adenosine (Adenocard)	A: Initially: 6 mg; then 12 mg in 1–2 min if needed; may repeat 12 mg × 1	Paroxysmal supraventricular tachycardia. *Pregnancy category:* C; PB: UK; t½: < 10 sec.
Atropine sulfate	IV: ETT: 0.5–1 mg; can repeat up to 0.03–0.04 mg/kg or 3 mg *(max)*	Symptomatic bradycardia; asystole. *Pregnancy category:* C; PB: 60%–80%; t½: 2–3 h
Bretylium tosylate (Bretylol)	IV: Initially: 5 mg/kg; then 10 mg/kg q10–30 min up to 30 mg/kg total *(max)* over 24 h	Ventricular tachycardia, ventricular fibrillation. *Pregnancy category:* C; PB: 1%–6%; t½: 4–18 h
Diltiazem	IV: 0.25 mg/kg; repeat in 15 min at 0.05 mg/kg IV: drip 5–15 mg/h	Supraventricular tachycardia, atrial fibrillation and flutter. *Pregnancy category:* C; PB: 80%; t½: 2–5 h
Epinephrine	IV: ETT: 0.5–1 mg; may be repeated q5min	Asystole, ventricular fibrillation. *Pregnancy category:* C; PB: UK; t½: UK
Lidocaine	See Prototype Drug Chart (Figure 47–1)	
Morphine sulfate	IV: 1–3 mg q5–30 min	Chest pain, unstable angina, pulmonary edema. *Pregnancy category:* C; PB: 35%; t½: 2–2.5 h
Nitroglycerin (Nitrostat, Tridil)	SL: 0.3–0.4 mg IV: Drip: 10–20 µg/min, increased 5–10 µg/min q5–10 min (titrated)	Chest pain, angina, unstable angina, MI. *Pregnancy category:* C; PB: 60%; t½: 1–4 min
Procainamide HCl (Pronestyl)	IV: 20–30 mg/min; max: 17 mg/kg *Recognize end points:* • Hypotension • QRS widens > 50% • Total dose of 17 mg/kg given Drip: 1–4 mg/min	PVCs, ventricular tachycardia, ventricular fibrillation, atrial dysrhythmias. *Pregnancy category:* C; PB: 20%; t½: 3–4 h
Sodium bicarbonate	IV: Initially: 1 mEq/kg; then 0.5 mEq/kg if needed	Metabolic acidosis. *Pregnancy category:* C; PB: UK; t½: UK
Verapamil HCl (Isoptin, Calan)	IV: Age- and weight-dependent dosages; should not exceed 5 mg; repeat doses may be needed	Paroxysmal supraventricular tachycardia. *Pregnancy category:* C; PB: 90%; t½: 3–8 h

KEY: *A:* adult; *ETT:* endotracheal tube; *IV:* intravenous; *PB:* protein-binding; *SL:* sublingual; *t½:* half-life; *UK:* unknown.

mEq/kg may be given every 10 min if blood gases are not available. Sodium bicarbonate is hyperosmolar and should be diluted from an 8.4% solution (1 mEq/mL) to a 4.2% solution (0.5 mEq/mL) for infants under 3 months of age (see Chapter 10).

EMERGENCY DRUGS FOR NEUROSURGICAL DISORDERS

The neurosurgical drugs discussed in this section are commonly administered in emergency, trauma, and critical care settings. For maximum benefit, these agents must be given as early as possible when clinically indicated. Knowledge of proper administration techniques and guidelines will enhance therapeutic effectiveness. These drugs are cross-referenced to the specialty chapters.

MANNITOL

Mannitol is an osmotic diuretic used in the emergency and neurosurgical setting to treat increased intracranial pressure, which may occur following head trauma, neurosurgery, and other types of intracranial pathology. Mannitol may be given as an intravenous bolus or via a continuous drip. The usual initial bolus dose of mannitol is 1.5 to 2.0 g/kg IV of a 25% solution. Subsequent dosing is highly variable. Mannitol is highly irritating to veins. The nurse must use a filter needle when administering mannitol, as crystals may form in the solution and be inadvertently injected. In addition, the nurse should monitor laboratory studies, including serum osmolality and keep accurate intake and output records to assess fluid volume status because diuresis may be substantial (see Chapters

FIGURE 47–2. Emergency Treatment of Neurosurgical States: Diuretic

Mannitol	Dosage	NURSING PROCESS Assessment and Planning

Mannitol
   (Osmitrol)
Osmotic diuretic
Pregnancy Category: C
	A: IV: Initially 1.5–2.0 g/kg of D 25%
	   sol as a bolus
	Highly individualized	

Contraindications	**Drug-Lab-Food Interactions**	
Hypersensitivity, severe dehydration *Caution:* Pregnancy, breast-feeding, current intracranial bleeding	May *decrease* effectiveness with lithium	
Pharmacokinetics	**Pharmacodynamics**	Interventions

Absorption: IV
Distribution: PB: Confined to extracellular space
Metabolism: t½: 100 min
Excretion: In urine
	Decrease in Intracranial Pressure:
	IV: Onset: 30–60 min
	         Peak: 1 h
	         Duration: 6–8 h
	Diuresis: Onset: 1–3 h
	         Peak: 1 h
	         Duration: 6–8 h	

Therapeutic Effects/Uses: To treat increased intracranial pressure, cerebral edema. *Mode of Action:* Inhibition of reabsorption of electrolytes and water by affecting pressure of glomerular filtrate.	Evaluation

Side Effects	Adverse Reactions
Temporary volume expansion, hypo/hypernatremia, hypo/hyperkalemia, dehydration, blurred vision, dry mouth	Pulmonary congestion, fluid/electrolyte imbalances *Life-threatening:* Convulsions

KEY: IV: intravenous; PB: protein-binding; t½: half-life; D: dextrose.

10 and 33). Drug data for mannitol are presented in Figure 47–2.

METHYLPREDNISOLONE

High-dose methylprednisolone (Solu-Medrol) recently has been reported to improve motor and sensory function in clients with traumatic spinal cord injuries from 6 weeks to 6 months after injury. A strict pharmacologic protocol must be followed. Methylprednisolone must be administered in the following manner within 8 hours of acute spinal cord injury: a loading dose of 30 mg/kg of client body weight is given intravenously in the first hour of therapy (mixed in 100 mL of normal saline solution); a maintenance infusion of 5.4 mg/kg/h is then initiated and continued for 23 hours.

Relative contraindications include pregnancy, uncontrolled diabetes mellitus, allergy to the drug, penetrating trauma to the spinal cord or spinal lesions below L2, HIV infection, severe infection, and a spinal cord injury more than 8 hours old. Adverse effects include transient hypertension with administration of the loading dose and elevation of blood sugar during the infusion. The nurse must monitor vital signs and blood sugar and perform frequent and accurate neurologic assessments pertinent to spinal cord injury. Table 47–2 lists neuro-

TABLE 47–2 Neurosurgical Emergency Drugs

Drug	Dosage	Uses & Considerations
Mannitol	See Prototype Drug Chart (Figure 47–2)	
Methylprednisolone (Solu-Medrol)	IV: Loading dose: 30 mg/kg in 100 mL NSS; then 5.4 mg/kg/h (23 h)	For treatment of acute spinal cord injury (within 8 h of injury). *Pregnancy category:* C; PB: 80%–90%; t½: 2–4 h

KEY: *IV: intravenous; NSS: normal saline solution.*

surgical emergency drugs and their dosages and indications (see Chapters 20 and 40).

EMERGENCY DRUGS FOR POISONING

Although there are numerous antidotes for specific types of poisoning, the drugs presented in this section are the most commonly prescribed agents in cases of drug overdose and ingestion of toxic substances, with pertinent exceptions noted. Particular attention must be given to administration guidelines to achieve the best possible clinical outcome for the client. These drugs are cross-referenced to the specialty chapters.

NALOXONE

Naloxone (Narcan) is classified as an opiate antagonist. It reverses the effects of all opiate drugs (common examples include morphine, meperidine, codeine, propoxyphene, and heroin) by competitively binding to opiate receptor sites in the body. Naloxone is indicated for individuals who have taken an overdose of opiate drugs, those experiencing respiratory or cardiovascular depression from therapeutic doses of opiates given in a health care setting, and those brought to the emergency department in a coma of unknown etiology (which may be drug-induced).

The typical dose of naloxone for actual or suspected opiate overdose in adults is 0.4 to 2 mg IV administered every 2 to 3 min until the client's condition improves to an acceptable level. If there is no improvement after 10 mg of the drug has been injected, nonopiate drugs or disease must be suspected. Although naloxone should be administered intravenously in emergency situations, it also may be given intramuscularly or subcutaneously if intravenous access is not obtainable.

Because most opiate drugs have a longer duration of action than naloxone, the nurse must monitor the client closely for signs and symptoms of recurrent opiate effects such as respiratory depression and hypotension. In this situation, naloxone admin-

istration may need to be repeated several times or a continuous IV infusion ordered. Naloxone has no major adverse effects but can precipitate withdrawal symptoms in clients addicted to opiate drugs. In addition, pulmonary edema has been reported following naloxone administration in clients who have had an overdose of morphine (see Chapter 14). Drug data for naloxone are presented in Figure 47–3.

IPECAC SYRUP

Ipecac syrup is an **emetic** (an agent used to induce vomiting of ingested poisons). It is a liquid, over-the-counter (OTC) medication that is taken orally. The standard dose of ipecac in children over the age of 1 year is 15 mL; in children over 12 years and in adults, the dose is 30 mL PO followed by 200 to 300 mL of water or milk to enhance the emetic effects (carbonated beverages may cause gastric distention). Administration of ipecac may be repeated once if vomiting has not occurred in 20 min.

Ipecac should be used with caution. The nurse should administer ipecac before activated charcoal (charcoal will inactivate ipecac). The nurse should also instruct clients and their family members to contact a poison control center prior to taking or giving ipecac in the home setting; they should then seek medical attention immediately. The nurse must know the following contraindications to administration: cardiac disease or shock (ipecac is potentially cardiotoxic); unconsciousness or semiconsciousness or impaired gag reflex (may lead to aspiration of vomitus); and ingestion of petroleum products or corrosive agents such as acids or alkalis (aspiration of these chemicals is extremely harmful). If the client does not vomit after two doses of ipecac syrup, gastric lavage is necessary. Cardiotoxic effects can occur if more than 30 mL of ipecac syrup is administered (e.g., cardiac dysrhythmias, hypotension, bradycardia, or fatal myocarditis). Other adverse effects include prolonged vomiting, diarrhea, and depression (see Chapter 36).

FIGURE 47–3. Emergency Treatment of Poisoning

Naloxone HCl	Dosage	**NURSING PROCESS** Assessment and Planning
Naloxone HCl (Narcan) Narcotic antagonist *Pregnancy Category:* B	IV/IM/SC: 0.4–2 mg; repeat every 2–3 min, as indicated	
Contraindications	**Drug-Lab-Food Interactions**	
Hypersensitivity, respiratory depression *Caution:* Opiate-dependent clients, cardiac disease, breast-feeding, neonates	Verapamil can precipitate withdrawal in a client dependent on narcotic analgesics *Lab:* Urine VMA, 5-HIAA, urine glucose	
Pharmacokinetics	**Pharmacodynamics**	Interventions
Absorption: IM/SC: Well absorbed *Distribution:* PB: UK *Metabolism:* t½: Adults 1–4 h; neonates: 1–3 h *Excretion:* In urine metabolites	SC/IM: Onset: 2–5 min Peak: UK Duration: 1–4 h IV: Onset: 1–2 min Peak UK Duration: 1–4 h	

Therapeutic Effects/Uses: To treat respiratory depression caused by narcotics; to treat narcotic-induced depressant effects and narcotic overdose.

Mode of Action: Blocks effects of narcotics by competing for the receptor sites.

Evaluation

Side Effects	Adverse Reactions
Negligible pharmacologic effect without narcotics in body	Nausea, vomiting, tremulousness, sweating, tachycardia, elevated blood pressure *Life-threatening:* Atrioventricular fibrillation, pulmonary edema (with overdose of morphine)

KEY: IV: intravenous; IM: intramuscular; SC: subcutaneous; PB: protein-binding; UK: unknown; t½: half-life.

ACTIVATED CHARCOAL

Activated charcoal is prescribed for poisoning because it adsorbs ingested toxins in the gastrointestinal (GI) tract and prevents their absorption into the body. In cases of known or suspected poisoning, activated charcoal is prepared as a slurry and given orally or via a gastric tube. The dose is dependent on the amount of poison ingested; the minimum dose is 30 g. Activated charcoal may be ordered every 6 hours for 1 or 2 days to aid elimination of toxins from the blood stream.

Vomiting is a common adverse reaction, and the nurse should use activated charcoal with extreme caution in the client with an impaired gag reflex or altered level of consciousness due to the risk of aspiration. Activated charcoal should not be administered with milk products because they decrease its adsorptive properties. A cathartic is often ordered following administration of activated charcoal to speed elimination of the charcoal-toxin complex from the body. The client should be told that charcoal produces black stools (see Chapter 36).

TABLE 47–3 Emergency Drugs for Poisoning

Drug	Dosage	Uses & Considerations
Naloxone (Narcan)	IV: 0.4–2 mg, q 2–3 min if needed (also may be given via ETT) See Figure 47–3	Opiate overdose; respiratory or cardiovascular depression from opiates; coma of unknown origin. *Pregnancy category:* C; PB: UK; t½: 1–4 h (adults)
Ipecac syrup	A and C >12 y: 30 mL PO; can repeat in 20 min (see text for precautions) C >1 y: 15 mL PO	Emetic agent; to treat poisoning. *Pregnancy category:* C; PB: UK; t½: UK
Activated charcoal	30 g PO (minimum dose)	Poisoning; decreases absorption of laxatives, ipecac; onset <1 min. *Pregnancy category:* C; PB: NA; t½: NA
Magnesium sulfate Magnesium citrate	PO: 5–15 g PO: 5–10 oz	Cathartic; poisoning. *Pregnancy category:* UK; PB: UK; t½: UK

KEY: *ETT: endotracheal tube; IV: intravenous; NA: not applicable; PB: protein-binding; PO: by mouth; t½: half-life; UK: unknown.*

MAGNESIUM SULFATE/MAGNESIUM CITRATE

In poisoning, magnesium sulfate or citrate is given orally or via a gastric tube as a **cathartic,** an agent that speeds elimination of stool and evacuates the bowel. It is often prescribed following administration of activated charcoal, as described earlier. The typical oral dose of magnesium sulfate is 5 to 15 g, administered in a glass of water. The oral dose of magnesium citrate is 5 to 10 oz. Cathartic action begins 1 to 2 hours after ingestion. Cathartics are contraindicated in clients with bowel obstruction, abdominal pain, nausea, or vomiting. If the use of cathartics is prolonged, the nurse should monitor the client for dehydration and electrolyte imbalances.

Table 47–3 lists the emergency drugs for poisoning, their dosages, and indications (see Chapters 10, 36, and 42).

EMERGENCY DRUGS FOR SHOCK

Drugs may be required to raise blood pressure and improve cardiac performance in various types of shock states. Therapeutic agents described in this section are indicated in conditions such as cardiogenic shock, neurogenic shock, septic shock, anaphylactic shock, and insulin shock. A noteworthy exception to the list of shock states is **hypovolemic shock** (shock due to loss of blood or fluid volume); drugs should not be used in an attempt to correct the hypotension associated with this condition. Administration of fluids or blood products or both is the only acceptable means to treat hypovolemic shock. These drugs are cross-referenced to the specialty chapters.

DOPAMINE

Dopamine (Intropin) is a sympathomimetic agent often used to treat hypotension in shock states that are *not* due to hypovolemia. Dopamine may also be used to increase heart rate (beta$_1$ effect) in bradycardic rhythms when atropine has not been effective at a dose range of 5 to 20 μg/kg/min. The actions of dopamine are dose-dependent: at low doses (1 to 2 μg/kg/min, dopamine dilates renal and mesenteric blood vessels, producing an increase in urine output (dopaminergic effect); at doses of 2 to 10 μg/kg/min, dopamine enhances cardiac output by increasing myocardial contractility and increasing heart rate (beta$_1$ effect) and elevates blood pressure through vasoconstriction (alpha-adrenergic effect). Alpha effects predominate at doses of 10 μg/kg/min and above: vasoconstriction of renal, mesenteric, and peripheral blood vessels occurs. Such vasoconstriction, although sometimes necessary to maintain adequate blood pressure in severe shock, can lead to poor organ and tissue perfusion, decreased cardiac performance, and reduction of urine output. The lowest effective dose of dopamine should be used. Clients must be weaned gradually from dopamine; abrupt discontinuation of the infusion can cause severe hypotension.

Dopamine is typically mixed as a concentration of 400 to 800 mg in 250 mL dextrose 5% in water and administered IV by a volumetric infusion pump for precision. Continuous heart and blood pressure monitoring is essential. The nurse must carefully document vital signs and intake and output as ordered. Significant adverse effects include tachycardia, dysrhythmias, myocardial ischemia, nausea, and vomiting. The IV site must be assessed hourly for signs of drug infiltration: **extravasation** (escape into tissues) of dopamine can produce tissue necrosis that can necessitate surgical debridement and skin grafting. If extravasation occurs, the site should be injected in multiple areas with phentolamine (Regitine), 5 to 10 mg diluted in 10 to 15 mL of normal saline to reduce or prevent tissue damage (see Chapter 18). Drug data for dopamine are presented in Figure 47–4.

DOBUTAMINE

Dobutamine (Dobutrex) is a sympathomimetic drug with beta$_1$-adrenergic activities. The beta$_1$ effects include enhancing the force of myocardial contraction (positive inotropic effect) and increasing heart rate (positive chronotropic effect). Dobutamine is indicated in shock states when improvement in cardiac output and overall cardiac performance is desired. Blood pressure is elevated only through the increase in cardiac output; dobutamine has no vasoconstriction effects. The usual IV dose range of dobutamine is 2.5 to 20 μg/kg/min administered via a volumetric infusion pump for precision. A typical concentration of dobutamine is 1000 mg mixed in 250 mL of dextrose 5% in water or normal

FIGURE 47–4. Emergency Treatment of Shock

Dopamine HCl	Dosage	NURSING PROCESS Assessment and Planning
Dopamine HCl (Intropin) Adrenegic *Pregnancy Category:* C	A: IV: Drip: 1–20 μg/kg/min (>10 μg/kg/min be ordered if lower doses are ineffective	
Contraindications	**Drug-Lab-Food Interactions**	
Hypersensitivity, tachydysrhythmias, ventricular fibrillation, pheochromocytomas *Caution:* Safety in children is not known	Use within 2 wk of MAOIs may result in hypertensive crisis; concurrent IV administration of phenytoin may result in hypotension and bradycardia; sodium bicarbonate solutions inactivate dopamine—do *not* administer through the same IV line	
Pharmacokinetics	**Pharmacodynamics**	Interventions
Absorption: IV *Distribution:* PB: UK *Metabolism:* t½: 2 min *Excretion:* In urine	IV: Onset: 1–2 min Peak <5 min Duration: <10 min	

Therapeutic Effects/Uses: To treat hypotension in shock states not due to hypovolemia; to increase heart rate in atropine-refractory bradycardia. To increase urine output at a "renal dose" (<5 mg/kg/min).

Mode of Action: Stimulation of receptors to cause cardiac stimulation and renal vasodiation. Increase systemic vascular resistance at higher dose ranges.

Evaluation

Side Effects	Adverse Reactions
Palpitations, tachycardia, hypertension, ectopic beats, angina, IV line site irritation, piloerection, nausea, vomiting	Cardiac dysrhythmias, azotemia, tissue sloughing (from extravasation) *Life-threatening:* MI, gangrene in extremities (from vasoconstriction)

KEY: IV: intravenous; MAOIs: monoamine oxidase inhibitors; PB: protein-binding; UK: unknown; t½: half-life; MI: myocardial infarction.

saline. Like dopamine, dobutamine administration should be tapered gradually as the client's condition warrants.

Continuous cardiac and blood pressure monitoring are required for clients receiving dobutamine infusions. Adverse effects are dose-related and include myocardial ischemia, tachycardia, dysrhythmias, headache, nausea, and tremors. The nurse must carefully monitor vital signs and intake and output and assess for any signs or symptoms of myocardial ischemia such as chest pain or development of dysrhythmias (see Chapter 18).

NOREPINEPHRINE

Norepinephrine (Levarterenol, Levophed) is a catecholamine with extremely potent vasoconstrictor actions (alpha-adrenergic effect). It is used in shock states, often when drugs such as dopamine and dobutamine have failed to produce adequate blood pressure. Like high-dose dopamine, the peripheral vasoconstriction that results has the potential to impair cardiac performance and decrease organ and tissue perfusion. In general, 4 to 8 mg of norepinephrine are added to 250 mL dextrose 5% in water or normal saline solution and infused at 2 to 12 μg/min for adults. Continuous cardiac monitoring and precise blood pressure monitoring are required. The drug must be tapered slowly; abrupt discontinuation can result in severe hypotension.

Nursing actions and considerations are the same as those for dopamine. Norepinephrine should not be used to treat hypotension in hypovolemic clients; fluid, blood, or both must be administered to restore adequate volume first. Adverse effects of norepinephrine include myocardial ischemia, dysrhythmias, and impaired organ perfusion. Extravasation of norepinephrine will cause tissue necrosis; therefore, attention to the IV site is essential. If extravasation occurs, the area should be infiltrated with phentolamine, as described for dopamine (see Chapter 18).

EPINEPHRINE

Epinephrine is the drug of choice in the treatment of **anaphylactic shock,** an allergic response of the most serious type brought about by an antibody-antigen reaction. Anaphylactic shock can prove fatal if prompt treatment is not initiated. Severe bronchoconstriction and hypotension due to cardiovascular collapse are its hallmarks. Epinephrine is also indicated for an acute, severe asthmatic attack.

Administration of epinephrine causes bronchodilation, enhanced cardiac performance, and vasoconstriction to increase blood pressure. In severe **asthma** and anaphylactic shock, epinephrine is given in a 0.1 to 0.5 mg dose range subcutaneously (SC) or intramuscularly (IM) for adults via a tuberculin syringe for accuracy (1:1000 solution). As an alternative, epinephrine can be given in a dose of 0.1 to 0.25 mg IV over 5 to 10 min (1:10,000 solution). Epinephrine administration can be repeated every 5 to 15 min if necessary.

The nurse must carefully monitor the client who receives epinephrine for tachycardia, cardiac dysrhythmias, hypertension, and angina. Clients who are given IV epinephrine must be on a cardiac monitor, with resuscitation equipment immediately available. Other adverse effects include excitability, fear, anxiety, and restlessness. In addition, the nurse should be alert to the possibility that the anaphylactic response may recur and necessitate repeated treatment. Client education should include strict avoidance of the agent(s) responsible for the anaphylactic reaction and follow-up care with a physician. For some clients, such as those with severe allergic responses to bee stings, the physician may prescribe an epinephrine kit to be carried with the client for self-medication in the event of contact with the antigen. Proper client education regarding the use of the kit is essential (see Chapters 18 and 31).

DIPHENHYDRAMINE HYDROCHLORIDE

Diphenhydramine (Benadryl), an antihistamine, is often administered with epinephrine in anaphylactic shock. This agent is effective for treating the histamine-induced tissue swelling and pruritus common to severe allergic reactions. The standard adult dose is 10 to 50 mg administered IV or deep IM. An oral form of the drug exists, but the parenteral form is preferred in emergency situations. Adverse effects include drowsiness, sedation, confusion, vertigo, excitability, hypotension, tachycardia, GI disturbances, and dry mouth (see Chapter 30).

DEXTROSE 50%

Dextrose 50% is a concentrated, high-carbohydrate solution given to treat insulin-induced hypoglycemia or insulin shock. When insulin shock is known or suspected and the client's state of consciousness is impaired such that oral administration of sugar solutions is contraindicated, 50 mL of dextrose 50% is commonly ordered and given as an IV bolus. Dextrose 50% is highly irritating to veins and should be administered in a large peripheral or central vein whenever possible. Phlebitis can occur. Extravasation of the solution can cause tissue sloughing and necrosis. The nurse must monitor the client's blood sugar carefully; hyperglycemia is common, especially after rapid injection. Urine output should be accurately recorded, because osmotic diuresis can occur when blood sugar is elevated, and a hyperosmolar state can result. Client education must be centered on teaching about diabetes and insulin administration.

Pediatric Implications

Glycogen stores in infants and children may be quickly depleted in stress states produced by severe illness. Because adequate amounts of glucose are essential to strong myocardial function, hypoglycemia must be corrected to provide the greatest chance for successful resuscitation. After determining that hypoglycemia is present by the finger- or heel-stick method of rapid blood glucose testing, dextrose 25% or less may be administered per physician order. Because glucose is supplied in a 50% concentration it must be diluted 1:1 in sterile water prior to administration to reduce its osmolarity and prevent sclerosis of peripheral veins. The standard dose is 0.5 to 1.0 g/kg IV (see Chapter 41).

GLUCAGON

Glucagon is a hormone produced by the pancreas that acts to raise blood sugar by stimulating glycogen breakdown **(glycogenolysis).** Glucagon, like dextrose 50%, is indicated in the treatment of severe insulin-induced hypoglycemia or insulin shock. In emergency situations in which dextrose 50% is unavailable or cannot be administered intravenously, glucagon is an effective agent. Glucagon may be given subcutaneously, intramuscularly, or intravenously. The standard dose for adults and children is 0.5 to 1 mg, which can be repeated in 20 min for persistent coma. If the coma has not resolved after two doses, dextrose 50% should be administered. Adverse effects from glucagon are uncommon but can include nausea and vomiting. Glucagon can be used as an agent to reverse the effects of beta blocker overdose as well as the persistent detrimental effects of ingested beta blockers for clients in shock states (beta blockers block the effects of the sympathetic nervous system; the sympathetic nervous system is the primary compensatory mechanism for clients in shock). Table 47–4 lists the emergency drugs for shock, their dosages, and indications (see Chapter 41).

EMERGENCY DRUGS FOR HYPERTENSIVE CRISES

A variety of pharmacologic agents may be prescribed to treat hypertensive crisis, generally defined as a diastolic blood pressure that exceeds 110 to 120 mmHg. One of the most commonly prescribed drugs is discussed in this section. This drug is cross-referenced to the specialty chapter.

TABLE 47–4 Agents for Emergency Treatment of Shock

Generic (Brand)	Route and Dosage	Uses & Considerations
Dextrose 50%	A: IV: 50 mL C: 0.5–1.0 g/kg IV of a D 25% sol	Insulin shock; severe hypoglycemia; altered mental status of unknown origin. *Pregnancy category:* C; PB: UK; t½: UK
Diphenhydramine (Benadryl)	IM/IV: 10–50 mg	Anaphylactic shock; acute allergic reaction. *Pregnancy category:* C; PB: 98%–99%; t½: 3–8 h
Dobutamine (Dobutrex)	IV: Drip: 2.5–10 μg/kg/min	Low cardiac output. Effects antagonized by beta blockers. *Pregnancy category:* C; PB: UK; t½: 2 min
Dopamine HCl (Intropin)	See Prototype Drug Chart (Figure 47–4)	
Epinephrine	SC/IM: 0.1–0.5 mg (1:1,000 sol) IV: 0.1–0.25 mg (1:10,000 sol) Intratracheal: 0.1 mg/kg q3–5 min)	Anaphylactic shock; severe acute asthmatic attack. Hypertensive crisis with MAOIs; increased dysrhythmias with cardiac glycosides. *Pregnancy category:* C; PB: UK; t½: UK
Glucagon	SC/IM/IV: 0.5–1 mg; may repeat × 1	Insulin shock; severe hypoglycemia; beta blocker overdose (reverses effects of beta blockers). *Pregnancy category:* B; PB: UK; t½: 3–10 min
Norepinephrine (Levophed)	IV: Drip: 2–12 μg/min	Hypotension not responsive to other therapies. *Pregnancy category:* D; PB: UK; t½: UK

KEY: A: adult; IV: intravenous; IM: intramuscular; SC: subcutaneous; C: child; MAOIs: monoamine oxidase inhibitors; PB: protein-binding; t½: half-life; UK: unknown.

SODIUM NITROPRUSSIDE

Sodium nitroprusside (Nipride) is an intravenous agent used to reduce arterial blood pressure in hypertensive emergencies. The mechanism of action is immediate direct arterial and venous vasodilation. Antihypertensive effects end when sodium nitroprusside is discontinued; blood pressure will rise as soon as drug administration is stopped. Continuous and accurate blood pressure measurement is required. In general, 50 mg of sodium nitroprusside is mixed in 250 mL dextrose 5% in water. The average dose range for adults and children is 0.5 to 10 μg/kg/min.

There are several important nursing considerations:

1. Sodium nitroprusside is rapidly inactivated by light; the IV bottle or bag must be wrapped with aluminum foil or another opaque material to protect the solution from degradation.
2. Although a faint brown tint is typical, blue or brown discoloration of the solution indicates degradation and mandates that the solution be discarded.
3. When sodium nitroprusside therapy is prolonged, clients are at risk for toxicity due to elevated serum thiocyanate and/or cyanide levels

FIGURE 47–5. Emergency Treatment of Hypertensive Crisis

Sodium Nitroprusside	Dosage	NURSING PROCESS Assessment and Planning
Sodium Nitroprusside (Nipride) *Pregnancy Category:* C	A: IV: Drip 0.5–10 μg/kg/min; begin at 0.1 mg/kg/min and titrate to desired effect up to 10 μg/kg/min	
Contraindications	**Drug-Lab-Food Interactions**	
Hypersensitivity, hypertension (compensatory), decreased cerebral perfusion, coarctation of aorta *Caution:* Increased intracranial pressure	Antihypertensives, general anesthetics Do not mix with any other drug in syringe or solution. *Lab:* Decrease in carbonate, P_{CO_2}, pH	
Pharmacokinetics	**Pharmacodynamics**	Interventions
Absorption: IV only *Distribution:* PB: UK *Metabolism:* t½: <10 min *Excretion:* In urine	IV: Onset: 1–2 min Peak: Rapid Duration: 1–10 min	

	Evaluation
Therapeutic Effects/Uses: To treat hypertensive crisis; to produce controlled hypotension to reduce surgical bleeding; and to decrease systemic vascular resistance to improve cardiac performance. *Mode of Action:* Stimulation of smooth muscle of veins and arteries; produces peripheral vasodilation.	

Side Effects	Adverse Reactions
Dizziness, headache, nausea, abdominal pain, sweating, palpitations, weakness, vomiting	Tinnitus, dyspnea, blurred vision *Life-threatening:* Severe hypotension, loss of consciousness, profound cardiovascular depression

KEY: IV: intravenous; P_{CO_2}: partial pressure of carbon dioxide; PB: protein-binding; UK: unknown; t½: half-life.

(byproducts of drug metabolism). Signs and symptoms include metabolic acidosis, profound hypotension, dizziness, and vomiting. Serum thiocyanate levels should be monitored at least every 72 hours. Clients with renal insufficiency or failure are at a higher risk because the metabolites are excreted in the urine.

4. Clients should be placed on an oral antihypertensive agent as soon as possible so that sodium nitroprusside can be tapered slowly (see Chapters 33 and 34). Drug data for sodium nitroprusside are presented in Figure 47–5.

STUDY QUESTIONS

1. What is the minimum dose of atropine that should be given to an adult with bradycardia?
2. Explain the actions of epinephrine and diphenhydramine for clients in anaphylactic shock? How are these drugs administered in this situation?
3. What are the signs and symptoms of lidocaine toxicity?
4. List common adverse effects of bretylium.
5. What guidelines should be followed when administering ipecac syrup? What client and family educational points should be emphasized?
6. Why are activated charcoal and magnesium sulfate given for poisoning? List the actions of each.
7. In what poisoning situations should vomiting not be induced?
8. Compare and contrast dextrose 50% and glucagon.
9. For what class of drug overdose is naloxone effective? What important precautions must be taken?
10. Describe the protocol for administering methylprednisolone to a client with an acute spinal cord injury. Would you expect the drug to produce a noticeable effect immediately?
11. What are the emergency indications for mannitol in the neurosurgical setting? Describe pertinent nursing considerations for its administration.

12. List the adverse effects of isoproterenol and the pertinent nursing considerations and actions.
13. List the end points of procainamide administration.
14. What is the antidote for extravasation of both norepinephrine and dopamine? How should it be administered?
15. List the signs and symptoms of thiocyanate toxicity in clients receiving sodium nitroprusside.
16. Explain how dobutamine increases blood pressure as compared with dopamine.
17. Describe the dose-dependent effects of dopamine.
18. List relevant nursing considerations and actions when administering verapamil.
19. Discuss indications for adenosine. What are pertinent nursing considerations when administering adenosine?
20. Compare and contrast intravenous diltiazem and verapamil.
21. What is the maximum total adult dose of intravenous atropine for the treatment of bradycardia? Why will additional doses of atropine be ineffective?
22. List at least three relative contraindications to methylprednisolone administration in acute spinal cord injury.
23. What are the relevant nursing considerations when administering sodium nitroprusside?
24. After administering the initial dose of adenosine, the nurse observes a short period of asystole. Does this represent an adverse drug effect?
25. Describe how to administer sublingual nitroglycerin tablets to the client experiencing chest pain.
26. What teaching points should be emphasized when a client is discharged to home with a prescription for sublingual nitroglycerin?
27. Name the drug that is indicated to reverse significant respiratory depressant effects of morphine sulfate.
28. What is the typical dose range of intravenous morphine?
29. Describe how to dilute a 50% dextrose solution for safe administration to pediatric clients.

APPENDIX A

*Generic Drugs with Corresponding Canadian Trade Drug Names**

Generic Drug Names	Canadian Trade/Brand Names
Acebutolol	Monitan
Acetaminophen	Abenol, Atasol, Campain, Exdol, Robigesic, Rounox
Acetazolamide	Acetazolam, Apo-Acetazolamide
Acetohexamide	Dimelor
Acetylcysteine	Airbron
Albuterol	Novosalmol, Salbutamol
Allopurinol	Alloprin, Apo-Allopurinol, Novopurinol, Purinol
Aminophylline	Gorophyllin, Paladron
Aminosalicylate sodium	Parasal Sodium
Amitriptyline hydrochloride	Apo-Amitriptyline, Levate, Meravil, Novotriptyn, Rolavil
Amoxicillin	Apo-Amoxi, Amoxican
Amoxicillin clavulanate K	Clavulin
Ampicillin	Ampilean, Novo-Ampicillin, Penbritin
Ascorbic acid	Apo-C, Ce-Vi-Sol, Redoxon
Asparaginase	Kidrolase
Aspirin	Ancasal, Astrin, Entrophen, Novasen, Supasa, Triaphen-10
Atenolol	Apo-Atenolol
Atropine sulfate	Atropair
Bacampicillin hydrochloride	Penglobe
Benzalkonium chloride	Pharmatex
Benztropine mesylate	Apo-Benzotropine, Bensylate, PMS Benzotropine
Betamethasone	Beban, Betaderm, Betanelan, Betnesol, Betnovate, Celestoderm, Novobetamet
Bisacodyl	Apo-Bisacodyl, Bisco-Lax, Laxit
Bretylium tosylate	Bretylate
Carbamazepine	Apo-Carbamazepine, Mazepine, PMS Carbamazepine
Carbenicillin disodium	Pyopen
Cephalexin	Ceporex, Novolexin
Cephalothin sodium	Ceporacin
Chloral hydrate	Novochlorhydrate
Chloramphenicol	Novochorocap, Pentamycetin
Chlordiazepoxide hydrocholoride	Medilium, Novopoxide, Solium
Chlorphenesin carbamate	Mycil
Chlorpheniramine maleate	Chlor-Tripolon, Novopheniram
Chlorpromazine hydrochloride	Chlorpromanyl, Largactil, Novochlorpromazine
Chlorpropamide	Apo-Chlorpropamide, Chloronase, Novopropamide
Chlorprothixene	Tarasan
Chlorthalidone	Novothalidone, Uridon
Cimetidine	Novocimetine, Peptol
Cisplatin	Abiplatin
Clindamycin	Dalacin-C
Clofibrate	Claripen, Claripex, Novofibrate
Clonazepam	Rivotril
Clonidine hydrochloride	Dixarit
Clorazepate dipotassium	Novoclopate
Clotrimazole	Canesten
Cloxacillin sodium	Apo-Cloxi, Bactopen, Novocloxin, Orbenin
Codeine phosphate	Paveral
Colchicine	Novocolchine
Colestipol hydrochloride	Cholestabyl, Lestid
Co-trimoxazole	Apo-Sulfatrim
Cromolyn sodium	Fivent, Intal p, Rynacrom, Vistacrom
Cyanocobalamin	Anacobin, Bedoz, Cyanabin, Rubion
Cyclizine hydrochloride	Marzine
Cyclophosphamide	Procytox
Cyproheptadine hydrochloride	Vimicon

Generic Drug Names	Canadian Trade/Brand Names
Danazol	Cyclomen
Dapsone	Avlosulfon
Dexamethasone	Deronil, Dexasone, Oradexon, Stress-Pam
Dextromethorphan	Balminil DM, Koffex, Ornex DM, Robidex, Sedatuss
Diazepam	Apo-Diazepam, Diazemuls, E-Pam, Meval, Novodipam, Vivol
Dicyclomine hydrochloride	Bentylol, Formulex, Lomine, Protylol, Viscerol
Diethylpropion hydrochloride	Nobesine
Diethylstilbestrol	Honval, Stilboestrol
Digitoxin	Digitaline, Purodigin
Dimenhydrinate	Apo-Dimenhydrinate, Gravol, Nauseatol, Novodimenate, Travamine
Dinoprostone	Prepidil Gel
Diphenhydramine hydrochloride	Allerdryl
Dipyridamole	Apo-Dipyridamole
Disopyramide	Rythmodan
Docusate sodium	Regulax
Dopamine hydrochloride	Revimine
Doxepin hydrochloride	Triadapin
Doxycycline hyclate	Doryx, Doxycin, Novodoxylin
Dyphylline	Protophylline
Econazole nitrate	Ecostatin
Epinephrine hydrochloride	SusPhrine, Eppy
Epinephrine racemic	Vaponefrin
Ergocalciferol	Ostoforte, Radiostol
Ergotamine tartrate	Gynergen
Erythromycin	Apo-Erythro Base, Erythromid, Novorythro, Ro-Mycin
Estradiol	Delestrogen
Estrogen, conjugated	C.E.S.
Estrogen, esterified	Climestrone, Neo-Estrone
Estrone	Femogen Forte
Ethambutol hydrochloride	Etibi
Ethopropazine hydrochloride	Parsitan
Fenfluramine hydrochloride	Ponderal
Ferrous fumarate	Neo-Fer-50, Novofumar, Palafer
Ferrous gluconate	Fertinic, Novoferrogluc
Ferrous sulfate	Novoferrosulfa
Flucytosine	Ancotil
Fluocinolone acetonide	Fluoderm
Fluocinonide	Lidemol, Lyderm, Topsyn
Fluoxymesterone	Ora T Estryl
Fluphenazine decanoate	Decanoate
Fluphenazine enanthate	Enanthate
Fluphenazine hydrochloride	Moditen HCl
Flurandrenolide	Drenison
Flurazepam	Apo-Flurazepam, Novoflupam, Somnol
Folic acid	Apo-Folic, Novofolacid
Furosemide	Fumide, Furomide, Luramide, Uritol
Gentamicin sulfate	Alcomicin, Cidomycin, Novosemide
Glyburide	DiaBeta, Euglucon
Griseofulvin, microsize	Grisovin-FP
Guaifenesin	Balminil, Resyl
Guanethidine sulfate	Apo-Guanethidine
Haloperidol	Haldol LA, Peridol
Heparin calcium	Calcilean, Calciparine
Heparin sodium	Hepalean
Hydrochlorothiazide	Apo-Hydro, Hydrozide, Neo-Codema, Urozide
Hydrocodone bitartrate	Hycodan, Robidone
Hydrocortisone	Cortamed, Cortiment, Rectocort
Hydroxocobalamin	Acti-B$_{12}$
Ibuprofen	Amersol
Imipramine hydrochloride	Impril, Novopramine
Indapamide	Lozide
Indomethacin	Indocid
Isoniazid (INH)	Isotamine
Isosorbide dinitrate	Coronex, Novosorbide
Iodoquinol	Diodoquin

Generic Drug Names	Canadian Trade/Brand Names
Kaolin/pectin	Donnagel-MB, Kao-Con
Ketoprofen	Rhodis, Orudis E
Lactulose	Lactulax
Levothyroxine sodium (T_4)	Eltroxin
Lidocaine hydrochloride	Xylocard
Lithium carbonate	Carbolith, Duralith, Lithizine
Lorazepam	Apo-Lorazepam, Novolorazepam
Loxapine hydrochloride	Loxapac
Magaldrate	Antiflux
Meclizine hydrochloride	Bonamine
Mefenamic acid	Ponstan
Meperidine hydrochloride	Pethadol, Pethidine Hydrochloride
Meprobamate	Apo-Meprobamate, Novomepro
Mesalamine	Salofalk
Methohexital	Brietal
Methotrimeprazine	Nozinan
Methylclothiazide	Duretic
Methyldopa	Apo-Methyldopa, Dopamet, Novomedopa
Methyltestosterone	Metandren
Metoclopramide	Maxeran
Metoprolol	Apo-Metoprolol, Betaloc, Novometoprol
Metronidazole	Neo-Metric, Novonidazol, PMS Metronidazole
Miconazole	Monistat
Mineral oil	Kondremul, Lansoyl
Morphine sulfate	Epimorph, Statex
Naphazoline	Vasocon
Naproxen	Apo-Naproxen, Naxen, Novonaprox
Niacin (vitamin B_3, nicotinic acid)	Novo-Niacin, Tri-B3
Nifedipine	Adalat P.A., Apo-Nifed, Novo-Nifedin
Nitrofurantoin	Apo-Nitrofurantoin, Nephronex, Novofuran
Norethindrone acetate	Aygestin, Norlutate
Nylidrin hydrochloride	Arlidin Forte, PMS Nylidrin
Nystatin	Nadostine, Nyaderm
Omeprazole	Losec
Oxazepam	Ox-Pam, Zapex, Apo-Oxazepam, Novoxapam
Oxtriphylline	Apo-Oxtriphylline, Novotriphyl
Oxycodone	Supeudol
Oxymetazoline hydrochloride	Nafrine
Oxymetholone	Anapolon
Penicillin G potassium	Megacillin, NovoPen-G, P-50, Crystapen
Penicillin G procaine	Ayercillin
Penicillin G sodium	Crystapen
Penicillin V	Apo-Pen-VK, Nadopen-V, Novopen-VK
Pentamidine isethionate	Pentacarinat
Pentobarbital	Novopentobarb
Perphenazine	Apo-Perphenazine, Phenazine
Phenazopyridine hydrochloride	Phenazo, Pyronium
Phentolamine mesylate	Rogitine
Phenazopyridine	Phenazo, Pyronium
Phenylephrine, ophthalmic	Minims Phenylephrine
Pilocarpine hydrochloride	Pilocarpine, Milocarpine
Piroxicam	Apo-Piroxicant
Potassium chloride	Apo-K, Kalium Durules, Klong, Novolente K, Roychlor 10% and 20%, Slo-Pot
Potassium gluconate	Potassium Rougier, Royonate
Potassium iodide	Thyro-Block
Pramoxine hydrochloride	Tronothane
Prednisone	Apo-Prednisone, Winpred
Primidone	Apo-Primidone, Sertan
Probenecid	Benuryl
Procarbazine hydrochloride	Natulan
Prochlorperazine maleate	Stemetil
Procyclidine hydrochloride	Procyclid
Progesterone	Progestilin
Promethazine hydrochloride	Histantil

Generic Drug Names	Canadian Trade/Brand Names
Propantheline bromide	Propanthel
Propoxyphene hydrochloride	642, Novopropoxyn
Propranolol hydrochloride	Apo-Propranolol, Detensol, Novopranol
Propylthiouracil (PTU)	Propyl-Thyracil
Protriptyline hydrochloride	Triptil
Pseudoephedrine hydrochloride	Eltor, Eltor 120, Pseudofrin, Robidrine
Psyllium hydrophilic muciloid	Karasil
Pyrantel pamoate	Combantrin
Pyrazinamide	Tebrazid, PMS Pyrazinamide
Pyridostigmine	Mestinon, Regonol
Quinidine sulfate	APO-Quinidine, Novoquinidin
Quinine sulfate	Novoquinine
Reserpine	Novoreserpine, Reserfia
Rifampin	Rofact
Scopolamine	Transderm-V
Secobarbital	Novosecobarb
Silver sulfadiazine	Flamazine
Simethicone	Ovol
Sodium fluoride	Fluor-A-Day
Sotalol	Sotacor
Spironolactone	Novospiroton, Sincomen
Sucralfate	Sulcrate
Sulfasalazine	PMS Sulfasalazine, Salazopyrin, SAS-Enema, SAS Enteric-500, S.A.S.-500
Sulfinpyrazone	Antazone, Anturan, Apo-Sulfinpyrazone, Novopyrazone
Sulfisoxazole	Novosoxazole
Tamoxifen citrate	Nolvadex-D, Tamofen
Testosterone	Malogen
Testosterone enanthate	Malogex
Testosterone propionate	Malogen in oil
Tetracycline hydrochloride	Novotetra, Apo-Tetra, Tetralean
Theophylline	PMS Theophylline, Pulmopylline, Somophyllin-12
Thiamine HCl (vitamin B_1)	Bewon, Betaxin
Thioguanine (TG, 6-thioguanine)	Lanvis
Thioridazine hydrochloride	Novoridazine
Timolol maleate	Apo-Timol
Tolbutamide	Mobenol, Novobutamide
Tolnaftate	Pitrex
Trifluoperazine hydrochloride	Novoflurazine, Solazine, Terfluzine
Trihexyphenidyl hydrochloride	Aparkane, Apo-Trihex, Novohexidyl
Trimeprazine tartrate	Panectyl
Tripelennamine hydrochloride	Pyribenzamine
Valproic acid (divalproex sodium, sodium valproate)	Epival
Vinblastine sulfate	Velbe
Warfarin sodium	Warfilone

*Many of the trade or brand names are used in both the United States and Canada. This appendix lists selected trade or brand names that are specific to Canada.

APPENDIX B

*Temperature Conversion: Celsius and Fahrenheit**

Two scales used to measure temperature are Fahrenheit (F) and Celsius (C), also called centigrade. Both temperature scales have boiling points and freezing points. The boiling point of Fahrenheit is 212°, and the freezing point is 32° with a range of 180 (212–32). The boiling point of Celsius is 100°, and the freezing point is 0° with a range of 100 (100–0). The difference of Fahrenheit to Celsius is 180 to 100 or $\frac{9}{5}$, and of Celsius to Fahrenheit is 100 to 180 or $\frac{5}{9}$.

Celsius is becoming the primary temperature scale for clinical use, so it may be necessary to convert Fahrenheit to Celsius, and Celsius to Fahrenheit. Two formulas may be used in the conversion of temperatures. Refer to the formulas as needed.

Formula A: To convert Celsius to Fahrenheit

$$F = \tfrac{9}{5}C + 32$$

EXAMPLE

35°C to Fahrenheit

$$F = \tfrac{9}{5}C + 32$$

$$F = \tfrac{9}{5} \times 35 + 32$$

$$F = \frac{9 \times 35}{5} + 32 = \frac{315}{5} + 32$$

$$F = 63 + 32$$

$$F = 95°$$

Formula B: To convert Fahrenheit to Celsius

$$C = \tfrac{5}{9}(F - 32)$$

EXAMPLE

99°F to Celsius

$$C = \tfrac{5}{9}(F - 32)$$

$$C = 5 \times \frac{(99 - 32)}{9}$$

$$C = \frac{5 \times 67}{9} = \frac{335}{9}$$

$$C = 37.2°$$

---

* *Source:* Kee, J. L., and Marshall, S. M.: *Clinical Calculations* (2nd ed). Philadelphia, WB Saunders, p. 250, 1992.

APPENDIX C
Alternative Pediatric Drug Calculations

In the past, pediatric drug dosages were calculated by adjusting the adult dose to the child's age or weight. The alternative methods for calculating the pediatric dose are seldom practiced; however, they are presented for those who may use the method(s) in a clinical situation.

AGE RULES

Fried's rule and Young's rule are two methods for determining pediatric drug doses based on the child's age. Fried's rule is primarily used for children younger than 1 year of age, whereas Young's rule is for children between 2 and 12 years of age. Because the maturational development of infants and children is variable, age cannot be an accurate basis for drug dosing.

Fried's Rule: <1 year old

$$\frac{\text{Age in months}}{150} \times \text{adult dose} = \text{infant's dose}$$

Young's Rule: 2 to 12 years old

$$\frac{\text{Child's age in years}}{\text{Age in years } + 12} \times \text{adult dose} = \text{child's dose}$$

BODY WEIGHT RULE

Clark's rule is a method used to derive a pediatric dosage based upon the child's weight in pounds and the average adult weight of 150 pounds. Population studies have shown an increase in the average weight of adults, therefore making 150 pounds an inaccurate constant in the rule. Using the fixed constant in Clark's rule can lead to underdosing of infants; consequently Clark's rule is being phased out as a method for determining drug dosage in children.

Clark's Rule: by weight

$$\frac{\text{Child's weight in pounds}}{150 \text{ pounds}} \times \text{adult dose} = \text{child's dose}$$

APPENDIX D

Recommended Daily Allowances for Vitamins and Minerals During Pregnancy

Nutrient	RDA for Pregnancy	Uses and Considerations
Fat-Soluble Vitamins		
A	4000 IU	Excessive intake can cause fetal bone malformations, cleft palate, renal anomalies and eye/ear anomalies if above 10,000 IU/d.
		Toxic level in mother can result in liver damage
		RDA same as for nonpregnant state.
		Due to high toxicity potential, client should take only when prescribed during first trimester for a specifically identified deficiency. Check multivitamin bottle that vitamin A levels do not exceed 5000 IU.
D	10 μg/d	Excessive maternal amounts can yield excessive calcium levels in the fetus and cause cardiac defects (aortic stenosis).
		Avoid intake > 25 μg/d due to toxic effects.
		Deficiency can affect fetal bone density and dental enamel and can cause neonatal hypocalcemia.
		Consider use in complete vegetarians, non–vitamin D fortified milk drinkers, those in northern latitudes in winter, and those with minimal sunlight exposure.
E	10 mg alpha-TE	Dietary sources should suffice; adequate amounts found in human milk (cow's milk level lower) for newborn.
Water-Soluble Vitamins		
C	70 mg/d	The need for ascorbic acid is increased in pregnancy; however, dietary sources should suffice if the diet is nutritious and C-foods are available to help in the formation of collagen and are cooked in only small amounts of water to only a crisp-tender state, not held too long, and not reheated.
		Maternal plasma levels of this vitamin at term are twice as low as midway through pregnancy due to placental concentration of the vitamin with elevated fetal levels as an outcome.
		Deficiency can include premature rupture of fetal membranes and PIH.
		Excessive maternal intake may manifest in the neonate as a rebound form of scurvy with muscle weakness, capillary hemorrhage, and progressive demise.
		Neonates fed mainly cow's milk are at higher risk of vitamin C deficiency.
B$_1$ (thiamine)	1.5 mg/d	Requirement increased in pregnancy proportional to caloric increases needed for energy metabolism.
		Serves as a coenzyme.
		Deficiency can result in congenital beriberi, but no adverse effects have been associated with excess intake.
B$_2$ (riboflavin)	1.6 mg/d	Increased need during pregnancy proportional to caloric increases needed for both energy and protein metabolism.
		Deficiency can result in fissuring and dry scaling of the lips and corners of the mouth, dermatitis, skin changes in the genital areas, and anemias.
		No effects have been associated with excess intake.
B$_6$ (pyridoxine)	2.2 mg/d	Increased need during pregnancy proportional to protein intake.
		Serves as a coenzyme in amino acid metabolism; dietary sources should be adequate.

Nutrient	RDA for Pregnancy	Uses and Considerations
		Deficiency has been associated with seizures, dermatitis, and anemia. Excess consumption has been associated with gait disturbances and sensory neuropathy.
		Prior to pregnancy, oral contraceptive users may have lower storage levels of this vitamin.
B₁₂ (cobalamin)	2.2 µg/d	Deficiency rarely found in childbearing-age women.
		Serves as a coenzyme in protein metabolism, especially red blood cell formation.
		Deficiency most likely to be found in complete vegetarians; otherwise, dietary sources should be adequate. Inability to absorb vitamin results in pernicious anemia, with some women experiencing infertility as an outcome.
		Excess consumption not associated with negative pregnancy outcome.
Niacin	17 mg/d	Serves as a coenzyme in metabolism. Need known to increase slightly in pregnancy although little is known; dietary sources should be adequate.
Minerals		
Calcium	1200 mg/d	Increased need exists during pregnancy due to fetal skeleton mineralization, especially during the third trimester.
		Important for women under age 25 whose daily calcium intake is less than 600 mg.
		No evidence that pregnant women older than 35 years of age need special supplements of calcium.
		If maternal deficiency, fetal needs will be met through maternal bone demineralization.
		Deficiency may be related to PIH, while excesses two times or more above the pregnancy RDA may be associated with constipation and kidney stone development.
		Should be taken at mealtime to augment absorption and diminish interaction with iron supplements.
Phosphorus	1200 mg/d	Need increases during pregnancy but must be kept in ratio with calcium. If excessive intake from snack foods, cola drinks, processed meats, calcium absorption may be altered especially in presence of inadequate amounts of vitamin D and magnesium.
Magnesium	320 mg/d	Little known about this mineral in pregnancy except that it has a relationship to calcium and potassium levels and serves as a coenzyme in energy and protein metabolism.
Zinc	15 mg/d	Need increased in pregnancy especially for complete vegetarians and pregnant diabetics (due to altered zinc metabolism).
		Women with a specific zinc metabolism disorder causing severe deficiency may have high fetal mortality or malformations.
		Excessive intake may be related to prematurity and/or stillbirth.
		If iron supplementation is given above 30 mg/d for anemia, zinc supplementation is recommended due to interference with zinc absorption.

KEY: PIH: pregnancy-induced hypertension; >: greater than.

(Reference: Brodsky, A. (1991). Nutrition and diet counseling. In Cohen, S. M., Kenner, C. A., and Hollingsworth, A. O.: Maternal neonatal and women's health nursing (pp 451–479). Springhouse, PA: Springhouse Corp. Moore, M. C. (1991). Maternal and fetal nutrition. In Bobak, I. M., and Jensen, M. O., Essentials of maternity nursing (3rd ed) (pp 290–313). St. Louis: Mosby–Year Book, Inc. Martin, L. L., and Reeder, S. J. (1991): Essentials of Maternity Nursing (Chapter 9, Nutrition and Pregnancy, pp 172–203). Philadelphia: J. B. Lippincott Co.)

APPENDIX E
Drugs that Discolor Urine and Feces

Discoloration of Urine Due to Drugs

Black
Cascara
Ferrous salts
Iron dextran
Levodopa
Methocarbamol
Methyldopa
Naphthalene
Phenacetin
Phenols
Quinine
Sulfonamides

Blue
Anthraquinone
Indigo blue
Indigo carmine
Methocarbamol
Methylene blue
Nitrofurans
Triamterene

Blue-Green
Amitriptyline
Anthraquinone
Indigo blue
Indigo carmine
Methylene blue

Brown
Anthraquinone dyes
Cascara
Levodopa
Methocarbamol

Methyldopa
Metronidazole
Nitrofurans
Nitrofurantoin
Phenacetin
Primaquine
Quinine
Rifampin
Senna
Sodium diatrizoate
Sulfonamides

Brown-Black
Quinine

Yellow-Brown
Cascara
Chloroquine
Methylene blue
Metronidazole
Nitrofurantoin
Primaquine
Quinacrine
Senna
Sulfonamides

Dark
Cascara
Levodopa
Metronidazole
Nitrites
Primaquine
Quinine
Senna

Green
Anthraquinone
Indigo blue
Indigo carmine
Indomethacin
Methocarbamol
Methylene blue
Nitrofurans
Phenols

Green-Yellow
Methylene blue

Milky
Phosphates

Orange
Chlorzoxazone
Dihydroergotamine
 mesylate
Heparin sodium
Rifampin
Sulfasalazine
Warfarin

Orange-Red
Chlorzoxazone
Doxidan
Rifampin

Orange-Yellow
Fluorescein sodium
Rifampin
Sulfasalazine

Pink
Anthraquinone dyes
Danthron
Deferoxamine
Phenolphthalein
Phenothiazines
Phenytoin
Salicylates

Yellow-Pink
Cascara
Senna

Red
Anthraquinone
Cascara
Daunorubicin
Dimethylsulfoxide
Doxorubicin
Heparin
Ibuprofen
Methyldopa
Oxyphenbutazone
Phenacetin
Phenolphthalein
Phenothiazines
Phenylbutazone
Phenytoin
Rifampin
Senna

Red-Brown
Cascara
Methyldopa

Oxyphenbutazone
Phenacetin
Phenolphthalein
Phenothiazines
Phenylbutazone
Phenytoin
Quinine

Red-Purple
Chlorzoxazone
Ibuprofen
Phenacetin
Senna

Rust
Cascara
Chloroquine
Metronidazole
Nitrofurantoin
Phenacetin
Riboflavin
Senna
Sulfonamides

Yellow
Nitrofurantoin
Phenacetin
Sulfasalazine

Discoloration of Feces Due to Drugs

Black
Acetazolamide
Alcohols
Alkalies
Aminophylline
Amphetamine
Amphotericin
Antacids
Anticoagulants
Aspirin
Betamethasone
Charcoal
Chloramphenicol
Chlorpropamide
Clindamycin
Corticosteroids
Cortisone
Cyclophosphamide
Cytarabine
Dicumarol

Blue
Chloramphenicol
Methylene blue

Dark Brown
Dexamethasone

Gray
Colchicine

Green
Indomethacin
Iron
Medroxyprogesterone

Green-Gray
Oral antibiotics
Oxyphenbutazone
Phenylbutazone

Light Brown
Anticoagulants
Digitalis
Ethacrynic acid
Ferrous salts
Floxuridine
Fluorouracil
Halothane
Heparin
Hydralazine
Hydrocortisone
Ibuprofen
Indomethacin
Iodine drugs

Iron salts
Levarterenol
Levodopa
Manganese
Melphalan
Methylprednisolone
Methotrexate

Orange-Red
Phenazopyridine
Rifampin

Pink
Anticoagulants
Aspirin
Heparin
Oxyphenbutazone
Phenylbutazone
Salicylates

Red
Anticoagulants
Aspirin
Heparin
Oxyphenbutazone
Phenolphthalein
Phenylbutazone

Salicylates
Tetracycline syrup
Methylene blue
Oxyphenbutazone
Paraldehyde
Phenacetin
Phenolphthalein
Phenylbutazone
Phenylephrine
Phosphorus
Potassium salts
Prednisolone
Procarbazine
Reserpine
Salicylates
Sulfonamides
Tetracycline
Theophylline
Thiotepa
Triamcinolone
Warfarin

Red-Brown
Oxyphenbutazone
Phenylbutazone
Rifampin

Tarry
Ergot preparations
Ibuprofen
Salicylates
Warfarin

White/Speckling
Aluminum hydroxide
Antibiotics (oral)
Indocyanine green

Yellow
Senna

Yellow-Green
Senna

Adapted from Drugdex—Drug Consults, Micromedex, *vol 62. Denver, CO: Rocky Mountain Drug Consultation Center, November 1989. Published by Lexi-Comp Inc. for Medical Center of Delaware:* Formulary and Drug Therapy Guide, 1993–1994. *With permission.*

APPENDIX F
Vaccines

NURSING IMPLICATIONS FOR THE ADMINISTRATION OF VACCINES

1. Obtain complete allergy and drug history.
2. Observe for signs and symptoms of adverse reactions.
3. Instruct parents or guardians about adverse reactions.
4. Keep epinephrine readily available for immediate use in the event of anaphylaxis.
5. Do not administer to pregnant individuals.
6. Instruct female clients to avoid pregnancy for at least 3 months after receiving vaccine prepared from live, attenuated virus.

STANDARDS FOR PEDIATRIC IMMUNIZATION PRACTICES

Recommended by the *National Advisory Committee* (April, 1992)
Approved by the *United States Public Health Service* (May, 1992)
Endorsed by the *American Academy of Pediatrics* (May, 1992)
Also endorsed by the *American Nurses Association* (January, 1992)

Standard 1. Immunization services are *readily available*.
Standard 2. There are *no barriers* or *unnecessary prerequisites* to the receipt of vaccines.
Standard 3. Immunization services are available *free* or for a minimal fee.
Standard 4. Providers utilize all clinical encounters to *screen* and, when indicated, *immunize* children.
Standard 5. Providers *educate* parents and guardians about immunization in general terms.
Standard 6. Providers *question* parents or guardians about *contraindications* and, before immunizing a child, *inform* them in specific terms about the risks and benefits of the immunizations that their child is to receive.
Standard 7. Providers follow only true *contraindications*.
Standard 8. Providers administer *simultaneously* all doses of vaccine for which a child is eligible at the time of each visit.
Standard 9. Providers use accurate and complete *recording procedures*.
Standard 10. Providers *coschedule* immunization appointments in conjunction with appointments for other child health services.
Standard 11. Providers *report adverse events* following immunization promptly, accurately, and completely.
Standard 12. Providers operate a *tracking system*.
Standard 13. Providers adhere to appropriate procedures for *vaccine management*.
Standard 14. Providers conduct semiannual *audits* to assess immunization coverage levels and to review immunization records in the client populations that they serve.
Standard 15. Providers maintain up-to-date, easily retrievable *medical protocols* at all locations where vaccines are administered.
Standard 16. Providers operate with *client-oriented* and *community-based* approaches.
Standard 17. Vaccines are administered by *properly trained* individuals.
Standard 18. Providers receive *ongoing education* and *training* on current immunization recommendations.

TABLE 1 Recommended Childhood Immunization Schedule United States—January, 1995*

Age Vaccine	Birth	2 mon.	4 mon.	6 mon.	12 mon.	15 mos.	18 mon.	4–6 y	11–12 y	14–16 y
Hepatitis B[1]	HB-1 ⟶									
		HB-2 ⟶								
				HB-3 ⟶						
Diphtheria, tetanus, pertussis[2]		DTP	DTP	DTP	DTP or DTaP at 15 + m			DTP or DTaP	Td ⟶	
Haemophilus influenzae type b[3]		Hib	Hib	Hib	Hib ⟶					
Polio		OPV	OPV	OPV ⟶				OPV		
Measles, mumps, rubella[4,5]					MMR ⟶			MMR	or MMR	

* Vaccines are listed under the routinely recommended ages. Shaded bars indicate the range of acceptable ages for vaccination.

[1] Infants born to HBsAg-negative mothers should receive the second dose of hepatitis B vaccine between 1 and 4 months of age provided that at least 1 month has elapsed since receipt of the first dose. The third dose is recommended between 6 and 18 months of age.

Infants born to HBsAg positive mothers should receive immunoprophylaxis for hepatitis B with 0.5 mL Hepatitis B immune globulin (HBIG) within 12 hours of birth, and 0.5 mL of either Merck Sharpe & Dohme vaccine (Recombivax H3) or of Smith-Kline Beecham vaccine (Engerix-B) at a separate site. In these infants, the second dose of vaccine is recommended at 1 month of age and the third dose at 6 months of age. All pregnant women should be screened for HBsAg in an early prenatal visit.

[2] The fourth dose of DTP may be administered as early as 12 months of age, provided that at least 6 months have elapsed since DTP3. Combined DTP-Hib products may be used when these two vaccines are to be administered simultaneously. DTaP (diphtheria and tetanus toxoids and acellular pertussis vaccine) is licensed for use for the fourth and/or fifth dose of DTP vaccine in children 15 months of age or older and may be preferred for these doses in children in this age group.

[3] Three H. influenzae type b conjugate vaccines are available for use in infants: HbOC [Hib TITER] (Lederle Praxis); PRP-T [ActHIB; OmniHIB] Pasteur Merieux, distributed by SmithKline Beecham; Connaught; and PRP-OMP [PedvaxHIB] (Merck Sharpe & Dohme). Children who have received PRP-OMP at 2 and 4 months of age do not require a dose at 6 months of age. After the primary infant Hib conjugate vaccine series is completed, any licensed Hib conjugate vaccine may be used as a booster dose at 12 to 15 months of age.

[4] The second dose of MMR vaccine should be administered either at 4 to 6 years of age or at 11 to 12 years of age.

[5] Vaccines recommended in the second year of life (12 to 15 months of age) may be given at either one or two visits.

Approved by the Advisory Committee on Immunization Practices (ACIP), the American Academy of Pediatrics (AAP), and the American Academy of Family Physicians (AAFP). (From Delaware Health and Social Services, Division of Public Health, Newark, DE. Document No. 35-05-20/94/12/21.)

SCHEDULE FOR CHILDREN BEGINNING IMMUNIZATION IN INFANCY

Recommended schedules for active immunization of normal infants and children.

TABLE 2

Recommended Age*	Vaccine(s)[†]	Comments
2 mon	DTP-1[‡], OPV-1[§], HbCV-1[11,¶]	Can be given earlier in areas of high endemicity. Haemophilus b conjugate vaccines (HbOC or PRP-OMP) can be administered at this age.
4 mon	DTP-2, OPV-2, HbCV-2	6-wk to 2-mon interval desired between OPV doses to avoid interference.
6 mon	DTP-3, HbCV-3	An additional dose of OPV at this time is optional for use in areas with a high risk of polio exposure.
15 mon**	DTP-4, MMR-1[††], OPV-3, HbCV-4	Completion of primary series. Any licensed HbCV may be given at 15 mon.
4–6 y	DTP-5[‡‡], OPV-4, MMR-2	Preferably at or before school entry.
14–16 y	Td[§§]	Repeat every 10 y throughout life.

* These recommended ages should not be construed as absolute; i.e., 2 months can be 6 to 10 weeks, etc.

† See chart on back of container: recommendations for storage and handling.

‡ DTP—diphtheria and tetanus toxoids and pertussis vaccine absorbed.

§ OPV—live oral poliovirus vaccine; contains poliovirus strains types 1, 2, and 3.
Haemophilus conjugate vaccine (HbCV) for use in the prevention of Haemophilus influenzae.

11 HbOC—Lederle/Praxis is given at 2, 4, 6 and 15 months.

¶ PRP-OMP—Merck, Sharp & Dohme is given at 2, 4, and 12 months.
PRP-D—Connaught is given at 15 months.

** Provided at least 6 months have elapsed since DTP-3 or, if fewer than three DTPs have been received, at least 6 weeks since previous dose of DTP or OPV. MMR vaccine should not be delayed just to allow simultaneous administration with DTP and OPV. Administering MMR at 15 months and DTP-4, OPV-3 and H. influenzae type b conjugate vaccine is acceptable.

†† MMR—measles, mumps, and rubella virus vaccine, live. A routine two-dose measles vaccination schedule is recommended for all children. The first dose should be administered at 15 months of age or older. The second dose should be administered between 4 and 6 years of age. MMR is the preferred vaccine to meet this requirement.

‡‡ Up to the seventh birthday; thereafter use of Td is appropriate.

§§ Td—tetanus and diphtheria toxoids absorbed (for adult use); contains the same dose of tetanus toxoid as DTP or DT and a reduced dose of diphtheria toxoid.

(Source: Immunization Practices Advisory Committee [ACIP], Bureau of Health Promotion and Disease Prevention, Delaware State Health Department, Newark, DE.)

SCHEDULE FOR CHILDREN NOT IMMUNIZED AS INFANTS

Recommended immunization schedule for infants and children up to the seventh birthday who are not immunized at the recommended time in early infancy.* (See individual recommendations of the Immunization Practices Advisory Committee [ACIP], April 7, 1989, for details.)

TABLE 3

Timing	Vaccine(s)	Comments
First visit	DTP-1, OPV-1, HbCV-1[†], if child is ≤ 15 mon of age, and MMR, if child is ≥ 15 mon of age	DTP, OPV, MMR, and HbCV can be given simultaneously to children at 15 mon of age. One dose of HbOC and PRP-OMP is recommended for infants 12 to 14 mon of age.
2 mon after first DTP, OPV, HbCV	DTP-2, OPV-2, HbCV-2	Two doses of HbOC and PRP-OMP are recommended for infants 7 to 11 mon of age. DTP, OPV, and HbCV can be administered together.
2 mon after second DTP, HbCV	DTP-3, HbCV-3	OPV is optional in high-risk; three doses of HbOC are recommended for infants 1 to 6 mon of age.
6–12 mon after third DTP	DTP-4, OPV-3, PRP-OMP-3	PRP-OMP booster is recommended at 12 mon of age.
Preschool[‡] (4–6 y)	DTP-5, OPV-4, MMR-2	Preferably at or before school entry (MMR can be administered as soon as 30 d after the first dose).
14–16 y	Td	Repeat every 10 y throughout life.

* If initiated in the first year of life, give DTP-1, 2 and 3, OPV-1, 2, and 3 according to this schedule, MMR and HbCV with either HbOC or PRP-OMP vaccine schedule.

† An additional dose of HbOC should be given to all children at 15 months of age, at an interval not less than 2 months after the previous date. (Any licensed HbCV may be given at 15 months).

‡ The preschool dose is not necessary if the fourth dose of DTP and third dose of OPV are administered after the fourth birthday.

(Source: Immunization Practices Advisory Committee [ACIP], Bureau of Health Promotion and Disease Prevention, Delaware State Health Department, Newark, DE.)

SCHEDULE FOR CHILDREN 7 YEARS OF AGE OR OLDER

Recommended immunization schedule for children 7 to 18 years of age. (See individual recommendations of the Immunization Practices Advisory Committee [ACIP] for details.)

TABLE 4

Timing	Vaccine(s)	Comments
First visit	Td-1*, OPV-1†, and MMR-1‡	OPV is not routinely administered to persons ≥ 18 y of age.
2 mon after first Td, OPV	Td-2, OPV-2, and MMR-2	MMR-2 may be administered as soon as 30 d after the first dose.
6–12 mon after Td, OPV	Td-3 and OPV-3	OPV-3 may be given as soon as 6 wk after OPV-2.
10 y after	Td	Repeat every 10 y throughout life.

* Td—tetanus and diphtheria toxoids (adult type) are used after the seventh birthday. The DTP doses given to children younger than 7 years of age who remain incompletely immunized at age 7 or older should be counted as a prior exposure to tetanus and diphtheria toxoids (e.g., a child who previously received two doses of DTP only needs one dose of Td to complete a primary series).

† OPV is contraindicated for persons 18 years and older. Enhanced IPC should be substituted for them and for individuals with immunodeficiency disorders who need to be vaccinated.

‡ MMR—Live measles, mumps, and rubella virus vaccines combined. Persons born prior to 1957 may generally be considered immune to measles and mumps and may not need routine immunization. Rubella vaccine may be given to persons of any age, particularly women of childbearing age. Prior to administering rubella vaccine to females past menarche, the client or her guardian must be asked if she is pregnant. Pregnant clients should not be given rubella vaccine (or other live virus vaccine) due to theoretical risks to the fetus. Females receiving vaccine should be informed of the importance of not becoming pregnant for 3 months following vaccination.

(Source: Immunization Practices Advisory Committee [ACIP], Bureau of Health Promotion and Disease Prevention, Delaware State Health Department, Newark, DE.)

APPENDIX G

Laboratory Tests Related to Drug Use

INTRODUCTION

Many drugs have an effect on blood and urine chemistry and hematologic parameters; therefore, drug therapy is frequently monitored by laboratory testing. Liver and cardiac enzymes, renal indicators, electrolytes, and complete blood count (CBC) are checked periodically to identify adverse drug effects. Selected drugs, such as aminoglycosides, may be hepatotoxic and cause the liver to release enzymes. Most drugs are metabolized by the liver; therefore, a liver dysfunction should be assessed to recognize adverse reactions. Usually, the drug dose is reduced when a liver disorder is present or a substitute drug is ordered. Individual liver enzyme test or liver profile group (laboratory) tests may be requested. Liver enzymes to be monitored include alkaline phosphatase (ALP) and ALP isoenzymes (ALP_1); alanine aminotransferase (ALT or SGPT); gamma-glutamyl transferase (GGT); leucine aminopeptidase (LAP); 5'nucleotidase (5'NT); and lactic dehydrogenase (LDH) and the isoenzyme LDH_3.

Serum electrolytes constitute another laboratory profile group that needs monitoring. Electrolytes are plentiful in body fluids, tissues, and cells. Certain drugs can adversely affect electrolytes. Potassium-wasting diuretics cause sodium, potassium, magnesium, and chloride losses. Abnormal serum electrolyte levels may be a factor in drug interactions. If a client is taking a digitalis preparation, such as digoxin, and has a low serum potassium level, the hypokalemic state enhances the effect of digoxin, and digitalis toxicity can occur.

Most drug elimination is through the kidneys. The drug may be toxic to the kidneys (nephrotoxicity), or kidney disorders or impairment may cause an adverse drug reaction. In either situation, the blood urea nitrogen (BUN) and the serum creatinine should be checked frequently. Elevation of these two laboratory values may indicate kidney dysfunction. In clients with kidney disorders, the drug dose is usually adjusted accordingly.

A CBC includes a white blood cell (WBC) count and differential, red blood cell (RBC) count and RBC indices, hemoglobin, and hematocrit. Many drugs can decrease the WBC count (leukopenia), especially when the drug is taken in large doses or over a prolonged period.

Urinalysis is an indicator of kidney function. If a drug impairs kidney function, proteinuria or glucosuria may be noted. Assessment of BUN and serum creatinine levels is indicated when urinalysis results are abnormal.

This appendix lists the reference values or normal ranges for a variety of laboratory tests.* The reference values given may vary among institutions. When a client is receiving a drug that can affect the body organs, such as the liver, kidneys, or heart, the nurse needs to check the client's serum laboratory values to determine whether they are within the normal range. The health care provider should be reminded if laboratory tests have not been performed within a "reasonable period of time."

---

* *Source:* Tabular material adapted from Kee, J. L. (1995). *Laboratory and Diagnostic Tests with Nursing Implications* (4th ed) (pp 640–665). Norwalk, CT: Appleton & Lange.

COMPLETE BLOOD COUNT (CBC)

	Reference Values	
Test	*Adult*	*Child*
Hematocrit (Hct)	Male: 40–54%; 0.40–0.54 SI units Female: 36–46%; 0.36–0.46 SI units	Newborn: 44–65%; 1–3 y old: 29–40%; 4–10 y old: 31–43%
Hemoglobin (Hb, Hgb)	Male: 13.5–18 g/dL Female: 12–16 g/dL	Newborn: 14–24 g/dL Infant: 10–15 g/dL Child: 11–16 g/dL
Red blood cells (RBCs)	Male: 4.6–6 mil/μL Female: 4–6 mil/μL	Newborn: 4.8–7.2 mil/μL Child: 3.8–5.5 mil/μL
RBC indices MCV	80–98 cu μ	Newborn: 98–108 cu μ Child: 82–92 cu μ
MCH	27–31 pg	Newborn: 32–34 pg Child: 27–31 pg
MCHC	32–36%	Newborn: 32–33% Child: 32–36%
RDW	11.5–14.5 Coulter S	
White blood cells (WBCs)	4500–10,000 μL	Newborn: 9000–30,000 μL 2 y old: 6000–17,000 μL

WBC differentials
  Neutrophils
    Segments
    Bands
  Eosinophils
  Basophils
  Lymphocytes
  Monocytes
	50–70% of total WBCs
	50–65%
	0–5%
	0–3%
	1–3%
	25–35%
	2–6%
		29–47%
		
		0–3%
		1–3%
		38–63%
		4–9%

Platelets	150,000–400,000 μL 0.15–0.4 × 10^{12}/L	Premature: 100,000–300,000 μL Newborn: 150,000–300,000 μL Infant: 200,000–475,000 μL Child: same as adult

KEY: MCV: mean corpuscular volume; MCH: mean corpuscular hemoglobin; MCHC: mean corpuscular hemoglobin concentration; RDW: RBC distribution width.

ELECTROLYTES

Electrolyte	Reference Values	
	Adult	*Child*
Sodium (Na)	135–145 mEq/L 135–142 mmol/L (SI units)	Infant: 134–150 mEq/L Child: 135–145 mEq/L
Potassium (K)	3.5–5.3 mEq/L	Infant: 3.6–5.8 mEq/L Child: 3.5–5.5 mEq/L
Calcium (Ca)	4.5–5.5 mEq/L or 9–11 mg/dL 2.3–2.8 mmol/L (SI units)	Newborn: 3.7–7 mEq/L or 7.4–14 mg/dL Infant: 5–6 mEq/L or 10–12 mg/dL Child: 4.5–5.8 mEq/L or 9–11.5 mg/dL
Ionized calcium (iCa)	2.2–2.5 mEq/L 4.4–5.9 mg/dL 1.1–1.24 mmol/L (SI units)	
Magnesium (Mg)	1.5–2.5 mEq/L	Newborn: 1.4–2.9 mEq/L Child: 1.6–2.6 mEq/L
Chloride (Cl)	90–105 mEq/L	Newborn: 94–112 mEq/L Infant: 95–110 mEq/L Child: 98–105 mEq/L
Phosphorus (P) (phosphate)	1.7–2.6 mEq/L or 2.5–4.5 mg/dL	Newborn: 3.5–8.6 mg/dL Infant: 4.5–6.7 mg/dL Child: 4.5–5.5 mg/dL
Carbon dioxide (CO_2)	22–30 mEq/L	20–28 mEq/L

CARDIAC PROFILE

Test	Reference Values	
	Adult	*Child*
Aspartate aminotransferase (AST, SGOT)	5–40 U/mL (Frankel) 4–36 IU/L 16–60 U/mL at 30°C 8–33 U/L at 37°C (SI units)	Newborn: 4 × adult level Child: same as adult
Creatine phosphokinase (CPK)	Male: 5–35 μg/mL, 30–180 IU/L, 55–170 U/L at 37°C (SI units) Female: 5–25 μg/mL, 25–150 IU/L, 30–135 U/L at 37°C (SI units)	Newborn: 65–580 IU/L at 30°C Male: 0–70 IU/L at 30°C Female: 0–50 IU/L at 30°C
CPK isoenzyme	CPK-MB: 0–6%	
Lactic dehydrogenase (LD, LDH)	100–190 IU/L, 70–250 U/L	Newborn: 300–1500 IU/L Child: 50–150 IU/L
LDH isoenzymes	LDH_1 14–26% LDH_2 27–37%	
Potassium (K)	3.5–5.3 mEq/L	*see* Electrolytes

KEY: CPK-MB: cardiac isoenzyme.

CORONARY PROFILE

Test	Reference Values	
	Adult	*Child*
Lipids (total)	400–800 mg/dL 4–8 g/L (SI units)	
LDL	60–160 mg/dL, Low risk for CHD: <130 mg/dL	
HDL	29–77 mg/dL, Low risk for CHD: 46–59 mg/dL Very low risk for CHD: >60 mg/dL	

Cholesterol	Desirable: <200 mg/dL
	Moderate risk: 200–240 mg/dL
	High risk: >240 mg/dL
	Pregnancy: high risk but returns to normal
		Infant: 90–130 mg/dL
		2–19 y old:
		   Desirable: 130–170 mg/dL
		   Moderate risk: 171–184 mg/dL
		   High risk: >185 mg/dL

Triglycerides	12–29 y old: 10–140 mg/dL 30–39 y old: 20–150 mg/dL 40–49 y old: 30–160 mg/dL >50 y old: 40–190 mg/dL	Infant: 5–40 mg/dL 5–11 y old: 10–135 mg/dL
Phospholipids	150–380 mg/dL	
Glucose (fasting blood sugar)	Serum: 70–110 mg/dL Blood: 60–100 mg/dL	Newborn: 30–80 mg/dL Child: 60–100 mg/dL

KEY: LDL: low-density lipoproteins; HDL: high-density lipoproteins; CHD: coronary heart disease.

HEPATIC PROFILE

Test	Reference Values	
	Adult	*Child*
Alkaline phosphatase (ALP)	30–120 IU/L; 25–97 U/L at 37°C (SI units); 2–4 U/dL (Bodansky); 4–13 U/dL (King-Armstrong); 0.8–2.3 U/dL (Bessey-Lowry)	Infant: 40–300 U/L Child: 60–270 U/L; 15–30 U/dL (King-Armstrong); 5–14 U/dL (Bodansky)
ALP$_1$ isoenzyme	20–120 U/L	
Alanine aminotransferase (ALT/SGPT)	5–25 mU/mL (Wroblewski) 4–36 U/L at 37°C (SI units) 5–35 U/mL (Frankel) 8–50 U/mL at 30°C (Karmen)	Infant: may be twice as high as adult Child: same as adult
Gamma-glutamyltransferase (GGT)	Male: 10–80 IU/L Female: 5–55 IU/L	
Lactic dehydrogenase (LDH/LD)	100–190 IU/L; 70–250 U/L	Newborn: 300–1500 IU/L Child: 50–150 IU/L

LDH isoenzymes
    LDH$_4$
    LDH$_5$
	8–16%
	6–16%	

Leucine aminopeptidase (LAP)	8–22 mU/mL, 12–33 IU/L	
5'Nucleotidase (5'NT)	<14 U/L	
Albumin	3.5–5 g/dL	
Protein	6–8 g/dL	Premature: 4.2–7.6 g/dL Newborn: 4.6–7.4 g/dL Infant: 6–6.7 g/dL Child: 6.2–8 g/dL
Bilirubin Total	0.1–1.2 mg/dL; 1.7–20.5 μmol/L (SI units)	Total, newborn: 1–12 mg/dL, 17.1–205 μmol/L (SI units) Total, child: 0.2–0.8 mg/dL
Direct	0.1–0.3 mg/dL 1.7–5.1 μmol/L (SI units)	
Prothrombin time (PT)	11–15 sec or 70–100%	

RENAL PROFILE

Test	Reference Values	
	Adult	*Child*
Albumin	3.5–5 g/dL	
Blood urea nitrogen (BUN)	5–25 mg/dL	Infant: 5–15 mg/dL Child: 5–20 mg/dL
Creatinine (Cr)	0.5–1.5 mg/dL 45–132.3 μmol/L (SI units)	Newborn: 0.8–1.4 mg/dL Infant: 0.7–1.7 mg/dL 2–6 y: 0.3–0.6 mg/dL; 24–54 μmol/L (SI units) 7–18 y: 0.4–1.2 mg/dL; 36–106 μmol/L (SI units)

Creatinine (urine)	Male: 20–26 mg/kg/24h
	  0.18–0.23 mmol/kg/24h (SI units)
	Female: 14–22 mg/kg/24h
	  0.12–0.19 mmol/kg/24h (SI units)
		Similar to adult

Creatinine clearance (urine)	85–135 mL/min	
Electrolytes	*see* Electrolytes	
Glucose (FBS)	70–110 mg/dL (serum) 60–100 mg/dL (blood)	Newborn: 30–80 mg/dL Child: 60–100 mg/dL
Protein	6–8 g/dL	Infant: 6–6.7 g/dL Child: 6.2–8 g/dL
urine	0–5 mg/dL/24h	
Uric acid	Male: 3.5–8 mg/dL Female: 2.8–6.8 mg/dL	Child: 2.5–5.5 mg/dL
urine	250–750 mg/24h (low purine diet)	

KEY: FBS: *fasting blood sugar.*

THYROID PROFILE

Test	Reference Values	
	Adult	*Child*
Calcitonin	Male: < 40 pg/mL Female: < 20 pg/mL	
Triiodothyronine (T₃)	80–200 ng/dL	Newborn: 90–170 ng/dL 6–12 y: 115–190 ng/dL
Thyroxine (T₄)	4.5–11.5 μg/dL 5–12 μg/dL (RIA) 1–2.3 ng/dL (thyroxine iodine)	Newborn: 11–23 μg/dL 1–4 mon: 7.5–16.5 μg/dL 4–12 mon: 5.5–14.5 μg/dL 1–6 y: 5.5–13.5 μg/dL 6–10 y: 5–12.5 μg/dL
Thyroid-binding globulin (TBG)	10–26 μg/dL	
T₃ resin uptake	25–35 relative % uptake	
Thyroid antibodies (TA)	Negative or < 1:20 titer	
Thyroid-stimulating hormone (TSH)	2–5.4 μIU/mL, < 3 ng/mL, < 10 μU/mL, < 10^{-3} IU/L (SI units)	Newborn: < 25 μIU/mL

FEMALE REPRODUCTIVE PROFILE

	Reference Values	
Test	*Adult*	*Child*
Estrogen	Early menstrual cycle: 60–400 pg/mL Midmenstrual cycle: 100–600 pg/mL Late menstrual cycle: 150–350 pg/mL Postmenopausal: <30 pg/mL Male: 40–115 pg/mL	
Estrogen (urine)	Female: Preovulation: 5–25 μg/24h Follicular: 24–100 μg/24h Luteal phase: 22–80 μg/24h Postmenopausal: 0–10 μg/24h Male: 4–25 μg/24h	
Estradiol (E_2)	Female: Follicular phase: 20–150 pg/mL Midcycle: 100–500 pg/mL Luteal phase: 60–260 pg/mL Male: 15–20 pg/mL	3–10 pg/mL
Progesterone	Preovulation: 20–150 ng/dL Midcycle: 250–2800 ng/dL	
Prolactin	Nonlactating female: 0–23 ng/dL Pregnancy: rise of 10–20 fold	
Follicle-stimulating hormone (FSH)	Female: Preovulation: 4–30 mU/mL Midcycle: 10–90 mU/mL Luteal phase: 4–30 mU/mL Postmenopausal: 40–250 mU/mL Male: 4–25 mU/mL	Child: 5–12 mU/mL
Follicle-stimulating hormone— urine (FSH-urine)	Female: Preovulation: 4–25 IU/24h Midcycle: 8–60 IU/24h Postmenopausal: 50–150 IU/24h Male: 4–18 IU/24h	Child: <10 IU/24h
Luteinizing hormone (LH)	Female: Follicular: 3–30 mIU/mL Midcycle: 30–100 mIU/mL Postmenopausal: 40–100 mIU/mL Male: 5–25 mIU/mL	Child: <10 mIU/mL
Pregnanediol (urine)	Female: Preovulation: 0.5–1.5 mg/24h Midcycle: 2–7 mg/24h Postmenopausal: 0.1–1 mg/24h Male: 0.1–1.5 mg/24h	Child: 0.4–1 mg/24h

URINALYSIS

Urine Content	Reference Values	
	Adult	*Child*
Color	Light straw to dark amber	Light straw to dark yellow
Appearance	Clear	Clear
Odor	Aromatic	Aromatic
pH	4.5–8.0	4.5–8.0
Specific gravity (SG)	1.005–1.030 Average: 1.015–1.024	1.005–1.030
Protein	Negative 2–8 mg/dL	
Glucose	Negative	Negative
Ketones	Negative	Negative
RBC	1–2 per low-power field	Rare
WBC	3–4 per low-power field	0–4
Casts	Occasional hyaline	Rare

KEY: *Units: mg: milligram; mEq: milliequivalent; L: liter; SI units: international system of units; g: gram; dL: deciliter; μL: microliter; cu μ: cubic micron; IU: international unit; mmol: millimole; ng: nanogram; pg: picogram; μg: microgram; μmol: micromole.*

APPENDIX H
Therapeutic Drug Monitoring *

Therapeutic drug monitoring (TDM), the client's serum and urine therapeutic drug ranges during drug therapy, is a common practice and is vitally important when the drug has a narrow therapeutic index and a high probability of adverse reactions. Digoxin and lithium have very narrow therapeutic ranges, and drug toxicities can occur when the drug therapeutic range is slightly above the norm. Drugs with a wide therapeutic index and range usually do not require TDM. TDM may be used for achieving and maintaining adequate drug dosage. For example, it is important that drug dosing of theophylline and phenytoin, with narrow therapeutic ranges, maintains an average serum level so that the desired therapeutic effects are achieved.

TDM has four additional purposes: (1) to evaluate the client's compliance with drug therapy, (2) to determine if other drugs have altered the drug concentration, (3) to identify a non-effective response to the prescribed drug therapy, and (4) to establish a new serum-drug level when the drug dose has been changed.

TDM is primarily associated with selected drug groups, including: (1) analgesics (aspirin, acetaminophen), (2) antibacterials and antibiotics, especially the aminoglycosides, (3) anticonvulsants, (4) anticancer drugs, (5) bronchodilators (theophyllines), (6) cardiac drugs (beta blockers, calcium blockers, antidysrhythmics), (7) oral antidiabetic agents, (8) sedatives, and (9) tranquilizers (benzodiazepines, phenothiazines). To determine that the drug dose is within the "normal range," blood may be drawn for peak levels, trough levels, or both. Peak serum drug levels are taken approximately 1 to 2 hours after the drug is given; trough levels are drawn within 1 hour prior to administration of the next dose. If the drug level is within the therapeutic range, the client has received a therapeutic dose.

To effectively conduct TDM, the laboratory must be provided with the following information: (1) the drug's name and daily dosage, (2) time administered, (3) amount of last drug dose, (4) time blood was drawn, (5) route of administration, and (6) client's age. Without complete information, serum drug reporting may be incorrect.

The following table alphabetically lists drugs, therapeutic range, peak time of action, and toxic level.

* Revised by Ronald J. Lefever, R.Ph., Pharmacy Services, Medical College of Virginia, Richmond, VA.

Drug	Therapeutic Range	Peak Time	Toxic Level
Acetaminophen (Tylenol)	10–20 μg/mL	1–2½ h	>50 μg/mL Hepatotoxicity: >200 μg/mL
Acetohexamide (Dymelor)	20–70 μg/mL (should be dosed according to blood glucose levels)	2–4 h	>75 μg/mL
Alcohol	Negative		Mild toxic: 150 mg/dL Marked toxic: >250 mgL
Alprazolam (Xanax)	10–50 ng/mL	1–2 h	>75 ng/mL
Amikacin (Amikin)	Peak: 20–30 μg/mL Trough: ≤10 μg/mL	Intravenously: ½ h Intramuscularly: ½–1½ h	Peak: >35 μg/mL Trough: >10 μg/mL
Aminocaproic acid (Amicar)	100–400 μg/mL	1 h	>400 μg/mL
Aminophylline (see Theophylline)			
Amiodarone (Cordarone)	0.5–2.5 μg/mL	2–10 h	>2.5 μg/mL
Amitriptyline (Elavil)	125–200 ng/mL	2–12 h	>500 ng/mL
Amobarbital (Amytal)	1–5 μg/mL	2 h	>15 μg/mL Severe toxicity: >30 μg/mL
Amoxapine (Asendin)	200–400 ng/mL	1½ h	>500 ng/mL
Amphetamine:			>0.2 μg/mL
Serum	20–30 ng/mL		
Urine		Detectable in urine after 3 h; positive for 24–48 h	>30 μg/mL urine
Aspirin (see Salicylates)			
Atenolol (Tenormin)	200–500 ng/mL	2–4 h	>500 ng/mL
Bromide	20–80 mg/dL		>100 mg/dL
Butabarbital (Butisol)	1–2 μg/mL	3–4 h	>10 μg/mL
Caffeine	Adult: 3–15 μg/mL Infant: 8–20 μg/mL	½–1 h	>50 μg/mL
Carbamazepine (Tegretol)	4–12 μg/mL	6 h (range 2–24 h)	>9–15 μg/mL
Chloral hydrate (Noctec)	2–12 μg/mL	1–2 h	>20 μg/mL
Chloramphenicol (Chloromycetin)	10–20 mg/L		>25 mg/L
Chlordiazepoxide (Librium)	1–5 μg/mL	2–3 h	>5 μg/mL
Chlorpromazine (Thorazine)	50–300 ng/mL	2–4 h	>750 ng/mL
Chlorpropamide (Diabinese)	75–250 μg/mL	3–6 h	>250–750 μg/mL
Clonidine (Catapres)	0.2–2 ng/mL (hypotensive effect)	2–5 h	>2 ng/mL
Clorazepate (Tranxene)	0.12–1 μg/mL	1–2 h	>1 μg/mL
Cimetidine (Tagamet)	Trough: 0.5–1.2 μg/mL	1–1½ h	Trough: >1.5 μg/mL
Clonazepam (Klonopin)	10–60 ng/mL	2 h	>80 ng/mL
Codeine	10–100 ng/mL	1–2 h	>200 ng/mL
Dantrolene (Dantrium)	1–3 μg/mL	5 h	>5 μg/mL
Desipramine (Norpramin)	125–300 ng/mL	4–6 h	>400 ng/mL
Diazepam (Valium)	0.5–2 mg/L 400–600 ng/mL therapeutic	1–2 h	>3 mg/L >3000 ng/mL
Digitoxin (rarely administered)	10–25 ng/mL	Noticeable: 2–4 h Peak: 12–24 h	>30 ng/mL
Digoxin	0.5–2 ng/mL	PO: 6–8 h IV: 1½–2 h	2–3 ng/mL
Dilantin (see Phenytoin)			
Diltiazem (Cardizem)	50–200 ng/mL	2–3 h	>200 ng/mL
Disopyramide (Norpace)	2–4 μg/mL	2 h	>4 μg/mL
Doxepin (Sinequan)	150–300 ng/mL	2–4 h	>500 ng/mL
Ethchlorvynol (Placidyl)	2–8 μg/mL	1–2 h	>20 μg/mL
Ethosuximide (Zarontin)	40–100 μg/mL	2–4 h	>150 μg/mL
Flecainide (Tambocor)	0.2–1 μg/mL	3 h	>1 μg/mL
Flurazepam (Dalmane)	20–110 ng/mL		>1500 ng/mL
Gentamicin (Garamycin)	Peak: 6–12 μg/mL Trough: <2 μg/mL	IV: 15–30 min	Peak: >12 μg/mL Trough: >2 μg/mL
Glutethimide (Doriden)	2–6 μg/mL	1–2 h	>20 μg/mL
Haloperidol (Haldol)	5–15 ng/mL	2–6 h	>50 ng/mL
Hydromorphone (Dilaudid)	1–30 ng/mL	½–1½ h	>100 ng/mL
Ibuprofen (Motrin, etc.)	10–50 μg/mL	1–2 h	>100 μg/mL
Imipramine (Tofranil)	150–300 ng/mL	PO: 1–2 h IM: 30 min	>500 ng/mL

Drug	Therapeutic Range	Peak Time	Toxic Level
Isoniazid (INH, Nydrazid)	1–7 μg/mL (dose usually adjusted based on liver function tests)	1–2 h	>20 μg/mL
Kanamycin (Kantrex)	Peak: 15–30 μg/mL Trough: 1–4 μg/mL	PO: 1–2 h IM: 30 min–1 h	Peak: >35 μg/mL Trough: >10 μg/mL
Lead	<20 μg/dL Urine: <80 μg/24 h		>80 μg/mL Urine: >125 μg/24 h
Lidocaine (Xylocaine)	1.5–5 μg/mL	IV: 10 min	>6 μg/mL
Lithium	0.8–1.2 mEq/L	½–4 h	>1.5 mEq/L
Lorazepam (Ativan)	50–240 ng/mL	1–3 h	>300 ng/mL
Maprotiline (Ludiomil)	200–300 ng/mL	12 h	>500 ng/mL
Meperidine (Demerol)	0.4–0.7 μg/mL	2–4 h	>1 μg/mL
Mephenytoin (Mesantoin)	15–40 μg/mL	2–4 h	>50 μg/mL
Meprobamate (Equanil, Miltown)	15–25 μg/mL	2 h	>50 μg/mL
Methadone (Dolophine)	100–400 ng/mL	½ to 1 h	>2000 ng/mL or >0.2 μg/mL
Methyldopa (Aldomet)	1–5 μg/mL	3–6 h	>7 μg/mL
Methyprylon (Noludar)	8–10 μg/mL	1–2 h	>50 μg/mL
Metoprolol (Lopressor)	75–200 ng/mL	2–4 h	>225 ng/mL
Mexiletine (Mexitil)	0.5–2 μg/mL	2–3 h	>2 μg/mL
Morphine	10–80 ng/mL	IV: immediately IM: ½–1 h SC: 1–1½ h	>200 ng/mL
Netilmicin (Netromycin)	Peak: 0.5–10 μg/mL Trough: <4 μg/mL	IV: 30 min	Peak: >16 μg/mL Trough: >4 μg/mL
Nifedipine (Procardia)	50–100 ng/mL	½–2 h	>100 ng/mL
Nortriptyline (Aventyl)	50–150 ng/mL	8 h	>200 ng/mL
Oxazepam (Serax)	0.2–1.4 μg/mL	1–2 h	
Oxycodone (Percodan)	10–100 ng/mL	½–1 h	>200 ng/mL
Pentazocine (Talwin)	0.05–0.2 μg/mL	1–2 h	>1 μg/mL Urine: >3 μg/mL
Pentobarbital (Nembutal)	1–5 μg/mL	½–1 h	>10 μg/mL Severe toxicity: >30 μg/mL
Phenmetrazine (Preludin)	5–30 μg/mL (urine)	2 h	>50 μg/mL (urine)
Phenobarbital (Luminal)	15–40 μg/mL	6–18 h	>40 μg/mL Severe toxicity: >80 μg/mL
Phenytoin (Dilantin)	10–20 μg/mL	4–8 h	>20–30 μg/mL Severe toxicity: >40 μg/mL
Pindolol (Visken)	0.5–6 ng/mL	2–4 h	>10 ng/mL
Primidone (Mysoline)	5–12 μg/mL	2–4 h	>12–15 μg/mL
Procainamide (Pronestyl)	4–10 μg/mL	1 h	>10 μg/mL
Procaine (Novocain)	<11 μg/mL	10–30 min	>20 μg/mL
Prochlorperazine (Compazine)	50–300 ng/mL	2–4 h	>1000 ng/mL
Propoxyphene (Darvon)	0.1–0.4 μg/mL	2–3 h	>0.5 μg/mL
Propranolol (Inderal)	>100 ng/mL	1–2 h	>150 ng/mL
Protriptyline (Vivactil)	50–150 ng/mL	8–12 h	>200 ng/mL
Quinidine	2–5 μg/mL	1–3 h	>6 μg/mL
Ranitidine (Zantac)	100 ng/mL	2–3 h	>100 ng/mL
Reserpine (Serpasil)	20 ng/mL	2–4 h	>20 ng/mL
Salicylates (Aspirin)	10–30 mg/dL	1–2 h	Tinnitis: 20–40 mg/mL Hyperventilation: >35 mg/dL Severe toxicity: >50 mg/dL
Secobarbital (Seconal)	2–5 μg/mL	1 h	>15 μg/mL Severe toxicity: >30 μg/mL
Theophylline (Thodur, Aminodur)	10–20 μg/mL	PO: 2–3 h IV: 15 minutes (depends on smoking or nonsmoking)	>20 μg/mL
Thioridazine (Mellaril)	100–600 ng/mL 1–1.5 μg/mL	2–4 h	>2000 ng/mL >10 μg/mL
Timolol (Blocadren)	3–55 ng/mL	1–2 h	>60 ng/mL

Table continued on following page

Drug	Therapeutic Range	Peak Time	Toxic Level
Tobramycin (Nebcin)	Peak: 5–10 μg/mL Trough: 1–1.5 μg/mL	IV: 15–30 min IM: ½–1½ h	Peak: >12 μg/mL Trough: >2 μg/mL
Tocainide (Tonocard)	4–10 μg/mL	½–3 h	>12 μg/mL
Tolbutamide (Orinase)	80–240 μg/mL	3–5 h	>640 μg/mL
Trazodone (Desyrel)	500–2500 ng/mL	1–2 wk	>4000 ng/mL
Trifluoperazine (Stelazine)	50–300 ng/mL	2–4 h	>1000 ng/mL
Valproic acid (Depakene)	50–100 μg/mL	½–1½ h	>100 μg/mL Severe toxicity: >150 μg/mL
Vancomycin (Vanocin)	Peak: 20–40 μg/mL Trough: 5–10 μg/mL	IV: Peak: 5 min IV: Trough: 12 h	Peak: >80 μg/mL
Verapamil (Calan)	100–300 ng/mL	PO: 1–2 h	>500 ng/mL
	1–10 μg/mL (dose usually		

(Source: *Kee, J. L. (1995). Laboratory and Diagnostic Tests with Nursing Implications (4th ed). (pp 618–623). Norwalk, CT: Appleton & Lange. With permission.)*

References

Abbott, C. (1987). The impaired nurse. Part II: Management strategies. *Association of Operating Room Nurses, 46* (6), 1104–1115.

Abel, E. L., and Sokol, R. J. (1988). Alcohol use in pregnancy. In J. R. Niebyl (Ed.), *Drug use in pregnancy* (2nd ed) (pp 193–202). Philadelphia: Lea & Febiger.

Abel, E. L., and Sokol, R. J. (1988). Marijuana and cocaine use in pregnancy. In J. R. Niebyl (Ed.), *Drug use in pregnancy* (2nd ed) (pp 223–230). Philadelphia: Lea & Febiger.

Abernathy, E. (1987). Biological response modifiers. *American Journal of Nursing, 87* (4), 458–459.

Abraham, W. T., and Schrier, R. W. (1994). Body fluid volume regulation in health and disease. *Advanced Internal Medicine, 39,* 23–47.

Abrams, A. C. (1987). *Clinical drug therapy* (2nd ed). Philadelphia: JB Lippincott.

Alexander, S. E., and Aksel, S. (1990). Estrogen replacement therapy: Which regimen to choose? In R. C. Cefalo, *Clinical decisions in obstetrics and gynecology* (pp 226–278). Rockville, MD: Aspen Publishers.

Allen, J. E. (1993). Drug-induced photosensitivity. *Clinical Pharmacy, 12* (8), 580–584.

American Association of Colleges of Pharmacology/Eli Lilly and Company Geriatric Curriculum Project (1985). B. Ameer ed, *Pharmacy practice for the geriatric patient.* Carrboro, NC: Health Sciences Consortium.

American College of Obstetricians and Gynecologists (1994). *Antenatal corticosteroid therapy for fetal maturation.* ACOG Committee Opinion, No. 147. Washington, D.C.: ACOG.

American College of Obstetricians and Gynecologists (1995). Menopause: emerging issues. *ACOG Update: An Approved System for Continuing Medical Education, 21* (3), 1–9.

American Heart Association (1992). Guidelines for emergency cardiac care. *Journal of the American Medical Association, 268,* 16, October 28.

American Heart Association (1987). *Textbook of advanced cardiac life support.* Dallas, TX: American Heart Association.

American Journal of Nursing (1992). OSHA stiffens bloodborne rules, decrees free hepatitis B vaccine. *American Journal of Nursing, 92* (1), 82–84.

American Medical Association, Division of Drugs and Toxicology (1993). *Drug evaluations annual.* Chicago: American Medical Association.

American Society of Hospital Pharmacists (1995) *AHFS drug information.* Bethesda, MD: American Society of Hospital Pharmacists.

Amgen, Inc. (1991). *Neupogen (Filgrastim) product monograph.* Thousand Oaks, CA: Amgen, Inc.

Amgen, Inc. (1992). *Procrit: epoetin alpha for injections.* Product monograph. Thousand Oaks, CA: Amgen, Inc.

Aral, S. O., and Holmes, K. K. (1991). Sexually transmitted diseases in the AIDS era. *Scientific American, 264* (2), 62–68.

Association of Women's Health, Obstetrics, and Neonatal Nursing (AWHONN). (1993). *Cervical ripening and induction and augmentation of labor.* [Practice Resource], December.

Association of Women's Health, Obstetrics, and Neonatal Nursing (AWHONN). (1994). *Issues in contraceptive method selection.* Independent study, monograph, module 2, 4–30.

Bachman, J. A. (1995). Management of discomfort. In I. M. Bobak, D. L. Lowdermilk, and M. D. Jensen. *Maternity nursing* (4th ed) (pp 221–245). St Louis: Mosby–Year Book, Inc.

Barbieri, R. L. (1991). The use of danazol as a treatment of endometriosis. In E. Thomas, and J. Rock (Eds.), *Modern approaches to endometriosis* (pp 239–255). Dordrecht, The Netherlands: Kluwer Academic Publishers.

Barnhart, E. R. (1995). *Physician's desk reference* (49th ed). Oradell, NJ: Medical Economics Company.

Barkauskas, V., Stoltenberg-Allen, K., Baumann, L., and Darling-Fisher, C. (1994). *Quick reference to health and physical assessment.* St Louis, CV Mosby.

Baylor College of Medicine (1995). Weighing the risks and benefits of hormone replacement therapy after menopause. *The Contraceptive Report, VI* (4), 4–14.

Bender, S. (1991). Personal communication. Letter from Professional Service Manager, Amgen, Inc. (February 20, 1991).

Benenson, A. S. (1990). *Control of communicable disease in man* (15th ed). Washington, DC: American Public Health Association.

Benson, M. D. (1994). *Obstetrical pearls: A practical guide for the efficient resident* (2nd ed). Philadelphia: FA Davis.

Berkowitz, G. S. (1988). Smoking and pregnancy. In J. R. Niebyl (Ed.), *Drug use in pregnancy* (2nd ed) (pp 173–191). Philadelphia: Lea & Febiger.

Besinger, R. E., and Niebyl, J. R. (1988). Tocolytic agents for the treatment of preterm labor. In J. R. Niebyl (Ed.), *Drugs used in pregnancy* (2nd ed) (pp 127–172). Philadelphia: Lea & Febiger.

Betz, C. L., and Poster, E. C. (1989). *Pediatric nursing reference.* St Louis: CV Mosby.

Biological Therapy Nurses of University of Chicago Hospital (1989). *Interleukin-2: A patient handbook.* Chicago: University of Chicago Hospital.

Blake, D. A., and Niebyl, J. R. (1988). Requirements and limitations in reproductive and teratogenic risk assessment. In J. R. Niebyl (Ed.), *Drug use in pregnancy* (2nd ed) (pp 1–9). Philadelphia: Lea & Febiger.

Bleck, T. P. (1990). Convulsive disorders: The use of anticonvulsant drugs. *Clinical Neuropharmacology, 13* (3), 198–209.

Blenner, J. L. (1991). Clomiphene-induced mood swings. *Journal of Obstetric, Gynecologic, and Neonatal Nursing; 20* (4), 321–327.

Blix, A. G. (1993). Environmental hazards. In S. Mattson, and J. E. Smith (Eds.), *NAACOG core curriculum for maternal newborn nursing* (pp 199–216). Philadelphia: WB Saunders.

Bobak, I. M. (1991). *Quick reference for maternity nursing.* St Louis: Mosby–Year Book, Inc.

Bobak, I. M., Jensen, M. O., and Zalar, M. K. (1989). *Maternity and gynecologic care: The nurse and the family* (4th ed). St Louis: CV Mosby.

Bobak, I. M., Lowdermilk, D. L., and Jensen, M. D. (1995). *Maternity nursing* (4th ed). St Louis: Mosby–Year Book, Inc.

Bond, L. (1993). Physiological changes. In S. Mattson, and J. E. Smith (Eds.), *NAACOG core curriculum for maternal newborn nursing* (pp 315–324). Philadelphia: WB Saunders.

Bortenschlager, L., and Zaloga, G. P. (1994). Vitamins. In B. Chernow (Ed.), *The pharmacologic approach to the critically-ill patient* (3rd ed) (pp 3–17). Baltimore: Williams & Wilkins.

Bozzette, S. A., Finkelstein, D. M., Spector, S. A., et al. (1995). Randomized trial of three antipneumocystis agents in patients with advanced human immunodeficiency virus infection. *New England Journal of Medicine, 332* (11), 593–639.

Brensilver, J. M., and Goldberger, E. (1996). *Water, electrolyte, and acid-base syndromes* (8th ed). Philadelphia: FA Davis.

Briggs, G. G., Freeman, R. K., and Yaffee, S. J. (1993). *Drugs in lactation*. Baltimore: Williams & Wilkins.

Briggs, G. G., Freeman, R. K., and Yaffe, S. J. (1994). *Drugs in pregnancy and lactation: A reference guide to fetal and neonatal risk* (4th ed). Baltimore: Williams & Wilkins.

Bristol-Myers Squibb Co. (1991). *Videx (didanosine) product* insert. Evansville, IN: Bristol-Myers Squibb Co.

Brogden, J. M., and Nevidjon, B. (1995). Vinorelbine tartrate (Navelbine): Drug profile and nursing implications of a new vinca alkaloid. *Oncology Nursing Forum, 22* (4), 635–646.

Bullock, B. L., and Rosendahl, D. P. (1988). *Pathophysiology: Adaptations and alterations in function* (2nd ed). Glenview, IL: Scott, Foresman.

Cargill, J. M. (1992). Medication compliance in elderly people: Influencing variables and interventions. *Journal of Advanced Nursing, 17*, 422–426.

Cashion, K., and Johnston, C. L. A. (1995). Nursing care during the postpartum period. In I. M. Bobak, D. L. Lowdermilk, and M. D. Jensen. *Maternity nursing* (4th ed) (pp 463–503). St Louis: Mosby–Year Book, Inc.

Caudell, K., and Whedon, M. B. (1991). Hematopoietic complications. In Whedon, M. B. (Ed.), *Bone marrow transplantation: Principles, practice and nursing insights* (pp 135–151). Boston: Jones and Bartlett Publishers.

Centers for Disease Control (1992). *1992 revised classification system for HIV infection and expanded AIDS surveillance case definition for adolescents and adults*. Draft of November 15, 1991. Atlanta: U.S. Department of Health and Human Services, Public Health Service, CDC.

Centers for Disease Control and Prevention (1991). Guidelines for prophylaxis against *Pneumocystis carinii* pneumonia for children infected with human immunodeficiency virus. *Morbidity and Mortality Weekly Report, 40* (RR-2), 1–13.

Centers for Disease Control and Prevention (1991). Pelvic inflammatory disease: Guidelines for prevention and management. *Morbidity and Mortality Weekly Report, 40* (RR-5), 1–25.

Centers for Disease Control and Prevention (1993). Recommendations for the prevention and management of *Chlamydia trachomatis* infections, 1993. *Morbidity and Mortality Weekly Report, 42* (RR-12), 1–39.

Centers for Disease Control and Prevention (1994). Recommendations of the U. S. Public Health Service task force on the use of zidovudine to reduce perinatal transmission of human immunodeficiency virus. *Morbidity and Mortality Weekly Report, 43* (RR-11), 1–20.

Centers for Disease Control and Prevention (1993). Sexually transmitted diseases treatment guidelines. *Morbidity and Mortality Weekly Report, 42* (No. RR-14), 1–73.

Chameides, L., and Hazinski, M. F. (Eds.). (1994). *Textbook of pediatric advanced life support*. Dallas, TX: American Heart Association.

Chasnoff, I. J. (1990). Cocaine in pregnancy. In R. C. Cefalo (Ed.), *Clinical decisions in obstetrics and gynecology* (pp 336–337). Rockville, MD: Aspen Publishers, Inc.

Chasnoff, I. J. (1988). Drug use in pregnancy: Parameters of risk. *Pediatric Clinics of North America, 35* (6), 1403–1411.

Chasse, R. (1994). Diuretics, erythropoietin, and other medications used in renal failure. In B. Chernow (Ed.), *The pharmacologic approach to the critically-ill patient* (3rd ed) (pp 632–637). Baltimore: Williams & Wilkins.

Chernecky, C. (1991). *Cancer diagnostics and chemotherapy*. Philadelphia: WB Saunders.

Chernow, B. (Ed.) (1994). *The pharmacologic approach to the critically-ill patient* (3rd ed). Baltimore: Williams & Wilkins.

Chiron Cetus Oncology Corporation (1994). Drug package insert for Proleukin. Emeryville, CA, The Chiron Corporation.

Clark, J., and Longo, D. (1986). Biological response modifiers. *Mediguide to Oncology, 6* (2), 1–5, 9, 10.

Clark, J., Queener, S., and Karb, V. (1990). *Pharmacologic basis of nursing practice* (3rd ed). St Louis: CV Mosby.

Colditz, G. A., Hankinson, S. E., Hunter, D. J., et al. (1995). The uses of estrogens and progestins and the risk of breast cancer in postmenopausal women. *The New England Journal of Medicine, 332* (24), 1589–1593.

Colfosceril (1995). *Drug evaluation monographs, 1974–1995*. Micromedex, Inc., 85, Aug 31, 1995.

Coltran, R. S., Kumar, V., and Robbins, S. L. (1994). *Robbins' pathologic basis of disease* (5th ed). Philadelphia: WB Saunders.

Colucci, R. D., and Somberg, J. C. (1994). Treatment of cardiac arrhythmias. In B. Chernow (Ed.), *The pharmacologic approach to the critically-ill patient* (3rd ed) (pp 445–463). Baltimore: Williams & Wilkins.

Committee on Practice of NAACOG (1988). *OGN nursing practice resource: The nurse's role in the induction/augmentation of labor*. Washington, DC: Committee on Practice of NAACOG.

Community Program for Clinical Research on AIDS (1991). *The human immunodeficiency virus (HIV) and protocol synopses*. Wilmington: Mid-Atlantic Regional Education and Training Center, HIV Grant Program, Medical Center of Delaware.

Conte, J. E. (1995). *Manual of antibiotics and infectious disease* (8th ed). Baltimore: Williams & Wilkins.

Cummins, R. O. (Ed.). (1994). *Textbook of advanced cardiac life support*. Dallas, TX: American Heart Association.

Cunha, B. S., and Ortega, A. M. (1995). Antibiotic failure. *Medical Clinics of North America, 79* (3), 663–671.

Davies, K. (1990). Genital herpes: An overview. *Journal of Obstetric, Gynecologic, and Neonatal Nursing, 19* (5), 401–406.

Davis, J. R., and Sherer, K. (1994). *Applied nutrition and diet therapy for nurses* (2nd ed). Philadelphia: WB Saunders.

DeVane, C. L. (1995). Brief comparison of the pharmacokinetics and pharmacodynamics of the traditional and newer antipsychotic drugs. *American Journal of Health-Systems Pharmacology, 52* (3), S15–S19.

Dickason, E. J. (1994). *Quick reference for maternal-infant assessment*. St Louis: Mosby–Year Book, Inc.

Dion, B. (1989). Hypertensive disorders in pregnancy. *International Journal of Childbirth Education, 4* (1), 29–30.

Dorr, R. T. (1992). *Hematopoietic colony stimulating factors*. Amgen Teleconference, February 21, 1992, Amgen, Inc.

Drug facts and comparisons (1995 updated monthly). St. Louis: J. B. Lippincott.

Dudjak, L. (1992). New roles of interferon-alpha. *American Journal of Nursing, 92* (2), 16.

Dutla, S. K., and Sood, R. (1994). Clinical pharmacology of drugs used in GI disorders of critically ill patients. In B. Chernow (Ed.), *The pharmacologic approach to the critically-ill patient* (3rd ed) (pp 614–628). Baltimore: Williams & Wilkins.

Ekbladh, L. (1995, June 7). *PMS*. Presentation presented as one of series on women's health through sponsorship of Wilmington Hospital, Medical Center of Delaware, Wilmington, DE.

Engel, N. S. (1989). Anabolic steroid use among high school athletes. *The American Journal of Maternal/Child Nursing, 14* (6), 417.

Engel, N. S. (1990). Update on cancer risks and oral contraceptives. *MCN: The American Journal of Maternal/Child Nursing, 15* (1), 37.

Fehring, R. J. (1990). Methods used to self-predict ovulation: A comparative study. *Journal of Obstetric, Gynecologic, and Neonatal Nursing, 19* (3), 233–237.

Finnegan, L. P., and Wapner, R. J. (1988). Narcotic addiction in pregnancy. In J. R. Niebyl (Ed.), *Drug use in pregnancy* (2nd ed) (pp 203–222). Philadelphia: Lea & Febiger.

Fisher, D., and Knobf, M. T. (1989). *The cancer chemotherapy handbook* (3rd ed) (pp 366–386). Chicago: Year Book Medical Publishers, Inc.

Forrest, D. E. (1994). Common gynecologic pelvic disorders. In E. Q. Youngkin, and M. S. Davis (Eds.), *Women's health: A primary care clinical guide* (pp 241–280). Norwalk, CT: Appleton & Lange.

Fry, S. T. (1989). Ethical issues in clinical research: Informed consent and risks versus benefits in the treatment of primary hypertension. *Nursing Clinics of North America, 24* (4), 1033–1039.

Fujisawa (1990). *Adenocard (adenosine) for rapid bolus intravenous use*. Product insert No. 45514A. Deerfield, IL: Fujisawa.

Garner, C. H. (1994). The climacteric, menopause, and the process of aging. In E. Q. Youngkin, and M. S. Davis (Eds.), *Women's health: A primary care clinical guide* (pp 309–343). Norwalk, CT: Appleton & Lange.

Garner, C. H. (1994). Uses of GRH agonists. *Journal of Obstetrical, Gynecological and Neonatal Nursing, 23* (7), 563–570.

Geissler, E. M. (1994). *Pocket guide to cultural assessments.* St Louis: Mosby–Year Book, Inc.

Gelone, S. (1995). *Therapy of opportunistic infections associated with the human immunodeficiency virus.* Philadelphia: Temple University Hospital.

Giamarellou, H. (1995). Empiric therapy for infections in the febrile, neutropenic compromised host. *Medical Clinics of North America, 79* (3), 559–571.

Gill, P., Smith, M., and McGregor, C. (1989). Terbutaline by pump to prevent recurrent preterm labor. *MCN: The American Journal of Maternal/Child Nursing, 14*, 163–167.

Gilman, A. G., Goodman, L. S., and Gilman, A. (1991). *Goodman and Gilman's The pharmacologic basis of therapeutics* (8th ed). New York: Pergamon Press.

Gliashan, R. (1990). A randomized controlled study of intravesicular alpha 2b-interferon in carcinoma in situ of the bladder. *The Journal of Urology, 144*, 658–661.

Goldfien, A. (1995). The gonadal hormones and inhibitors. In B. G. Katzung (Ed.), *Basic and Clinical Pharmacology* (6th ed) (pp 608–636). Norwalk, CT: Appleton & Lange.

Goldzieher, J. W. (1994). Menopause: A deficiency disease. In J. A. Rock, S. Faro, N. F. Gant, et al. (Eds.), *Advances in obstetrics and gynecology 1* (pp 159–177). St Louis: Mosby–Year Book, Inc.

Gravell, C. (1990). Progression of HIV infection in women: Asymptomatic state to frank AIDS. *NAACOG's Clinical Issues in Perinatal and Women's Health Nursing, 1* (1), 20–27.

Green, M. R. (1991). *The role of colony-stimulating factors in chemotherapy-induced neutropenia.* Seattle, WA: Immunex Corporation.

Griffin, J. E., and Wilson, J. D. (1992). Disorders of the testes and the male reproductive tract. In J. D. Wilson, and D. W. Foster (Eds). *Williams' textbook of endocrinology* (8th ed) (pp 799–852) Philadelphia: WB Saunders.

Groenwald, S., Frogge, M., Goodman, M., et al. (1990). *Cancer nursing: Principles and practice* (2nd ed). Boston: Jones and Bartlett Publishers.

Groer, M. W., and Shekleton, M. E. (1989). *Basic pathophysiology: A holistic approach.* St Louis: CV Mosby.

Groopman, J. (1989). Clinical experience with hematopoietic growth factors. *Biotherapy and Cancer, 2* (4), 1, 4, 5.

Grothe, J. U. (1985). Nursing in research and clinical testing of drugs. Chapter 9 in Wiener, M. B., and Pepper, G. A., *Clinical pharmacology and therapeutics in nursing* (2nd ed). New York: McGraw-Hill.

Gullatte, M. M., and Graves, T. (1990). Advances in antineoplastic therapy. *Oncology Nursing Forum, 17* (6), 867–876.

Gurevich, I. (1989) AIDS in critical care. *Heart and Lung, 18* (2), 107–112.

Guyton, A. C. (1987). *Human physiology and mechanisms of disease* (4th ed). Philadelphia: WB Saunders.

Haeuber, D. (1989). Recent advances in the management of biotherapy-related side effects: Flu-like syndrome. *Oncology Nursing Forum, 16* (6), 35–41.

Haeuber, D., and Dijulio, J. E. (1989). Hematopoietic colony-stimulating factors: An overview. *Oncology Nursing Forum, 16* (2), 247–255.

Hahn, M. B., and Jassak, P. T. (1988). Nursing management of patients receiving interferon. *Seminars in Oncology Nursing, IV* (2), 132–141.

Handbook of nonprescription drugs (1992). (10th ed). Washington, DC: American Pharmaceutical Association.

Haney, A. F. (1991). The pathogenesis and aetiology of endometriosis. In E. Thomas, and J. Rock (Eds.) *Modern Approaches to Endometriosis* (pp 3–19). Dordrecht, The Netherlands: Kluwer Academic publishers.

Hardy, R. I. and Friedman, A. J. (1994). The role of gonadotropin-releasing hormone agonists in gynecology. In J. A. Rock, S. Faro, N. F. Gant, et al. (Eds.). *Advances in obstetrics and gynecology 1* (pp 179–209). St Louis: Mosby–Year Book, Inc.

Harvey, C. J., and Burke, M. E. (1992). Hypertensive disorders in pregnancy. In L. K. Mandevill, and N. H. Troiano (Eds.). *High risk intrapartum nursing* (pp 147–164). Philadelphia: JB Lippincott.

Hatcher, R. A., Trussell, J., and Stewart, F., et al. (1994). *Contraceptive technology* (16th rev. ed). New York: Irvington Publishers, Inc.

Hayes, E. R., and Kee, J. L. (1996). *Pharmacology: Pocket companion for nurses.* Philadelphia: WB Saunders.

Hayes, J. E. (1982). Normal changes in aging and nursing implications of drug therapy. *Nursing Clinics of North America, 17* (2), 253–261.

Hellerstein, D. K., and Lipshultz, L. I. (1993). Male infertility. In L. J. Copeland (Ed.), *Textbook of gynecology* (pp 347–368). Philadelphia: WB Saunders.

Henke-Yarbro, C. (Ed.), (1994). Management of patients receiving interleukin-2 therapy. *Seminars in Oncology Nursing, 9* (3), Suppl. 1, 1–35.

Heslin, J. A. (1990). Guide to caffeine consumption. *Childbirth Educator, 9* (2), 11, 36.

Higgs, D., Nagy, C., and Einhorn, L. (1989). Ifosfamide: A clinical review. *Seminars in Oncology Nursing, 5* (2) Suppl. 1 (May), 70–77.

Hirsch, M. S. (1992). The treatment of cytomegalovirus in AIDS—more than meets the eye. *New England Journal of Medicine, 326* (January 23, 1992), 264–266.

Hirschel, B., Lazzarin, A., Chorpard, P., et al. (1991). A controlled study of inhaled pentamidine for primary prevention of *Pneumocystis carinii* pneumonia. *New England Journal of Medicine, 324* (April 18, 1991), 1079–1083.

HIV Digest (1991). Update: HIV infection among health care workers in 1991. *HIV Digest, 1* (1), 1, 6. Publication of the Pennsylvania AIDS Education and Training Center.

Hodgson, B. B., Kizior, R. J., and Kingdon, R. T. *Nurse's Drug Handbook 1995.* Philadelphia: WB Saunders.

Hoechst-Roussel Pharmaceuticals, Inc. (1991). *Myeloid growth factors.* Somerville, NJ: Hoechst-Roussel Pharmaceuticals, Inc.

Hoechst-Roussel Pharmaceuticals (1991). *Prokine (Sargramostim),* Product Monograph. Somerville, NJ: Hoechst-Roussel Pharmaceuticals, Inc.

Holmes, J., and Maglera, L. (1987). *Maternity nursing.* New York: Macmillan Publishing.

Hood, L. E. (1987). Interferon. *American Journal of Nursing, 87* (4), 459–464.

Howards, S. S. (1995). Treatment of male infertility. *New England Journal of Medicine, 332*, (5), 312–317.

Immunex Corporation (1991). *Leukine (Sargramostim).* Product Monograph. Seattle, WA: Immunex Corporation.

Intramuscular injections: A guide to sites and technique (1989). Philadelphia: Wyeth-Ayerst Laboratories.

Irwin, M. M. (1987). Patients receiving biologic response modifiers: Overview of nursing care. *Oncology Nursing Forum, 14* (6), Supplement, 32–37.

Irwin, R. P., and Nutt, J. G. (1992). Principles of neuropharmacology I. Pharmacokinetics and Pharmacodynamics. In H. L. Klawans, et al. (Eds.). *Textbook of clinical neuropharmacology and therapeutics* (2nd ed) (pp 1–28). New York: Raven Press.

Jackson, B., Strauman, J., Frederickson, K., et al. (1991). Long-term biopsychosocial effects of interleukin-2 therapy. *Oncology Nursing Forum, 18* (4), 683–690.

Jassak, P. (1991). Knowledge deficit related to biotherapy. In J. McNally, E. Somerville, C. Miakowski, et al. (Eds.). *Guidelines for cancer nursing practice* (2nd ed). Philadelphia: WB Saunders.

Jawetz, E. (1995). Penicillins and cephalosporins. In B. G. Katzung (Ed.). *Basic and clinical pharmacology* (6th ed) (pp 680–692). Norwalk, CT: Appleton & Lange.

Johnson, T. R. B., and Niebyl, J. R. (1988). Caffeine in pregnancy. In J. R. Niebyl (Ed.), *Drug use in pregnancy* (2nd ed) (pp 231–234). Philadelphia: Lea & Febiger.

Kaliner, M., Eggleston, P. A., and Mathews, K. P. (1987). Rhinitis and asthma. *JAMA, 258* (20), 2851–2873.

Kee, J. L., and Paulanka, B. (1994). *Fluids and electrolytes with clinical applications* (5th ed). New York: John Wiley & Sons.

Kee, J. L. (1995), *Laboratory and diagnostic tests* (4th ed), Norwalk, CT: Appleton & Lange.

Kee, J. L. (1987). Potassium imbalance. *Nursing '87, 17*(9), 32K, 32M, 32P.

Kee, J. L., and Hayes, E. R. (1990). Assessment of patient laboratory data in the acutely ill. *Nursing Clinics of North America, 25* (4), 751–759.

Kee, J. L., and Marshall, S. M. (1996). *Clinical calculations* (3rd ed). Philadelphia: WB Saunders.

Kelley, W. N. (Ed.) (1992). *Textbook of internal medicine.* Vols. I and II (2nd ed). Philadelphia: JB Lippincott.

Kimmel, D. C. (1990). *Adulthood and aging* (3rd ed). New York: John Wiley & Sons.

Klawans, H. L., Goetz, C. G., and Tanner, C. M. (Eds.) (1992). *Textbook of clinical neuropharmacology and therapeutics* (2nd ed). New York: Raven Press.

Knuppel, R. A., and Drukker, J. E. (1986). Hypertension in pregnancy. In R. A. Knuppel and J. E. Drukker (Eds.), *High risk pregnancy: A team approach* (pp 362–398). Philadelphia: WB Saunders.

Koll, B. S., and Armstrong, D. (1995). Acquired immune deficiency syndrome (AIDS). In Rakel, R. E. (Ed.). *1995 Conn's current therapy* (pp 42–52). Philadelphia: WB Saunders.

Kuhn, M. M. (1991). *Pharmacotherapeutics* (2nd ed). Philadelphia: FA Davis.

Ladewig, P. W., London, M. L., and Olds, S. B. (1990). *Essentials of maternal-newborn nursing* (2nd ed). Redwood City, CA: Addison-Wesley Nursing.

LaGodna, G., and Hendrix, M. (1989). Impaired nurses: A cost analysis. *Journal of Nursing Administration, 19* (9), 13–18.

Lauver, D., and Welch, M. B. (1990). Sexual response cycle. In C. I. Fogel and D. Lauver (Eds.), *Sexual health promotion* (pp 39–52). Philadelphia: WB Saunders.

Lehne, R. A. (1994). *Pharmacology for nursing care* (2nd ed). Philadelphia: WB Saunders.

Levin, R. H. (1991). Advances in pediatric drug therapy of asthma. *Nursing Clinics of North America, 26* (2), 263–269.

Lipton, S. A., and Gendelman, H. E. (1995). Dementia associated with the acquired immunodeficiency syndrome. *New England Journal of Medicine, 332* (14), 934–940.

Lowdermilk, D. L. (1995). *Quick reference for maternity nursing* (2nd ed). St Louis: Mosby–Year Book, Inc.

MacLaren, A. (1994). *Maternal-neonatal nursing: Concepts and activities.* Springhouse, PA: Springhouse Corp.

Malinowski, J. S. (1989). Fetal well-being in preterm and postterm gestation. In J. S. Malinowski, C. G. Pedigo, and C. R. Philips (Eds.), *Nursing care during the labor process* (3rd ed) (pp 309–353). Philadelphia: FA Davis.

Malinowski, J. S. (1989). Labor stimulation. In J. S. Malinowski, C. G. Pedigo, and C. R. Phillips (Eds.), *Nursing care during the labor process* (3rd ed) (pp 158–184). Philadelphia: FA Davis.

Marshall, C. (1985). The art of induction/augmentation of labor. *Journal of Obstetric, Gynecologic, and Neonatal Nursing, 14* (1), 22–28.

Martin, E. J. (1990). Module 5: Care of the laboring woman. In E. J. Martin (Ed.), *Intrapartum management modules: A perinatal education program* (pp 119–150). Baltimore: Williams & Wilkins.

Martin, L. L., and Reeder, S. J. (1991). *Essentials of maternity nursing.* Philadelphia: JB Lippincott.

Masten, Y. (1993). *The Skidmore-Roth outline series: Obstetric nursing.* El Paso, TX: Skidmore Roth Publishing, Inc.

Masters, W. H., Johnson, V. E., and Kolodny, R. C. (1988). *Human sexuality,* (3rd ed). Glenview, IL: Scott, Foresman and Co.

Mattson, S. (1993). Ethnocultural considerations in the childbearing period. In S. Mattson, and J. E. Smith (Eds.), *NAACOG core curriculum for maternal newborn nursing* (pp 81–97). Philadelphia: WB Saunders.

McCance, K. L., and Huether, S. E. (1990). *Pathophysiology: The biologic basis for disease in adults and children.* St Louis: CV Mosby.

McCloskey, J. C., and Bulechek, G. M. (Eds.) (1992). *Iowa intervention project: Nursing interventions classification (NIC).* St Louis: Mosby–Year Book, Inc.

McDonald, L. Y. (1994). Personal communication regarding IL-2 administration. Emeryville, CA, The Cetus Oncology Corporation.

McEvoy, G. K. (Ed.) (1995). *AHFS '95 drug information.* Bethesda, MD: American Society of Health-System Pharmacists.

McGregor, J. A. (1990). Trichomoniasis: A continuing challenge.

In R. C. Cefalo (Ed.), *Clinical decisions on obstetrics and gynecology* (pp 289–295). Rockville, MD: Aspen Publishers, Inc.

McKay, M. (1990). Recurrent vulvar pruritus. In R. C. Cefalo (Ed.), *Clinical decisions in obstetrics and gynecology* (pp 296–298). Rockville, MD: Aspen Publishers, Inc.

McKenry, L. M., and Salerno, E. (1992). *Mosby's pharmacology in nursing* (18th ed). St Louis: CV Mosby.

McKeon, V. A. (1993). Hormone replacement therapy: Evaluating the risks and benefits. *Journal of Obstetric, Gynecologic and Neonatal Nursing, 23* (8), 647–657.

McManus, M. T. (1990). Module 7: Induction and augmentation of labor. In E. J. Martin (Ed.), *Intrapartum management modules: A perinatal education program* (pp 235–258). Baltimore: Williams & Wilkins.

McMurdo, M. E. T., Jarvis, A., Fraser, C. G., and Ghosh, U. K. (1991). A novel approach to the assessment of drug compliance in the elderly. *Gerontology, 37,* 339–344.

Medical Center of Delaware (1995). *Formulary and drug therapy guide 1995–1996.* Hudson, OH: Lexi-Comp, Inc.

Melone, L., Anderson-Drevs, K., Jassak, P., et al. (1991). A teaching booklet for patients receiving GMCSF-therapy. *Oncology Nursing Forum 18* (3), 593–597.

Miller, E. P., and Armstrong, C. L. (1990). Surfactant replacement therapy: Innovative care for the premature infant. *Journal of Obstetric, Gynecologic and Neonatal Nursing, 19* (1), 14–17.

Miller-Slade, D. (1994). Ask the experts: Is suppression of lactation in postpartum patients still an indication for the use of bromocriptine mesylate (Parlodel)? *AWHONN Voice, 2* (11), 11.

Minoff, H. (1990). HIV infection in pregnancy. In R. C. Cefalo (Ed.), *Clinical decisions in obstetrics and gynecology* (pp 34–36). Rockville, MD: Aspen Publishers, Inc.

Monahan, F. D., Drake, T., and Neighbors, M. (1994). *Nursing care of adults.* Philadelphia: WB Saunders.

Monier, M., and Laird, M. (1989). Contraceptives: A look at the future. *American Journal of Nursing, 89* (4), 496–499.

Moroso, G., and Holman, S. (1990). Counseling and testing women for HIV. *NAACOG's clinical issues in perinatal and women's health nursing, 1* (1), 10–19.

Moss, A. (1992). *HIV and AIDS: Management by the primary team.* Oxford: Oxford University Press.

Mott, S. R., and Fazekas, A. (1987). *Nursing care of children and families* (2nd ed). Menlo Park, CA: Addison-Wesley Publishing Co.

Murphy, R. (1992). Infection in the compromised host. In S. T. Shulman, J. P., and H. M. Somers (Eds.). *The biologic and chemical basis of infectious diseases* (pp 394–405). Philadelphia: WB Saunders.

Nadler, J. L., and Rude, R. K. (1995). Disorders of magnesium metabolism. *Endocrinology and Metabolism Clinics of North America, 24* (3), 623–637.

Nayduch, D., Lee, A., and Butler, D. (1994). High-dose methylprednisolone after acute spinal injury. *Critical Care Nurse, 14* (4), 69–78.

Neibyl, J. R., and Maxwell, K. D. (1988). Treatment of the nausea and vomiting of pregnancy. In J. R. Niebyl, (Ed.), *Drug use in pregnancy* (2nd ed) (pp 11–20). Philadelphia: Lea & Febiger.

Newman, V., Fullerton, J. T., and Anderson, P. O. (1993). Clinical advances in the management of severe nausea and vomiting during pregnancy. *Journal of Obstetric, Gynecologic and Neonatal Nursing, 22* (6), 483–490.

Newton, E. R. (1989). The use of mechanical dilators for cervical ripening. In R. H. Petrie (Ed.). *Perinatal pharmacology* (pp 303–312). Oradell, NJ: Medical Economics Books.

Nicolau, D. P., Quintiliani, R., and Nightingale, C. H. (1995). Antibiotic kinetics and dynamics for the clinician. *Medical Clinics of North America, 79* (3), 477–493.

Nolan, L., and O'Malley, K. (1988). Prescribing for the elderly: Part II. *Journal of American Geriatrics Society, 38,* 245–254.

Noronha, S., and Arnason, B. G. W. Multiple sclerosis. In H. L. Klawans, *Textbook of clinical neuropharmacology and therapeutics* (2nd ed) (pp 287–296). New York: Raven Press.

Norton, B. A., and Miller, A. M. (1986). *Skills for professional nursing practice.* Norwalk, CT: Appleton-Century-Crofts.

Notterman, D. A. (1994). Pediatric Pharmacotherapy. In B. Chernow (Ed.). *The Pharmacologic Approach to the Critically-Ill Patient* (3rd ed) (pp 139–151). Baltimore: Williams & Wilkins.

Nursing Drug Handbook (1994). Springhouse, PA: Springhouse Corp.

Olds, S. B., London, M. L., and Ladewig, P. W. (1996). *Maternal-newborn nursing: A family-centered approach.* Menlo Park, CA: Addison-Wesley.

Olin, B. R. (Ed.) (1994). *Drug facts and comparisons.* St Louis: Facts and Comparisons.

Oncology Nursing Society (1989). *Biologic response modifier guidelines: Recommendations for nursing education and practice.* Pittsburgh: Oncology Nursing Society.

Pedigo, C. G. (1989). Management of pain with drugs. In J. S. Malinowski, C. G. Pedigo, and C. R. Phillips (Eds.), *Nursing care during the labor process* (3rd ed) (pp 185–231). Philadelphia: FA Davis.

Pepping, P. B. (1994). Endometriosis: A nursing perspective. *Innovations in Women's Health Nursing, 1* (1), 2–8.

Pepping, P. B., and Fitzgerald, K. (1994). Treating endometriosis. *Innovations in Women's Health Nursing, 1* (1), 11–12.

Perry, S. E. (1995). Nursing care of the newborn. In I. M. Bobak, D. L. Lowdermilk, and M. D. Jensen. *Maternity Nursing* (4th ed) (pp 361–405). St Louis: Mosby–Year Book, Inc.

Petree, B., and Mattson, S. (1993). Hypertensive states in pregnancy. In S. Mattson, and J. E. Smith (Eds.). *NAACOG core curriculum for maternal-newborn nursing* (pp 412–433). Philadelphia: WB Saunders.

Phair, J. P., and Chadwick, E. G. (1992). Human immunodeficiency virus infection and AIDS. In S. T. Shulman, J. P. Phair, and H. M. Somers (Eds.). *The biologic and chemical basis of infectious diseases* (pp 380–393). Philadelphia: WB Saunders.

Phipps, W. J., Long, B. C., and Woods, N. F. (1995). *Medical-surgical nursing* (5th ed). St Louis: CV Mosby.

Plachetka, J. R. (1980). Sympathomimetic pharmacology. *Critical Care Quarterly, 3,* 27–34.

Porth, C. M. (1994). *Pathophysiology* (4th ed). Philadelphia: JB Lippincott.

Rainey, T. G., and Read, C. A. (1994). Pharmacology of colloids and crystalloids. In B. Chernow (Ed.), *The Pharmacologic Approach to the Critically-Ill Patient* (3rd ed) (pp 272–288). Baltimore: Williams and Wilkins.

Rakel, R. E. (Ed.). (1991). *Conn's current therapy 1991.* Philadelphia: WB Saunders.

Ramin, S. M., Maberry, M. C., and Cox S. M. (1993). Lower genital tract infections. In L. J. Copeland (Ed.), *Textbook of gynecology* (pp 505–516). Philadelphia: WB Saunders.

Rayburn, W. F., and Engdahl, K. L. (1989). Antiemetic agents for gestational nausea. In R. H. Petrie (Ed.). *Perinatal pharmacology* (pp 43–51). Oradell, NJ: Medical Economics Books.

Redman, B. K. (1988). *The process of patient education.* St Louis: CV Mosby.

Reiss, B. S., and Evans, M. E. (1990). *Pharmacologic aspects of nursing care* (3rd ed). Albany, NY: Delmar Publishers, Inc.

Rittenberg, C., Grallo, R., and Rehmeyer, T. (1995). Assessing and managing venous irritation associated with vinorelbine tartrate (Navelbine). *Oncology Nursing Forum, 22* (4), 707–710.

Robinson, W. (1988). Clinical use of colony-stimulating factors. *Mediguide to Oncology, 8* (3), 1–4.

Roche Laboratories (1986). *Roferon-A in the treatment of hairy cell leukemia.* Nutley, NJ: Roche Laboratories.

Roche Laboratories (1987). *Roche oncology report #2: Tips on teaching self-administration techniques to the cancer patient.* Nutley, NJ: Roche Laboratories.

Rogers, A. (1990). Drugs and disturbed sexual functioning. In C. I. Fogel, and D. Lauver (Eds.), *Sexual health promotion* (pp 485–497). Philadelphia: WB Saunders.

Rogove, H. J., and Moore, K. A. (1993). *Critical Care Medicines: Handbook of intravenous pharmacotherapeutics.* Columbus, OH: Contemporary Critical Care Resources, Inc.

Romanczuk, A. N., and Brown, J. P. (1994). Folic acid will reduce risk of neural tube defects. *MCN: The American Journal of Maternal/Child Nursing, 19* (6), 331–334.

Rowland, M., and Tozer, T. N. (1989). *Clinical pharmacokinetics: concepts and applications* (2nd ed). Philadelphia: Lea & Febiger.

Rudy, A. C., and Brater, D. C. (1994). Drug interactions. In B. Chernow (Ed.). *The pharmacologic approach to the critically-ill patient* (3rd ed) (pp 18–32). Baltimore: Williams & Wilkins.

Rudy, A. C., and Brater, D. C. (1994). Pharmacokinetics. In B. Chernow (Ed.), *The pharmacologic approach to the critically-ill patient* (3rd ed) (pp 3–17). Baltimore: Williams & Wilkins.

Santos, A. C., and Pedersen, H. (1989). Local anesthetics in obstetrics. In R. H. Petrie (Ed.) *Perinatal pharmacology* (pp 371–383). Oradell, NJ: Medical Economics Books.

Scavone, J. M. (1994). Pharmacotherapy in the elderly. In B. Chernow (Ed.), *The pharmacologic approach to the critically-ill patient* (3rd ed) (pp 202–219). Baltimore: Williams & Wilkins.

Schad, R. F., and Rayburn, W. F. (1986). Antiemetics, iron preparations, vitamins, and OTC drugs. In W. F. Rayburn and F. P. Zuspan (Eds.), *Drug therapy in obstetrics and gynecology* (2nd ed) (pp 24–36). Norwalk, CT: Appleton-Century-Crofts.

Schwertz, D. W. (1991). Basic principles of pharmacologic action. *Nursing Clinics of North America, 26* (2), 245–262.

Schwertz, D. W., and Buschmann, M. G. T. (1989). Pharmacogeriatrics. *Critical Care Nursing Quarterly, 12* (1), 26–37.

Seligman, M. (1994). Bronchodilators. In B. Chernow (Ed.), *The pharmacologic approach to the critically-ill patient* (3rd ed) (pp 567–575). Baltimore: Williams & Wilkins.

Seymour, F. J. (1991). A new program for the management of the chemically impaired nurse in Delaware. Unpublished manuscript; an executive position paper.

Sharts-Engel, N. C. (1990). Syphilis in pregnancy: Centers for Disease Control guidelines. *American Journal of Maternal/Child Nursing, 15* (6), 342.

Shattuck, J. C., and Schwarz, K. K. (1991). Walking the line between feminism and infertility: Implications for nursing, medicine, and client care. *Health Care for Women International, 12* (3), 331–340.

Shaw, N. K. (1991). Pharmacotherapeutics for the obstetrical patient. In M. M. Kuhn (Ed.), *Pharmacotherapeutics: A nursing process approach* (2nd ed) (pp 326–356) Philadelphia: FA Davis.

Shaw, R. W. (1991). GrRH analogues in the treatment of endometriosis: Rationale and efficacy. In E. Thomas, and J. Rock (Eds.), *Modern approaches to endometriosis* (pp 257–274). Dordrecht, The Netherlands: Kluwer Academic Publishers.

Sibai, B. M., and Armon, E. A. (1989). Aspirin safety during pregnancy. In R. H. Petric (Ed.), *Perinatal pharmacology* (pp 53–60). Oradell, NJ: Medical Economics Books.

Simchak, M. (1989). Medications for labor pain. *International Journal of Childbirth Education, 4* (4), 15–17.

Simpson, C., Seipp, D., and Rosenberg, S. (1988). The current status and future application of interleukin-2 and adaptive immunotherapy in cancer treatment: Seminars. *Oncology Nursing, IV* (2), 132–141.

Skidmore-Roth, L. (1994). *Nursing Drug Reference.* St Louis: CV Mosby.

Smith, K. V. (1993). Normal childbirth. In S. Mattson, and J. E. Smith (Eds.), *NAACOG core curriculum for maternal newborn nursing* (pp 255–283). Philadelphia: WB Saunders.

Soules, M. R. (1990). Endometriosis: New facets of treatment for an old disease. In R. C. Cefalo (Ed.), *Clinical decisions in obstetrics and gynecology* (pp 208–212). Rockville, MD: Aspen Publishers, Inc.

Spector, R. E., (1991). Cultural diversity in health and illness (3rd ed). Norwalk, CT: Appleton & Lange.

Spratto, G. R., and Woods, A. L. (1995). *Nurse's drug reference.* New York: Delmar Publishers, Inc.

Stevens, D. A. (1995). Coccidioidomycosis. *New England Journal of Medicine, 332* (16), 1077–1082.

Stratton, P., and McGregor, J. A. (1993). Human immunodeficiency virus infection in women. In L. J. Copeland (Ed.), *Textbook of gynecology* (pp 576–585). Philadelphia: WB Saunders.

Swonger, A. K., and Matejski, M. P. (1991). *Nursing pharmacology* (2nd ed). Philadelphia: JB Lippincott.

Taylor, P. J., and Kredenster, J. V. (1993). Investigation of the infertile couple, In L. J. Copeland (Ed.), *Textbook of gynecology* (pp 261–275) Philadelphia: WB Saunders.

Theodore, W. H. (1990). Basic principles of clinical pharmacology. *Neurologic Clinics, 8* (1), 1–13.

Timmons, M. C. (1990). The use of estrogen replacement therapy. In R. C. Cefalo (Ed.), *Clinical decisions in obstetrics and gynecology* (pp 229–231). Rockville, MD: Aspen Publishers, Inc.

Tinkle, M. B. (1990). Genital human papillomavirus infection: A growing health risk. *Journal of Obstetric, Gynecologic, and Neonatal Nursing, 19* (6), 501–507.

Trissel, L. A. (1994). *Handbook on injectable drugs.* Bethesda, MD, American Society of Hospital Pharmacists.

Tucker, S. M. (1988). *Pocket nurse guide to fetal monitoring.* St Louis: CV Mosby.

Understanding lung medications: How they work–how to use them (1993). New York, American Lung Association.

Understanding the immune system (1991). N.I.H. Publication No. 88–529.

USDA's food guide pyramid (April, 1992). Prepared by Human Nutrition Information Service. Home and Garden Bulletin.

U.S. Department of Health and Human Services. *Final regulations amending basic HHS policy for the protection of human subjects: final rule: 45 CFR 46. Federal register: rules and regulations 46* (No. 16, January 26, 1981): 8366–8392.

U.S. Department of Health and Human Services. *1992 revised classification system for HIV infection and expanded AIDS surveillance case definition for adolescents and adults.* CDC, November 15, 1991.

U.S. Department of Health and Human Services (1989). *Understanding the immune system.* Bethesda, MD: National Cancer Institute.

United States Pharmacopeia Drug Information (USP-DI) for the Health Care Professional (1995), Vol I, 15th ed. Rockville, MD, The US Pharmacopeial Convention, Inc.

U.S. Public Health Service Task Force on Antipneumocystis Prophylaxis for the Patient with Human Immunodeficiency Virus Infection (1992). *Recommendations for prophylaxis against Pneumocystis carinii pneumonia for adults and adolescents infected with human immunodeficiency virus.* Washington, DC, US Public Health Service.

Weiss, H. D. (1994). Parkinson's disease and other disorders of movement and tone. In B. Chernow (Ed.), *The pharmacologic approach to the critically-ill patient* (3rd ed) (pp 548–558). Baltimore: Williams & Wilkins.

Whaley, L. F., and Wong, D. L. (1995). *Essentials of pediatric nursing* (4th ed). St Louis: CV Mosby.

Whitley, N. (1985). *A manual of clinical obstetrics.* Philadelphia: JB Lippincott.

Wilcox, S. M., Himmelstein, D. U., and Woolhandler, S. (1994). Inappropriate drug prescribing for the community-dwelling elderly. *Journal of American Medical Association, 272* (4), 292–296.

Williams, B. R., and Baer, C. L. (1990). *Essentials of clinical pharmacology.* Springhouse, PA: Springhouse Corp.

Wilson, B. A., Shannon, M. T., and Stang, C. L. *Nurses Drug Guide 1996.* Norwalk, CT: Appleton & Lange.

Wilson, J. D., Tinskey, R., Harrison, A., et al. (1990). *Harrison's principles of internal medicine*, Volumes I and II. 12th ed. New York: McGraw-Hill.

Winter, M. E. (1994). *Basic clinical pharmacokinetics* (3rd ed). Vancouver, WA: Applied Therapeutics, Inc.

Woods, N. F., Olshansky, E., and Draye, M. A. (1991). Infertility: Women's experiences. *Health Care for Women International, 12,* 179–190.

Yarbro, C. (1989). Carboplatin: A clinical review. *Seminars in oncology nursing, 5* (2) Suppl 1 (May) 63–69.

Yasko, J., and Dudjak, L. (1990). *Biological response modifier therapy-symptom management.* Pittsburgh: Park Row Publishers.

Young, T. E., and Manqum, O. B. (1994). *NeoFax '94: A manual of drugs used in neonatal care* (7th ed). Columbus, OH: Ross Products Division, Abbott Laboratories.

Yuen, B. H., Fluker, M., and Urman, B. (1993). Infertility: Medical management of ovulation induction. In L. J. Copeland (Ed.), *Textbook of gynecology* (pp 292–301). Philadelphia: WB Saunders.

Zaloga, G. P. (1994). Enteral nutrition in critically ill. In B. Chernow (Ed.), *The pharmacologic approach to the critically-ill patient* (3rd ed) (pp 1034–1046). Baltimore: Williams & Wilkins.

Zaloga, G. P., and Chernow, B. (1994). Insulin and oral hypoglycemics. In B. Chernow (Ed.), *The pharmacologic approach to the critically ill patient* (3rd ed) (pp 758–771). Baltimore: Williams & Wilkins.

Ziegler, M. G., and Ruiz-Ramon, P. F. (1994). Antihypertensive therapy. In B. Chernow (Ed.), *The pharmacologic approach to the critically ill patient* (3rd ed) (pp 405–425). Baltimore: Williams & Wilkins.

Zuspan, F. P., and Rayburn, W. F. (1986). Drug abuse during pregnancy. In W. F. Rayburn and F. P. Zuspan, *Drug therapy in obstetrics and gynecology* (2nd ed) (pp 37–52). Norwalk, CT: Appleton-Century-Crofts.

Glossary

abortifacient: agent that promotes removal of conception products.

absorption: movement of drug particles from the gastrointestinal tract to body fluids.

abstinence syndrome: withdrawal symptoms.

acetylcholine: neurotransmitter at cholinergic synapses in central, sympathetic, and parasympathetic nervous systems.

acetylcholinesterase inhibitors: the group of drugs used to slow the destruction of acetylcholine, such as in the treatment of myasthenia gravis.

acidosis: abnormal condition as the result of increased acid and decreased alkaline reserve in blood and body tissues; decrease in pH (<7.35).

acne vulgaris: formation of papules, nodules, and cysts on the face, neck, shoulders, and back resulting from keratin plugs at the base of the pilosebaceous follicles.

acquired bacterial resistance: resistance caused by prior exposure to the antibacterial.

acrocyanosis: cyanosis of the extremities.

acromegaly: enlargement of the jaw, nose, feet, and hands as the result of hypersecretion of growth hormone from the pituitary gland.

activated partial thromboplastin time (APTT): commonly used to monitor heparin therapy; more sensitive in detecting clotting factor defects than PTT.

active absorption: requires a carrier to move the particles against a concentrated gradient; e.g., an enzyme or protein can carry drugs.

acute rhinitis: inflammation of the mucous membrane of the nose.

addiction: psychologic or physiologic dependence on an agent with an increase in its use.

Addison's disease: condition resulting from inadequate production of hormones from the cortex of the adrenal glands (glucocorticoids and mineralocorticoids). Fluid and electrolyte imbalance and marked hypoglycemia are major associated problems.

additive action: the drug has an increased effect.

adenohypophysis: the anterior portion of the pituitary gland.

adrenal glands: glands composed of adrenal medulla and adrenal cortex that secrete hormones.

Adrenalin: trademark for epinephrine.

adrenergic: relating to the sympathetic portion of the autonomic nervous system.

adrenergic agonists: drugs that stimulate the sympathetic nervous system. Also called adrenergics or sympathomimetics.

adrenergic blockers: drugs that block secretion of epinephrine and norepinephrine.

adrenergic neuron blockers: drugs that block the release of norepinephrine from sympathetic terminal neurons.

adrenergic receptors: receptors for epinephrine and norepinephrine.

adrenocorticotropic hormone (ACTH): released in response to the corticotropin-releasing factor (CRF) from the hypothalamus.

adsorbents: substances that attract other materials to their surface; e.g., charcoal.

adverse reactions or effects: a range of undesirable effects (unintended and occurring at normal doses) of drugs that cause mild to severe reactions, including anaphylaxis.

affective disorder: (mood disorder) disturbance of mood manifested by manic and/or depressive symptoms.

afterload: the force/tension developed by the heart contracting; the arterial force opposing ventricular ejection.

aggregation: clumping of cells/materials.

agonist: drug that is attracted to receptors of another drug that causes a physiologic effect.

agranulocytosis: a sudden drop in leukocytes that renders the body defenseless against bacterial invasion.

AIDS: acquired immune deficiency syndrome. A fatal condition caused by a retrovirus, human immunodeficiency virus (HIV); spread primarily by sexual contact, sharing IV needles and syringes, and blood transfusions; predisposition to opportunistic infections.

akathisia: motor restlessness, muscle quivering; a common side effect of neuroleptic drugs.

alkalosis: abnormal condition as a result of loss of acid and increased alkaline reserve; increase in pH (> 7.35).

allergic rhinitis: inflammation of the mucous membrane of the nose caused by pollen or foreign substances.

alopecia: absence or loss of hair.

alpha blockers: group of drugs that selectively inhibits the activity of the alpha receptors in the sympathetic nervous system.

amblyopia: impairment of vision unrelated to organic defect or refractive error; "lazy eye."

amenorrhea: absence of menses.

amphetamine: major drug group of CNS stimulants that act on the brain stem. Long-term use can produce psychological dependence and tolerance.

ampule: small glass container with a tapered neck for "snapping" open; designed for single-dose drug use.

anabolic: building up of body tissues.

anabolic agent: steroids that stimulate a positive nitrogen balance, protein storage, and tissue, particularly muscle, buildup.

analeptic: drug that acts as a central nervous system stimulant.

analgesia: drug that relieves pain without any loss of consciousness.

analgesic: drug that relieves pain.

anaphylactic shock: the most serious type of allergic response due to antibody-antigen reaction. Prompt medical attention required.

anaphylaxis: severe allergic hypersensitivity reaction due to drug or foreign protein; life-threatening.

androgens: natural and synthetic steroids responsible for expression of primary and secondary male sex characteristics.

anesthesia: loss of sensation or feeling with or without loss of consciousness depending on agent(s) used; may be total or partial.

angina: (angina pectoris) severe pain in the heart due to inadequate oxygenation of the muscle.

angioedema: localized edematous reaction appearing as wheals.

anion: ion carrying a negative charge.

anorexia: loss or lack of appetite.

anorexiants: drugs that act as appetite suppressants.

anovulation: failure of the ovaries to produce, mature, or release eggs.

anoxia: lack of oxygen in the tissues; hypoxia.

antacids: agents that neutralize hydrochloric acid and pepsin activity, which promotes ulcer healing.

antagonistic action: effect of either or both drugs is decreased; drugs that block a response. A drug interaction that has a decreased pharmacologic effect as an outcome.

antiandrogens: drugs that interfere with androgen production or compete with androgens at receptor sites to block their actions.

antianginal drugs: agents that cause vasodilation (especially venous), thereby decreasing the amount of blood returning to the heart and thus decreasing cardiac workload; agents that decrease symptoms of angina.

antibacterials: substances that inhibit the growth of or kill bacteria or other microorganisms, including bacteria, viruses, fungi, protozoa, and rickettsiae.

anticancer: another term for antineoplastic and chemotherapeutic agent used to treat cancer.

anticholinergic: drug that blocks the impulses through the parasympathetic nerves.

anticholinesterase: drugs that inhibit or inactivate the enzyme cholinesterase, thus permitting acetylcholine to accumulate at receptor sites.

anticoagulant: agent used to delay blood clotting.

anticonvulsant: agent used to prevent or treat seizures.

antidepressant: agent used as central nervous system stimulant or mood elevator.

antidiarrheal: drug that counteracts diarrhea.

antidiuretic hormone (ADH): secreted by the posterior pituitary gland and increases the reabsorption of water from the renal tubules.

antidysrhythmic: agent that prevents or alleviates cardiac arrhythmias.

antiemetic: agent that prevents vomiting.

antiestrogen: agent that blocks action of estrogen.

antihistamines: drugs that counteract the effects of histamine; used to treat allergic reactions. Some drugs are useful in the relief of motion sickness; some have sedative–hypnotic action.

antihypertensives: agents used to treat high blood pressure.

antilipemics: agents used to lower abnormal blood lipid levels.

antimicrobials: substances that inhibit the growth of or kill bacteria or other microorganisms, including bacteria, viruses, fungi, protozoa, and rickettsiae.

antimycotic: agent destructive to fungus.

antineoplastic: agent used to treat cancer.

antipsychotic: agent that is effective in management of clinical manifestations caused by psychiatric disorders.

antitussive: agent that suppresses coughing.

anuria: absence of urine formation.

anxiolytics: agents that act as mild sedatives; used for relief of anxiety.

aphakia: absence of the lens of the eye.

aphasia: loss or impairment of speech.

aplastic anemia: anemia due to impairment of the bone marrow.

apnea: cessation of breathing.

APTT (activated partial thromboplastin time): laboratory test to be monitored in clients receiving heparin.

aqueous: prepared with water.

Arabic numerals: expressed as 1, 2, 3, 4, 5, 6, 7, 8, 9. Each has an increasing place value reading from left to right.

ARC: AIDS-related complex.

arthralgia: joint pain.

artificial rupture of the membranes (AROM): rupture of the amniotic sac by other than spontaneous means, usually with an amniotic hook.

ascites: fluid accumulation in the peritoneal cavity.

assessment: the first step in the nursing process; collection of both subjective and objective data and formulation of nursing diagnosis.

asthma: a condition characterized by bronchospasm, wheezing, and dyspnea.

asystole: cardiac arrest.

ataractics: tranquilizing drugs; may be used alone; often used to potentiate effects of narcotics.

atonic seizures: head drop, loss of posture.

atrial fibrillation: cardiac dysrhythmia with rapid uncoordinated contractions of atrial myocardium.

atrial flutter: cardiac dysrhythmia with rapid contractions of 200 to 300 beats per minute.

attention deficit disorder (ADD): a mental disorder affecting children and adolescents, characterized by inattention, impulsiveness, and hyperactivity.

autoimmune: response against body's own tissues; may be a hypersensitivity reaction.

autoinoculate: organism spread via hands to other body parts.

automaticity: spontaneous depolarization to initiate cardiac beat.

autonomic nervous system (ANS): branch of the nervous system that works without conscious control.

axon: path of nerve cell traveled by impulses as they travel away from body cell.

azotemia: increased nitrogen or urea in the blood.

bacteremia: abnormal presence of microorganisms in the blood stream.

bactericidal: agent that kills bacteria.

bacteriostatic: decreases or inhibits growth of bacteria.

balanced anesthesia: anesthesia using a combination of drugs, resulting in decreased anesthesia-related problems and increased recovery from anesthesia.

barbiturates: group of organic compounds available by prescription only; commonly known as sleeping pills.

beta blockers: drugs that block action of epinephrine and at beta-adrenergic receptors on cells of effector organs; $beta_1$ receptors in myocardium and $beta_2$ receptors in the bronchioles and vascular smooth muscle.

bevel: the angular pointed tip of a needle.

biologic half-life: the time it takes for one half of the drug to be excreted from the blood.

biologic response modifiers (BRMs): class of agents used to enhance the body's immune system.

bipolar affective disorder: disorder with both manic and depressive episodes.

blastocyst: the inner, solid mass of cells, early in cell replication of the fertilized ovum, that will become in the embryo.

blepharospasm: twitching of the eyelid.

blood dyscrasias: blood cell disorders.

body surface area: amount of exposed body surface area relative to height and weight; may be used for calculating fluid and drug administration.

bolus: concentrated mass of drug.

bone marrow: spongelike material within bones; primary function is manufacture of erythrocytes.

bradycardia: slowness of heart rate in relation to expected norm. Frequently associated with heart rate of <60 bpm in adults, <100 bpm in newborns.

bradykinesia: slow movement.

brand name: usually a registered trademark owned by a specific manufacturer; also known as trade name or proprietary name.

broad-spectrum antibiotic: effective against both gram-positive and gram-negative organisms; frequently used when offending microorganisms are not identified by culture and sensitivity.

bronchial asthma: congestive obstructive pulmonary disease (COPD) characterized by periods of bronchospasm resulting in wheezing and difficulty in breathing.

bronchiectasis: abnormal dilation of the bronchi and bronchioles secondary to frequent infection and inflammation.

bronchodilator: agent that causes dilatation of the bronchi.

bronchospasm: spasmodic contraction of the bronchioles.

buccal: fleshy inner portion of the cheek. For selected drugs, the tablet is placed between the gum and cheek to obtain systemic absorption across the oral mucosa.

calcium channel blocker: drug that selectively blocks movement of calcium ions through specific ion channel (slow, or calcium channel) of cardiac and smooth muscle cells.

cannabinoids: an active ingredient of cannabis.

capsule: dissolvable container surrounding a dose of medication.

carbonic anhydrase inhibitor: agent used primarily in the treatment of glaucoma that inhibits the action of carbonic anhydrase enzyme.

cardiac dysrhythmias (arrhythmias): any deviation from the normal rate or pattern of the heartbeat; includes heart rates that are too slow, too fast, or irregular.

cardiac glycosides: drugs that increase the force of myocardial contraction and decrease the heart rate.

cardiotonics: agents that have a tonic effect on the heart; old term for cardiac glycoside.

carminative: agent used to rid gastrointestinal tract of gas.

catabolism: breakdown of complex body substances with release of energy.

catecholamines: chemical structures of a substance that can produce a sympathomimetic response.

cathartic: agent that causes evacuation of the bowel.

cations: positively charged ions.

caudal anesthetic: local anesthetic injected into the spinal canal near the sacrum.

cell-cycle nonspecific (CCNS): agents that act on any phase during the cell cycle.

cell-cycle specific (CCS): agents that act on specific phase of the cell cycle.

cellulitis: inflammation of cellular or connective tissue.

central nervous system (CNS): portion of the nervous system consisting of the brain and spinal cord.

cephalopelvic disproportion (CPD): condition in which the shape or size of the head of the fetus is incompatible with the shape or size of the maternal pelvis, causing inability of the fetus to pass through the pelvis.

cerebrovascular insufficiency: lack of oxygenated blood flow to the brain.

cerumen: waxy secretion of the glands of the external meatus of the ear; ear wax.

cerumenolytic: agent that dissolves cerumen.

cervical dilatation: the enlarging of the cervical os (opening) during labor from 0 to 10 cm, allowing for the descent and birth of the fetus.

cervical ripeness: a ripe cervix is partially dilated, shorter, softer, and centered (anterior) as compared to an unripe cervix, which is not dilated (closed), centered (posterior) and firm; ripeness is an important factor to consider when induction of labor is contemplated.

cervix: the lowermost portion of the uterus that extends into the vaginal canal.

chemical name: describes the drug's chemical structure.

chemoreceptor trigger zone (CTZ): center in the medulla of the brain that when stimulated can cause vomiting.

chemotherapy: treatment of an illness with medication; commonly associated with anticancer drugs.

chloasma: hyperpigmentation in circumscribed areas of the skin.

cholelithiasis: stones or calculi in the gallbladder or bile ducts.

cholinergic: relating to the parasympathetic portion of the autonomic nervous system.

cholinergic agonist: drugs that mimic acetylcholine and initiate a cholinergic response. Also called parasympathomimetics.

cholinergic blocking agents: drugs that inhibit the action of acetylcholine by occupying the acetylcholine receptors; also called anticholinergics.

cholinergic crisis: condition caused by overdosing with acetylcholinesterase inhibitors that requires emergency medical intervention. Characterized by increased salivation, tears, and sweating, and miosis.

cholinesterase: enzyme that separates acetylcholine into acetic acid and choline.

chronic bronchitis: a progressive lung disease caused by smoking and/or chronic lung infections. Bronchial inflammation and excessive mucous secretion result in airway obstruction.

chronic obstructive pulmonary disease (COPD): one of two major disease categories that affect the lower respiratory tract. Caused by airway obstruction with increased airway resistance to airflow to lung tissue.

chronotropics: mediations affecting time or rate, such as the heart beat.

chrysotherapy: gold therapy.

chylomicrons: one of four classifications of lipoproteins.

cirrhosis: a degenerative disease of the liver.

clinical trials: investigational studies that test the usefulness of drugs or treatments.

clonic seizures: dysrhythmic muscle contractions.

colitis: inflammation of the colon.

colony stimulating factors (CSFs): proteins that stimulate and regulate the growth, maturation, and differentiation of bone marrow stem cells.

common cold: most frequent upper respiratory infection; caused by rhinovirus and affects primarily the nasopharyngeal tract.

conception: fertilization of an ovum by a sperm.

congenital rubella syndrome: fetus infected transplacentally due to maternal infection, resulting in various multiple developmental abnormalities in the newborn.

congestive heart failure: condition occurring when the compensatory mechanisms of heart failure are not successful and the peripheral and lung tissues are congested.

conjunctivitis: inflammation of the conjunctiva of the eye.

contact dermatitis: (exogenous dermatitis) characterized by a skin rash with itching, swelling, blistering, oozing, or scaling at the affected sites caused by chemical or plant irritation.

contraceptive (oral): pills that contain estrogen, progestin, or a combination for the purpose of preventing conception through inhibition of ovulation.

control group: subjects who do not receive the experimental treatment and whose performance provides the baselines against which the treatment is measured.

controlled substance: a drug regulated by law(s) relative to use and prescribing.

corpus luteum: structure that develops during menstrual cycle after graafian follicle ruptures; atrophies prior to menstrual flow but provides progesterone in interim; helps to maintain pregnancy through progesterone production until placental function is well established.

corticosteroid: any of the hormones produced by the adrenal cortex.

cretinism: arrested physical and mental development due to congenital lack of thyroid gland secretion.

cross resistance: occurs between antibacterial drugs that have similar structure and action, such as penicillin and cephalosporins.

cryptorchidism: undescended testes.

crystalluria: crystals in the urine.

cumulative effect: occurs when a drug is metabolized or excreted more slowly than the rate at which it is being administered.

Cushing's disease: symptoms resulting from an excess of free circulating cortisol from the adrenal cortex.

Cushing syndrome: excess of free circulating cortisol from adrenal cortex, resulting in the following signs and symptoms: painful swelling in face (moon face) and interscapular area (buffalo hump), abdominal distention, ecchymoses, hypertension, impotence, amenorrhea, and general weakness.

cyanosis: a bluish coloration of the mucous membrane and skin related to an excessive concentration of reduced hemoglobin in the blood.

cycloplegia: paralysis of the ciliary muscles of the eye.

DEA: Drug Enforcement Agency.

decongestant: a drug that reduces swelling or congestion, usually of the nasal membranes.

deep vein thrombosis (DVT): blood clot in deep vein, usually in leg or pelvis.

delayed puberty: the failure of secondary sex characteristics to begin to appear in the male by the age of 14.

dependence: state of compulsion to take a drug to experience its psychic effects or to avoid the discomfort associated with the absence of the drug.

depolarization: the process of neutralizing polarity as occurs as part of cardiac contraction.

diabetes insipidus: disorder characterized by urinary output of 2 to 10 L/24 h with noncorresponding fluid intake, a result of a lack of antidiuretic hormone.

diabetes mellitus: chronic disease resulting from lack of glucose metabolism caused by insufficient insulin secretion by the beta cells of the islets of Langerhans. Characterized by polyuria, polydipsia, and polyphagia.

differentiation: ability to take on different forms; maturation.

digitalization: the process of administering digitalis on a dosage schedule to produce and maintain therapeutic concentration of the cardiac glycosides.

diluent: an agent that dilutes.

diplopia: double vision.

direct-acting cholinergics: drugs that act on the receptors to activate a tissue response.

disease-modifying antirheumatic drugs (DMARDs): groups of drugs, including gold drug therapy, immunosuppressive agents, and antimalarials.

disintegration: the process of breaking up; the breakdown of the tablet or pill into smaller particles.

dissolution: process whereby one substance is dissolved into another; the smaller particles from disintegration are dissolved in gastrointestinal fluid for absorption.

distribution: process by which a drug becomes available to body fluids and tissues.

diuresis: increased excretion of urine.

diuretics: drugs that promote urine excretion.

dividend: in mathematical division, such as 16 divided by 8 (16 ÷ 8), 16 in this example is the dividend.

divisor: in mathematical division, such as 16 divided by 8 (16 ÷ 8), 8 in this example is the divisor.

DNA: deoxyribonucleic acid.

dopamine: a neurotransmitter in the central nervous system.

dose: the amount of drug administered.

doubling time: the time required for a number of cancer cells to double in mass; related to the growth fraction.

dram: a unit of fluid volume in the apothecary system.

dromotropic: conductivity of a nerve fiber.

drop factor: the number of drops per milliliter.

drug abuse: use of drug(s) for other than prescribed or recommended purpose.

drug interaction: altered or modified action or effect of a drug as a result of interaction with one or more other drugs.

drug parameters: the calculated safe dosage range based on client weight.

duodenal ulcer: peptic ulcer located in the duodenum.

duration of action: the length of time a drug has a pharmacologic effect.

dyscrasia: condition relating to imbalance of parts; synonym for disease.

dyskinesia: impairment of movement of the voluntary muscles.

dysmenorrhea: difficult or painful menstruation.

dyspareunia: painful sexual intercourse.

dyspepsia: difficult or disturbed digestion.

dysphagia: difficulty or inability to swallow.

dysphoria: deep depression.

dyspnea: labored or difficult breathing.

dysrhythmias: irregular heartbeats such as premature ventricular contractions (PVDs), ventricular tachycardia, and ventricular fibrillation.

dystocia: prolonged, painful, or difficult labor and delivery due to interference from such factors as uterine dysfunction or anomalies, cephalopelvic disproportion, malpresentation or malposition of the fetus, or insufficient uterine and accessory muscle empowerment.

dystonia: impairment of muscle tone.

dysuria: difficult or painful urination.

ecchymosis: hemorrhagic area producing discoloration of the skin varying from blue-black to green-brown to yellow.

eclampsia: a serious condition in pregnancy-induced hypertension characterized by seizures and generally preceded by headache, visual changes, severe epigastric pain, decreased urinary output, increased hematocrit, and hyperreflexia; occurs in approximately 5% of women with pre-eclampsia.

ectopic: at a site other than normal; frequently refers to heart beat or pregnancy.

ED$_{50}$: median effective dose.

edema: abnormal collection of fluid in the tissue spaces.

efficacy: the ability of an agent to produce a biologic or clinical response.

ejaculation: emission of semen during the orgasmic phase of the male sexual response cycle.

ejaculatory dysfunction: sexual difficulty characterized by premature, delayed, or absent ejaculation.

electroencephalogram: instrument used in the recording of abnormal electrical discharges of the cerebral cortex; useful in diagnosing epilepsy.

electrolytes: substances capable of conducting an electric current when dissolved in water; electrically charged particles.

elimination: the process by which a drug is excreted from the body. The major route of drug elimination is via the kidneys; other routes include bile, feces, lungs, saliva, sweat, and breast milk.

embolus: blood clot that has traveled from the site of formation via the blood stream to another location.

embryo: the human developmental state from 2 weeks post-conception through 8 weeks when skeletal ossification begins together with cellular differentiation.

emetic: agent used to induce vomiting.

emollients: agents that soothe or soften.

emphysema: progressive lung disease in which air is trapped in the overexpanded alveoli, leading to inadequate oxygen and carbon dioxide exchange.

encephalography: a radiographic technique to show intracranial fluid–containing spaces.

endocrine: cell groups or organs that secrete regulatory substances such as hormones, directly into the circulation.

endocrine gland: gland that secretes a regulatory substance directly into the circulation.

endometriosis: abnormal location of endometrial tissue outside of the uterus in the pelvic cavity resulting in symptoms of pressure in the pelvis, painful menstruation, abnormal bleeding from the uterus or rectum, and infertility.

engorgement: breast tissue swelling lasting approximately 48 hours postpartum due to an increase in breast blood and lymph supply prior to the establishment of true lactation.

enteral nutrition: a nutrient preparation taken by mouth if the client is able to swallow, or via a tube inserted into the stomach or small intestine if the client is not able to swallow.

enteric coating: special coating on capsules or tablets that prevents release of contents until it reaches the intestines.

enteritis: inflammation of the intestines.

enuresis: urinary incontinence, particularly while asleep.

epidural anesthesia: local anesthetic solution injected into the epidural space (outside the dura mater) of the spinal column.

episiotomy: surgical incision made in the perineum to facilitate delivery of the fetus and avoid laceration; grade 1–4 depending on degree of extension, with 4 being the most severe.

epistaxis: bleeding from the nose.

erectile dysfunction: the inability to establish or maintain an erection for sexual intercourse.

ergot: a drug extracted from a fungus, used for its pharmacologic action of stimulating smooth muscles (blood vessels/uterus), causing vasoconstriction and uterine contraction.

ergotism: toxic condition caused by chronic or excessive use of ergot drug.

eructation: belching.

erythema: redness of the skin.

erythema multiforem: reaction of the skin and mucous membranes secondary to various factors and characterized by sudden onset of macular or vesicular eruptions.

erythrocyte: red blood cell that transports oxygen; average life span is 21 days.

erythrocytic phase: a phase of malaria in which the protozoan parasite invades the red blood cells, causing the symptoms of chills, fever, and sweating.

erythropoietin: a glycoprotein produced by the kidney in response to hypoxia that stimulates blood cell production.

esophageal ulcer: ulcer resulting from reflux of acidic gastric secretion into the esophagus due to a defective or incompetent cardiac sphincter.

estrogen: female sex hormone produced by the ovaries and placenta.

estrogen replacement therapy (ERT): hormones used to relieve symptoms of menopause.

evaluation: fourth phase of the nursing process; effectiveness of health teaching about drug therapy and attainment of goals. The time at which the evaluation of a goal occurs depends on the time frame specified in the statement of the goal.

exfoliative dermatitis: condition that causes the skin to come off in scales or layers.

exocrine: cell groups or glands that secrete externally via a duct.

exocrine gland: gland that secretes a regulatory substance via a duct.

exogenous dermatitis. See *contact dermatitis.*

expectorant: a drug that promotes expectoration, the raising and spitting out of mucous material from the trachea, bronchi, and lungs.

experimental group: subjects who receive the experimental treatment/intervention.

extrapyramidal symptoms: abnormal involuntary movements or alterations in muscle tone and posture.

extravasation: escape into tissue of an agent that is administered intravenously; may result in tissue necrosis that requires surgical debridement and tissue grafting.

FDA: Food and Drug Administration.

fertilization: penetration of an ovum by a sperm.

fetal distress: significant change in parameters of fetal well-being (reassuring signs) (e.g., fetal heart patterns), indicating fetus is in jeopardy.

fetal period: time from 8 weeks postconception until birth.

fetus: developing conceptus from eighth week of conception until birth.

fibrillation: muscle contraction due to spontaneous action of single muscle cells; e.g., atrial and ventricular fibrillation (cardiac dysrhythmias).

fibrinolysis: breakdown of fibrin.

first-line drugs: drugs considered to be more effective and less toxic than second-line drugs such as in treating tuberculosis.

first-pass effect: the process by which the drug passes to the liver first.

flatus: gas in the gastrointestinal tract.

flutter: a rapid regular vibration; e.g., atrial flutter (a cardiac dysrhythmia).

follicle-stimulating hormone (FSH): hormone secreted by the anterior lobe of the pituitary gland that stimulates production of graafian follicles in the ovary and spermatogenesis in the testes.

fundus (uterine): the uppermost portion of the uterus between the insertion points of the fallopian tubes into the uterus.

gastric mucosal barrier (GMB): a thick viscous mucous material that provides a barrier between the mucous lining and the acidic gastric secretions.

gastric ulcer: ulcer occurring in the stomach.

gastritis: inflammation of the stomach.

gauge: diameter of the lumen of the needle; the larger the gauge, the smaller the diameter of the lumen.

generic name: the official or nonproprietary name of a drug; a universal name.

gigantism: childhood condition caused by hypersecretion of growth hormone from the anterior pituitary gland.

gingivitis: inflammation of the gums.

glaucoma: an eye condition manifested by increased intraocular pressure.

glossitis: inflammation of the tongue.

glucocorticoid: a substance that raises the concentration of liver glycogen and blood sugar; secreted from the adrenal cortex.

gluten-free diet: diet in which wheat, oats, barley, and rye must be avoided; used in the treatment of celiac disease.

glycogenolysis: stimulation of glycogen breakdown.

glycosuria: glucose in the urine.

goal setting: based on assessment data, the identification of expected outcomes. Stated in such a way as to include the following: client-centered, realistic, measurable, realistic deadline, acceptable to both client and nurse, and shared with other health care providers.

gout: excessive uric acid deposited in joints and tissues; hereditary form of arthritis.

graafian follicle: small egg-containing sac embedded in the ovary.

granulocyte: any cell with granules; commonly a leukocyte.

granulocyte colony stimulating factor (GCSF): a glycoprotein produced by monocytes, fibroblasts, and endothelial cells that regulates the production of neutrophils within the bone marrow.

granulocyte macrophage colony stimulating factor (GMCSF): a group of growth factors that support survival, clonal expression, and differentiation of hematopoietic progenitor cells.

Graves' disease: the most common type of hyperthyroidism; a clinical syndrome characterized by tachycardia, palpitations, excessive perspiration, heat intolerance, exophthalmos, and weight loss; thyrotoxicosis.

growth fraction: the percentage of the cancer cells that are actually dividing.

gumma: large bulbous lesion on the skin.

gynecomastia: unusual enlargement of the breasts in males.

habituation: desire for continued use but with little or no increase in dose; results from repeated consumption of drug.

half-life: time required for one half of a substance (e.g., a drug) to be eliminated from a system.

hangover: residual drowsiness and impaired reaction time frequently caused by intermediate and long-acting hypnotics.

heart block: alteration in cardiac conduction system. Frequently applied to atrioventricular heart block when excitation is prolonged or does not reach ventricle.

heart failure: a condition in which the weakened and enlarged heart muscle loses its ability to pump blood through the heart and into the systemic circulation.

HELLP syndrome: a syndrome named in 1982 that includes hemolysis, elevated liver enzymes, and low platelet count that can develop in preeclampsia; also manifested by anemia, liver disease, coagulation deficiencies, and multiple organ involvement.

helminthiasis: worm infestation.

helminths: parasitic worms that feed on host tissue.

hematemesis: vomiting of blood.

hematuria: blood in the urine.

hemolytic: destruction of red blood cells.

hemoptysis: coughing of blood due to bleeding in the respiratory tract.

hemorrhoid: swollen distended vein inside or protruding outside the rectum.

hepatotoxicity: damage to the liver.

high-density lipoprotein (HDL): a conjugated protein that removes cholesterol from the blood stream and delivers it to the liver for breakdown; "friendly" lipoprotein.

high therapeutic index: these drugs have a wide margin of safety with less danger of producing toxic effects.

hirsutism: excessive growth of hair.

histamine$_2$ receptor antagonists: agents that prevent reflux acid in the esophagus by blocking the H$_2$ receptors of the parietal cells in the stomach.

holistic nursing approach: an approach in which the client is viewed as a biopsychosocial being interacting within the environment.

hybridoma technology: process to mass-produce monoclonal antibodies using mice.

hydantoins: one of several groups of anticonvulsant drugs.

hydrochloric acid: a component of gastric juice.

hypercalcemia: excessive calcium in the blood (>11 mg/100 mL).

hypercapnia: excessive carbon dioxide in the blood.

hyperglycemia: excessive blood sugar.

hyperhidrosis: excessive sweating.

hyperkalemia: excessive potassium in the blood (>5.5 mEq/L).

hyperkinesia: abnormally increased motor activity.

hyperlipidemia: elevated concentrations of any or all of the lipids in the plasma.

hypernatremia: excessive sodium in the blood (>147 mEq/L).

hyperplasia: excessive growth of normal cells of an organ.

hyperpyrexia: increased body temperature.

hypersensitivity: abnormally increased response to a drug or other substance.

hypertension (essential): elevated blood pressure of unknown cause that accounts for 95% of all cases of hypertension; contributing factors include age, obesity, smoking, heredity, and an aggressive, hyperactive personality.

hypertension (pregnancy-induced): see *pregnancy-induced hypertension.*

hypertension (secondary): elevated blood pressure that results from an underlying disease, such as stenosis of the renal artery.

hypertensive crisis: a medical emergency characterized by marked rapid increase in systolic and diastolic blood pressure.

hyperthyroidism: excessive activity of the thyroid gland.

hypertrichosis: excess growth of hair.

hyperuricemia: increased uric acid in the blood.

hypnotic effect: inducing hypnosis or sleep.

hypocalcemia: decreased calcium in the blood (<8.5 mg/100 mL).

hypocapnia: decreased carbon dioxide in the blood.

hypoglycemia: decreased sugar in the blood.

hypoglycemic reaction: (insulin shock) occurs when more insulin is administered than is needed for glucose metabolism; characterized by nervousness, trembling, cold and clammy skin, and headache.

hypogonadism: inadequate function of the gonads to produce gonadal hormones or viable germ cells.

hypokalemia: decrease of potassium in the blood (<3.5 mEq/L).

hyponatremia: decrease of sodium in the blood (<135 mEq/L).

hypophysis: (pituitary gland) endocrine gland located at the base of the brain, composed of anterior and posterior lobes that secrete several hormones.

hypothyroidism: deficiency in activity of the thyroid gland; extreme form is myxedema.

hypovolemic shock: shock due to loss of blood or fluid volume.

hypoxia: lack of oxygen to body tissues.

IDDM: insulin-dependent diabetes mellitus.

idiopathic: of unknown origin.

ileus: obstruction of the intestine.

immune system: an intricate network of specialized cells and organs that defend the body against attacks by invaders.

immunocompetence: the ability to demonstrate an immune response following exposure to an antigen.

immunoglobulin: a protein with known antibody material.

immunosuppressives: agents capable of suppressing immune response.

implantation: the burrowing into the endometrial lining of the uterus of a blastocyst.

indirect-acting cholinergics: drugs that inhibit the action of the enzyme cholinesterase by forming a chemical compound, thus allowing acetylcholine to persist and attach to receptor.

infection: a condition caused by microorganisms that results in inflammation; not all inflammations are caused by infection.

infertility: the inability to become pregnant following 1 year of regular unprotected intercourse during fertile periods.

infertility, primary, secondary: considered primary if a couple has never borne a live infant; secondary if couple has borne a live infant.

infiltration anesthesia: diluted drug solution can be injected into the skin area to be anesthetized.

inflammation: response to injury and/or infection; vascular reaction that occurs at the site; a protective mechanism by which the body attempts to neutralize and destroy harmful agents at the site and establish conditions for tissue repair.

inhalation: drug administration by oral or nasal respiratory route.

inherent resistance: bacterial resistance that occurs without previous exposure to the antibacterial drug.

inhibited sexual desire: lack of interest in sexual intercourse in a healthy adult with a partner.

inotropic: affecting the force of muscular contractions.

insomnia: difficulty in falling and/or remaining asleep; abnormal wakefulness.

instillation: administration of a liquid drop by drop.

insulin: hormone released by the pancreatic islets of Langerhans in response to an increase in blood sugar.

insulin-dependent diabetes mellitus (IDDM): type

I diabetes mellitus; condition requires injection of insulin.

insulin shock: may occur when more insulin is administered than is needed for glucose metabolism; individual may become nervous, tremulous, and uncoordinated, with cold and clammy skin, and may complain of headache.

insulin syringe: 1-mL syringe calibrated in units; used only for administration of insulin.

interferons (IFNs): a family of naturally occurring proteins discovered in the 1950s; regulates cell growth and has effects on the immune system.

interleukins: hormone-like glycoproteins manufactured by lymphocytes with antitumor activities.

intermittent claudication: pain in the calf muscles when walking or climbing stairs and relieved by resting.

intradermal injection: injection in which the drug is delivered within the dermis; intracutaneous injection.

intramuscular injection: injection in which the drug is delivered into the muscle tissue.

intravenous: within a vein.

in vitro: observable in an artificial environment.

irritant: an agent that may cause aching and phlebitis along the vein/injection site; inflammatory reaction may occur.

ischemia: abnormal reduction of blood supply to a tissue or organ.

jaundice: yellow pigmentation of the skin, mucous membranes, whites of the eyes, and body fluids due to excess bilirubin.

ketosis: (ketoacidosis) accumulation of ketone bodies in the blood resulting in metabolic acidosis.

KVO: keep vein open.

labor augmentation: acceleration of labor progress and performance using artificial means such as pharmacologic agents.

labor induction: artificial stimulation of labor progress using pharmacologic agents.

laceration: a wound due to tearing of body tissues, differentiated from incision or cut.

lacrimation: secretion of tears.

lactation: milk formation and secretion.

laryngitis: inflammation of vocal cords resulting in weak or husky voice.

laxative: agent that promotes evacuation of the bowels.

LD$_{50}$: median lethal dose.

least common denominator (LCD): smallest whole number that contains the denominator of each of the fractions.

let-down reflex: process by which milk moves from the breast alveoli into the milk ducts (under oxytocin stimulation) to be available for the nursing baby.

lethargic: drowsy, sluggish.

leukopenia: abnormal decrease in white blood cells.

libido: sexual drive.

lipodystrophy: disturbance of fat metabolism.

lipoproteins: complexes in which lipids are transported in the blood.

lithiasis: calculi formation in the body.

loading dose: for immediate drug response, a large initial dose is given to achieve minimum effective concentration in the plasma; e.g., digitalis preparations, selected antibiotics, and anticonvulsants.

local infiltration anesthesia: injection of an anesthetic agent into the subcutaneous tissue in the pattern of a fan.

lochia: blood, mucus, and tissue discharge from the uterus in the puerperal period; discharge changes from red (rubra) to pink (serosa) to creamy white (alba) over a period of about 3 weeks.

low-density lipoprotein (LDL): lipoprotein related to risk of coronary heart disease; transports 60%–75% of the serum cholesterol.

low therapeutic index: drugs with a narrow margin of safety.

L/S ratio (lecithin/sphingomyelin ratio): test for fetal lung maturity.

lumen: the inner hollow portion of a needle through which the drug passes.

luteal phase: the second half of the menstrual cycle from ovulation to menstruation.

luteinizing hormone (LH): one of the three hormones secreted from the anterior pituitary gland that acts with follicle-stimulating hormone to promote ovulation of mature ovarian follicles and stimulates secretion of testosterone by the testes.

lymphadenopathy: disease involving the lymph nodes.

lymphokines: fat-soluble protein mediators from sensitized lymphocytes involved in macrophage activation.

macrophage: phagocytic cells derived from monocytes; originate in bone marrow; function in cytotoxic, antigen, and inflammatory response.

macule: a flat skin lesion.

malaise: nonspecific, generalized discomfort.

malfeasance: giving the correct drug by the wrong route, causing the client to die.

manic depression: a psychiatric condition characterized by alternating periods of mania and depression.

maturation: a stage in cell division when the number of chromosomes in the germ cells is reduced to half the number associated with the specific species.

median effective dose: least amount of drug needed to produce a stated effect in one half the subjects receiving the drug.

median lethal dose: least amount of drug needed to kill one half of the subjects receiving the drug.

megavitamin therapy: massive doses of vitamins far beyond the recommended daily allowances.

melena: black, tarry stools due to presence of blood.

meniscus: concave or convex surface of a column of liquid.

menopause: the actual permanent cessation of menstruation as a cyclic process.

menorrhagia: excessive menstrual bleeding.

metabolism: process by which living organisms are created, maintained, and make energy available.

metabolites: substances produced during the process of metabolism.

metered dose: specific dose of medication automatically delivered from a multiple dose source; frequently used for inhaled bronchodilators.

methadone treatment program: a program that helps the narcotic-addicted person to withdraw from heroin or similar narcotics without causing withdrawal symptoms.

microorganisms: microscopic organisms: microscopic organisms, including bacteria, viruses, fungi, rickettsiae, spirochetes, and protozoa; some may cause disease.

micturition: urination.

mineralocorticoid: any one of several hormones secreted from the adrenal cortex with effects on sodium, chloride, and potassium in the extracellular fluid.

minerals: naturally occurring inorganic substances that are essential to body function.

minim: a unit of fluid volume in the apothecary system.

miosis: constriction of the pupils of the eye.

miotic: agent used to lower intraocular pressure in open-angle glaucoma, thereby increasing blood flow to retina and decreasing retinal damage and loss of vision.

misfeasance: negligence; giving the wrong drug or dosage, resulting in client death.

mixed narcotic agonist-antagonist: a narcotic antagonist is added to a narcotic agonist for the purpose of decreasing narcotic abuse.

monoamine oxidase (MAO) inhibitors: drugs used as antidepressants and antihypertensives; cause increase in catecholamine and serotonin levels in the brain.

mucolytic: agent that dissolves or destroys mucus.

multipara: a woman who has carried two or more pregnancies to the age of viability (20 weeks), regardless of whether they resulted in a live birth or stillbirth.

multiple sclerosis: a chronic disease characterized by patches of demyelinization throughout the central nervous system, causing weakness, incoordination, speech and visual disturbances, and parasthesias.

muscarinic receptors: cholinergic receptors of autonomic receptor cells that are blocked by atropine.

muscle relaxants: agents that relieve muscle spasm and pain associated with traumatic injuries and chronic debilitating disorders such as multiple sclerosis, stroke, cerebral palsy, and spinal cord injuries.

myalgia: muscle tenderness or pain.

myasthenia crisis: profound muscle weakness with difficulty in breathing and swallowing in clients diagnosed with myasthenia gravis.

myasthenia gravis: condition in which a lack of nerve impulses and muscle responses at the myoneural junction cause fatigue and weakness of the respiratory and facial muscles.

mydriasis: dilation of the pupils of the eye.

myocardial infarction (MI): necrosis of cells in a portion of the heart muscle as the result of a lack of oxygen due to obstruction of the blood supply; "heart attack."

myocardial ischemia: lack of blood supply to the heart muscle.

myxedema: hypofunction of the thyroid gland in adults.

nadir: the point at which the white blood cell count is the lowest after chemotherapy administration.

narcolepsy: uncontrollable desire to sleep.

narcotic: habit-forming drug that produces insensibility or stupor; legally, requires health care provider's prescription.

narcotic agonist: narcotic analgesic prescribed for moderate and severe pain.

narcotic antagonist: antidote for overdoses of narcotic analgesics; agent such as naloxone (Narcan) is mixed with a narcotic agonist to decrease narcotic abuse.

narrow-spectrum antibiotics: primarily effective against one type of organism.

natriuresis: sodium loss in the urine.

necrosis: cell death.

neonate: the newborn baby during the first 28 days after a live birth.

neoplasm: a tumor or unnatural growth in the body.

nephrotoxicity: damage to the kidneys.

nerve block anesthesia: local anesthetics administered near or into the nerve.

neuritis: inflammation of the nerve.

neurohypophysis: the posterior lobe of the pituitary gland.

neuroleptic: any drug that modifies psychotic behavior.

neurons: nerve cells.

neuropathy: functional disturbances in the peripheral nervous system.

neurotoxicity: ability to have a destructive effect upon nerve tissue.

neurotransmitters: a substance (e.g., norepinephrine, acetylcholine, dopamine) that excites or inhibits the target cell.

neutropenia: abnormal decrease of neutrophils in the blood.

neutrophil: type of granulocyte that functions in chemotaxis and phagocytosis; constitutes about 60–70% of total leukocytes.

nicotinic receptors: cholinergic receptors that are stimulated by low doses of nicotine.

NIDDM: non–insulin-dependent diabetes mellitus.

nitrates: agents used in the treatment of angina pectoris.

nocturia: excessive urination during the night.

noncompliance: client's informed decision not to follow a prescribed health-related recommendation.

nonfeasance: omission; omitting a drug dose resulting in client death.

non–insulin-dependent diabetes mellitus (NIDDM): type II diabetes mellitus; deficient or delayed response to glucose load; more likely to develop later in life than type I.

nonionized: not electrically charged; neutral.

non-narcotic analgesic: analgesic that is not addictive and is less potent than narcotic analgesics; used to treat mild to moderate pain.

nonreassuring FHR response: fetal heart rate patterns that indicate fetal distress and that suggest a nonpositive fetal outcome in the absence of prompt intervention.

nonselective drug response: drugs that affect various receptors.

nonselectivity: a drug that acts on several receptors.

nonspecific drug response: drugs that affect various sites.

nonsteroidal antiinflammatory drugs (NSAIDs): agents that inhibit the synthesis of prostaglandins and are used as analgesics, antipyretics, and antiinflammatory agents.

nonvesicants: agents that do not cause blistering of the skin.

norepinephrine: a catecholamine neurotransmitter found in most sympathetic postganglionic neurons and selected tracts of the central nervous system.

nosocomial infection: infection acquired while client is hospitalized.

NREM (non-rapid eye movement) sleep: one of four stages of sleep that is restful and recuperative. Accounts for 75% of sleep.

nursing diagnoses: clinical judgements about individual, family, or community responses to actual or potential health problems/life processes. Nursing diagnoses provide the basis for selection of nursing interventions to achieve outcome for which the nurse is accountable (NANDA, 1990).

nystagmus: involuntary oscillatory movement of the eyeball.

oliguria: decrease in the amount of urine excreted.

onset of action: begins when the drug enters the plasma and continues until it reaches minimum effective concentration (MEC).

open-label study: all parties—data collectors, prescribing health care provider, and subject—know the treatment group assignment.

ophthalmic: relating to the eye.

opiate: a sedative narcotic that contains opium or its derivatives.

opisthotonos: in the dorsal position, the body is arched with head and feet touching the surface.

opportunistic infection: an infection caused by an organism that does not usually cause disease but becomes pathogenic under selected conditions.

optic: relating to the eye.

oral contraceptives. See *contraceptive (oral)*.

oral hypoglycemic drugs: chemical preparations that stimulate insulin release.

orchitis: inflammation of the testes.

organogenesis: the origin or development of the organs.

orthostatic hypotension: sudden drop in blood pressure when arising quickly from a reclining or sitting position.

osmolality: concentration of solution in regard to osmoles of solutes per kilogram of solvent.

osmotic: passage of solvent from a solution of lesser concentration to one of greater concentration when two solutions are separated by a selectively permeable membrane that allows passage of solvent.

osteitis: inflammation of the bone.

otic: relating to the ear.

otitis: inflammation of the ear.

ototoxicity: damage to hearing.

ounce: a unit of fluid volume in the apothecary system.

over-the-counter (OTC) drugs: nonprescription preparations.

ovulation: the expulsion of the egg from the ovary when a mature graafian follicle ruptures at the midpoint of an approximately 28-day cycle.

oxytocics: drugs given to stimulate uterine contractions; used to augment childbirth and to contract the uterus to prevent postpartum hemorrhage; also enhance the let-down reflex.

oxytocin: hormone from the posterior pituitary that stimulates uterine contractions and let-down reflex.

palliative: agent that improves the client's condition but does not cure.

palpitations: throbbing or rapid pulsations of the heart.

pancreatitis: inflammation of the pancreas.

papilledema: edema and inflammation of the optic nerve where it enters the eyeball.

papule: a raised skin lesion that is palpable and <1 cm in diameter.

parasympathetic nervous system: part of the autonomic nervous system; predominant secretion of nerve endings is acetylcholine.

parasympatholytics: anticholinergics; agents that have a destructive effect on parasympathetic fibers or block their impulses.

parasympathomimetics: agents that produce effects similar to those achieved by stimulation of the parasympathetic nerve supply.

parathyroid hormone: secreted by the parathyroid gland; regulates calcium levels in the blood.

parenteral: generally refers to subcutaneous, intramuscular, or intravenous injections or infusions, not through the alimentary canal.

parenteral nutrition: involves administering high caloric nutrients through a large vein (e.g., subclavian vein).

paresis: partial paralysis.

parkinsonism: a symptom complex that may occur secondary to another disorder. Symptoms include masklike facies, tremors of resting muscles, shuffling gait, and muscular weakness.

paroxysmal: a sudden intensification of symptoms, spasm, or seizure.

partial thromboplastin time (PTT): useful for monitoring heparin therapy; heparin doses are adjusted according to this test. Screening test to detect deficiencies in all clotting factors except factors VII and XIII.

passive absorption: absorption mostly by diffusion (movement from higher concentration to lower concentration).

pathogen: disease-producing microorganism or agent.

patient-controlled analgesia (PCA): intravenous analgesia controlled by client within prescribed parameters. Usually client pushes and releases control button for medication administration.

PDR (Physician's Desk Reference): annual reference volume containing pharmacologic data supplied by pharmaceutical companies on their drugs.

peak action: occurs when the drug reaches its highest blood or plasma concentration.

peak drug level: the highest plasma concentration of drug at a specific time according to the route of administration; can indicate the rate of absorption of the drug.

pepsin: primary digestive enzyme in gastric juice; also has milk clotting action.

peptic ulcer: inclusive term for ulcers occurring in the esophagus, stomach, or duodenum.

perinatal: pertaining to the time period surrounding and the process of giving birth or being born; generally 20th week of pregnancy to 28 days postdelivery.

perinatal infection: the transmission of an infection (e.g., STD) to the infant during pregnancy or birth.

peripheral nervous system (PNS): the nerves and ganglia outside the brain and spinal cord.

peripheral vasocilators: drugs that increase blood flow to the extremities.

peristalsis: involuntary contractions of the gastrointestinal tract.

petechiae: purplish red spots on the skin or mucous membranes caused by intradermal or submucosal bleeding.

petit mal: a mild epileptic attack with momentary loss of consciousness usually occurring in children.

pharmaceutic phase: for a drug taken orally, the first of three phases that is required for the drug action to occur.

pharmacodynamics: the study of a drug's effect on cellular physiology and biochemistry and its mechanism of action.

pharmacogenetics: the study of the relationships between genetic factors and the responses to drugs.

pharmacokinetics: process of drug movement to achieve drug action; involves four processes: absorption, distribution, metabolism/biotransformation, and excretion.

pharmacology: science that deals with the origin, nature, chemistry, effects, and use of drugs.

pharyngitis: inflammation of the throat, "sore throat"; caused by virus or bacteria.

phenothiazine: denotes a group of anxiolytics.

phlebitis: inflammation of a vein.

photophobia: intolerance of bright light; frequently caused by drugs that dilate the pupils.

photosensitivity: excessive sensitivity to sunlight.

pinocytosis: cellular engulfment of a drug to carry it across the cellular membrane.

placebo: a substance that produces a response but is without biologic activity.

placenta: structure through which oxygen, nutrients, and metabolic wastes pass between maternal and fetal circulation during pregnancy; begins to function by fourth week of pregnancy.

placental barrier: an aspect of placental function whereby it acts to decrease the transmission of certain drugs or other substances from the maternal to the fetal system.

planning: second phase of the nursing process characterized by goal setting or identification of expected client outcomes.

plaque: a skin lesion that is hard, rough, raised, and flat on top.

plasma: fluid portion of the blood; 55% of the total blood volume.

platelet: blood component (thrombocyte) associated with coagulation and clotting of blood; normal value: $250,000/cm^2$ of blood.

pluripotent stem cell: primitive blood-forming cell found in the bone marrow; has the potential to change into any blood cell.

polydipsia: excessive thirst.

polyphagia: excessive appetite.

polyuria: excessive formation and discharge of urine.

postpartum: (puerperium) after delivery; from the third stage of labor through 6 weeks after delivery during which time the reproductive system returns to the prepregnant state.

potassium-sparing diuretic: diuretics that promote potassium retention.

potassium-wasting diuretic: diuretics that promote potassium excretion.

pre-eclampsia: entity included in pregnancy-induced hypertension; demonstrated by increase in blood pressure, proteinuria, and edema occurring after the 20th week of gestation.

pregnancy-induced hypertension (PIH): a leading cause of maternal illness and death; includes a variety of entities (pre-eclampsia, eclampsia, chronic hypertension with superimposed pre-eclampsia, late or transient hypertension); appears after 20th gestational week; manifests as proteinuria, hypertension, and edema.

preload: the volume of blood in the ventricle at the end of diastole.

premature rupture of membranes (PROM): rupture of the amniotic sac more than 24 hours before the onset of labor.

premenstrual syndrome (PMS): syndrome in which a woman experiences irritability, depression, mood swings, breast tenderness and swelling, and emotional tension at a certain point in the menstrual cycle.

presbyopia: age-related loss of accommodation of the eyes.

presentation: the part of the fetus that first enters the maternal pelvis and covers the inlet; *malpresentation* is an abnormal presentation, such as transverse lie or breech.

preterm labor: labor that occurs before the 38th week of gestation.

priapism: continuous and often painful penile erection.

primary infertility: infertility in an individual who has never parented a live infant.

primipara: a woman who carries her first pregnancy to the age of viability (20 weeks) without regard to status (alive/stillborn) at the time of birth.

progenitor cell: immature bone marrow cell that develops from the pluripotent stem cell; progenitor cells can further differentiate into mature functional blood cells.

progesterone: hormone produced by the corpus luteum that prepares the uterus for implantation of the fertilized ovum; maintains pregnancy and develops glandular tissue in breasts.

progestins: synthetic forms of progesterone.

prolactin: anterior pituitary hormone responsible for stimulating milk production.

prophylaxis: preventive treatment.

proportion: the relationship between two ratios; expressed with a double colon or equal sign separating the ratios; e.g. 3:4 (:: or =) 6:8.

prostaglandins: naturally-occurring complex lipid compounds that stimulate uterine contractions.

protein-binding: substance that binds to protein receptors; when drugs bind to protein sites they become inactive.

proteinuria: protein (albumin) in the urine.

prothrombin time (PT): test to measure clotting factors; used to establish and maintain anticoagulant therapy.

pruritus: severe itching.

pseudoparkinsonism: drug-induced parkinsonism; a side effect of the phenothiazide antipsychotic drug group.

psoriasis: chronic skin disorder that affects 1–2% of the U.S. population; characterized by erythematous papules and plaques covered with silvery scales.

psychologic dependence: intense desire for drug when it is not available; habituation.

psychosis: any major mental disorder characterized by loss of contact with reality.

puerperium: the period from the delivery of the baby and the placenta until 6 weeks post partum.

purgative: agent that stimulates peristalsis, causing evacuation of the bowel.

purpura: hemorrhagic areas in the mucous membrane or skin.

rales: abnormal sound due to the movement of air through the bronchi that contain secretions or are constricted.

rate limiting: refers to the time required for the drug to disintegrate and be available for the body to absorb.

ratio: relationship between two numbers that is expressed with a colon separating the numbers; e.g., 1:2. See also *proportion*.

RDA: recommended daily allowance.

reactive depression: depression caused by some external situation and relieved by removal from the situation.

reassuring FHR response: normal expected fetal heart rate patterns that indicate fetus is not distressed and predict a positive fetal outcome.

rebound nasal congestion: results from excessive use of nasal spray decongestant.

receptors: molecules within or on the cell surface that bind with other specific molecules.

recombinant DNA: genetic engineering process whereby genes from an organism are combined with genes from another organism to produce mass quantities of human proteins.

regional anesthesia: anesthesia of a body area accomplished by injecting a local anesthetic agent in areas surrounding nerves to block a group of sensory nerve fibers; types used for labor pain include epidural block, pudendal block, spinal block, saddle block, and paracervical block.

REM sleep: rapid eye movement sleep. Accounts for 25% of all sleep; dreams occur during this cycle.

repolarization: return of cell membrane resting potential after depolarization.

respiratory distress syndrome (RDS): neonatal condition related to prematurity in which decreased gas exchange occurs due to a lack of pulmonary surfactant and lung immaturity. Examples of causes include asphyxia in prenatal period and maternal diabetes.

restrictive lung disease: a decrease in total lung capacity due to fluid accumulation or loss of lung elasticity.

rhinitis: inflammation of the mucosa of the nose.

rhinorrhea: watery nasal discharge.

Rho (D) immune globulin (RhoGAM): an anti-Rh (D) gamma globulin used for passive immunization of an Rh-negative mother to avoid Rh sensitization from an Rh-positive fetus; prevents the development of active immunity to the Rh antigen.

rhonchi: sounds produced owing to mucous secretions in lung tissue or accumulation of secretions in the lungs.

Rh sensitization: development of protective antibodies against Rh-positive blood.

right client: an essential component of correct administration of medications.

right documentation: an essential component of correct administration of medications.

right drug: an essential component of correct administration of medications.

right dose: an essential component of correct administration of medications.

right route: an essential component of correct administration of medications.

right time: an essential component of correct administration of medications.

RNA: ribonucleic acid.

Roman numerals: numbers expressed by capital or lower case letters; e.g., I, V, X, i, v, x.

saluretic: sodium-losing.

SASH procedure: procedure associated with the administration of an intravenous medication followed by heparin flush: S = solution (saline) flush (2 mL); A = administer drug in to rubber stopper; S = solution (saline) flush (2 mL); H = heparin 1:100 solution.

schizophrenia: general term for a large group of mental disorders characterized by mental deterioration and disturbances of multiple psychological processes.

sclerosis: hardening of an organ or tissue.

scurvy: vitamin C deficiency.

secondary infertility: infertility in an individual who has previously parented a live infant.

second-generation antidepressants: first marketed in the 1980s; cause fewer anticholinergic symptoms than the tricyclics, e.g., amoxapine (Ascendin).

second-line drugs: drugs that are less effective and may be more toxic than first-line drugs such as in treating tuberculosis.

sedation: decreasing or allaying of excitement or irritability.

sedative–hypnotic: sedatives depress the central nervous system and calm nervousness and excitement; hypnotics induce sleep.

seizure: involuntary focal or generalized muscle contractions associated with brain dysfunction.

selectivity: effects of drugs that affect specific receptors.

sepsis: condition that results from the presence of pathogenic microorganisms or their toxins.

sexually transmitted disease (STD): any disease that can be transmitted through sexual contact.

sialorrhea: excessive salivation.

side effects: effects other than those for which an agent is taken.

single-blind study: only the subject knows to which treatment group he or she is assigned.

sinusitis: inflammation of the mucous membrane of one or more maxillary, frontal, ethmoid, or sphenoid sinuses.

somatic: relating to the body.

spacer: device to improve the delivery of medication from the metered dose inhaler (MDI).

spermatogenesis: the development of mature sperm.

spinal anesthesia: local anesthetic solution injected into the subarachnoid space to produce anesthetic effect of the lower portion of the spinal cord. Also called subarachnoid nerve block.

splenomegaly: enlargement of the spleen.

status epilepticus: a rapid succession of generalized seizures without consciousness that can result in brain damage or death.

steady state: maintenance of the average therapeutic effect of drug.

stenosis: narrowing of an orifice or duct.

stepped-care approach: various levels of drug therapy for treatment of hypertension.

Stevens-Johnson syndrome: life-threatening allergic drug reaction with inflammation of internal organs; hypotension may result in shock and death.

stimulant: agent that promotes activity of a body tissue or organ.

stomatitis: inflammation of the mouth.

stress ulcer: ulcer that results from a critical situation such as extensive trauma or major surgery.

subcutaneous: fatty tissue layer of the skin.

sublingual: beneath the tongue.

superinfection: overgrowth of bacteria other than those causing the original infection.

suppositories: have both local and systemic absorption.

surfactant: a surface-active phosphoprotein produced by type II epithelial alveolar lung cells; helps respiratory function by decreasing surface tension alveoli and preventing alveolar collapse.

sustained-release: a drug prepared to provide a relatively constant and long-lasting effect.

sympathetic nervous system: postganglionic fibers distributed to the heart, smooth muscle, and glands.

sympatholytic: antiadrenergic; sympathetic depressant.

sympathomimetic: $beta_2$ adrenergic; drug that suppresses uterine motility by stimulating the $beta_2$ receptors found in the smooth muscle, causing muscle relaxation.

syncope: fainting.

synergistic action: cooperative action by two or more drugs.

systemic analgesia: drugs given IM or IV including narcotics, narcotic agonists and antagonists, sedatives and tranquilizers.

$t\frac{1}{2}$: symbol for half life

T_3: symbol for triiodothyronine.

T_4: symbol for thyroxine.

tablets: a solid dosage form of a drug.

tachycardia: abnormal increase in heart rate.

tardive dyskinesia: extrapyramidal reaction, including protrusion of the tongue, chewing motion, and involuntary movement of the body and extremities.

teratogenic: capable of causing a deformity in the developing embryo.

teratogens: agents that can cause malformation in the fetus; examples are drugs, viruses, and radiation.

testosterone: the primary natural male sex hormone, which in its metabolized state is primarily responsible for most androgenic effects.

tetanic contraction: a prolonged uterine contraction, generally over 90 sec in duration.

tetany: continuous tonic spasm of a muscle.

therapeutic index (TI): an estimate of the margin of safety of a drug using a ratio that measures the effective therapeutic dose in 50% of animals (ED_{50}) and lethal dose in 50% of animals (LD_{50}); TI $= LD_{50}/ED_{50}$.

therapeutic range: drug concentration in plasma between the minimum effective concentration (MEC) and the toxic effect.

thrombocytopenia: abnormal decrease in circulating blood platelets.

thromboembolism: obstruction of a blood vessel with material carried by the blood from a distant site.

thrombolytics: agents that split or dissolve a thrombus.

thrombosis: presence of thrombus; an aggregation of blood factors that can cause vascular obstruction.

thyroid-stimulating hormone: hormone that stimulates release of thyroid hormones (T_3 and T_4) from the thyroid gland.

thyrotoxicosis: condition resulting from excess thyroid hormones due to overproduction, loss of storage, leakage, or any other reason.

thyroxine (T_4): iodine-containing hormone of the thyroid gland; acts as a catalyst and influences metabolic rate, growth and development, vitamin requirements, reproduction, and resistance to infection.

time response curve: evaluates three parameters of drug action (onset, peak, and duration).

tinea capitis: ringworm of the scalp.

tinea pedis: athlete's foot.

tinnitus: ringing in the ears.

tissue phase: a phase of malaria that produces no clinical symptoms in humans.

TKO: to keep (vein) open.

tocolysis: drug therapy to suppress premature labor.

tolerance: ability to take unusually high doses of a drug; acquired drug tolerance is a decreasing response to repeated drug doses or a need for increasing doses to maintain consistent response.

tonic seizures: sustained muscle contractions.

tonsillitis: inflammation of the tonsils.

topical: applied to a certain area of the skin; medications that are applied to the skin.

total parenteral nutrition (TPN): also called hyperalimentation or intravenous hyperalimentation (IVH) is the primary method for providing complete nutrients by intravenous route. An infusion of hyperosmolar glucose, amino acids, vitamins, electrolytes, minerals, and trace elements.

toxicity: quality of being poisonous.

toxin: poisonous substance released by microorganisms.

transdermal: administration of drug to the skin.

transmission: the mechanism of spread of an infection.

trichinosis: Condition caused by pork roundworm. Parasite is destroyed by thorough cooking of pork.

tricyclic antidepressants: most common type of drug used for relief of symptoms of depression.

triiodothyronine (T_3): iodine containing thyroid hormone; several times stronger than thyroxine.

trophoblast: the outer layer of cells in a differentiating fertilized egg that becomes the fetal portion of the placenta and the chorion.

trough level: lowest plasma concentration of a drug; measures the rate at which the drug is eliminated.

tube feeding: administration of nutrients through a nasogastric tube in a solution form.

tuberculin syringe: a 1-mL syringe calibrated in tenths and hundredths used for administration of amounts less than 1 mL and for pediatric and heparin drugs.

tumoricidal: destructive to cancer cells.

unipolar depression: depression characterized by loss of interest and inability to complete tasks; can be either primary or secondary.

unit dose: system of packaging a medication dosage in accord with a single ordered dose.

uricosuric: relating to excretion of uric acid in the urine.

urinary analgesics: drugs that are used to relieve pain, burning, frequency, and urgency in lower urinary tract infections.

urinary antiseptics: drugs that act on the renal tubules and bladder to prevent bacterial growth.

urinary antispasmodics: drugs used to treat spasms due to infection or injury with a direct action on the smooth muscle of the urinary tract.

urinary stimulants: drugs that act to increase bladder tone.

urinary tract infection: infection in the urinary tract, most commonly the bladder and urethra (lower urinary tract). Upper urinary tract infection involves the kidneys.

urticaria: vascular reaction of the skin characterized by red or pale wheals associated with severe itching; hives.

USP/NF: United States Pharmacopeia/National Formulary, the current authoritative source for drug standards.

uterine atony: the absence of muscle tone in the uterus.

uterine dysfunction: abnormal, difficult, or faulty performance of the uterus in relation to anticipated norms.

uterine hyperstimulation: labor contractions less than 2 min in frequency or greater than 90 sec in duration or elevation in uterine resting tone over previous baseline.

uterine inertia: the presence of weak or absent uterine contractions during labor.

uterine motility: the ability of the uterus to contract or move to facilitate the descent of the fetus during labor and to help prevent postpartal hemorrhage.

uterine resting tone: intrauterine pressure between contractions; state of relaxation between contractions.

uveitis: inflammation of the iris, choroid, and/or ciliary body of the eye.

Valsalva maneuver: performed by the client as the nurse changes the parenteral nutrition bags/bottles to prevent air embolism. The client takes a deep breath and holds it, and bears down during the procedure.

vertical transmission: transmission of an infection, particularly an STD, from the mother to her fetus or infant.

vertigo: dizziness or lightheadedness.

very low-density lipoproteins (VLDL): lipoprotein related to risk of coronary heart disease.

vesicant: an agent that can destroy tissue.

vesicle: a raised skin lesion filled with fluid and <1 cm in diameter.

vial: a small glass container with a self-sealing rubber top used for administration of multiple doses of drug.

vinca alkaloids: antineoplastic agents that are cell-cycle specific and act on the M phase (blocking cell division).

virilization: the emergence of secondary male sex characteristics.

visceral: relating to a viscus (any large organ in body cavity).

vitamins: essential substances found in foods and needed for health and life; major vitamins include A, C, D, E, K, and B complex. Vitamins B and C are water-soluble; the rest are fat-soluble.

vomiting center: located in the medulla of the brain, causes vomiting when stimulated.

wasting: catabolic processes characterized by negative nitrogen balance, weight loss, muscular atrophy, and flaccidity.

wheals: localized area of edema on skin associated with severe itching; typical lesion of urticaria.

withdrawal symptoms: group of symptoms associated with abrupt withdrawal of narcotic or other drug to which the person was addicted. Therapy is the provision of a substitute drug along with treatment of symptoms.

xerophthalmia: dryness of the conjunctiva of the eye.

xerostomia: dryness of the mouth associated with lack of normal salivation.

Z-tract technique: manner of administering an intramuscular injection that prevents the medication from leaking back into the subcutaneous tissue.

zygote: the fertilized egg.

Index

Note: Page numbers in **boldface** refer to main discussions; page numbers followed by the letter t refer to tables.

A

A. S. A., 332t, 649t
Abbreviations, inside front cover
Absorption, 4, 5
　active, 4, 5
　bioavailability, 4, 5
　passive, 4
　pinocytosis, 5
acarbose (Precose), 636t, 637
Accutane, 598t
ACE inhibitors, **513–516**, 515t
acebutolol HCl (Sectral), 289t, 485t, 508t
acetaminophen (Tylenol), 230–232, 231t,
　648, 649
　nursing process, 232
　prototype drug chart for, 230
acetazolamide (Diamox), 248t, 498t, 585t
acetic acid and aluminum acetate (Otic
　Domeboro), 592t
acetohexamide (Dymelor), 635, 636t
acetophenazine maleate (Tindal), 257t
acetylcholine Cl (Miochol), 585t
acetycholinesterase (AChE) inhibitors,
　313–315
achromycin, 592t
Acquired immunodeficiency syndrome
　(AIDS), **739–746**
　common complications of advanced HIV
　　infection, 743t
　current CDC criteria for staging and
　　diagnosis, 743t
　diseases complicating HIV infection in
　　women, 744t
　drugs used in management of selected
　　complications, 745t
　guidelines for antiretroviral treatment,
　　744t
　prevention and management of common
　　opportunistic infections, 744t
Acthar, 612t
Actifed, 449t
Actinomycin, 420t
Activan, 263t
activated charcoal, 760, 761t
Activated partial thromboplastin time
　APTT, 519
Acular, 583t
Acute rhinitis, drug(s) for, 445–454
　Chlor-Trimeton as, 448t
Acute laryngitis, 453
Acute tonsillitis, 453
Acute pharyngitis, 453
acyclovir sodium (Zovirax), 387, 388, 389t
ADD (attention deficit disorder), 208–210
Addictive drug effect, 141, 142
Adenocard, 486, 754, 757t
Adenohypophysis. See *Pituitary gland,
　anterior.*

adenosine (Adenocard), 486, 754, 757t
Adrenalin, 281–283, 284t
Adrenals, 609, **621–626**
　glucocorticoids, 621–625
　hypo-hypersecretion effects, 622
　nursing process, 625, 626
Adrenergic agonists. See *Adrenergics.*
Adrenergic antagonists. See *Adrenergic
　blockers.*
Adrenergic blockers, **275, 287–291**
　adrenergic neuron blockers, 290
　alpha-adrenergic blockers, 287
　beta-adrenergic blockers, 287, 288, 290
　drug table for, 289t
　nursing process, 290, 291
　prototype drug chart for, 288
　receptor response, 287
Adrenergic neuron blockers, 510, 511t
Adrenergics, **280–287**
　drug table, 284t, 285t
　beta adrenergic, 283, 284
　epinephrine, 281–283
　nursing process, 286, 287
　physiologic reponses, 280
　prototype drug charts, 282, 283
　sympathetic responses, 280
Adrenocorticotropic hormone, drugs for,
　611–614, 612t
　prototype drug chart for, 613
Adriamycin, 418, 419, 420t
Adsorbents, 552, 553t
Adverse drug reaction, 11, 139
Advil, 231t
Aerosporin, 400t
Aged. See *Geriatric pharmacology; Older
　adults*
Agonist drug, 8
Agoral, 687t
AIDS. See *Acquired immunodeficiency
　syndrome (AIDS).*
Akineton, 303t
albuterol (Proventil), 283, 285t, 460t
　prototype drug chart for, 283
Aldactazide, 501t
Aldactone, 500t
Aldomet, 508t
Aliphatic phenothiazines, 252, 252t, 254,
　257t
Alkeran, 412t
Alkylating drugs, **410–414**
　drug table for, 412t, 413t
　nursing process, 413, 414
　prototype drug chart for, 411
allopurinol (Zyloprim), 338t, 339
　prototype drug chart for, 339
Alpha and beta (adrenergic) blockers, 510,
　511t
Alpha (adrenergic) blockers, 507, **509–513**,
　511t

Alpha (adrenergic) blockers *(Continued)*
　nursing process, 512, 513
　prototype drug chart for, 510
alprazolam (Xanax), 263t
Alteplase, 527t
altretamine (Hexalen), 412t
aluminum hydroxide (Amphojel), 567,
　568t, 649t
aluminum carbonate (Basaljel), 568t
Alupent, 285t
amantadine HCl (Symmetrel), 309t, 311t,
　387, 389t
ambenonium Cl (Mytelase), 296t, 313t
Amen, 714t
Americaine, 682t
American Diabetes Association, 629, 630
American Hospital Formulary, 135
Amicar, 527t
amikacin sulfate (Amikin), 364t
Amikin, 364t
amiloride HCl (Midamor), 500t
aminocaproic acid (Amicar), 527t
aminoglutethimide (Cytadren), 421t
Aminoglycosides, **362–365**
　case study, 369
　drug table for, 364t–365t
　nursing process, 365
　prototype drug chart for, 363
aminosalicylate sodium (P.A.S. sodium),
　378
amiodarone HCl (Cordarone), 486t
amitriptyline HCl (Elavil), 265–267, 268t
　prototype drug chart for, 266, 267
amlodipine (Norvasc), 481t
amobarbitol sodium (Amytal), 217t, 246t
amoxapine (Asendin), 265–267, 269t
amoxicillin (Amoxil), 346, 347t, 592t
amoxicillin-clavulanate (Augmentin), 346,
　347t, 593t
Amoxil, 346, 347t, 592t
Amphetamines, **208–210**, 208t
　amphetamine-like drugs, 208
　prototype drug, 209
　side effects/adverse reactions, 208
Amphojel, 568t, 649t
amphotericin B (Fungizone), 382
ampicillin trihydrate (Polycillin), 347t, 592t
ampicillin-sulbactam (Unasyn), 347t
amrinone lactate (Inocor), 476t
amyl nitrite, 480t
Amytal sodium, 217t
Anabolic steroids, 725–727
Anadrol-50, 724t
Analeptics, 211t, 212
　side effects/adverse reactions, 212
Analgesics, **229–241**, 231t
　narcotic, 233–238
　narcotic agonist-antagonists, 238–240,
　　239t–240t

Analgesics (*Continued*)
　narcotic antagonists, 239t–240t, 241
　nonnarcotic, 229–232
　nursing process, 232, 234, 237, 238
Ancef, 351, 352t
Andro-Cyp, 724t
Androgens, 721–725
　contraindications to, 722
　drug table for, 724t
　indications for therapy, 723
　nursing process, 726, 727
　prototype drug chart for, 722
Androgens, 421t, 422
Android, 724t
Androlone-D, 724t
Andronate, 724t
Andropository, 724t
Anesthetics, **223–226,** 224t
　inhalation, 223
　intravenous, 223
　local, 224, 225
　nursing process, 226
　spinal, 225
　stages of, 223t
Angiotensin antagonists. See *Angiotensin converting enzyme (ACE) inhibitors.*
Angiotensin-converting enzyme (ACE) inhibitors, **513–516,** 515t
　nursing process, 515, 516
　prototype drug chart for, 514
anistreplase (APSAC), 525, 526t
Anorexiants, **210–212,** 211t
Antacids, **566–569**
　drug table for, 568t
　nursing process, 569
　prototype drug chart for, 567t
Antacids, commonly used in pregnancy, 649t
Antagonist, drug, 8
Antagonistic drug effect, 142
Antepar, 394t
Antepartum drugs, 644–651
　nursing process, 650, 651
Anterior pituitary gland. See *Pituitary gland, anterior.*
Anthelmintic drugs, **394–395**
　drug table for, 394t
　nursing process, 395
anthralin (Anthra-Derm), 598t
Antiandrogens, 727
　drug table for, 727t
Antianginal drugs, **477–482**
　beta blockers, 478, 480
　drug table, 480t
　nitrates, 478
　prototype drug chart for, 479
Antibacterial drugs, **342–345**
　broad-spectrum, 344, 345
　definition, 342
　general adverse reactions, 344t
　mechanisms of actions, 342, 343
　narrow-spectrum, 344
　pharmacodynamics of, 343, 344
　resistance to, 344
Antibiotics, 342. See also *Antibacterial drugs.*
Anticancer drugs, **407–423**
　alkylating drugs, 410–414
　antimetabolites, 414–418
　antitumor antibiotics, 418–420, 420t
　case study, 423
　cell cycle and phases, 408, 409
　cell-cycle nonspecific (CCNS), 408, 409, 409t
　cell-cycle specific (CCS), 408, 409, 409t

Anticancer drugs (*Continued*)
　combination chemotherapy, 409
　drug resistance, 409
　general adverse reactions, 410, 410t
　hormones and hormone antagonists, 419, 421t, 422
　miscellaneous antineoplastics, 422
　vinca alkaloids, 419, 420t
Anticholinergics, **298–304,** 306–308, 566, 566t
　antiemetics, 543, 546t
　antihistamines, 301, 302
　antiparkinsonism-anticholinergics, 300, 301
　drug table for, 302t, 303t, 307t
　nursing process, 303, 304
　prototype drug chart for, 299, 300
　responses of, 298, 299
Anticholinesterase. See *Cholinesterase inhibitors.*
Anticoagulants, **519–525**
　action of heparin, 519
　case study for, 536
　comparison of oral and parenteral, 522t
　coumarin group (oral), 520–524
　drug interactions, 522
　drug table for, 523t
　heparin, 519, 520
　nursing process, 524, 525
　prototype drug chart for, 521
Anticonvulsants, **243–250**
　barbiturates, 244
　benzodiazepines, 248
　case study, 250
　hydantoins, 243–245, 248, 249
　iminostibenes, 248
　nursing process, 249
　oxazolidones, 245
　seizures, classification of, 243
　succinimides, 245
　valproate, 248
Antidepressants, **264–270**
　drug table for, 268t, 269t
　monoamine oxidase inhibitors, 268, 269t
　nursing process, 265, 267
　prototype drug chart for, 266, 267
　second generation of, 265–267
　tricyclic antidepressants (TCA's), 265–267
Antidiabetic drugs, **629–630**
　case study, 638, 639
　insulins, 629–634
　nursing process, 633, 634, 637, 638
　oral hypoglycemic drugs, 634–637
　sulfonylureas, 634–636
Antidiarrheal drugs, **551–554**
　adsorbents, 552, 553t
　nonpharmacologic measures, 551
　nursing process, 554
　opiates and opiate-related, 551, 552, 553t
　prescriptive antidiarrheals, 551
　prototype drug chart for, 552
Antidysrhythmics, **483–487**
　beta blockers, 483, 485t
　calcium channel blockers, 486t
　drug table for, 485t, 486t
　fast sodium channel blockers, I, II, III, 483, 485t
　nursing process, 487
　pharmacodynamics, 483t, 484
　pharmacokinetics, 483, 484
　prototype drug chart for, 484, 486
　prolongation of repolarization, 483, 486t

Antiemetics, 543–548
　anticholinergics, 543, 546t
　antihistamines, 543, 546t
　cannabinoids, 546
　nonprescriptive, 542, 543, 543t
　nursing process, 548
　phenothiazine, 544, 545
　prescriptive, 543–547, 546t, 547t
Antiestrogens, 422
Antifungal drugs, **380–383**
　antimetabolite, 382
　drug table for, 382t
　imidazole group, 381
　nursing process, 382, 383
　polyenes, 380
　prototype drug chart for, 381
Antigout drugs, **337–340**
　antiinflammatory, 338, 338t
　drug table for, 338t
　nursing process, 340
　uric acid inhibitor, 338, 338t
　uricosurics, 338, 338t
Antihistamines, **445–449,** 448t
　antiemetics, 543, 546t
　drug table for, 448t
　nursing process, 447
　prototype drug chart for, 446
Antihypertensive drugs, **503–517**
　adrenergic neuron blockers, 510, 511t
　alpha-adrenergic blockers, 507, 509, 510, 511t
　alpha- and beta-adrenergic blockers, 510, 511t
　angiotensin-converting enzyme (ACE) inhibitor, 513–516, 515t
　beta-adrenergic blockers, 504–507, 508t
　calcium channel blockers, 513–516
　case study, 516
　centrally-acting sympatholytics, 507, 508t
　direct-acting arteriolar vasodilators, 511t, 512t, 513
　nonpharmacologic control of hypertension, 503
　stepped-care approach, 503, 504
Antiinflammatory drugs, **327–340**
　antigout drugs, 337–340
　antimalarials, 337
　corticosteroids, 334
　disease-modifying antirheumatic drugs, 335–337
　immunosuppressive agents, 337
　nonsteroidal (NSAIDs), 327–334
Antilipemics, **528–533**
　drug table for, 531t
　lipid serum values, 529t
　lipoprotein groups, 528t
　lipoprotein phenotype, 529t
　nicotinic acid, 529, 532
　nursing process, 532, 533
　prototype drug chart for, 530
Antimalarial drugs, **377, 391–393**
　drug table for, 391t, 393t
　nursing process, 393
　prototype drug chart for, 392
Antimanic, **270–272**
　lithium, 269t, 270–272
　nursing process, 270, 272
Antimetabolites, **414–418**
　drug table for, 415t, 416t
　nursing process, 417, 418
　prototype drug chart for, 415
Antimicrobials. See *Antibacterial drugs.*
Antiminth, 394t
Antineoplastic agents. See *Anticancer drugs; Biologic response modifiers.*

Antiparkinsonism-anticholinergics, 300, 301
  prototype drug chart for, 301
Antipsychotics, **252–260**
  drug table for, 257t, 258t
  nonphenothiazines, 253, 256
  nursing process, 258–260
  phenothiazines, 252–255
Antithyroid drugs, 617t, 618, 619
  nursing process, 618, 619
Antitubercular drugs, **377–380**, 384
  case study, 384
  drug table for, 378
  first-line drugs, 379
  nursing process, 379, 380
  prototype drug chart for, 377
  second-line drugs, 379
  side effects/adverse reactions, 379
Antitumor antibiotics, **418–420**
  drug table for, 420t
  prototype drug chart for, 418, 419
Antitussives, **450–453**
  drug table for, 452t
  prototype drug chart for, 451
Antiulcer drugs, **564–575**
  antacids, 566–569, 568t
  anticholinergics, 566, 566t
  gastric acid secretion inhibitor, 572, 574t
  GI stimulants, 565, 574t
  histamine$_2$ blockers, 570–572, 571t
  nonpharmacologic measures, 564, 565
  pepsin inhibitor, 572–574, 574t
  prostaglandin analog, 574, 574t
  tranquilizers, 565
Antivert, 647t
Antiviral drugs, **387–390**
  drug table for, 389t
  nursing process, 390
  prototype drug chart for, 388
Anturane, 338t, 523t
Anxiolytics, **260–264**
  benzodiazepines, 260, 261
  drug table for, 263t
  nursing process, 264
  prototype drug chart for, 262, 263
Apomorphine, 550, 550t
Apothecary system, 43, 44
  conversion within, 44
  equivalents, 43t
Appendicies, 767–794
Apresoline, 662t
Apresoline HCl, 511t
aprobarbital, 217t
AquaMEPHYTON, 692t
Aramine, 284t
Aristocort, 624t
Artane, 300, 301, 303t
Asendin, 265–267, 269t
asparaginase (Elspar), 421t
aspirin (A.S.A., Bayer, Astrin, Ecotrin), 229, 231t, 332t, 523t, 649t. See also *Salicylates.*
Assessment, 15
  objective data, 15
  subjective data, 15
astemizole (Hismanal), 449t
Astrin, 649t
Atarax, 263t, 448t, 546t
atenolol (Tenormin), 289t, 480t, 508t
Ativan, 222t
atovaquone (Mepron), 382
Atromid-S, 531t
atropine sulfate, (BufOpto-atropine, Isopto-atropine opthalmic) 298–300, 302t, 303, 304, 591t

atropine sulfate *(Continued)*
  nursing process, 303, 304
  prototype drug chart for, 299
Atrovent, 461t, 752, 753, 757t
Attention deficit disorder (ADD), 208–210
Augmentin, 592t
auranofin (Ridaura), 335t
aurothioglucose (Solganal), 335t
Autonomic nervous system (ANS), 204, **275–278**
  comparison, 277t
  parasympathetic nervous system, 275–277
  sympathetic nervous system, 275
Aventyl, 268t
Axid, 571t
Azactam, 367t, 369, 400t
azatadine maleate (Optimine), 448t
azithromycin (Zithromax), 357t
aztreonam (Azactam), 367t, 369, 400t
azulfidine (sulfasalazine), 593t

B

bacampicillin HCl (Spectrobid), 347t
bacitracin (Bactrin USP), 384
Bactericidal drugs, 342
Bacteriostatic drugs, 342
Bactrim, 371, 372, 400t, 593t
Bactrin, 384
Barbiturates, 216–220, 217t
  intermediate-acting, 216, 217t
  nursing process, 219, 220
  prototype drug, 218
  short-acting, 216, 217, 217t
Basic formula, drug calculation, 53
Bayer, 649t
beclomethasone dipropionate (Vanceril), 624t
belladonna tincture, 566t
Benadryl, 763, 764t
benazepril HCl (Lotensin), 515t
bendroflumethiazide (Naturetin), 491t
Benemid, 338t
Benylin DM, 451, 452t
benzocaine (Americaine, Dermaplast), 682t
Benzodiazepines, **220–222**, 222t, 246, 248, **260–263**
  nursing process, 221, 222
  prototype drug, 221t
benzonatate (Tessalon), 449t
benzoquinamide HCl, 547t
benzoyl peroxide (Benzac), 598t
benzphetamine HCL (Didex), 211t
benzthiazide (Aquatag), 491t
benztropine mesylate (Cogentin), 303t, 307t
bepridil HCl (Vascor), 481t
Beta adrenergic, 283, 284, 653t, 654–656
Beta (adrenergic) blockers, 287, 288, 290, 478, 480t, 483, 485t
  nursing process, 290, 291
  prototype drug chart for, 288
Beta blockers (antihypertensive), **504–507**, **508t**
  nursing process, 506, 507
  prototype drug chart for, 505
beta-adrenergic agonists, 283, 284, 653t, 654–656
betamethasone (Celestone), 624t, 657t
betaxolol HCl (Detoptic, Kerlone), 508t, 585t
bethanechol Cl (Urecholine), 296t, 404t
Betoptic, 585t

Biaxin, 357t, 593t
Biologic response modifiers, **425–439**
  case study, 439
  colony-stimulating factors, 429, 430
  erythropoietin, 430–432
    prototype drug chart for, 431
  granulocyte colony–stimulating factor, 432, 433
    prototype drug chart for, 432
  granulocyte macrophage colony–stimulating factor, 433–435
    prototype drug chart for, 434
  interferons, 426–430
    drug table for, 428t
  interleukins, 435, 436t, 437t
  nursing process, 437, 438
Biotransformation, 7
biperiden lactate, HCl (Akineton), 303t, 307t
bisacodyl USP (Dulcolax), 557t, 686t
bismuth salts (Pepto-Bismol), 553t
bisoprolol fumarate (Zebeta), 508t
bitolterol mesylate (Tornalate), 460t
bleomycin sulfate (Blenoxane), 420t
blood-borne pathogens, occupational exposure of health workers, 746
Body fluids, 178, 178t
Body surface area, 57, 58
Body weight, 56, 57
boric acid (Ear-Dry), 592t
Brand drug name, 134, 135
Brethine, 285t
bretylium tosylate (Bretylol) 486t, 756, 757t
Bretylol, 486t, 756, 757t
bromocriptine mesylate (Parlodel), 309t, 311t, 735t
brompheniramine maleate (Bromphen), 448t
Bronchodilators, **457–462**
  aerosol inhalor, use of, 459, 460
  drug table for, 460t, 461t
  methylxanthine, 462–465
  nursing process, 461, 462, 466, 467
  prototype drug chart for, 458
Bronkosol, 285t
BufOpto-atropine, 591t
Bulk-forming laxatives, **558–560,** 560t
  nursing process, 561
  prototype drug chart for, 559
bumetanide (Bumex), 497t
bupivacaine HCl, 225t
buprenorphine HCl (Buprenex), 239t
bupropion HCl (Wellbutrin), 269t
Burns, **601–604**
  degree of, 601t
  drug table for, 603
  nursing process, 603, 604
  prototype drug chart for, 602
  tissue depth of, 601t
buspirone HCl (BuSpar), 263t
busulfan (Myleran), 412t
butabarbital sodium (Butisol), 217t
Butisol sodium, 217t
butorphanol tartrate (Stadol), 239t
Butyrophenone 253, 258t

C

Caffeine, 211t
Calan, 757t, 481t, 486t, 515t
calcifediol (Calderol), 619t
calcitonin (human, salmon), 620t
calcitriol (Rocaltrol), 619t, 620

Calcium, **188–191**
 functions, 188, 189
 hypocalcemia, 190
 nursing process, 190, 191
 prototype drug for, 189
calcium blockers. See *Calcium channel blockers.*
calcium carbonate (Tums), 568t
Calcium channel blockers, **480–482**, 486t, 513–515
 drug table, 481t
 nursing process, 482
Calculations, drugs, **42–128.** See also *Drug calculations.*
 injectable dosages, 88–110
 oral dosages, 66–86
Canadian drug names, **767–770**
Canadian Drug Regulation, 134
 Schedule F, 134
 Schedule G, 134
 Schedule H, 134
Cancer drugs. See *Anticancer drugs.*
Cannabinoids, 546, 547t
Cantil, 302t
Capoten, 515t
captopril (Capoten), 515t
 nursing process, 515, 516
 prototype drug chart for, 514
Carafate, 573, 574t
carbachol intraocular (Miostat), 296t, 585t
carbamazepine (Tegretol), 247t
carbamide peroxide (Debrox), 592t
carbenicillin disodium, 347t
carbidopa-levodopa, 308–310, 311t
 nursing process, 312
 prototype drug chart for, 310
Carbonic anhydrase inhibitors, 497, 498t, 499, 588, 589
carboplatin (Paraplatin), 412t
Cardene, 481t
Cardiac glycosides, **474–477**
 case study, 488
 digitalis toxicity, 474, 475
 digoxin, 474–476, 486t
 drug interactions, 474
 drug table for, 476t
 nursing process, 476, 477
 prototype drug chart for, 470
Cardiac physiology, **470–472**
 afterload, 471
 blood, 472
 cardiac output, 471
 circulation, 471
 conduction of electrical impulses, 470
 heart structure, 470
 preload, 471
 regulation of heart rate and blood flow, 471
 vascular structures, 470
Cardizem, 481t, 486t, 515t
carisoprodol Cl (Soma), 317t, 318, 319
 nursing process, 319, 320
carmustine (Bi-CNU), 412t
carteolol HCl (Cartrol), 508t
casanthranol with docusate potassium (Dialose Plus), 686t
casanthranol with docusate sodium (Peri-Colace), 686t
Cascara sagrada, 557t
Castor oil, 557t
Catapres, 508t
CCNS. See *Cell-cycle nonspecific (CCNS).*
CCS. See *Cell-cycle specific (CCS).*
Ceclor, 351, 352t, 592t
cefaclor (Ceclor), 351, 352t, 592t

cefadroxil (Duricef), 352t
Cefadyl, 352t
cefamandole (Mandol), 352t
cefazolin sodium (Ancef), 351, 352t
cefixime (Suprax), 353t
cefmetazole sodium (Zefazone), 352t
cefonicid sodium (Monocid), 352t
cefoperazone (Cefobid), 353t
ceforanide (Precef), 352t
cefotaxime (Claforan), 353t
cefotetan (Cefotan), 353t
cefoxitin sodium (Mefoxin), 353t
cefpodoxime (Proxetil), 352t
cefprozil monohydrate (Cefzil), 352t
ceftazidime (Fortaz), 353t
ceftizoxime sodium (Cefizox) 353t
ceftriaxone (Rocephin), 353t
cefuroxime (Zinacef), 353t
Celestone, 657t
Cell-cycle nonspecific (CCNS), 408, 409, 422
 drug groups, 408, 422
 effects of, 409t
Cell-cycle specific (CCS), 408, 409, 422
 drug groups, 408, 422
 effects of, 409t
Celsius, conversion, 771
Central nervous system (CNS), 204
Central nervous system depressants, **215–227**
 anesthetics, 223
 narcotics, 232–238
 sedative-hypnotics, 215–222
Central nervous system stimulants, **208–213**
 amphetamines, 208–210, 208t
 analeptics, 212
 anorexiants, 210–212
 nursing process, 212, 213
Centrally-acting (adrenergic blockers) sympatholytes, 507
Centrax, 263t
cephalexin (Keflex), 352t
Cephalosporins, **350–354**
 drug table for, 352t, 353t
 first, second, third generations of, 350
 nursing process, 353, 354
 prototype drug chart for, 351
cephalothin (Keflin), 352t
cephapirin sodium (Cefadyl), 352t
cephradine (Velosef), 352t
Cesamet, 547t
Charcoal, 550t
chlorambucil (Leukeran), 412t
chloral hydrate, 217t, 220
chloramphenicol (Chloromycetin), 367t, 369
chloramphenicol (Chloromycetin Otic), 592t
Chloramphenicol (AK-Chlor, Chlor-omycetin Ophthalmic), 582t
chlordiazepoxide HCl (Librium), 263t
Chloromycetin, 367t, 369
chloroprocaine, 225t
chloroquine HCl (Aralen HCl), 391t, 392
chlorothiazide (Diuril), 491t
chlorotrianisene (Tace), 714t
chlorphenesin carbamate (Maolate), 317t
chlorpheniramine maleate (Chlor-Trimeton), 448t
chlorpromazine HCl (Thorazine), 252–255, 257t, 546t
 prototype drug chart for, 254, 255
chlorpropamide (Diabinese), 636t
chlorprothixene HCl (Taractan), 258t

chlorthalidone (Hygroton), 492t
cholestyramine resin (Questran), 531t
cholinergic receptors, 9
Cholinergic blocking agents. See *Anticholinergics.*
Cholinergic agonists. See *Cholinergics.*
Cholinergic antagonists, 277. See also *Anticholinergics.*
Cholinergics, **293–298**, 275, 277
 cholinesterase inhibitors, 293, 294
 direct-acting drugs, 293–295
 drug table for, 296t
 effects of, 294
 indirect-acting drugs, 293–296
 irreversible cholinesterase inhibitors, 297
 nursing process, 297, 298
 prototype drug chart for, 295
 responses of, 293
 reversible cholinesterase inhibitors, 296, 297
Cholinesterase inhibitors, 293, 294, 296, 297
 irreversible, 297
 reversible, 296, 297
chorzoxazone (Paraflex), 317t
cimetidine (Tagamet), 570, 571t
Cinobac, 367t, 399t
cinoxacin (Cinobac), 367t, 399t
Cipro, 366–368, 367t, 399t, 582t
ciprofloxacin HCl (Cipro), 366–368, 367t, 399t, 582t
 nursing process, 368
 prototype drug chart for, 366
cisapride (Propulsid), 574t
cisplatin (Platinol), 413t
cladribine (Leustatin), 417t
clarithromycin (Biaxin), 357t, 593t
Claritin, 449t
clemastine fumarate (Tavist), 448t
Client teaching, 17, 18
 diet, 17
 general, 17
 side effects, 17
 skill, 17
 teaching plan, 18
clindamycin HCl (Cleocin), 358t, 598t
Clinoril, 332t
clofibrate (Atromid-S), 531t
Clomid, 735t
clomiphene citrate, 735t
 prototype drug chart, 734
clomipramine HCl (Anafranil), 268t
clonazepam (Klonopin), 246t
clonidine HCl (Catapres), 508t
clorazepate dipotassium (Tranxene), 247t, 263t
cloxacillin (Tegopen), 346, 347t
clozapine (Clozaril), 258t
coal tar (Estar), 598t
codeine sulfate and phosphate, 236t, 452t
Cogentin, 303t
Colace, 686t
colchicine (Novocolchine), 338, 338t
colestipol HCl (Colestid), 531t
colistimethate sodium (Coly-Mycin M), 384
colistin sulfate (Coly-Mycin S), 384, 553t
Colony-stimulating factors, 429, 430
Coly-Mycin S, 384, 553t
Common cold, drugs for, 445–454
Compazine, 253–255, 547t
Conjugated estrogens, 713
 prototype drug chart for, 713
Constipation, 555

Contact laxatives, **555–558,** 557t
  nursing process, 558
  prototype drug chart for, 556
Continuous intravenous administration,
    112–116
  flow rate, 114
  practice problems, 115, 116
Controlled Substance Act, 1970, 133
  nursing interventions, 133
  schedule categories, 133t
Corgard, 289t, 508t
Correctal, 557t
Cortef, 624t
corticosteroid therapy in preterm labor,
    656–658
  nursing process, 657, 658
corticotropin (Acthar), 612t
corticotropin repository (Acthar gel), 612t
cortisone acetate, 624t
Cortrosyn, 612t
cosyntropin (Cortrosyn), 612t
Co-trimoxazole, 400t
Co-Tylenol, 284t
Creatinine clearance, 7, 8
Critical care drug calculation, 126–128
cromolyn sodium (Intal), 449t, 465
Crystodigin, 476t
Cultural considerations, 136
Curretab, 714t
cyclandelate (Cyclospasmol), 535t
cyclobenzaprine HCl (Flexeril), 317t
cyclopentolate HCl (Cyclogyl), 303t, 591t
cyclophosphamide (Cytoxin), 410–414, 412t
  nursing process, 413, 414
  prototype drug chart for, 411
Cycloplegics, **589–591**
  drug table, 591t
Cyclopropane, 224t
Cycrin, 714t
Cylert, 208t, 209 ,210
cyproheptadine HCl (Periactin), 448t
cytarabine HCl (Cytosar-U), 416t
Cytomel, 617t
Cytoxan, 410–414, 412t

D

dacarbazine (DTIC), 413t
dactinomycin (Actinomycin), 420t
Dalmane, 222t
dalteparin sodium (Fragmin), 523t
danazol (Danocrine), 706t, 707, 724t
Danocrine, 706t, 724t
Dantrium, 318, 318t, 319
dantrolene Cl (Dantrium), 318, 318t, 319
Darbid, 302t
Darvon, 236t
Darvon-N, 236t
Datril, 648, 649
daunorubicin HCl (Cerubidine), 420t
Deca Durabolin, 724t
Decadron, 624t
Declomycin, 360t
Decongestants, 449, 450
  nasal, 449, 450, 450t
  systemic, 449, 450, 450t
Delatest, 724t
Delatestryl, 724t
demecarium bromide (Humorsol), 296t,
    585t
demeclocycline HCl (Declomycin), 360t
depoAndro, 724t
Depo-Estradiol Cypionate, 714t

Depo-Provera, 714t
Depo-Testosterone, 724t
Dermatologic disorders, **597–604**
  acne vulgaris, 597
  burns, 601–604
  contact dermatitis, 600
  drug table for, 598t, 601t
  drug-induced dermatitis, 600
  hair loss and baldness, 600, 601
  nursing process, 599, 600
  psoriasis, 597
Dermoplast, 682t
Desflurane, 224t
desipramine HCl (Norpramin, Pertofrane),
    268t
desmopressin (Stimate), 612t
desmopressin acetate (DDAVP), 612t
Desyrel, 269t
dexamethasone (AK-Dex Opthalmic,
    Maridex Opthalmic), 583t
dexamethasone (Decadron), 624t
dexchlorpheniramine maleate (Dexchlor),
    448t
Dexedrine, 208t, 211t
dextroamphetamine sulfate, 208t, 211t
dextromethorphan hydrobromide
    (Robitussin DM), 451, 452t
Dextrose 50%, 763, 764, 764t
dezocine (Dalgan), 240t
Diabetes mellitus, 629
  case study, 638, 639
Diabinese, 636t
Dialose, 686t
Dialose Plus, 686t
Diamox, 497t, 585t
diazepam (Valium), 224t, 247t, 261, 262,
    263t, 317t
  prototype drug chart for, 262, 263
diazoxide (Hyperstat), 511t
Diazoxide, 637
Dibenzoxazepine, 258t
Dibucaine HCl, 225t
dibucaine ointment (Nupercaine), 682t
dichlorphenamide (Daranide), 498t, 588t
diclofenac sodium (Voltaren), 583t
dicloxacillin sodium (Dynapen), 347t
dicumarol (bishydroxycoumarin), 523t
dicyclomine HCl (Bentyl), 302t
didanosine (Videx), 389t
dienestrol (DV), 714t
diethylcarbamazine (Hetrazan), 394t
diethylpropion (Dospan), 211t
diethylstilbestrol, 714t
difenoxin and atropine (Motofen), 553t
Diflucan, 382
diflunisal (Dolobid), 231t, 332t
Digitalis toxicity, 474, 476
digitoxin, 476t
digoxin, 474–476, 476t, 486t
dihydroxyaluminum sodium carbonate
    (Rolaids), 568t
Dilantin, 244–246, 486t
Dilaudid, 236t
diltiazem HCl (Cardizem), 481t, 486t, 515t,
    753, 754, 757t
dimethyl sulfoxide (DMSO), 404t
dinoprostone cervical gel (Prepidil Gel),
    673t
diphenhydramine HCl (Benadryl),
    445–447, 448t, 763, 764t
  nursing process, 447
  prototype drug chart for, 446
diphenidol HCl (Vontrol), 547t
diphenoxylate with atropine (Lomotil),
    553t

dipivefrin HCl (Propine), 591t
dipyridamole (Persantine), 531t
Direct-acting ateriolar vasodilators, 511t,
    512t, 513
Disease-modifying antirheumatic drug
    (DMARD), **335–337**
  drug table for, 335t
  nursing process, 336, 337
  prototype drug chart for, 336
Disipal, 307t
disopyramide phosphate (Norpace), 485t
Distribution (drug), 5, 6
  protein binding, 6, 6t
Diuretics, **490–501**
  carbonic anhydrase inhibitors, 497t,
    499
  effects on renal tubules, 490
  loop (high-ceiling), 495–498
  mercurial, 499
  osmotic, 497, 497t
  potassium-sparing, 499–501
  thiazides and thiazide-like, 491–495
dobutamine HCl (Dobutrex), 285t, 762,
    764t
Dobutrex, 762, 764t
docusate sodium (Colace), 682t
docusate potassium (Dialose), 686t
docusate calcium (Surfak), 686t
dopamine HCl (Intropin), 284t, 761, 764t
  prototype drug chart, 762
Dopaminergics, **308–312**
  drug table for, 311t
  nursing process, 312
  prototype drug chart for, 310
Doriden, 222t
dorzolamide (Trusopt), 588t
doxapram HCl (Dopram), 211t
doxazosin mesylate (Cardura), 289t, 511t
doxepin HCl (Sinequan), 268t
doxorubicin (Adriamycin), 418, 419, 420t
doxycycline (Vibramycin), 360t
dronabinol (Marinol), 547t
droperidol (Inapsine), 224t, 258t, 547t
Drug abuse, **144–146**
  addiction, 144
  chemical impairment in nurses, 144,
    145
  nursing process, 145, 146
Drug action, **3–13**
  nursing process, 12, 13
  pharmaceutic phase, 4
  pharmacodynamics, 8–11
  pharmacokinetics, 4–8
Drug addiction, 144
Drug administration, **22–39**
  factors modifying drug response, 27–29
  forms for, 29–33
    drops, ear, 30, 30t
    liquids, 30
    ointment, eye, 30, 30t
    suppositories, 32
    tablets, 29, 30
  guidelines for, 28t, 29t
  medication record, 27
  nursing implications, 37, 38
  order, drug, 24, 25, 25t
  routes of, 29–37
    inhalations, 31, 32, 33t
    instillation, 31
    nasal, 32, 32t
    nasogastric/gastrostomy tubes, 31,
      32
    oral, 29, 30
    parenteral, 33–37
    topical, 30, 31

Drug administration (Continued)
  transdermal, 30
  vaginal, 33
  z-track, 36
  sites for intramuscular injections, 36, 37
  ten rights in, 23
Drug calculations, 42–128
  apothecary system, 43, 44
    conversion within, 44
  conversion between metric, apothecary and household systems, 46–48, 47t, 54t
    equivalents, 47t
  household system, 44
    conversion within, 45
  injectable dosages, 88–110
  intravenous fluid calculations, 112–128
  methods for, 53–64
  metric system, 42, 43
    conversion within, 42, 43
  nomograms, 58, 59
    West nomogram, 58
    adult nomogram, 59
  oral dosages, 66–86
Drug differentiation, 67, 68
Drug distribution methods, 25, 25t
Drug Enforcement Administration (DEA), 133
Drug enzyme inducer, 140, 140t
Drug enzyme inhibitor, 140, 140t
Drug facts and comparisons, 135
Drug incompatibility, 139
Drug interactions, 139–146
  pharmacodynamic interaction, 141, 142
  pharmacokinetic interaction, 141, 142
  nursing process, 143
Drug label, interpretation, 53, 67, 92
Drug names, 134, 135
Drug orders, 24, 25, 25t
Drug reaction, adverse, 11, 139
Drug research, 158–161
  approved (recently) drugs, 161
  basic ethical principles, 158
  basic sequence of new drug, 158t
  human clinical experimentation, 159
  informed consent, 158, 160t
  nursing process, 160, 161
  study designs, 159, 160
Drug resources, 135
  American Hospital Formulary, 135
  Drug Facts and Comparisons, 135
  Physicians' Desk Reference, 135
Drug response, factors modifying, 27–29
Drug standards, 132
Drug-food interactions, 142
Drug-induced photosensitivity, 143, 144, 144t
Drug-laboratory interactions, 142
  brand, 134
  generic, 134
Dulcolax, 557t, 686t
Durabolin, 724t
Duragesic, 236t
Duratest, 724t
Durathate, 724t
Duration of drug action, 8
Durham-Humphrey Amendment (1952), 132, 133
Duricef, 352t
DV, 714t
Dyazide, 501t
Dymelor, 635, 636t
DynaCirc, 481t

E

E-Mycin, 592t
Ear, drugs for, 591–594
  antibacterials, 592t, 593t
  antihistamine-decongestants, 594
  case study, 594
  ceruminolytics, 594
  combination products, 594
  health teaching, 594
  overview of, 578, 579
echothiophate iodide (Phospholine Iodide), 585t
Econopred, 584t
Ecotrin, 649t
Edecrin, 497t
edrophonium Cl (Tensilon), 296t, 313t
Elavil, 265–267, 268t
Electrolytes, 183–193
  calcium, 188–191
  case study, 193
  magnesium, 191, 192
  potassium, 183–187
  sodium, 187, 188
Electronic intravenous regulators, 117
Elimination, 7, 8
Emergency drugs, 752–766
  cardiac disorders, 752–757
    drug table for, 757t
    prototype drug chart, 755
  hypertensive crises, 764–766
    prototype drug chart for, 765
  neurosurgical disorders, 757–759
    drug table for, 759t
    prototype drug chart, 758
  poisoning, 759–761
    drug table for, 761t
    prototype drug chart for, 760
  shock, 761–764
    drug table for, 764t
    prototype drug chart for, 762
Emetics, 548–551
  drug chart for, 550t
  ipecac, 548
  nursing process, 550, 551
  prototype drug chart for, 549
Emollient laxatives, 560, 560t
enalapril maleate (Vasotec), 515t
encainide HCl, 485t
Endocrine system, 606–609
  adrenal glands, 609
  pancreas, 609
  parathyroid glands, 608
  pituitary gland, 606–608, 611
    anterior, 607, 608
    posterior, 608
  thyroid gland, 608
Endometriosis, 707–710
  drug table for, 706t
  nursing process, 708–710
Enflurane, 224t
Engerix B, 693t
enoxacin (Penetrex), 367t, 399t
enoxaparin sodium (Lovenox), 523t
Enteral medications, 197, 198
  osmolality of, 198t
Enteral nutrition, 195–199
  complications, 197
  medications, 197, 198
  methods for delivery, 196, 197
  nursing process, 198, 199
  routes for, 195, 196
  solutions for, 195–197, 197t
ephedrine HCl, 284t, 460t

ephedrine sulfate, 284t, 460t
Ephedsol, 284t, 460t
epinephrine borate (Epinal, Eppy/N), 591t
epinephrine (Adrenalin), 281–283, 284t, 460t, 591t, 756, 757t, 763, 764t
  nursing process, 286, 287
  prototype drug chart for, 282
Equanil, 263t, 317t
ergocalciferol (Drisdol), 619t
ergoloid mesylates (Hydergine), 535t
ergonovine maleate (Ergotrate), 676t
Ergotrate, 676t
erythromycin, (E-Mycin, Ilotycin), 356–359, 357t–358t, 582t, 592t, 598t
  nursing process, 358, 359
  prototype drug chart for, 357
erythromycin ophthalmic, 692t
Erythropoietin, 430–432
  prototype drug chart for, 431
estazolam (ProSom), 222t
esterified estrogens (Estratab, Menest), 714t
Estrace, 714t
Estraderm, 714t
estradiol (Estrace, Estraderm), 714t
estradiol cypionate (Depo-Estradiol Cypionate), 714t
estramustine phosphate sodium (Encyt), 412t
Estratab, 714t
Estrogen therapy, 422
estrone (Theelin, Kestrone 5), 714t
estropipate SO_4 (Ogen, Ortho-Est), 714t
Estrovis, 714t
ethacrynic acid (Edecrin), 497t
ethambutol HCl (Myambutol), 378
ethchlorvynol (Placidyl), 217t
Ether, 224t
ethopropazine HCl (Parsidol), 307t
ethosuximide (Zarontin), 247t
ethotoin (Peganone), 247t
Etidocaine, 225t
etidronate (Didronel), 620t
etodolac (Lodine), 333t
Etomidate, 224t
etoposide (Ve Pesid), 416t, 422
etretinate (Tegison), 598t
Eulexin, 421t
Evaluation, 19
Everone, 724t
Excretion, 7, 8
  creatinine clearance, 7, 8
  half-life, 6t, 7t, 7, 8
Ex-Lax, 557t
Exosurf Pediatric, 659t
Expectorants, 452, 453
  drug table for, 452t
Extra Strength Maalox Plus Suspension, 649t
Eye, drugs for, 582–591
  antiinfectives, 582, 582t, 583t
  antiinflammatories, 583t, 584t
  diagnostic aids, 582, 582t
  health teaching, 590, 591
  lubricants, 582, 583
  topical anesthetics, 582
  overview of, 578
Eye disorders, suggestions for client teaching, 590, 591

F

Fahrenheit, conversion, 771
famciclovir (Famvir), 389t

famotidine (Pepcid), 571t
FDA Pregnancy Categories, 135, 136, 136t
  classification system, 135, 136t
Feces, drugs that discolor, 776
Federal Legislation, 132, 133
  Controlled Substance Act, 133
  Durham-Humphrey Amendment, 132, 133
  Food, Drug and Cosmetic Act of 1938, 132
  Kefauver-Harris Amendment, 133
Feldene, 333t
felodipine (Plendil), 515t
Femiron, 646t
Fenfluramine HCl (Pondimin), 211t
fenofibrate (Lipidil), 531t
fenoprofen calcium (Nalfon), 333t
fentanyl (Duragesic), 236t
Feosol, 646t
Feostat, 646t
Fergon, 646t
Fer-In-Sol, 646t
Fer-Iron, 646t
ferrous fumarate (Fumasorb, Feostat, Simron, Fetinic), 646t
ferrous sulfate, 646t
ferrous gluconate (Fergon, Ferralet, Simron, Fetinic), 646t
Fetinic, 646t
flavoxate HCl (Urispas), 404t
flecainide (Tambocor), 485t
Florinef acetate, 624t
Floxin, 367t, 400t
floxuridine (FUDR), 416t
fluconazole (Diflucan), 382
flucytosine (Ancobon), 382
fludarabine (Fludara), 417t
fludrocortisone acetate (Florinef acetate), 624t
Fluid replacements, **178–183**
  intravenous solutions, 180–182
  nursing process, 182, 183
  osmolality, 178, 179
Fluoroquinolones, **366–368,** 400
  drug table for, 367t–368t
  nursing process, 368
  prototype drug chart for, 366
fluorouracil (5-FU), 414–418, 416t
  nursing process, 417, 418
  prototype drug chart for, 415
fluoxetine (Prozac), 269t
fluoxymesterone (Halotestin), 724t
fluphenazine HCl (Prolixin), 257t
Flurazepam HCl (Dalmane), 222t
  prototype drug chart for, 221
flurbiprofen sodium (Ansaid), 333t, 583t
flutamide (Eulexin), 421t
fluvastatin (Lescol), 531t
folic acid, 646
Food, Drug and Cosmetic Act of 1938, 132
5-FU, 414–418, 416t
Fumerin, 646t
furosemide (Lasix), 495–498, 497t

G

gabapentin (Neurontin), 248t
ganciclovir sodium (Cytovene), 389, 389t
Gantanol, 372t
Gantrisin, 372t, 593t
Gastric acid secretion inhibitor, 572, 574t
Gastroesophageal reflux disease (GERD), 564

Gaviscon, 568t
Gelusil I, II, 568t
gemfibrozil (Lopid), 531t
Generic drug name, 134
gentamicin sulfate (Garamycin), **362–365,** 364t
  nursing process, 365
  prototype drug chart for, 363
gentamicin sulfate (Garamycin Ophthalmic), 582t
GERD (gastroesophageal reflux disease), 564
Geriatric pharmacology, **150–156**
  drugs that affect, 152–154
  noncompliance, 154, 155t
  nursing process, 155, 156
  pharmacodynamics, 152
  pharmacokinetics, 150–152, 151t
  physiologic changes, 150, 150t
GI stimulants, 564, 574t
glipizide (Glucotrol), 636t
Glossary, 801–818
glucagon, 764, 764t
Glucagon, 637
Glucocorticoid, **621–626,** 465
  case study, 626
  nursing process, 625, 626
  prototype drug chart for, 623
  topical, 601t
Glucophage, 636t, 636t, 637
glutethimide (Doriden), 222t
glyburide micronized (Glynase), 636t
glyburide nonmicronized (Dia Beta), 636t
glycerin, 590t
glycopyrrolate (Robinul), 302t, 566t
GnRH (gonadotropin-releasing hormone), 735t
gold sodium thiomalate (Myochrysine), 335t
Gold, **335–337,** 335t
  nursing process, 336, 337
  prototype drug chart for, 336
gonadotropin-releasing hormone (GnRH), 735t
gonadotropin-releasing hormone (GnRH) agonists, 706t
goserelin acetate (Zoladex), 421t
Granulocyte macrophage colony-stimulating factor, 433–435
  prototype drug chart for, 434
Growth hormone, drugs for, 612t
Granulocyte colony–stimulating factor, 432, 433
  prototype drug chart for, 432
guaifenesin and dextromethorphan, 449t
guaifenesin (Robitussin), 449t
guanabenz acetate (Wytensin), 508t
guandrel sulfate (Hylorel), 511t
guanethedine monosulfate (Ismelin sulfate), 511t
guanfacine HCl (Tenex), 508t

H

Halcion, 222t
Haldol, 253, 256
Haley's M-O, 686t
haloperidol (Haldol), 253, 256
  prototype drug chart for, 256
Halotestin, 724t
Halothane, 224t
halzepam (Paxipam), 263t
Helicobacter pylori, predisposing factor, 564

Heparin, **519–525,** 523t
  action of, 519
  nursing process, 524, 525
  prototype drug chart for, 521, 522
hepatitis B vaccine, 693t
Histamine$_2$ (H$_2$) blockers, **570–572**
  drug table for, 571t
  nursing process, 572
  prototype drug chart for, 570
Histerone, 724t
homotropine hydrobromide (Isopto Homatropine), 303t, 591t
Hormone replacement therapy, **711–716**
  contraindications, 712
  estrogens and progestins, 714t
  nursing process, 715, 716
  prototype drug chart, 713
Hormones and hormone antagonists, 419, 421t, 422
Household system, 44, 45
  conversion within, 45
  equivalents, 45t
human menopausal gonadotropin, 735t
  mentropin and FSH, 735t
Humorsol, 296t
Humulin insulins, 632t
Hybolin Decanoate, 724t
Hybolin Improved, 724t
hydralazine HCl (Apresoline), 511t, 662, 662t, 663
  nursing process, 662–664
hydrochlorothiazide (HydroDIURIL), 491t
hydrocodone bitartrate (Hycodan), 449t
hydrocortisone (Cortef), 624t
hydrocortisone acetate (Anusol HC, Anusol Ointment), 682t
hydrocortisone acetate 1% and promazine HCl, 682t
HydroDIURIL, 491t
hydroflumethiazide (Saluron), 491t
hydromorphine HCl (Dilaudid), 236t
hydroxychloroquine sulfate (Plaquenil), 391t
hydroxyurea (Hydrea), 416t
hydroxyzine HCl (Atarax, Vistaril), 263t, 448t
Hygroton, 492t
hyoscyamine sulfate (Anaspaz), 302t
Hyperglycemic drugs, 637
  diazoxide, 637
  glucagon, 637
Hyperstat, 511t
Hypertension, control of, **503–517**
  antihypertensive drugs, 503–517
  diuretics, thiazides, 491t–495
  nonpharmacologic, 503
  stepped-care approach, 503, 504
Hypnotics. See *Sedatives-hypnotics.*
Hypoglycemic (oral) drugs, **634–638**
  guidelines for use of, 637
  nonsulfonylureas, 636, 637
  nursing process, 637, 638
  prototype drug chart for, 635
  sulfonylureas 634–636, 636t
    first generation, 634–636
    second generation, 634–636

I

ibuprofen (Motrin), 231t, 330, 331, 333t
idarubicin (Idamycin), 420t
idoxuridine (IDU, Herplex, Liquifilm), 583t
ifosfamide (Ifex), 412t

Imdur, 480t
Iminostilbenes, 246, 247, 247t
imipenem/cilastatin, sodium (Primaxin), 368t, 369, 400t
imipramine HCl (Tofranil), 268t
Immunosuppressive agents, 337
Implementation, 17
indapamide (Lozol), 492t
Inderal, 288, 480t, 508t
Indocin, 332t
indomethacin (Indocin), 332t
Infection, 324
Infertility, **732–738**
   case study, 748
   causes, 733t
   common tests for, 733t
   male, 736
   management, 733–739
   nursing process, 736, 737
   process of fertilization, 732
Inflammation, 324
   cardinal signs of, 327, 327t
INH (isoniazid), 377–379
Inhalation anesthesia, 223
Inhalations, 31, 32, 33t
Injectable dosages for calculations, **88–110**
   angles for injection, 91
   insulin injections, 94–98
   interpreting injectable drug label, 92
   intradermal injections, 92, 93
   intramuscular injections, 98–110
   needles, 90t, 91
   subcutaneous injections, 93, 94
   syringes, 89, 90
   vials and ampules, 88
Innovar, 224t
Inocor, 476t
INR (international normalized ratio), 520
Insulins, 94–97, **629–634**
   drug table for, 632t
   hypoglycemic reactions, 633
   injection of, 94–96
   nursing process, 633, 634
   prototype drug chart for, 631
   sites for insulin injection, 630
   syringe for, 90
   types of, 95, 96, 630, 632t
Insulin syringe, 90
Interferons, **426–429**
   drug table for, 428t
Interleukins, 435, 436t, 437t
Intermittent intravenous administration, 116, 117
   answers, 123–126
   electronic IV regulators, 117
   practice problems, 120–122
   secondary IV sets, 116
Interpretation of drug labels. See *Drug label.*
Intradermal injections, 92, 93
Intramuscular injections, 35–37, **97–107**
   answers, 104–109
   mixing drugs, 99, 100
   pediatric calculations, 102–104
   practice problems, 100–104
   powdered drug reconstitution, 98
Intravenous anesthesia, 223
Intravenous fluids, calculations, **112–128**
   continuous IV administration, 112–116
   drug calculations, 119
   electronic IV regulators, 117
   flow rate calculation, 113
   intermittent IV administration, 116
   intravenous sets, 112, 112t
   mixing drugs, 113
   patient-controlled analgesic, 118, 119

Intravenous fluids, calculations (*Continued*)
   practice problems, 115, 116, 120–122
   solution types, 114t
Intravenous injections, 37, 38
Intravenous solutions, 180–182, 182t
   osmolality, 178–180, 182t
Intropin, 284t, 761, 764t
iodinated glycerol (Isophen), 449t
iodine (Lugol solution), 617t
ipecac syrup, 759, 761t
ipratropium bromide (Atrovent), 461t
Iron, 174, 175, 646
   prototype drug for, 174
Iron products, 646t
Ismelin, 511t
isocarboxazid (Marplan), 269t
isoetharine HCl (Bronkosol), 460t
Isoflurane, 224t
isoflurophate (Floropryl), 585t
isoniazid (INH), 377–379
   first-line drugs, 379
   prototype drug chart for, 377
   second-line drugs, 379
isopropamide iodide (Darbid), 302t
isoproterenol HCl (Isuprel), 285t, 461t, 753
Isopt Hyoscine, 591t
Isoptin, 515t, 753, 757t
Isopto Carpine, 585t
Isopto Eserine, 585t
Isopto Homatropine, 591t
Isordil, 480t
isosorbide dinitrate (Isordil), 480t, 590t
isotretinoin (Accutane), 598t
isoxsuprine (Vasodilan), 533–536, 534t
   nursing process, 535, 536
   prototype drug chart for, 534
isradipine (DynaCirc, Plendil), 481t, 515t
Isuprel, 285t, 461t, 753
itraconazole (Sporanox), 382

K

kanamycin sulfate (Kantrex), 364t
Kantrex, 364t
Keflex, 352t
Keflin, 352t
Kemadrin, 303t
Kestrone 5, 714t
Ketamine HCl, 224t
ketoconazole (Nizoral), 382
ketoprofen (Orudis), 333t
ketorolac tromethamine (Acular, Toradol), 333t, 583t
Konakin, 693t

L

labetalol HCl (Trandate), 511t
labor pain control, **664–672**
   analgesia, 664–668
      drug table for, 665t, 666t
      nursing process, 667, 668
   anesthesia, 668–672
   regional anesthesia, 668–672
      caudal, 670
      local infiltration, 670
      lumbar epidural, 669, 670
      nursing process, 671, 672
      paracervical block, 670
      pudendal, 670
      saddle block, 669
      subarachnoid block, 669

Laboratory tests for drug use, **782–790**
lansoprazole (Prevacid), 574t
Lasix, 497t
Laxatives, contact. See *Contact laxatives.*
Lente insulin, 632t
Lescol, 531t
Leukeran, 412t
leuprolide acetate (Lupron Depot 3.75), 706t, 707
Levarterenol, 763
levobunolol HCl (Betagan, Liquifilm), 585t
Levodopa, 308, 311t
Levo-Dromoran, 236t
levomethadyl acetate (Orlaam), 236t
Levophed, 284t, 763, 764t
levorphanol tartrate (Levo-Dromoran), 236t
levothyroxine sodium (Synthroid), 616, 617t
Librax, 566t
Librium, 269t, 270–272
   prototype drug chart for, 271, 272
lidocaine (Xylocaine), 225t, 485t, 754, 757t
   prototype drug chart, 755t
lincomycin (Lincorex), 358t, 359
   minocycline HCl (Minocin), 360t
liothyronine sodium (Cytomel), 617t
liotrix (Euthroid, Thyrolar), 617t
Lipid values, 529t
Lipoprotein groups, 528t
Lipoprotein phenotype, 529t
lisinopril (Prinivil), 515t
Loading dose, 11
Local anesthesia, 224, 225, 225t
lomefloxacin HCl (Maxaquin), 367t, 499t
lomustine (CeeNu), 412t
Loop (high-ceiling) diuretics, **495–498**
   drug table for, 497t
   nursing process, 498
   prototype drug chart for, 496
Lopid, 531t
Lopressor, 289t, 480t
Lorabid, 593t
loracarbef (Lorabid), 353t, 593t
loratadine (Claritin), 449t
lorazepam (Activan), 222t, 247t, 263t
Lorelco, 531t
lovastatin (Mevacor), 529–533, 531t
   nursing process, 532, 533
   prototype drug chart for, 530
low molecular weight heparins (LMWHs), 520
Lower respiratory disorders, **456–467**
   bronchial asthma, 456
   chronic obstructive pulmonary disease (COPD), 456
   factors contributing to, 457
   sympathomimetics, 457
loxapine (Loxitane), 258t
Loxitane, 258t
Lozol, 492t
lypressin (Diapid), 612t

M

Maalox, 568t
Maalox Plus, 649t
Macrodantin, 397, 398, 399t
Macrolides, **356–359**
   drug table for, 357t, 358t
   erythromycin, 356, 357, 358t
   nursing process, 358, 359
   prototype drug chart for, 357

mafenide acetate (Sulfamylon), 373, 602, 603, 603t
  prototype drug chart for, 602
magaldrate with simethicone (Riopan Plus Tablets, Riopan Plus Suspension), 568t, 649t
Magnesium, **191, 192**
  functions, 191
  hypomagnesemia, 192
  nursing process, 192
magnesium citrate, 761, 761t
magnesium hydroxide (Milk of Magnesia), 686t
magnesium hydroxide with mineral oil (Haley's M-O), 686t
magnesium hydroxide with simethicone, 649t
magnesium sulfate, 248t, 653t, 654, 655, 661, 662t, 761, 761t
magnesium trisilicate (Gaviscon), 568t
Malfeasance, 134
Mandol, 352t
mannitol (Osmitrol), 497t, 590t, 757, 758, 759t
  prototype drug chart, 758
MAO inhibitors, 268, 269t
maprotiline HCl (Ludiomil), 269t
Marplan, 269t
Maxaquin, 367t, 399t
Mazindol (Sanorex), 211t
mebendazole (Vermox), 394t
mechlorethamine (Mustargen), 412t
Meclizine (Antivert, Bonamine, Vertol), 647t
meclocycline (Meclan), 598t
meclofenamate (Meclomen), 333t
Medication record, 27
Medroxyprogesterone acetate (Amen, Curretab, Provera, Cycrin, Depo-Provera), 714t
Medrysone (HMS Liquifilm), 584t
mefenamic acid (Ponstel), 333t
mefloquine HCl (Lariam), 393t
megestrol acetate (Megace), 714t
Megace, 714t
megestrol acetate, 421t
Mellaril, 258t
melphalan (Alkeran), 412t
Menest, 714t
Menopause, **710–716**
mepenzolate bromide (Cantil), 302t
meperidine (Demerol), 235–238, 236t
  case study, 241
  nursing process, 237, 238
  prototype drug chart for, 237
mephenytoin (Mesantoin), 247t
mephobarbital (Mebaral), 246t
Mepivacaine, 225t
meprobamate (Equanil, Miltown), 263t, 317t
6-Mercaptopurine, 416t
mesoridazine besylate (Serentil), 258t
Mestinon, 296t, 315t
Metaprel, 457–459, 461t
metaproterenol sulfate (Alupent, Metaprel), 285t, **457–459**, 461t
  prototype drug chart for, 458
metaraminol bitartrate (Aramine), 284t
metformin (Glucophage), 636, 636t, 637
methadone treatment program, 241
Methamphetamine (Desoxyn), 208t
methazolamide (Neptazane), 498t, 588t
methdilazine HCl (Tacaryl), 449t
methenamine (Hiprex) 397, 399t
Methergine, 676t

methicillin (Staphcillin), 347t
methimazole (Tapazole), 617t
methocarbamol (Robaxin), 317t
Methods for calculations, **53–64**
  answers, 62–64
  basic formula, 53–55
  body surface area, 57, 58
  body weight, 56, 57
  interpreting drug labels, 53
  practice problems, 59–61
  ratio and proportion, 55–57
methotrexate (MTX), 416t
methotrimeprazine HCl (Levoprome), 231t, 232t
methoxsalen (Oxsoralen), 598t
Methoxyflurane, 224t
methscopolamine bromide (Pamine), 302
methsuximide (Celontin), 247t
methyclothiazide (Enduron), 491t
Methyl Testred, 724t
methyldopa (Aldomet), 508t, 509t
methylene blue, 400t
methylergonovine maleate (Methergine), 676t
methylphenidate (Ritalin), 208–210, 208t
  nursing process, 212, 213
  prototype drug chart for, 209
methylprednisolone (Solu-Medrol), 624t, 758, 759, 759t
methyltestosterone (Android, Oreton Methyl, Testred, Virilon), 724t
Methylxanthine (Xanthine) derivatives, **462–465**
  drug chart for, 464t
  nursing process, 466, 467
  theophylline, 462–464
    prototype drug chart for, 463
metolazone (Zaroxolyn), 492t
metoprolol tartrate (Lopressor), 289t, 480t, 505, 506
  nursing process, 506, 507
  prototype drug chart for, 505
Metric system, 42, 43
  conversion within, 42, 43
  equivalents, 42t
Metrodin, 735t
mexiletine HCl (Mexitil), 485t
mezlocillin sodium (Mezlin), 348t
Micatin, 382
miconazole nitrate (Monistat, Micatin), 382
Microsulfon, 372t
Midazolam, 224t
Milk of Magnesia, 686t
milrinone lactate (Primacor), 476t
Miltown, 263t
mineral oil (Agoral), 687t
Minerals, **173–175**
  iron, 174, 175
  nursing process, 175
Minipress, 289t, 511t
Minocin, 360t
minoxidil (Rogaine, Loniten), 512t
Miotics, **584–587**
  beta-adrenergic blockers, 58t
  direct-acting cholinergics, 585t
  indirect-acting cholinesterase inhibitors, 585t
  nursing process, 587
  prototype drug chart for, 586
Misfeasance, 134
misoprostol (Cytotec), 574t
Mithracin, 418, 419, 420t
mitomycin (Mutamycin), 420t
mitotane (Lysodren), 421t
mitoxantrone (Novantrone), 420t

Moduretic, 501t
molindone HCl (Moban), 258t
Mol-Iron, 646t
Monistat, 382
Morphine sulfate, **233–235, 752**
  nursing process, 234–235
  prototype drug chart for, 233
Motrin, 231t, 330, 331, 333t
Mucolytics, 466
Multiple vitamins, 646, 647
Multiple sclerosis, 315, 316, 316t
  treatment stratagies, 316t
Muscle relaxants, skeletal. See *Skeletal muscle relaxants.*
Myasthenia gravis, **313–315**
  acetylcholinesterase inhibitors, 313–315
  drug table for, 313t, 314t
  nursing process, 315
  prototype drug chart for, 314
Mydriacyl Ophthalmic, 591t
Mydriatics, 589, 590
  drug table, 591t
Myidyl, 449t
Mylanta II, 649t
Mylanta Liquid, 649t
Myleran, 412t
Mylicon, 687t
Mytelase, 296t, 314t

N

nadolol (Corgard), 289t, 508t
nafaralen acetate (Synarel Nasal Solution), 706t, 709, 710
nafcillin (Nafcin), 348t
nalbuphine HCl (Nubain), 240t
nalidixic acid (NegGram), 367t, 399t
naloxone HCl (Narcan), 240t, 759, 761t
  prototype drug chart, 760
Nandrobolic, 724t
nandrolone deconate (Androlone-D, Deca Durabolin, Hybolin Decanoate, Neo-Durabolic), 724t
nandrolone phenpropionate (Durabolin, Hybolin Improved, Nandrobolic), 724t
naproxen (Naprosyn), 333t
Narcan, 240t, 759, 761t
Narcolepsy, 208–210
Narcotic agonist-antagonists, **238–240**
  drug table for, 239t, 240t
  nursing process, 240
  prototype drug chart for, 239
Narcotic analgesics, **233–238**
  case study, 241
  drug table for, 236t
  meperidine, 235–238
    nursing process, 237, 238
    prototype drug chart for, 237
  morphine, 233–235
  nursing process, 234
    prototype drug chart for, 233
Nasogastric and gastrostomy tubes, 31, 32
natamycin (Natacyn Ophthamalic), 583t
Navane, 257t
Nebcin, 365t
Needle sizes for injection, 90
nefazodone HCl (Serzone), 269t
NegGram, 367t, 399t
Nembutal sodium, 217t
Neo-Durabolic, 724t
Neo-Synephrine, 284t

neomycin sulfate (Mycifradin), 364t
neostigmine (Prostigmin), 296t, 313t
netilmicin sulfate (Netromycin), **362–365,** 364t
  nursing process, 365
  prototype drug chart for, 363
Niacin, 531t
nicardipine HCl (Cardene), 481t
niclosamide (Niclocide), 394t
nicotinic acid (Niacin), 531t
nifedipine (Procardia), 481t, 515t
Nipride, 512t
Nitrates, 478–480
Nitro-Bid, 479
nitrofurantoin (Macrodantin), 397, 398, 399t
  nursing process, 401, 402
  prototype drug chart for, 398
nitrofurazone (Furacin), 603t
nitroglycerin (Nitrostat, Tridil), **478–480,** 752, 757t
  nursing process, 482
  prototype drug chart for, 479
Nitropress, 512t
nitroprusside sodium (Nipride), 512t
Nitrosoureas, 412t
Nitrostat, 479, 757t
Nitrous oxide, 224t
nizatidine (Axid), 571t
Nomograms, 58, 59
Non-rapid eye movement, 215
Noncompliance, drug regimen, 154, 155t
Nonfeasance, 134
Nonnarcotic analgesics, **229–232**
  acetaminophen, 230–232
    nursing process, 232
    prototype drug chart for, 230
  drug table for, 231t, 232t
  nonsteroidal antiinflammatory drugs (NSAIDs), 239, 240
Nonphenothiazines, 253, 256, 258t
  butyrophenones, 253, 258t
  dibenzoxazepine, 258t
  nursing process, 258–260
  prototype drug chart for, 256
  thioxanthenes, 258t
Nonsteroidal antiinflammatory drugs (NSAIDs), **327–334**
  drug table for, 332t, 333t
  fenamates, 331
  nursing process, 333, 334
  oxicams, 331
  para-chlorobenzoic acid, 330
  phenylacetic acid derivatives, 332
  propionic acid derivatives, 330, 331
  prototype drug chart for, 328, 329, 331
  pyrazolone derivatives, 330
  salicylates, 328–330
Nonsteroidal estrogens, 714t
nonsulfonylureas, 636, 637
  acarbose (Precose), 637
  metformin (Glucophage), 636, 637
norepinephrine bitartrate (Levarterenol, Levophed), 284t, 763, 764t
norethindrone (Norlutin), 714t
Norflex, 317t
norfloxacin (Noroxin, Chibroxin), 367t, 399t, 582t
Norlutin, 714t
Norpramin, 268t
nortriptyline HCl (Aventyl), 268t
Novocain, 225t
NPH insulin, 632t
NSAIDs, **327–334.** See also *Nonsteroidal antiinflammatory drugs (NSAIDs).*

Nupercaine, 225t, 682t
Nurse Practice Act, 134
Nursing process, **15–19**
Nursing diagnosis, **15–19,** 16t
Nutritional support, **195–202**
  case study, 201–202
  enteral nutrition, 195–199
  parenteral nutrition, 199
nylindrin (Arlidin), 534t
nystatin (Mycostatin), 380–382
  prototype drug chart for, 381

O

octreotide acetate (Sandostatin), 553t
Ocusert Pilo-20, Pilo-40, 585t
ofloxacin (Floxin), 367t, 400t
Ogen, 714t
Older adults, drugs that affect, **152–154**
  antibacterials, 154
  anticoagulants, 154
  antidepressants, 154
  antihypertensives, 153
  cardiac glycosides, 153, 154
  diuretics, 153
  hypnotics, 153
  narcotic analgesics, 154
omeprazole (Prilosec), 574t
Onset of drug action, 8
Oral contraceptive products, **698–704**
  contraindications, 701t
  dosage schedule, 700
  drug interactions, 701t
  drug table, 699t
  estrogen-progestin combination, 698
    biphasic, 699t
    monophasic, 699t
    triphasic, 699t
  nursing process, 702–704
  progestin, 698
Oral dosages, calculations of, **66–86**
  answers, 80–86
  interpreting drug labels, 67
  pediatric drug calculations, 73–80
  percentage of solutions, 73
  practice problems, 70–73
Oreton, 724t
orphenadrine citrate (Norflex), 307t, 317t
orphenadrine HCl (Disipal), 307t
Ortho-Est, 714t
Osmitrol, 590t
Osmolality, 178
  IV fluids, 178, 179
  plasma/serum, 178
Osmotic laxatives, 555, 557t
Osmotics, 497, 497t, 589, 590
  drug table, 590t
  nursing process, 589
OTC (over-the-counter) drugs, 19, 20t
Otic Domeboro, 592t
Over-the-counter (OTC) drugs, 19, 20t
ovulation stimulant, 734, 735
  drug table for, 735t
  prototype drug chart, 734
ovulation, induction of 734–736
oxacillin sodium, 348t
oxamniquine (Vansil), 394t
Oxandrin, 724t
oxandrolone (Oxandrin), 724t
oxaprozin (Daypro), 333t
oxazepam (Serax), 263t
Oxazolidones/oxazolidinedione, 245, 247t

Oxsoralen, 598t
oxybutynin (Ditropan), 404t
oxycodone HCl with acetaminophen (Percocet), 236t
oxycodone with aspirin (Percodan), 236t
oxymetholone (Androl-50), 724t
oxyphencyclimine HCl (Daricon), 302t
oxytetracycline HCl (Terramycin), 360t
oxytocin (Pitocin, Syntocinon), 676t

P

paclitaxel (Taxol), 416t
Pains, type of, 229
pancuronium bromide, (Pavulon), 317t
papaverine (Pavabid), 535t
paraldehyde, 217t
paramethadione (Paradione), 247t
paramethasone acetate (Haldrone), 624t
Parasympathetic nervous system, 275–277
Parasympatholytics, 277. See also *Anticholinergics.*
Parasympathomimetics 275. See also *Cholinergics.*
Parathyroids, 608, **619–621**
  drug table for, 619t, 620t
  nursing process, 621
  prototype drug chart for, 620
Parenteral drug administration, **33–37**
  intradermal, 33
  intramuscular, 34t, 35t, 36t, 35–37
  intravenous, 37, 38
  subcutaneous, 34
Parepectolin, 553t
Parkinsonism, **306–312**
  anticholinergics, 306–308
    drug table for, 307t
    nursing process, 307, 308
  case study, 320
  dopamine agonists, 398
  dopaminergics, 308
    carbidopa and levodopa, 308, 311t
    levodopa, 308, 311t
    nursing process, 312
  drug table for, 309t, 311t
  MAO-B inhibitor, 309, 319
  purpose of drugs in, 309t
Parlodel, 309t, 311t, 735t
Parnate, 269t
paromomycin sulfate (Humatin), 364t
paroxetine HCl (Paxil), 269t
Partial thromboplastin time (PTT), 519
Pathilon, 566t
Patient-controlled analgesia, 118, 119
PDR (Physicians' Desk Reference), 135
Peak and trough levels, 10, 11
Peak drug action, 8
Pediatric drug calculations, 73–80, 93, 94, 103–105
  injectables, 103–105
  orals, 73–80
Pediatric drug conversion, alternative methods, 772
Pediatric pharmacology, **148–150**
  nursing process, 149, 150
  pharmacodynamics, 148
  pharmacokinetics, 148, 149t
pemoline (Cylert), 208t, 209, 210
  pharmacodynamics, 210
  pharmacokinetics, 210
Pen-V, 592t
penbutolol (Levatol), 508t
Penetrex, 399t

penicillin (Pentids, Pen-V), 592t
penicillin G procaine, 347t
penicillin G benzathine (Bicillin), 347t
penicillin G sodium/potassium, 347t
penicillin V potassium (V-Cillin K), 347t
Penicillins, **345–349**
  antipseudomonal, 348
  broad-spectrum, 345
  case study, 354
  drug table for, 347t, 348t
  nursing process, 349
  penicillinase-resistant, 345
  prototype drug chart for, 346
pentaerythritol tetranitrate (Peritrate),
  480t
pentazocine lactate (Talwin), 238–240, 240t
  nursing process, 240
  prototype drug chart for, 239
Pentids, 592t
Pentobarbital sodium (Nembutal), 217t
  prototype drug for, 218
pentostatin (Nipent), 416t, 422
pentoxifylline (Trendal), 535t
Pepcid, 571t
Pepsin inhibitor, **572–574**
  drug table for, 574t
  nursing process, 575
  prototype drug chart for, 573
Peptic ulcers, 564, 565
  case study, 574, 575
  predisposing factors, 564, 565t
Peptides, **383, 384**
  drug table for, 384
  side effects/adverse reactions, 384
Pepto-Bismol, 553t
Percocet, 236t
Percodan, 236t
pergolide mesylate (Permax), 309t, 311t
Pergonal, 735t
Periactin, 448t
Peri-colace, 686t
Peripheral vasodilators, **533–536**
  drug table for, 534t, 535t
  nursing process, 535, 536
  prototype drug chart for, 534
Peripherally acting sympatholytics. See
  Adrenergic neuron blockers.
Peritrate, 480t
perphenazine (Trilafon), 257t
Pertofrane, 268t
Pharmaceutic phase, 4
Pharmacodynamic drug interactions, 141,
  142, 141t
  addictive drug effect, 141, 142
  antagonistic drug effect, 142
  synergistic drug effect, 142
Pharmacodynamics, **8–11**
  duration, 8
  onset, 8
  peak, 8
  peak and trough levels, 10, 11
  receptor theory, 8–10
  side effects, 11
  therapeutic index, 10, 11
  therapeutic range, 10, 11
Pharmacokinetic drug interaction, **139–141,**
  141t
  absorption, 139
  biotransformation, 140
  distribution, 139, 140
  excretion, 140, 141
  metabolism, 140
Pharmacokinetics, **4–8**
  absorption, 4, 5
  distribution, 5, 6

Pharmacokinetics *(Continued)*
  excretion, 7, 8
  metabolism, 7
Pharmacology, 132
  history, 132
phenazopyridine HCl (Pyridium), 402–404,
  404t
  nursing process, 402, 403
  prototype drug for, 403
phendimetrazine tartrate (Adipost), 211t
phenelzine sulfate (Nardil), 269t
Phenergan, 448t
phenmetrazine HCl (Preludin), 211t
phenobarbital (Luminal), 246t
phenolphthalein (Ex-Lax), 557t
phenosuximide (Milontin), 248t
Phenothiazines, **252–255,** 257t
  aliphatics, 252, 252t, 257t
  nursing process, 258–260
  piperazines, 252, 252t, 254, 257t
  piperidines, 252, 252t, 258t
  prototype drug chart for, 254, 255
phenoxybenzamine HCl (Dibenzyline),
  511t
Phentermine HCl, 211t
phentolamine mesylate (Regitine), 289t,
  511t
Phenylacetic acid, 333t
phenylbutazone (Butazolidin), 333t
phenylephrine HCl (Neo-Synephrine),
  284t, 591t
phenylpropanolamine HCl (Acutrim), 211t
phenytoin (Dilantin), **244–246,** 247t, 249,
  486t
  nursing process, 249
  prototype drug chart for, 245
Physicians' Desk Reference (PDR), 135
physostigmine salicylate (Isopto Eserine),
  296t, 585t
phytonadione (AquaMEPHYTON,
  Konakion, Mephyton, Vitamin K),
  692t
PIH. See *Pregnancy induced hypertension
  (PIH).*
pilocarpine nitrate (Ocusert Pilo-20, Pilo-
  40), 585t
pilocarpine HCl (Isopto Carpine, Pilocar),
  296t, 585t
  nursing process, 587
  prototype drug chart, 586
pindolol (Visken), 289t, 508t
piperacillin sodium (Pipracil), 348t
piperazine citrate (Antepar), 394t
Piperazine phenothiazines, 252, 252t, 254,
  257t
Piperidine phenothiazines, 252, 252t,
  258t
Piperidinediones, 220
pipobroman (Vercyte), 413t
pirbuterol acetate (Maxair), 461t
piroxicam (Feldene), 333t
Pitocin, 676t
Pitressin, 612t
Pituitary gland, 606–608, **611–615**
  anterior, 607, 608, 611–614
    adrenocorticotropic hormone, 607, 611,
    612t
    growth hormone, 608, 611, 612t
    thyroid-stimulating hormone, 607, 611,
    612t
  nursing process, 614, 615
  posterior, 608, 612t, 614
Placidyl, 217t
Planning, 17
Plasminogen inactivator, 527t

Platinol, 413t
plicamycin (Mithracin), 418, 419, 420t
Polycillin, 592t
polyestradiol phosphate (Estradurin), 421t
polymyxin B SO$_4$ (Aerosporin), 384, 400t,
  592t
polythiazide (Renese-R), 492t
Pontocaine, 225t
Posterior pituitary gland, 608, 614
  drugs for, 612t
Postpartum, **680–694**
  bowel function, 686t, 687t
    nursing process: laxatives, 687, 688
  lactation suppression, 685
  immunization, 689–694
    nursing process: hepatitis B vaccine
    (newborn), 694
    nursing process: Rh$_o$(D) immune
    globulin, 689, 690
    nursing process: rubella vaccine, 691
  perineal wounds and hemorrhoids, 683
    nursing process, 683, 684
  self medication, pain relief, 682t
  systemic analgesics, 682t
  uterine contractions, 682, 683
Potassium, **183–187**
  case study, 193
  corrections, 186
  functions, 183, 184
  hyperkalemia, 185
  hypokalemia, 184
  nursing process, 186, 187
  prototype drug for, 185
  supplements, 184
potassium iodide (SSKI), 452t
Potassium-sparing diuretics, **499–501**
  drug table for, 500t, 501t
  nursing process, 499, 501
  prototype drug chart for, 500
prazepam (Centrax), 263t
praziquantel (Biltricide), 394t
prazosin HCl (Minipress), 289t, 511t
Predforte, 584t
prednisolone acetate (Econopred,
  Predforte), 584t
prednisolone (Delta-Cortef), 624t
prednisolone Na phosphate (AK-
  PredInflamase), 584t
prednisone (Meticorten), 622–626, 624t
  case study, 626
  prototype drug chart for, 623
Pregnancy, drugs for minor discomfort of,
  647–658
  nausea and vomiting, 647, 648
  heartburn, 648
  pain, 648–650
  substances abused during, 654t
  vitamins and minerals, 773, 774
Pregnancy categories, 135, 136, 136t
Pregnancy induced hypertension (PIH),
  660–664
  comparison of mild vs severe
    preclampsia and eclampsia, 661t
  drug table, 661t
  nursing process, 662–664
  predisposing factors, 660t
Pregnancy physiology, 644
Preludin, 211t
Premarin, 713
  prototype drug chart, 713
Premenstrual syndrome, 704, 705
  nursing process, 708
  physical and psychobehavioral
    symptoms, 705t
Primacor, 476t

primaquine phosphate, 393t
Primaxin, 367t, 400t
primidone (Mysoline), 246t
Priscoline HCl, 511t
Pro-Banthine, 302t, 404t, 566t
probenecid (Benemid), 338t
probucol (Lorelco), 531t
procainamide HCl (Pronestyl), 485t, 754, 755, 757t
  prototype drug chart for, 484
Procaine HCl (Novocain), 225t
Procan, 485
procarbazine HCl (Matulane), 416t
Procardia, 481t, 515t
prochlorperazine (Compazine), 253–255
  prototype drug chart for, 254, 255
Proctofoam-HC, 682t
procyclidine HCl (Kemodrin), 303t, 307t
progesterone (Gesterol 50), 421t
progestins, 422, 714t
Prolixin, 257t
Proloprim, 397, 399t, 400
promazine HCl (Sparine), 257t
promethazine HCl (Phenergan), 448t
Pronestyl, 485t, 754, 755, 757t
propafenone HCl (Rythmol), 485t
propantheline bromide (Pro-Banthine), 302t, 404t, 566t
Propionic acid derivatives, 330–334
  drug table for, 333t
  nursing process, 333, 334
  prototype drug chart for, 331
propofol, 224t
propoxyphene napsylate (Darvon-N), 236t
propoxyphene HCl (Darvon), 236t
propranolol HCl (Inderal), 288, 289t, 480t, 508t
propylthiouracil (PTU), 617t
ProSom, 222t
Prostaglandin analog, 574, 574t
Prostigmin, 296t, 314t
protamine sulfate, 523t
Prothrombin time (PT), 520
protriptyline HCl (Vivactil), 268t
provastatin sodium (Pravachol), 531t
Proventil, 285t
Provera, 714t
Prozac, 269t
pseudoephedrine HCl (Sudafed), 284t
Psychological drug dependence, 144
PT (prothrombin time), 520
PTT (partial thromboplastin time), 519
pyrantel pamoate (Antiminth), 394t
pyrazinamide (Tebrazid), 378
Pyridium, 402–404, 404t
pyridostigmine bromide (Mestinon), 296t, 314t
  prototype drug chart for, 314
pyrimethamine (Daraprim), 393t
PZI insulin, 632t

Q

quazepam, 222t
Questran, 531t
quinacrine HCl (Atabrine HCl), 393t
quinestrol (Estrovis), 714t
quinethazone (Hydromox), 492t
quinidine sulfate, 485t
quinine sulfate (Quiphile), 393t
Quinolones. See Fluoroquinolones.

R

ramipril (Altrace), 515t
ranitidine (Zantac), 570, 571t
Rapid eye movement, 215
Ratio and proportion, 55–57
Receptor theory, 8–10
  agonist, 8
  antagonists, 8
recuronium bromide (Flumadine), 317t
References, 795–800
Regitine, 511t
Regular insulin, 95, 96, 632t
Renin-angiotensin system, 503
Reproductive disorders, male, developmental, 728
  drugs causing sexual dysfunction, 729t
  drugs for, 728, 729
  malignant and benign tumors, 729
  nonsexually transmitted infections, 728, 729
  pituitary, thyroid and adrenal, 728
  sexual dysfunction, 728
Reproductive processes, male, 719–721
  anatomy and physiology, 719
  hormonal regulation, 719
  sexual function, 720, 721
Research. See Drug research.
reserpine (Serpasil), 511t
resorcinol (Bicozene), 598t
  sulfur with, 598t
Respiratory system, 442, 443
  bronchial smooth muscle, 443
  control of respiration, 443
  lung compliance, 442
  upper, infections of. See Upper respiratory infections.
Restoril, 222t
Retrovir, 387, 389t
Rh₀(D) immune globulin, 689
  nursing process, 689–691
ribavirin (Virazole), 389t
Ridaura, 335t
rifabutin (Mycobutin), 378
rifampin (Rimactane), 378
Rights of drug administration, 23–26
rimantadine HCl (Flumadine), 389t
Riopan Plus Tablets, 649t
Riopan Plus Suspension, 649t
risperidone (Risperdal), 258t
Ritalin, 208–210
ritodrine (Yutopar), 285t, 652–656
  nursing process, 655, 656
  prototype drug chart, 654
Robaxin, 317t
Robitussin DM, 452t
Rocephin, 353t
Rogaine, 511t
Rolaids, 568t
rubella vaccine, 690, 691
  nursing process, 691

S

Salicylates, 229, 231t, 328–330
  nursing process, 329, 330
  prototype drug chart for, 328, 329
salicylic acid (Sebulex), 598t
salmeterol (Serevent), 461t
scopolamine hydrobromide (Isopto Hyoscine), 302t, 591t

secobarbital sodium (Seconal), 217t
Seconal sodium, 217t
Second-generation antidepressants, 265–267
Sectral, 289t, 485t, 508t
Sedative-hypnotics, 215–222
  adverse reaction, 216t
  barbiturates, 216–220
  benzodiazepines, 220–222, 222t
  side effects, 216t
  stages of sleep, 215
Seizures, 243
  classification of, 243, 243t
Seldane, 448t
selegiline HCl (Eldepryl), 309t, 311t
Self-medication administration, 26, 27
senna (Senokot), 557t, 687t
Senokot, 557t, 687t
Septra, 371, 372, 400t
Serax, 263t
sermorelin acetate (Geref), 612t
Serophene, 735t
Serpasil, 511t
sertraline HCl (Zoloft), 269t
sexually transmitted diseases, common, and their causative pathogens, 740t
  guidelines for primary therapies for, 741t, 742t
  drug table for, 741t, 742t
  drugs for, 738–748
  nursing process, 747
  pathogens causing, 739t
  risk reducing behaviors, 739t
  transmission and risk, 738, 739
Side effects, 11
Silvadene, 603t
Silver nitrate, 603t
silver nitrate 1% (Dey-Drop), 583t
silver sulfadiazine (Silvadene), 373, 603t
simethicone (Mylicon), 687t
simvastatin (Zocor), 531t
Sinemet, 309t, 310, 311t
Sinequan, 268t
Sinusitis, 453
Skeletal muscle relaxants, 316–320
  centrally acting, 316
  drug table for, 317t, 318t
  nursing process, 319, 320
  peripherally acting, 318, 318t
  prototype drug chart for, 318, 319
Skin, overview of, 579, 580
Sodium, 187, 188
  functions, 187, 188
  hypernatremia, 188
  hyponatremia, 188
  nursing process, 188
sodium bicarbonate, 568t, 756, 757t
sodium nitroprusside, 765, 766
  prototype drug chart, 765
Solu-Medrol, 624t, 758, 759, 759t
Soma, 317t, 318, 319
Somatic nervous system (SNS), 204
somatrem (Protropin), 612t
somatropin (Humatrope), 612t
Sorbitrate, 480t
sotalol HCl (Betapace), 485t
Sparine, 257t
spectinomycin HCl (Trobicin), 368t, 369
Spinal anesthesia, 225
  caudal block, 225
  epidural block, 225
  saddle block, 225
spironolactone (Aldactone), 500t

Stages of sleep, 215
stanozolol (Winstrol), 724t
Stelazine, 258t
Steroidal estrogens, 714t
Stimulant laxatives. See *Contact laxatives.*
streptokinase (Streptase), 525, 526, 526t, 527t
  prototype drug chart for, 526
streptomycin sulfate, 364t, 378
streptozocin (Zanosar), 412t
Subcutaneous injections, 34, 93, 94
  calculations, 93, 94
  practice problems, 93, 94
Succinimides, 245, 247t
succinylcholine Cl, 317t
sucralfate (Carafate), 573, 574t
Sudafed, 284t
sulfacetamide sodium, 372
sulfadiazine (Microsulfon), 372t
sulfalmethizole (Sulfasol), 372t
sulfamethoxazole (Gantanol), 372t
sulfamethoxazole-trimethoprim (Bactrim, Septra), 400t
sulfasalazine (Azulfidine), 372t
sulfentanil citrate (Sulfenta), 236t
sulfinpyrazone (Anturane), 338t, 523t
sulfisoxazole (Gantrisin), 372t, 593t
Sulfonamides, **371–375**, 593t
  case study, 374
  drug table for, 372t
  nursing process, 373, 374
  topical and ointment, 372
Sulfonylureas, **634–638**, 636t
  nursing process, 637, 638
sulindac (Clinoril), 332t
sumatriptan succinate (Imitrex), 211t
Suprax, 353t
suprofen (Profenal), 583t
Surfactant therapy in preterm birth, 658–660
  nursing process, 659, 660
  drug table, 659t
Surfak, 686t
Survanta (beractant) Intratracheal Suspension, 659t
Symmetrel, 309t, 311t, 389t
Sympathetic nervous system, 275–277
Sympatholytics, 275, **504–511**. See also *Adrenergic blockers.*
  adrenergic neuron blockers, 510, 511t
  alpha blockers, 507, 509, 510, 511t
  alpha and beta adrenergic blockers, 510, 511t
  beta (adreneregic) blockers, 504–507
  centrally-acting, 507, 508t
Sympathomimetic, 275. See also *Adrenergics.*
  bronchodilators, 460t, 461t
Sympathomimetic amines, 449, 450
Synarel nasal solution, 706t, 707, 709, 710
Synergistic drug effect, 142
Synthetic surfactant, 658–660
Synthroid, 616, 617t
Syntocinon, 676t
Syringes, 89, 90

T

t-PA (tissue-type plasminogen activator), 527t
T_4, 616
Tacaryl, 449t

Tace, 714t
tacrine HCl (Cognex), 296t
Tagamet, 571t
Tambocor, 485t
tamoxifen citrate (Nolvadex), 421t
Tapazole, 617t
Taractan, 258t
Tavist, 448t
Taxol, 416t
TDM, 791–794
Teaching plan, 19t
Tegison, 598t
Tegopen, 346, 347t
Tegretol, 247t
Temaril, 448t
temazepam (Restoril), 222t
Temperature conversion, 771
  Celsius, 771
  Fahrenheit, 771
  Tenex, 508t
teniposide (Vumon), 416t
Tenormin, 289t, 480t, 508t
Tensilon, 296t, 314t
terazosin HCl (Hytrin), 289t, 511t
terbinafine HCl (Lamisil), 382
terbutaline sulfate (Brethine), 285t, 461t, 653t
terfenadine (Seldane), 448t
Tesamone, 724t
Testex, 724t
testolactone (Teslac), 421t
Testopel pellets, 724t
testosterone (Histerone, Tesamone, Testopel pellets), 724t
testosterone propionate (Testex), 724t
testosterone enanthate (Andro L.A., Andropository, Delatest, Delatestryl, Durathate, Everone, Testrin), 724t
testosterone cypionate (Andro-Cyp, Andronate, depAndro, Depotest, Depo-estosterone, Duratest, Testred Cypionate, Virilon), 724t
Testred Cypionate, 724t
Testrin, 724t
tetracaine HCl (Pontocaine), 225t
tetracycline HCl (Achromycin Ophthalmic) 583t
tetracyclines, **359–362**, 592t, 598t
  demeclocycline HCl, 360t
  doxycycline hyclate, 360t
  drug table for, 360t
  minocycline HCl, 360t
  nursing process, 361, 362
  oxytetracycline, 360t
  prototype drug chart for, 361
Theelin, 714t
theophylline (Theo-Dur), 211t, **462–464**, 464t
  nursing process, 466, 467
  prototype drug chart for, 463
Therapeutic drug monitoring (TDM), 791–794
Therapeutic index, 10, 11
Therapeutic range, 10, 11
Therapeutic window, 10, 11
thiabendazole (Mintezol, Minzolum), 394t
Thiamylal sodium (Surital), 224t
Thiazides and thiazide-like diuretics, **491–495**
  drug table for, 491t, 492t
  nursing process, 494, 495
  prototype drug chart for, 493
  serum laboratory abnormalities, 494t
thioguanine, 416t

Thiopental sodium (Pentothal) 224t
thioridazine HCl (Mellaril), 258t
Thiotepa, 413t
thiothixene (Navane), 257t
Thorazine, 252–255, 257t
Thrombolytics, **525–528**
  drug table for, 526t, 527t
  nursing process, 527, 528
  prototype drug chart for, 526
Thrombus formation, 519
thyroglobulin (Proloid), 617t
Thyroid extract, 617t
Thyroid gland, 608, **615–619**
  hyperthyroidism, 616–619
    drug table for, 617t
  hypothyroidism, 615–617
    drug table for, 617t
  nursing process, 618, 619
Thyroid hormone replacement, 615–619, 617t
  nursing process, 618, 619
Thyroid-stimulating hormone, drugs for, 611, 612t
Thyrolar, 617t
thyrotropin (Thytropar), 612t
Ticar, 348t
ticarcillin disodium (Ticar), 348t
ticarcillin-clavulanate (Timentin), 348t
Tigan, 647t
Timenton, 348t
timolol maleate (Blocadren), 289t, 508t
timolol maleate (Timoptic Ophthalmic), 585t
Timoptic, 585t
Tissue injury, response of, 324
tissue-type plasminogen activator (t-PA, alteplase), 525, 527t
tobramycin sulfate (Nebcin, Tobrex), 365t, 583t
tocainide HCl (Tonocard), 485t
Tocolytic therapy, 651–656
  nursing process, 655, 656
  prototype drug chart, 654
Tofranil, 268t
tolazamide (Tolinase), 636t
tolazoline HCl (Priscoline), 289t, 511t, 534t
tolmetin (Tolectin), 332t
torsemide (Demadox), 497t
Total parenteral nutrition (TPN), **199–202**
  complications, 200, 200t
  nursing process, 200, 201
Toxic effects, 11, 12
Trade drug name, 134
tramadol (Ultram), 231t
Tranxene, 263t
tranylcypromine sulfate (Parnate), 269t
trazodone HCl (Desyrel), 269t
tretinoin (Retin-A), 598t
triamcinolone (Aristocort), 624t
triamterene (Dyrenium), 500, 500t
triazolam (Halcion), 222t
trichlormethiazide (Metahydrin), 492t
Tricyclic antidepressants (TCAs), 265–267
tridihexethyl Cl (Pathilon), 566t
Tridil, 757t
triethylenethiophosphoramide (Thiotepa), 413t
trifluoperazine HCl (Stelazine), 258t
triflupromazine (Vesprin), 257t
trifluridine (Viroptic), 583t
trihexyphenidyl HCl (Artane), 300, 301, 303t, 307t
  prototype drug chart for, 301
Trilafon, 257t

trimeprazine tartrate (Temaril), 448t
trimethadione (Tridione), 247t
trimethobenzamide (Tigan, T-Gen), 647t
trimethoprim (Proloprim), 397, 399t, 400
trimethoprim-sulfamethoxazole (Co-trimoxazole) 371, 372, 372t, 593t
  prototype drug chart for, 373
trimetrexate glucuronate (NeuTrexin), 416t
trimipramine maleate (Surmontil), 268t
tripelennamine HCl (Pelamine), 448t
triprolidine HCl (Alleract), 449t
Trobicin, 369
trolamine polypeptide oleate-condensate (Cerumenex), 592t
tropicamide (Mydriacyl Ophthalmic) 591t
Trough levels, 11
Tube feedings, calculations, **73–75**
Tuberculin syringe, 90
Tucks, 682t
Tums, 568t
Tylenol, 230–232, 231t, 648, 649

U

Ulcers, 564
  duodeneral, 564
  gastric, 564
  Helicobacter pylori, 564
  peptic, 564
  predisposing factors, 564, 565t
United States Pharmacopeia—Drug Information, 135
Upper respiratory infections, agents for, **445–454**
  antihistamines, 445–449, 448t
    drug table for, 448t
    nursing process, 447
    prototype drug chart for, 446
  antitussives, 450–453
    drug table for, 452t
    prototype drug chart for, 451
  expectorants, 452t, 453
  nasal and systemic decongestants, 449, 450
  common cold and acute rhinitis, 445–454
    nursing process, 453, 454
uracil mustard, 412t
urea (Ureaphil), 497t, 590t
urecholine, 294, 295, 296t, 404t
  nursing process, 297, 298
  prototype drug chart, 295
Uric acid inhibitor, 338, 338t, 339
  prototype drug chart for, 339
Urinary analgesics, 402–404
  nursing process, 402, 403
  prototype drug chart for, 403

Urinary antiseptics/antiinfectives, **397–402**
  drug table for, 399t, 400t
  fluoroquinolones, 400
  methenamine, 397
  nitrofurantoin, 397, 398
  trimethoprim, 397, 400
Urinary antispasmodics, 404
  drug table for, 404t
Urinary stimulants, 404
Urinary tract disorders, drugs for, **397–404**
  analgesics, 402–404, 404t
  antiinfectives, 397–402
  antiseptics, 397–402
  antispasmodics, 404, 404t
  stimulants, 404, 404t
Urine, drugs that discolor, 775
urofollitropin (Pergonal, Metrodin), 735t
urokinase (Abbokinase), 527t
Uterine dysfunction, drugs for, 704
  menstrual cycle, 704
  nursing process: endometriosis, 704
  nursing process: premenstrual syndrome, 704

V

Vaccines, 689–694, **777–781**
  newborn, immediately after delivery, 694
  post partum, 689–691
  schedule recommendations, 778–781
Valium, 261–263
valproic acid (Depakene), 247t, 248, 248t
Vanceril, 624t
vancomycin HCl (Vanocin), 358t, 359
Vasodilators (peripheral). See *Peripheral vasodilators.*
vasopressin (Pitressin), 612t
  oil in, 612t
Vasotec, 515t
vecuronium bromide (Norcuron), 317t
verapamil HCl (Calan, Isoptin), 481t, 486t, 515t, 753, 757t
Vermox, 394t
Vesprin, 257t
Vibramycin, 360t
vidarabine monohydrate (Vira-A), 387, 389, 389t
vidarabine (Vira-A Ophthalmic), 583t
vinblastine sulfate (Velban), 420t
Vinca alkaloids, 419, 420t
vincristine sulfate (Oncovin), 420t
vinorelbine (Navelbine), 420t
Virilon, 724t
Vistaril, 263t, 448t

Vitamins, **166–173**, 172t, 173t
  fat-soluble, 169–171
  food source, 172t
  justification for, 166t
  nursing process, 171, 172
  water soluble, 169–171
Vitamin A, 167
  prototype drug for, 168
Vitamin B_{12}, 170, 171
Vitamin C, 169
  prototype drug for, 170
Vitamin D, 167
Vitamin E, 167, 168
Vitamin K, 168, 169, 692t
Vitamin K_1 (AquaMEPHYTON), 523t
Vitamin K_4 (menadiol sodium diphosphate), 523t
Voltaren, 583t

W

warfarin sodium (Coumadin), 521–525, 523t
  nursing process, 524, 525
  prototype drug chart for, 521, 522
Winstrol, 724t
Witch hazel pads, 682t

X

Xanax, 263t
Xylocaine, 225t, 485t

Y

Yutopar, 652–656

Z

Z-track injection technique, 36
zalcitabine (Hivid), 389t
Zantac, 571t
Zarontin, 247t
zidovudine (Retrovir), 387, 389t
Zocor, 531t
Zolpidem tartrate, 222t
Zovirax, 388, 389t
Zyloprim, 338t

IV Flow Rate: Continuous
Method II:

a. Amount of fluid ÷ hours to administer = mL/hr

b. $\dfrac{\text{ml/hr} \times \text{gtt/mL (IV set)}}{60 \text{ min/hr}} = \text{gtt/min}$

Example:
Order: 1000 mL, $D_5/\frac{1}{2}$ NSS in 8 hours.
IV Set: Macrodrip: 10 gtt/mL.

a. 1000 mL ÷ 8 hours = 125 mL/hr

b. $\dfrac{125 \text{ mL/hr} \times \overset{1}{\cancel{10}} \text{gtt/mL}}{\underset{6}{\cancel{60}} \text{ min/hr}} = 21 \text{ gtt/min}$

IV Flow Rate: Intermittent
Secondary Sets: Buretrol and Add-A-Line

$\dfrac{\text{Amount of solution} \times \text{gtt/mL (set)}}{\text{Minutes to administer}} = \text{gtt/min}$

Order: Administer 5 mL of drug solution in 50 mL of D_5W in 30 minutes.
IV set: Buretrol (60 gtt/mL)

$\dfrac{55 \text{ mL} \times \overset{2}{\cancel{60}} \text{gtt}}{\underset{1}{\cancel{30}} \text{ minutes}} = 110 \text{ gtt/min}$

Drug Category

Drug Name	Dosage
Pregnancy Category:	
Contraindications	**Drug-Lab-Food Interactions**
Pharmacokinetics	**Pharmacodynamics**

Absorption:
Distribution: PB:
Metabolism: t½:
Excretion:
	PO: Onset:
	      Peak:
	      Duration:

Therapeutic Effects/Uses: Mode of Action:

Side Effects	Adverse Reactions
	Life-threatening:

KEY: PO: by mouth, PB: protein-binding, t½: half-life.

Therapeutic Drug Monitoring (TDM)

Drug	Therapeutic Range	Peak Time	Toxic Level
Acetaminophen (Tylenol)	10–20 µg/mL	1–2½ hours	>50 µg/mL Hepatotoxicity: >200 µg/mL
Amikacin (Amikin)	Peak: 20–30 µg/mL Trough: ≤10 µg/mL	Intravenously ½ hour Intramuscular: ½–1½ hours	Peak: >35 µg/mL Trough: >10 µg/mL
Aspirin (see Salicylates)			
Carbamazepine (Tegretol)	4–12 µg/mL	6 hours (Range 2–24 hours)	>9–15 µg/mL
Chlorpromazine (Thorazine)	50–300 ng/mL	2–4 hours	>750 ng/mL
Clonidine (Catapres)	0.2–2.0 ng/mL	2–5 hours	>2.0 ng/mL
Cimetidine (Tagamet)	Trough: 0.5–1.2 µg/mL	1–1½ hours	Trough: >1.5 µg/mL
Codeine	10–100 ng/mL	1–2 hours	>200 ng/mL
Diazepam (Valium)	0.5–2 mg/L 400–600 ng/mL Therapeutic	1–2 hours	>3 mg/L >3000 ng/mL
Digoxin	0.5–2 ng/mL	PO: 6–8 hours IV: 1½–2 hours	2–3 ng/mL
Dilantin (see Phenytoin)			
Ethosuximide (Zarontin)	40–100 µg/mL	2–4 hours	>150 µg/mL
Flurazepam (Dalmane)	20–110 ng/mL		>1500 ng/mL
Haloperidol (Haldol)	5–15 ng/mL	2–6 hours	>50 ng/mL

IV Flow Rate: Intermittent Volumetric Pump:

$$\text{Amt of solution} \div \frac{\text{minutes to administer}}{60 \text{ min/hr}} = \text{mL/hr}$$

Order: Administer 5 mL of drug solution in 100 mL of D_5W in 45 minutes.

$$105 \text{ mL} \div \frac{45 \text{ minutes}}{60 \text{ min/hr}} \quad \text{(Invert divisor and multiply)}$$

$$= 105 \times \frac{\overset{4}{\cancel{60}}}{\underset{3}{\cancel{45}}} = 140 \text{ mL/hr}$$

Set volumetric pump at 140 mL/hr to deliver 105 mL in 45 minutes.

IV Flow Rate: Continuous Method III:

$$\frac{\text{Amount of fluid} \times \text{gtt/mL (IV set)}}{\text{Hours to administer} \times \text{min/hr (60)}} = \text{gtt/min}$$

Example:

Order: 1000 mL of D_5W in 10 hours.
IV Set: Microdrip: 60 gtt/mL.

$$\frac{\overset{100}{\cancel{1000}} \text{ mL} \times \overset{1}{\cancel{60}} \text{ gtt/mL}}{\underset{1}{\cancel{10}} \text{ hours} \times \underset{1}{\cancel{60}} \text{ min/hr}} = 100 \text{ gtt/min}$$

Therapeutic Drug Monitoring (TDM)

Drug	Therapeutic Range	Peak Time	Toxic Level
Lidocaine (Xylocaine)	1.5–5 μg/mL	IV: 10 minutes	>6 μg/mL
Lithium	0.8–1.2 mEq/L	$\frac{1}{2}$–4 hours	>1.5 mEq/L
Lorazepam (Ativan)	50–240 ng/mL	1–3 hours	>300 ng/mL
Methyldopa (Aldomet)	1–5 μg/mL	3–6 hours	>7 μg/mL
Metoprolol (Lopressor)	75–200 ng/mL	2–4 hours	>225 ng/mL
Nifedipine (Procardia)	50–100 ng/mL	$\frac{1}{2}$–2 hours	>100 ng/mL
Pentazocine (Talwin)	0.05–0.2 μg/mL	1–2 hours	>1.0 μg/mL
Phenytoin (Dilantin)	10–20 μg/mL	4–8 hours	>20–30 μg/mL Severe toxicity: >40 μg/mL
Procainamide (Pronestyl)	4–10 μg/mL	1 hour	>10 μg/mL
Propranolol (Inderal)	>100 ng/mL	1–2 hours	>150 ng/mL
Ranitidine (Zantac)	100 ng/mL	2–3 hours	>100 ng/mL
Salicylates (Aspirin)	10–30 mg/dL	1–2 hours	Tinnitis: 20–40 mg/mL Severe toxicity: >50 mg/dL
Theophylline (Thodur)	10–20 μg/mL	PO: 2–3 hours IV: 15 minutes	>20 μg/mL
Verapamil (Calan)	100–300 ng/mL	PO: 1–2 hours IV: 5 minutes	>500 ng/mL
Warfarin (Coumadin)	1–10 μg/mL	$1\frac{1}{2}$–3 days	>10 μg/mL

Nursing Process
Assessment and Planning

Interventions

Evaluation